Breast Cancer Treatment

A Comprehensive Guide to Management

Breast Cancer Treatment

A Comprehensive Guide to Management

Barbara Fowble, MD
Professor of Radiation Oncology at the Hospital of the University of Pennsylvania
Department of Radiation Oncology
University of Pennsylvania School of Medicine
Philadelphia, Pennsylvania

Robert L. Goodman, MD
Professor and Chairman
Department of Radiation Oncology
University of Pennsylvania School of Medicine
Philadelphia, Pennsylvania

John H. Glick, MD
Director, University of Pennsylvania Cancer Center
Professor of Medicine
University of Pennsylvania School of Medicine
Madlyn and Leonard Abramson Professor of Clinical Oncology
Philadelphia, Pennsylvania

Ernest F. Rosato, MD
Professor of Surgery
Department of Surgery
University of Pennsylvania School of Medicine
Philadelphia, Pennsylvania

with 180 illustrations

Mosby Year Book

St. Louis Baltimore Boston Chicago London Philadelphia Sydney Toronto

Mosby Year Book
Dedicated to Publishing Excellence

Sponsoring Editor: Susan M. Gay
Assistant Editors: Janet R. Livingston/Sandra E. Clark
Project Manager: Lilliane Anstee
Book and Cover Design: Julie Taugner

Printed in the United States of America

Mosby–Year Book, Inc.
11830 Westline Industrial Drive
St. Louis, Missouri 63146

Library of Congress Cataloging-in-Publication Data

Breast cancer treatment : a comprehensive guide to management / Barbara Fowble . . . [et al.].
p. cm.
Includes bibliographical references and index.
ISBN 0-8016-6207-9
1. Breast—cancer. I. Fowble, Barbara.
[DNLM: 1. Breast Neoplasms—therapy. WP 870 B8243]
RC280.B8B6895 1991
616.99'44906 dc20
DNLM/DLC
for Library of Congress 91-19565
CIP

GW/MY/MY 9 8 7 6 5 4 3 2 1

For Kate, Frank, G.E., and Mannix

Contents

Contributors

MARY E. COOLEY, RN, MSN, OCN
Oncology Clinical Nurse Specialist
Veterans Affairs Medical Center
Philadelphia, Pennsylvania

PAUL G. CURCILLO II, MD
Instructor in Surgery
Jefferson Medical College
Thomas Jefferson University
Philadelphia, Pennsylvania

F. ANDREW DORR, MD
Senior Investigator
National Cancer Institute
Bethesda, Maryland

BERNADETTE ERIKSON, PT
Department of Physical Therapy
Hospital of the University of Pennsylvania
Philadelphia, Pennsylvania

BARBARA FOWBLE, MD
Professor of Radiation Oncology at the Hospital of the University of Pennsylvania
Department of Radiation Oncology
University of Pennsylvania School of Medicine
Philadelphia, Pennsylvania

KEVIN R. FOX, MD
Assistant Professor of Medicine at the Hospital of the University of Pennsylvania
University of Pennsylvania School of Medicine
Assistant Director of Clinical Affairs
University of Pennsylvania Cancer Center
Philadelphia, Pennsylvania

JOHN H. GLICK, MD
Director, University of Pennsylvania Cancer Center
Professor of Medicine
University of Pennsylvania School of Medicine
Madlyn and Leonard Abramson Professor of Clinical Oncology
Philadelphia, Pennsylvania

DONNA GLOVER, MD
Clinical Associate Professor of Medicine at the Hospital of the University of Pennsylvania
Chief of Hematology Oncology
Presbyterian Medical Center
Philadelphia, Pennsylvania

ROBERT L. GOODMAN, MD
Professor and Chairman
Department of Radiation Oncology
University of Pennsylvania School of Medicine
Philadelphia, Pennsylvania

GLORIA A. HAGOPIAN, RN, EdD
Associate Professor of Oncology Nursing
University of Pennsylvania School of Nursing
Clinician Educator
Department of Radiation Oncology
Hospital of the University of Pennsylvania
Philadelphia, Pennsylvania

DANIEL G. HALLER, MD
Associate Professor of Medicine at the Hospital of the University of Pennsylvania
Hematology Oncology Section
Department of Medicine
University of Pennsylvania School of Medicine
Philadelphia, Pennsylvania

GERALD E. HANKS, MD
Professor of Radiation Oncology
University of Pennsylvania School of Medicine
Vice Chairman, Department of Radiation Oncology
Hospital of the University of Pennsylvania
Chairman, Department of Radiation Oncology
Fox Chase Cancer Center
Philadelphia, Pennsylvania

MICHELE L. HARTIGAN, Esquire
Associate, Litigation Department
Duane, Morris, & Heckscher
Philadelphia, Pennsylvania

MARTIN L. KELSTEN, MD
Pathologist
Department of Pathology
Riverside Methodist Hospital
Clinical Assistant Professor
Ohio State University
College of Medicine
Columbus, Ohio

DON LaROSSA, MD
Professor of Surgery at the Hospital of the University of Pennsylvania
Department of Plastic Surgery and Reconstruction
University of Pennsylvania School of Medicine
Philadelphia, Pennsylvania

VIRGINIA A. LiVOLSI, MD
Professor of Pathology and Laboratory Medicine
University of Pennsylvania School of Medicine
Director of Surgical Pathology
Hospital of the University of Pennsylvania
Philadelphia, Pennsylvania

GERALD MARGOLIS, MD
Clinical Professor of Psychiatry at the Hospital of the University of Pennsylvania
Department of Psychiatry
University of Pennsylvania School of Medicine
Philadelphia, Pennsylvania

JAMES J. McCABE, Esquire
Chairman, Litigation Department
Duane, Morris & Heckscher
Philadelphia, Pennsylvania

RUTH McCORKLE, PhD, FAAN
American Cancer Society Professor of Oncology Nursing and Director, Serious Illness Center
Professor of Nursing
University of Pennsylvania School of Nursing
Philadelphia, Pennsylvania

MARY DEE McEVOY, RN, PhD
Clinical Director
Ambulatory Oncology
Hospital of the University of Pennsylvania
Philadelphia, Pennsylvania

JEANNIE PASACRETA, MSN, RN
Teaching Assistant
University of Pennsylvania School of Nursing
Philadelphia, Pennsylvania

ELIZABETH A. PATTERSON, MD
Assistant Professor of Radiology at the Hospital of the University of Pennsylvania
Department of Radiology
University of Pennsylvania School of Medicine
Philadelphia, Pennsylvania

ROSEMARY C. POLOMANO, MSN, RN
Oncology/Pain Clinical Nurse Specialist
Hospital of the University of Pennsylvania
Philadelphia, Pennsylvania

ERNEST F. ROSATO, MD
Professor of Surgery
Department of Surgery
University of Pennsylvania School of Medicine
Philadelphia, Pennsylvania

LYNN M. SCHUCHTER, MD
Assistant Professor of Medicine at the Hospital of the University of Pennsylvania
Hematology Oncology Section
Department of Medicine
University of Pennsylvania School of Medicine
Philadelphia, Pennsylvania

DELRAY J. SCHULTZ, MA
Biostatistics Unit
University of Pennsylvania Cancer Center
University of Pennsylvania School of Medicine
Philadelphia, Pennsylvania

FREDERICK SCHWAIBOLD, DO
Director
Radiation Care Incorporated
Atlanta, Georgia

ELISE E. SINGER, JD
Partner
Duane, Morris & Heckscher
Philadelphia, Pennsylvania

LAWRENCE J. SOLIN, MD
Associate Professor of Radiation Oncology at the Fox Chase Cancer Center
Department of Radiation Oncology
University of Pennsylvania School of Medicine
Philadelphia, Pennsylvania

EDWARD A. STADTMAUER, MD
Assistant Professor of Medicine at the Hospital of the University of Pennsylvania
Hematology Oncology Section
Department of Medicine
University of Pennsylvania School of Medicine
Associate Director, Bone Marrow Transplant Program
University of Pennsylvania Cancer Center
Philadelphia, Pennsylvania

ROSALIND H. TROUPIN, MD
Professor of Radiology
University of Pennsylvania School of Medicine
Department of Radiology
Chief, Breast Imaging Section
Hospital of the University of Pennsylvania
Philadelphia, Pennsylvania

MARY JO VIGLIONE, MD
Resident
Department of Pathology and Laboratory Medicine
University of Pennsylvania School of Medicine
Philadelphia, Pennsylvania

MARISA C. WEISS, MD
Assistant Professor of Radiation Oncology at the Hospital of the University of Pennsylvania
Department of Radiation Oncology
University of Pennsylvania School of Medicine
Philadelphia, Pennsylvania

I-TIEN YEH, MD
Assistant Professor of Pathology and Laboratory Medicine
University of Pennsylvania School of Medicine
Staff, Surgical Pathology Section of the Hospital of the University of Pennsylvania
Philadelphia, Pennsylvania

Introduction

In the latter half of the twentieth century major changes in the diagnosis and treatment of breast cancer have occurred. One of the most important changes relates to the perception of the natural history of the disease. In the late 1960s and early 1970s laboratory and clinical investigations provided increasing evidence that the spread of breast cancer was not orderly. The "alternative hypothesis" proposed that breast cancer has the potential for systemic dissemination from its inception, and that changes in local-regional treatment were unlikely to impact on outcome. This philosophy, accompanied by mounting evidence from retrospective series and results from prospective clinical trials, provided the impetus for the use of surgical procedures less than the radical mastectomy. The two most commonly employed local treatment options for early stage breast cancer now include the modified radical mastectomy and conservative surgery and radiation.

Concurrent with the changing perception of the natural history of breast cancer has been an increased emphasis on screening and early detection, resulting in an increased frequency of patients with in situ breast cancer. The clinical challenge remains to determine optimal treatment for this group of patients.

The concept of occult metastases or undetectable micrometastases as a source of treatment failure also was introduced in the early 1970s and provided the rationale for the use of adjuvant systemic therapy. The clinical importance of adjuvant chemotherapy and/or hormonal therapy for node-positive breast cancer patients was established by multiple prospective randomized trials. A consistent benefit in terms of survival has been demonstrated in selected patients. The role of adjuvant therapy in node-negative breast cancer patients is currently under investigation, and preliminary results suggest at least a disease-free survival benefit in certain subsets of this patient population.

The prospective randomized clinical trial has provided a means to test biologic principles systematically, to resolve clinical dilemmas, and to evaluate new treatment strategies. Its importance in establishing treatment alternatives to mastectomy and the role of adjuvant systemic chemotherapy cannot be overestimated. The results from these clinical trials have provided a scientific basis for making treatment decisions, as opposed to a reliance on intuition. Future trials will test some of the recent advances in molecular and cellular biology.

Measures of the effectiveness of one treatment versus another routinely have included an assessment of overall survival, disease-free suvival, and local-regional recurrence. However, the importance of the long-term effects of treatment recently has been recognized. Various methods of quantifying the benefits of treatment, i.e., reduction in symptoms from recurrent or persistent disease versus its toxic effects, have been proposed.

Increasing attention also has been drawn toward determining prognostic factors that can predict outcome reliably and identify patients at high risk for recurrence despite current treatment. While many factors have been evaluated, the relative importance of each remains to be determined. The goal is to identify prognostic factors that can aid the physician and patient in making intelligent treatment decisions.

It is clear that our knowledge related to breast cancer treatment and outcome is expanding rapidly. The ability to remain current with the most recent advances has become increasingly difficult. In an attempt to narrow the gap between research and clinical practice, the National Institutes of Health established the Consensus Development Program. There have been five consensus conferences related to breast cancer. Topics have included breast cancer screening (1977), management of local disease (1979, 1990), and adjuvant systemic therapy (1980, 1985, 1990). The consensus conferences have provided the means for ensuring public exposure at an early stage to state of the art knowledge. Their ability to impact on clinical practice was demonstrated by the increasing use of tamoxifen in postmenopausal node-positive patients following the 1985 conference. A precedent for the rapid dissemination of the preliminary results of clinical trials was set by the National Cancer Institute in 1988 with a mailing of the Clinical Alert to practicing physicians. The Alert addressed the issue of adjuvant therapy in node-negative breast cancer patients. However, the formal mechanism for the dissemination of results remains publication of data in peer-reviewed journals.

Progress in breast cancer research depends on the ability to identify important scientific questions, to design appropriate trials to test these questions, and to obtain answers within a reasonable period of time. In the past, most clinical trials have required at least 6 years for completion. The recognition of this fact, as well as the desire to keep trials current with our knowledge base, has resulted in major cooperative efforts on both a national and an international basis. Conceptual duplication of studies has been minimized, and priorities have been established by those sponsoring the trials. The metaanalysis or overview process of data from large numbers of clinical trials has further attempted to estimate the benefit of various treatments. The overview has the advantage of detecting potential real treatment differences in a large number of patients that, in smaller trials, may not have appeared significant.

Despite these efforts, uncertainty in clinical research continues to exist and to generate controversy. Decision-making in breast cancer treatment has become increasingly more complex. The goal is delivery of optimal therapy in any setting, although the concept of optimal therapy at any given time may change with the expanding knowledge base. The current approach to treatment is clearly multidisciplinary and involves the efforts of the diagnostic radiologist, surgeon, pathologist, radiation oncologist, medical oncologist, nurse oncologist, rehabilitation specialist, and plastic surgeon. Treatment options are numerous, and more often the patient chooses to participate in the decision-making process. Each member of the multidisciplinary team must possess the knowledge to aid the patient in making an intelligent decision. Within this context the present text was conceived.

The multidisciplinary approach to the treatment of breast cancer was initiated at the University of Pennsylvania in the late 1970s. This experience has become the foundation for the present text. We provide the reader with the rationale for treatment strategies, the outcome of treatment, and a comprehensive review of the literature, so that a comparison of results can be performed. While the emphasis is on the University of Pennsylvania treatment approach, we encourage the reader to formulate his or her own conclusions. We purposely have confined our discussions to treatment-related issues concerning the patient with known breast cancer. Therefore we have omitted sections related to epidemiology or prevention, screening and detection, benign disease, and basic pathology. We concentrate, however, on a detailed discussion of treatment options for in situ breast cancer, early invasive breast cancer, and locally advanced breast cancer. Pathology is discussed in terms of prognostic factors that are important in determining treatment outcome in terms of both overall and disease-free survival as well as local and regional recurrence. The role of mammography in the pretreatment evaluation of patients with breast cancer is presented, as well as its role in the posttreatment evaluation of patients who have undergone conservative surgery and radiation. The technical aspects of surgery and radiation for breast preservation are presented. Adjuvant therapy is discussed for node-positive and node-negative patients, and the role of postmastectomy adjuvant radiotherapy is described. Special considerations include Paget's disease, the axillary lymph node presentation, pregnancy and breast cancer, male breast cancer, breast cancer in patients who have undergone augmentation or reduction mammoplasty, and bilateral breast cancer. The treatment of local-regional recurrence following either conservative surgery and radiation or mastectomy is reviewed, and the role of systemic chemotherapy and hormonal therapy in the treatment of metastatic disease is discussed. The discussion of rehabilitation covers both psychosocial and physical rehabilitation, including the role of reconstructive surgery. The nursing management of the effects of treatment and progressive disease also is presented. We have devoted a chapter to the medicolegal aspects of the treatment of breast cancer, especially timely in light of the recent report from the Physician Insurers Association of America identifying breast cancer as a major area for malpractice claims. We also present the patterns of care in breast cancer treatment in the United States, documenting variations throughout the country, and we review international patterns of care. A discussion of current ongoing randomized trials and the future direction of breast cancer research has been provided by Dr. Andrew Dorr of the National Cancer Institute. In summary, our goal is to provide the practicing physician with state of the art knowledge as it relates to the clinical decision-making process.

There are many individuals who have contributed to the preparation of this text. Foremost are our patients, who have provided us with the basis for our clinical experience and entrusted us with their care. We would also like to express our gratitude to the many colleagues who have participated in the management of these patients. We would like to acknowledge the efforts of our staff, including the radiation oncology technologists, social workers, and nurses whose expertise has contributed to the favorable outcome of our patients. We would especially like to acknowledge the efforts of Vikki Goodstein, whose superb secretarial support has withstood our many revisions and deadlines. The monumental task of data management, computer programming, and statistical analysis has been performed by Cindy Rosser, Ellen Zaleta, and Delray Schultz. Finally, we would like to pay tribute to the memory of Carrie Solin, whose sudden and untimely death served to remind us of the role of ongoing clinical research and the importance of expanding our knowledge in all fields.

Barbara Fowble
Robert L. Goodman
John H. Glick
Ernest F. Rosato

1 Staging of Breast Cancer

Barbara Fowble

Staging of breast cancer refers to the classification of patients according to the extent of their disease. This results in the grouping of patients with a similar prognosis. Staging is important in that it provides consistency when describing the extent of breast cancer, it defines prognostic subgroups for whom various treatment options are appropriate, and it provides a reference base for eligibility criteria for clinical trials. Results of treatment from individual institutions and prospective randomized trials both nationally and internationally can be compared more readily when patients have been staged similarly.

Staging may be based on clinical or pathologic information or on a combination of both types of information. Clinical staging includes information obtained from physical examination of the primary tumor and regional nodes as well as x-rays or radionuclide scans. Pathologic staging includes information used for clinical staging as well as histologic evaluation of the primary tumor, ipsilateral breast, and regional nodes. Clinical staging is determined before definitive treatment and is most useful in determining initial treatment options.

While many different staging classifications have been employed for breast cancer, the following three appear to have achieved more general acceptance: the Manchester classification, the Columbia Clinical Classification (CCC), and the American Joint Commission on Cancer (AJCC) TNM classification.

The Manchester system[5] was introduced in 1940 by the Christie Hospital and Holt Radium Institute in Manchester, England. The classification is based exclusively on clinical evaluation, dividing patients into four stages. Tumor size is not employed to distinguish between stages, and patients with locally advanced breast cancer may be placed in either stage III or stage IV. The primary distinction between stage I and stage II disease is the presence of palpable nonfixed nodes in the axilla. The Manchester classification is presented at right.

The Columbia Clinical Classification[3] is also based on clinical evaluation. Four stages are employed (see p. 2). Stages A and B are considered operable breast cancer and stages C and D inoperable breast cancer as defined by Haagensen. Again, tumor size is not employed and locally advanced breast cancer may be placed in either stage C or stage D. The distinction between stage A and stage B disease is the presence of palpable axillary nodes <2½ cm in transverse diameter. The Columbia Clinical Classification has become accepted widely and was employed in 1974 to compare results in an international cooperative study.[4]

In 1954 the International Union against Cancer (UICC) initiated an effort to develop a staging classification that would achieve world-wide acceptance. A TNM system was adopted based on an

---

MANCHESTER CLASSIFICATION[5]

Stage I

The growth is confined to the breast. Involvement of the skin directly over and in continuity with the tumor does not affect staging provided the area involved is small in relation to the size of the breast.

Stage II

The growth is confined to the breast but there are palpable, mobile lymph nodes in the axilla.

Stage III

The growth extends beyond the corpus mammae.
Signs:

- The skin is invaded or fixed over an area that is large in relation to the size of the breast or is ulcerated.
- The tumor is fixed to the underlying muscle or fascia.
- Axillary glands may or may not be palpable, but if glands are present, they must be mobile.

Stage IV

The growth has extended beyond the breast area, as shown by:

- Fixation or matting of the axillary nodes
- Complete fixation of tumor to chest wall
- Secondary lymph nodes in supraclavicular region
- Secondary deposits in skin wide of tumor
- Secondary deposits in the opposite breast
- Distant metastases

COLUMBIA CLINICAL CLASSIFICATION (CCC)[3]

Stage A

No skin edema, ulceration, or solid fixation of tumor to chest wall. Axillary nodes not clinically involved.

Stage B

No skin edema, ulceration, or solid fixation of tumor to chest wall. Clinically involved nodes, but <2.5 cm in transverse diameter and not fixed to overlying skin or deeper structures of axilla.

Stage C

Any of five grave signs of advanced breast cancer:

- Edema of skin of limited extent (involving less than one third of the skin over the breast)
- Skin ulceration
- Solid fixation of tumor to chest wall
- Massive involvement of axillary lumph nodes (measuring ≥ 2.5 cm in transverse diameter)
- Fixation of the axillary nodes to overlying skin or deeper structures of the axilla

Stage D

All other patients with advanced breast cancer, including:

- A combination of any two or more of the five grave signs listed under stage C
- Extensive edema of the skin (involving more than one third of the skin over the breast)
- Satellite skin nodules
- The inflammatory type of carcinoma
- Clinically involved supraclavicular lymph nodes
- Internal mammary metastases, as evidenced by a parasternal tumor
- Edema of the arm
- Distant metastases

evaluation of the primary tumor, regional nodes, and distant metastases. Four stages of breast cancer were defined by the grouping of various combinations of tumor extent, nodal involvement, and the presence or absence of distant metastases. The TNM UICC staging system was first published in 1960. It was adopted by the American Joint Committee for Cancer Staging and End Results Reporting (AJCC) in a revised form and published in 1962. Zippin,[7] however, demonstrated that this AJC version failed to give adequate consideration to tumor size, and subsequent revisions were published in 1972 and 1977. The 1983 version (see pp. 3-4), which was agreed upon in 1978, represents the most widely accepted staging system at the present time.

The American Joint Committee on Cancer 1983 staging classification includes a clinical diagnostic stage (cTNM), a surgical-evaluative stage (sTNM), and a postsurgical resection pathologic stage (pTNM). *Clinical staging* is based on information obtained from physical examination of the breast and regional lymph nodes as well as x-ray examination including chest x-ray, mammography, and radionuclide scans. It requires a tissue diagnosis of cancer. *Pathologic staging* includes all information employed in the clinical diagnostic staging as well as histologic evaluation of the primary cancer, ipsilateral breast, and axillary lymph nodes. The *surgical-evaluative staging* includes information employed in the clinical diagnostic staging as well as pathologic examination of the primary tumor and the axillary lymph nodes. This staging is employed when the definitive treatment is less than a mastectomy, i.e., conservative surgery with or without radiation. For both the pathologic staging and the surgical-evaluative staging, the pathologic size of the primary tumor is that of the invasive component of the tumor. The noninvasive component of the tumor is not included in the overall tumor size.

There are four stages in the TNM classification. Stages I and II are considered early breast cancer. Stage I includes primary tumors ≤ 2 cm in diameter with clinically negative axillary nodes. Stage II disease includes primary tumors ≤ 2 cm with clinically positive axillary nodes and primary tumors 2 to 5 cm in diameter regardless of the axillary nodal status. Patients with no evidence of a primary tumor in the breast (T_0) and positive axillary nodes are classified as stage II. Stage III has been defined as locally advanced breast cancer and includes both operable and inoperable patients, and stage IV represents distant metastatic disease. Stage T_{is} represents in situ noninvasive breast cancer.

In 1986 the AJCC revised the 1983 TNM classification and the current classification is presented on pp. 4-6. The essential differences between the 1983 and 1986 classifications are: the omission of surgical-evaluative stage, the classification of supraclavicular nodes as M_1 instead of N_3, and the grouping of $T_3N_0M_0$ into stage II, which was previously stage IIIA disease. The latter change was based on survival data from the Surveillance Epidemiology and End Results (SEER) program of the National Cancer Institute indicating that the 5-year survival of $T_3N_0M_0$ disease was more characteristic of stage II, i.e., approximately 75% rather than that of stage IIIA disease of 56%.[6] The 1986 classification also excludes consideration of fixation to the pectoral fascia as an influence on stage. Inflammatory carcinoma in the 1986 classification has received a separate designation of T_{4d}.

1983 TNM CLASSIFICATION[2]

Primary tumor (T)

Definitions for the primary tumor (T) for clinical-diagnostic classification are the same as those for postsurgical resection-pathologic classification.

T_x Minimum requirements to assess primary tumor cannot be met
T_0 No evidence of primary tumor
T_{is} In situ cancer (in situ lobular, pure intraductal, and Paget's disease of the nipple without palpable tumor)
T_1 Tumor ≤2 cm in greatest dimension
- T_{1a} No fixation to underlying pectoral fascia or muscle
- T_{1b} Fixation to underlying pectoral fascia or muscle
  - i Tumor ≤0.5 cm
  - ii Tumor >0.5, ≤1.0 cm
  - iii Tumor >1.0, ≤2.0 cm

T_2 Tumor >2 cm but not >5 cm in its greatest dimension
- T_{2a} No fixation to underlying pectoral fascia or muscle
- T_{2b} Fixation to underlying pectoral fascia or muscle

T_3 Tumor >5 cm in its greatest dimension
- T_{3a} No fixation to underlying pectoral fascia or muscle
- T_{3b} Fixaton to underlying pectoral fascia or muscle

T_4 Tumor of any size with direct extension to chest wall or skin (chest wall includes ribs, intercostal muscles, and serratus anterior muscle, but not pectoral muscle)
- T_{4a} Fixation to chest wall
- T_{4b} Edema (including peau d'orange), ulceration of the skin of the breast, or satellite skin nodules confined to the same breast
- T_{4c} Both of the above

Nodal involvement (N)

The definition of N categories varies somewhat as to time period of staging.

Definitions for clinical-diagnostic stage

N_x Regional lymph nodes cannot be assessed clinically
N_0 Homolateral axillary lymph nodes not considered to contain growth
N_1 Movable homolateral axillary nodes considered to contain growth
N_2 Homolateral axillary nodes considered to contain growth and fixed to one another or to other structures
N_3 Homolateral supraclavicular or infraclavicular nodes considered to contain growth or edema of the arm (edema of the arm may be caused by lymphatic obstruction and lymph nodes may not then be palpable)

Definitions for surgical-evaluative and postsurgical resection–pathologic stage

N_x Regional lymph nodes cannot be assessed (not removed for study or previously removed)
N_0 No evidence of homolateral axillary lymph node metastasis
N_1 Metastasis to movable homolateral axillary nodes not fixed to one another or to other structure
N_{1a} Micrometastasis ≤0.2 cm in lymph node(s)
N_{1b} Gross metastasis in lymph node(s)
- I Metastasis >0.2 cm but <2.0 cm in one to three lymph nodes
- II Metastasis >0.2 cm but <2.0 cm in four or more lymph nodes
- III Extension of metastasis beyond the lymph node capsule (<2.0 cm in dimension)
- IV Metastasis in lymph node ≥2.0 cm in dimension

N_2 Metastases to homolateral axillary lymph nodes that are fixed to one another or to other structures
N_3 Metastasis to homolateral supraclavicular or infraclavicular lymph node(s). Edema of the arm may be caused by lymphatic obstruction, and lymph nodes may not then be palpable. Homolateral internal mammary nodes considered to contain growth are included in N_3 for surgical-evaluative classification and postsurgical resection–pathologic classification.

Continued.

Distant metastasis (M)

All time periods

M_x Minimum requirements to assess the presence of distant metastasis cannot be met

M_0 No (known) distant metastasis

M_1 Distant metastasis present

Specify ______________________

Specify sites according to the following notations:

Pulmonary	PUL	Bone marrow	MAR
Osseous	OSS	Pleura	PLE
Hepatic	HEP	Skin	SKI
Brain	BRA	Eye	EYE
Lymph nodes	LYM	Other	OTH

Stage grouping

Always indicate time of classification

Clinical-diagnostic (cTNM), surgical-evaluative (sTNM), and postsurgical resection–pathologic (pTNM) staging

Stage T_{is}	In situ	Stage IIIA	T_0, N_2, M_0
Stage x	Cannot stage		T_0, or T_{1b}, N_2, M_0
Stage I	T_{1ai}, N_0, M_0		T_{2a}, or T_{2b}, N_2, M_0
	T_{1aii}, N_0, M_0		T_{3a}, or T_{3b}, N_0, M_0
	T_{1aiii}, N_0, M_0		T_{3a}, or T_{3b}, N_1, M_0
	T_{1bi}, N_0, M_0		T_{3a}, or T_{3b}, N_2, M_0
	T_{1bii}, N_0, M_0	Stage IIIB	Any T, N_3, M_0
	T_{1biii}, N_0, M_0		Any T_4, and N, M_0
Stage II	T_0, N_{1a}, or N_{1B}, M_0	Stage IV	Any T_4, any N, M_1
	T_{1a}, or N_{1b}, N_{1a}, or N_{1b} M_0		
	T_{2a}, or T_{2b}, N_0, M_0		
	T_{2a}, or T_{2b}, N_{1a}, or N_{1b} M_0		

1986 TNM CLASSIFICATION[1]

Primary tumor

The clinical measurement used for classifying the primary tumor (T) should be the one judged most accurate (e.g., physical examination or mammogram). Pathologically, the tumor size for classification (T) is a measurement of the invasive component. For example, if there is a large in situ component (4 cm) and a small invasive component (0.5 cm), the tumor is classified T_{1a}. The size of the primary tumor should be measured before any tissue is removed for special studies, such as for estrogen receptors.

Multiple simultaneous ipsilateral primary cancers

The following guidelines should be used when classifying multiple simultaneous ipsilateral primary (infiltrating, grossly measurable) carcinomas. These criteria do not apply to one grossly detected tumor associated with multiple separate microscopic foci.

1. Use the largest primary carcinoma to classify T.
2. Enter into the record that this is a case of multiple simultaneous ipsilateral primary carcinomas. Such cases should be analyzed separately.

Simultaneous bilateral breast carcinomas

Each carcinoma should be staged separately.

Inflammatory carcinoma

Inflammatory carcinoma is a clinicopathologic entity characterized by diffuse brawny induration of the skin of the breast with an erysipeloid edge, usually without an underlying palpable mass. Radiologically there may be a detectable mass and characteristic thickening of the skin over the breast. This clinical presentation is related to tumor embolization of dermal lymphatics. The tumor inflammatory carcinoma is classified T_{4d}.

Paget's disease of the nipple

Paget's disease of the nipple without an associated tumor mass (clinical) or invasive carcinoma (pathologic) is classified T_{is}. Paget's disease with a demonstrable mass (clinical) or an invasive component (pathologic) is classified according to the size of the tumor mass or invasive component. Note: Paget's disease associated with a tumor is classified according to the size of the tumor.

Skin of breast

Dimpling of the skin, nipple retraction, or any other skin change except those described under inflammatory carcinoma (T_{4b}) may occur in T_1, T_2, or T_3 without changing the classification.

Primary tumor (T)

Definitions for classifying the primary tumor (T) are the same for clinical and for pathologic classification. The telescoping method of classification can be applied. If the measurement is made by physical examination, the examiner will use the major headings (T_1, T_2, or T_3). If other measurements, such as mammographic or pathologic, are used, the telescoped subsets of T_1 can be used.

- T_x Primary tumor cannot be assessed
- T_0 No evidence of primary tumor
- T_{is} Carcinoma in situ: intraductal carcinoma, lobular carcinoma in situ, or Paget's disease of the nipple with no tumor
- T_1 Tumor ≤2 cm in greatest dimension
  - T_{1a} ≤0.5 cm in greatest dimension
  - T_{1b} >0.5 cm but not >1 cm in greatest dimension
  - T_{1c} >1 cm but not >2 cm in greatest dimension
- T_2 Tumor >2 cm but not >5 cm in greatest dimension
- T_3 Tumor >5 cm in greatest dimension
- T_4 Tumor of any size with direct extension to chest wall or skin
  - T_{4a} Extension to chest wall
  - T_{4b} Edema (including peau d'orange) or ulceration of the skin of the breast or satellite skin nodules confined to the same breast
  - T_{4c} Both (T_{4a} and T_{4b})
  - T_{4d} Inflammatory carcinoma (see definition of inflammatory carcinoma in the introduction)

Note: Chest wall includes ribs, intercostal muscles, and serratus anterior muscle but not pectoral muscle.

Regional lymph nodes (N)

- N_x Regional lymph nodes cannot be assessed (e.g., previously removed)
- N_0 No regional lymph node metastasis
- N_1 Metastasis to movable ipsilateral axillary lymph node(s)
- N_2 Metastasis to ipsilateral axillary lymph node(s) fixed to one another or to other structures
- N_3 Metastasis to ipsilateral internal mammary lymph node(s)

Pathologic classification (pN)

- pN_x Regional lymph nodes cannot be assessed (e.g., previously removed or not removed for pathologic study)
- pN_0 No regional lymph node metastasis
- pN_1 Metastasis to movable ipsilateral axillary lymph node(s)
  - pN_{1a} Only micrometastasis (none >0.2 cm)
  - pN_{1b} Metastasis to lymph node(s), any >0.2 cm
    - pN_{1bi} Metastasis in 1 to 3 lymph nodes, any >0.2 cm and all <2 cm in greatest dimension
    - pN_{1bii} Metastasis to four or more lymph nodes, any >0.2 cm and all <2 cm in greatest dimension
    - pN_{1biii} Extension of tumor beyond the capsule of a lymph node metastasis <2 cm in greatest dimension
    - pN_{1biv} Metastasis to a lymph node ≥2 cm in greatest dimension
- pN_2 Metastasis to ipsilateral axillary lymph nodes that are fixed to one another or to other structures
- pN_3 Metastasis to ipsilateral internal mammary lymph node(s)

Continued.

1986 TNM CLASSIFICATION—cont'd

Distant metastasis (M)

M_x	Presence of distant metastasis cannot be assessed
M_0	No distant metastasis
M_1	Distant metastasis [includes metastasis to ipsilateral supraclavicular lymph nodes(s)]

Staging grouping

Stage 0	T_{is}	N_0	M_0	Stage IIIA	T_0	N_2	M_0
Stage I	T_1	N_0	M_0		T_1	N_2	M_0
Stage IIA	T_0	N_1	M_0		T_2	N_2	M_0
	T_1	N_1*	M_0		T_3	N_1, N_2	M_0
	T_2	N_0	M_0	Stage IIIB	T_4	Any N	M_0
Stage IIB	T_2	N_1	M_0		Any T	N_3	M_0
	T_3	N_0	M_0	Stage IV	Any T	Any N	M_1

*The prognosis of patients with pN_{1a} is similar to that of patients with pN_0.

T_1 tumors are now subdivided into those $\leq$0.5 cm (T_{1a}), those 0.5 cm to 1 cm (T_{1b}), and those >1 cm but $\leq$2 cm (T_{1c}). Metastases to the ipsilateral internal mammary nodes are now classified as N_3. For the most part, current literature reflects the 1983 staging system, although the reporting of results according to the 1986 classification certainly will appear in the future.

There are obvious limitations to the current staging system. It is recognized that clinical assessment of the axilla is in error in approximately 30% of patients. Discrepancies between the clinical and pathologic size of the tumor also may influence the stage. The pathologic tumor size includes only that of the invasive component of the disease, whereas the clinical size may be related to both components. Pathologic tumor size may be also difficult to determine in patients whose initial biopsy is incisional rather than excisional. Prognostic factors such as patient age, tumor grade or histologic subtype, and estrogen or progesterone receptor status are not included. Although information from the newer biologic markers, including ploidy and proliferative rate, oncogenes and cathepsin D, provide a guide for clinical practice, it does not influence staging. However, it must be emphasized that accurate staging allows for the uniform reporting of results and facilitates communication among breast cancer specialists.

Throughout the text results of treatment are represented in terms of staging criteria. For the most part the TNM classification is based upon the 1983 staging system. As the body of knowledge relating to prognostic factors in breast cancer increases, refinements in the staging system may become necessary. While these changes are important, retrospective comparisons of results from individual institutions or prospective randomized clinical trials may be made more difficult. It is most important in clinical practice that a uniform system be employed.

REFERENCES

1. Beahrs OH, Henson DE, Hutter RVP, and Myers MH, editors: Manual for staging of cancer: American Joint Committee on Cancer, ed 3, Philadelphia, 1988, JB Lippincott, pp 145-150.
2. Beahrs OH and Myers MH, editors: Manual for staging of cancer: American Joint Committee on Cancer, ed 2, Philadelphia, 1983, JB Lippincott, pp 127-133.
3. Haagensen CD: Diseases of the breast, ed 3, Philadelphia, 1971, WB Saunders Co, p 630.
4. Haagensen CD, Cooley E, Miller E, et al: Treatment of early mammary carcinoma: a cooperative international study, Ann Surg 170:875, 1969.
5. Windeyer BW: Cancer of the breast, Am J Roentgenol Radium Ther Nucl Med 62:345, 1949.
6. Yorkshire Breast Cancer Group: Critical assessment of the clinical TNM system in breast cancer, Br Med J 281:134, 1980.
7. Zippin C: Comparison of the International and American systems for staging of breast cancer, J Natl Cancer Inst 36:53, 1966.

2 The Role of Mammography in the Pretreatment Evaluation of the Patient with Breast Cancer

Rosalind H. Troupin** and **Elizabeth A. Patterson

Mammography plays a contributory and at times decisive role in the management of the breast cancer patient at several points in the decision-making process. Patient selection for conservative surgery and radiation is based on many factors. Mammography provides a readily measured tumor volume to assist clinical judgment in anticipating the cosmetic consequences of wide excision and irradiation. Perhaps more important, it also serves to detect or exclude other suspicious lesions. Chapter 6 focuses on the special problems of mammographic follow-up of treated patients after lumpectomy and irradiation. In this chapter two distinct clinical points in time are considered: the initial evaluation of a patient with clinically or mammographically suspected neoplasm, and the pretreatment reevaluation after a positive biopsy.

In all three instances, mammograms of excellent technical quality must be obtained and be interpreted with insight into the specific questions being asked. At times this requires a tailored, problem-solving examination utilizing special views to clarify important issues. Although it is not within the scope of this text to elaborate at length on mammographic diagnosis, an overview of basic principles is required in order to understand the special problems of these patients.

TECHNICAL FACTORS DETERMINING IMAGE QUALITY

Modern, dedicated mammographic equipment is now widely available, replacing the former option of modifying standard x-ray equipment for part-time use in mammography. High quality mammographic images can be achieved utilizing either film-screen or xeroradiographic technology, providing that meticulous attention is given to equipment, positioning, exposure, and processing. While both film and xerox methods can yield excellent images, they can be difficult to compare to one another in that the very high contrast of film greatly accentuates differences between fat and water density (Fig. 2-1). This can lead to the incorrect impression that a new density is developing or that a scar is unstable.

The x-ray tube

High-contrast screen film mammography utilizes an x-ray tube with a molybdenum target and filtration, operating in the 25 to 28 kVp range. Xeromammography is done in the 40 to 55 kVp range using a tungsten target with aluminum filtration. Dual focal spots in mammography units include an extremely fine (0.1 mm, nominal) spot to minimize unsharpness when supplemental air-gap magnification imaging is needed.

X-ray grids

These devices improve contrast and definition of the x-ray image by selectively transmitting the primary beam while reducing secondary scatter from the breast that would otherwise contribute to film exposure. Grids are constructed of parallel, alternating, very fine strips of absorbing and transmitting material that block the entry of scattered radiation striking from nonparallel directions. Reciprocating (Bucky) devices are grids that move at the instant of exposure so that no distracting grid lines are visible on the film.

Phototiming

Modern units have sensitive photoreceptor cells that are designed to provide automatic control of the exposure time when kilovoltage and photocell density have been set. For most mammographic examinations this works very well. There are instances, particularly with extremely dense or very heterogeneous breasts, where automatic exposure does not result in optimal images. In such situations, the technologist must have the skill to proceed with supplemental views using manual settings.

A

B

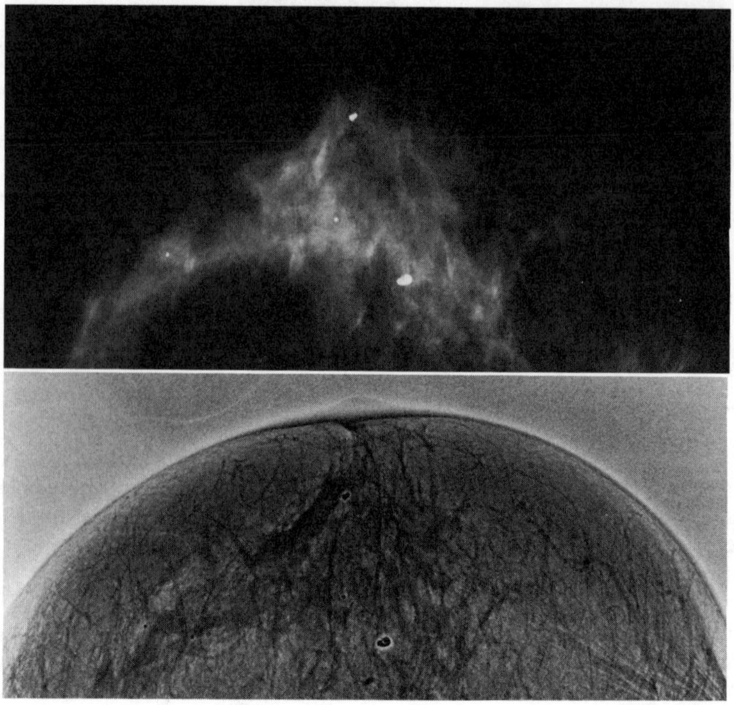

Fig. 2-1 Cephalocaudad views in film screen mammography **(A)** and **B,** xeromammography. In **A,** the soft tissues are highly contrasted against the radiolucent fat but the basic interface shapes are no different. On the film image posterior coverage is better but the skin is difficult to see without a hot-light.

Breast positioning and compression

The two basic views are the craniocaudad (CC) and an oblique modification of the mediolateral view. To include and penetrate the thicker posterior tissues, the base of the breast must be drawn anteriorly from the chest wall while vigorous compression (to the point of discomfort but not of pain) is applied for a few moments. Compression reduces fibroglandular tissue overlap in addition to minimizing geometric and motion unsharpness. A rigid plastic compression device utilized by a technologist with excellent interpersonal as well as technical skills is essential for high quality images.

Image recording systems

Enormous improvements in image detail and dose reduction have occurred since the early low-kilovoltage, nonscreen industrial film techniques of the 1950s. In the early 1970s, at the same time that film mammography was being improved, xeromammography was developed. This is an electrostatic imaging process utilizing a selenium semiconductor plate, altered by x-rays to produce a latent image, which is then made visible by development with charged pigmented particles. Subsequently, however, as xeromammography was being improved, a major breakthrough in film mammography occurred with the introduction of film-screen technique. In this photographic process the film is exposed by light output from a very sensitive intensifying screen, rather than directly by the x-ray beam. This results in very significant reductions in radiation dose while maintaining high resolution and high contrast. The spectral response of the specific film must be matched to the screen and coordinated with the proper cassettes and film processing chemicals.

Processing

Meticulous dark room technique must include attention to proper processing temperatures, clean solutions, and gentle film handling, as well as dust and static precautions. Mammographic image contrast benefits from higher temperatures and slower processing than standard x-rays, and many large institutions with large volumes have a dedicated processor for mammography.

Constant supervision and attention to quality control are clearly mandatory. Frequent testing utilizing breast phantoms provides ongoing checks of dosimetry, image detail, and processor performance. At any point in this fastidious technical chain, fine-detail image quality can be lost, effectively negating the interpretive skills of the mammographer.

THE PREOPERATIVE MAMMOGRAM

There are two types of patients to be considered: patients with a palpable lesion and those undergoing screening mammography. In both types of patients mammographic coverage and scrutiny of all parts of both breasts are needed, and an understanding of factors that contribute to the detectability of lesions is pertinent to film interpretation.

Lesion detection

With increasingly widespread use of screening mammography, nonpalpable, and in many instances noninvasive lesions are being detected, many of which have an excellent prognosis. Several factors contribute to the detectability of a small malignancy, some but not all of which are controllable.

The breast tissue background. If, as is true in 50% of cases, a tumor does not contain calcium particles large enough to be mammographically visible, detectability is dependent on the tumor being perceived as a dense focus against a more lucent fatty background. The subcutaneous, retromam-

A

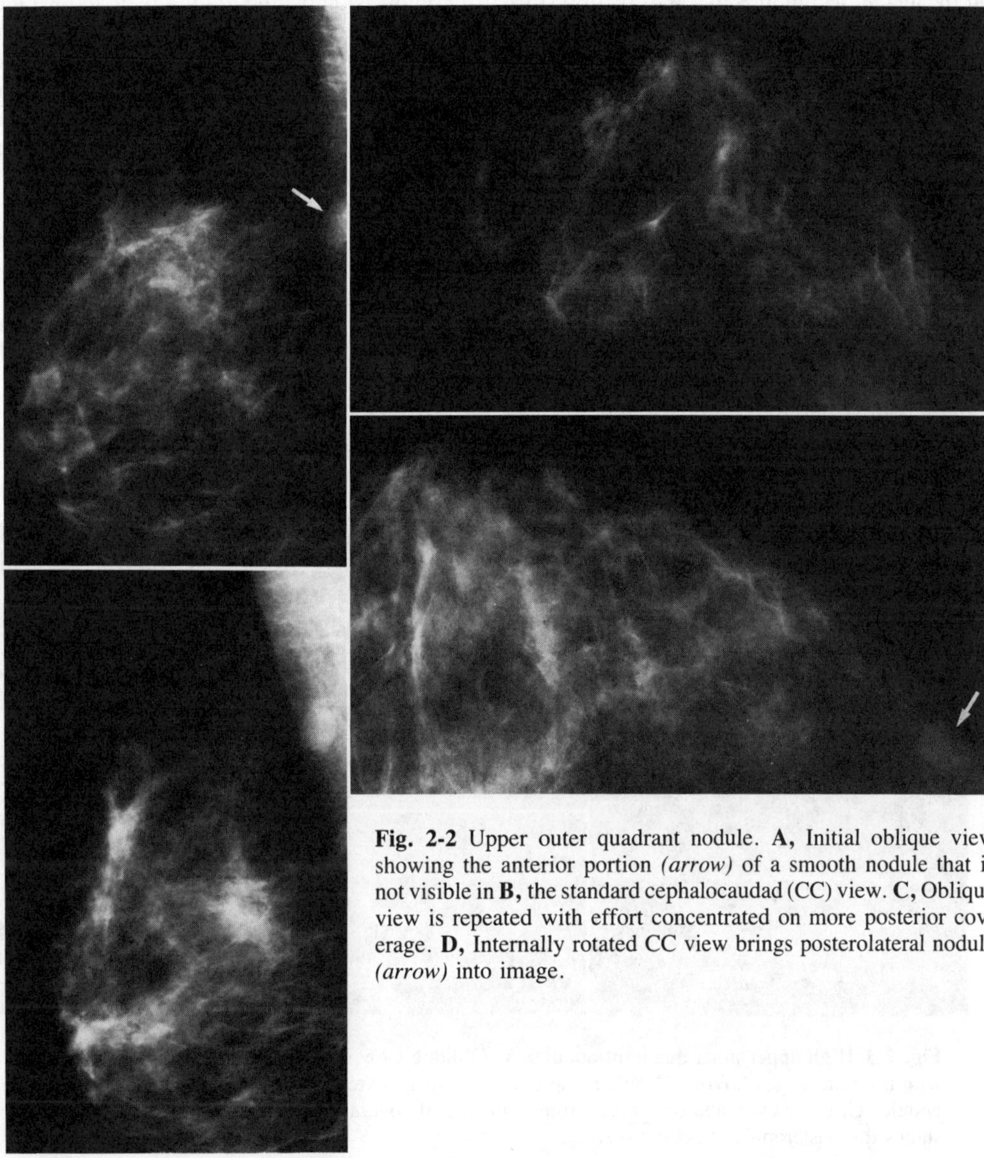

B

C

D

Fig. 2-2 Upper outer quadrant nodule. **A,** Initial oblique view showing the anterior portion *(arrow)* of a smooth nodule that is not visible in **B,** the standard cephalocaudad (CC) view. **C,** Oblique view is repeated with effort concentrated on more posterior coverage. **D,** Internally rotated CC view brings posterolateral nodule *(arrow)* into image.

mary and interlobular fat content of a breast determines this background mammographic appearance. The glands and ducts (parenchyma) and the supporting fibrous tissue (stroma) are basically all of "water density" on mammography. The mammographically dense breasts of a young woman have high proportions of glandular elements, while the elderly or cachectic breast also may appear dense if composed of sheets of fibrous tissue with relatively little fat. The frustrating reality is that a noncalcified tumor will be mammographically invisible in any uniformly dense, fibroglandular breast.

Detectability also can be reduced in a mixed background where fibroglandular islands are randomly interspersed with zones of more radiolucent fat. Subtle clues, if perceived, can initiate clarification by special techniques that will be described later in the chapter. Unfortunately, however, some early cancers will be indistinguishable from benign heterogeneous fibroglandular islands, and only later will it become apparent that one focal density was progressing while the others remained stable.

The completeness of tissue coverage. Because of the broad-based attachment of most breasts to the curving chest wall, routine craniocaudad and mediolateral oblique views may fail to include the very peripheral edges of breast tissue. This is more likely to occur with a firm conical breast that is tightly adherent to the chest wall than in a flabby, malleable breast that the technologist can draw forward more readily into the compression field. Special projections have been developed to overcome these geometric/anatomic problems, for use if the lesion is suspected clinically or the radiologist sees a hint of it on one view.

The most common example requiring tailored problem solving is a peripheral upper outer quadrant focus, partially visible on mediolateral oblique and totally absent on the basic craniocaudad view (Fig. 2-2). A special CC view made with the patient's breast and chest rotated medially displays the lateral tissue and abnormality, while sacrificing coverage medially. A supplementary oblique might sacrifice a perfectly profiled nipple to achieve greater depth posterolaterally.

A second problem zone occurs very high and posteriorly, particularly in the superomedial or superocentral areas. This results from the CC compression paddle gliding over and excluding the most superior tissue as compression is applied. If something is suspected from other views, however, a modified CC view can be made in which the breast is rotated under, sacrificing lower coverage but accentuating the upper zone (Fig. 2-3).

Problems in perception. In studies that attempt to analyze the causes of mammographic failure to diagnose carcinomas, there is ample evidence that dense fibroglandular breasts, very peripheral lesions, and tumors hiding in heterogeneous backgrounds were the major causes. When these are excluded, two additional categories of false negatives emerge. In one, a subtle but real finding was not appreciated or pursued by an inadequately ex-

A

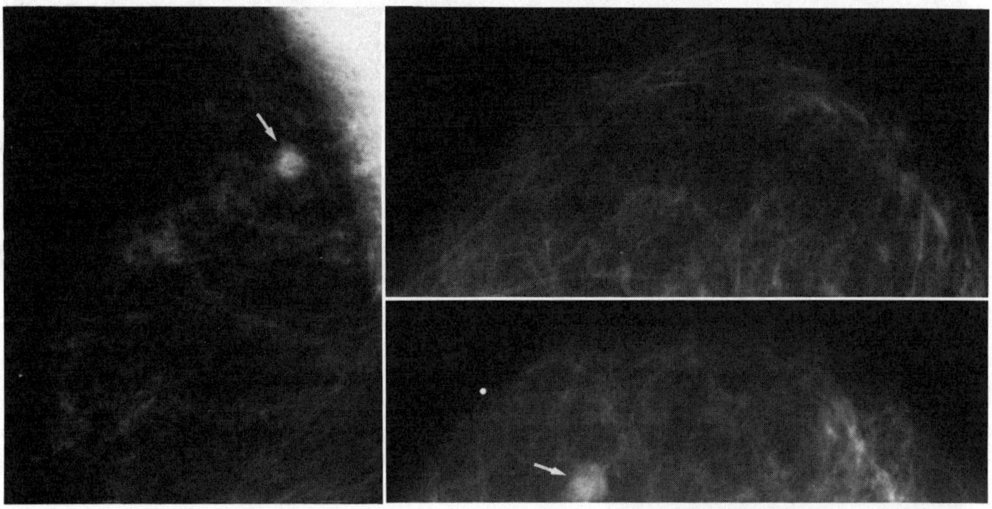

B

C

Fig. 2-3 High upper inner quadrant nodule. **A,** Oblique view showing a superiorly located nodule with irregular edges *(arrow)*. Neither traditional CC or **B,** externally rotated CC views showed the nodule. **C,** CC view made with breast rolled under and coverage accentuating the upper quadrants shows the posteromedial nodule *(arrow)*.

perienced interpreter. In the other, a relatively obvious focus was inexplicably missed.[8] This type of perceptual failure can originate in a setting where haste, fatigue, distractions by other cases, ongoing activities in the reading room, or internal preoccupation were to blame. Obvious solutions relate to controlling the reading room environment, providing adequate staffing for clinician consultations and case-load management, or, ideally, utilizing a double reading system.

Lesion analysis

Only after a dominant or potentially worrisome focus has been detected can its analysis proceed. Because certain benign and malignant breast lesions can overlap in their mammographic appearances, image interpretation must be expressed in terms of probabilities. At either end of the spectrum are appearances virtually pathognomonic of malignant or of benign lesions, with a central range spanning the "very high" to "very low" likelihood of cancer range. A threshold level for recommending biopsy evolves in each clinical setting, as interpreters strive to detect early cancers while avoiding excessive numbers of benign biopsies. Multiple studies published in the United States[2,20] find positive predictive values averaging in the 20% to 30% range for the general mammographic population, such that three or four negative biopsies are done for each true positive. Less commonly, a center practicing more aggressive screening[10] deliberately sets a threshold to detect subtler malignancies and accepts nine negative biopsies for each cancer. In Sweden, in a stable screening population where compliance with follow-up is reliable, medicolegal issues are rare and cost containment is a reality, thresholds resulting in 60% or 70% positive predictive values can be set.[18]

Mammographic interpretation and recommendation should obviously employ more aggressive thresholds in patients with suspected, proven, or treated breast cancer. In this high-risk group, borderline or mildly suspicious features that could be followed closely in a reliable screening population will generally be biopsied.

In 20% of nonpalpable malignancies detected mammographically by Sickles,[16] diagnosis was based on a subtle finding such as focal asymmetry, gradually developing focal density, mild architectural distortion (Fig. 2-4), or localized duct dilatation. The more commonly utilized parameters, alone or in combination, are nodules and calcifications.

The mammographic nodule. In analyzing water-density mass lesions, the more irregular the margins, the higher the probability of malignancy.

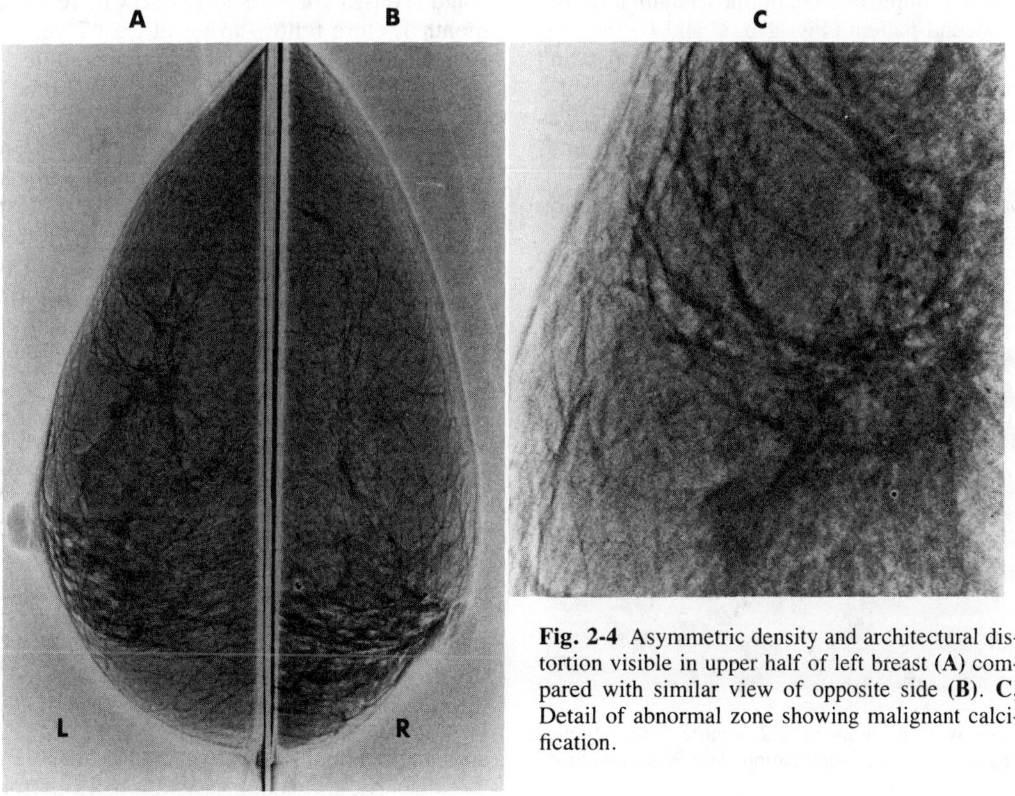

Fig. 2-4 Asymmetric density and architectural distortion visible in upper half of left breast (**A**) compared with similar view of opposite side (**B**). **C,** Detail of abnormal zone showing malignant calcification.

Invasive ductal or lobular carcinomas, extending in an infiltrating manner into adjacent fat, and evoking a fibrotic response, result in a macroscopic image of radiating, spiculated, or corona-like margins. While this appearance is highly suspicious, it is not, of itself, pathognomonic because a resolved abscess, hematoma, surgical scar, fat necrosis, radial scar, or intensely fibrous focus of sclerosing adenosis could all simulate the stellate nodule. By the same token, carcinomas can advance with a pushing, broader front resulting in relatively smooth or knobby margins (Fig. 2-5). This is certainly true of mucinous, medullary, and papillary carcinomas, but also can be seen with ordinary duct carcinomas. This appearance would have macroscopic overlap with benign breast lesions, particularly fibroadenomas and cysts.

Evaluating the margins. Because margin irregularity can be simulated by overlapping or adjacent tissue, mammographers often use spot compression views of the area in question. A small circular paddle firmly applied to the area of suspicion can often spatially rearrange overlying and adjacent fibroglandular tissue and permit a more valid assessment of margin characteristics. In Fig. 2-6, three patients with suspected focal densities on mammography have undergone clarification by spot compression views. In the first patient (Fig. 2-6, *A* and *B*) the "lesion" disappeared, indicating that it was a simple overlap of fibroglandular tissue. In the second patient (Fig. 2-6, *C* and *D*) the stellate density was confirmed, leading to biopsy and the diagnosis of invasive carcinoma. In the third patient (Fig. 2-6, *E* and *F*) a smooth outline was demonstrated, prompting the use of ultrasound, which showed a simple cyst.

Combining spot compression and magnification

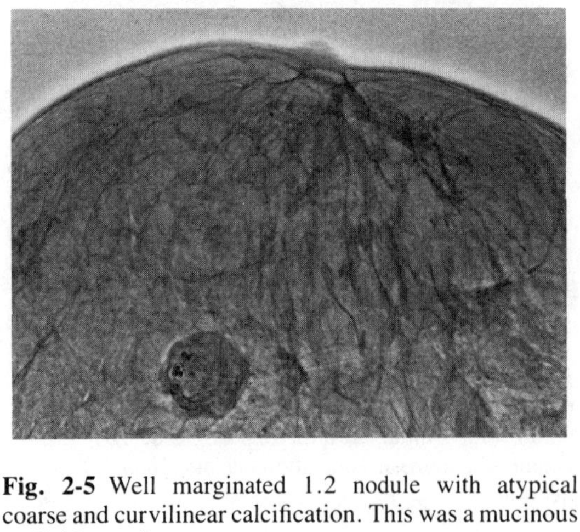

Fig. 2-5 Well marginated 1.2 nodule with atypical coarse and curvilinear calcification. This was a mucinous (colloid) carcinoma.

techniques to clarify the margins of a nodule and to search for fine calcification within it can guide the decision to biopsy or to follow a small nodular density closely (Fig. 2-7).

Ultrasound for cyst/solid differentiation. Strict sonographic criteria for identifying cysts have been developed and tested. If the lesion is anechoic, smooth walled, and shows a sharp back wall and enhanced through-transmission,[3] it is a simple cyst and in most clinical settings can be left alone. Lingering anxiety in the high-risk patient can be alleviated by aspiration. If the fluid is not unusual and the mammographic "nodule" disappears, many would not subject the fluid to cytologic analysis[14] unless it is bloody. Others would prefer to do cytology on all aspirated fluid. At least one author[19] advocates injecting air into the aspirated cyst for additional imaging of the cyst lining and because it may decrease the incidence of recurrence. Further investigation of the therapeutic benefits of pneumocystography is in progress.

Short-interval follow-up. Solid spherical or ovoid nodular densities with absolutely sharp margins on all projections have a very high probability of being benign; 95% according to Meyer[9]; 98% quoted by Moskowitz.[11] In a general population a small (<1 cm), smooth, solid nodule could be biopsied, stipulating an extremely low level of suspicion, in an anxious patient. Alternatively, management could consist of a short interval recheck (6 months), close follow-up for at least 2 years, and yearly check-ups thereafter.[4] Probabilities and thresholds would be appropriately modified in a breast cancer patient.

Mammographic calcifications: general diagnostic guidelines. There are a great many kinds of easily dismissed, obviously benign calcifications that can occur in the breast, caused by fibroadenomas, duct stasis, fat necrosis, and atherosclerosis. While these pose only rare problems in differentiation from malignant calcification, calcifications seen in entities within the fibrocystic spectrum may be more difficult to distinguish.

Character. Because tumor calcification occurs primarily within the luminal debris of duct carcinoma, in its pathognomonic form it may exhibit linear, cast-like, or branching features, often with angular, irregular, or pleomorphic morphology. Incompletely developed calcium casts are interrupted, showing a more granular "dot-dash" linear array (Fig. 2-8). These linear calcifications are finer than the benign stasis calcifications seen commonly in larger ducts. When concretions form in benign adenosis or within the microcystic dilated terminal lobules, they tend to be spherical and smooth, without individual linear shapes. Fig. 2-9 displays six examples of biopsies performed

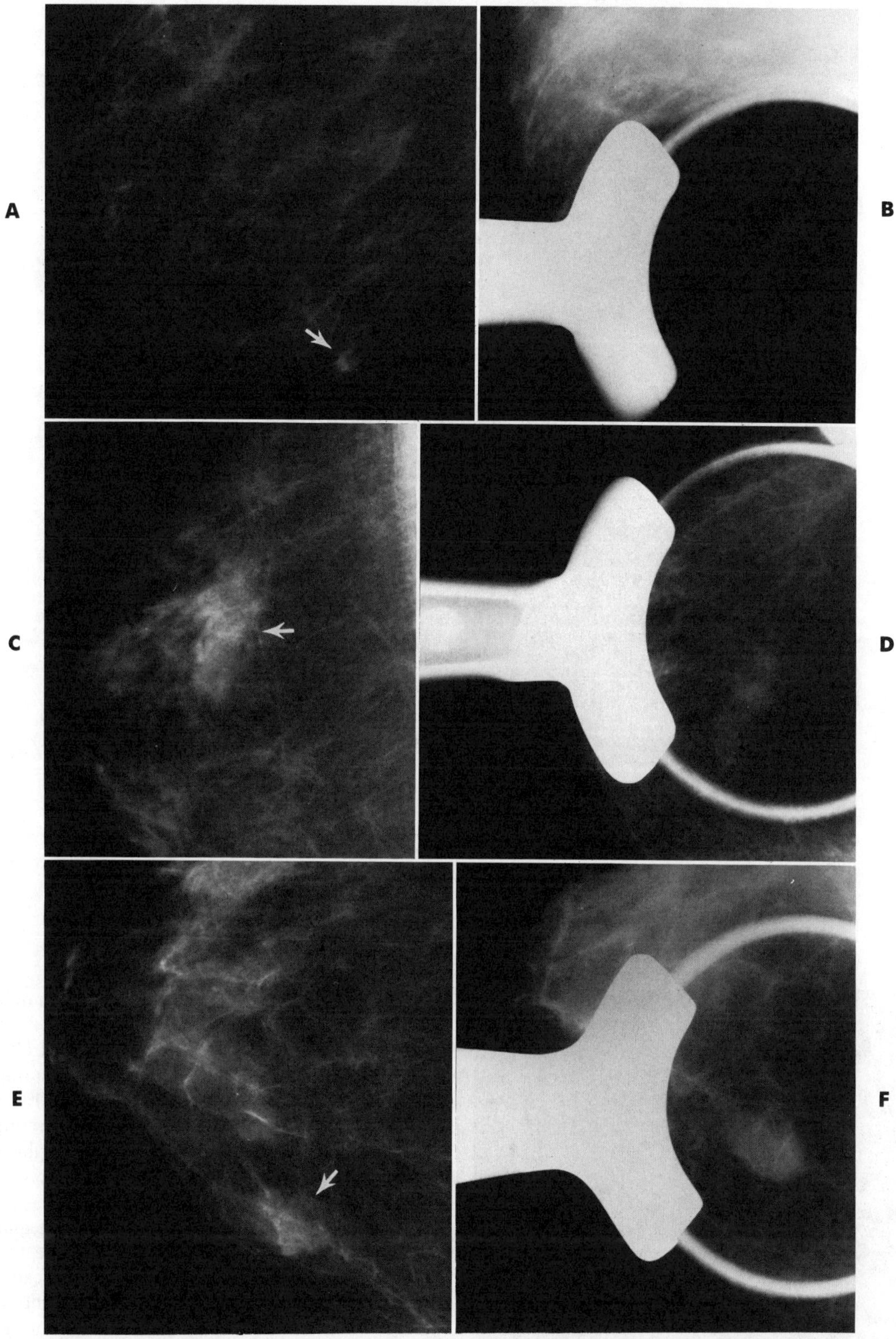

Fig. 2-6 Use of spot compression views to clarify suspected abnormality. Patient 1, stellate focus *(arrow)* inferiorly in **A,** disappears entirely on compression in **B,** indicating a fibroglandular overlap. Patient 2, irregular central density *(arrow)* in **C,** maintains stellate nodular configuration with compression in **D.** Localization and biopsy showed infiltrating carcinoma. Patient 3, ill-defined density *(arrow)* in **E,** shows smoother edges in **F,** prompting ultrasound, which demonstrated a simple cyst.

A

B

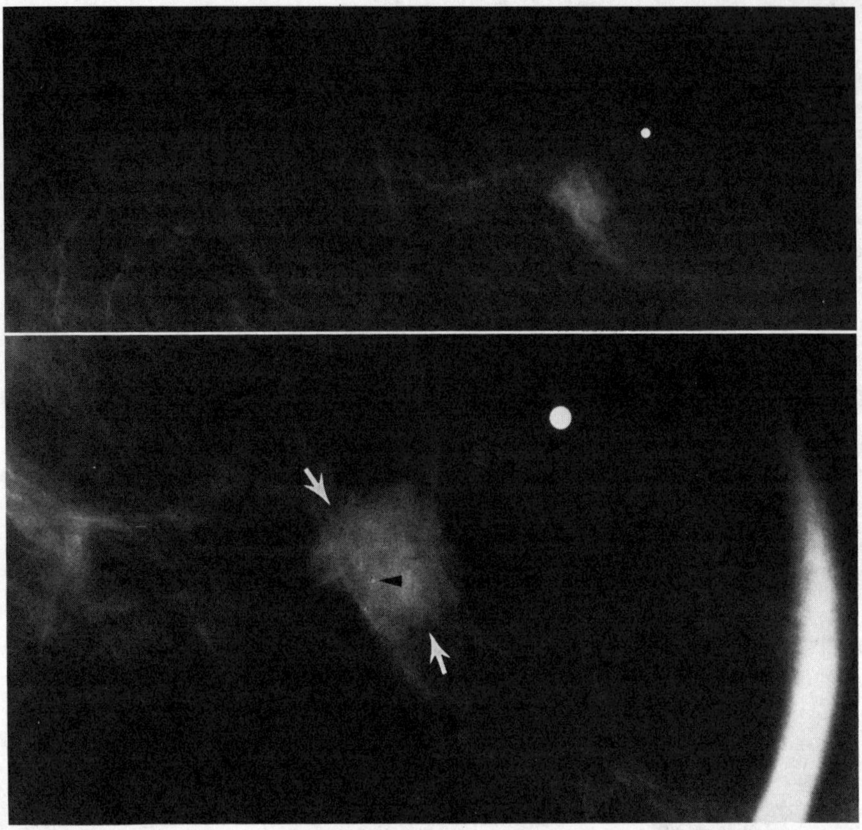

Fig. 2-7 Combining spot compression and magnification techniques. **A,** Defined nodule of 1 cm on routine mammogram. **B,** Spot compression magnification view shows zones of poor margination *(white arrows)* as well as several internal calcifications *(black arrowhead)*. Biopsy demonstrated infiltrating carcinoma.

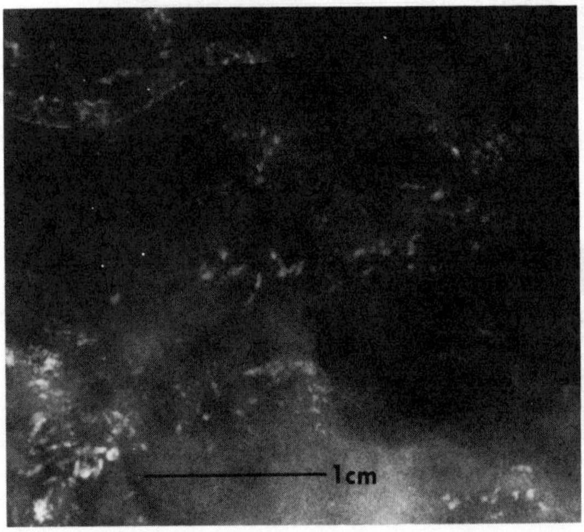

Fig. 2-8 Malignant-appearing calcifications in 4-cm zone showing pleomorphism, irregular shapes, linear casts, branching, and interrupted dot-dash patterns.

for clustered calcifications showing a range of suspicious and ambiguous appearances.

Number. Four or five particles in a tight cluster would trigger a positive call from most mammographers, and result in approximately a 20% true positive rate. More aggressive screening programs and interpretations in high-risk patients might take action in a three- or four-particle cluster, accepting an 11% positive rate.[10]

Distribution. Particle number is more meaningful in the context of the remainder of the breast tissue. If there are innumerable, diffusely scattered calcifications from benign disease, a concentration greater than three or four per cubic centimeter would be required to be considered suspicious. Three or four particles in a breast with no other areas of calcification could be significant. Magnification filming can clarify the texture and number of the particles as well as reveal more widespread calcification than could be appreciated on standard

A B C D E F

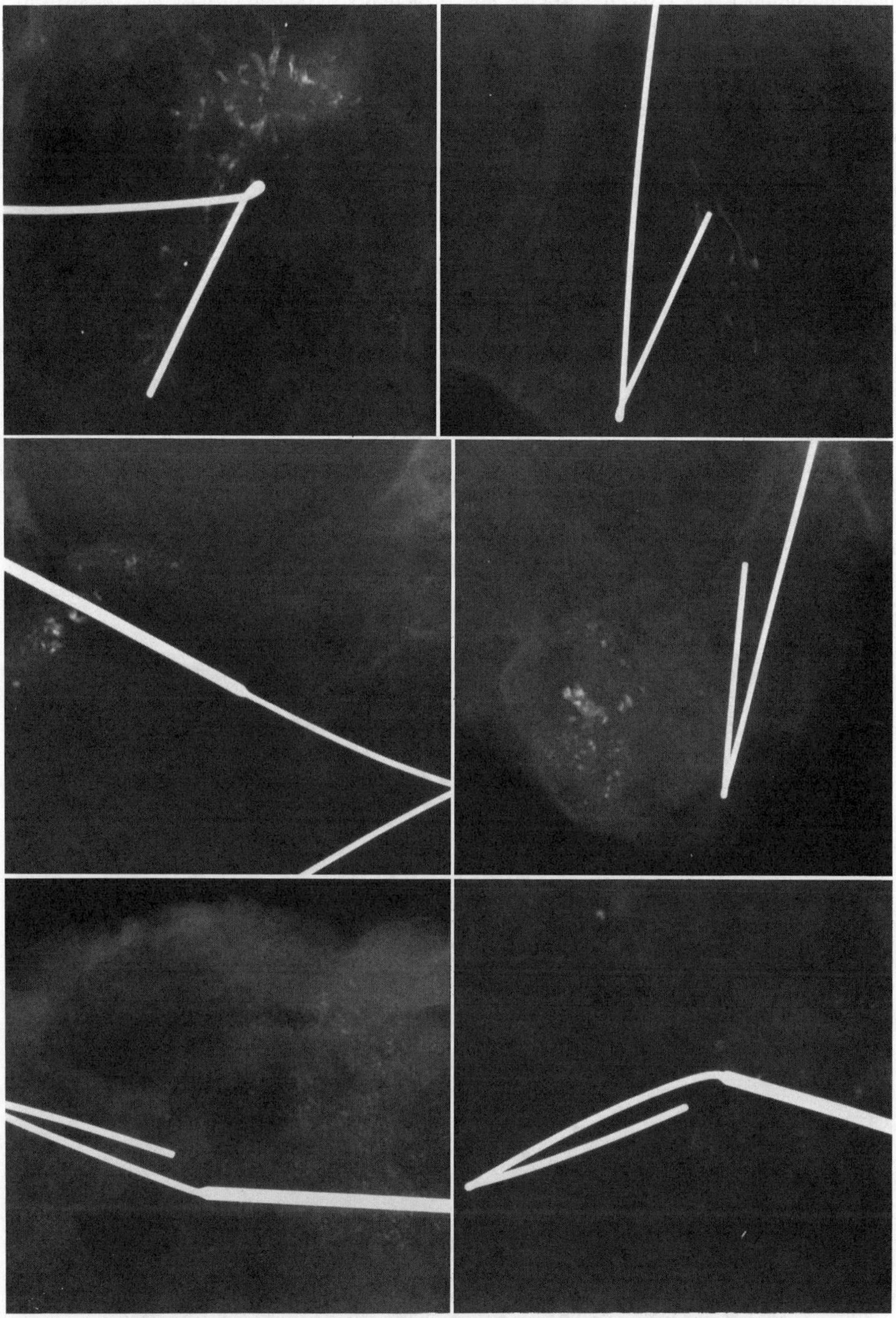

Fig. 2-9 Six examples of calcifications for which biopsy was performed. For reference, the hook is 1 cm long. In **A** and **B** the linear branching indicates an extremely high probability of malignancy, which was confirmed. The calcification in **C** and **D** appear similar to one another but that in **C,** proved malignant while that in **D** was benign. **E,** An extremely fine, uniform zone of calcium caused by sclerosing adenosis. **F,** Amorphous groupings, an ambiguous mammographic appearance that in this instance was benign.

films.[17] Calcifications clustered into a tightly spherical group are much more likely to be benign than when the same number and type of particles are distributed in a linear or geographic grouping.[7]

Stability. If calcifications in one area of the breast are increasing while other zones remain stable, biopsy should be considered. Stability, however, may not always be easily judged, as some images are not comparable. Continuing technical improvements in fine-definition images may make it difficult to be certain whether the calcifications are unchanged relative to older baseline films.

Calcifications: special considerations. In general, decisions regarding the suspicion level for a focus of calcification are based on morphology, distribution, number, and stability. Magnification filming techniques help in this analysis by providing high-detail imaging. In the patient with suspected or known neoplasm, the probability thresholds for a positive call must be modified based on experience derived from long-term collaboration with surgical pathologists and careful correlation on a case-by-case basis. It is not sufficient to note that a given biopsy, done for mammographic calcium, did show microscopic tumor and was, therefore, called a true positive. If the calcium was actually in benign disease and the histologic tumor was an incidental finding, it is incorrect to "learn" that this type of calcification can be produced by malignant ducts. These juxtapositions of calcification and microscopic tumor are in all probability accidental, but theoretically might result if duct neoplasm downstream caused obstructed benign lobules to precipitate benign calcification. This concept of benign calcification as a marker for adjacent neoplasm is not widely accepted.[5]

Some sources suggest that when invasive carcinoma is accompanied by extensive intraductal carcinoma (EIC), there is a greater likelihood of tumor recurrence in the treated breast.[13] Other studies have not confirmed this.[15] However, because most malignant calcification does occur within the intraductal portion of the tumor, if it is visible mammographically, it could serve to predict widespread or multifocal in situ carcinoma. This preoperative information can be used to influence decisions regarding the number and extent of biopsies (Fig. 2-10).

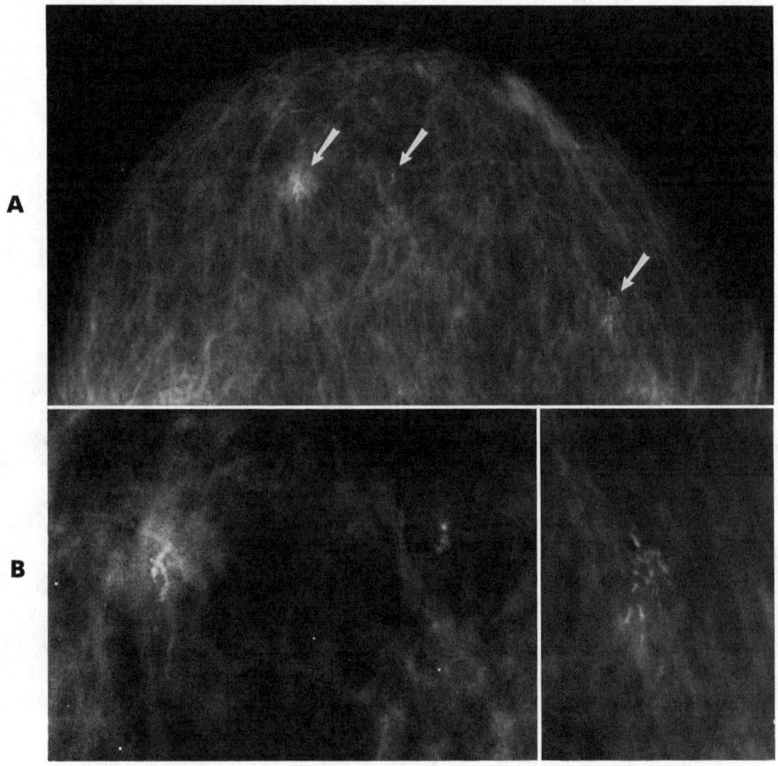

Fig. 2-10 Multifocal malignant calcifications. **A,** Craniocaudad view of mammogram done for screening. Several widely separated, multiquadrant areas of calcification are present, three of which *(arrows)* are shown in photographic magnifications (**B** and **C**). Breast-conserving management was not an option.

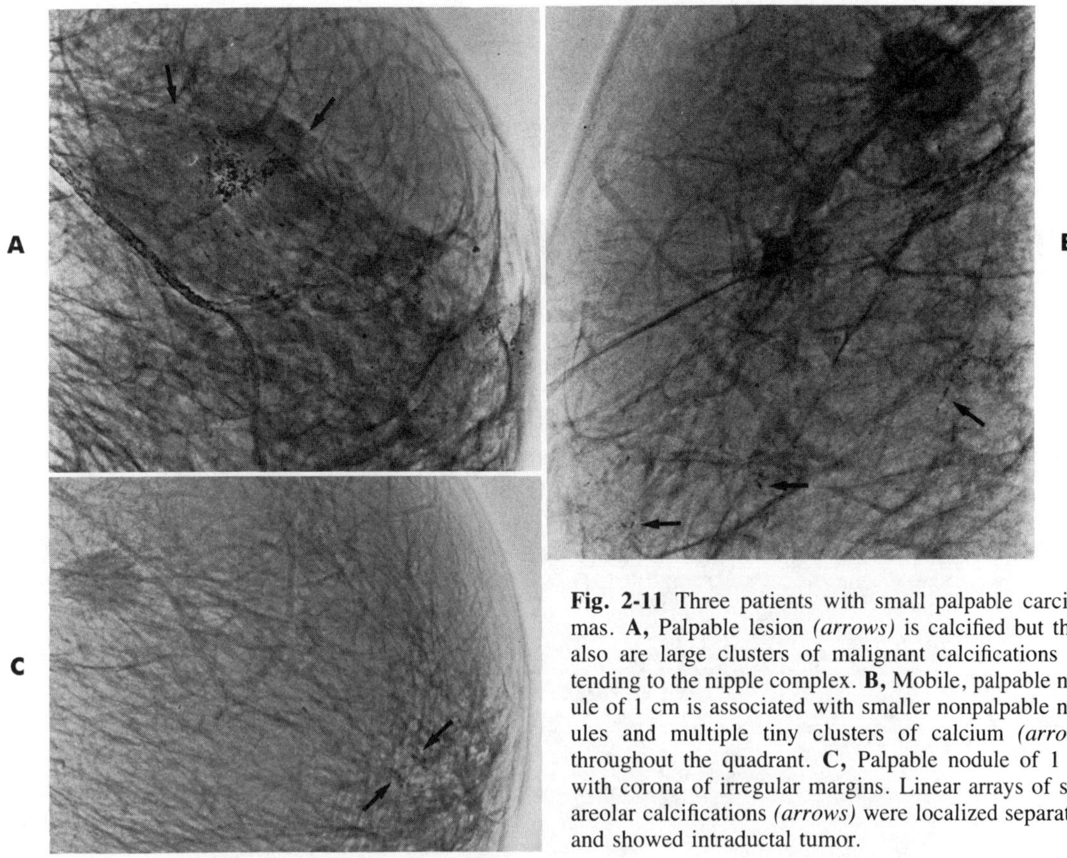

Fig. 2-11 Three patients with small palpable carcinomas. **A,** Palpable lesion *(arrows)* is calcified but there also are large clusters of malignant calcifications extending to the nipple complex. **B,** Mobile, palpable nodule of 1 cm is associated with smaller nonpalpable nodules and multiple tiny clusters of calcium *(arrows)* throughout the quadrant. **C,** Palpable nodule of 1 cm with corona of irregular margins. Linear arrays of subareolar calcifications *(arrows)* were localized separately and showed intraductal tumor.

Evaluation of the remainder of the breast tissue

Once detection and analysis of the dominant focus are completed, meticulous scrutiny of the tissues elsewhere in that breast and contralaterally is mandatory. Distraction by the dominant site is a very real pitfall in the detection of additional areas of suspicion. Failure to note more extensive disease in the same or other quadrants will result in errors in patient selection for lumpectomy and primary irradiation. Fig. 2-11 depicts three patients in whom mammographic disclosure of clinically unsuspected additional disease resulted in a decision for mastectomy. In other patients, ambiguous lesions remote from the dominant focus were biopsied and found negative, permitting breast conservation management to be pursued. Concretions of a clearly benign nature in the parenchyma or within the skin, milk-of-calcium layering in tiny microcysts on lateral views, and small intramammary lymph nodes with lucent hila are all examples of findings that should not be biopsied, even in these very high-risk breasts.

BIOPSY PLANNING AND PREOPERATIVE NEEDLE LOCALIZATION

In the instance of the clinically palpable lesion, the mammogram functions not only to survey the remainder of the breast but to determine whether the visible abnormality is actually larger than its palpable component. If so, this can reveal the need for wider excision (Fig. 2-12, *A* and *B*) or for needle localization of an adjacent, nonpalpable focus (Fig. 2-12, *C* and *D*). A very large zone of extremely suspicious calcification (see Fig. 2-11, *A*) suggests that diagnostic biopsy can be relatively small, as mastectomy rather than breast conservation will be the management plan. If a moderately large zone is present, but the management plan is to await microscopic assessment, the surgeon may want to attempt a complete excision with clear margins. Localizing two separate foci independently (Fig. 2-13, *A* and *B*) or using flanking, paired localization wires to show the mammographic boundaries (Fig. 2-13, *C* and *D*) is more effective than placing a single hook wire in the midst of the calcifications.

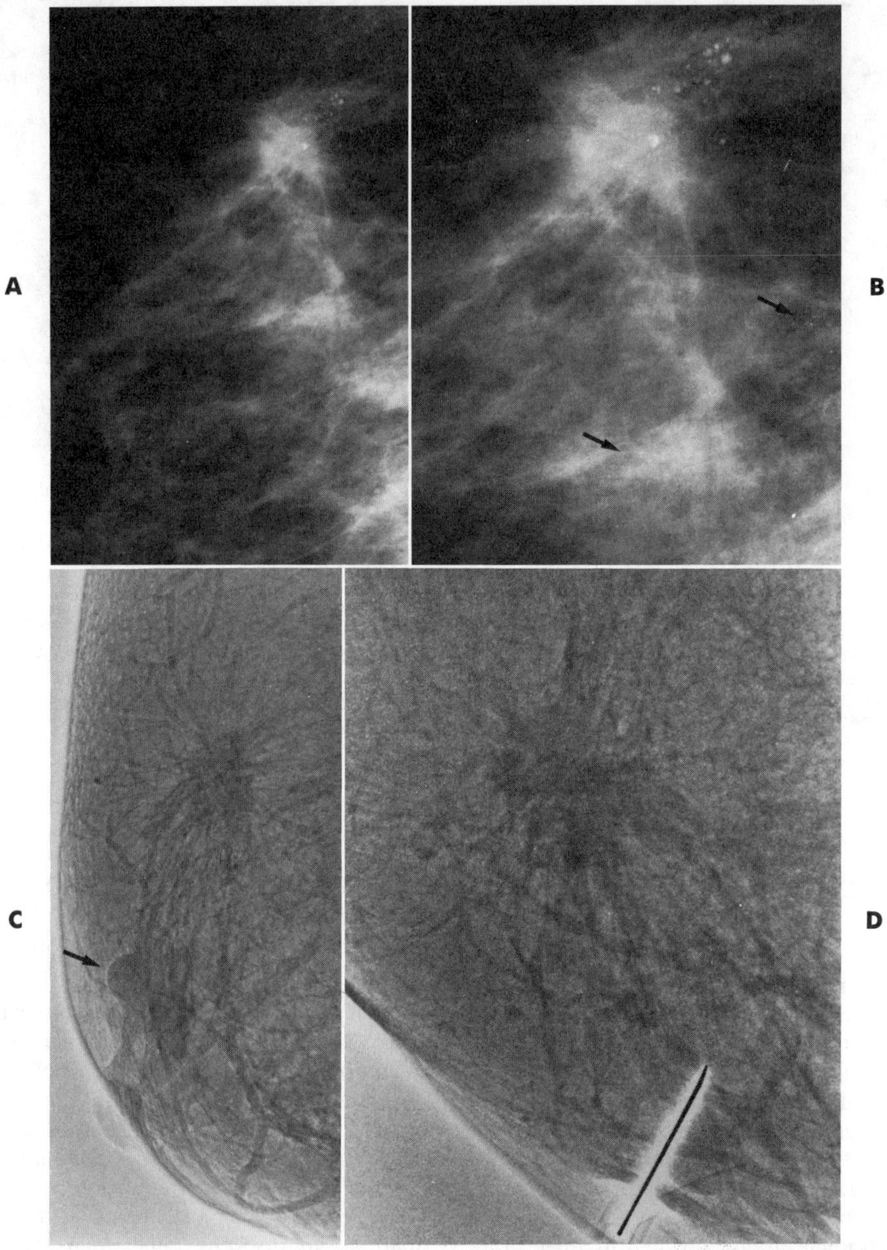

Fig. 2-12 Two patients, each with a 2-cm clinically suspicious mass in the upper outer quadrant. **A** and **B,** First patient. **A,** Stellate carcinoma with pleomorphic calcifications. **B,** Additional groups of suspicious calcifications *(arrows)* indicate need for much wider resection and poor cosmesis if lumpectomy is to be considered. **C** and **D,** Second patient. **C,** Stellate carcinoma corresponds to area palpated. Nonpalpable smooth nodule *(arrow)* deep to areola. **D,** Smooth nodule was localized and shown to be a fibroadenoma.

A

B

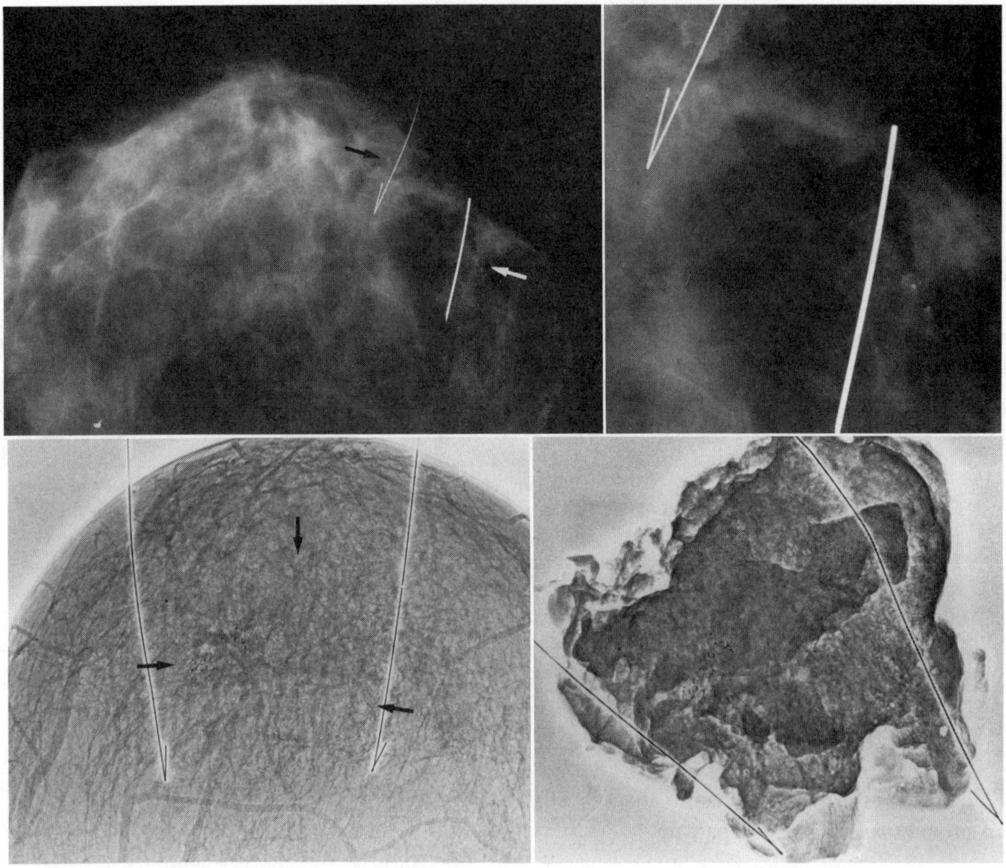

C

D

Fig. 2-13 Two patients with wide zone of malignant calcification. **A** and **B,** First patient. Two separate foci of calcification (*arrows* in **A**) localized individually with hook wire and needle. **C** and **D,** Second patient. Localization films and specimen radiograph showing use of paired flanking wires to mark boundaries of calcifications (*arrows* in **C**). Mastectomy was required.

A careful correlation between clinical and mammographic findings is obligatory; it must be certain that the clinically palpable and mammographically visible focus are the same. This can be accomplished by marking the palpable area with stick-on metallic skin dots before mammography (Fig. 2-14). The radiation oncologist, surgeon, and radiologist make the decision conjointly. If needle localization is needed preoperatively, decision regarding needle placement should take into consideration the planned surgical approach. This is particularly important if more than one focus is being localized and if the radiologic approach will influence the number and placement of biopsy incisions.

The technical aspects of preoperative needle localization are of only modest interest in a clinical management text. There is a wide variety of devices available. In skilled hands a simple hypodermic needle often suffices, providing that judgment is employed in selecting length and direction, as well as in modifying patient motion between the localization procedure and the biopsy. In more popular use now are devices consisting of a 20- or 21-gauge needle, within which is loaded a fine wire with a distal hook. Guided by the mammographic films, the radiologist inserts the needle, confirms its location on cephalocaudad and lateral views, advances and engages the hook, and then removes the needle. The approach can be parallel or perpendicular to the chest wall, utilizing an alphanumeric or perforated target grid or a free-hand approach. The procedure is brief and generally very easily tolerated. The wire is taped to the skin, a dressing is applied, and the patient goes to the operating room with films showing the precise final relationship of the wire and the lesion.

Gentle surgical dissection using the wire for guidance, but with care to avoid traction or tran-

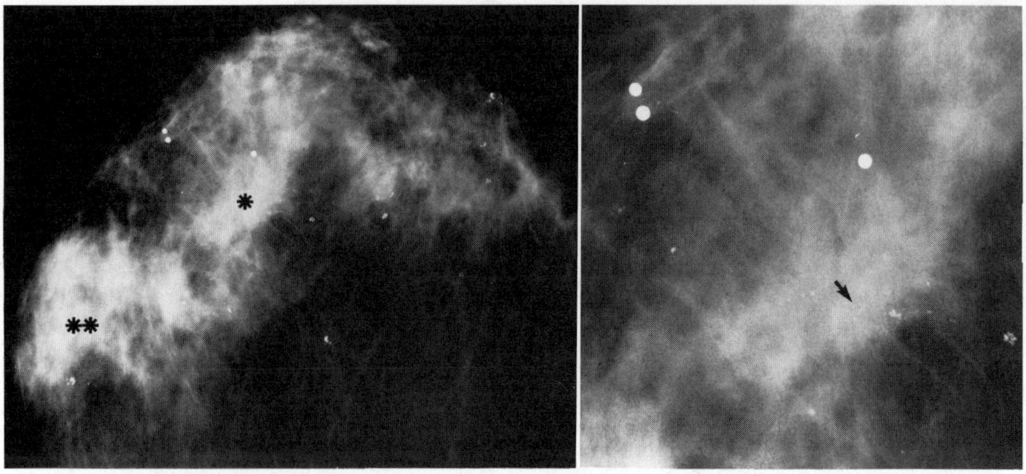

Fig. 2-14 Clinical requisition says "palpable mass laterally." **A,** Craniocaudad mammogram shows at least two zones of density *(asterisks)* and widespread coarse calcium that appears benign. **B,** The more central of the lateral zones (*single asterisk* in **A**) showed architectural distortion and what appeared to be malignant calcification *(arrow)*. To be certain that the mammographically suspicious area corresponded to the palpable focus, metallic dots *(single and paired)* were placed by the radiologist at the margins of the palpable area after the initial films were viewed. This illustration shows the second set of images.

section, allows excision of a tissue specimen that is then brought to the x-ray department.

SPECIMEN RADIOGRAPHY

The tissue containing the wire is compressed on the mammography x-ray unit between layers of clear plastic or in a specimen cassette, and a specimen radiograph is made. This is carefully compared to the mammography films to make certain that the lesion is completely contained within the specimen. At our institution, if the abnormality involved calcification, a magnification film also is obtained. If the wire is not closely adjacent to the focus, a hypodermic needle is inserted into the specimen to assist the pathologist to concentrate attention on that portion of the specimen (Fig. 2-15, *A* and *B*) that prompted the biopsy. If needed, the specimen can be refilmed at right angles or with altered orientation to simulate more closely the lesion in vivo. This may help to ascertain that the area has been completely excised. The presence and location of the lesion within the specimen are communicated to the surgeon, who can then close the biopsy wound. If the specimen radiograph shows that the lesion abuts the biopsy margin, additional tissue is excised (Fig. 2-15, *C*). The tissue specimen and the specimen radiograph are brought to pathology, where orientation is facilitated by reference to the x-ray, the protruding wire, and, at times, the secondary needle.

POSTBIOPSY EVALUATION

This section concerns the patient with a recent positive biopsy who is now being evaluated for possible breast conservation management. In the woman who had prebiopsy high-quality bilateral mammograms showing a single nodule, which was subsequently excised with verified negative margins, no further images are needed after biopsy. If the technical quality of the preoperative mammogram had been suboptimal, or if the original lesion contained multiple calcifications, postbiopsy mammography is indicated. In such a patient, mammographic evaluation has specific problems and can make potential contributions. The first issue is a technical one. There is an understandable wish to perform the examination promptly and to proceed with decision making and definitive management. This must be balanced by concern that wound tenderness will make it impossible to apply the vigorous compression needed for high-definition mammographic images. There are no obstacles to mammography contralaterally; however, failure to compress the postoperative breast will result in artifactually dense, indistinct images, adding to the true indistinctness caused by blood and edema fluid in the breast. For most patients, 2 weeks is the minimum interval possible between biopsy and mammogram.

Study of this new mammogram includes careful appraisal of both breasts for additional areas of

A

B

C

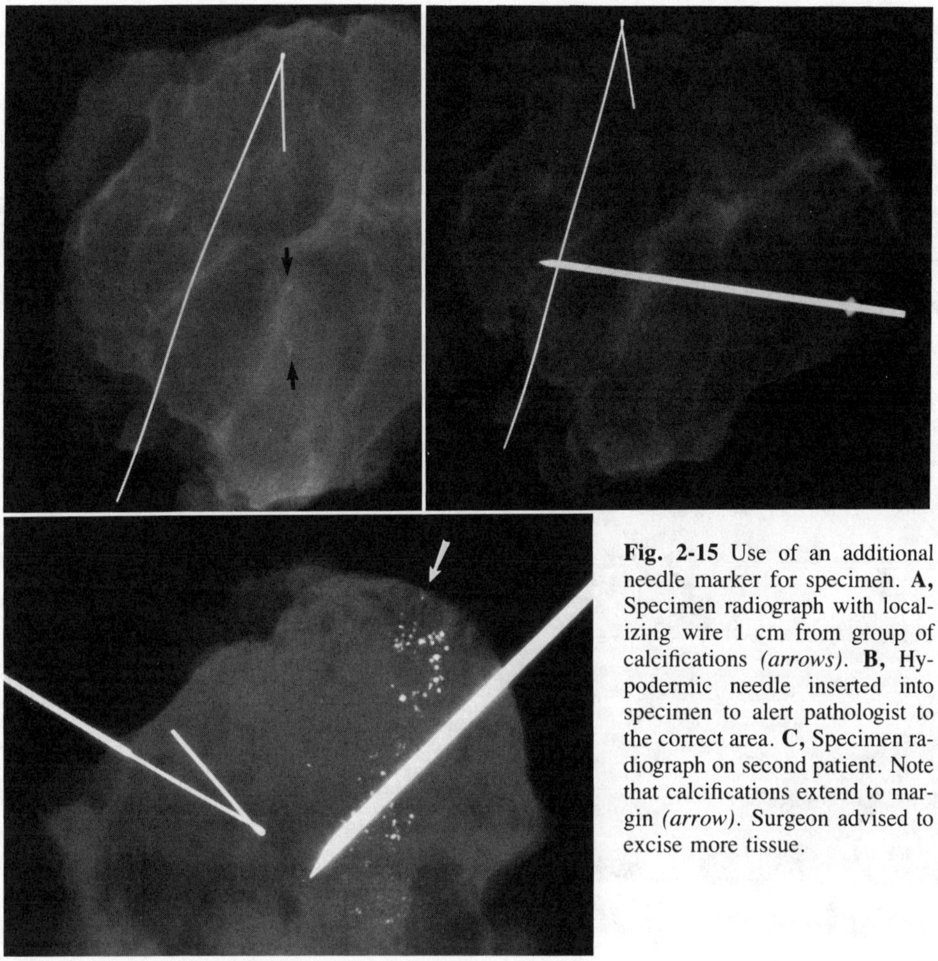

Fig. 2-15 Use of an additional needle marker for specimen. **A,** Specimen radiograph with localizing wire 1 cm from group of calcifications *(arrows)*. **B,** Hypodermic needle inserted into specimen to alert pathologist to the correct area. **C,** Specimen radiograph on second patient. Note that calcifications extend to margin *(arrow)*. Surgeon advised to excise more tissue.

suspicion. Analysis of the biopsy site is greatly facilitated by comparison with the original prebiopsy study. A localized hematoma, sometimes containing air, is present in most instances and will generally be much larger than the original abnormality. This postoperative hematoma will make it exceedingly difficult to judge whether a portion of a noncalcified nodule has been completely excised. Attempts have been made using ultrasound; however, clotted blood and debris are still indistinguishable from a residual tumor nodule (Fig. 2-16). Residual calcifications should be carefully searched for, utilizing magnification filming if necessary. If extensive calcification was present originally, it may be impossible to document that all of it was accounted for in the specimen radiograph (Fig. 2-17). Additionally, however, the specimen x-ray portrays such fine detail that at times other calcifications may be seen within it that were not necessarily the ones visible on the preoperative mammogram.

Many authors cite the usefulness of mammography at this point in the patient's course.[12] In 1982, reporting from the Hospital of the University of Pennsylvania on 38 postbiopsy mammograms, Gefter et al.[1] described positive findings including residual mass or calcifications, adenopathy, or contralateral calcification in eight instances. In 1989, however, a study by Homer et al.[6] in 21 patients undergoing tumor bed reexcision showed that of the 12 patients showing residual tumor on reexcision pathology, mammograms and palpation were negative in 7. The postbiopsy mammogram is, therefore, useful if it is positive; however, a negative result provides no assurance of complete excision.

A B C

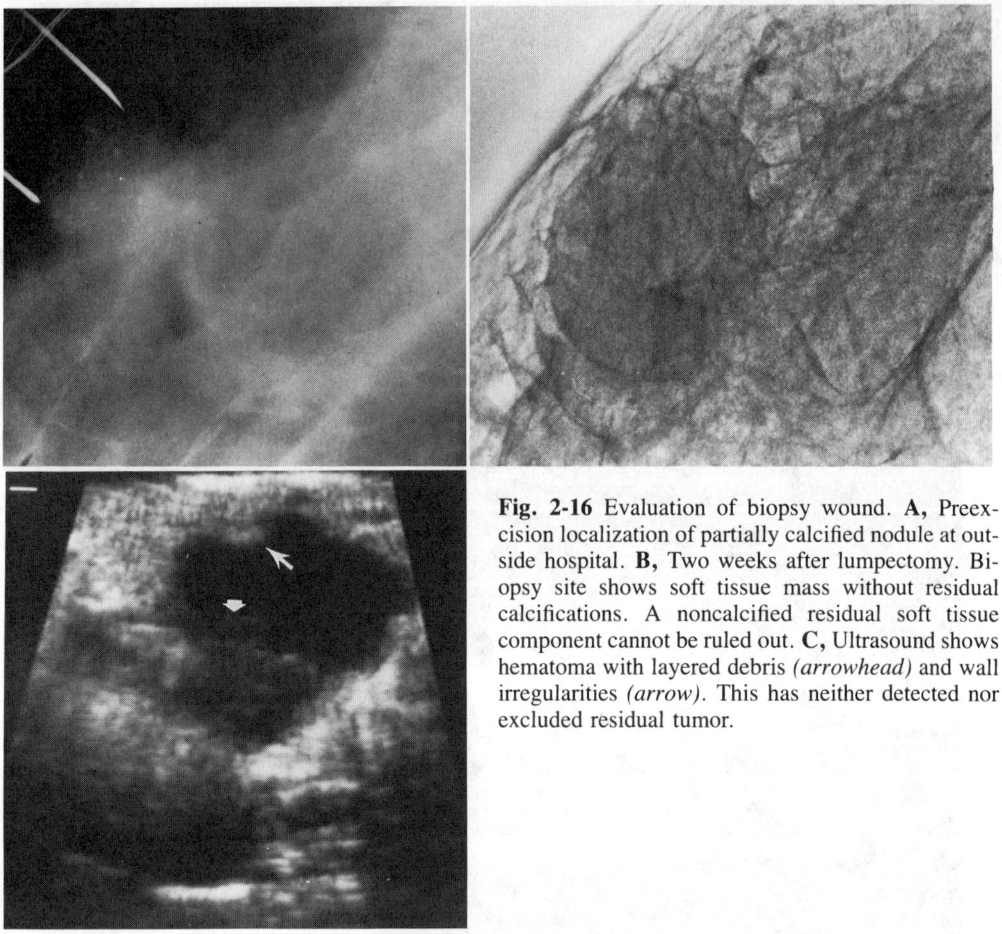

Fig. 2-16 Evaluation of biopsy wound. **A,** Preexcision localization of partially calcified nodule at outside hospital. **B,** Two weeks after lumpectomy. Biopsy site shows soft tissue mass without residual calcifications. A noncalcified residual soft tissue component cannot be ruled out. **C,** Ultrasound shows hematoma with layered debris *(arrowhead)* and wall irregularities *(arrow)*. This has neither detected nor excluded residual tumor.

A B

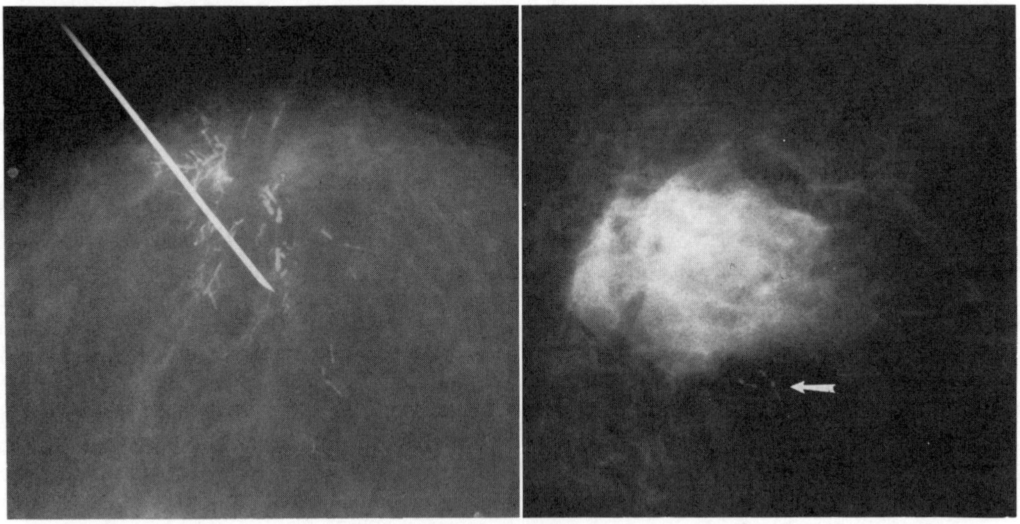

Fig. 2-17 Evaluation of biopsy wound. **A,** Outside film of preexcision localization of a zone of malignant calcification. **B,** Postlumpectomy film showing wound hematoma and residual malignant calcification *(arrow)*. Residual tumor was present in the reexcision specimen.

REFERENCES

1. Gefter WB, Friedman AK, and Goodman RL: The role of mammography in evaluating patients with early carcinoma of the breast for tylectomy and radiation therapy, Radiology 142:77, 1982.
2. Hall FM, Storella JM, Silverstone DZ, and Wyshak G: Non-palpable breast lesions: recommendations for biopsy based on suspicion of carcinoma at mammography, Radiology 167:353, 1988.
3. Hilton SV, Leopold G, Olson KL, and Willson SA: Real-time breast sonography: application in 300 consecutive patients, AJR 174:479, 1986.
4. Homer MJ: Nonpalpable mammographic abnormalities: timing the followup studies, AJR 136:923, 1981.
5. Homer MJ, Safaii H, Smith TJ, and Marchant DJ: The relationship of mammographic microcalcifications to histologic malignancy: radiologic pathology correlation, AJR 153:1187, 1989.
6. Homer MJ, Schmidt-Ullrich R, Safaii H, et al: Residual breast carcinoma after biopsy: role of mammography in evaluation, Radiology 170:75, 1989.
7. Lanyi M: Diagnosis and differential diagnosis of breast calcifications, Berlin, 1986, Springer-Verlag, pp 91-98.
8. Martin JE, Moskowitz M, and Milbrath JR: Breast cancer missed by mammography, AJR 132:737, 1979.
9. Meyer JE, Kopans DB, Stomper PF, and Lindfors KK: Occult breast abnormalities: percutaneous preoperative needle localization, Radiology 150:335, 1984.
10. Moskowitz M: Impact of a priori medical decisions on screening for breast cancer, Radiology 171:605, 1989.
11. Moskowitz M: The predictive value of certain mammographic signs in screening for breast cancer, Cancer 51:1007, 1983.
12. Paulus DD: Conservative treatment of breast cancer mammography in patient selection and followup, AJR 143:483, 1984.
13. Recht A, Connolly JL, Schnitt SJ, et al: The effect of young age on tumor recurrence in the treated breast after conservative surgery and radiotherapy, Int J Radiat Oncol Biol Phys 14:3, 1988.
14. Rosen PP: The pathology of breast carcinoma. In Harris JR, Hillman S, Henderson IC, and Kinne DW, editors: Breast disease, Philadelphia, 1987, JB Lippincott, p 191.
15. Ryoo MC, Kagan AR, Wollen M, et al: Prognostic factors for recurrence and cosmesis in 393 patients after radiation therapy for early mammary carcinoma, Radiology 172:555, 1989.
16. Sickles EA: Mammographic features of "early" breast cancer, AJR 143:461, 1984.
17. Sickles EA: Further experience with microfocal spot magnification mammography in the assessment of clustered breast microcalcifications, Radiology 137:9, 1980.
18. Tabar L, Fagerberg CJ, Gad A, et al: Reduction in mortality from breast cancer after mass screening with mammography, Lancet i:829, 1985.
19. Tabar L, Pentek Z, and Dean P: The diagnostic and therapeutic value of breast cyst puncture and pneumocystography, Radiology 141:659, 1981.
20. Wolfe JN, Buck KA, Salane M, and Parekh NJ: Xeroradiography of the breast: overview of 21,057 consecutive cases, Radiology 165:305, 1987.

3 Local-Regional Treatment Options for Early Invasive Breast Cancer

Barbara Fowble

HISTORY

The goal of local-regional treatment is to eradicate the primary tumor in the breast and any extension to regional lymph nodes. The role of local-regional therapy in the overall treatment of breast cancer has varied with changes in the clinician's perception of the natural history of the disease.

The earliest recorded reference to breast cancer appears in the Edwin Smith papyrus written between 3000 and 2500 BC.[34] In the pre-Christian era breast cancer was perceived as an incurable disease for which surgical intervention was not warranted. Hippocrates (400 BC) recommended no treatment for deep-seated cancers, and Theophilus in his commentary on Hippocrates stated that "even if the disease is eradicated by cutting or burning, many untoward symptoms follow."[77] The first surgical treatment of breast cancer has been attributed to Galen (200 AD)[77] who recommended excision for early lesions. Local excision was practiced during the 10th and 11th centuries by Rhazes, Haly Ben-Abbas, Avicenna, and Albucasis, and during the 14th century by Henri De Mondeville and Guy de Chauliac.[77] The 16th century witnessed the introduction of the mastectomy and in 1590 Cabrol performed what has become the standard radical mastectomy.[77] However, Jean Louis Petit (1674-1750) has been credited with developing the first unified approach for the surgical treatment of breast cancer including wide excision, en bloc resection, axillary dissection, and assessment of the pectoral fascia.[282] In the mid-19th century, in the absence of sterile techniques and anesthesia, aggressive surgery was greeted with pessimism by James Syme, James Paget, and Samuel D. Gross. Women not infrequently presented with locally advanced disease and treatment was deemed palliative at best. However, proponents of radical surgery remained, including Joseph Pancoast, Charles H. Moore, Mitchell Banks, and Samuel W. Gross.

It must be emphasized that during this period the approach to the treatment of breast cancer was not based on any universally accepted concept regarding the natural history or spread of the disease. Random efforts and the individual experience of multiple physicians contributed to the divergent philosophies. A perceptible change occurred with the introduction of the radical mastectomy in 1882 by W.S. Halsted[163] and in 1894 by Willy Meyer.[250] The scientific basis for the radical mastectomy was derived from an accumulation of knowledge regarding the lymphatic spread of breast cancer. As detailed in Silvergirl's *Surgery: The Breast,*[282] the efforts of Heidenhain, Grossman, Rotter, Stiles, and Sappey helped to establish the local and regional patterns of the spread of breast cancer. Heidenhain demonstrated the dissemination of breast cancer through lymphatics into the retromammary tissue, pectoral fascia, and pectoralis major muscle. He recommended basing the extent of the surgical procedure on these anatomic considerations. Grossman and Rotter described the interpectoral nodes and their association with blood vessels. Sappey established the axilla as being the primary lymphatic drainage of the breast.

The Halstedian concept of the biology of breast cancer developed from these findings as well as from Virchow's studies,[352] which suggested that regional lymph nodes effectively filtered cancer cells, and from Handley's report[167] that spread along lymphatic channels was by direct extension instead of embolization. The basic tenets of the Halsted theory include the orderly spread of cancer in a contiguous manner from the breast to regional nodes and subsequently to distant sites, the ability of regional nodes to function as barriers to the spread of cancer cells, and the role of lymphatic extension as the source of distant metastases rather than the blood stream. Outcome was determined by the extent of the surgical procedure and the ability to intercept the cancer at a local-regional stage before distant metastases occurred.

The Halstedian hypothesis was accepted readily because it was both credible and practical. It was based on the available knowledge of the spread of breast cancer, and it coincided with advances in surgical and anesthetic techniques that reduced the morbidity and mortality of the radical procedure. Halsted's results with the radical mastectomy in 50 patients were also the best reported at that time, with a local recurrence rate of 6% and a 3-year survival of 38% to 42%.[162,163] Halsted subsequently extended the procedure to include dissection of the supraclavicular and internal mammary nodes in an attempt to encompass all possible regional node extensions. This superradical mastectomy was later advocated by Wangensteen.[355] Proponents of the dissection of the internal mammary nodes in conjunction with the radical mastectomy included Dahl-Iversen,[72] Margottini,[241] Urban,[338] and Handley.[167]

A national survey by the American College of Surgeons[360] indicated that as of 1972 the radical mastectomy was the most commonly practiced (48%) surgical procedure for breast cancer. Haagensen refined this approach, developing the Columbia Clinical Staging System in an attempt to select the appropriate patients for the procedure, and he continued to recommend the radical mastectomy as the treatment of choice in his 1986 textbook.[154]

A conservative response to the radical mastectomy was noted as early as 1924. Geoffrey Keynes[199,200] employed a radium needle implant technique to treat initially inoperable patients and later operable cases. He rationalized that radical surgery was unnecessary in those with early disease and futile in those with advanced disease. In 1948 McWhirter reported the results of simple mastectomy with postoperative radiotherapy.[245] He advocated radiotherapy alone for the treatment of the axilla based on the hypothesis that surgical removal of the axillary nodes precipitated distant metastases, that the results of surgical removal in patients with positive nodes were disappointing, and that surgical removal in patients with negative nodes was unnecessary. Also in 1948, Patey and Dyson[269] described the modified radical mastectomy with preservation of the pectoralis major muscle. The American College of Surgeons survey[360] indicates that it was not until 1976 that the modified radical mastectomy became the most frequently employed surgical treatment for breast cancer. Each of these conservative approaches subsequently has been proven in prospective randomized trials[10,13,24,38,41,103,113,114,220,234,236,237,295,296,333,334,345,347] to produce results comparable to those of the radical mastectomy. However, they stemmed from a dissatisfaction with the results of the radical mastectomy and not from a disbelief in the Halstedian concept of the spread of breast cancer. Their individual experiences remained unconvincing for many.

In 1968 Bernard Fisher and his colleagues[100] synthesized an alternative hypothesis for the biology of breast cancer. Through a series of laboratory investigations they demonstrated that lymph nodes are not barriers to tumor cell dissemination,[107] that tumor cells traverse lymphatics and disseminate through the blood stream,[106] that lymph nodes can destroy tumor cells,[116] that the pattern of tumor cell dissemination is not orderly,[109] that the presence of tumors as well as their removal can[101,102] evoke host responses,[108] and that host factors play a role in the development of metastases.[108] They proposed "that a tumor is a systemic disease, probably from its inception."[100] Therefore, "variations in local-regional therapy are unlikely to substantially affect survival."[100]

Clinical investigations also supported this alternative hypothesis. Devitt,[82] in a retrospective review of 922 patients with curable breast cancer, found no difference in survival when comparing patients with histologically positive axillary nodes treated by radical mastectomy or simple mastectomy, despite a higher incidence of axillary recurrences in the latter group. The author concluded that the regional lymph nodes were not a source of metastases but rather a marker of the biologic activity of the tumor. A similar observation was made by Crile[66] who noted no difference in 5-year survival in patients with stage I breast cancer who underwent radical mastectomy vs. simple mastectomy with axillary dissection delayed until the appearance of positive nodes. Again the author suggested that the axillary nodes were not responsible for metastases but were a manifestation of the aggressiveness of the tumor. Data from the National Surgical Adjuvant Breast Project (NSABP) B-01 protocol[117] demonstrated a treatment failure rate of 24% for axillary node-negative patients and 75% for axillary node-positive patients at 10 years when treated with radical mastectomy. Patients with apparently localized or regional disease developed distant metastases in a significant percentage despite aggressive local-regional treatment.

In 1971 a clinical trial was begun by the NSABP to test simultaneously the Halstedian and alternate hypothesis. The results of this trial demonstrated that variations in local-regional therapy did not affect overall treatment failure, distant metastases, or survival after a mean follow-up of 10.5 years for either clinically positive axillary node patients or clinically negative axillary node patients.[113] Node-negative patients were randomized to radical mastectomy vs. total mastectomy with axillary dissection reserved until the time of axillary recurrence vs. total mastectomy and postoperative radiation to the chest wall and regional nodes. Node-positive patients were randomized to radical mastectomy vs. total mastectomy and radiation. In node-negative patients the failure to remove axillary nodes that may have been microscopically positive did not result in an increased incidence of distant metastases or a decreased survival; however, axillary recurrences were higher. The findings from this study affirmed the alternative hypothesis.

The concept of occult metastases or undetectable micrometastases as a source of treatment failure in early breast cancer gained increasing acceptance in the early 1970s and became the basis for adjuvant systemic therapy.[242,299,307] Because chemotherapeutic agents killed a constant fraction of cells, and cure was dependent on total cell kill, the theoretical advantage of initiating treatment at a time when the tumor burden was the smallest seemed appropriate. Prospective randomized trials evaluating perioperative[111,117,263] and postoperative chemotherapy[30,110] were begun. It was within this milieu that randomized trials evaluating surgical procedures less than mastectomy for early breast cancer were initiated.[10,103,296,348] The impetus for these trials included the accumulation of data from prospective randomized trials that failed to demonstrate the superiority of the extended radical or radical mastectomy over the modified radical or simple mastectomy with or without radiation, an improved understanding of the biology of breast cancer from laboratory and clinical investigations, an increased emphasis on screening and early diagnosis with a resultant change in the patient population from one with primarily advanced disease to one with early disease, and the promising initial results from adjuvant chemotherapy trials.[30,104]

In summary, the prevailing hypothesis regarding the natural history of breast cancer or lack of one not only directed individual endeavors but also influenced the design of prospective randomized trials. In the 1960s and early 1970s the Halstedian concept of centrifugal spread was responsible for trials that compared radical mastectomy to the extended radical mastectomy or radical mastectomy to radical mastectomy with radiation to the chest wall and/or regional nodes. The challenge of the alternative hypothesis, which had a basis both in the clinic and the laboratory, as well as the concept of micrometastases prompted the implementation of randomized trials in the 1970s and early 1980s comparing radical mastectomy to the modified radical mastectomy or to conservative surgery with or without radiation. The randomized clinical trial has increasingly become the mechanism for testing the relevance of biologic principles in the clinical setting as well as the potential means for resolving clinical dilemmas. Future efforts in evaluating local-regional treatment options will be directed toward identifying the minimum treatment in the presence or absence of systemic therapy that will not compromise relapse-free or overall survival.

THE CONCEPT OF CURE AND THE RELEVANCE OF LOCAL-REGIONAL CONTROL

Concept of cure

Breast cancer is a heterogeneous disease that manifests a variable biologic behavior resulting in diverse natural histories. Analysis of survival curves has suggested that at least two patient populations exist.[137,290] Fox plotted the relative survival of breast cancer patients treated from 1950 to 1973 collected by the End Results Section, Biometry Branch of the National Cancer Institute.[137] A semilogarithmic presentation was employed with relative survival plotted logarithmically (Fig. 3-1). A relative mortality of approximately 25% per year was exhibited by 40% of the population, while the remaining 60% exhibited a relative mortality of 2.5% per year. These data suggested the presence of two populations, one of which manifested aggressive disease. Rutqvist et al[290] found that the log-normal model in which the logarithms of the survival times were assumed to be distributed normally best approximated the patterns of breast cancer survival noted in a long-term follow-up study of 14,731 women. The model was compatible with the observed decreasing mortality with increasing time from diagnosis and treatment. The model also suggested that there was a group of patients who continued to manifest late excess mortality when compared to a normal population as well as a group of patients whose mortality was equal to that of the normal population, i.e., a fraction that had been cured.

The existence of a population of breast cancer patients who have experienced a cure has been the focus of numerous investigations that have produced variable results. Evidence or the lack thereof for a cured population, however, depends on the period of follow-up, the comparability of the control or normal population, the method chosen to present survival curves, and the magnitude of the effect of the confounding influence of mortality from contralateral breast cancer and second nonbreast cancer malignancies. The demonstration of a cured population with local-regional treatment only attests to the importance of such treatment.

Assessing mortality. In general cure implies a mortality from all causes—including intercurrent disease, contralateral breast cancer, and second nonbreast cancer malignancies in patients treated for breast cancer equal to that of an age-adjusted normal female population. Comparisons of actuarial survival curves for the patient population with those for women in the general population adjusted

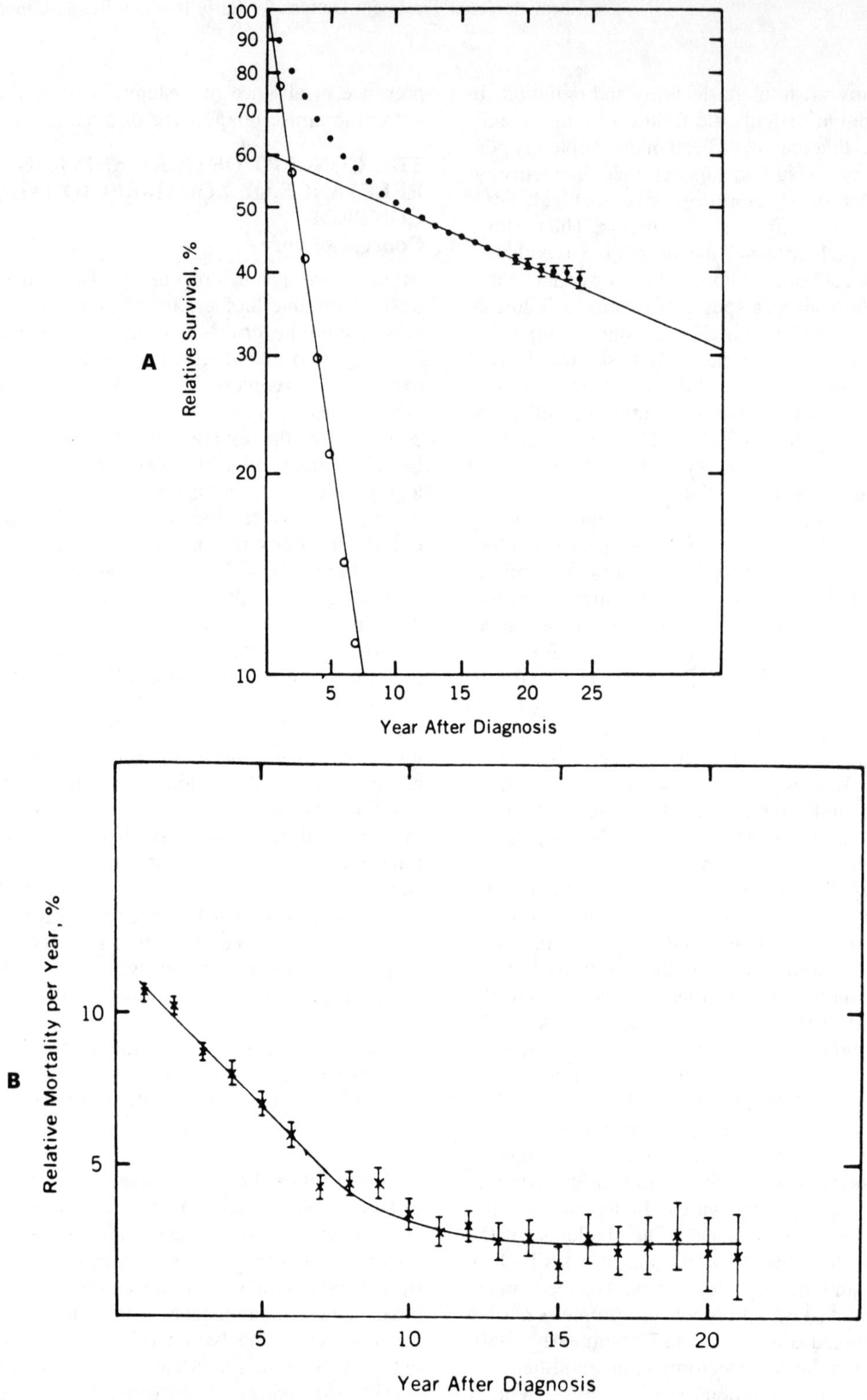

Fig. 3-1 A, Relative survival of patients with histologically confirmed breast cancer, all stages (1950-1973) after correction for other causes of death for U.S. mortality data *(closed circle)*. Vertical lines represent SE of calculated values. (Unpublished data, End Results Section, Biometry Branch, National Cancer Institute, 1977.) *Open circles* represent survival of that portion of population that dies at a relative rate >2½% per year. **B,** Relative mortality per year from data displayed in **A.** Vertical lines represent SE of calculated values. (From Fox MS: JAMA 241:491, 1979. Copyright 1979, American Medical Association.)

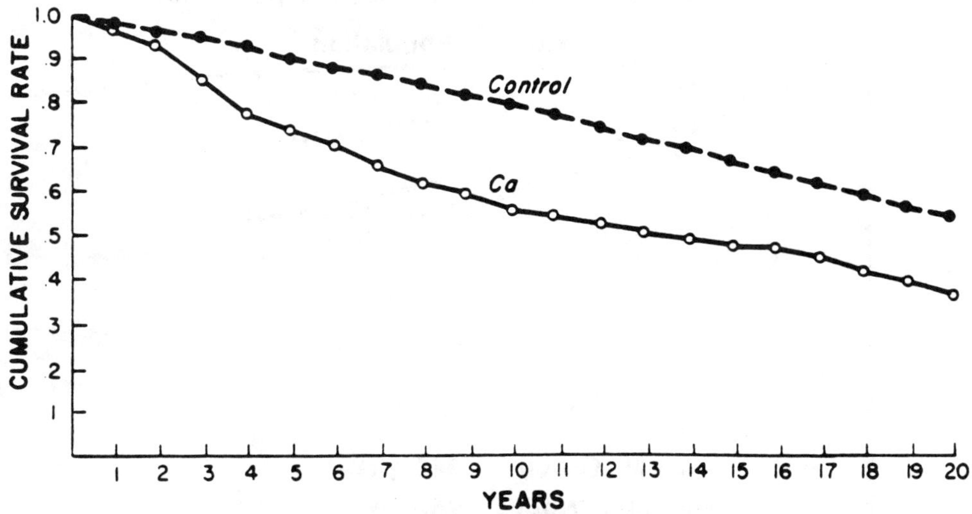

Fig. 3-2 Cumulative probabilities of survival in 622 women treated by radical mastectomy for carcinoma of one breast, compared to age-adjusted survival rates for women in the general population of New York State. (From Haagensen CD: Diseases of the breast, ed 2, Philadelphia, 1971, WB Saunders Co.)

for age offer one method of assessing mortality. In this instance, survival and time usually are plotted in a linear fashion. Parallelism of the curves after a certain point in time indicates a mortality in the treated group similar to that of the control group and suggests that a certain fraction are cured. An example of such a comparison is demonstrated in Fig. 3-2. Harris and Hellman,[172] however, argue that the linear plot may give a false impression of a "tail" or cured population in the survival curve. They recommend the semilogarithmic display of survival curves with survival plotted logarithmically and time linearly. The slope of the curve describes the mortality rate. A change in the slope indicates a change in the mortality rate. Back extrapolation to the y-axis at the point at which this change occurs indicates the percentage of the population to which this new rate applies. Cure occurs when the patient population experiences the same mortality rate as that of an age-adjusted normal population. On a semilogarithmic plot the slopes of the curves would be the same and the curves would be parallel. Back extrapolation to the y-axis at the point the curves become parallel indicates the percentage of the population cured. An example of parallel survival curves on a semilogarithmic plot is shown in Fig. 3-3. An alternative approach is to calculate relative survival rates for specific time periods.[169] The relative survival rate[91] is the ratio between the observed survival rate for the patient population and the expected rate calculated for an age-adjusted female population. Cure, i.e., normal mortality, occurs in the patient population when the relative survival curve parallels the time axis. The relative survival rate minimizes the effect of intercurrent disease, but does not eliminate the effect of excess mortality from diseases associated with breast cancer such as second malignancies.

Evidence for a statistical cure. The above considerations relate to statistical cure, which is defined by Haybittle[175] as the demonstration of a mortality rate from all causes in the treated group equal to that of a normal population matched for age and sex. Evidence for a statistical cure is conflicting and is related to the period of follow-up and the extent of disease at presentation. Brinkley and Haybittle[37] reported the results of a long-term follow-up study of 704 breast cancer patients treated from 1947 to 1950. Of the patients, 41% had stage III or stage IV disease.[39] With a minimum follow-up of 22 years, the actuarial survival rate of the patients paralleled that of the age-adjusted normal population after 21 years in a semilogarithmic plot. Extrapolation back to the y-axis at the time the curves became parallel suggested that 18% of all patients were cured, with a 30% cure rate for stages I and II. However, in a subsequent update[36] with a minimum follow-up of 31 years, the curves were noted to diverge between 25 and 30 years (Fig. 3-4) with breast cancer patients exhibiting an increased mortality rate. Rutqvist and Wallgren[289] reported the long-term survival of 458 young women (age ≤40 years) with operable breast cancer who

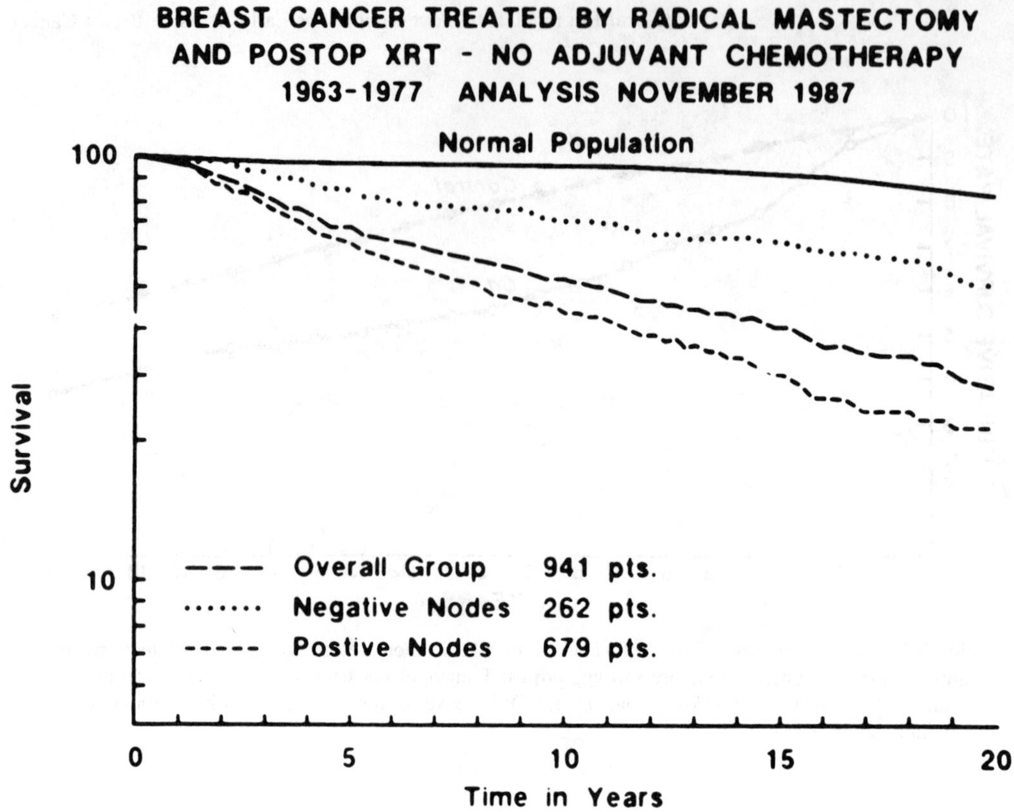

Fig. 3-3 Survival rates for patients with breast cancer compared with the survival experience of the normal white female population beginning at age 53 (mean age of the M.D. Anderson Cancer Center patients). Data obtained from Vital Statistics of the United States, 1970. (From Fletcher GH et al: Int J Radiat Oncol Biol Phys 17:12, 1989.)

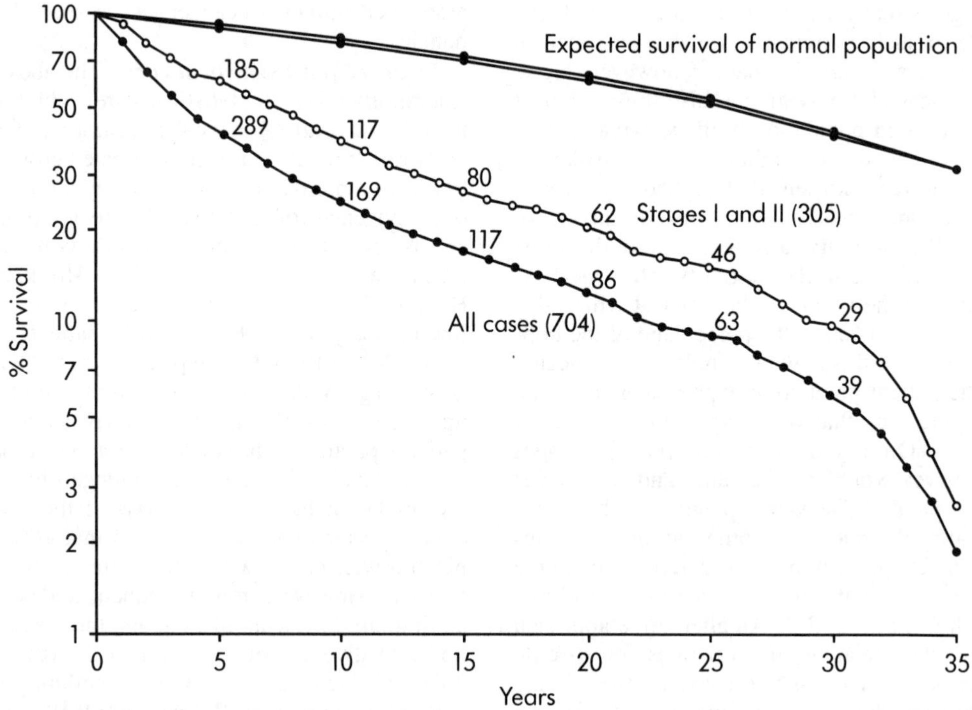

Fig. 3-4 Survival curves for all patients and for patients with stages I and II disease only. (From Brinkley D and Haybittle JL: Lancet i:1118, 1984.)

were followed from 20 to 51 years. An excess mortality rate for the patients was observed throughout the follow-up period when compared to that of the general population. The curves in a semilogarithmic plot never became parallel (Fig. 3-5). Similarly, a plot of the relative survival failed to demonstrate parallelism with the x-axis. Hibberd et al.[184] retrospectively analyzed the 30-year survival of 2019 women with breast cancer treated in public hospitals or cancer consultation clinics in New Zealand from 1950 to 1954. The analysis included all stages of disease, but excluded patients treated in private hospitals. Comparison of crude survival curves plotted linearly over 30 years of the patient population with a similar group of normal women demonstrated parallelism of the curves only for the 20- to 34-year age group (Fig. 3-6). However, the relative survival rate appeared to flatten after 10 years in the 20- to 34-year age group and after 20 years in all patients. This finding, and the extremely small excess mortality rate after 20 years (one excess death per 100 women with breast cancer a year) suggested that the mortality of women with breast cancer approached normal after 20 years. Langlands et al.[219] reported an increased mortality from all causes in a group of 3878 women with breast cancer (all stages) up to 20 years after initial treatment, when compared to an age-adjusted normal population. The excess mortality was 58% at 15 to 20 years; however, it decreased to 28% for patients disease-free after 15 years. The excess mortality was noted for all stages, for all tumor sizes, and for both premenopausal and postmenopausal patients.

Duncan and Kerr[90] compared the survival rates of 982 women with localized breast cancer treated primarily with simple mastectomy and radiation and followed for a minimum of 20 years to those of the normal population. In a linear plot the age-corrected survival rate became parallel to the x-axis after 12 years in all patients except those with primary tumors ≤2 cm in diameter. In this latter group the curve appeared parallel from the 6th to the 15th year, but declined from the 15th to 20th year, emphasizing the importance of long-term follow-up in the smaller tumors. Rosen et al.[286] studied the probability of cure in 644 women with T_1 tumors treated by mastectomy. The median follow-up was 18.2 years. For patients with primary tumors ≤1 cm and pathologically negative axillary nodes, the observed survival curve seemed to parallel the expected after 13 years. For patients

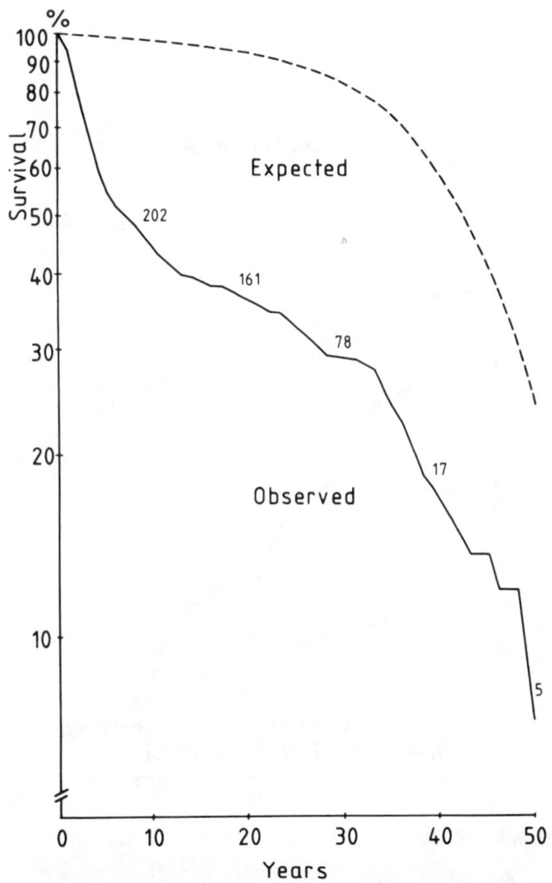

Fig. 3-5 Observed and expected survival of 458 young patients with breast cancer. Figures denote the number of patients at risk. (From Rutquist LE and Wallgren A: Cancer 55:660, 1985.)

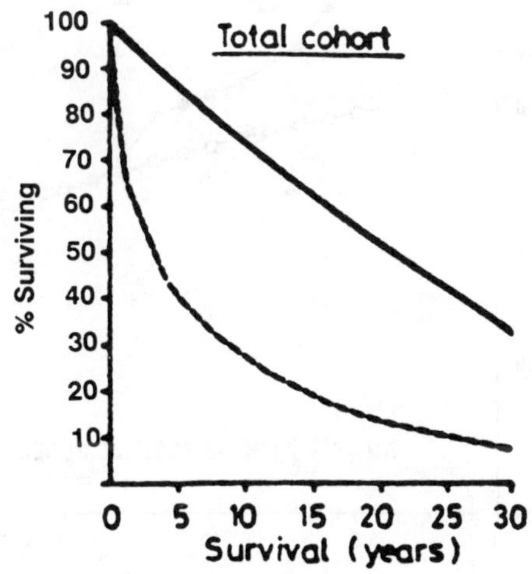

Fig. 3-6 Cumulative percentage survival curves for total cohort of women with breast cancer. For comparison each graph shows survival of equivalent cohort of normal women. *Lower line,* Women with breast cancer. *Upper line,* Normal women. (From Hibberd AD et al: Br Med J 286:1778, 1983.)

with primary tumors 1.1 to 2.0 cm in diameter and pathologically negative nodes, the observed survival curve paralleled the expected after 18 years. For T_1 pathologically node-positive patients the curves did not become parallel during the follow-up period (Fig. 3-7). Again the importance of long-term follow-up was emphasized, especially for smaller tumors (≤1 cm), which tended to manifest late recurrences. Fletcher et al.[129] compared the survival of 941 patients with operable breast cancer who underwent mastectomy and postoperative radiation with that of an age-adjusted white female population. In a semilogarithmic plot the curves became parallel at 17 years, suggesting a cured fraction (see Fig. 3-3). Peters[270] compared the survival of patients with early breast cancer ($T_1T_2N_0$) treated by wide excision and radiation or mastectomy and radiation with that of a normal popula-

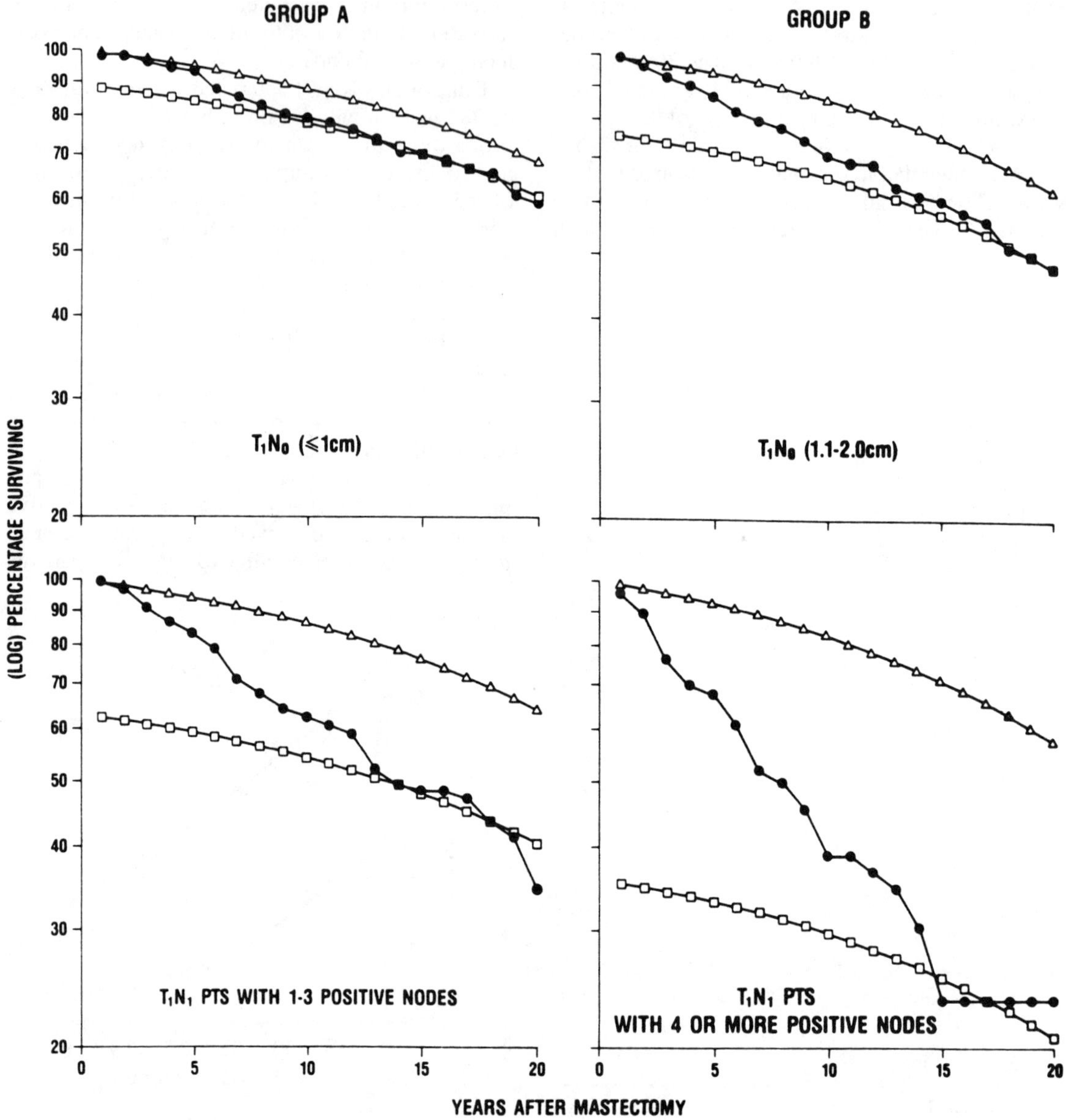

Fig. 3-7 Comparison of observed and expected hazard for dying. Observed and expected survival compared by the method of Brinkley and Haybittle. A logarithmic scale is used. ●, observed; △, expected; extrapolation to zero line of the portion of the observed curve that is approximately parallel to the normal population (□). Vertical intercept of □, estimates size of cured group. (From Rosen PP et al: J Clin Oncol 7:360, 1989.)

tion. Deaths from intercurrent disease within 10 years were excluded in an attempt to minimize the effect of early noncancer deaths. In a semilogarithmic plot the survival of the treated patients paralleled that of normal population from 12 to 30 years (Fig. 3-8). Haagensen[151] compared the survival of 662 women treated by radical mastectomy with an age-adjusted female population in New York State. In a linear plot up to 20 years the curves became parallel after 15 years (Fig. 3-2). Hankey and Steinhorn[169] examined long-term survival patterns in patients collected from the National Cancer Institute's End Results Program. By analyzing conditional 5-year relative survival rate patterns for 8149 patients with localized or regional disease, evidence for a cured fraction was demonstrated only in the subgroup of patients <35 years of age at diagnosis with localized disease. This group achieved a normal mortality at 20 years.

Therefore there appears to be evidence for a statistical cure in certain subsets of patients; however, the strength of this conclusion may depend upon follow-up of >20 years in some of the series. Also, as noted by Sutherland and Mather,[320] mortality from all causes may not be the same in the treated group as in the general population. To minimize differences in nonbreast cancer deaths, the comparability of the control population to the treated population should be analyzed not only in terms of age and sex but also in terms of race, socioeconomic status, and geographic area, as these factors can affect deaths from other causes.

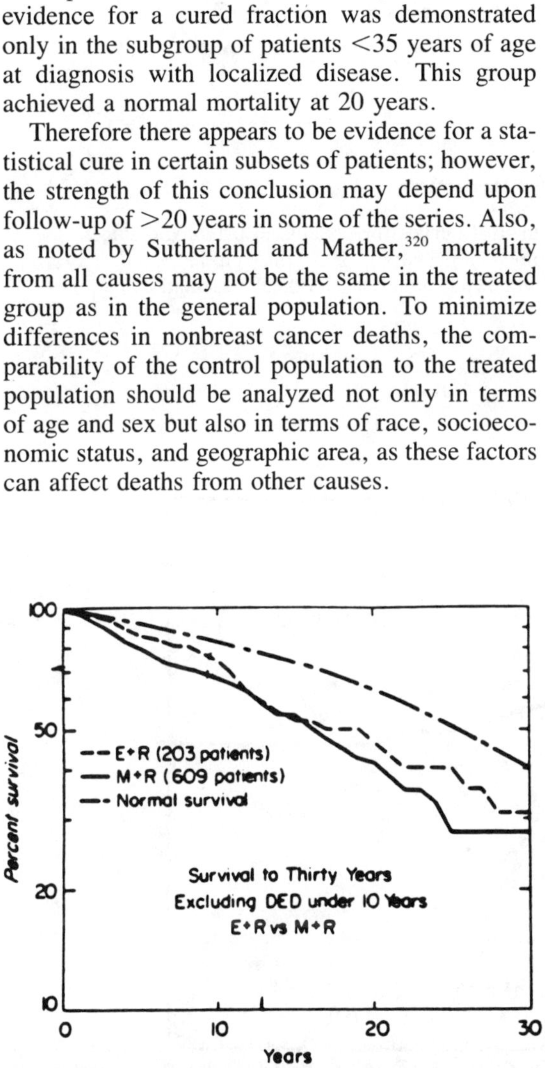

Fig. 3-8 Comparison of survival of patients treated by wide excision and radiation (E + R) or mastectomy and radiation (M + R) with that of the normal population. DED, death from extraneous disease. (From Peters MV: Int J Radiat Oncol Biol Phys 2:1152, 1977.)

Evidence for a clinical cure. The potentially confounding influence of nonbreast cancer deaths can be avoided by assessing results in terms of clinical cure. Clinical cure as defined by Haybittle[175] is achieved when eradication of all tumor results in a mortality rate from breast cancer in the treated group that is the same as that of a matched control population. However, use of this definition requires precise information regarding the cause of death that may be missing or inaccurate. Available evidence for a clinical cure is less convincing than that for a statistical cure. Sutherland and Mather[320] noted a five times greater excess mortality from breast cancer at 25 years in the treated group as compared to that of a general population adjusted for sex, age, race, and year of diagnosis. The treated group consisted of patients with operable breast cancer. Duncan and Kerr[90] noted an excess mortality from breast cancer in the treated group compared to the control with 20 year follow-up. This excess was evident for all tumor sizes. Brinkley and Haybittle[37] reported deaths after 20 years from breast cancer in the treated population to be 16 times the expected number from breast cancer in the normal population. Langlands et al.[219] noted a 20-fold excess in breast cancer deaths after 15 years. Ederer et al.,[92] in an analysis of 4100 5-year survivors from breast cancer in the Connecticut Tumor Registry, noted an excess mortality for deaths from breast cancer after 20 years of follow-up. Mortality for all causes other than breast cancer, however, was normal. The authors concluded that the overall excess mortality in these long-term survivors was related almost exclusively to the excess mortality from breast cancer. Rutqvist et al.[290] observed excess mortality from breast cancer in 11,997 women with stage I and stage II breast cancer followed from 5 to 18 years compared to that expected for an age-matched general population. For stages III and IV there was no excess mortality after the 13th year. In a follow-up study, Rutqvist and Wallgren[289] limited their analysis to 458 women ≤40 years of age at diagnosis with operable breast cancer in an attempt to reduce mortality from other causes and eliminate advanced disease. An excess mortality from breast cancer was observed with follow-up extended to 40 years. After 40 years there were no breast cancer deaths; however, there were only 17 patients at risk. Adair et al.[1] also reported no deaths caused by breast cancer from the 29th to 33rd year of follow-up. Ferguson et al.[99] reported the long-term survival of 1259 patients with stages I, II, and III breast cancer who underwent radical mastectomy. Deaths from intercurrent disease without evidence of recurrent breast cancer were censored. The control population was adjusted for sex, age, race, and calendar

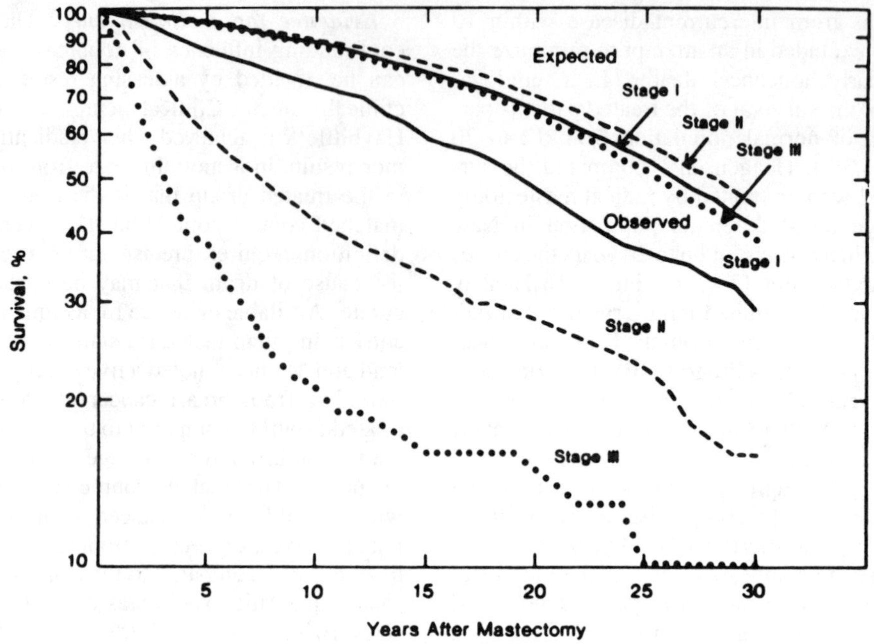

Fig. 3-9 Comparison of expected and observed survival curves for patients in pathologic stages I, II, III (modified 1962 criteria of American Joint Commission), 1927 through 1978. (From Ferguson DJ et al: JAMA 248:1339, 1982. Copyright 1982, American Medical Association.)

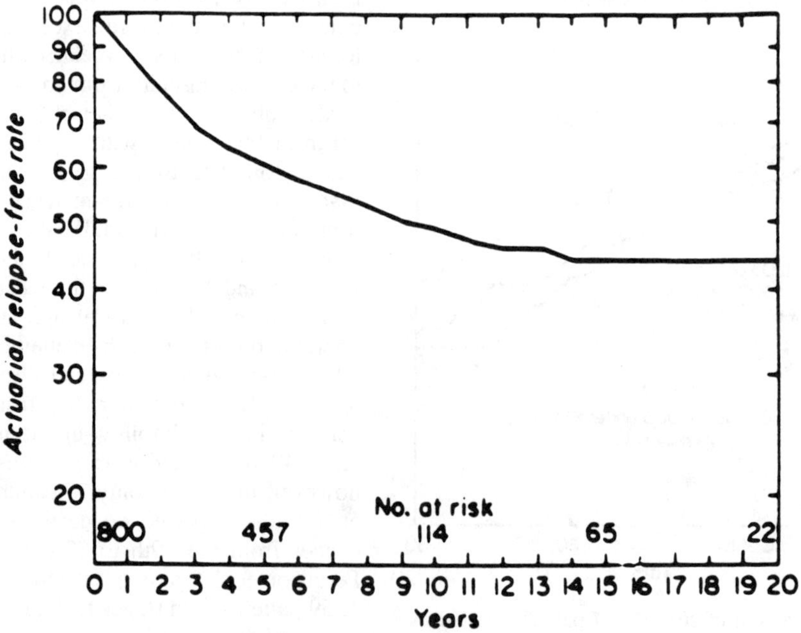

Fig. 3-10 Overall relapse-free rate. (From Clark RM: Alternatives to mastectomy: the Princess Margaret Hospital experience. In Harris JR et al, editors: Conservative management of breast cancer, Philadelphia, 1983, JB Lippincott.)

Table 3-1 Percentage of deaths from other causes in breast cancer patients

Author	Deaths from other causes (%)	Follow-up (yr)
Rutqvist and Wallgren[289]	18	20-51
Adair et al.[1]	30	30.6 (mean)
Brinkley and Haybittle[36]	26	20-30
Fentiman et al.[97]	15	20
Clark et al.[56]	31	20

period, and comparisons were made for each stage. In a semilogarithmic plot the observed survival curves paralleled the expected curves for each stage between 15 and 20 years (Fig. 3-9). Clark[55] analyzed the relapse-free survival of 800 women with $T_1T_2N_0$ breast cancer treated at the Princess Margaret Hospital. In a semilogarithmic plot the actuarial relapse-free survival paralleled the time axis after 14 years, suggesting a clinically cured fraction (Fig. 3-10).

Evidence for a personal cure. A final definition of cure is that of personal cure. Personal cure occurs when the patient dies of causes other than breast cancer without evidence of disease.[175] The percentage of deaths from other causes in breast cancer patients as reported by various series is listed in Table 3-1. While the majority of patients die of breast cancer, approximately 20% to 30% of the deaths are from causes other than breast cancer. This percentage varies with the period of follow-up and the initial extent of disease. Approximately two thirds of the deaths after 20 years result from other causes.[36,90,289] Ederer et al.[92] reported breast cancer as a cause of death in 32% of all patients followed for 15 to 20 years after diagnosis. The percentage of breast cancer deaths during this interval was 22% for patients with localized disease, as compared to 36% for patients with regional disease.

Estimates of breast cancer patients cured

From the above discussion there appears to exist a group of patients whose tumors demonstrate a limited metastatic potential and whose disease is apparently cured by local-regional treatment alone. Table 3-2 demonstrates long-term survival rates for patients with operable breast cancer treated by mastectomy with or without postoperative radiation. At 30 to 40 years approximately one third of the patients are alive. Estimates of the percentage of patients cured from semilogarithmic plots of survival curves, which have suggested a statistical cure, range from 40% to 89%, depending on the patient population and the follow-up period (Table 3-3). In the log-normal model of Rutqvist et al.[290] the estimated fraction of patients cured for all stages was 35% with 54% for stage I and 27% for stage II. These figures are quite comparable to those in Table 3-2.

Factors predicting long-term survival

The status of the axillary nodes and primary tumor size are the most important predictors for long-term survival (i.e., ≤20 years). Adair et al.[1] noted that 67% of their long-term survivors (minimum follow-up 28 years) had negative axillary nodes. Dawson et al.[76] found that 60% of the 93 patients with invasive breast cancer who survived ≥25 years had negative axillary nodes. However, patients with positive axillary nodes represent approximately 30% of the long-term survivors (Table 3-4). Dawson et al.[76] noted that 11% of long-term survivors had ≥4 positive nodes. Fletcher et al.[129] demonstrated a statistical cure for both node-positive and node-negative patients at 17 years. Rosen et al.,[286] however, failed to demonstrate a statistical cure for T_1 pathologically node-positive patients at 20 years. Small primary tumor size is also most com-

Table 3-2 Long-term survival (≥20 years) in operable breast cancer patients treated by mastectomy with or without radiation

Author	Total no. pts.	Survival (%)			Follow-up (yr)
		All pts.	Axillary node-negative pts.	Axillary node-positive pts.	
Rutqvist and Wallgren[289]	458	32	53	19	40
Adair et al.[1]	1458	38	60	—	30
Peters[270]	609	37			30
Fletcher et al.[129]	941	[50]	[75]	[40]	20
Fentiman et al.[97]	227	22			20

[ ], disease-free survival.

Table 3-3 Estimates from semilogarithmic plots of survival curves of the percentage of breast cancer patients cured

Author	No. pts.	Clinical stage	Pts. cured (%)	Follow-up (yr)
Rosen et al.[286]	171	T_1 ≤1 cm	89	20
	303	T_1 1.1-2.0 cm	77	20
	170	T_1 pathologic N_1	—	20
Peters[270]	812	$T_1T_2N_0$	65*	30
Fletcher et al.[129]	941	Stages I-II		20
	262	Pathologic N_0	70	20
	679	Pathologic N_1	40	20

—, curves not parallel, therefore no evidence for cure.
*Approximated from curves.

patible with long-term survival. Approximately 40% of long-term survivors have primary tumors ≤2 cm.[1,76] Long-term survival results for primary tumor size ≤2 cm and negative axillary nodes are presented in Table 3-5. While Rosen et al.[286] demonstrated a cured fraction of 77% to 89% for T_1 pathologic N_0 tumors at 20 years, Duncan and Kerr[90] and Langlands et al.[219] failed to demonstrate a statistical cure for these small tumors and emphasized the necessity for long-term follow-up. Duncan and Kerr[90] noted a significant drop in the survival curve for tumors ≤1 cm in diameter between the 15th and 20th year. The authors suggested, however, that patients with tumors ≤2 cm would achieve a normal mortality between 25 and 30 years of follow-up. A long latent period for recurrences with smaller tumors also has been observed by Rosen et al.[286] Therefore the majority of long-term survivors have negative axillary nodes and/or primary tumors ≤2 cm in diameter.

This observation correlates well with the relationship between primary tumor size and distant metastases. Duncan and Kerr[90] reported that 27% of patients with tumors ≤1 cm in diameter developed metastases during a 20-year follow-up compared to 38% with 2-cm tumors, 37% with 3-cm tumors, 47% with 4-cm tumors, 51% with 5-cm tumors, and 58% with 6-cm tumors. The mean time to the development of metastases was 10.2 years for tumors ≤1 cm. Koscielny et al.[205] reported that 27% of patients with tumors 1 to 2.5 cm in diameter presented with or developed distant metastases over a period of 25 years. Distant metastases occurred in 50% of patients with tumors 3.56 cm in diameter. In patients with negative axillary nodes a tumor size of 11 cm was associated with a 50% metastatic rate compared to a tumor diameter of 3.87 for patients with one to three positive nodes and 2.4 cm for ≥4 positive nodes for a similar rate. Distant metastases occurred in 16% of patients with tumors ≤2 cm in diameter with negative axillary nodes. The interval between diagnosis and the detection of distant metastases was related to primary tumor size and axillary node status. Patients with larger tumors or positive nodes had a shorter interval. The data suggested that a threshold volume of tumor must exist before distant metastases occur, and that a group of patients who did not develop distant metastases clearly exists. In a subsequent report[204] the authors correlated tumor size with axillary node involvement. The mean tumor diameter for the initiation of the first axillary node metastasis was 1.32 cm. The mean tumor volume for initiation of axillary node metastases was smaller than that for initiation of distant metastases with wide variations noted. This observation suggested a continuum in the progression of breast cancer, again indicating the presence of an isolated local-regional stage without distant metastases.

Table 3-4 Percentage of long-term survivors with positive axillary nodes

Author	Pts. with positive axillary nodes (%)	Follow-up (yr)
Rutqvist and Wallgren[289]	30.7	40
Adair et al.[1]	32.6	30.6 mean
Brinkley and Haybittle[37]	26	20+
Fentiman et al.[97]	35	20+
Rosen et al.[286]	20.5	20

Other factors associated with long-term survival include age and histology. The incidence of patients with colloid carcinoma, mucinous carcinoma, or tubular, medullary, or papillary carcinoma in long-term survivors is greater than that of the general breast cancer population.[76,90] An improved long-term survival has been reported in patients with these histologic subtypes.[1,286] In their analyses for

Table 3-5 Long-term survival $T_1N_0M_0$ breast cancer following mastectomy ± radiation

Size of tumor and axillary node status	Author	Survival (%)	Follow-up (yr)
T_1 pathologic N_0	Adair et al.[1]	75	30
	Rosen et al.[286]	53 [75]	20
$T_1 \leq 1$ cm pathologic N_0	Rosen et al.[286]	61 [86]	20
$T_1 \leq 1$ cm clinical N_0	Duncan and Kerr[90]	80	20
T_1 1.1-2.0 cm pathologic N_0	Rosen et al.[286]	49 [69]	20
T_1 1.1-2.0 cm clinical N_0	Duncan and Kerr[90]	62	20

[ ], relapse-free survival.

evidence of statistical cure both Hibberd et al.[184] and Hankey and Steinhorn[169] identified young women (age ≤35) as the only group whose mortality paralleled that of the control population. For Hankey and Steinhorn[169] this finding was confined to young women with localized disease. Fentiman et al.[97] noted a significant effect of age on long-term survival from 10 to 20 years with patients <50 years of age achieving a better survival rate.

In summary, there is evidence to suggest that a portion of the breast cancer patient population achieves a mortality equal to that of an age-matched normal population, i.e., cure with local treatment alone. The size of this cured fraction is dependent on tumor size, histology, axillary node status, and age. Approximately one third of all patients with operable breast cancer are alive 30 to 40 years following treatment. Long-term survivors (i.e., ≥20 years) are most likely to have small primary tumors (≤2 cm), negative axillary nodes, initial age ≤35 years, and histologic subtypes including colloid mucinous, tubular, medullary, or papillary carcinoma. Approximately 30% of long-term survivors, however, had positive axillary nodes. It is estimated that approximately two thirds of patients with T_1T_2 tumors and histologically negative axillary nodes are cured (Table 3-3). The importance of local-regional treatment is most apparent in this group of patients.

Impact of inadequate local-regional treatment on survival

Efforts directed toward local-regional control in the treatment of early breast cancer have been for the most part successful. While a review of retrospective series may demonstrate differences in outcome related to inadequate local treatment,[230] these comparisons suffer from their retrospective nature and inconsistencies in the patient populations, staging, period of treatment, and treatment techniques. Evidence to support the assumption that uncontrolled local-regional disease promotes distant metastases resulting in decreased survival is best obtained from prospective randomized trials. Unfortunately, few trials have compared adequate local-regional treatment with inadequate treatment.

Perhaps the best example of such a trial is the Guy's Hospital trials.[177,178] In the first trial begun in 1961 and completed in 1971, patients ≥50 years of age with operable breast cancer (T_1, T_2, T_3, N_0, N_1, M_0) were randomized to either radical mastectomy and postoperative radiation to the regional nodes or wide excision and postoperative radiation to the breast and regional nodes. Axillary dissection was not performed in the latter group. In the second trial (1971 to 1975), the treatment options were unchanged; however, patients of all ages were now included, and those with clinically positive axillary nodes were excluded. None of the patients received adjuvant systemic treatment. It is generally agreed that in both trials, radiotherapy was inadequate when compared to current standards, especially in terms of low total dose employed.[178] The results of the trials are presented in Table 3-6. For both trials, all patients randomized to wide excision and radiation experienced a statistically significant increase in local-regional recurrence, especially in the axilla. For node-negative patients in the first trial, this increase in local-regional recurrence did not result in a statistically significant increase in distant metastases or a significant decrease in survival. However, in the second trial the increase in local-regional recurrence in this group of patients resulted in a statistically significant increase in distant metastases and a significant decrease in survival. The discrepancies in the results between these two trials were explained by a significant improvement in survival in the radical mastectomy patients between the first and second trials. A similar improvement was not observed in the wide excision and radiation patients. An additional significant difference between the two trials was the percentage of patients with T_1 tumors. In the first trial T_1 patients represented 19% of the radical

Table 3-6 Ten-year results of Guy's Hospital trials[178]

	Treatment	$T_1T_2T_3N_0$ First trial		$T_1T_2T_3N_0$ Second trial		$T_1T_2T_3N_1$ First trial	
Local-regional recurrence	RM	14%	[p<.003]	8%	[p<.000009]	24%	[p<.00003]
	WE and R	31%		30%		57%	
Distant metastases*	RM	37%		30%		50%	[p<.003]
	WE and R	42%		45%		68%	
10 year actuarial survival*	RM	52%		67%	[p<.002]	51%	[p<.05]
	WE and R	57%		58%		35%	

RM, radical mastectomy; WE and R, wide excision and radiation; [ ], p values for comparison (RM vs. WE and R).
*Percentages interpreted from actuarial curves.

mastectomy group and 18% of the wide excision and radiation group. These figures increased to 37% and 38% respectively for the second trial. In a subsequent analysis[177] combining patients with T_1 and T_2 tumors from the two trials, the investigators noted that significant survival differences were confined to the T_1 patients with those undergoing radical mastectomy doing significantly better. Therefore the impact of local-regional treatment on survival was most obvious in the second trial, in which a greater percentage of patients had earlier tumors. For patients with clinically positive axillary nodes, inadequate local-regional treatment resulted in a significant decrease in survival and an increase in distant metastases that was not statistically significant.

A second trial with similar findings is the Southeast Scotland trial (1964 to 1971).[220] This trial randomized patients with operable breast cancer ($T_1T_2T_3N_0N_1$) to radical mastectomy versus simple mastectomy and postoperative radiotherapy. Patients <60 years of age also underwent bilateral oophorectomy or ovarian ablation by radiation. The postmastectomy radiotherapy technique has been considered inadequate,[130,229] and the high daily fractions employed may have contributed to the increased frequency of nonbreast cancer deaths in the irradiated patients. While differences in local-regional recurrence rates and distant metastases were not analyzed for statistical significance, local-regional recurrences were greater in the simple mastectomy and radiation group for stage I and stage II (Table 3-7). These primarily axillary recurrences occurred in 3% of the radical mastectomy patients vs. 12% of the simple mastectomy patients. Distant metastases were not increased. Overall survival was significantly better in the radical mastectomy patients; however, this difference was confined to stage I ($T_1T_2N_0$) patients.

The Guy's Hospital trials and the Southeast Scotland (Edinburgh) trial suggest that the impact of local-regional control on survival is especially significant in patients with small primary tumors and a clinically negative axilla. These trials clearly demonstrate an adverse impact on survival with inadequate local-regional treatment. Their findings correlate well with the previous discussion regarding the identification of patient subsets for whom local-regional treatment alone has resulted in cure.

There are, however, trials that demonstrate significantly increased local-regional recurrence rates but fail to demonstrate a significant decrease in

Table 3-7 Ten-year results of the Southeast Scotland Trial for operable breast cancer[220]

	Treatment	Stage I		Stage II	Stage III	All pts.	
Local-regional recurrence (%)	RM	15		25	40	23	
	SM and R	25		33	23	27	
Distant metastases (%)	RM	28		43	46	38	
	SM and R	25		41	42	36	
10-year crude survival (%)	RM	70*	[p<.05]	58*	48*	61	[p<.05]
	SM and R	50*		58*	51*	51.5	

RM, radical mastectomy; SM and R, simple mastectomy and radiation; [ ], p values for comparison (RM vs. SM and R).
*Percentages interpreted from survival curves.

overall survival. These include the Cape Town Trial (1968 to 1971),[181] the Cancer Research Campaign Trial (1970 to 1975),[22,48] the Manchester Regional Breast Study (1970 to 1975),[234] the NSABP B-06 trial (1976 to 1984),[103,114] and the NSABP B-04 trial (1971 to 1974).[113]

The Cape Town Trial[181] randomized 95 patients with $T_1T_2N_0N_1M_0$ breast cancer to radical mastectomy or simple mastectomy. Clinically enlarged axillary nodes were removed with the simple mastectomy but a formal axillary node dissection was not performed. No adjuvant treatment was given. Patients undergoing simple mastectomy had a significantly increased incidence of local-regional recurrence (23.5% vs. 2.3%), however; there was no difference in overall survival or distant disease-free survival. The study was terminated after 3 years because of the significant difference in local-regional recurrence, and the concern that this could translate into a survival difference with longer follow-up.

The Cancer Research Campaign[22,48] randomized 2268 patients with clinical stage I or stage II breast cancer to simple mastectomy or simple mastectomy and radiation. At 14 years there was a statistically significant decrease in local-regional recurrence with radiation (43% vs. 22%); survival, however, was not affected. Five-year analysis revealed no differences between the two treatments in terms of survival or freedom from distance recurrence for either stage I or stage II patients. Unfortunately, long-term results have not been presented separately for stage I and stage II, although a separate analysis of 418 patients in whom axillary nodes were identified in the mastectomy specimen revealed no significant survival differences between the two treatment groups for node-positive or node-negative patients.[94]

The Manchester trial[234] randomized 714 patients with clinical stage I ($T_{1\text{-}2}N_0M_0$) breast cancer to simple mastectomy or simple mastectomy and radiation. Premenopausal or perimenopausal patients were offered oophorectomy or ovarian irradiation. The addition of local-regional radiation resulted in a significant decrease in local-regional recurrence (42% vs. 23%) and a nonsignificant improvement in 10-year overall and metastasis-free survival. The study, however, found a significant improvement in disease-free survival at 10 years (52% vs. 36%) with radiation.

The NSABP B-06 trial[103,114] randomized 1843 women with stage I or stage II breast cancer to lumpectomy (segmental mastectomy) and axillary dissection with or without breast irradiation or total mastectomy and axillary dissection. For statistical considerations, a breast recurrence following lumpectomy was not included in the disease-free survival analysis. Nonetheless, patients undergoing segmental mastectomy without radiation had a statistically significant increase in breast recurrence resulting in a statistically significant decrease in disease-free and distant disease-free survival in axillary node–negative patients, when compared to segmental mastectomy and radiation at 5 years (Table 3-8).[103] Distant disease-free survival was also significantly worse in node-negative lumpec-

Table 3-8 Results of NSABP B-06 trial of histologically node-negative patients[114]

Result	Total mastectomy		Lumpectomy		Lumpectomy and breast irradiation
Disease-free survival*					
5 yr	75%		68%		77%
8 yr	66%		61%		66%
Overall p value		.05		.02	
Distant disease-free survival					
5 yr	82%		75%		81%
8 yr	74%		70%		71%
Overall p value		.03		0.1	
Overall survival					
5 yr	88%		87%		88%
8 yr	79%		77%		82%
Overall p value		0.5		0.5	
Breast recurrence	–		37%		12%
Overall p value			<.001		

*Excludes patients with ipsilateral breast recurrence.
Modified from Fisher B et al: N Engl J Med 320:822, 1989.

tomy patients who did not receive radiation when compared to total mastectomy patients.[114] There was no significant difference in overall survival for any of the treatment groups. At 8 years the lumpectomy patients continued to manifest a significantly increased breast recurrence, resulting in a persistent significant decrease in disease-free survival but not in distant disease-free survival when compared to patients undergoing lumpectomy and radiation.[114] In a comparison with total mastectomy patients, lumpectomy patients given no radiation also demonstrated a significant decrease in distant disease-free survival. Again no differences were seen in overall survival. At both 5 and 8 years all patients undergoing lumpectomy without radiation had a significantly decreased disease-free survival when compared to patients undergoing lumpectomy and radiation. For patients with positive axillary nodes, no differences in disease-free, distant disease-free, or overall survival were observed for the three treatment groups, despite a significant difference in breast recurrence for patients undergoing lumpectomy and chemotherapy without radiation (6% vs. 43%, $p<.001$). This trial, while demonstrating the effect of breast recurrence on disease-free or distant disease-free survival depending on the comparison group and axillary nodes status, failed to demonstrate an effect on overall survival.

An additional trial that has addressed the significance of local-regional control in the treatment of early breast cancer is the NSABP B-04 trial.[113] This trial evaluated the adequacy of surgical procedures less than radical mastectomy in the treatment of operable breast cancer. Patients with clinically negative axillary nodes were randomized to radical mastectomy, total mastectomy, or total mastectomy and local-regional radiation. Clinically node-positive patients underwent radical mastectomy or total mastectomy and radiation. The subsequent appearance of positive axillary nodes was not deemed a treatment failure unless surgical salvage was impossible. Of axillary node–negative patients, 17.8% required a delayed axillary dissection for the development of palpable nodes. The exclusion of these patients as a treatment failure resulted in no significant differences in local-regional recurrence among the three treatment groups for node-negative patients, although the total mastectomy group had the highest incidence. Similarly there was no difference in distant disease-free or overall survival at 10 years. There was a significant difference in disease-free survival at 10 years ($p=.05$) with the total mastectomy patients having the lowest 10-year disease-free survival. Because the definition of treatment failure chosen for statistical analysis affected the reported incidence of local-regional recurrence and disease-free survival, it is difficult to draw conclusions regarding the impact of local-regional control in node-negative patients, though clearly, overall survival was not affected. For node-positive patients the two treatments yielded no significant differences in local-regional control or in distant disease-free, disease-free, or overall survival rates.

The contradictory results of these randomized trials are difficult to explain. Differences may be related to patient selection, follow-up procedures, methods employed to detect recurrence, definitions of treatment failure, and statistical considerations as well as the actual magnitude of local-regional recurrence. There appears to be some consistency in the findings that local-regional recurrence rates of 30% to 40% in node-negative patients adversely affect distant disease-free and/or disease-free survival[103,113,114,178,220,234] that in some studies translates into a decrease in overall survival.[178,220]

Survival gain from improved local-regional control

The survival gain that can be expected from improved local-regional control can be calculated by determining the difference between local-regional control for two treatments, multiplying this difference by the percentage of patients with local control who develop distant metastases, and subtracting this number from the first.[319] This calculation requires detailed information about sites of first failure, which is not always available. It assumes virtually no long-term salvage for isolated local-regional recurrences. This latter assumption is appropriate for most local-regional recurrences postmastectomy because 80% to 90% will develop distant metastases, and 5 year survival rates following recurrence are approximately 30%.[18,87,98,143,238,330] Suit and Westgate[319] have applied this calculation to data from the NSABP B-04 study.[113] The local-regional recurrence rate (excluding salvageable axillary recurrences) in node-negative patients who underwent total mastectomy was 13.9%, compared to 6% for total mastectomy and radiation. Approximately 30% of patients with local control developed distant metastases, and prevention of local-regional recurrence in this group would not result in a survival benefit. Therefore the expected survival benefit would be 5.5%. The observed difference in disease-free survival was 6%. It can be seen from this example that large differences in local-regional control, with a small percentage of controlled patients developing distant metastases, result in the greatest potential for a survival benefit. However, the magnitude of this benefit can be decreased by the development of distant metastases in a significant percentage of patients with local-regional control or by the successful salvage of local-regional recurrences.

Local-regional recurrences that are salvageable are less likely to have a significant impact on disease-free or overall survival and may require a longer period of follow-up to demonstrate such an effect. The ability to salvage axillary failures in the clinically negative undissected axilla has been demonstrated by the Cancer Research Campaign trial,[47] the NSABP B-04 trial,[113] and a retrospective review reported by Crile.[65] In the Cancer Research Campaign trial,[47] 75 of 110 patients who experienced an axillary failure were alive after salvage treatment. In the NSABP B-04 trial, patients with clinically negative axillary nodes who underwent total mastectomy had a 17.8% incidence of axillary failures without an adverse effect on overall survival.[113] Crile[65] reported that patients who developed an axillary recurrence following simple mastectomy and were salvaged by a subsequent axillary dissection had a 5-year survival rate of 75%. The ability to salvage axillary failures decreases the potential gain in survival from initial treatment to this region and may be responsible for the lack of a significant survival benefit in the NSABP B-04 and Cancer Research Campaign trials.[47,113] Also, as previously noted, axillary failures that were surgically salvaged were not included in disease-free calculations in the NSABP B-04 study. Similarly, surgical salvage of isolated breast recurrences following conservative surgery and radiation has resulted in 5-year survival rates of 50% to 80%.[57,59,89,136,159,208,264] In the NSABP B-06 study the difference between breast recurrences in the lumpectomy versus lumpectomy and radiation patients was 29%.[114] Approximately 20% of patients developed distant metastases without a local-regional failure. Therefore the maximum anticipated survival gain would be 23%. However, this figure must be adjusted by the fact that at least 50% of breast failures are salvaged. The corrected potential survival gain is at best 11.5%. The minimum time required to express the overall mortality of nonsalvageable local recurrences (assuming a 5-year survival of 50% following treatment for recurrence) would be 7½ years from initial treatment, because the median time to a breast recurrence was approximately 2½ years. Currently, at 8 years, the trial has demonstrated a 5% overall and disease-free survival benefit for lumpectomy and radiation patients when compared to lumpectomy alone. Longer follow-up, therefore, has the potential of demonstrating a significant impact on overall survival. Applying the above considerations to the Guy's Hospital second trial,[178] the difference in local-regional recurrence was 22% (30% vs. 8%), approximately one third of patients developed distant metastases and, assuming a 50% salvage of local-regional recurrences in the conservatively treated group, the expected survival gain would be 7.5%. The actual benefit was 9% at 10 years, which was statistically significant; the benefit was most marked after 8 years.[178] In mastectomy trials where local-regional recurrences (other than axillary as noted above) frequently are not salvageable and where the interval to recurrence is relatively short (i.e., majority within 2 to 3 years)[87,330] the impact of inadequate local-regional control is seen earlier, and survival differences have the potential for being greater.

Local-regional control may significantly impact on survival, especially in patients with small primary tumors and negative axillary nodes. It is important to all patients because uncontrolled local-regional disease may be the source of distant metastases and chemotherapy-resistant cell lines.[81] It can produce significant problems for the patient including pain, ulceration, bleeding, arm edema, and brachial plexopathy. Local-regional control is important in node-positive patients not only for the above reasons but also because approximately one third of long-term survivors (≥20 years) had positive nodes. The argument that breast or axillary recurrences are salvageable in a significant proportion of patients should not deter the physician from initial efforts at optimal local-regional control. Not all of these recurrences are salvageable. The psychologic impact of a preventable recurrence and the need for further surgery and/or systemic therapy may be devastating to the patient.

COMPARISONS OF LOCAL-REGIONAL TREATMENT OPTIONS

In evaluating the success of local-regional treatment, outcome commonly is measured in terms of overall survival, disease-free or relapse-free survival, local-regional recurrence, and complications. Evaluation of overall survival takes into consideration deaths from breast cancer as well as other causes and may be presented as crude or actuarial survival. Actuarial survival curves allow the use of data from patients followed for variable time periods, while crude survival curves restrict the analysis to all patients followed for the same time period or a specified minimum period. Disease-free survival includes patients with no evidence of disease. Patients who experience a recurrence and undergo successful salvage treatment renders them alive without disease are included in the disease-free survival curve. Relapse-free survival censors patients at the time of first relapse. Local recurrence following mastectomy is defined as a recurrence on the chest wall. In some series, axillary recurrences after mastectomy also are classified as local recurrences. Local recurrence following lumpectomy or segmental mastectomy is defined as a recurrence in the treated breast. Regional recurrences include those in the ipsilateral axilla, supraclavicular nodes, or internal mammary nodes. In general the definition of a local-regional recurrence includes those that present as isolated recurrences or simultaneously with distant metastases. Patients who first present with distant metastases and subsequently develop a local-regional recurrence are excluded in many series from local-regional recurrence calculations, as they may represent a reseeding phenomenon.

The comparative effectiveness of treatment alternatives is best evaluated in a prospective randomized clinical trial. Defined eligibility criteria, detailed treatment regimens, and strict follow-up procedures contribute to the objective assessment of treatment outcome in a relatively homogeneous patient population. Bias as well as the influence of various prognostic factors other than the treatment itself can be minimized. The 1970s witnessed the emergence of randomized clinical trials to evaluate treatment regimens objectively and to test biologic principles. The well-designed and analyzed trial that addresses pertinent clinical questions can provide meaningful results and significantly enhance our knowledge. Retrospective comparisons suffer from variations in the period of treatment, patient selection, and therapy as well as in follow-up procedures, and such comparisons should be interpreted with caution. However, the nonrandomized efforts of individual institutions have provided the fundamental clinical basis for the development of randomized clinical trials, and their contribution should not be ignored.

Definitions of local-regional treatment options

Radical mastectomy. The radical mastectomy removes all breast tissue through a skin incision that incorporates the nipple and biopsy site. The skin around the tumor and biopsy site is excised widely; a skin graft may be required to close the defect. The pectoralis major and minor muscles are removed, and a complete axillary dissection is performed.

Extended radical mastectomy. The extended radical mastectomy removes the internal mammary nodes at the time of the radical mastectomy or modified radical mastectomy. The internal mammary nodes can be removed by an extrapleural discontinuous dissection or an en bloc resection of the bony chest wall.

Superradical mastectomy. The superradical mastectomy incorporates the removal of the internal mammary and supraclavicular nodes with the radical mastectomy. The supraclavicular nodes are removed by resection of the first rib in a discontinuous manner[356] or by en bloc resection including the clavicle, medial portion of the first and second ribs, and adjacent sternum.[350]

Modified radical mastectomy. The Patey[269] modified radical mastectomy removes all breast tissue, the fascia of the pectoralis major muscle, and the pectoralis minor muscle and is accompanied by a complete axillary node dissection. The Auchincloss[8] and the Madden[235] modified radical mastectomy preserves the pectoralis major and minor muscles. The axillary dissection is usually that of levels I and II unless the pectoralis minor muscle is divided and level III nodes are removed. For both procedures a transverse skin incision incorporating the nipple and biopsy site is employed, and the skin is closed primarily.

Total (simple) mastectomy. The total mastectomy removes all breast tissue, preserves the pectoralis major and minor muscles, and is not accompanied by an axillary node dissection.

Partial mastectomy. Partial mastectomy implies resection of only a portion of the breast. Lumpectomy, tumorectomy, or excisional biopsy result in gross excision of the primary tumor without regard to microscopic margins.[173] In a wide excision the primary tumor is resected with a 1- to 2-cm margin of normal adjacent breast tissue. Quadrantectomy removes the primary tumor as well as its quadrant of origin, including the overlying skin and the underlying pectoral fascia.

Postoperative radiation may be employed as an adjuvant to any of the above surgical procedures. It may be directed to the chest wall, breast, and/or regional (axillary, supraclavicular, or internal mammary) nodes. The term *conservative surgery and radiation* generally has been reserved for patients undergoing partial mastectomy, axillary dissection, and radiation to the remaining breast with or without regional node irradiation.

Treatment with mastectomy

The results of local-regional treatment for early breast cancer from retrospective reviews, intrainstitutional nonrandomized comparisons, and prospective randomized trials are presented in the following sections. For each study the period of treatment is indicated as well as the number of patients treated and the use of adjuvant therapy. Results are presented in terms of overall survival, disease-free or relapse-free survival, local-regional recurrence, and distant metastases, where available. For comparison p values are provided when they have been reported.

Retrospective reviews

Radical mastectomy. The results of radical mastectomy from retrospective reviews are presented in Tables 3-9 to 3-11. Comparisons are difficult

Table 3-9 Results of radical mastectomy from retrospective series stage I or A and stage II or B

Author	No. pts.	Treatment period	Adjuvant therapy	Survival (%) 5 yr I/A	Survival (%) 5 yr II/B	Survival (%) 10 yr I/A	Survival (%) 10 yr II/B
Ferguson et al.[99]	960	1927-1978	±R, C, H	84	62	73	42
Ariel[6]	887	1930-1965	±R	82	64	60	47
Haimov et al.[160]	479	1933-1965	±R, C, H	64	50	54	28
Haagensen and Cooley[155]	482	1935-1951	±R	85	59	70	40
Anglem and Leber[5]	188	1939-1959	NS	—	—	57	57
Donegan[85]	561	1940-1970	NS	77	57	70	43
Lee and Lambley[224]	402	1947-1959	None	—	—	60	29
Butcher[42]	351	1950-1955	±R	76	48	56	30
Schottenfeld et al.[300]	242	1960	±R	96	72	91	57
Baker et al.[11]	152	1969-1972	±R	85	83	—	—
Wilson et al.[360]	4248	1976	None	61	78	—	—

NS, not stated; R, radiation therapy; C, chemotherapy; H, hormonal management including oophorectomy.

Table 3-10 Incidence of local regional recurrence following radical mastectomy

Author	Adjuvant therapy	Stage	Local-regional recurrence (%)	Follow-up (yr)
Schottenfeld et al.[300]	None	I	0	10
Haagensen and Cooley[155]	±R	A	7	10
		B	18	
Donegan[85]	NS	A	16	5-24
		B	27	
Lee and Lambley[224]	±R	I and II	5	10
Papatestas and Lesnick[267]	±R	I and II	7	5
Ferguson et al.[99]	±R, C, H	I-III	10	4-30
Valagussa et al.[340]	None	T_{1-3} pathologic N_0	6	10
		T_{1-3} pathologic N_1	17	
Fisher et al.[113]	None	I-III	14	10

NS, not stated; R, radiation; C, chemotherapy; H, hormonal management including oophorectomy.

Table 3-11 Sites of local-regional recurrence following radical mastectomy

Author	Local-regional recurrences (%) Chest wall	Axilla	Internal mammary node	Supraclavicular node	Total incidence of local-regional recurrence (%)
Haagensen and Cooley[155]	59	2	39	—	10
Baker et al.[11]	88	12	—	—	10
Lee and Lambley[224]	74	—	26	—	5
Ferguson et al.[99]	56	—	14	30	10
Fisher et al.[119]	82	0	0	18	19
Veronesi and Valagussa[349]					
Pathologic N_0	21	0	28	51	8
Pathologic N_1	38	2	16	41	29

because of the use of different staging systems (Manchester classification, Columbia Clinical Classification, or TNM classification) and different treatment periods, and the nonstandard use of adjuvant therapy. In general postmastectomy radiation was used selectively in patients with histologically positive axillary nodes, medial or centrally located tumors regardless of the nodal status, or large primary tumors. Although it is impossible to assure comparability of the groups, the results appear similar, with 5- and 10-year survival rates of 70% to 80% and 60% to 70% respectively for stage I/A and 60% to 70% and 40% to 50% respectively for stage II/B. A 1982 national survey by the American College of Surgeons reported a 5-year actuarial survival rate of 93% for 3058 breast cancer patients with localized disease treated by radical mastectomy without adjuvant therapy and a 5-year survival rate of 78% for 1190 women with regional disease.[360] Localized disease was defined as tumors confined to the breast, whereas regional disease included patients with tumor extension to the axillary nodes. Valagussa et al.[340] reported a 5-year survival rate of 70% and a 10-year survival rate of 58% in a group of 716 patients with operable breast cancer who underwent radical mastectomy in a randomized trial comparing this procedure to the extended radical mastectomy. No adjuvant therapy was given. Fisher et al.[119] reported a 5-year survival rate of 62% in 317 patients who underwent radical mastectomy alone in the NSABP B-02 randomized trial, which compared radical mastectomy alone, radical mastectomy and regional node irradiation, and radical mastectomy and thiotepa.

Local-regional recurrence rates following radical mastectomy vary with the stage, length of follow-up, and use of adjuvant radiation (see Tables 3-10 and 3-11) with overall rates of 10% (Table 3-12). The most common sites of recurrence are the chest wall and supraclavicular nodes (see Table 3-11). The axillary nodes are an infrequent site following a complete axillary dissection.

Modified radical mastectomy. The modified radical mastectomy with preservation of the pectoralis major muscle is a cosmetically less deforming procedure. It was not until 1976 that it became the surgical procedure employed in the majority of breast cancer patients in the United States.[360] By 1981 only 3.4% of patients underwent the radical mastectomy compared to 25.5% in 1976. Results of the modified radical mastectomy are presented in Tables 3-12 to 3-14. Five- and 10-year survival rates of 75% to 90% and 60% to 80% respectively are reported for stage I/A patients. For stage II/B patients, the 5- and 10-year survival rates are 70% to 80% and 30% to 40%. The 1982 survey by the American College of Surgeons reported a 5-year survival rate of 92% for localized disease and an 80% survival rate for regional disease in patients who underwent a modified radical mastectomy without adjuvant therapy.[360] Donegan,[85] in a review of patients treated at the Medical College of Wisconsin, found no difference in disease-free survival by stage or axillary nodal status between the Patey modified radical mastectomy (complete axillary dissection) and the Auchincloss procedure (limited axillary dissection), although axillary recurrences were more common with the Auchincloss mastectomy in patients with four or more positive nodes.

Local regional recurrence rates following modified radical mastectomy range from 0 to 30% with the most common site being the chest wall (see Tables 3-13 and 3-14). Axillary recurrences are somewhat more frequent than those reported following radical mastectomy.

Table 3-12 Results of modified radical mastectomy from retrospective series stage I or A and stage II or B

Author	No. pts.	Treatment period	Adjuvant therapy	Survival (%) 5 yr I/A	5 yr II/B	10 yr I/A	10 yr II/B
Handley and Thackray[166]	135	Before 1969	±R	75	57	61	25
Donegan[85]*	512	—	±R	83	72	79	48
Leis[225]	730	1950-1977	±R	—	—	72	40
Baker et al.[11]	113	1969-1972	±R	90	73	—	—
Wilson et al.[360]	8668	1976	None	92	80	—	—
Donegan[85]	305	1967-1979	±R, C	87	81	78	36
Hermann et al.[182]	793	1957-1979	None	76		59	

R, radiation; C, chemotherapy.
*Donegan's review of Handley's pts.

Table 3-13 Local-regional recurrence following modified radical mastectomy

Author	Adjuvant therapy	Local-regional recurrence (%)			Follow-up (yr)
		I/A	II/B	I/A and II/B	
Baker et al.[11]	±R	13	9		5
Delarue et al.[78]	NS	0	12		5
Handley and Thackray[166]	±R	16	26		10
Leis[225]	±R	5	14		10
Papatestas and Lesnick[257]	±R			6	5
Donegan[85]	±R, C			18	10

NS, not stated; R, radiation; C, chemotherapy.

Table 3-14 Sites of local-regional recurrence following modified radical mastectomy

Author	Local-regional recurrences (%)				Total incidence of local-regional recurrence (%)
	Chest wall	Axilla	Internal mammary node	Supraclavicular node	
Handley and Thackray[166]	60	13	27	—	22
Baker et al.[11]	88	12	—	—	14

Simple mastectomy with or without radiation. Simple or total mastectomy with postoperative radiotherapy was originally advocated by McWhirter in 1948.[245] He postulated that the surgical removal of axillary nodes promoted the development of distant metastases and that their removal was unnecessary in patients with clinically negative nodes and produced disappointing results in patients with clinically positive nodes. Consequently, he employed radiation to treat the regional nodes. In the 1960s, Crile,[66] Devitt,[82] and Fisher et al.[106,107] recognized through clinical observations and laboratory investigations that the axillary nodes were not a source of distant metastases, and they predicted that variations in treatment would not result in survival differences. The simple or total mastectomy leaves the axillary nodes untreated because it does not involve an axillary dissection. When this type of procedure is combined with postoperative radiation, the regional nodes are treated solely by radiation. Results of retrospective series employing simple mastectomy with or without postoperative radiotherapy are presented in Tables 3-15 and 3-16. The American College of Surgeons' 1982 survey reported a 5-year survival rate of 87% for localized disease and 66% for regional disease in patients treated by simple mastectomy without adjuvant therapy.[360]

Local-regional recurrence rates following simple mastectomy from retrospective series range from 10% to 29% (see Table 3-16). The axilla is a common site for recurrence in patients who are treated by simple mastectomy alone. The axillary recurrence rate in the clinically negative undissected or unirradiated axilla ranges from 16% to 41%.[67,82,113,133,234] For patients with clinically positive axillary nodes, 48% will experience progression in these nodes within 8 months.[14] The second most common site for local-regional recurrence is the chest wall.[48,113,234]

Additional data regarding outcome in patients undergoing simple mastectomy is obtained from four prospective randomized trials that compared simple mastectomy to simple mastectomy and postoperative radiation (Table 3-17). Five-year and 10-year survival rates of 69% to 74% and 55% to 62% are reported. There is no significant survival advantage for the addition of postoperative radiotherapy in any of these studies. However, local-regional recurrences are reduced significantly by the addition of radiation. In both the Manchester Regional Breast Study[234] and the Cancer Research Campaign Study[22] the addition of radiation decreased the local-regional recurrence rate at 10 years from approximately 40% to 20%. In the Southampton Study[333] patients with positive axillary nodes had a decrease in local-regional recurrence at 4 years with the addition of radiation (43% vs. 15%, $p<.05$); however, there was no associated survival benefit.

The concept of the lack of an effect on survival of untreated axillary nodes while evaluated in the

Table 3-15 Results of simple mastectomy from retrospective series

				Survival (%)					
				5 yr			10 yr		
Author	No. pts.	Treatment period	Adjuvant therapy	I/A	II/B	I/A and II/B	I/A	II/B	I/A and II/B
Kaae and Johansen[196]	187	1951 – *	+R	70	50		50	32	
Wilson et al.[360]	1217	1976	None	87	66		—	—	
Hermann et al.[182]	544	1957-1979	±R			84			74

R, radiation.
*Not stated.

Table 3-16 Incidence of local-regional recurrence following simple mastectomy

Author	Adjuvant therapy	Stage	Local-regional recurrence (%)	Follow-up (yr)
Crile[64]	±R	I and II	10	10
Williams et al.[359]	None	A, B, C	27	4-10
Kaae and Johansen[196]	+R	A	19	10
		B	29	

R, radiation.

Table 3-17 Results of randomized trials comparing simple mastectomy (SM) with simple mastectomy and radiation (SM and R)

	Cancer Research Campaign[22,48]		Southamptom[333]		Manchester Regional[234]		Edinburgh I[133]	
Treatment period	1970-1975		1973-1976		1970-1975		1974-1979	
No. pts.	2800		150		714		342	
Stage	I and II		I and II		I		I and II	
Adjuvant therapy	None		None		None		None	
	SM	SM and R	SM	SM and R	SM	SM and R	SM	SM and R
Survival (%)								
5-yr overall	70	73	78*	81*	69	74	80†	73†
			[>.05]					
5-yr DFS					49	65		
10-yr overall	55	55			55	62		
	[.88]				[.20]			
10-yr DFS					36	52		
					[<.0001]			
Distant metastases (%)	35	33	—	—	—	—	—	—
Local-regional recurrence	39	17	28	9	42	22	24	14
	[<.001]		[<.05]		[<.0001]			
Followup	10 yr		4 yr		10 yr		4 yr	

DFS, disease-free survival; [ ], p value for comparison (adjacent columns).
*3-yr survival.
†4-yr survival.

trials comparing simple mastectomy to simple mastectomy and radiation was best tested in the NSABP B-04 randomized trial.[113] Patients with clinically negative axillary nodes were randomized to radical mastectomy, total mastectomy and radiation, or total mastectomy with axillary dissection delayed until the time of axillary recurrence. Results are presented in Table 3-18. The axillary recurrence rate was 17.8% for patients who underwent total mastectomy alone, compared to 1.4% for radical mastectomy and 3.1% for total mastectomy and radiation. There was no significant difference in the incidence of chest wall or supraclavicular recurrences among the three treatment groups, although the recurrence rate was lowest in the irradiated patients. Overall survival rates at 5 and 10 years were not significantly different. There was, however, a significant difference ($p = .05$) in 10 year disease-free survival, with total mastectomy patients having the lower survival. The Cape Town trial also attempted to address this issue.[181] Ninety-five patients with stages I and II breast cancer were randomized to radical mastectomy or simple mastectomy with gross excision of clinically positive axillary nodes. The study was terminated after 3 years because of a significant increase in local-regional recurrence in the simple mastectomy patients (23.5% vs. 2.3%). However, there was no difference in overall or distant disease-free survival.

While treatment of the axillary nodes offers no advantage in terms of survival, the axillary dissection is important for staging purposes, and it provides prognostic information, removes grossly positive nodes, and reduces the incidence of axillary recurrence. At the present time axillary dissection is performed routinely in patients with early breast cancer. (For further discussion see Treatment of Regional Nodes—Axillary Nodes, p. 67.)

Comparison of results for mastectomy

Intrainstitutional comparisons. Comparisons of outcome with variations in local-regional treatment within a single institution frequently suffer from differences in patient selection, the accumulation of patients over different periods of time, differences in the number of patients treated, and lack of a statistical analysis. Conclusions drawn from these studies are limited in their clinical application; they are cited frequently as justification for a particular treatment preference, however. They are presented here for completeness, especially as the number of intrainstitutional comparisons of radical mastectomy to modified radical mastectomy exceeds the number of prospective randomized trials.

The results of intrainstitutional comparisons of radical mastectomy with modified radical mastectomy are presented in Table 3-19. None of these studies has suggested a survival advantage for the radical mastectomy either for all patients or for those with histologically positive or negative axillary nodes.[85,283]

Results of intrainstitutional comparisons of radical or modified radical mastectomy with simple mastectomy with or without radiation are presented in Table 3-20. Despite the limitations of such comparisons, there appears to be no advantage in terms of survival for the more aggressive surgical procedure.

Prospective randomized trials. There have been two prospective randomized trials that have compared radical mastectomy to modified radical mastectomy (Table 3-21). None of the patients in the Manchester trial received adjuvant therapy,[334] whereas in the University of Alabama study[236,237] patients with histologically positive axillary nodes received adjuvant chemotherapy consisting of cyclophosphamide, methotrexate, and fluorouracil (CMF) or melphalan. The Manchester trial[334] reported no significant differences in 5-year overall or disease-free survival rates or the incidence of local-regional recurrence or distant metastases. In a subset analysis, there were also no differences for patients with histologically positive or negative axillary nodes. The University of Alabama trial[236,237] with a smaller number of patients noted similar findings at 5 and 10 years; however, the incidence of local-regional recurrence was significantly less with the radical mastectomy. In a subset analysis, patients with T_{2a} tumors and clinically

Table 3-18 Results of the NSABP B-04 randomized trial in clinically axillary node negative patients[113]

Treatment period	1971-1974		
No. pts.	1079		
Stage	$T_{1\text{-}3}$ clinical N_0		
Adjuvant therapy	None		
	RM	**TM**	**TM and R**
Survival (%)			
5-yr overall	75	74	75
5-yr disease-free*	60	56	65
10-yr overall	58	54	59 [.2]
10-yr disease-free*	47	42	48 [.05]
Distant metastases (%)	30	34	32
Local regional recurrence (%)*	9	14	5

RM, radical mastectomy; TM, total mastectomy; R, radiation; [ ], p value for comparison (RM vs. TM vs. TM and R).
*Excludes patients with operable axillary recurrences.

Table 3-19 Results of intrainstitutional comparisons of radical mastectomy (RM) with modified radical mastectomy (MRM)

Author	Treatment period	No. pts. RM	No. pts. MRM	Stage	Survival (%) 5 yr RM	Survival (%) 5 yr MRM	Survival (%) 10 yr RM	Survival (%) 10 yr MRM
St. Bartholomew's Hospital[358]	1930-1939	269	117	I	65	54	38	46
				II	41	38	22	19
Rockford, Ill.[247]	1924-1972	1127	176	I-IV	66	74	45	43
Ontario Cancer Institute[78]	1950-1960	1793	743	I-IV	51	51	—	—
Mt. Sinai, N.Y.[267]	1964-1968	83	51	I and II	84	81	—	—
Mayo Clinic[243]	1965-1968	322	208	I-III	82	87	74	74
Hopkins[11]	1969-1972	152	113	I	85	90	—	—
				II	83	73	—	—
Medical College of Wisconsin[85]	1967-1979	403	362	I-III	76	80	47	54

positive axillary nodes or T_{3a} tumors had an improved 10-year survival rate with the radical mastectomy (59% vs. 38%, p = .05).

Two randomized trials have compared radical mastectomy to simple or total mastectomy. The Cape Town trial[181] randomized 95 patients with stages I and II breast cancer to radical mastectomy or simple mastectomy with selective removal of clinically positive nodes. As previously noted the trial was terminated after 3 years because of a significant difference in local-regional recurrence between the two treatments favoring the radical mastectomy (23.5% vs. 2.3%). However, no survival differences were noted. The NSABP B-04 study[113] randomized patients with clinically negative axillary nodes to radical mastectomy, total mastectomy, or total mastectomy and radiation. Results are presented in Table 3-18. No significant differences in overall survival rates at 5 or 10 years, or in the incidence of distant metastases were demonstrated, although a significant difference (p = .05) in 10-year disease-free survival was noted. These two studies not only address the impact of surgical procedures less than radical mastectomy on survival but also the impact of untreated axillary nodes on survival.

There has been a single trial comparing modified radical mastectomy to simple mastectomy with

Table 3-20 Results of intrainstitutional comparisons of radical (RM) or modified radical mastectomy (MRM) with simple mastectomy (SM)

Author	Treatment period	Stage	Treatment	No. pts.	Survival (%) 5 yr	Survival (%) 10 yr
Ontario Cancer Foundation[82]	1946-1954	I and II	RM ± R	243	63	43
			SM ± R	62	66	45
Cleveland Clinic[182]	1957-1979	I and II	MRM	793	76	59
			SM ± R	544	84	74
University of Iowa[80]	1938-1960	I-III	RM	318	42*	—
					31†	—
			SM	228	56*	—
					34†	—
Rockford, Ill.[305]	1929-1954	I-III	RM	237	55	33
			SM	103	51	31

R, radiation.
*Clinical N_0.
†Clinical N_1.

Table 3-21 Results of prospective randomized trials comparing radical mastectomy (RM) with modified radical mastectomy (MRM)

	Trial					
	Manchester[334]			University of Alabama[236,237]		
Treatment period	1969-1976			1975-1978		
No. pts.	534			311		
Stage	I, II			$T_{1-3}N_0N_1$		
Adjuvant therapy	None			CMF or melphalan		
	RM		**MRM**	**RM**		**MRM**
Survival (%)						
5-yr overall	70		70	84	[.14]	76
5-yr DFS	58	[.8]	58	72	[.10]	57
10-yr overall	—		—	71	[.14]	64
Distant metastases (%)	37	[.9]	37	—		—
Follow-up		5 yr				
Local-regional recurrence (%)	25	[.4]	21	6	[.04]	11
Follow-up		5 yr			10 yr	

DFS, disease-free survival; [ ], p value for comparison (adjacent columns).

pectoral node biopsy. The Cardiff trial[132,133] randomized 200 patients with clinical stage I or II breast cancer between 1967 and 1973. Patients with histologically positive axillary nodes who underwent modified radical mastectomy received postoperative radiation to the chest wall and regional nodes, whereas those who underwent simple mastectomy received radiation only to the axilla. At 5 years there was no significant difference in overall or disease-free survival between the two treatments. The 5-year overall survival rate was 69% for modified radical mastectomy and 77% for simple mastectomy with disease-free survival rates of 50% and 55% respectively. There were no significant differences in local-regional recurrence in patients with negative or unidentified axillary nodes; however, in node-positive patients a higher incidence of local-regional recurrence was found in those treated by simple mastectomy and axillary radiotherapy (29% vs. 8%).[132]

Results of prospective randomized trials comparing radical mastectomy with simple mastectomy and radiation are presented in Table 3-22. Only one of the trials has demonstrated a significant survival advantage for the radical mastectomy.[220] Details of the Southeast Scotland trial can be found in Table 3-7. The radiotherapy has been deemed inadequate,[130,229] and any advantage in terms of survival was limited to stage I ($T_1T_2N_0$) patients. The remaining four studies failed to demonstrate a significant difference in 5- or 10-year overall or disease-free survival rates, local-regional recurrence, or distant metastases.

Adequate radiotherapy to the chest wall and regional nodes following simple or total mastectomy therefore achieves results in terms of survival or local-regional recurrence equal to those of radical mastectomy. An overview[71] of the Southeast Scotland trial, Manchester Regional trial, NSABP B-04 trial, and the Copenhagen trial (randomized patients to extended radical mastectomy or simple mastectomy and radiation—see discussion on treatment of internal mammary nodes) concluded that there was no significant difference in survival in a comparison of radical mastectomy to simple mastectomy and radiation. A nonsignificant trend toward an improved survival rate was noted in the radical mastectomy patients, limited to the first 5 years of follow-up and primarily related to the results of the Southeast Scotland trial, in which radical mastectomy patients did significantly better. The fact that inadequate radiotherapy was employed in this trial was not accounted for in the overview and, as noted by Simon,[306] substantial differences among studies in the treatment delivered, patient population, or data quality can significantly affect the validity of conclusions drawn from the pooling of these studies.

In summary, radical mastectomy, modified radical mastectomy, and simple mastectomy plus radiation result in equivalent survival rates and local-regional control in women with early breast cancer. Simple mastectomy without radiation results in an increased incidence of local-regional recurrence, but a survival rate that is probably equivalent to the above three treatments.

Table 3-22 Results of prospective randomized trials comparing radical mastectomy (RM) with simple (SM) or total mastectomy (TM) and radiation (R)

	NSABP B-04[113]			Southeast Scotland trial[220]			Manchester[234]			Addenbrook[38]		Hammersmith[41]	
Treatment period	1971-1974			1964-1971			1970-1975			1958-1965		1965-1970	
No. pts.	586			498			308			204		195	
Stage	$T_{1-3}N_1$			$T_{1-3}N_0N_1$			II			II		$T_{1-3}N_0N_1$	
Adjuvant therapy	None			Ovarian ablation			Ovarian ablation			None		Oophorectomy	
	RM		**TM and R**	**RM**		**SM and R**	**RM**		**SM and R**	**RM and R**	**SM and R**	**RM and R**	**SM and R**
Survival (%)													
5-yr overall	62		58	75		68	57		55	62	64	70	65
5-yr DFS	45		40				38		39	53	58		
10-yr overall	29	[.2]	25	61	[<.05]	52	35	[.9]	31	49	46		
10-yr DFS	38	[.07]	39				19	[.56]	28	42	46		
Distant metastases (%)	46		50	38		36	—		—	—	—	—	—
Follow-up		10 yr											
Local-regional recurrence (%)	20		18	23		27	51		42	—	—	13	14
Follow-up		10 yr			10 yr			10 yr				5 yr	

DFS, disease-free survival; [ ], p value for comparison (adjacent columns).

Table 3-23 Incidence of residual carcinoma following excisional biopsy in patients undergoing mastectomy

Author	No. pts.	Margin	Positive residual tumor (%)	
			T_1	T_1+T_2
Holland et al.[187]	282	>2 cm	42	43
		3 cm	17	18
		4 cm	10	11
Gump et al.[149]	657	>2 cm	18	27
Rosen et al.[287]	573	Separate quadrant	22	26
Lagios[216]	85	Separate quadrant	—	21
Lesser et al.[226]	687	Separate quadrant	—	27
Cahill et al.[44]	107	Separate quadrant	—	20
Fisher et al.[123]	904	Separate quadrant	—	13
Morgenstern et al.[258]	500	Separate quadrant	—	31

Treatment with partial mastectomy

Partial mastectomy by definition involves removal of only a portion of the breast. It may be accompanied by an axillary dissection and/or breast irradiation, which also may include the regional nodes. The partial mastectomy may vary from simple gross excision of the primary tumor (lumpectomy, tylectomy, local excision) to wide excision in which normal adjacent breast tissue also is removed, to quadrantectomy in which the entire quadrant is removed along with the overlying skin and underlying fascia.

For the most part surgical procedures less than mastectomy have been followed by radiation to the remaining breast. The rationale for treatment of the entire breast either by complete surgical removal (mastectomy) or radiation following partial mastectomy is based on the concept of multicentricity of breast cancer. As noted in Table 3-23 the incidence of residual cancer in the breast following an excisional biopsy in patients undergoing mastectomy ranges from 13% to 43% and varies with the distance from the primary tumor and the thoroughness of the pathologic sampling and examination of the mastectomy specimen. The random section technique provides less information than Egan's technique of serial subgross and correlated mammographic examination,[93] which was employed by Holland et al.,[187] Lagios,[216] and Tinnemans et al.[327] Approximately one half to two thirds of the residual cancer is noninvasive, and one third is invasive cancer.[187,226,285] The incidence of multicentricity is unrelated to tumor size for T_1 and T_2 tumors (see Table 3-23). It is also not lower for clinically occult primary tumors (Table 3-24).[302,322,327] It is, however, related to histology (Table 3-25). It is more common with invasive lobular cancer than invasive ductal cancer. Holland et al.[186] correlated the presence of an extensive intraductal component (EIC+) in an invasive ductal cancer with the incidence of residual tumor following an excisional biopsy. Their findings are presented in Table 3-26. The EIC+ tumors were significantly more likely to have residual tumor and tumor at greater distances from the primary than EIC− tumors. The residual tumor was predominantly noninvasive. Lesser et al.[226] also have correlated the incidence of multicentricity with the location of the primary tumor and the histologic status of the axillary nodes. The incidence of multicentricity was 48% for central tumors compared to 26% for inner quadrant tumors and 30% for those

Table 3-24 Incidence residual carcinoma following excisional biopsy in patients with *occult* primary tumors

Author	No. pts.	Margin	Positive residual tumor (%)
Tinnemans et al.[327]	57	Separate quadrant	47
Schwartz et al.[302]	53	Separate quadrant	40
Symmonds and Roberts[322]	65	Outside biopsy site	24

in outer quadrants. Patients with positive axillary nodes had a 45% incidence of multicentricity compared to 27% for those with negative axillary nodes. Based on the above findings, surgical and radiotherapeutic techniques have been designed to treat the entire breast as well as the primary tumor site.

The concept of conservative surgery and radiation for the treatment of early breast cancer involves surgical removal of the primary tumor followed by moderate doses of radiation to the remaining breast. A boost dose of irradiation may be given to region of the primary tumor. Surgical removal of the primary tumor is essential for local control. Limiting the dose of radiation to one that is compatible with an excellent cosmetic result is also desirable. The goals of this approach are eradication of the primary tumor as well as any microscopic foci of multicentric cancer in the breast resulting in a minimal risk of breast recurrence, an acceptable cosmetic result, and a maximal benefit in terms of quality of life with an uncompromised survival.

Retrospective reviews of conservative surgery and radiation. Among the earliest reports of the use of conservative surgery and radiation for operable breast cancer are those of Hirsch[185] and Keynes[201] in 1927 and 1929. Biopsy or local excision of the tumor was followed by radium treatment. Five-year survival rates of 69%[199] and 78%[185] were reported for disease limited to the breast and were comparable to results achieved with mastectomy at the time. The early efforts of Keynes and Hirsch were expanded by Baclesse at the Curie Foundation,[9] Peters at the Princess Margaret Hospital,[270] and Mustakallio in Helsinki[259] in the 1930s and 1940s. Radium treatment eventually was supplanted by external beam irradiation, and with the development of modern megavoltage equipment in the 1950s the frequency of reports employing conservative surgery and radiation increased. Fletcher[127,128,131] demonstrated that a dose of 4500 to 5000 cGy given over a period of approximately 5 weeks was capable of controlling subclinical or multicentric disease in the breast in 90% of patients. This treatment regimen became the basis for modern series. The efforts of Pierquin,[272] initially at the Institut Gustave-Roussy and later at the Hospital Henri Mondor, Amalric and Spitalier in Marseille,[313] Calle at the Institut Curie,[46] Hellman at the Harvard Joint Center for Radiation Therapy,[180] Montague at the M.D. Anderson Hospital,[252] Prosnitz at Yale,[275] and Clark at the Princess Margaret Hospital[57] provided the extensive clinical experience upon which randomized trials comparing conservative surgery and radiation with mastectomy

Table 3-25 Incidence of residual carcinoma related to histology of invasive cancer

	Incidence of residual tumor (%)				
Author	**Ductal cancer**	**Ductal cancer and EIC**	**Lobular cancer**	**Medullary cancer**	**Colloid cancer**
Holland et al.[186]	42 [151]	74 [66]			
Shah et al.[303]	55 [359]		77 [39]	42 [12]	55 [9]
Gump et al.[149]	19 [496]		50 [92]		
Rosen et al.[285]	33 [165]		50 [10]		
Lagios[216]	14 [56]		22 [9]		
Tinnemans et al.[327]	52 [44]		83 [6]		
Lesser et al.[226]	26 [635]		54 [70]	10 [58]	

[ ], total no. pts.

Table 3-26 Incidence of residual carcinoma related to EIC and distance from primary tumor

	Distance from primary tumor				
	>0.5 cm	**>2 cm**	**>4 cm**	**>6 cm**	**>8 cm**
EIC+	74 [36]	59 [20]	32 [12]	21 [2]	9 [2]
EIC−	42 [19]	29 [12]	12 [7]	8 [4]	3 [1]

[ ], percent of invasive residual tumor.
Modified from Holland R, Connolly J, Gelman R, et al: J Clin Oncol 8:113, 1990.

subsequently were based. The 1970s witnessed a resurgence of interest in the conservative approach concurrent with the changing concept of the natural history of breast cancer and thc initiation of randomized trials evaluating surgical procedures less than mastectomy.

Results of retrospective series employing conservative surgery and radiation are presented in Tables 3-27 and 3-28. Despite differences in the period of treatment, selection criteria, and the use of adjuvant systemic therapy the results are quite similar, with a 5-year survival rate of 90% and a 10-year survival rate of 70%. Axillary dissection was performed in all patients in only three of the series.[89,191,311] However, it was performed in ≥80% of the patients in an additional four.[142,183,277,294]

The incidence of breast recurrence following conservative surgery and radiation is presented in Table 3-29. The variation noted among the series reflects different selection criteria, the adequacy of surgical resection of the primary tumor, and the adequacy of the radiotherapy employed. Late local failures have been observed with inadequate radiotherapy both in terms of low total dose and prolonged treatment times.[210,264] Incisional biopsies or excisional biopsies with grossly positive margins of resection result in high breast recurrence rates.[19,52,134,278,343] The role of complete surgical excision of the primary tumor, with attention to margins of resection placing an emphasis on reexcision when margins are unknown or positive, was acknowledged only in the 1980s. Regional node recurrence following conservative surgery and radiation occurs in ≤5% of patients treated with the most common sites being the axillary and supraclavicular nodes.[135]

Table 3-27 Survival following conservative surgery and radiation for early breast cancer—North American experience

Author	No. pts.	Treatment period	Adjuvant therapy	Survival (%) 5 yr I	5 yr II	10 yr I	10 yr II
Ray et al.[277]	120	1970-1979	C	95	65		
Chu et al.[52]	146	1956-1978	C, H	93	73		
Haffty et al.[159]	278	1962-1982	C, H	92	68	73	58
Clark et al.[57]	456	1958-1984	NS	83	63	71	62
Stotter et al.[316]	490	1955-1985	C, H	92	85	78	65
Harris et al.[174]	525	1968-1981	C, H	93	85	85	57
University of Pennsylvania	697	1977-1985	C, H	93	87	87	77

C, chemotherapy; H, hormones; NS, not stated.

Table 3-28 Survival following conservative surgery and radiation for early breast cancer—European experience

Author	No. pts.	Treatment period	Adjuvant therapy	Survival (%) 5 yr	10 yr	15 yr
Hunig et al.[191]	105	1977-1982	None	99		
Hery et al.[183]	108	1975-1980	None	90		
Gerard et al.[142]	195	1973-1982	C, H	87		
Van Limbergen et al.[343]	235	1966-1979	C	80	61	
Dubois et al.[89]	392	1972-1982	None	86	78	
Sarrazin et al.[294]	592	1970-1982	C, H	92	80	
Fourquet et al.[134]	518	1960-1980	None	93	86	
Delouche et al.[79]	410	1956-1979	C, H	82	62	45
Pierquin et al.[271,272]	1200	1961-1982	NS	84	67	63
Spitalier et al.[313]	1133	1961-1979	O	86	80	62
Greco et al.[146]	1232	1970-1983	C	—	80	—

C, chemotherapy; H, hormones; O, oophorectomy; NS, not stated.

Table 3-29 Breast recurrence following conservative surgery and radiation at 5, 10, and 15 years

Author		No. pts.	Breast recurrence (%) 5 yr	10 yr	15 yr
Clarke et al.[59]		436	5	7	
Recht et al.[280]		607	10	16	
Haffty et al.[159]		278	9	20	
Leung et al.[227]		493		10	
Clark et al.[57]		1130	10	14	
Pierquin[271]	T_1	99	3	8	
	T_2	235	6	7	
Kurtz et al.[206]		1593	7	14	18
Fourquet et al.[134]		518	7	11	18
Stotter et al.[316]		490	9	19	
Greco et al.[146]		1232	—	7	
University of Pennsylvania		697	8	18	

Comparison of results: mastectomy vs. conservative surgery and radiation

Intrainstitutional comparisons. Intrainstitutional comparisons of conservative surgery and radiation with mastectomy are presented in Table 3-30. While caution is again advised in interpreting these results, their strength lies in the long-term follow-up, especially in the series reported by Vera Peters from the Princess Margaret Hospital.[270] Initially, patients selected for radiation were those who refused mastectomy or in whom radical surgery was medically contraindicated. Despite this selection bias there appears to be no difference in survival or local-regional recurrence at 10, 20, or 30 years.

Prospective randomized trials. The first prospective randomized trial to compare mastectomy with conservative surgery and radiation was the Guy's Hospital trial.[177,178] The first trial was begun in 1961 and was completed in 1971. Women ≤50 years of age with operable breast cancer ($T_{1\text{-}3}N_0N_1M_0$) were randomized to radical mastectomy or wide excision and postoperative radiation to the breast and regional nodes. Axillary dissection was not performed in the latter group. The second trial (1971 to 1975) continued the same randomization but included patients of all ages and excluded those with clinically positive axillary nodes. The results were previously presented in detail in Table 3-6. In both trials local-regional recurrence, especially in the axilla, was increased significantly in the conservatively treated group resulting in a significant decrease in survival rates and an increase in distant metastases in node-negative patients in the second but not the first trial and in node-positive patients in the first. In a subsequent analysis[177] the significant advantage in terms of survival for radical mastectomy in patients with clinically negative axillary nodes was confined to T_1 tumors and was

Table 3-30 Results of intrainstitutional comparisons mastectomy (M) versus conservative surgery and radiation (CS and R) for stages I and II breast cancer

	Peters[270]		Montague and Fletcher[254]		Komaki et al.[202]	
Treatment period	1939-1972		1955-1980		1980-1986	
No. pts.	812		885		2140	
Adjuvant therapy	None		None		C, H	
	M	**CS and R**	**M**	**CS and R**	**M**	**CS and R**
Overall survival (%)						
Stage I						
5 yr					[88]*	[96]*
10 yr	75	70	80	78		
20 yr	43	50				
30 yr	28	30				
Stage II						
5 yr					[77]†	[96]†
10 yr			65	73		
Local-regional recurrence (%)	5	8	6	5		

[ ], disease-free survival.
*Pathologic node-negative patients.
†Pathologic node-positive patients.

accounted for by an increased percentage of T_1 tumors in the second trial and an overall improvement in survival for radical mastectomy patients in the second trial. The radiotherapy in these trials was inadequate by contemporary standards. These trials are among the few that demonstrate the adverse effect of inadequate local-regional treatment on survival and distant metastases. The trials provide a historical perspective but do not accurately reflect results obtained with appropriate doses of radiation combined with excision of the primary tumor and axillary node dissection.

To date seven modern prospective randomized trials[10,13,23,24,32,103,114,144,157,296,342,345,348] comparing mastectomy to conservative surgery and radiation have been initiated or completed. Published results are available from six of these trials and are presented in Table 3-31. Eligibility for the trials varied from a primary tumor size of ≤2 cm to ≤5 cm. Only the Danish Breast Cancer Cooperative Group[24] extended the criteria for the conservative approach to operable tumors ≥5 cm. The role of lumpectomy and radiation in the treatment of T_3 tumors is discussed in detail in the chapter on locally advanced breast cancer. The Milan trial[348] accepted only patients with clinically negative axillary nodes, whereas in the remaining trials patients with clinically positive axillary nodes also were accepted, provided the primary tumor size was appropriate. An axillary dissection was performed in all treatment groups. Surgery for the primary tumor in the conservatively treated group varied from quadrantectomy (Milan)[348] to wide excision with negative margins (NSABP B-06)[103] to wide excision or lumpectomy without specification of microscopic margins (National Cancer Institute,[144] Danish Breast Cancer Cooperative Group,[24] Institut Gustave-Roussy,[296] EORTC,[13] and Guy's Hospital[157]). In six of the seven trials the mastectomy performed was the modified radical or total mastectomy. Only in the Milan trial[348] was the radical mastectomy performed. In six of the seven trials, patients with histologically positive axillary nodes received adjuvant systemic chemotherapy as follows: Milan—CMF for 1 year; NSABP B-06—melphalan and 5-fluorouracil for 1 year; National Cancer Institute (NCI)—Adriamycin and cyclophosphamide for nine to eleven cycles; European Organization for Research and Treatment of Cancer (EORTC)—CMF; Danish Breast Cancer Cooperative Group (DBCG)—premenopausal patients with positive nodes or primary tumors ≥5 cm received CMF for eight cycles and postmenopausal patients received tamoxifen for 1 year; Guy's Hospital—CMF for 1 year. In the Institut Gustave-Roussy (IGR) trial patients with positive axillary nodes were randomized to receive postoperative radiotherapy to the regional nodes or no further treatment. A similar randomization was carried out in the Milan trial from 1973 to 1975. Beginning in 1976, however, all node-positive patients received adjuvant chemotherapy.

With follow-up at 5, 6, 8, and 10 years, none of the reported trials has demonstrated a significant advantage for mastectomy in terms of overall survival, disease-free survival, or distant metastases. The NCI trial is the only trial that reported a significant increase in local recurrence at 8 years for the conservatively treated patients when compared to mastectomy patients.[144] None of the other trials has noted significant differences in local-regional control between the two treatments. While it was expected by some that patients with histologically positive axillary nodes would do better with mastectomy, the Milan trial[345] demonstrated an advantage for the conservative procedure in this group of patients (Table 3-32). The NSABP B-06 trial[103,114] demonstrated equivalent overall and disease-free survival rates at 5 and 8 years in node-positive patients. One additional trial has been completed, although 5-year results have not been published. In the Guy's Hospital trial[157] between 1981 and 1986 patients with T_1 or T_2 tumors <4 cm with clinically positive or negative axillary nodes were randomized to modified radical mastectomy or conservative surgery and radiation. Node-positive patients received CMF for 1 year.

The conservative approach as evaluated in six prospective randomized trials clearly represents an alternative equal to mastectomy in appropriately selected patients. While it can be argued that long-term results are not available (i.e., >17 years),[344] the three trials with results at periods greater than 5 years have demonstrated that the 5-year results were predictive of the 8- and 10-year results.[103,114,144,295,296,345,348] Kurtz et al.[209] have reported the long-term results of conservative surgery and radiation for 300 women with clinical stage I and II breast cancer with a minimum follow-up of 10.5 years. The actuarial survival at 15 years was 86% and at 20 years 78%. After 10 years, 5.3% of patients developed a breast recurrence. None of the two randomized trials comparing radical mastectomy to modified radical mastectomy has reported results beyond 10 years.[236,237,334] The National Institutes of Health Consensus Development Conference (June 1990) for the treatment of early breast cancer concluded that breast conservation treatment is preferable to mastectomy in appropriately selected patients with stage I and II breast cancer because it provides an equivalent chance for survival and preserves the breast.

Table 3-31 Results of modern randomized trials comparing conservative surgery and radiation (CS and R) with mastectomy for early breast cancer

	Milan[344,345,351]		Institut Gustave-Roussy[295,296]		NSABP B-06[103,114]		National Cancer Institute[10,144]		European Organization for Research and Treatment of Cancer[13,342]		Danish Breast Cancer Group[23,24]	
Treatment period	1973-1980		1972-1980		1976-1984		1979-1989		1980-1986		1983-1989	
No. pts.	701		179		1843		237		874		905	
Stage	I		I & II		I & II		I & II		I & II		I-II	
Adjuvant therapy	CMF		None		Melphalan, 5-FU		AC		CMF		CMF, T	
	RM	**Q and R**	**MRM**	**CS and R**	**TM**	**CS and R**	**MRM**	**CS and R**	**MRM**	**CS and R**	**TM**	**CS and R**
Survival (%)												
5-yr overall	90	92	92	92	86	85	85	89	85	85	82*	79*
5-yr DFS	86	88	77	83	65	69	82	72			66*	70*
10-yr overall	78 [.27]	79	80	78	77† [.3]	76†	79* [>.05]	85†			13	
10-yr DFS	76 [.13]	77	60	69	58† [.2]	59†	76* [>.05]	66†			4	
Distant metastasis (%)	21	16	27	26	19	23						
Breast/chest wall recurrence (%)	2	4	7	9	8	10	6 [.01]	19	8	9	2	
Regional recurrence (%)	3	2	5	1	4	4	—	—	<1	<1		

Q, quandrantectomy; RM, radical mastectomy; TM, total mastectomy; MRM, modified radical mastectomy; CS, conservative surgery; R, radiation; DFS, disease-free survival; [ ], p values for comparison (adjacent columns).
*6-yr results.
†8-yr results.

Table 3-32 Conservative surgery and radiation (CS and R) versus mastectomy: outcome in node-*positive* patients receiving chemotherapy

	CS and R		Mastectomy
Milan[345] survival (%)			
5-yr overall	88		83
5-yr DFS	84		71
10-yr overall	73	[.08]	57
10-yr DFS	71	[.03]	57
NSABP B-06[103,114] survival (%)			
5-yr overall	77		72
5-yr DFS	59		54
8-yr overall	68	[0.3]	60
8-yr DFS	47	[0.2]	44

DFS, disease-free survival; [ ], p value for comparison (adjacent columns).

Retrospective reviews of partial mastectomy without radiation. Several authors have evaluated the concept of excision of the primary tumor without radiation as adequate local treatment. One of the earliest proponents of this procedure was George Crile, Jr., from the Cleveland Clinic. Beginning in 1955, Crile advocated the use of partial mastectomy without radiation for small (≤2 cm) peripherally located tumors with clinically negative axillary nodes. The surgical procedure included resection of the primary tumor with at least 2 to 3 cm of surrounding breast tissue, including the overlying skin and the underlying fascia.[68] It was not uncommon to remove 25% to 50% of the breast.[68] A breast recurrence rate of 6% initially was reported in this carefully selected group of patients.[65] This figure included only those recurrences at the original site of the primary tumor and excluded those elsewhere in the breast. In a subsequent update the figure increased to 12%.[63] The incidence of breast recurrence following surgical excision alone from other series is presented in Table 3-33. Approximately 30% of patients with T_1 or T_2 tumors treated with excision only will develop a breast recurrence. The extent of the surgical resection may impact on the incidence of this recurrence. With a quadrantectomy alone for T_1 tumors the reported incidence of recurrence ranges from 12% to 15%.[147,222] However, Kantorowitz et al.[197] reported a 22% incidence for T_1 and T_2 tumors treated with quadrantectomy alone. This incidence was similar to that noted following local excision alone (30%) or wide excision alone (27%). Breast recurrence also is related to margins of resection. Lagios et al.[217] reported a rate of 71% in seven patients with positive margins of resection compared to 9.5% in 21 patients with negative margins ($p<.0005$). Recurrence was more likely if only in situ ductal cancer was at the margin (two of two patients) than if both in situ ductal cancer and invasive cancer were at the margin (three of five patients). Freeman et al.[140] also noted a higher recurrence rate for T_2 tumors (47%) than for T_1 (16%). None of 12 patients whose primary tumor was nonpalpable developed a breast recurrence. Moffat et al.[251] reported a breast recurrence rate of 10% in 51 patients with primary tumors <2.5 cm, negative margins of resection, no in situ component, and no lymphatic or vascular invasion. The median follow-up was 6 years. The mean time to a recurrence following excision alone ranges from 17 to 30 months.[140,217,256,323] While the overall incidence of breast recurrence following excision alone correlates well with the incidence of multicentricity as previously noted (see Table 3-23), 90% or greater of the recurrences occur in the vicinity of the original primary tumor.[57,323] This clinical observation has raised the question as to the

Table 3-33 Breast recurrence following conservative surgery *without* radiation for early breast cancer.

Author	No. pts.	Primary tumor size (cm)	Surgical procedure	Breast recurrence (%)	Follow-up (yr)
Greening et al.[147]	81	≤2	Q	15	5
Kantorowitz et al.[197]	99	2 mean	LE, WE, Q	26	3.2 (median)
Moffat et al.[251]	51	<2.5 cm	WE	10	6 (median)
Lash et al.[222]	130	≤4	≥Q	12	4.8-10.7
Clark et al.[57]	374	≤5	WE	29	10
Lagios et al.[217]	25	≤5	WE	20	0.5-4
Freeman et al.[140]	47	≤5	LE	26	1.5-9.5
Montgomery et al.[256]	31	≤5	WE	33	5
Tagart[323]	44	≤5	WE	54	9-13

WE, wide excision; Q, quadrantectomy; LE, local excision.

Table 3-34 Survival following conservative surgery *without* radiation for early breast cancer

Author	No. pts.	Stage	Survival (%) 5 yr	Survival (%) 10 yr
Wilson et al.[360]	301	$T_{1\text{-}3}N_0$	83	—
Tagart[323]	44	I, II	78	36
Greening et al.[147]	81	T_1 pathologic N_0	87	73
Hermann et al.[182]	444	T_1N_0	78	56
Clark et al.[57]	374	I, II	73	55

biologic significance of multicentric breast cancer.

The incidence of axillary recurrences in patients with clinically negative axillary nodes who undergo partial mastectomy as the sole treatment is similar to that reported following simple mastectomy. Clark et al.[57] reported an axillary recurrence rate of 13% at 5 years and 19% at 10 years in this group of patients.

Survival rates following partial mastectomy without radiation are reported in Table 3-34. Overall survival varies significantly at 10 years among the series and may reflect differences in patient selection.

Comparison of results: segmental mastectomy without radiation vs. conservative surgery and adiation or mastectomy

Intrainstitutional comparisons. Retrospective comparisons of outcome for conservative surgery with and without radiation are available from the 1982 survey of the American College of Surgeons,[360] the Princess Margaret Hospital,[57] the Cleveland Clinic,[182] and the University of Rochester[197] (Table 3-35). There are no apparent survival differences at 5 or 10 years. The discrepancy between the 5-year survival rates in the University of Rochester series are caused by a significantly younger patient population in the group receiving radiation.[197] It is clear that the addition of radiation decreases the incidence of local-regional recurrences.

Prospective randomized trials. Two prospective randomized trials have been completed comparing segmental mastectomy with or without radiation to total mastectomy. The NSABP B-06 trial[103,114] randomized 1843 women with primary tumors ≤4 cm and clinically positive or negative axillary nodes between 1976 and 1984. All patients underwent an axillary node dissection and all node-positive patients received melphalan and 5-fluorouracil for 1 year. Patients undergoing segmental mastectomy had negative margins of resection. The results at 8 years are presented in Table 3-36. There was no overall advantage in terms of survival for any treatment. The addition of radiation to lumpectomy re-

Table 3-35 Results of intrainstitutional comparisons of conservative surgery (CS) with or without radiation (R)

	Princess Margaret Hospital[57]		American College of Surgeons[360]		Cleveland Clinic[182]		University of Rochester[197]	
Treatment period	1958-1984		1976		1957-1979		1971-1984	
No. pts.	1504		382		684		245	
Stage	I and II		Localized		I and II		I-III	
Adjuvant therapy	None		None		None		C, H	
	CS*	CS and R*	CS	CS and R	CS	CS and R	CS	CS and R
Survival (%)								
5-yr overall	82	85	83	84	78	80	58	82
10-yr overall	71	73	—	—	56	—	—	—
Local-regional recurrence (%)	29	14	—	—	—	—	35	12

C, chemotherapy; H, hormones.
*Absolute survival censoring nonbreast cancer deaths.

Table 3-36 Eight-year results of the NSABP B-06 trial comparing segmental mastectomy with or without radiation to mastectomy

	Total mastectomy		Lumpectomy		Lumpectomy and radiation
No. pts.	590		636		629
Disease-free survival (%)*					
All pts.	58	—	54	[.01]	59
Node-negative pts.	66	[.05]	61	[.02]	66
Node-positive pts.	44	[.6]	43	[.3]	49
Distant disease-free survival (%)					
All pts.	65	—	62	[.2]	64
Node-negative pts.	74	[.03]	70	[.1]	71
Node-positive pts.	51	[.4]	49	[.7]	56
Overall survival (%)					
All pts.	71	—	71	[.3]	76
Node-negative pts.	79	[.5]	77	[.5]	82
Node-positive pts.	60	[.7]	62	[.5]	70
Breast recurrence (%)					
All pts.	8†	—	39	[<.001]	10
Node-negative pts.	—	—	37	[<.001]	12
Node-positive pts.	—	—	43	[<.001]	6
Regional recurrence (%)	4	—	7	—	4

[ ], p value for comparison (adjacent columns).
*Excludes patients with ipsilateral breast recurrence.
†Chest wall recurrence.
Modified from Fisher B et al: N Engl J Med 320:822, 1989.

sulted in a significant improvement in disease-free survival for all patients and for node-negative patients. Mastectomy resulted in a significant improvement in distant disease-free survival in node-negative patients when compared to lumpectomy without radiation. A significant reduction in breast recurrence was noted with the addition of radiation, demonstrating the ability of radiation to sterilize microscopic disease. Overall, 39% of patients undergoing segmental mastectomy alone experienced a breast recurrence despite negative margins of resection. Chemotherapy in node-positive patients did not alter the rate of this recurrence in patients undergoing lumpectomy without radiation. In fact the incidence was highest in this group (43%). This trial again demonstrates the lack of an adverse effect of local recurrences on survival; however, differences in disease-free and distant disease-free survival exist in certain subgroups.

Between 1984 and 1989 the Ontario Clinical Oncology Group randomized 837 patients with primary tumors ≤4 cm in diameter and histologically negative axillary nodes[54,57] to segmental mastectomy with or without radiation. With a median followup of 31 months, the risk of a breast recurrence was significantly decreased with radiation (14.3% vs. 2.2%) although there was no difference in 3-year survival rates (93% vs. 91%). A second trial (1983 to 1987) randomized node-positive patients to a 12-week chemohormonal regimen (cyclosphosphamide, methotrexate, 5-fluorouracil, vincristine, and prednisone [CMFVP] and Adriamycin and tamoxifen [AT]) or 36 weeks of CMFVP.[228] One hundred and twenty patients in this trial had lumpectomy, axillary dissection, and no radiation. Three hundred and seventeen patients had a modified radical mastectomy. The breast recurrence rate in the lumpectomy patients was 27%. There were no differences in distant disease-free survival or overall survival when comparing the lumpectomy patients to the modified radical mastectomy patients. However, the randomization was for chemotherapy and not the treatment of the primary tumor. This trial again demonstrates a high breast recurrence rate in patients with positive nodes who receive adjuvant chemotherapy and undergo lumpectomy without radiation.

Two additional prospective randomized trials have compared segmental mastectomy with or without radiation. The Milan trial was carried out between 1988 and 1989, comparing quadrantectomy and axillary dissection with or without radiation.[344,346] A total of 601 patients were entered. Early results revealed four local recurrences in the quadrantectomy group (301 patients) and none in the quadrantectomy plus radiotherapy group (300 patients). The Uppsala-Orebro Cancer Study Group randomized 381 patients with T_1 tumors and histologically negative axillary nodes to quadrantectomy with or without postoperative breast irradiation.[336] Negative margins of resection were required for entry into the trial. The actuarial 3-year local recurrence rate was 2.9% in the quadrantectomy and radiation group compared to 7.6% in the quadrantectomy alone group. A local recurrence developed in 15 patients, 4 in women assigned to radiation and 11 in the surgery alone group. However, 2 of the recurrences in the radiotherapy group occurred in women who did not actually receive radiation. The 5-year overall and regional or distant relapse-free survival rates were 88.9% and 86.5% for the radiotherapy group and 86.6% and 84.7% for the surgery alone group. None of these differences was statistically significant, although the 3% survival benefit is what would be expected from a two-thirds reduction in local recurrence. The long-term results of these trials may further clarify the role of breast irradiation following conservative surgery in selected patients.

The results of the NSABP B-06 study and Ontario Clinical Oncology Group along with those from retrospective series have stimulated an interest in identifying a subset of patients in whom the omission of breast irradiation would result in a breast recurrence rate equal to that with radiation.

A review of NSABP B-06 (Tables 3-37 and 3-38) study[125,361] suggested that the only subset of patients that did not benefit from radiation were those with primary tumors ≤1 cm. The presence of intralymphatic extension and primary tumor size >1 cm were associated with a >30% risk of breast recurrence in the absence of radiation. Based on this analysis a new trial (NSABP B-21) was initiated. Patients with primary tumors ≤1 cm and histologically negative axillary nodes are randomized to treatment with tamoxifen for 5 years, breast irradiation, or breast irradiation and tamoxifen for 5 years. The rationale for tamoxifen is based on the observation that patients with negative axillary nodes and positive estrogen receptors who received tamoxifen in addition to lumpectomy and radiation experienced a significant decrease in ipsilateral recurrences when compared to the placebo group in the NSABP B-14 study.[105] A significant decrease in contralateral breast cancer also was noted with the addition of tamoxifen. However, a recent study from the Guy's Hospital in which elderly women (≥70 years) were randomized to tumorectomy and tamoxifen vs. modified radical mastectomy reported an 18% breast recurrence in the tamoxifen

Table 3-37 Five-year results of the NSABP B-06 study in patients undergoing conservative surgery *without* radiation for early breast cancer

	Breast recurrence (%)	p value
All pts.	28	—
T size		
T_1	26	
T_2	30	
Pathologic nodal status		
N_0	24	—
N_1	36	—
Intralymphatic extension		
No	12	.0004
Yes	41	
Nuclear grade		
1	4	.002
2	8	
3	13	
Histologic grade		
1	2	.01
2	9	
3	12	

Adapted from Fisher ER et al: Cancer 57:1717, 1986; and Fisher B et al: N Engl J Med 312:665, 1985.

Table 3-38 Results of the NSABP B-06 study involving breast recurrence related to tumor size and nodal status

		6-yr breast recurrence rate (%)		
Tumor size	Treatment	All pts.	Pathologic N_0	Pathologic N_1
0-1 cm	CS	14	18	8
	CS and R	11	13	6
1-2 cm	CS	38	32	48
	CS and R	6	9	0
2-3 cm	CS	39	36	42
	CS and R	8	11	2
3-4 cm	CS	53	29	57
	CS and R	14	19	3

CS, conservative surgery; R, radiation.
From Wolmark N: Scripps 20th Annual Cancer Symposium, San Diego, November 1988.

group, although not all of the original tumors were small.[51] Greening et al.,[147] in an attempt to identify pathologic stage T_1N_0 patients with a low risk or breast recurrence following quadrantectomy alone, noted a 36% incidence in patients <46 years of age compared to 15% for all patients. Age as a predictor of breast recurrence in lumpectomy only patients was not a factor in the NSABP B-06 study.[103]

The available data suggests that patients with primary tumors >1 cm,[140,361] intralymphatic extension,[125] positive margins of resection,[217] or age <46 years of age,[147] when treated with segmental mastectomy alone, experience a significant incidence of breast recurrence (i.e., >30%). Data regarding the multicentricity of invasive cancer indicate that the greatest incidence of multicentric foci is associated with centrally located tumors,[226] those patients with positive axillary nodes[226] or histology demonstrating invasive lobular cancer[149,285,303,327] or the presence of an extensive intraductal component in association with an invasive ductal cancer[186] and consequently these patients may not be candidates for treatment directed to less than the entire breast. While the clinical significance of multicentricity can be questioned, patients who are at greatest risk for developing a breast recurrence following conservative surgery alone coincidentally are often those in whom multicentricity is most common. In summary, patients who may be candidates for conservative surgery alone include those with primary tumors ≤1 cm, negative axillary nodes, negative margins of resection, histology other than invasive lobular cancer or infiltrating ductal cancer with an extensive intraductal component, the absence of intralymphatic extension, a noncentral primary tumor location, and age >46 years. Given the above exclusions it is likely that this subset will represent a relatively small percentage of the patients diagnosed with early breast cancer.

The question arises regarding the optimal surgical procedure for the primary tumor in patients undergoing conservative surgery alone. As noted by Holland et al.[187] the incidence of residual tumor following excisional biopsy decreases to approximately 10% with a 4-cm margin. This is the equivalent of a quadrantectomy, and it appears that this procedure best minimizes the risk of residual tumor. It is of note that the Milan trial and the Uppsala-Orebro Cancer Study Group have chosen quadrantectomy for the group of patients randomized to no radiation. It is uncertain as to whether more limited resections with negative margins in a very select group of patients such as in the NSABP B-21 study will offer the same benefit.

Ultimately the impact of local treatment directed only to the region of the primary tumor on long-term survival will need to be assessed. Table 3-39 demonstrates survival rates of patients with T_1 tumors with histologically negative axillary nodes, i.e., a potential subgroup for conservative surgery alone. While survival rates at 5 years seem comparable there is a trend towards decreased survival at 10 years with the omission of radiation. These are retrospective comparisons and are, therefore, limited. As previously noted, however, this subgroup experienced a significantly lower survival with inadequate local-regional treatment in the Guy's Hospital trials.[177] The minimal local-regional treatment that is compatible with an acceptable incidence of local-regional recurrence and overall or disease-free survival has yet to be determined. Ten-year analysis of the NSABP B-06 study, especially for patients with tumors of pathologic stage T_1N_0 will provide significant information that may impact on future clinical decisions.

Complications

The above discussion has presented results in terms of overall and disease-free survival and local-regional recurrence for the various treatment options for early breast cancer. A final area of comparison is that of complications.

Complications following mastectomy. Postoperative complications following mastectomy include wound infection, skin flap necrosis, and seroma formation. Danforth and Lippman[75] tabulated the incidence of these complications from several series. The mean incidence of skin flap necrosis was 31.2% following radical mastectomy, compared to 21.4% for the modified radical mastectomy and 9.3% for total mastectomy. An increased

Table 3-39 Retrospective comparisons of survival of patients with tumors of pathologic stage T_1N_0 given conservative surgery with or without radiation

Author	Radiation	5-yr actuarial survival (%)	10-yr actuarial survival (%)
Greening et al.[147]	No	87	73
Veronesi et al.[345]	Yes	93	82
University of Pennsylvania	Yes	97	88

incidence of skin flap necrosis has been noted with vertical incisions as opposed to transverse incisions, the omission of drains or the use of Penrose drains rather than suction catheters, the use of primary closure rather than skin grafts, the use of thin skin flaps, and in elderly or obese patients.[40,297,332] Seroma formation results from drainage from transected lymphatics or other small vessels and may occur in the axilla or chest wall. Suction catheters are used to prevent this complication. Approximately 10% to 15% of patients undergoing a modified radical or total mastectomy will develop seromas, compared to 30% to 40% of those undergoing a radical mastectomy.[40,75,297] Treatment of seromas is by aspiration. Wound infection occurs in approximately 10% of patients undergoing mastectomy.[40] Prolonged catheter drainage, skin-flap necrosis, and seroma formation may increase the incidence of infection.[2] Treatment usually involves the administration of antibiotics.

Complications related specifically to axillary node dissection include nerve injury and axillary vein thrombosis. Injury to the long thoracic nerve of Bell results in a winged scapula. Sacrifice of the thoracodorsal nerve, which innervates the latissimus dorsi, results in an almost imperceptible weakness in internal rotation and abduction.[40] Division of the intercostobrachial nerve results in decreased sensation along the medial aspect of the arm. Removal of the medial pectoral nerve with the pectoralis minor muscle results in atrophy of the lateral portion of the pectoralis major muscle.

Long-term complications following mastectomy: lymphedema, pain syndrome, lymphangiosarcoma. Long-term complications of mastectomy include lymphedema, postmastectomy pain syndrome, and lymphangiosarcoma. The reported incidence of lymphedema following mastectomy is quite variable and depends upon the definition chosen. For the most part, circumferential measurements >2 to 2.5 cm between the affected and nonaffected arm are classified as lymphedema. Lymphedema may be transient or permanent and may occur relatively early in the postoperative period or later. Danforth and Lippman[75] reported the mean incidence of arm edema to be 19.9% following radical mastectomy, 8.2% following modified radical mastectomy, and 4.7% after total mastectomy. Factors predisposing to arm edema include infection, seroma formation, skin flap necrosis, and obesity.[40,193,297] Division of the intercostobrachial nerve may result in a disabling pain syndrome in a small percentage of patients.[362] Stewart and Treves[314] reported the incidence of lymphangiosarcoma following radical mastectomy to be 4 in 894 women alive after more than 5 years, with an incidence of 0.045%.

Complications associated with radiation. Complications associated with conservative surgery and radiation or postmastectomy radiation include symptomatic pneumonitis, rib fracture, arm edema, pericarditis, brachial plexopathy, severe breast or chest wall fibrosis, and soft tissue or bone necrosis. The acute complications are similar to those described with surgery and include wound infection and axillary seromas.

Breast edema. Breast edema is unique to patients undergoing conservative surgery and radiation. It

Table 3-40 Complications following conservative surgery and radiation for breast cancer in early stages

	University of Pennsylvania[311]	Joint Center for Radiation Therapy[171]	M.D. Anderson[316]	University of Chicago[161]	Yale[275]	Institut Gustave-Roussy and Henri Mondor[272]	Centre Charlebourg[79]
Total no. pts.	548	735	536	219	179	330	494
Complications							
Arm edema	11*	13*	8	4*	—	5	9
Symptomatic pneumonitis	1	1	5	3	2	—	—
Rib fracture	1	3	3	0	—	—	—
Pericarditis	0	<1	—	0	<1	—	0
Brachial plexopathy	0	<1	—	0	<1	0	<1
Severe breast fibrosis	<1		10	—	—	5	7
Soft tissue/bone necrosis	0	<1	—	<1	—	—	—

*Arm edema in patients undergoing axillary dissection.

appears during the period of radiation treatment or within 1 to 2 months following it. It is almost always transient, although it may take as long as 3 years to resolve,[58] and the addition of adjuvant systemic chemotherapy may prolong its resolution. It is related to the extent of axillary dissection and is most frequent in patients who have undergone an axillary dissection with ≥11 nodes removed.[15,58] At 6 months following radiation treatment approximately one third of patients will have mild breast edema.[15,255,277]

Arm edema. The incidence of complications occurring with conservative surgery and radiation as reported by various series are presented in Table 3-40. The most common complication is arm edema. The incidence of arm edema is related to the extent of the axillary surgery as well as to the addition of radiation (Table 3-41). In patients in whom an axillary dissection is not performed and the axilla is treated with radiation alone, the incidence of arm edema ranges from 2% to 4%. The incidence of arm edema following a limited axillary dissection without radiation is 2% to 3%. The addition of radiation to a limited axillary dissection increases the incidence of arm edema to 8% to 10%. The addition of radiation to a complete axillary dissection results in a significant incidence of arm edema. The role of axillary irradiation in patients with positive nodes who have undergone a complete axillary dissection can be questioned. Veronesi et al.[351] and Dewar et al.[83] reported no axillary recurrences in this group of patients when axillary irradiation was omitted. There is also no benefit to axillary irradiation in patients with negative nodes who have undergone a complete axillary dissection.[83,351] Therefore the overall incidence of arm edema should be in the range of 2% to 10% for patients undergoing conservative surgery and

Table 3-41 Incidence of arm edema related to extent of axillary surgery and radiation

	Incidence of arm edema %				
	No R		R		
Author	LAD	CAD	None	LAD	CAD
Veronesi et al.[348]		3			
Larson et al.[221]			4	8	43
Solin et al.[311]	3			10	
Delouche et al.[79]			3	9	
Clarke et al.[58]			3		
Groupe European[273]	2		2	9	
Lichter et al.[231]					18

R, radiation; LAD, limited axillary dissection; CAD, complete axillary dissection.

radiation. This figure is quite comparable to that reported following modified radical mastectomy.[75]

Symptomatic pneumonitis. Symptomatic pneumonitis is characterized by a dry cough, low-grade fever, and shortness of breath. Symptoms typically appear within 2 to 3 months following treatment and may require steroids for relief.[148] Infiltrates or a haziness within the radiation treatment fields can appear as early as a few weeks following treatment. These changes gradually progress to radiation fibrosis. The incidence of symptomatic pneumonitis is ≤5% and is related to the volume of lung treated and the radiation dose. Larger volumes of lung are less tolerant of high doses. The concurrent use of methotrexate and 5-fluorouracil during radiation also has been associated with an increased incidence of radiation pneumonitis.[33] With current techniques and an emphasis on placing a minimal amount of lung within the treatment field, the incidence of radiation pneumonitis should be 1% to 2%.

Cardiac complications. Radiation pericarditis is uncommon in patients treated for breast cancer. The reported incidence is <1%. Techniques that treat the internal mammary nodes with a direct photon beam field may increase the incidence of pericarditis or myocardial infarction. In the Oslo trial of postmastectomy radiation, patients with stage I disease who received cobalt-60 irradiation to the internal mammary nodes had an increased risk of death related to acute myocardial infarction.[190] Jones and Ribeiro[194] reported an increased mortality after 15 years in the Manchester trial in the group of patients receiving postmastectomy irradiation. This increase appears to be the result of cardiovascular disease. Radiation-induced coronary artery disease is caused by vascular endothelial damage, degeneration, and occlusion of arteries.[293,331] The combination of internal mammary node irradiation with chemotherapy regimens employing Adriamycin in the treatment of locally advanced breast cancer resulted in cardiac toxicity in 25% of the patients in one series.[233] This occurred primarily in patients with left-sided tumors. Variations in the radiation technique employed in the treatment of breast cancer clearly have an impact on the incidence and severity of pulmonary and cardiac complications, and in patients receiving systemic chemotherapy these effects may be compounded. Therefore careful attention to technical detail is important in minimizing these complications.

Brachial plexopathy. Brachial plexopathy is a rare occurrence following radiation in moderate doses, i.e., 4500 to 5000 cGy. Symptoms include paresthesias with or without weakness of the arm and hand, usually in the C5-6 distribution.[203] They may be transient or permanent. Permanent changes are related to fibrosis of the adjacent soft tissues, usually in the supraclavicular or infraclavicular regions, and the resultant decreased vascularity. Transient changes have been noted more commonly in patients receiving adjuvant chemotherapy.[171] An increased incidence of brachial plexopathy has been noted with higher doses per fraction of radiation[274] as well as with higher total doses.[203]

Rib fractures. Rib fractures occur in <5% of patients undergoing conservative surgery and radiation. They may be asymptomatic with detection occurring on a follow-up chest x-ray or bone scan. One series has suggested that they are more frequent in patients receiving adjuvant chemotherapy.[231] Treatment is conservative management.

Soft tissue and bone necrosis. Soft tissue and bone necrosis is rare with moderate doses of radiation. However, severe breast fibrosis occurs in approximately 10% or less of cases and is related to the total breast dose and daily fraction. Patients with a preexisting history of collagen vascular disease may be especially prone to the development of marked soft-tissue changes following radiation.[126,276]

Radiation carcinogenicity. Perhaps the greatest concern with radiation in the treatment of breast cancer is the potential for carcinogenicity. This includes contralateral breast cancer, sarcomas in the treated breast or chest wall, and second nonbreast cancer malignancies, especially leukemia. While a number of studies have addressed the issue of radiation carcinogenicity,[20,62,84,218,240,310,329] their relevance to the present discussion is questionable as they differ significantly in age of the population exposed, the dose of radiation used, and the region(s) exposed. The risk of a radiation-induced malignancy is related to age at exposure and dose. With doses up to 1000 cGy, the risk increases linearly[12]; however, there appears to be a negligible risk with therapeutic doses of radiation, i.e., ≥4500 cGy.[12,27] The breast cancer risk in survivors of the atom bomb was greatest in those exposed at a young age.[329] Similarly, Boice and Monson[28] demonstrated the greatest risk for breast cancer in women undergoing multiple fluoroscopies to be in those exposed before age 30. Because the majority of patients treated for breast cancer receive therapeutic doses of radiation and are >30 years of age, it is not surprising to find studies failing to document a substantial risk of radiation carcinogenesis in this population.

A number of isolated case reports have documented radiation-induced sarcomas either in bone or soft tissue. The overall incidence of radiation-induced sarcomas in long-term survivors has been estimated to be 0.03%.[198] Sarcomas arising in the irradiated breast or chest wall following treatment for breast cancer have been infrequent with the first report appearing in 1936.[357] Three of the largest series are those from the M.D. Anderson Hospital,[312] Memorial Sloan-Kettering Cancer Center,[192] and the Northern Israel Oncology Center.[212] During the period from 1944 to 1984, ten chest wall sarcomas were observed at M.D. Anderson Hospital following therapeutic breast irradiation.[312] Doses of radiation ranged from 4000 to 6500 cGy, and the median latent period was 10 years. The most common histologic type was malignant fibrous histiocytoma. Six cases of osteogenic sarcoma of bone or soft tissues following radiation for breast cancer were reported by the Memorial Sloan-Kettering Cancer Center from 1921 to 1983. The median interval again was 10 years. Kuten et al.[212] reported seven cases of soft tissue sarcoma observed at the Northern Israel Oncology Center. Radiation doses ranged from 2200 to 5400 cGy, and the median latent period was 9 years. To date seven cases of radiation-induced sarcoma have been reported in a minimum of 4255 patients undergoing conservative surgery and radiation.[26,79,206,207,288,304,316] Kurtz et al.[206] have estimated that two radiation-induced sarcomas will be observed for every 1000 five-year

Table 3-42 Incidence of contralateral breast cancer related to initial treatment

	Incidence of contralateral breast cancer (%)		
	M.D. Anderson[253]	**UCLA[268]**	**London, Ontario[244]**
Mastectomy	5 [567]	5 [648]	17 [369]
Mastectomy plus postoperative R	4 [1102]	2 [836]	23 [1120]
Regional nodes	5 [553]		
CW plus regional nodes	2 [549]		
Preoperative R plus mastectomy	4 [473]		
Follow-up period (yr)	4-36	5-30	20

R, radiation; CW, chest wall; [ ], total no. pts.

Table 3-43 Conservative surgery and radiation for early breast cancer

Author	Incidence of metachronous contralateral breast cancer (%)	Follow-up (yr)
Delouche et al.[79]	5.4	11 (median)
Leung et al.[227]	7	10 (median)
Sarrazin et al.[294]	10	10
Spitalier et al.[313]	7	5-23
Clark et al.[57]	3	2-28
Calle et al.[45]	6	≥5
Recht et al.[278]	9	10 (actuarial)
Kurtz et al.[207]	6	20 (actuarial)

survivors of the conservative treatment for each decade of follow-up. The risk of a radiation-induced sarcoma is, therefore, lower than that of a lymphangiosarcoma following radical mastectomy.[314]

The incidence of contralateral breast cancer following either postmastectomy radiation or conservative surgery and radiation is of concern, because the contralateral breast receives approximately 100 to 300 cGy in a conventional course of treatment.[138] Several studies have compared the incidence of contralateral breast cancer in patients who have received radiation as part of their primary treatment to those who have not. These cohort studies can be divided into institutional reviews, reports from cancer registries, and those from prospective randomized trials. Table 3-42 presents data from institutional reviews. There is no evidence from these three series[244,253,268] that patients who received radiation experienced a higher risk of contralateral breast cancer. Data from the cancer registry of Connecticut[168] also demonstrate no long-term effect of radiation exposure on the risk of contralateral breast cancer. A nonsignificant, age-adjusted relative risk of 1.2 to 1.4 was observed in the irradiated patients within the first 5 years of follow-up. Because the latent period between radiation exposure and the induction of malignancy is typically ≥10 years, these findings are not consistent with a radiation effect. In the Danish Cancer Registry,[315] however, a significant increase in the relative risk of contralateral breast cancer was demonstrated for irradiated patients as compared to nonirradiated patients only after 10 to 15 years (2.6 vs. 2.0). The overall risk, however, was lower in the irradiated patients. The incidence of contralateral breast cancer in series reporting the results of conservative surgery and radiation with long-term follow-up is presented in Table 3-43. Results from three prospective randomized trials comparing conservative surgery and radiation to mastectomy have failed to demonstrate an increased incidence of contralateral breast cancer in patients receiving radiation (Table 3-44).

An additional method of examining the issue of radiation-induced malignancy is by case-control studies in which patients with a second cancer are compared to matched controls to eliminate the possibility of confounding variables. Horn and Thompson[189] performed a case-control study of 556 women with breast cancer obtained from the Connecticut Tumor Registry. There was no increased risk of contralateral breast cancer in patients who received radiation. In particular there was no association between the area(s) irradiated or the age of the patient at diagnosis. Younger women treated with radiation did not have a significantly increased risk of developing a contralateral breast cancer.

The issue of second nonbreast cancer malignancies in patients receiving radiation for breast cancer includes consideration of acute nonlymphocytic leukemia (ANLL) and other solid tumors. Curtis et al.[70] reviewed the data from the Surveillance, Epidemiology and End Results Program (SEER) regarding the risk of leukemia as related to the initial therapy in 59,115 patients with breast cancer. The highest risk for leukemia was observed in patients receiving chemotherapy and surgery as initial treatment (relative risk 6.7). There was no significant increase in the risk of leukemia for patients receiving radiation when all types were considered. However, the relative risk was 3.7 for acute non-

Table 3-44 Randomized trials of stage I and II breast cancer: incidence of second malignancy

Treatment	Series	Contralateral breast cancer (%)	Second cancer (%)
Conservative surgery and radiation	Institut Gustave-Roussy[295]	9	
	Milan[344,363]	5	2
	NSABP B-06[114]	3	3
Mastectomy	Institut Gustave-Roussy[295]	9	
	Milan[344,363]	6	2
	NSABP B-06[114]	2	2

lymphocytic leukemia. The elevated risk occurred after 3 years and was confined to the group of patients with regional disease. There was no increased risk in patients with localized disease. The authors postulated that some of the increased risk in patients with regional disease who received radiation may be attributed to chemotherapy that was given but not reported. Fisher et al.[115] reviewed the risk of leukemia in 8483 women with breast cancer entered into seven (B-04 through B-10) of the NSABP adjuvant radiation or chemotherapy trials from 1971 to 1984. The cumulative risk of leukemia or myeloproliferative syndrome at 10 years following surgery was 1.39% for patients receiving regional node irradiation, as compared to 1.29% following chemotherapy and 0.27% after surgery alone. It should be noted that one of the five cases of leukemia in patients receiving regional node irradiation was chronic lymphocytic leukemia, which is not considered to be a radiation-induced disease.[260] The relative risk for development of leukemia was determined by comparing the observed with the expected incidence obtained from SEER data. The relative risk for developing any type of leukemia was 11.0 for chemotherapy, 6.1 for radiation, and 1.5 for surgery alone. The first two were significant. The relative risk for acute myelogenous leukemia (AML) was 24 for chemotherapy, 10.3 for radiation and 2.5 for surgery alone. The first two again were significant. There was no increased risk of leukemia for patients who received radiation to the breast only (B-06), perhaps because of the limited volume of bone marrow treated. Similar to the SEER findings, the risk of leukemia was greatest in the period of 3 to 7 years following initial surgery. There were no instances of leukemia after 7 years. The authors conclude that the benefits of adjuvant therapy in high-risk patients outweigh the potential risk of leukemia. Lavey and Prosnitz,[223] in a review of 407 breast cancer patients treated at Duke University Medical Center with a median follow-up of 5.4 years, found no increase in the 10-year actuarial risk of leukemia or second nonbreast cancer malignancy in patients receiving chemotherapy and/or radiation. Curtis et al.[69] in a case-controlled study from the Connecticut Tumor Registry of 22,753 breast cancer patients, found no significant association between radiation and the risk of leukemia when comparing 48 cases of leukemia with 97 controls matched for age, calendar year of diagnosis, and survival time. Subgroup analysis revealed no increased risk for women <50 years of age or for doses of radiation to the total active bone marrow ranging from 0 to >500 cGy. The authors emphasize that they could not confirm the tenfold increase as reported by Fisher et al.[115] and suggest that the NSABP findings based on only four cases of acute myelogenous leukemia in 1116 irradiation patients may have been influenced by chance. Haas et al.,[156] in a case-controlled study from the National Cancer Registry of the German Democratic Republic, also found no increased risk of acute leukemia in patients receiving radiation. A single case control study[29] from the tumor registries of California, Connecticut, Kansas, and Massachusetts demonstrated a significantly increased relative risk (2.2) for leukemias other than chronic lymphocytic leukemia in patients with breast cancer receiving radiotherapy.

A single case of ANLL has been reported in patients undergoing conservative surgery and radiation for early breast cancer.[278] However, this patient also received 2 years of adjuvant therapy with melphalan. Of the 470 patients undergoing conservative surgery and radiation in the NSABP B-06 study, the only patient to develop leukemia had chronic lymphoctyic leukemia, which is not known to be radiation-induced subtype.[260]

There is little evidence to support an increased risk of second nonbreast cancer solid malignancies in patients receiving radiation for breast cancer. As previously noted, three prospective randomized trials (see Table 3-44) and a single cohort study[223] have found no association. Retrospective studies of patients undergoing conservative surgery and radiation have reported a 2% to 3% incidence of second nonbreast cancer malignancies.[25,313] Bluming et al.[25] reported a 3% incidence of second malignancies in patients receiving radiation, as compared to 2% in a comparable group of mastectomy patients.

Data supporting the carcinogenic effect of therapeutic doses of radiation employed in the treatment of breast cancer are, therefore, minimal. Cohort studies from the long-term results of prospective randomized trials will provide additional information on patients treated with contemporary regimens. As noted by Harris and Coleman,[170] registry studies may not have accurate patient data, and institutional reviews often have small patient numbers limiting the interpretation of their findings. An additional consideration involves what the most clinically meaningful expression of the true risk of a treatment-induced malignancy is. Harris and Coleman[170] justifiably suggest absolute risk rather than relative risk, which may exaggerate the significance to the individual patient. In the NSABP study the relative risk for radiation-associated leukemia was 6.1, while the 10-year actuarial risk was 1.39%.[115] At this time the potential risk for carcinogenesis from therapeutic irradiation should not impact on treatment decisions for early breast cancer.

Table 3-45 Incidence of positive axillary nodes related to primary tumor size

Author	Positive nodes (%) in relation to primary tumor sizes				
	<1 cm	1-1.9 cm	2-2.9 cm	3-4.9 cm	≥5 cm
Haagensen[154]	28 [25]	27 [96]	28 [214]	45 [350]	52 [222]
Fisher et al.[118]	22 [52]	39 [375]	42 [611]	53 [996]	53 [665]
Nemoto et al.[262]	25 [1107]	34 [4044]	43 [3546]	52 [3052]	65 [1232]
Carter et al.[49]	21 [1335]	33 [6985]	45 [7282]	55 [6441]	70 [2698]
University of Pennsylvania	20 [81]	26 [284]	33 [298]	41 [196]	
Reger et al.[281]	8 [178]	27 [356]			
Say and Donegan[298]	33 [101]		51 [196]		

[ ], total no. pts.

TREATMENT OF THE REGIONAL LYMPH NODES

Axillary nodes

Factors correlating with axillary node involvement. The axillary nodes comprise 75% of the lymphatic drainage of the breast.[335] The incidence of axillary node involvement is related directly to the primary tumor size (Table 3-45). Koscielny et al.[204] developed a method for computing the distribution of breast tumor size at the time of development of the first, second, third, etc., axillary node metastasis based on a study population of 2408 women treated for invasive breast cancer at the Institut Gustave-Roussy between 1954 and 1979. The authors found a progressive increase in both the incidence of axillary involvement and the number of positive nodes with increasing tumor size. The mean tumor volume for the initiation of the first axillary node metastasis was 1.21 ml corresponding to a tumor diameter of 1.32 cm. From Table 3-45 it can be seen that even tumors <1 cm have a 20% to 25% incidence of positive nodes. Data from the American College of Surgeons[16] and the Surveillance, Epidemiology and End Results program of the National Cancer Institute[49] demonstrate a 23% and 21% incidence of axillary node metastases respectively for tumors ≤5 mm. The incidence of positive axillary nodes for occult primary tumors demonstrated solely by mammography or detected incidentally at the time of biopsy for a benign lesion is presented in Table 3-46. Again, for these nonpalpable tumors the incidence of positive nodes is related to tumor size.

Histologically positive axillary nodes are more common in patients who present with clinically positive axillary nodes. Approximately 70% to 80% of patients with clinically positive axillary nodes will have histologically positive nodes, as compared to 30% to 40% of patients with clinically negative nodes (Table 3-47).

Table 3-48 demonstrates the relationship between tumor location and the incidence of positive nodes. There appears to be a higher incidence of positive nodes in outer quadrant tumors, although the magnitude of this increase is variable. Koscielny et al.[204] noted a smaller tumor volume at the time of first axillary node involvement for outer quadrant tumors when compared to inner quadrant tumors despite tumor volumes for initiation of distant metastases that were equal for the two locations.

Histologic grade II or III tumors have a higher incidence of positive axillary nodes than histologic grade I tumors.[124,188,281] However, there appears to be no consistent relationship between increasing histologic grade from II to III and the incidence of positive axillary nodes, especially for small primary tumors (≤2 cm).[188,266,281]

Additional pathologic factors that correlate with nodal positivity include the presence of intralymphatic or blood vessel invasion, perineural space

Table 3-46 Incidence of positive axillary nodes in patients with occult *invasive* primary tumors

Author	Total no. pts.	Positive axillary nodes (%)
Pagana et al.[266]	21	14
Haagensen[154]	38	29
Symmonds and Roberts[322]	52	13
Strax[317]	54	35
Meyer et al.[248]	75	22
Frankl and Rosenfeld[139]	75	27
Schwartz et al.[301]	105	32
Tinnemans et al.[326]	81	21
≤5 mm	13	8
6-10 mm	24	12
>1 cm	44	29

Table 3-47 Incidence of false positive or false negative axillary nodes

Author	False negative (%)	False positive (%)
Butcher[42]	32	25
Haagensen[153]	28	31
Schottenfeld et al.[300]	27	26
Danforth et al.[74]	37	7
Fisher et al.[121]	39	27
Sacre[291]	41	22
Smart et al.[308]	34	12

invasion, high nuclear grade, absent sinus histiocytosis, histology other than mucinous carcinoma, and a stellate tumor border.[124]

There appears to be no consistent relationship between estrogen or progesterone receptor status and the incidence of positive axillary nodes,[53,95,120,281] although estrogen receptor–negative tumors tend to have a greater incidence of positive nodes.[4]

Recent efforts have been directed towards identifying prognostic factors related to alterations of protooncogenes or measures of cell kinetics including proliferative rate and DNA ploidy status. The relationship between these factors and axillary node status has been variable. Both amplication and expression of the HER-2/neu oncogene have been correlated with axillary node status.[21,60,325] Other studies have demonstrated no correlation with nodal status.[341] DNA flow cytometry provides both a measurement of DNA content abnormalities and calculations of the cell cycle distribution. Node-positive patients more frequently have aneuploid tumors and high S-phase fractions.[88,265] However, significant correlations between DNA content and nodal status have not been found.[96,141,211,257,353] Meyer et al.[249] also found no significant correlation between nodal status and thymidine labeling index.

A recent discovery has been the presence of several growth factors in human breast cancer. Epidermal growth factor is more commonly present in node-positive patients,[292] although Toi and others[328] found no correlation between epidermal growth factor and axillary lymph node status. Cathepsin D is an estrogen-induced lysosomal protease whose activity in growth promotion and extracellular proteolysis may facilitate the spread of breast cancer. Higher levels of mature 34-kd cathepsin D have been found in node-positive patients.[324]

The extent of nodal involvement (i.e., ≥4 positive nodes) has been correlated with a clinically positive axilla,[124] primary tumor size >4 to 5 cm,[49,118,124] the presence of extracapsular extension,[124] histologic or nuclear grade III,[124] multicentric foci of cancer,[124] intralymphatic or perineural space invasion,[124] nipple involvement,[124] expression of the HER-2/neu oncogene[325] and aneuploid tumors.[179]

Rationale for treatment of axillary nodes. The rationale for treatment of the axillary nodes is related to the Halstedian concept of the spread of breast cancer with emphasis on interception of the disease at a local-regional stage before distant dissemination. The recognition that the axillary nodes were not a source of distant metastases[66,82,106,107] prompted a reassessment of the role of their treatment. Four prospective randomized trials have compared simple mastectomy to simple mastectomy and radiation for stages I and II breast cancer.[22,48,133,234,333] In these trials treatment of the ax-

Table 3-48 Incidence of positive axillary nodes related to primary tumor location

Author		Positive axillary nodes (%) Outer quadrant	Central/inner quadrant
Haagensen[153]		45 [460]	33 [457]
Nemoto et al.[262]		43 [6948]	34 [2417]
Carter et al.[49]		46 [8850]	37 [3075]
Handley[165]		56 [475]	51 [525]
Lacour et al.[213]		58 [796]	52 [630]
Fisher et al.[122]		52 [373]	48 [360]
University of Pennsylvania		37 [508]	23 [404]
	Primary tumor size		
Veronesi and Valagussa[349]	T_{1-2}	54 [392]	50 [241]
	T_3	58 [38]	66 [44]

[ ], total no. pts.

illa was by radiation. Results were previously presented in Table 3-17. None of the trials has shown a significant improvement in 5- or 10-year overall survival rates with the addition of radiation, although a significant improvement in 10-year disease-free survival was demonstrated by the Manchester Regional Breast Study.[234] Three of the trials have demonstrated a significant reduction in local-regional recurrence with the addition of radiation.[22,48,234,333] The NSABP B-04 trial[113] was specifically designed to test the effect of untreated axillary nodes on survival. Patients with clinically negative axillary nodes were randomized to radical mastectomy, total mastectomy and radiation, or total mastectomy. Despite a 17.8% incidence of axillary recurrence in the untreated axilla, there was no adverse effect on overall survival at 5 or 10 years (see Table 3-18), although there was a significant difference in 10-year disease-free survival. The incidence of axillary recurrence in this trial was less than expected based on the finding of positive nodes in 40% of the patients undergoing radical mastectomy.[121] Presumably a similar incidence could be found in the patients undergoing total mastectomy, yet the axillary recurrence rate was less than half this figure. The incidence of axillary recurrence in the NSABP B-04 trial is, however, comparable to that reported by others in patients with clinically negative nodes in whom either axillary dissection or radiation was omitted (Table 3-49) although higher rates have been reported. In the NSABP B-04 trial approximately 35% of patients who were assigned to total mastectomy actually underwent limited axillary dissection. The axillary recurrence in patients in whom no nodes were obtained was 21%.[121] A similar finding was noted in the Edinburgh trial[133] in which the axillary recurrence was 41% if no nodes were identified, as compared to 16% when nodes were identified at the time of pectoral biopsy and were negative. Crile[64] reported 5- and 10-year survival rates of 75% and 33% in patients who developed an axillary recurrence following simple mastectomy and underwent an axillary dissection at the time of recurrence, comparing favorably to the 5- and 10-year survival rates of 64% and 29% for patients with clinically negative but histologically positive nodes who underwent modified radical mastectomy initially. Both of these studies demonstrate the lack of an adverse effect of axillary recurrences on survival in patients with clinically negative axillary nodes. In the Cardiff-St. Mary's trial[133] an attempt was made to determine the histological status of the axillary nodes by a pectoral node biopsy. Patients with negative biopsies underwent simple mastectomy or modified radical mastectomy. The trial was designed to determine the effect of the untreated axilla on survival in patients whose axillary nodes were clinically negative as well as histologically negative, as determined by biopsy or gross inspection. The ability of the pectoral node biopsy to be used for accurate staging of the axilla can be questioned because the axillary recurrence was 16% in those who underwent simple mastectomy. This rate is comparable to the NSABP B-04 trial in which no surgical procedure on the axilla was performed. The Cardiff trial again demonstrated no survival advantage at 5 or 10 years for the modified radical mastectomy (i.e., dissection of the axillary nodes).

Table 3-49 Incidence of axillary recurrence in patients with clinically negative axillary nodes and an undissected axilla

Author	Axillary recurrence (%)	Follow-up (yr)
Edinburgh trial[133]	41	2-7
Baum and Coyle[14]	21	≤4
Devitt[82]	17	5
Crile[67]	30	6
Clark et al.[57]	19	10
Forrest et al.[133]	16	10
Fisher et al.[113]	17.8	10
Lythgoe and Palmer[234]	37	10

The recent study of Koscielny et al.[204] correlating tumor size with axillary node involvement also lends support to the concept that axillary nodes are not the exclusive source of distant metastases. While the authors noted a definite correlation between the propensity for axillary node metastases and the probability of distant spread, inner quadrant tumors demonstrated a greater mean tumor volume for initiation of axillary node metastases and a smaller mean tumor volume for initiation of distant metastases as compared to outer quadrant tumors. This discrepancy suggests that positive axillary nodes function to indicate the potential for distant spread. However, in comparison with a previous study,[205] it was noted that the mean tumor volume for initiation of axillary node metastases was smaller than that for distant dissemination, indicating an earlier pattern of axillary node involvement. The difference noted in the mean tumor volume for the initiation of axillary nodal involvement and distant metastases were consistent with a continuum in the progression of breast cancer from slow growing disease without early nodal or distant dissemination to rapidly progressive disease. This latter observation helps to reconcile the findings of the Guy's Hospital trial II[177] and the Southeast Scotland trial[220] with those of the NSABP B-04 trial.[113]

In the former two trials inadequate local-regional treatment resulted in a significant increase in axillary recurrences and a significant decrease in survival for stage I patients. There appears to be a subset of patients for whom optimal axillary node treatment may be beneficial.

Treatment options and comparison of results. Treatment of the axillary nodes may include axillary dissection, radiation, or a combination of the two. Axillary recurrence as related to the type of treatment and the clinical axillary node status is presented in Table 3-50. The data are collected from prospective randomized trials and retrospective series. Axillary dissection for the most part results in axillary recurrence rates of ≤5% in patients with clinically positive or negative axillary nodes. Radiation alone is comparable to surgical dissection in clinically node-negative patients. However, for patients with clinically positive axillary nodes the use of radiation alone to control disease in a significant percentage of patients requires doses in the range of 6000 to 7000 cGy, which are associated with an increased risk of brachial plexopathy, radiation fibrosis, and lymphedema. Axillary recurrence rates following radiation alone for clinically positive nodes are variable, but in general are higher than those for surgical dissection. Therefore in patients with clinically positive nodes an axillary dissection is the preferred treatment. The relative merits of the various axillary procedures employed in the conservative treatment of early breast cancer are discussed in Chapter 5.

Radiotherapy alone to the axilla results in an incidence of arm edema of 2% to 4%,[58,79,221,273] which is comparable to that following surgical dissection alone.[273,311,348] However, the combination of radiation and a complete axillary dissection either at the time of mastectomy or lumpectomy results in an increase in the incidence and severity of arm edema.[3,35,132,221,321]

Table 3-50 Axillary recurrence related to treatment and clinical nodal status

	Axillary recurrence (%)			
	Clinical N_0		Clinical N_1	
Author	AD	R	AD	R
NSABP B-04[113]	1	3	1	12
Southeast Scotland[220]	1	14	5	14
Manchester[234]	—	—	29	28
Haffty et al.[158]		3		
Fletcher[127]		2		
Leung et al.[227]		2		6
Haagensen[154]	0		1	
Handley[164]	2		1	
Pierquin et al.[273]	1	2	6	4

AD, axillary dissection; R, radiation.

In summary, the therapeutic benefit of an axillary dissection or radiation is the prevention of an axillary recurrence. While prospective randomized trials have shown no survival benefit for prophylactic treatment in patients with clinically negative axillary nodes, approximately 20% to 40% (see Table 3-49) of these patients will ultimately require treatment for an axillary recurrence. In patients with untreated clinically positive nodes, almost 50%[14] will develop progressive axillary disease that may or may not be resectable.

Perhaps the most important aspect of an axillary dissection is its value as a staging procedure and its ability to provide prognostic information. Clinical staging of the axilla (see Table 3-47) is associated with a false negative rate of 30% to 40% (i.e., clinically negative axilla, histologically positive) and a false positive rate of 20% to 30% (i.e., clinically positive axilla, histologically negative). Therefore the most accurate information regarding nodal status is obtained from histologic examination. The pathologic status of the axillary nodes remains the most important prognostic factor for outcome. The status of the axillary nodes (i.e., positive vs. negative) and the extent of nodal positivity are the primary determinant of eligibility for adjuvant systemic therapy and the primary indicator for the aggressiveness of the regimen(s) employed. Axillary dissection, therefore, remains an important component of the treatment of early breast cancer.

Internal mammary nodes

Factors correlating with node involvement. Approximately 25% of the lymphatic channels of the breast drain primarily to the internal mammary nodes.[335] The internal mammary lymph nodes are located in decreasing order of frequency from the first to the fifth interspaces and may lie either medially or lateral to the internal mammary blood vessels. Metastases to the internal mammary nodes, however, occur most frequently to the second interspace, followed by the third and first.[339] The fourth and fifth interspaces are involved least often.[339]

The recognition of this pathway of spread resulted in the development of various techniques designed to treat the internal mammary nodes based on the concept that interception of the disease at a regional stage would prevent metastases to distant sites, decrease regional recurrence, and result in an improved cure rate. The extended radical mastectomy includes a surgical dissection of the internal mammary nodes either en bloc or in a discontinous manner with the radical or modified radical mastectomy. External beam irradiation may be employed to treat the internal mammary nodes either as the sole modality or as adjuvant treatment following the extended radical mastectomy.

Information regarding the incidence of internal mammary node involvement is obtained from histologic review of nodes removed either by a selective biopsy procedure or a formal dissection. The average number of internal mammary nodes removed by a formal dissection ranges from two to six.[214,246] The overall incidence of positive nodes is approximately 20%.[43,86,165,213,232,349] The frequency of positive nodes is related to the primary tumor size, the age of the patient, and the pathologic status of the axillary nodes. Veronesi and others[347] reported the highest incidence of involvement (44.3%) in women <40 years of age with histologically positive axillary nodes and a primary tumor >2 cm in diameter. The lowest incidence (6.8%) was observed in women >50 years of age with negative axillary nodes and a primary tumor <2 cm. The incidence of positive internal mammary nodes related to pathologic axillary node status, location of the primary tumor, and primary tumor size is presented in Table 3-51. The incidence of positive nodes is relatively low for T_1T_2 inner or outer quadrant lesions with negative axillary nodes (5% to 10%) and is highest for inner quadrant lesions with positive axillary nodes. Urban[337] also related the incidence of positive internal mammary nodes to the level of involvement of axillary nodes. For inner or central quadrant primary tumors the incidence of positive internal mammary nodes was 23% if only level I axillary nodes were positive, compared to 47% with positive level II nodes and 67% with positive level III nodes. The majority of patients with positive internal mammary nodes have positive axillary nodes. Less than 10% of all patients will have positive internal mammary nodes with negative axillary nodes (Tables 3-52 and 3-53).

Despite what appears to be a relatively high incidence of occult metastases to internal mammary nodes in certain subgroups, the incidence of clinical internal mammary recurrence is extremely low (Table 3-54) and is not significantly higher in patients with positive internal mammary nodes (10%) than in those with negative nodes (6%).[86] Similarly it is slightly higher in patients with positive axillary nodes compared to negative. Urban reported the highest incidence of clinical internal mammary node recurrence in patients with inner quadrant tumors and positive axillary nodes (11/45).[337]

Treatment options and comparison of results. Surgical dissection and radiation are equally effective in the treatment of internal mammary nodes. A single randomized trial in Copenhagen[195] compared the extended radical mastectomy (ERM) to simple mastectomy (SM) and radiation (R) to the regional nodes and chest wall. Between 1951 and

Table 3-51 Incidence of positive internal mammary nodes related to pathologic status of axillary nodes and location of the primary tumor

		Positive internal mammary nodes (%)						
			Negative axillary nodes			Positive axillary nodes		
Author		**Overall**	**Outer**	**Inner**	**Central**	**Outer**	**Inner**	**Central**
Urban[339]		30		11			48	
Handley[164]		22	4	12	6	22	50	46
Caceres[43]		19				19	44	33
Livingston and Arlen[216]		18	5	14	10	23	59	43
Donegan[86]		22	4	12	0	31	54	29
	Primary tumor							
Lacour[213]		16	8	11	—	22	37	—
	T_1T_2		4	11	—	17	32	—
	T_3		19	8	—	31	42	—
Veronesi and Valagussa[349]		20						
	T_1T_2		8	9	—	22	35	—
	T_3		25	18	—	64	43	—

Table 3-52 Incidence of positive internal mammary nodes related to pathologic status of axillary nodes

	Positive internal mammary nodes (%)	
Author	Negative axillary nodes	Positive axillary nodes
Livingston and Arlen[216]	8	34
Handley[165]	11	40
Donegan[86]	6	34
Veronesi and Valagussa[349]	9	30

1957, 559 patients with operable breast cancer were randomized to one of these two treatments. There were no differences in overall survival at 5 years (67% ERM vs. 66% SM and R), 10 years (50% ERM vs. 46% SM and R), or 15 years (37% ERM vs. 36% SM and R), or in the incidence of distant metatases (46% ERM vs. 47% SM and R) or local-regional recurrences (27% ERM vs. 22% SM and R) at 10 years. A separate analysis for patients with only stage I disease yielded similar results.

Surgery, radiation, or both. Arriagada and colleagues[7] analyzed the results of treatment of the internal mammary nodes with surgical resection, radiation, or both in 1060 patients with histologically positive axillary nodes and primary tumors ≤7 cm in diameter. There was no difference in 10-year overall survival rates or in the incidence of

Table 3-53 Incidence of positive axillary and internal mammary nodes in patients undergoing extended radical mastectomy

	Pts. (%)			
	Negative axillary nodes		Positive axillary nodes	
Author	IMN−	IMN+	IMN−	IMN+
Urban[339]	46	7	25	22
Handley[165]	37	5	35	23
Livingston and Arlen[232]	57	5	25	13
Donegan[86]	40	3	38	19
Veronesi and Valagussa[349]	43	4	37	16

IMN− , negative internal mammary nodes; IMN+ , positive internal mammary nodes.

Table 3-54 Incidence of clinical internal mammary node recurrence

			Clinical internal mammary node recurrence (%)		
Author	Total no. pts.	Primary treatment	All pts.	Axilla negative	Axilla positive
Urban[339]	786	RM ± R	5	5	5
Handley[164]	424	MRM ± R	2	—	—
Fisher et al.[113]	654	RM	0	0*	0*
	646	TM and R	0	0*	0*
Fisher et al.[119]	269	RM	0	0	0
	406	RM and R	0	0	0
Meier et al.[246]	56	RM	4	—	—
	56	ERM	0	—	—
Veronesi and Valagussa[349]	374	RM	4	2	6
	342	ERM	0.3	0	0.6
Donegan[86]	113	ERM ± R	7	4	9

RM, radical mastectomy; MRM, modified radical mastectomy; TM, total mastectomy; ERM, extended radical mastectomy; R, radiation.
*Clinical assessment of axilla.

Table 3-55 Results of treatment of internal mammary nodes by surgery, radiation, or both

	Institute Gustave-Roussy			
Treatment period	1958-1978			
No. pts.	1195			
Stage	T_{1-3} pathologic N_1			
Adjuvant therapy	None			
	RM/MRM	**ERM**	**ERM and R**	**RM/MRM and R**
10-yr survival rate (%)	50	52	58	58
Distant metastases (%)	46	44	40	42
Local-regional recurrence (%)	32	22	8	6

RM, radical mastectomy; MRM, modified radical mastectomy; ERM, extended radical mastectomy; R, radiation.
From Arriagada A et al: Radiother Oncol 11:213, 1988.

distant metastases at 10 years among the three treatment groups (Table 3-55). However, patients who received radiation either as the sole treatment of the internal mammary nodes or as adjuvant treatment following the extended radical mastectomy had a lower incidence of local-regional recurrence at 10 years.

Extended radical mastectomy and radical mastectomy. The results of retrospective series employing the extended radical mastectomy for the treatment of operable breast cancer are presented in Table 3-56. Overall survival is approximately 80% at 5 years and 60% at 10 years. Local-regional recurrence is less than 10%. A number of institutions have compared their own results with extended radical mastectomy to the radical or modified radical mastectomy through the retrospective review process (Table 3-57). None of these series has demonstrated a statistically significant benefit in terms of survival at 5 or 10 years, local-regional recurrence, or distant metastases for the overall group of patients receiving treatment to the internal mammary nodes.

Two prospective randomized trials have compared the radical mastectomy with the extended radical mastectomy (Table 3-58).[213,214,246] Both have failed to demonstrate the superiority of the extended procedure in terms of survival at 5 or 10 years for all patients entered. The International Cooperative Trial[213,214] also found no difference in the incidence of distant metastases at 10 years, although there was a lower incidence of local-regional recurrence in the group of patients undergoing the extended radical mastectomy ($p = .05$). The University of Chicago trial found no difference in local-regional recurrence rates between the two treatments.[246] Neither of these trials employed postoperative radiation. Five cancer centers (Lima, Milan, Reme, Villejuif, and Warsaw) participated in the International Cooperative Trial and two of these (Milan, Villejuif) have chosen to present separately the results of their own patients entered into the trial (see Table 3-58).[215,349] While patients entered into the trial did not receive postmastectomy irradiation, premenopausal patients entered by Villejuif underwent ovarian ablation by pelvic irradiation. Again, no significant differences in survival rates (overall or disease-free) at 5 or 10 years, distant metastases, or local-regional recurrence were observed for all patients entered.

Table 3-56 Results of extended modified radical mastectomy from retrospective series

	Urban[337,339]	Caceres[43]	Livingston and Arlen[232]
Treatment period	1951-1964	1954-1963	1955-1970
No. pts.	455	425	373
Stage	I-III	NS	I-III
Adjuvant therapy	±R	±R	NS
5-yr survival rate (%)	73	61	75 [68]
10-yr survival rate (%)	61	42	63 [60]
Local-regional recurrence (%)	6	—	8

NS, not stated; [ ], disease-free survival.

Table 3-57 Results of intrainstitutional comparisons of radical mastectomy (RM) with extended radical mastectomy (ERM)

	Urban[337]		Caceres[43]		Sugarbaker[318]		Meier[246]	
Treatment period	1955-1964		1954-1963		1947-1957		1960-1978	
No. pts.	507		425		248		390	
Stage	I-III		NS		NS		I, II	
Adjuvant therapy	±R		±R		NS		±R, C, H	
	RM	ERM	RM	ERM	RM	ERM	RM	ERM
5-yr survival (%)	—	—	58	61	57	70	75	82
10-yr survival (%)	54 [51]	62 [60]	44	42	—	—	60	68
			p=.52				p=.287	
Local-regional recurrence (%)	0	8	10	10	—	—	—	—

R, radiation; NS, not stated; C, chemotherapy; H, hormones; [ ], disease-free survival.

Table 3-58 Results of prospective randomized trials comparing radical mastectomy (RM) to extended radical mastectomy (ERM)

	University of Chicago[246]		International cooperative trial					
			Entire trial[213,214]		Villejuif[215]		Milan[349]	
Treatment period	1973-1982		1963-1968		1963-1968		1964-1968	
No. pts.	112		1453		243		737	
Stage	I, II		T_{1-3}, N_0N_1					
Adjuvant therapy	C, H		None		Ovarian R		None	
	RM	ERM	RM	ERM	RM	ERM	RM	ERM
5-yr survival (%)								
Overall	70	82	69	72	69	75	—	—
Disease-free			55	57				
10-yr survival (%)								
Overall	60 [.13]	74	53 [.40]	56	60	60	61 [.51]	57
Disease-free			46 [.20]	50			49	47
Distant metastasis (%)	—	—	49 [.10]	44	60	57		
Local-regional recurrence (%)	4	0	24 [.05]	14	21	17	22	19

C, chemotherapy; H, hormones; R, radiation; [ ], p values for comparison (adjacent columns).

Table 3-59 NSABP B-02 results of radical mastectomy (RM) versus radical mastectomy and regional node irradiation (RM and R)[119]

	All pts.		Negative axillary nodes		Positive axillary nodes	
	RM	RM and R	RM	RM and R	RM	RM and R
5-yr survival (%)	62	56	74	80	47	48
5-yr NED survival (%)	49	50	71	79	32	38
Regional recurrence (%)	7	0.5	4	0	3	0.8
Distant metastases (%)	32	40	21	12	40	52

Mastectomy with radiation. A number of trials have evaluated the addition of postoperative radiation to the various types of mastectomy (simple, modified radical, radical) and found no survival advantage.[48,61,113,133,190,234,333,354] However, in most of these trials radiation was directed to the chest wall and regional nodes. A single trial (NSABP B-02) evaluated the addition of regional node irradiation to radical mastectomy.[119] Treatment included the internal mammary, apical axillary, and supraclavicular nodes, but excluded the chest wall. At 5 years there was no significant difference in overall or no evidence of disease (NED) survival (Table 3-59). Regional recurrences as first site of relapse were decreased by the addition of radiation. In axillary node-negative patients, the incidence of distant metastases was also decreased in the irradiated group; however, in axillary node-positive patients the incidence of distant metastases was higher in the irradiated group.

Subgroup analysis for treatment of internal mammary nodes. In summary, none of the randomized trials has demonstrated a survival advantage for all patients receiving treatment to the internal mammary nodes despite several retrospective intrainstitutional comparisons suggesting a benefit. The question arises as to whether a subgroup of patients who may benefit from treatment of the internal mammary nodes can be identified. Results of subgroup analysis from retrospective series and prospective randomized trials are presented in Tables 3-60 and 3-61. There is uniform agreement that lateral tumors with negative axillary nodes do not benefit from treatment of the internal mammary nodes. In fact, patients in the International Cooperative Trial with lateral tumors and negative axillary nodes had a significant survival advantage when treated by radical mastectomy as opposed to the extended radical mastectomy.[213] None of the prospective randomized trials has shown a benefit for medial or central primary tumors with negative axillary nodes. The University of Chicago randomized trial demonstrated a significant survival benefit at 5 and 10 years for all medial tumors, although a separate analysis was not performed for axillary node-negative vs. node-positive patients.[246] Roseman and James,[284] in a retrospective review of 76 patients with stage I or II disease, histologically negative axillary nodes, and medial tumors, reported a significant decrease ($p < .01$) in overall recurrences, local recurrence, and distant metastases in the 17 patients who received postmastec-

Table 3-60 Results of subgroup analysis for treatment of internal mammary nodes in pathologic axillary node-*negative* patients

						Survival (%)			
						5 yr		10 yr	
Subgroup	**Author**	**Series**		**Total no. pts.**	**p value**	**M**	**ERM or R**	**M**	**ERM or R**
All patients	Sugarbaker[318]	RS		178	None	69	69		
	Caceres[43]	RS		227	.65	74	83	65	67
	Meier et al.[246]	RS		58	.35	87	93	77	84
		PRT		175	.19	88	91	76	84
Lateral	Fisher et al.[113]*	PRT		467	.6	75	75	67	64
	Nemoto et al.[261]	RS		3979	>.05	87	84	—	—
	Lacour et al.[213]	PRT	T_{1-2}	239	.05	87	78	—	—
			T_3	78	>.05	92	88	—	—
	Veronesi and Valagussa[349]	PRT	T_{1-2}	182	>.05	94	81	85	78
			T_3	16	>.05	92	75	92	75
	Chahbazian et al.[50]	RS		97	>.05	—	—	61	63
Medial	Urban[337]	RS		281	None	—	—	72	68
	Fisher et al.[113]	PRT		231	.6	75	79	63	56
	Lacour et al.[213]	PRT	T_{1-2}	214	>.05	89	88	—	—
			T_3	74	>.05	77	85	—	—
	Veronesi and Valagussa[349]	PRT	T_{1-2}	121	>.05	82	93	79	80
			T_3	16	>.05	60	100	60	85
	Nemoto et al.[261]	RS		1583	>.05	88	90	—	—
	Chahbazian et al.[50]	RS		128	.05	—	—	58	76

RS, retrospective series; PRT, prospective randomized trial; M, mastectomy; ERM, extended radical mastectomy; R, radiation.

*Clinical assessment of axilla.

Table 3-61 Results of subgroup analysis treatment of internal mammary nodes in pathologic axillary node-*positive* patients

						Survival (%)			
						5 yr		10 yr	
	Author	Series		Total no. pts.	p value	M	ERM or R	M	ERM or R
All patients	Sugarbaker[318]	RS		178	None	69	69		
	Caceres[43]	RS		227	.65	74	83	65	67
	Meier et al.[246]	RS		215	.27	64	74	48	53
		PRT		54	.14	50	71	41	63
Lateral	Fisher et al.[113]*	PRT		397	.8	60	60	36	39
	Lacour et al.[213]	PRT	T_{1-2}	297	>.05	63	68	—	—
			T_3	160	>.05	51	48	—	—
	Veronesi and Valagussa[349]	PRT	T_{1-2}	210	>.05	63	61	46	45
			T_3	22	>.05	50	23	25	8
	Nemoto et al.[261]	RS		2957	>.05	64	58	—	—
Medial	Urban[337]	RS		226	None	60	70	33	54
	Arriagada et al.[7]	RS		588	.01	—	—	45	60
	Nemoto et al.[261]	RS		823	>.05	62	57	—	—
	Lacour et al.[213,214]	PRT	T_{1-2}	192	.01	52	71	—	—
			T_3	137	>.05	49	48	—	—
	Lacour et al.[215]	PRT		70	.02	42	79	39	56
	Veronesi and Valagussa[349]	PRT	T_{1-2}	120	>.05	58	52	46	38
			T_3	29	>.05	43	31	29	15
	Fisher et al.[113]*	PRT		180	.3	65	56	44	36
	Oslo trial[190]	PRT		72	>.05	63	79	42	59
	Stockholm trial[17]	PRT		31	>.05	52	65	38	65

RS, retrospective series; PRT, prospective randomized trial; M, mastectomy; ERM, extended radical mastectomy; R, radiation.
*Clinical assessment of axilla.

tomy irradiation. It is difficult to interpret these results in the absence of survival data and given the small number of patients who received radiation. Chahbazian et al.[50] reported a significant improvement ($p = .05$) in 10-year survival for patients with medial or central tumors and histologically negative axillary nodes who received postoperative internal mammary node irradiation (76% vs. 58%). These are the only two studies that demonstrate a benefit for treatment of the internal mammary nodes in patients with medial lesions and negative axillary nodes, and both are retrospective. Nemoto et al.[261] in a retrospective review of 1583 patients with medial tumors and negative axillary nodes obtained from the 1978 American College of Surgeons survey, found no difference in 5-year survival rates between patients treated by mastectomy (84%) and mastectomy and radiation (86%). However, the authors caution that interpretation of their results is limited by the fact that radiotherapy data regarding dose, areas treated, and timing of the treatment were lacking. Fisher et al.,[113,122] found no significant benefit for postmastectomy radiation in terms of 5- or 10-year survival rates, the incidence of any first treatment failure, or distant metastases for lateral, medial, or central tumors with clinically negative axillary nodes. In the Cancer Research Campaign trial the addition of postmastectomy irradiation that included the internal mammary nodes did not result in an improvement in survival up to 8 years for patients with medial tumors and clinically positive or negative nodes.[48] Therefore there is little convincing data to support treatment of the internal mammary nodes in patients with medial or lateral tumor and negative axillary nodes.

The role of treatment for the internal mammary nodes in patients with positive axillary nodes is controversial, especially for medial tumors. None of the retrospective series or prospective randomized trials has demonstrated a benefit for lateral tumors with histologically positive axillary nodes or for all patients with positive axillary nodes. Data supporting treatment of the internal mammary nodes in patients with central or medial lesions and histologically positive axillary nodes is conflicting. The International Cooperative Trial,[213,214] while failing to demonstrate a survival or disease-free survival benefit at 5 or 10 years for all patients, identified this subgroup consisting of 192 patients as having a statistically significant improved survival at 5 years with the extended radical mastectomy (71% vs. 52%, p=.01). In the 10-year update,[214] however, no subgroup analysis was performed. The authors state the analysis was omitted because of a lack of significant overall survival differences and the fact that there were major differences in the number of axillary and internal mammary nodes examined among the treatment centers that could affect the subgroup analysis. In contrast to the latest report of the complete trial, the cancer centers at Villejuif and Milan performed a subset analysis of their own patients entered into the trial.[215,349] There were 70 patients with medial tumors and positive axillary nodes entered in Villejuif and 72 in Milan. As previously noted, neither group demonstrated a significant survival advantage with the extended radical mastectomy for all patients. However, the Villejuif[215] analysis noted a significant survival and disease-free survival advantage at 5, 10, and 15 years for patients with medial tumors and positive axillary nodes who underwent the extended radical mastectomy. These patients also experienced a significant decrease in local-regional recurrence and distant metastases. The Milan analysis,[349] however, failed to demonstrate a significant overall or disease-free survival at 10 years for any subgroup of patients. The major differences between the results of these two institutions appear to be related to the outcome of patients undergoing the extended radical mastectomy. Survival for patients undergoing radical mastectomy is comparable; however, at 5 and 10 years, patients in the Villejuif trial who underwent the extended radical mastectomy did better than those undergoing the radical mastectomy, whereas in the Milan trial they did worse. A subgroup analysis of the 192 patients entered into the complete trial at 10 years would have provided additional useful information. Fisher et al.[113] noted no benefit to postmastectomy irradiation in patients with medial lesions and clinically positive axillary nodes. Two additional randomized trials evaluating the role of postmastectomy irradiation have suggested a nonsignificant trend towards improved survival with internal mammary node irradiation in patients with positive axillary nodes and medial or central tumors.[17,190] In the Oslo trial[190] the 10-year survival rate was 59% for those patients receiving cobalt-60 radiation (38 patients) compared to 42% for those treated by radical mastectomy alone (34 patients). The difference was not statistically significant because of the small number of patients. In the Stockholm trial,[17] with only 31 patients, the 10-year survival rate was 65% for the irradiated patients, as compared to 38% for the controls. Again, statistical significance was not achieved because of the small number of patients. Only one of the retrospective series has demonstrated a significant improvement in survival with internal mammary node treatment in this subgroup of patients. Arriagada et al.[7] reported a 10-year survival rate of 45% for patients with medial lesions and histologically positive axillary nodes who received no treatment to the internal mammary nodes, compared to 60% for those whose internal mammary nodes were treated by surgery, radiation, or a combination of both. Similar results were obtained at 15 and 20 years, and internal mammary node treatment resulted in a significant decrease in distant metastases (p=.05). There were a total of 588 patients in this subgroup, which also included patients who had been entered into the International Cooperative Trial and treated at the Institut Gustave-Roussy. Nemoto et al.[261] noted no improvement in 5-year survival rates with postmastectomy irradiation in a group of 823 patients with medial lesions and positive axillary nodes.

In summary, there appears to be no benefit from internal mammary node treatment in patients with lateral tumors and positive axillary nodes. For patients with medial tumors and positive axillary nodes, the largest prospective randomized trial[213,214] demonstrated a benefit in this group of patients at 5 years, but did not perform a subset analysis at 10 years. However, two of the institutions participating in the trial performed a subset analysis of their own patients and arrived at divergent conclusions. In the Villejuif patients[215] a survival benefit was observed, whereas in the Milan patients[349] no benefit could be demonstrated. Similar disparities exist in a review of the two largest retrospective series.[7,261] There appears to be no clear resolution of the issue of internal mammary node treatment in this group of patients.

Survival related to pathologic status of axillary and internal mammary nodes. Survival as related to the pathologic status of the axillary and internal mammary nodes in patients undergoing the extended radical mastectomy is presented in Table 3-62. Patients with positive internal mammary nodes only appear to have a prognosis similar to those with positive axillary nodes only. Patients with positive axillary and internal mammary nodes have the worst prognosis. These results have been achieved without the benefit of adjuvant systemic therapy.

Evidence of survival benefit and prevention of recurrence. The value of internal mammary node treatment either by surgical removal, radiation, or a combination of both can be measured in terms of survival, disease-free survival, and/or prevention of a parasternal recurrence. A review of pro-

Table 3-62 Results of extended radical mastectomy: survival related to pathologic status of axillary and internal mammary node (IMN)

	Negative axillary node (%)				Positive axillary node (%)			
	Negative IMN node		Positive IMN node		Negative IMN node		Positive IMN node	
Author	5 yr	10 yr	5 yr	10 yr	5 yr	10 yr	5 yr	10 yr
Urban[337]	87	76 [73]	64	56 [53]	68	60 [57]	54	29 [25]
Livingston and Arlen[232]	89 [85]	82 [78]	60 [53]	38 [38]	61 [52]	54 [50]	50 [32]	17 [17]
Veronesi et al.[347]		80 [73]		53 [52]		55 [47]		30 [25]
Donegan[86]	67	40	0	0	35	21	28	6
Caceres[43]	85	67	56	—	52	31	24	10
Sugarbaker[318]	86		14		70		51	
Lacour et al.[214]				43				25
Handley[165]		[64]		[39]		[36]		[7]
Dahl-Iversen and Tobiassen[73]			64	28				

[ ], disease-free survival.

spective randomized trials as well as retrospective series demonstrates no convincing evidence for a survival benefit in patients with negative axillary nodes or in those with lateral tumors and positive axillary nodes. For patients with medial tumors and positive axillary nodes the evidence is contradictory and arguments for or against treatment clearly exist. Treatment of the internal mammary nodes does not result in a significant decrease in the incidence of internal mammary node recurrences. Veronesi and Valagussa[349] reported a 3.7% incidence of internal mammary node recurrences at 10 years in patients undergoing radical mastectomy without postoperative irradiation, as compared to an incidence of 0.3% for those undergoing extended radical mastectomy. Urban and Marjani[339] found no advantage to postoperative radiation in terms of survival or local-regional recurrence in patients with positive internal mammary nodes who underwent the extended radical mastectomy. The overall incidence of clinical internal mammary node recurrence is <10% (see Table 3-54) despite an overall incidence of occult involvement of 20%. Donegan[86] reported a 10% incidence of internal mammary node recurrence in patients with positive internal mammary nodes who underwent extended radical mastectomy compared to an incidence of 6% for patients with negative internal mammary nodes. The incidence of internal mammary node recurrences is still less than 10% for patients with positive axillary nodes. Urban and Marjani[339] reported the highest incidence of parasternal recurrences in patients with inner quadrant tumors and positive axillary nodes who underwent radical mastectomy with or without radiation (24%). However, in a review of regional node recurrences in patients undergoing conservative surgery and radiation at the University of Pennsylvania, there were no internal mammary node recurrences in patients with medial tumors and positive axillary nodes whose internal mammary nodes were untreated.[135] Because the overall incidence of clinical internal mammary node recurrence is low despite the presence of positive axillary nodes, it is difficult to demonstrate a significant reduction in parasternal recurrences with treatment.

Complications. Finally, the benefits of treatment of the internal mammary nodes must be weighed against the complications of such treatment. In the Oslo trial a significant increase in deaths related to myocardial infarction was observed in stage I patients who received radiation.[190] An increased incidence of cardiovascular deaths was noted in the Manchester trial[194] and in the Cancer Research Campaign trial[176] in patients who received orthovoltage radiation. It is postulated that these deaths were related to the technique employed to treat the internal mammary nodes, which also irradiated the heart. Arriagada et al.[7] employing a different technique, reported no major complications in patients who received internal mammary node irradiation. Complications related to the surgical resection of the internal mammary nodes include a longer operating time, increased transfusion requirements, and a higher incidence of seroma formation and wound infection when compared to the radical or modified radical mastectomy.[246] The operative mortality is <1.0%.

Internal mammary node dissection as a staging procedure. It has been suggested that internal mammary node dissection may be useful as a staging procedure in identifying patients with negative axillary nodes and positive internal mammary nodes; these patients may be candidates for adjuvant systemic therapy as their prognosis is similar to that of axillary node-positive patients. However, of all patients undergoing an internal mammary node dissection <7% will have negative axillary nodes and positive internal mammary nodes (see Table 3-53). Approximately 10% of patients with negative axillary nodes will have positive internal mammary nodes (see Table 3-52). Indications for adjuvant systemic therapy have now been extended to patients with negative axillary nodes. Eligibility criteria for entry into the randomized trials evaluating adjuvant chemotherapy in axillary node-negative patients have included negative estrogen receptors, high-risk flow cytometry or thymidine labeling index, and primary tumor size ≥3 cm for estrogen receptor–positive tumors.[31,112,239] As noted by Veronesi et al.[347] the greatest frequency of internal mammary node positivity in axillary node-negative patients is seen with primary tumors ≥2 cm and/or with ages <40 years. It therefore appears that axillary node-negative patients identified by noninvasive procedures as candidates for adjuvant systemic therapy also may be those most likely to have positive internal mammary nodes. With the identification of newer prognostic factors the role of internal mammary node dissection merely as a staging procedure certainly can be questioned.

Supraclavicular nodes

Factors correlating with node involvement. The supraclavicular lymph nodes represent the nodal station adjacent to the apical axillary nodes. The incidence of positive supraclavicular nodes is related to the status of the internal mammary and axillary nodes. In patients with negative axillary or internal mammary nodes the incidence is 2%.[150,356] In patients with positive axillary or internal mammary nodes the incidence increases to 17% to 43%.[150,356,357]

The incidence of supraclavicular recurrence ranges from 10% to 26% for patients with positive axillary nodes to ≤5%[119,349] for patients with negative axillary nodes. The majority of supraclavicular recurrences are associated with positive axillary nodes at multiple levels and extensive involvement.[309] The supraclavicular nodes are the most common site for a regional node recurrence in patients undergoing a radical or modified radical mastectomy[119,349] and are the second most common site (the axillary being the most common) for patients undergoing conservative surgery and radiation.[59,79,135,237,279]

Treatment options and comparison of results. The superradical mastectomy was an extension of the extended radical mastectomy in which the supraclavicular nodes were dissected. Dahl-Iversen and Tobiassen[73] reported a 5-year survival rate of 78% and a 10-year survival rate of 59% for patients with clinical stage A breast cancer undergoing the superradical mastectomy. For clinical stage B patients the rates were 46% and 21% at 5 and 10 years. These results are comparable to those of the extended radical procedure. Others have confirmed the lack of a survival benefit for surgical treatment of the supraclavicular nodes and the procedure virtually has been abandoned.[356] Prophylactic irradiation of the supraclavicular nodes results in a significant decrease in supraclavicular recurrences without a demonstrable survival benefit.[119] The incidence of supraclavicular recurrences in patients with positive axillary nodes who receive prophylactic irradiation to this region is 1.5%.[127] Supraclavicular node irradiation is not indicated in patients with negative axillary nodes; however, it may be useful in decreasing the incidence of supraclavicular recurrences in patients with extensive axillary nodal involvement.

There is currently no role for dissection of the supraclavicular nodes as a staging procedure because involvement of these nodes without involvement of axillary or internal mammary nodes is rare.

REFERENCES

1. Adair F, Berg J, Joubert L, and Robbins GF: Long-term followup of breast cancer patients: the 30-year report, Cancer 33:1145, 1974.
2. Aitken DR and Minton JP: Complications associated with mastectomy, Surg Clin North Am 63:1331, 1983.
3. Aitken RJ, Gaze MN, Rodger A, et al: Arm morbidity within a trial of mastectomy and either nodal sample with selective radiotherapy or axillary clearance, Br J Surg 76:568, 1989.
4. Allegra JC, Lippman ME, Simon R, et al: Association between steroid hormone receptor status and disease-free interval in breast cancer, Cancer Treat Rep 63:1271, 1979.
5. Anglem TJ and Leber RE: Characteristics of 10 year survivors after radical mastectomy for cancer of the breast, Am J Surg 121:363, 1971.
6. Ariel IM: Results of treating 1178 patients with breast cancer by radical mastectomy and post-operative irradiation where metastases to axillary lymph nodes occurred, J Surg Oncol 12:137, 1979.
7. Arriagada A, Le MG, Mouriesse H, et al: Long-term effect of internal mammary chain treatment: results of a multivariate analysis of 1195 patients with operable breast cancer and positive axillary nodes, Radiother Oncol 11:213, 1988.
8. Auchincloss H: Significance of location and number of axillary metastases in carcinoma of the breast: a justification for a conservative operation, Ann Surg 158:36, 1963.
9. Baclesse F: Roentgenotherapy as the sole method of treatment of cancer of the breast, Am J Roentgenol 62:311, 1949.
10. Bader J, Lippman M, Swain S, et al: Preliminary report of the NCI early breast cancer study: a prospective randomized comparison of lumpectomy and radiation to mastectomy for Stage I and II breast cancer, Int J Radiat Oncol Biol Phys 13:160, 1987 (abstract).

11. Baker RR, Montague AC, and Childs JN: A comparison of modified radical mastectomy to radical mastectomy in the treatment of operable breast cancer, Ann Surg 189:553, 1979.
12. Baral E, Larsson LE, and Mattson B: Breast cancer following irradiation of the breast, Cancer 40:2905, 1977.
13. Bartelink H and von Donegan JA: Randomized clinical trial to assess the value of breast conserving therapy (BCT) in stage I and stage II breast cancer: EORTC trial 10801. Proceedings of the fifth European Conference on Clinical Oncology, London, September 1989 (abstract).
14. Baum M and Coyle PJ: Simple mastectomy for early breast cancer and the behavior of the untreated axillary nodes, Bull Cancer 64:603, 1977.
15. Beadle GF, Harris JR, Silver B, et al: Cosmetic results following primary radiation therapy for early breast cancer, Cancer 54:2911, 1984.
16. Bedwani R, Vana J, Rosner D, et al: Management and survival of female patients with "minimal" breast cancer: as observed in the long-term and short-term surveys of the American College of Surgeons, Cancer 47:2769, 1981.
17. Bedwinek J: Adjuvant irradiation for early breast cancer: an on-going controversy, Cancer 53:729, 1984.
18. Bedwinek JM, Lee J, Fineberg B, and Ocwieza M: Prognostic indicators in patients with isolated local-regional recurrence of breast cancer, Cancer 47:2232, 1981.
19. Bedwinek JM, Perez CA, Kramer S, et al: Irradiation as the primary management of stage I and II adenocarcinoma of the breast, Cancer Clin Trials 3:11, 1980.
20. Beebe GW, Kato H, and Land CE: Studies of the mortality of A-bomb survivors, Radiat Res 75:138, 1978.
21. Berger MS, Locher GW, Sauer S, et al: Correlation of C-erb-B2 gene amplication and protein expression in human breast carcinoma with nodal status and nuclear grade, Cancer Res 48:1238, 1988.
22. Berstock DA, Houghton J, Haybittle J, and Baum M: The role of radiotherapy following total mastectomy for patients with early breast cancer, World J Surg 9:667, 1985.
23. Blichert-Toft M: A Danish randomized trial comparing breast preservation with mastectomy in mammary carcinoma. Proceedings of the NIH Consensus Development Conference Early Stage Breast Cancer, June 1990, pp 28-31.
24. Blichert-Toft M, Brincker H, Andersen JA, et al: A Danish randomized trial comparing breast-preserving therapy with mastectomy in mammary carcinoma, Acta Oncol 27:671, 1988.
25. Bluming AZ, Dosik G, Lowiz B, et al: Treatment of primary breast cancer without mastectomy: the Los Angeles community experience and review of the literature, Ann Surg 204:136, 1986.
26. Body G, Sauvanet E, Calais G, et al: Angiosarcome cutane du sein apres adenocarcinome mammaire opere et irradie, J Gynecol Obstet Biol Reprod 16:479, 1987.
27. Boice JD Jr and Hutchinson GB: Leukemia in women following radiotherapy for cervical cancer, J Natl Cancer Inst 65:115, 1980.
28. Boice JD Jr and Monson RR: Breast cancer in women after repeated fluoroscopic examinations of the chest, J Natl Cancer Inst 59:823, 1977.
29. Boivin J-F, Hutchinson GB, Evans FB, Abou-Daoud KT, and Juned B: Leukemia after radiotherapy for first primary cancers of various anatomic sites, Am J Epidemiol 123:993, 1986.
30. Bonadonna G, Brusamolino E, Valagussa P, et al: Combination chemotherapy as an adjuvant treatment in operable breast cancer, N Engl J Med 294:405, 1976.
31. Bonadonna G, Valagussa P, Tancini G, et al: Current status of Milan adjuvant chemotherapy trials for node-positive and node-negative breast cancer, NCI Monographs 1:45, 1986.
32. Bonadonna G, Valagussa P, Zucali R, DelVecchio M, and Veronesi U: Feasibility of adjuvant chemotherapy plus radiotherapy in operable breast cancer. In Harris J, Hellman S, and Silen W, editors: Conservative management of breast cancer, Philadelphia, 1983, JB Lippincott, pp 329-338.
33. Botnick L, Come S, Rose C, et al: Primary breast irradiation and concomitant adjuvant chemotherapy. In Harris J, Hellman S, and Silen W, editors: Conservative management of breast cancer, Philadelphia, 1983, JB Lippincott, pp 321-328.
34. Breasted JH: The Edwin Smith papyrus, Chicago, 1930, University of Chicago Press.
35. Bretton RC and Nelson PA: Causes and treatment of postmastectomy lymphedema of the arm, JAMA 180:95, 1962.
36. Brinkley D and Haybittle JL: Long term survival of women with breast cancer, Lancet i:1118, 1984.
37. Brinkley D and Haybittle JL: The curability of breast cancer, Lancet ii:95, 1975.
38. Brinkley D and Haybittle JL: Treatment of stage two cancer of the female breast, Lancet ii:1086, 1971.
39. Brinkley D and Haybittle JL: Results of treatment of carcinoma of the breast, Lancet i:86, 1959.
40. Budd DC, Cochran RC, Sturtz DL, and Fouty WJ: Surgical morbidity after mastectomy operations, Am J Surg 135:218, 1978.
41. Burn JI: "Early" breast cancer: the Hammersmith trial, Br J Surg 61:762, 1974.
42. Butcher HR: Radical mastectomy for mammary carcinoma, Ann Surg 170:883, 1969.
43. Caceres E: An evaluation of radical mastectomy and extended radical mastectomy for cancer of the breast, Surg Gynecol Obstet 125:337, 1967.
44. Cahill CJ, Gibbs NM, Boulter PS, et al: Invasive breast cancer: the tip of an iceberg, Ann R Coll Surg Engl 65:356, 1983.
45. Calle R, Vilcoq JR, Zafrani B, et al: Local control and survival of breast cancer treated by limited surgery followed by irradiation, Int J Radiat Oncol Biol Phys 12:873, 1986.
46. Calle R, Vilcoq R, Pilleron JP, et al: Conservative treatment of operable breast carcinoma by irradiation with or without limited surgery: ten year results. In Harris J, Hellman S, and Silen W, editors: Conservative management of breast cancer, Philadelphia, 1983, JB Lippincott, pp 3-10.
47. Cancer Research Campaign: Management of early breast cancer of the breast: report of a international multicentric trial, Br Med J 1:1035, 1976.
48. Cancer Research Campaign Working Party: Cancer Research Campaign (King's/Cambridge) trial for early breast cancer: a detailed update at the tenth year, Lancet ii:55, 1980.
49. Carter CL, Allen C, and Henson DE: Relation of tumor size, lymph node status and survival in 24,740 breast cancer cases, Cancer 63:181, 1989.
50. Chahbazian C, Del Regato J, and Wilson F: Post-operative radiation therapy for "early" carcinoma of the breast, Cancer 42:1126, 1978.
51. Chaudary MA, Doran Z, and Fentiman IS: A randomized trial comparing tumorectomy plus tamoxifen with modified radical mastectomy for elderly patients with operable breast cancer, Breast Cancer Res Treat 14:137, 1989 (abstract).
52. Chu AM, Cope O, Russo R, and Lew R: Patterns of local-regional recurrence and results in stages I and II breast cancer treated by irradiation following limited surgery, Am J Clin Oncol 7:221, 1984.
53. Clark GM, Osborne CK, and McGuire WL: Correlations

between estrogen receptor, progesterone receptor, and patient characteristics in human breast cancer, J Clin Oncol 2:1102, 1984.

54. Clark R, McCulloch P, Levine M, Lipa M, and Wilkinson R: A randomized clinical trial to assess the effectiveness of breast irradiation following lumpectomy and axillary dissection for node negative breast cancer, Proc Am Soc Clin Oncol 9:21, 1990 (abstract).
55. Clark RM: Alternatives to mastectomy: the Princess Margaret Hospital experience. In Harris J, Hellman S, and Silen W, editors: Conservative management of breast cancer, Philadelphia, 1983, JB Lippincott, pp 35-46.
56. Clark RM, Wilkinson RH, Mahoney LJ, Reid JG, and MacDonald WD: Breast cancer: a 21 year experience with conservative surgery and radiation, Int J Radiat Oncol Biol Phys 8:967, 1982.
57. Clark RM, Wilkinson RH, Miceli PN, and MacDonald WD: Breast cancer: experiences with conservation therapy, Am J Clin Oncol 10:461, 1987.
58. Clarke D, Martinez A, Cox RS, and Goffinet DR: Breast edema following staging axillary node dissection in patients with breast carcinoma treated by radical radiotherapy, Cancer 49:2295, 1982.
59. Clarke DH, Le MG, Sarrazin D, et al: Analysis of local-regional relapse in patients with early breast cancers treated by excision and radiotherapy: experience of the Institut Gustave-Roussy, Int J Radiat Oncol Biol Phys 11:137, 1985.
60. Cline MJ, Battifora H, and Yokota J: Proto-oncogene abnormalities in human breast cancer: correlations with anatomic features and clinical course of disease, J Clin Oncol 5:999, 1987.
61. Cole MP: The place of radiotherapy in the management of early breast cancer: a report of two clinical trials, Br J Surg 51:216, 1964.
62. Court-Brown WM and Doll R: Mortality from cancer and other causes after radiotherapy for ankylosing spondylitis, Br Med J 2:1327, 1965.
63. Crile G: The incidence of local recurrence of carcinoma of the breast, Surg Gynecol Obstet 156:497, 1983.
64. Crile G: Managment of breast cancer: limited mastectomy, Int J radiat Oncol Biol Phys 2:969, 1977.
65. Crile G: Results of conservative treatment of breast cancer at 10 and 15 years, Ann Surg 181:26, 1975.
66. Crile G: Metastases from involved lymph nodes after removal of various primary tumors: evaluation of radical and of simple mastectomy for cancers of the breast, Ann Surg 163:267, 1966.
67. Crile G: Results of simplified treatment of breast cancer, Surg Gynecol Obstet 118:517, 1964.
68. Crile G, Esselstyn CB, Hermann RE, and Hoerr SO: Partial mastectomy for carcinoma of the breast, Surg Gynecol Obstet 136:929, 1973.
69. Curtis RE, Boice JD, Stovall M, Flannery JT, and Moloney WC: Leukemia risk following radiotherapy for breast cancer, J Clin Oncol 7:21, 1989.
70. Curtis RE, Hankey BF, Myers MH, and Young JL: Risk of leukemia associated with first course of cancer treatment: an analysis of the surveillance, epidemiology, and end results program experience, J Natl Cancer Inst 72:531, 1984.
71. Cuzick J, Stewart H, Peto H, et al: Overview of randomized trials comparing radical mastectomy without radiotherapy against simple mastectomy with radiotherapy in breast cancer, Cancer Treat Rep 71:7, 1987.
72. Dahl-Iversen E: Recherches sur les metastases microscopique des ganglions lymphatigues parasternaux dans le cancer du sein, Int J Chir 11:492, 1951.
73. Dahl-Iversen E, and Tobiassen T: Radical mastectomy with parasternal and supraclavicular dissection for mammary carcinoma, Ann Surg 170:889, 1969.
74. Danforth DM, Findlay PA, McDonald HD, et al: Complete axillary lymph node dissection for Stage I-II carcinoma of the breast, J Clin Oncol 4:655, 1986.
75. Danforth DN and Lippman ME: Surgical treatment of breast cancer. In Lippman ME, Lichter A, and Danford DN, editors: Diagnosis and management of breast cancer, Philadelphia, 1988, WB Saunders, pp 95-154.
76. Dawson PJ, Ferguson DJ, and Karrison T: The pathologic findings of breast cancer in patients surviving 25 years after radical mastectomy, Cancer 50:2131, 1982.
77. Degenshein GA and Ceccarelli F: The history of breast cancer surgery. Part I: Early beginnings to Halsted, Breast 3:28, 1977.
78. Delarue NC, Anderson WD, and Starr J: Modified radical mastectomy in the individualized treatment of breast carcinoma, Surg Gynecol Obstet 129:79, 1969.
79. Delouche G, Bachelot F, Premont M, and Kurtz JM: Conservation treatment of early breast cancer: long term results and complications, Int J Radiat Oncol Biol Phys 13:29, 1987.
80. Den Besten L and Ziffren SE: Simple and radical mastectomy, Arch Surg 90:755, 1965.
81. DeVita VT: The relationship between tumor mass and resistance to chemotherapy: implications for surgical adjuvant treatment of cancer, Cancer 51:1209, 1983.
82. Devitt JE: The significance of regional lymph node metastases in breast carcinoma, Can Med Assoc J 93:289, 1965.
83. Dewar JA, Sarrazin D, Benhamou E, et al: Management of the axilla in conservatively treated breast cancer: 592 patients treated at Institut Gustave-Roussy, Int J Radiat Oncol Biol Phys 13:475, 1987.
84. Doll R and Smith PG: The long-term effects of x-irradiation in patients treated for metropathia haemmorrhagica, Br J Radiol 41:362, 1968.
85. Donegan WL: Staging and primary treatment. In Donegan WL and Spratt JS, editors: Cancer of the Breast, ed 3, Philadelphia, 1988, WB Saunders, pp 336-402.
86. Donegan WL: The influence of untreated internal mammary metastases upon the course of mammary cancer, Cancer 39:533, 1977.
87. Donegan WL, Perez-Mesa CM, and Watson RF: A biostatistical study of locally recurrent breast carcinoma, Surg Gynecol Obstet 122:529, 1966.
88. Dressler LG, Seamer LC, Owens MA, et al: DNA flow cytometry and prognostic factors in 1331 frozen breast cancer specimens, Cancer 61:420, 1988.
89. Dubois JB, Gary-Bobo J, Pourquier H, and Pujol H: Tumorectomy and radiotherapy in early breast cancer: a report on 392 patients, Int J Radiat Oncol Biol Phys 15:1275, 1988.
90. Duncan W and Kerr GR: The curability of breast cancer, Br Med J 2:781, 1976.
91. Ederer F, Axtell LM, and Cutler SJ: The relative survival rate: a statistical methodology, Natl Cancer Inst Monogr 6:101, 1961.
92. Ederer F, Cutler SJ, Goldenberg IS, and Eisenberg H: Causes of death among long-term survivors from breast cancer in Connecticut, J Natl Cancer Inst 30:933, 1963.
93. Egan RL: Multicentric breast carcinomas: clinical-radiographic-pathologic whole organ studies and 10 year survival, Cancer 49:1123, 1982.
94. Elston CW, Gresham GA, Rao GS, et al: The Cancer Research Campaign (King's/Cambridge) Trial for Early Breast Cancer: clinico-pathologic aspects, Br J Cancer 45:655, 1982.
95. Elwood JM and Godolphin W: Estrogen receptors in breast tumors: associations with age, menopausal status and epidemiological and clinical features in 735 patients, Br J Cancer 42:635, 1980.

96. Fallenus AG, Franzen SA, and Auer GU: Predictive value of nuclear DNA content in breast cancer in relation to clinical and morphologic factors: a retrospective study of 227 consecutive cases, Cancer 62:521, 1988.
97. Fentiman IS, Cuzick J, Millis RR, and Hayward JL: Which patients are cured of breast cancer? Br Med J 289:1108, 1984.
98. Fentiman IS, Mathews PN, Davison OW, et al: Survival following local skin recurrence after mastectomy, Br J Surg 72:14, 1985.
99. Ferguson DJ, Meier P, Karrison T, et al: Staging of breast cancer and survival rates: an assessment based on 50 years of experience with radical mastectomy, JAMA 248:1337, 1982.
100. Fisher B: The revolution in breast cancer surgery: science or anecdotalism? World J Surg 9:655, 1985.
101. Fisher B: The changing role of surgery in the treatment of cancer. In Becker F, editor: Cancer: a comprehensive treatise—radiotherapy, surgery, and immunotherapy, vol 6, New York, 1977, Plenum, pp 401-421.
102. Fisher B: Surgery of primary breast cancer. In McGuire W, editor: Breast cancer: advances in research and treatment—current approaches to therapy, vol 1, New York, 1977, Plenum, pp 1-42.
103. Fisher B, Bauer M, Margolese R, et al: Five-year results of a randomized clinical trial comparing total mastectomy and segmental mastectomy with or without radiation in the treatment of breast cancer, N Engl J Med 312:665, 1985.
104. Fisher B, Carbone P, Economou SG, et al: L-phenylalanine mustard (L-PAM) in the management of primary breast cancer: a report of early findings, N Engl J Med 292:117, 1975.
105. Fisher B, Costantino J, Redmond C, et al: A randomized clinical trial evaluating tamoxifen in the treatment of patients with node-negative breast cancer who have estrogen-receptor-positive tumors, N Engl J Med 320:479, 1989.
106. Fisher B and Fisher ER: The interrelationship of hematogenous and lymphatic tumor cell dissemination, Surg Gynecol Obstet 122:791, 1976.
107. Fisher B and Fisher ER: The barrier function of lymph node to tumor cells and erythrocytes. I. Normal nodes, Cancer 20:1907, 1967.
108. Fisher B and Fisher ER: Host-tumor relationship in the development and growth of hepatic metastases. In Wissler RW, Dao TL, Wood SW Jr, editors: Endogenous factors in influencing host-tumor balance, International Symposium sponsored by the Argonne Cancer Research Hospital, University of Chicago (1966), Chicago, 1967, University of Chicago Press, pp 149-166.
109. Fisher B and Fisher ER: The organ distribution of disseminated 51Cr-labeled tumor cells, Cancer Res 27:412, 1967.
110. Fisher B, Glass A, Redmond C, et al: L-phenylalanine mustard (L-PAM) in the management of primary breast cancer: an update of earlier findings and a comparison with those utilizing L-PAM plus 5-fluorouracil (5-FU), Cancer 39:2883, 1977.
111. Fisher B, Ravdin RG, Ausman RK, et al: Surgical adjuvant chemotherapy in cancer of the breast: results of a decade of cooperative investigation, Ann Surg 168:337, 1968.
112. Fisher B, Redmond C, Dimitrov NV, et al: A randomized clinical trial evaluating sequential methotrexate and fluorouracil in the treatment of patients with node-negative breast cancer who have estrogen-receptor-negative tumors, N Engl J Med 320:473, 1989.
113. Fisher B, Redmond C, Fisher ER, et al: Ten year results of a randomized clinical trial comparing radical mastectomy and total mastectomy with or without radiation, N Engl J Med 312:674, 1985.
114. Fisher B, Redmond C, Poisson R, et al: Eight-year results of a randomized clinical trial comparing total mastectomy and lumpectomy with or without irradiation in the treatment of breast cancer, N Engl J Med 320:822, 1989.
115. Fisher B, Rockette H, Fisher ER, et al: Leukemia in breast cancer patients following adjuvant chemotherapy or postoperative radiation: the NSABP experience, J Clin Oncol 3:1640, 1985.
116. Fisher B, Safer E, and Fisher ER: Studies concerning the regional lymph nodes in cancer. IV. Tumor inhibition by regional lymph node cells, Cancer 33:631, 1974.
117. Fisher B, Slack N, Katrych DL, and Wolmark N: Ten year follow-up of patients in a cooperative clinical trial evaluating surgical adjuvant chemotherapy, Surg Gynecol Obstet 140:528, 1975.
118. Fisher B, Slack NH, and Bross IDJ: Cancer of the breast: size of neoplasm and prognosis, Cancer 24:1071, 1969.
119. Fisher B, Slack NH, Cavanaugh PJ, et al: Post-operative radiotherapy in the treatment of breast cancer: results of the NSABP clinical trial, Ann Surg 172:711, 1970.
120. Fisher B, Wickerham DL, Brown A, and Redmond CK: Breast cancer estrogen and progesterone receptor values: their distribution, degree of concordance, and relation to number of positive axillary nodes, J Clin Oncol 1:349, 1983.
121. Fisher B, Wolmark N, Bauer M, et al: The accuracy of clinical nodal staging and of limited axillary dissection as a determinant of histologic nodal status in carcinoma of the breast, Surg Gynecol Obstet 152:765, 1981.
122. Fisher B, Wolmark N, Redmond C, et al: Findings from NSABP protocol no. B-04: comparison of radical mastectomy with alternative treatments. II. The clinical and biologic significance of medial-central breast cancers, Cancer 48:1863, 1981.
123. Fisher ER, Gregorio R, Redmond C, et al: Pathologic findings from the National Surgical Adjuvant Breast Project (protocol 4). I. Observations concerning the multicentricity of mammary cancer, Cancer 35:247, 1975.
124. Fisher ER, Sass R, and Fisher B: Pathologic findings from the National Surgical Adjuvant Project for breast cancers (protocol 4). X. Discriminants for tenth year treatment failure, Cancer 53:712, 1984.
125. Fisher ER, Sass R, Fisher B, et al: Pathologic findings from the National Surgical Adjuvant Breast Project (Protocol 6). II. Relation of local breast recurrence to multicentricity, Cancer 57:1717, 1986.
126. Fleck RS, McNeese MD, Ellerbrock NA, et al: Consequences of breast irradiation in patients with pre-existing collagen vascular disease, Int J Radiat Oncol Biol Phys 17:829, 1989.
127. Fletcher GH: Subclinical disease, Cancer 53:1274, 1984.
128. Fletcher GH: Clinical dose-response curves of human malignant epithelial tumors, Br J Radiol 46:1, 1973.
129. Fletcher GH, McNeese MD, and Oswald MJ: Long-range results for breast cancer patients treated by radical mastectomy and postoperative radiation without adjuvant chemotherapy: an update, Int J Radiat Oncol Biol Phys 17:11, 1989.
130. Fletcher GH and Montague E: Does adequate irradiation of the internal mammary chain and supraclavicular nodes improve survival rates? Int J Radiat Oncol Biol Phys 4:481, 1978.
131. Fletcher GH and Shukovsky LJ: The interplay of radiocurability and tolerance in the irradiation of human cancers, J Radiol Electrol 56:383, 1975.
132. Forrest APM, Robers MM, Cant ELM, et al: Simple mastectomy and pectoral node biopsy: the Cardiff-St. Mary's Trial, World J Surg 1:320, 1977.

133. Forrest APM, Stewart HJ, Roberts MM, and Steele RJC: Simple mastectomy and axillary node sampling (pectoral node biopsy) in the management of primary breast cancer, Ann Surg 196:371, 1982.
134. Fourquet A, Campana F, Zafrani B, et al: Prognostic factors in the conservative management of early breast cancer: a 25 year follow-up at the Institut Curie, Int J Radiat Oncol Biol Phys 17:7199, 1989.
135. Fowble B, Solin LJ, Schultz DJ, and Goodman RL: Frequency, sites of relapse and outcome of regional node failures following conservative surgery and radiation for early breast cancer, Int J Radiat Oncol Biol Phys 17:703, 1989.
136. Fowble B, Solin LJ, Schultz DJ, et al: Breast recurrence following conservative surgery and radiation: patterns of failure, prognosis and pathologic findings from mastectomy specimens with implications for treatment, Int J Radiat Oncol Biol Phys 19:833, 1990.
137. Fox MS: On the diagnosis and treatment of breast cancer, JAMA 241:489, 1979.
138. Fraass BA, Roberson PL, and Lichter AS: Dose to the contralateral breast due to primary breast irradiation, Int J Radiat Oncol Phys 11:485, 1985.
139. Frankl G and Rosenfeld DD: Xeroradiographic detection of occult breast cancer, Cancer 35:542, 1975.
140. Freeman CR, Belliveau NJ, Kim TH, and Boivin J: Limited surgery with or without radiotherapy for early breast carcinoma, J Can Assoc Radiol 32:125, 1981.
141. Gentili G, Sanfilippo O, and Silvestrini R: Cell proliferation and its relationship to clinical features and relapse in breast cancers, Cancer 48:974, 1981.
142. Gerard JP, Montbarbon JF, Chassard JL, et al: Conservative treatment of early carcinoma of the breast: significance of axillary dissection and iridium implant, Radiother Oncol 3:17, 1985.
143. Gilliland MD, Barton RM, and Copeland EM: The implications of local recurrence of breast cancer as the first site of therapeutic failure, Ann Surg 197:284, 1983.
144. Glatstein E, Straus K, Lichter A, et al: Results of the NCI early breast cancer trial. Proceedings of the NIH Consensus Development Conference Early Stage Breast Cancer, June 1990, pp 32-33.
145. Glick JH, Danoff B, Weiler C, and Goodman R: The administration of adjuvant chemotherapy in node-positive patients undergoing definitive irradiation: the University of Pennsylvania experience. In Harris J, Hellman S, and Silen W, editors: Conservative management of breast cancer, Philadelphia, 1983, JB Lippincott, pp 311-320.
146. Greco M, Sacchini V, Merson M, and Galimberti V: Risk of local failure in conservative treatment of breast cancer, Breast Cancer Res Treat 12:116, 1988.
147. Greening WP, Montgomery ACV, Gordon AB, and Gowing NFC: Quadrantic excision and axillary node dissection without radiation therapy: the long-term results of a selective policy in the treatment of Stage I breast cancer, Eur J Surg Oncol 14:221, 1988.
148. Gross NJ: Pulmonary effects of radiation therapy, Ann Interm Med 86:81, 1977.
149. Gump FE, Shikora S, Habif DV, et al: The extent and distribution of cancer in breasts with palpable primary tumors, Ann Surg 204:384, 1986.
150. Haagensen CD: Diseases of the breast, ed 2, Philadelphia, WB Saunders Co, 1971, pp 412-413.
151. Haagensen CD: Diseases of the breast, ed 2, Philadelphia, WB Saunders, 1971, pp 455-457.
152. Haagensen CD: My personal technique for the Halsted radical mastectomy. In Haagensen CD, editor: Diseases of the breast, ed 3, Philadelphia, 1986, WB Saunders Co, pp 872-902.
153. Haagensen CD: The natural history of breast carcinoma. In Haagensen CD, editor: Diseases of the breast, ed 3, Philadelphia, 1986, WB Saunders Co, pp 635-718.
154. Haagensen CD: Results with Halsted's radical mastectomy. In Haagensen CD, editor: Diseases of the breast, ed 3, Philadelphia, 1986, WB Saunders Co, pp 903-932, 933-938.
155. Haagensen CD and Cooley E: Radical mastectomy for mammary carcinoma, Ann Surg 170:884, 1969.
156. Haas JF, Kittelman B, Mehnert WH, et al: Risk of leukaemia in ovarian tumor and breast cancer patients following treatment by cyclophosphamide, Br J Cancer 55:213, 1987.
157. Habibollahi F, Fentiman IS, Chaudary MA, et al: Conservation treatment of operable breast cancer, Proc Am Soc Clin Oncol 6:59, 1987 (abstract).
158. Haffty BG, Fisher DB, and Fisher JJ: Regional node irradiation in the conservative treatment of breast cancer, Int J Radiat Oncol Biol Phys 19:859, 1990.
159. Haffty BG, Goldberg NB, Fischer D, et al: Conservative surgery and radiation therapy in breast carcinoma: local recurrence and prognostic implications, Int J Radiat Oncol Biol Phys 17:727, 1989.
160. Haimov M, Kark AE, and Lesnick GJ: Carcinoma of the breast: thirty years' experience with radical mastectomy, Am J Surg 115:341, 1968.
161. Hallahan DE, Michel AG, Halpern HJ, et al: Breast conserving surgery and definitive irradiation for early breast cancer, Int J Radiat Oncol Biol Phys 17:1211, 1989.
162. Halsted WS: The results of radical operations for the cure of carcinoma of the breast, Ann Surg 46:1, 1907.
163. Halsted WS: The results of operation for the cure of cancer of the breast performed at the Johns Hopkins Hospital from June 1889 to January 1894, Johns Hopkins Hosp Bull 4:297, 1894.
164. Handley RS: The conservative radical mastectomy of Patey: 10 year results in 425 patients, Breast 2:16, 1976.
165. Handley RS: Carcinoma of the breast, Ann R Coll Surg Engl 57:59, 1975.
166. Handley RS and Thackray AC: Conservative radical mastectomy (Patey's operation), Ann Surg 170:880, 1969.
167. Handley WS: Parasternal invasion of the thorax in breast cancer and its suppression by the use of radium tubes as an operative precaution, Surg Gynecol Obstet 45:721, 1927.
168. Hankey BF, Curtis RE, Naughton MD, et al: A retrospective cohort analysis of second breast cancer risk for primary breast cancer patients with an assessment of the effect of radiation therapy, J Natl Cancer Inst 70:797, 1983.
169. Hankey BF and Steinhorn SC: Long-term patient survival for some of the more frequently occurring cancers, Cancer 50:1904, 1982.
170. Harris JR and Coleman CN: Estimating the risk of second primary tumors following cancer treatment, J Clin Oncol 7:5, 1989.
171. Harris JR and Hellman S: Conservative surgery and radiotherapy. In Harris JR, Hellman S, Henderson IC, and Kinne DW, editors: Breast diseases, Philadelphia, 1987, JB Lippincott, pp 299-324.
172. Harris JR and Hellman S: Observations on survival curve analysis with particular reference to breast cancer treatment, Cancer 57:925, 1986.
173. Harris JR, Hellman S, and Kinne DW: Limited surgery and radiotherapy for early breast cancer, N Engl J Med 21:1365, 1985.
174. Harris JR, Recht A, Schnitt, et al: Current status of conservative surgery and radiotherapy as primary local treatment for early carcinoma of the breast, Breast Cancer Res Treat 5:245, 1985.

175. Haybittle JL: The curability of breast cancer, Experientia (suppl) 41:145, 1983.
176. Haybittle JL, Brinkley D, Houghton J, et al: Postoperative radiotherapy and late mortality: evidence from the Cancer Research Campaign trial for early breast cancer, Br Med J 298:1611, 1989.
177. Hayward J: The significance of local control in the primary treatment of breast cancer, Arch Surg 122:1244, 1987.
178. Hayward JL: The Guy's Hospital trials on breast conservation. In Harris J, Hellman S, and Silen W, editors: Conservative management of breast cancer, Philadelphia, 1983, JB Lippincott, pp 77-90.
179. Hedley DW, Friedlander ML, and Taylor IW: Application of DNA flow cytometry to paraffin-embedded archival material for the study of aneuploidy and its clinical significance, Cytometry 6:327, 1985.
180. Hellman S, Harris JR, and Levine MB: Radiation therapy of early carcinoma of the breast without mastectomy, Cancer 46:988, 1980.
181. Helman P, Bennett MB, Leuw JH, et al: Interim report on trial of treatment for operable breast cancer, S Afr Med J 46:1374, 1972.
182. Hermann RE, Esselstyn CB, and Grundfest-Broniatowski S: The treatment of curable breast cancer: the Cleveland Clinic experience. In Grundfest-Broniatowski S and Esselstyn CB, editors: Controversies in breast disease: diagnosis and management, New York, 1988, Marcel Dekker Inc, pp 287-306.
183. Hery M, Namer M, Verschoore J, et al: Conservative treatment of breast cancer: a report of 108 patients, Int J Radiat Oncol Biol Phys 10:2185, 1984.
184. Hibberd AD, Horwood LJ, and Wells JE: Long term prognosis of women with breast cancer in New Zealand: study of survival to 30 yrs, Br Med J 286:1777, 1983.
185. Hirsch J: Radiumchirurgie des Brust Krebses, Dtsch Med Wochenschr 53:1419, 1927.
186. Holland R, Connolly J, Gelman R, et al: The presence of an extensive intraductal component following a limited excision correlates with prominent residual disease in the remainder of the breast, J Clin Oncol 8:113, 1990.
187. Holland R, Veling S, Mravunac M, and Hendriks J: Histologic multifocality of Tis T1-2 breast carcinomas. Implications for clinical trials of breast-conserving surgery, Cancer 56:979, 1985.
188. Hopton DS, Thorogood J, Clayden AD, and MacKinnon D: Histologic grading of breast cancer: significance of grade on recurrence and mortality, Eur J Surg Oncol 15:25, 1989.
189. Horn PL and Thompson D: Risk of contralateral breast cancer: associations with histologic clinical and therapeutic factors, Cancer 62:413, 1988.
190. Host H, Brennhoud IO, and Loeb M: Post-operative radiotherapy in breast cancer: long term results from the Oslo study, Int J Radiat Oncol Biol Phys 12:727, 1986.
191. Hunig R, Walther E, Harder F, et al: The Basel lumpectomy protocol: 5 year experience with a prospective study for conservative treatment of breast cancer. In Harris JR, Hellman S, and Silen W, editors: Conservative management of breast cancer, Philadelphia, 1983, JB Lippincott, pp 23-35.
192. Huvos AG, Woodard HQ, Cahan WG, et al: Post-irradiation osteogenic sarcoma of bone and soft tissues: a clinicopathologic study of 66 patients, Cancer 55:1244, 1985.
193. Jolly PC and Viar W: Reduction of morbidity after radical mastectomy, Am Surg 47:377, 1981.
194. Jones JM and Ribeiro GG: Mortality patterns over 34 years of breast cancer patients in a clinical trial of post-operative radiotherapy, Clin Radiol 40:204, 1989.
195. Kaae S and Johansen H: Does simple mastectomy followed by irradiation offer survival comparable to radical procedures? Int J Radiat Oncol Biol Phys 2:1163, 1977.
196. Kaae S and Johansen H: Simple mastectomy plus postoperative irradiation by the method of McWhirter for mammary carcinoma, Ann Surg 170:895, 1969.
197. Kantorowitz DA, Poulter CA, Rubin P, et al: Treatment of breast cancer with segmental mastectomy alone or segmental mastectomy plus radiation, Radiother Oncol 15:141, 1989.
198. Karaparkar AP, Pandya SK, and Desai AP: Radiation induced sarcoma, Surg Neurol 13:419, 1980.
199. Keynes G: Conservative treatment of cancer of the breast, Br Med J 2:643, 1937.
200. Keynes G: The radium treatment of carcinoma of the breast, Br J Surg 19:425, 1931.
201. Keynes G: The treatment of primary carcinoma of the breast with radium, Acta Radiol 10:393, 1929.
202. Komaki R, Cox JD, Kister SJ, et al: Stage I and II breast carcinoma: treatment with limited surgery and radiation versus mastectomy, Radiology 174:255, 1990.
203. Kori SH, Foley KM, and Posner JB: Brachial plexus lesions in patients with cancer: 100 cases, Neurology 31:45, 1981.
204. Koscielny S, Le MG, and Tubiana M: The natural history of human breast cancer: the relationship between involvement of axillary lymph nodes and the initiation of distant metastases, Br J Cancer 59:775, 1989.
205. Koscielny S, Tubiana M, Le MG, et al: Breast cancer: relationship between size of the primary tumor and probability of metastatic dissemination, Br J Cancer 49:709, 1984.
206. Kurtz JM, Amalric R, Brandone H, et al: Local recurrence after breast-conserving surgery and radiotherapy: frequency, time course and prognosis, Cancer 63:1912, 1989.
207. Kurtz JM, Amalric R, Brandone H, et al: Contralateral breast cancer and other second malignancies in patients treated by breast-conserving therapy with radiation, Int J Radiat Oncol Biol Phys 15:277, 1988.
208. Kurtz JM, Amalric R, Brandone H, et al: Results of salvage surgery for mammary recurrence following breast-conserving therapy, Ann Surg 207:347, 1988.
209. Kurtz JM, Amalric R, Delouche G, et al: The second ten years: long-term risks of breast conservation in early breast cancer, Int J Radiat Oncol Biol Phys 13:1327, 1987.
210. Kurtz JM, Spitalier J, Amalric R, et al: The prognostic significance of late local recurrence after breast conserving therapy, Int J Radiat Oncol Biol Phys 18:87, 1990.
211. Kute TE, Muss HB, Hopkins M, et al: Relationship of flow cytometry results to clinical and steroid receptor status in human breast cancer, Breast Cancer Res Treat 6:113, 1985.
212. Kuten A, Sapir D, Cohen Y, et al: Post-irradiation soft tissue sarcoma occurring in breast cancer patients: report of seven cases and results of combination chemotherapy, J Surg Oncol 28:168, 1985.
213. Lacour J, Bucalossi P, Caceres E, et al: Radical mastectomy vs. radical mastectomy plus internal mammary dissection: five year results of an international cooperative study, Cancer 37:206, 1976.
214. Lacour J, Le M, Caceres E, et al: Radical mastectomy versus radical mastectomy plus internal mammary dissection: ten year results of an international cooperative trial in breast cancer, Cancer 51:1941, 1983.
215. Lacour J, Le MG, Hill C, et al: Is it useful to remove internal mammary nodes in operable breast cancer? Eur J Surg Oncol 13:309, 1987.
216. Lagios MD: Multicentricity of breast carcinoma demonstrated by routine correlated serial subgross and radiographic examination, Cancer 40:1726, 1977.

217. Lagios MD, Richards UE, Rose MR, and Yee E: Segmental mastectomy without radiotherapy: short-term follow-up, Cancer 52:2173, 1983.
218. Land CE: Low-dose irradiation: a cause of breast cancer? Cancer 46:868, 1980.
219. Langlands AO, Pocock SJ, Kerr GR, and Gore SM: Long-term survival of patients with breast cancer: a study of the curability of the disease, Br Med J 2:1247, 1979.
220. Langlands AO, Prescott RJ, and Hamilton T: A clinical trial in the management of operable cancer of the breast, Br J Surg 67:170, 1980.
221. Larson P, Weinstein M, Goldberg I, et al: Edema of the arm as a function of the extent of axillary surgery in patients with Stage I-II carcinoma of the breast treated with primary radiotherapy, Int J Radiat Oncol Biol Phys 12:1575, 1986.
222. Lash RH, Bauer TW, Hermann RE, and Esselstyn CB: Partial mastectomy: pathologic findings and prognosis, Hum Pathol 17:813, 1986.
223. Lavey RS and Prosnitz LR: Impact of radiation therapy and/or chemotherapy on the risk for a second malignancy following breast cancer. Proceedings of the European Society for Therapeutic Radiology and Oncology, Seventh Annual Meeting, Den Haag, 1988, p 38.
224. Lee RO and Lambley DG: Radical mastectomy in the treatment of breast cancer, Br J Surg 58:137, 1971.
225. Leis HP: Modified radical mastectomy: definition and role in breast cancer surgery, Int Surg 65:211, 1980.
226. Lesser ML, Rosen PP, and Kinne DW: Multicentricity and bilaterality in invasive breast carcinoma, Surgery 91:234, 1982.
227. Leung S, Otmezguine Y, Calitchi E, et al: Local regional recurrences following radical external beam irradiation and interstitial implantation for operable breast cancer: a twenty three year experience, Radiother Oncology 5:1, 1986.
228. Levine M, Goodyear M, Gent M, et al: Systemic adjuvant chemotherapy reduces ipsilateral breast recurrence following lumpectomy: results from a randomized trial, Proc Am Soc Clin Oncol 9:33, 1990 (abstract).
229. Levitt SH: Is there a role for post-operative adjuvant radiation in breast cancer? Beautiful hypothesis versus ugly facts: 1987 Gilbert H. Fletcher lecture, Int J Radiat Oncol Biol Phys 14:787, 1988.
230. Levitt SH, Potish RA, Boen JR, and Lindgren B: The effect of definitive irradiation on local control and disease free survival in breast cancer, Int J Radiat Oncol Biol Phys 12:673, 1986.
231. Lichter AS, Lippman ME, Gorrell CR, et al: Adjuvant chemotherapy in patients treated primarily with irradiation for localized breast cancer. In Harris J, Hellman S, and Silen W, editors: Conservative management of breast cancer, Philadelphia, 1983, JB Lippincott, pp 299-310.
232. Livingston SF and Arlen M: The extended extrapleural radical mastectomy: its role in the treatment of carcinoma of the breast, Ann Surg 179:260, 1974.
233. Loprinzi CL, Carbone PP, Tormey DC, et al: Aggressive combined modality therapy for advanced local-regional breast carcinoma, J Clin Oncol 2:157, 1984.
234. Lythgoe JP and Palmer MK: Manchester regional breast study: 5 and 10 year results, Br J Surg 69:693, 1982.
235. Madden JL: Modified radical mastectomy, Surg Gynecol Obstet 121:1221, 1965.
236. Maddox WA, Carpenter JT, Laws HT, et al: Does radical mastectomy still have a place in the treatment of primary operable breast cancer? Arch Surg 122:1317, 1987.
237. Maddox WA, Carpenter JT, Laws HL, et al: A randomized prospective trial of radical (Halsted) mastectomy versus modified radical mastectomy in 311 breast cancer patients, Ann Surg 198:207, 1983.
238. Magno L, Bigrardi M, Micheletti E, et al: Analysis of prognostic factors in patients with isolated chest wall recurrence of breast cancer, Cancer 60:240, 1987.
239. Mansour EG, Gray R, Shattle AH, et al: Efficacy of adjuvant chemotherapy in high risk node-negative breast cancer: an intergroup study, N Engl J Med 320:485, 1989.
240. March HC: Leukemia in radiologists, ten years later, Am J Med Sci 242:137, 1961.
241. Margottini M: Recent developments in the surgical treatment of breast carcinoma, Acta Union Int Cancer 8:176, 1952.
242. Martin DS: An appraisal of chemotherapy as an adjuvant to surgery for cancer, Am J Surg 97:685, 1959.
243. Martin JK, van Heerden JA, Taylor WF, and Gaffey TA: Is modified radical mastectomy really equivalent to radical mastectomy in treatment of carcinoma of the breast? Cancer 57:510, 1986.
244. McCredie JA, Inch WR, and Alderson M: Consecutive primary carcinomas of the breast, Cancer 35:1472, 1975.
245. McWhirter R: The value of simple mastectomy and radiotherapy in the treatment of cancer of the breast, Br J Radiol 21:599, 1948.
246. Meier P, Ferguson DJ, and Karrison T: A controlled trial of extended radical versus radical mastectomy: ten-year results, Cancer 63:188, 1989.
247. Meyer AC, Smith SS, and Potter M: Carcinoma of the breast: a clinical study, Arch Surg 113:364, 1978.
248. Meyer JE, Kopans DB, Stomper PC, and Lindfors KK: Occult breast abnormalities: percutaneous preoperative needle localization, Radiology 150:335, 1984.
249. Meyer JS, Prey MU, Babcock DS, and McDivitt RW: Breast carcinoma cell kinetics, morphology, stage and host characteristics: a thymidine labeling study, Lab Invest 54:41, 1986.
250. Meyer W: An improved method of the radical operation for carcinoma of the breast, Med Rec 46:746, 1894.
251. Moffat FL, Ketcham AS, Robinson DS, et al: Segmental mastectomy without radiotherapy for T_1 and small T_2 breast carcinomas, Arch Surg 125:364, 1990.
252. Montague ED: Conservative surgery and radiation therapy in the treatment of operable breast cancer, Cancer 53:700, 1984.
253. Montague ED, Ames FC, Schnell SR, and Romsdahl MM: Conservative surgery and irradiation as an alternative to mastectomy in the treatment of clinically favorable breast cancer, Cancer 54:2668, 1984.
254. Montague ED and Fletcher GH: Local regional effectiveness of surgery and radiation therapy in the treatment of breast cancer, Cancer 55:2266, 1985.
255. Montague ED, Schell SR, Romsdahl MD, and Ames FS: Conservative surgery and irradiation in clinically favorable breast cancer: the M.D. Anderson experience. In Harris J, Hellman S, and Silen W, editors: Conservative management of breast cancer, Philadelphia, 1983, JB Lippincott, pp 53-60.
256. Montgomery ACV, Greening WP, and Levene AL: Clinical study of recurrence rate and survival time of patients with carcinoma of the breast treated by biopsy excision without any other therapy, J R Soc Med 71:339, 1978.
257. Moran RE, Black MM, Alpert L, and Straus MJ: Correlation of cell-cycle kinetics, hormone receptors, histopathology and nodal status in human breast cancer, Cancer 54:1586, 1984.
258. Morgenstern L, Kaufman PA, and Friedman NB: The case against tylectomy for carcinoma of the breast: the factor of multicentricity, Am J Surg 130:251, 1975.
259. Mustakallio S: Conservative treatment of breast carcinoma: review of 25 years follow-up, Clin Radiol 23:110, 1972.

260. National Academy of Sciences Committee on the Biologic Effects of Ionizing Radiations: The effects on populations of exposure to low levels of ionizing radiation: 1980, Washington, DC, National Academy Press, 1980, p 524.
261. Nemoto T, Natarajan N, Bedwani R, et al: Breast cancer in the medial half: results of 1978 national survey of the American College of Surgeons, Cancer 51:1333, 1983.
262. Nemoto T, Vana J, Bedwani RN, et al: Management and survival of female breast cancer: results of a national survey by the American College of Surgeons, Cancer 45:2917, 1980.
263. Nissen-Meyer R, Kjellgren K, Malmio K, et al: Surgical adjuvant chemotherapy: results with one short course with cyclophosphamide after mastectomy for breast cancer, Cancer 41:2088, 1978.
264. Osborne MP, Ormiston N, Harmer CL, et al: Breast conservation in the treatment of early breast cancer, Cancer 53:349, 1984.
265. Owens MA, Beardslee S, Wenger CR, et al: DNA flow cytometry correlates with other prognostic factors for breast cancer, Breast Cancer Res Treat 14:134, 1989 (abstract).
266. Pagana TJ, Lubbe WJ, Schwartz SM, and Sprechini GD: A comparison of palpable and non-palpable breast cancers, Arch Surg 124:26, 1989.
267. Papatestas AE and Lesnick GJ: Treatment of carcinoma of the breast by modified radical mastectomy, Surg Gynecol Obstet 140:22, 1975.
268. Parker RG, Grimm P, and Enstrom JE: Contralateral breast cancers following treatment for initial breast cancers in women, Am J Clin Oncol 12:213-216, 1989.
269. Patey DH and Dyson WH: The prognosis of carcinoma of the breast in relation to the type of operation performed, Br J Cancer 2:7, 1948.
270. Peters MV: Wedge resection with or without radiation in early breast cancer, Int J Radiat Biol Phys 2:1151, 1977.
271. Pierquin B: Conservative treatment for carcinoma of the breast: experience of Creteil—ten year results. In Harris J, Hellman S, and Silen W, editors: Conservative management of breast cancer, Philadelphia, 1983, JB Lippincott, pp 11-14.
272. Pierquin B and Marin L: The past and future of conservative treatment of breast cancer, Am J Clin Oncol 9(6):476, 1986.
273. Pierquin B, Mazeron J, and Glaubiger D: Conservative treatment of breast cancer in Europe: report of the groupe Europeen du Curietherapie, Radiother Oncol 6:187, 1986.
274. Powell S and Cooke J: Radiation induced brachial plexus injury: follow-up of two different fractionation schedules. Proceedings of the Fifth European Conference on Clinical Oncology, London, England, September 1989 (abstract).
275. Prosnitz LR, Weshler Z, and Goldenberg IS: Primary radiotherapy for breast carcinoma instead of mastectomy: the Yale experience. In Harris J, Hellman S, and Silen W, editors: Conservative management of breast cancer, Philadelphia, 1983, JB Lippincott, pp 61-70.
276. Ransom DT and Cameron FG: Scleroderma: a possible contra-indication to lumpectomy and radiotherapy in breast carcinoma, Australas Radiol 31:317, 1987.
277. Ray GR, Fish VJ, Lee RH, et al: Biopsy and definitive radiation therapy in stages I and II carcinoma of the female breast, Int J Radiat Oncol Biol Phys 9:23, 1983.
278. Recht A, Connolly JL, Schnitt SJ, et al: Conservative surgery and radiation therapy for early breast cancer: results, controversies, and unsolved problems, Semin Oncol 13:434, 1986.
279. Recht A, Schnitt SJ, Connolly JL, et al: Prognosis following local or regional recurrence after conservative surgery and radiotherapy for early stage breast carcinoma, Int J Radiat Oncol Biol Phys 16:3, 1989.
280. Recht A, Silen W, Schnitt SJ, et al: Time course of local recurrence following conservative surgery and radiotherapy for early stage breast cancer, Int J Radiat Oncol Biol Phys 15:255, 1988.
281. Reger V, Beito G, and Jolly PC: Factors affecting the incidence of lymph node metastases in small cancers of the breast, Am J Surg 157:501, 1989.
282. Robbins GF, editor: Silvergirl's surgery: the breast, Austin, Texas, 1984, Silvergirl Inc.
283. Robinson GN, van Heerden JA, Payne WS, et al: The primary surgical treatment of carcinoma of the breast: a changing trend toward modified radical mastectomy, Mayo Clin Proc 51:433, 1976.
284. Roseman JM and James AG: The significance of internal mammary lymph nodes in medially located breast cancer, Cancer 50:1426, 1982.
285. Rosen PP, Fracchia AA, Urban JA, et al: "Residual" mammary carcinoma following simulated partial mastectomy, Cancer 35:739, 1975.
286. Rosen PP, Groshen S, Saigo PE, et al: A long-term follow-up study of survival in stage I (T1N0M0) and stage II (T1N1M0) breast carcinoma, J Clin Oncol 7:355, 1989.
287. Rosen PP, Kinne DW, Lesser M, and Hellman S: Are prognostic factors for local control of breast cancer treated by primary radiotherapy significant for patients treated by mastectomy? Cancer 57:1415, 1986.
288. Rubin E, Maddox WA, and Mazur MT: Cutaneous angiosarcoma of the breast 7 years after lumpectomy and radiation therapy, Radiology 174:258:1990.
289. Rutqvist LE and Wallgren A: Long-term survival of 458 young breast cancer patients, Cancer 55:658, 1985.
290. Rutqvist LE, Wallgren A, and Nilsson B: Is breast cancer a curable disease? A study of 14,731 women with breast cancer from the cancer registry of Norway, Cancer 53:1793, 1984.
291. Sacre RA: Clinical evaluation of axillary lymph nodes compared to surgical and pathologic findings, Eur J Surg Oncol 12:169, 1986.
292. Sainsbury JRC, Needham GK, Farndon JR, et al: Epidermal-growth-factor receptor status as predictor of early recurrence of and death from breast cancer, Lancet i:1398, 1987.
293. Sams A: Histologic changes in the larger blood vessels of the hind limb of the mouse after x-irradiation, Int J Radiat Biol 9:165, 1965.
294. Sarrazin D, Dewar JA, Arriagada R, et al: Conservative management of breast cancer, Br J Surg 73:604, 1986.
295. Sarrazin D, Le MG, Arriagada R, et al: Ten-year results of a randomized trial comparing a conservative treatment to mastectomy in early breast cancer, Radiother Oncol 14:177, 1989.
296. Sarrazin D, Le MG, Fontaine MF, and Arriagada R: Conservative treatment versus mastectomy in T_1 or small T_2 breast cancer: a randomized clinical trial. In Harris J, Hellman S, and Silen W, editors: Conservative management of breast cancer, Philadelphia, 1983, JB Lippincott, pp 101-111.
297. Say CC and Donegan W: A biostatistical evaluation of complications from mastectomy, Surg Gynecol Obstet 138:370, 1974.
298. Say CC and Donegan WL: Invasive carcinoma of the breast: prognostic significance of tumor size and involved axillary lymph nodes, Cancer 34:468, 1974.
299. Schabel FM: Concepts for treatment of micrometastases developed in murine systems, Am J Roentgenol Radium Ther Nucl Med 126:500, 1976.
300. Schottenfeld D, Nash AG, Robbins GF, and Beattie EJ: Ten-year results of the treatment of primary operable breast carcinoma, Cancer 38:1001, 1976.

301. Schwartz GF, Feig SA, Rosenberg AL, et al: Staging and treatment of clinically occult breast cancer, Cancer 53:1379, 1984.
302. Schwartz GF, Patchefsky AS, Feig SA, et al: Clinically occult breast cancer: multicentricity and implications for treatment, Ann Surg 191:8, 1980.
303. Shah JA, Rosen PP, and Robins GF: Pitfalls of local excision in the treatment of carcinoma of the breast, Surg Gynecol Obstet 136:721, 1973.
304. Shaikh NA, Beaconsfield T, Walker M, and Ghilchik NW: Postirradiation angiosarcoma of the breast: a case report, Eur J Surg Oncol 14:449, 1988.
305. Shimkin MB, Koppel M, Connolly RR, and Cutler SJ: Simple and radical mastectomy for breast cancer: a re-analysis of Smith and Meyer's report from Rockford, Illinois, J Natl Cancer Inst 27:1197, 1961.
306. Simon R: Overviews of randomized clinical trials, Cancer Treat Rep 71:3, 1987.
307. Skipper HE: Kinetics of mammary tumor cell growth and implications for therapy, Cancer 28:1479, 1971.
308. Smart CR, Myers MH, and Gloecker LA: Implications from SEER data on breast cancer management, Cancer 41:787, 1978.
309. Smith JA, Gamez-Araujo J, Gallagher HS, et al: Carcinoma of the breast: analysis of total lymph node involvement versus level of metastases, Cancer 39:527, 1977.
310. Smith PG: Leukemia and other cancers following radiation treatment of pelvic disease, Cancer 39:1901, 1977.
311. Solin LJ, Fowble B, Martz KL, and Goodman RL: Definitive irradiation for early stage breast cancer: the University of Pennsylvania experience, Int J Radiat Oncol Biol Phys 14:235, 1988.
312. Souba WW, McKenna RJ Jr, Benjamin R, et al: Radiation-induced sarcomas of the chest wall, Cancer 57:610, 1986.
313. Spitalier JM, Gambarelli J, Brandone H, et al: Breast conserving surgery with radiation therapy for operable mammary carcinoma: a 25 year experience, World J Surg 10:1014, 1986.
314. Stewart FW and Treves N: Lymphangiosarcoma in post-mastectomy lymphedema: a report of six cases in elephantiasis chirurgica, Cancer 1:64, 1948.
315. Storm HH and Jensen OM: Risk of contralateral breast cancer in Denmark 1943-1980, Br J Cancer 54:483, 1986.
316. Stotter AT, McNeese MD, Ames FC, et al: Predicting the rate and extent of locoregional failure after breast conservation therapy for early breast cancer, Cancer 64:2217, 1989.
317. Strax P: Results in mass screening for breast cancer in 50,000 examinations, Cancer 37:30-35, 1976.
318. Sugarbaker ED: Extended radical mastectomy: its superiority in the treatment of breast cancer, JAMA 187:96, 1964.
319. Suit HD and Westgate SJ: Impact of improved local control on survival, Int J Radiat Oncol Biol Phys 12:453, 1986.
320. Sutherland CM and Mather FJ: Long term survival and prognostic factors in breast cancer patients with localized (no skin, muscle or chest wall attachment) disease with and without positive lymph nodes, Cancer 57:622, 1986.
321. Swedborg I and Wallgren A: The effect of pre- and post-mastectomy radiotherapy on the degree of edema, shoulder joint mobility and gripping force, Cancer 47:877, 1981.
322. Symmonds RE and Roberts JW: Management of nonpalpable breast abnormalities, Ann Surg 205:520, 1987.
323. Tagart REB: Partial mastectomy alone in early breast cancer, Br Med J 290:434, 1985.
324. Tandon AK, Clark GM, Chamness GC, et al: Cathepsin D and prognosis in breast cancer, N Engl J Med 322:297, 1990.
325. Tandon AK, Clark GM, Chamness GC, et al: HER-2/neu oncogene protein and prognosis in breast cancer, J Clin Oncol 7:1120, 1989.
326. Tinnemans JGM, Wobbes T, Holland R, et al: Treatment and survival of female patients with nonpalpable breast carcinoma, Ann Surg 209:249, 1989.
327. Tinnemans JGM, Wobbes T, van der Sluis RF, et al: Multicentricity in nonpalpable breast carcinoma and its implications for treatment, Am J Surg 151:334, 1986.
328. Toi M, Nakamura T, Mukaida H, et al: Relationship between epidermal growth factor receptor status and various prognostic factors in human breast cancer, Cancer 65:1980, 1990.
329. Tokunaga M, Norman JE Jr, Asano M, et al: Malignant breast tumors among atomic bomb survivors, Hiroshima and Nagasaki 1950-74, J Natl Cancer Inst 62:1347, 1979.
330. Toonkel LM, Fix I, Jacobson UH, and Wallach CB: The significance of local recurrence of carcinoma of the breast, Int J Radiat Oncol Biol Phys 9:33, 1983.
331. Tracy GP, Brown DE, Johnson LW, and Gottlieb J: Radiation induced coronary artery disease, JAMA 228:1660, 1974.
332. Tubiana M, Arriagada R, and Sarrazin D: Human cancer natural history, radiation induced immunodepression and post-operative radiation therapy, Int J Radiat Oncol Biol Phys 12:477, 1986.
333. Turnbull AR, Chant ADB, Buchanan RB, et al: Treatment of early breast cancer, Lancet ii:7, 1978.
334. Turner L, Swindell R, Bell WGT, et al: Radical versus modified radical mastectomy for breast cancer, Ann R Coll Surg Engl 63:239, 1981.
335. Turner-Warnick RT: Lymphatics of the breast, Br J Surg 46:524, 1959.
336. Uppsala-Orebro Breast Cancer Study Group: Sector resection with or without postoperative radiotherapy for Stage I breast cancer: a randomized trial, J Natl Cancer Inst 82:277, 1990.
337. Urban JA: Management of operable breast cancer: the surgeon's view, Cancer 42:2066, 1978.
338. Urban JA and Baker HW: Radical mastectomy in continuity with en block resection of the internal mammary lymph node chain, Cancer 5:992, 1952.
339. Urban JA and Marjani MA: Significance of internal mammary lymph node metastases in breast cancer, Am J Roentgenol Radium Ther Nucl Med 3:130, 1971.
340. Valagussa P, Bonadonna G, and Veronesi U: Patterns of relapse and survival following radical mastectomy: analysis of 716 consecutive patients, Cancer 41:1170, 1978.
341. Van de Vijver MJ, Peterse JL, Mooi WJ, et al: Neu-protein overexpression in breast cancer: association with comedo-type ductal carcinoma in situ and limited prognostic value in stage II breast cancer, N Engl J Med 319:1239, 1988.
342. Van Dongen JA: Randomized clinical trial to assess the value of breast conserving therapy in stage I and II breast cancer; EORTC trial 10801. Proceedings of the NIH Consensus Development Conference—Early Stage Breast Cancer, June 1990, pp 25-27.
343. Van Limbergen E, Van der Bogaert W, Van der Schueren E, and Rijnders A: Tumor excision and radiotherapy as primary treatment of breast cancer analysis of patient and treatment parameters and local control, Radiother Oncol 8:1, 1987.
344. Veronesi U: Breast conservation trials of the NCI-Milan. Proceedings of the NIH Consensus Development Conference—Early Stage Breast Cancer, June 1990, pp 19-22.
345. Veronesi U, Banfi A, DelVecchio M, et al: Comparison of Halsted mastectomy with quadrantectomy, axillary dissection and radiotherapy in early breast cancer: long-term results, Eur J Cancer Clin Oncol 22:1085, 1986.

346. Veronesi U, Cascinelli N, Greco M, et al: Prognosis of breast cancer patients after mastectomy and dissection of internal mammary nodes, Ann Surg 202:702, 1985.
347. Veronesi U, Cascinelli N, and Luini AL: The surgical treatment of curable breast cancer: the Milan experience. In Grundfest-Broniatowski S and Esselstyn CB, editors: Controversies in breast disease: diagnosis and management, New York, 1988, Marcel Dekker Inc, pp 307-318.
348. Veronesi U, Saccozzi R, DelVecchio M, et al: Comparing radical mastectomy with quadrantectomy, axillary dissection and radiotherapy in patients with small cancers of the breast, N Engl J Med 305:6, 1981.
349. Veronesi U and Valagussa P: Inefficacy of internal mammary nodes dissection in breast cancer surgery, Cancer 47:170, 1981.
350. Veronesi U and Zingo L: Extended mastectomy for cancer of the breast, Cancer 20:677, 1967.
351. Veronesi U, Zucali R, and Del Vecchio M: Conservative treatment of breast cancer with the Q.U.A.R.T. technique, World J Surg 9:767, 1985.
352. Virchow R: Cellular pathology, Philadelphia, JB Lippincott Co, 1863 (Translated by Frank Chase).
353. von Rosen A, Rutgvist LE, Carstensen J, et al: Prognostic value of nuclear DNA content in breast cancer in relation to tumor size, nodal status and estrogen receptor content, Breast Cancer Res Treat 13:23, 1989.
354. Wallgren A, Arner O, Bergstrom J, et al: Radiation therapy in operable breast cancer: results from the Stockholm trial on adjuvant radiotherapy, Int J Radiat Oncol Biol Phys 12:533, 1986.
355. Wangensteen OH: Remarks on extension of the Halsted operation for cancer of the breast, Ann Surg 130:315, 1949.
356. Wangensteen OH, Lewis FJ, and Arhelger SW: The extended or superradical mastectomy for carcinoma of the breast: a justification for a conservative operation, Surg Clin North Am 36:1051, 1956.
357. Warren S and Sommer GM: Fibrosarcoma of the soft parts with special reference to recurrence and metastasis, Arch Surg 33:425, 1936.
358. Williams JG, Murley RS, and Curwen MP: Carcinoma of the female breast: conservative and radical surgery, Br Med J 2:788, 1953.
359. Williams MR, Hinton CP, Todd JH, et al: The prediction of local or regional recurrence after simple mastectomy for operable breast cancer, Br J Surg 72:721, 1985.
360. Wilson RE, Donegan WL, Mettlin C, et al: The 1982 national survey of carcinoma of the breast in the United States by the American College of Surgeons, Surg Gynecol Obstet 159:309, 1984.
361. Wolmark N: Current generation of NSABP studies. Paper presented at the Scripps 20th Annual Cancer Symposium, San Diego, November 1988.
362. Wood KM: Intercostobrachial nerve entrapment syndrome, S Afr Med J 71:662, 1978.
363. Zucali R, Luini A, Del Vecchio M, et al: Contralateral breast cancer after limited surgery plus radiotherapy of early mammary tumors, Eur J Surg Oncol 13:413, 1989.

4 Surgical Considerations in the Management of Breast Cancer

Ernest F. Rosato and Paul G. Curcillo II

This chapter reviews various surgical procedures and techniques used in the management of breast cancer, including fine needle aspiration, biopsy for palpable masses or mammographic abnormalities, modified radical mastectomy, total mastectomy, and partial mastectomy and axillary dissection. The emphasis is on surgical procedures currently used at the University of Pennsylvania. A more detailed analysis of the history of surgical procedures for breast cancer, as well as the results of retrospective series, intrainstitutional comparisons and prospective randomized trials, is presented in Chapter 3. Complications related to the various procedures also are presented in Chapter 3. The role of mastectomy in the treatment of ductal carcinoma in situ and breast cancer presenting as axillary adenopathy are reviewed briefly in this chapter. Additional information may be found in Chapters 13 and 20. The technical aspects of breast conservation surgery also are presented. Details of patient selection, radiotherapy technique, and integration with chemotherapy, however, are outlined in Chapter 5. The role of surgery in the treatment of locally advanced breast cancer is presented in Chapter 14.

FINE NEEDLE ASPIRATION

Fine needle aspiration was introduced in 1930,[43] but its acceptance among general surgeons has been relatively slow. Originally, concerns were voiced about needle track implantations. However, many studies have shown no difference in treatment outcome in cases where fine needle aspiration has been initially employed.[53] Despite these assurances, accurate records should be kept of the site of needle track placement and the track should take the shortest and most direct course to the tumor mass. If these precautions are followed, the needle track can be subsequently removed whether the patient has mastectomy or breast conserving surgery/radiotherapy for definitive treatment.

Aspiration techniques utilizing a stereotactic device or using mammographic localization techniques have been described and have the potential for eliminating many biopsies now performed for mammographic abnormalities. We have not utilized these techniques. Mammographic abnormalities have been treated by excision and not fine needle aspiration because of the risk of a false-negative aspiration. Fine needle aspiration in our practice has been limited to palpable masses. Provided that a satisfactory specimen has been obtained, the diagnostic accuracy of a needle aspirate positive for carcinoma is quite high.[73] The false-negative rate of the procedure is low but is estimated at up to 10% even with good specimen quality. It should be emphasized that tissue that does not contain epithelial cells cannot be relied upon for diagnostic purposes. Smith et al.[66] evaluated fine needle aspiration utilizing a 22-gauge needle with immediate smear preparation and review by the cytopathologist. Of 133 carcinomas, 68% were identified as malignant and 17% as suspicious by the aspirate. Of these malignant tumors, 6% were interpreted as benign and 9% were unsatisfactory cell preparations. Conversely, all cytopathologically identified carcinomas were confirmed by biopsy. There were therefore no false-positive studies in this particular report. A contrasting analysis by Wolberg[75] was reported for 378 patients in whom epithelial cells were obtained. In this group of aspirates, three false-negative (no tumor seen) and 16 false-positive (tumor identified but subsequent biopsy benign) identifications were made. Therefore a fine needle aspirate cannot be relied upon to have 100% accuracy in either confirming the presence of carcinoma or excluding its presence. The rate of accuracy will be determined not only by the technique, but by the cytopathologists involved in the interpretation.

Because of the possibility of an incorrect diagnosis, careful follow-up examination is required whenever the diagnosis is benign. Additionally, the presence of a benign diagnosis should not outweigh other clinical parameters that are suspicious for carcinoma. These standard criteria for diagnosis should not be discarded because of the presence of a benign cytopathologic aspirate. If the lesion is reported as benign, more than one aspirate should be performed to reduce sampling error problems. Attention to technical preparation of the specimen should be intensified. In our institution, the cytopathologist actually is present at the time of aspiration for immediate and optimal preparation of the cytologic smear. In situations where all clinical parameters are consistent with a benign diagnosis and the cytopathologist obtains a good epithelial smear that is benign, follow-up can be recommended with a fair degree of safety. However, this follow-up should be arranged definitely and should include follow-up aspiration if the area of suspicion remains. Finally, it should be kept in mind that open biopsy is the "gold standard" of diagnosis. Persistent abnormalities in most cases should be removed, even when the weight of evidence is strongly in favor of it being a benign lesion.

When the fine needle aspirate results in a positive diagnosis for malignancy, our practice has been to confirm this finding by open biopsy at the time of definitive treatment. However, given the extreme accuracy of positive fine needle aspiration, the definitive treatment is arranged as a single procedure, following counseling of the patient, appropriate staging studies, and consultation with both radiation and medical oncologists where indicated. At this single operation, an open biopsy is performed to confirm the diagnosis of carcinoma. Assuming that the frozen section diagnosis of carcinoma is definite, then the definitive procedure can be performed.

The technique of fine needle aspiration used at this institution is designed to minimize the risk of obtaining a poor specimen for analysis. The cytopathologist is present to prepare the air-dried slides immediately and to assess the quality of the cellular aspirate. Repeat aspirates are performed if the initial aspirate is not satisfactory in terms of cell numbers or quality. A 23-gauge needle attached to a 10-ml syringe is utilized. Local anesthesia generally is not used because fine needle aspiration is not particularly painful, and nothing should be injected into the mass itself. The needle is inserted into the mass and forceful suction pressure applied with the syringe. The needle is then moved in several directions within the mass, making three to six passes into the area in different directions while maintaining negative syringe pressure. The pressure is released from the syringe before the needle is withdrawn in order to leave the specimen within the hub of the needle. For instances where a cytopathologist cannot be present, the technique of slide preparation is an important feature. Techniques are described in many standard texts, but it is best to confer with the cytopathologist who will be interpreting the slides prepared and utilize the technique favored by him or her.

BREAST BIOPSY

Indications for biopsy

The diagnosis of breast cancer generally is made by self-examination of the breast, mammography, or physician examination. Biopsy of the breast is utilized liberally because of the relative insensitivity of laboratory methods such as mammography, ultrasonography, and thermography. As many as 80% of these biopsies prove benign because the biopsy is a diagnostic test as well as possible therapy. Because biopsy has a relatively low morbidity rate and can be performed utilizing local anesthesia and sedation, this continued liberal application seems to be in the best interests of the patient. The presence of a dominant mass is an indication for a biopsy and removal of that mass. In very young women with a slippable, firm, smooth mass that is clinically and mammographically characteristic of a fibroadenoma, observation may be appropriate. In this instance, fine needle aspiration should be carried out and the patient warned of the importance of close follow-up observation by self-examination and continued physician evaluation. Increase in the size of the nodule should prompt excision. Except for this circumstance, a persistent dominant solid mass should be removed, even if fine needle aspiration is negative for malignancy. Secondary signs of malignancy such as skin dimpling, and peau d'orange make biopsy mandatory even though such signs are occasionally secondary to fat necrosis or trauma. Occasionally, a red, indurated breast may be secondary to localized infection and may initially be treated by diagnostic aspiration and antibiotics. However, failure of the problem to resolve promptly and completely should lead to early biopsy to rule out an underlying inflammatory type of carcinoma.

Nipple discharge may occasionally be the presenting symptom of breast disease. When associated with a mass, the mass always should be biopsied. The nipple discharge should be examined for blood and also subjected to cytologic inspection. Factors associated with increased malignancy include a bloody nipple discharge and the presence of an associated mass. In the absence of a mass, age is an important consideration in assessing the risk of malignancy.[64] A persistent discharge from a single duct, particularly unilaterally, should prompt excision of that duct whether the discharge is bloody or nonbloody. Leis[42] reported that nipple discharge was the chief complaint in 7.4% of patients undergoing surgery in a series of 8703 breast operations. He analyzed the multiple types of discharge present, dividing them into seven types: (1) milky, (2) multicolored and sticky, (3) purulent, (4) clear/watery, (5) yellow or serous, (6) pink or serosanguinous, and (7) bloody or sanguinous. The first three types were generally benign. While the others were usually benign, he recommended surgery to obtain tissue for diagnosis. An important point of emphasis is that the discharge must be spontaneous and persistent and not be occurring during lactation. Many women firmly manipulate the nipple during self-examination and obtain a "discharge" that has no significance. An increasing likelihood of cancer associated with discharge occurs in order of increasing frequency as follows: with yellow, pink, bloody, or watery discharge, when it is accompanied by a mass, when it is unilateral and from a single duct, when mammogram or cytology results are positive, and when the patient is >50 years of age. While these statistical analyses are helpful, the end result is that a patient with a nipple discharge from a single duct requires excision of that duct for definite diagnosis.

Devitt[13] emphasizes the low rate of cancer in patients with a nipple discharge without any other signs of carcinoma. He recommends excision of the duct in the absence of other signs if the discharge is from a single duct or if it is yellow, serous, bloody, or black. If nipple discharge is associated with excoriation of the nipple's skin, then Paget's disease with a subareolar carcinoma should be suspected, and the biopsy should include a small portion of the abnormal skin for diagnosis.

Mammographic indications for biopsy have been covered earlier. In general these include clustered microcalcifications, distortion of breast parenchymal architecture, and the presence of suspicious solid masses. It is important to reaffirm that a negative mammogram should not dissuade the surgeon from recommending biopsy in the presence of a palpable abnormality. Equally important, our practice has been to never perform an open biopsy without first obtaining a mammogram. When biopsy is performed, the mammogram may identify additional lesions that require removal and that might alter the ultimate treatment plan. Such additional lesions could be biopsied at the time of the first surgery. It remains surprising that some surgeons will biopsy a palpable mass utilizing an open biopsy without the additional information that a presurgical mammogram might provide.

Technique of breast biopsy

Biopsy of a palpable lesion. The biopsy incision should be made with consideration of the potential morbidity, cosmetic outcome, and effect upon subsequent procedures if the mass is malignant. Circumareolar incisions are the most cosmetic and are used when possible, particularly when there is a low risk of malignancy. If the tumor is malignant, it can be excised fully through such an incision and the patient treated by radiation therapy without further surgery. Conversely, if mastectomy is required, the skin overlying the dissection between the circumareolar incision and the most distal part of the resection margin can be excised as a single ellipse including the nipple/areolar complex. Much is made of the variously described mastectomy incisions, associated with the proponents who described them (e.g., Halsted, Kocher, Stewart, etc.). However, if one analyzes these incisions, they all represent a circle or an ellipse with an additional extension by skin incision where appropriate. Our current approach for mastectomy is to use an ellipse as required to remove the nipple/areolar complex and the area directly overlying the tumor. Any previous biopsy incision should be included in this ellipse, which requires planning of the incision with this subsequent removal in mind. No matter in what quadrant the ellipse is placed, the skin will stretch sufficiently after mobilization of the skin flaps to allow a full mastectomy and axillary dissection if required.

In performing the biopsy, the skin incision descends through the fat layer to the superficial plane of the breast. The plane of dissection then should be developed just superficial to the breast tissue until the area of abnormality is reached. The fatty tissue surrounding the abnormality can then be freed from the breast, preserving the fatty tissue overlying the breast itself. The suspicious breast tissue can be removed widely by scalpel excision through normal breast tissue. If possible, the posterior plane of the breast should not be breached in order not to open tissue planes above the pectoral fascia. However, at times this cannot be avoided as the tumor might extend close to the posterior margin. The margin of resection should be wide enough that one would expect normal histologic margins as well as normal gross margins, avoiding the need for reexcision if carcinoma is present. Circumstances may alter this initial approach. If the lesion is benign by all appearances, smaller margins are taken, even though reexcision for positive margins may be needed. If the lesion is suspicious for carcinoma, a 2-cm margin of excision within the breast tissue is planned. Significant amounts of breast tissue can be removed without cosmetic distortion when the overlying fatty tissue of the breast is preserved. While scalpel excision of the breast tissue is my personal preference, scissors or cautery can be used effectively. Thermocautery has the theoretic disadvantage of denaturing tumor receptors, which are heat labile. Early reports of direct cautery application to the tumor surface producing various protein receptor levels[58] have been challenged recently by studies comparing scalpel and cautery excision with no substantial change in estrogen assay results.[26] The resected tissue should be placed immediately in ice and transported to the pathologist. If the initial procedure was a needle localization, then an x-ray of the specimen should be obtained first, again keeping the specimen on ice. Several studies have demonstrated hormone receptor levels to be lower in mastectomy specimens than in biopsy specimens.[31] This finding suggests that even short periods of warm ischemia lead to changes in labile hormone receptors. This lability also supports the use of preliminary biopsy even when the mass is clearly a carcinoma and has been confirmed by fine needle aspiration (see earlier discussion in this chapter). The preliminary biopsy at the time of definitive surgery allows for confirmation of the diagnosis by whole tissue frozen section analysis and also allows for a more accurate assessment of hormone receptor sites.

The most important cosmetic aspect of a breast biopsy is the preservation of an intact fat layer. Significant amounts of breast tissue can be removed without any noticeable defect if the fat layer has been well preserved. The breast tissue is generally not approximated because it will tend to produce distortion of the overlying skin and fat and may produce fixation to the chest wall, which does not allow the breast to fall freely with changes in body position. Almost all significant cosmetic failures are caused by this type distortion/fixation and not to a defect in the underlying breast tissue that might occur by leaving the breast tissue unopposed. Hemostasis should be meticulous and generally is achieved by electrocautery. Any visible small arteries require ligation to prevent significant hemorrhage. Drainage is not used unless a very large defect has been created, in which case a small Penrose drain is brought out through the incision and is removed the following day. The skin incision is closed with a subcuticular type of suture to avoid the tracking seen with skin sutures. It is imperative to close the underlying preserved fat layer loosely to avoid skin stretching, a wide scar, and a palpable defect in the breast itself. While a breast biopsy is considered a minor procedure, it is imperative to obtain the best cosmetic result, particularly in view of the high percentage of biopsies that are benign.

Local anesthesia is used for all breast biopsies. Epinephrine is added to prolong the anesthetic effect and reduce bleeding, provided there is no medical contraindication to local epinephrine. Intravenous sedation is used in virtually all cases. This combination of local anesthesia and intravenous sedation allows for wide dissection of any portion of the breast tissue, including wide resection required for local removal of the tumor so that patients who are candidates for radiation therapy require no further surgical procedure. A general anesthetic clearly is not required for this type of surgery. The anesthesiologist administers the sedation and monitors the patient, providing analgesia and sedation to allow a wide resection of tissue with excellent safety and allowing the surgeon to pay full attention to the details of the surgical procedure.

Because only 15% to 20% of biopsies are malignant, it is not appropriate to do a full-scale cancer evaluation and consultation before biopsy. Whenever possible, however, the operation is performed as a one-stage procedure, combining the biopsy and the definitive procedure following frozen section analysis. This approach is usually not possible except in those situations where the abnormality is clearly a carcinoma or the use of fine needle aspiration has allowed documentation of a malignant process before the initial biopsy. Although in the majority of biopsy cases this information will not be available, planning for a one-stage procedure is advisable wherever possible. Too often, obvious breast carcinoma is subjected to a preliminary biopsy in a short stay unit to establish a diagnosis that is obvious and could have been established by preoperative needle aspiration and confirmed by frozen section examination. In such a situation, any complications such as extensive bleeding or infection might delay subsequent surgery and would at least lead to the theoretic dissemination of tumor cells through the tissue planes of the breast. Pathologic examination of frozen section specimens by an experienced pathologist allows detection of breast cancer in almost all cases with few (and hopefully none) false-positive examinations.[54] In this regard, the surgeon must not abdicate complete responsibility to the pathologist. If the tumor is not clearly malignant during the surgeon's gross examination, then permanent section results should be awaited rather than placing reliance on frozen section examination. Conversely, the pathologist should make a diagnosis of carcinoma using frozen section examination only when there is no doubt at all. Any marginal pathologic abnormality should be deferred to permanent section examination. If the tumor is malignant by both gross and microscopic frozen examination, then the procedure can be performed without the potential for a tragic false-positive diagnosis. However, realizing the possibility of the above, all minimal carcinomas are subjected to a preliminary biopsy with local anesthesia/sedation. Only obvious carcinomas or those with a positive fine needle aspiration are treated as single-stage procedures. Timing of the subsequent procedure after open biopsy remains important but does not have the urgency originally attributed to it. Fisher et al. noted no difference in survival rates for patients treated within 2 weeks of initial biopsy as compared to those treated more than 2 weeks after surgery.[21] This finding was not altered even in those patients in whom residual tumor was left in the breast at the time of initial biopsy.

Biopsy of a mammographically detected lesion. Mammographically guided biopsy is required for the removal of any mammographically suspect mass, architectural distortion, or microcalcifications that may represent a nonpalpable carcinoma. The presurgical needle localization is used to guide the surgical procedure to the abnormal area. This insures that the suspicious area is removed, the most cosmetic incision is utilized, and the smallest amount of tissue consistent with total removal of the area is sacrificed. Many variations have been described since the early descriptions utilizing direct needle placement.[52] In direct needle placement a hypodermic needle is inserted as close as possible to the abnormal area. Although the patient is sent directly to the operating room, there is concern that the needle will become displaced during preparation for surgery or during the operative dissection itself. To avoid these problems, the technique of needle wire placement[34] is used at the University of Pennsylvania. A malleable wire with a hooked end is inserted through the hypodermic needle. The needle is then withdrawn and the securely placed wire is used for operative guidance. Other variations include the injection of methylene blue dye through the needle with subsequent excision of the stained tissue.[14] Further variations of these basic techniques have been described. One technique utilized injection of both a vital stain for surgical identification and a radiopaque dye for radiographic confirmation of the excision of the suspicious area. Kwasnik et al. have advocated the use of a stiff teflon catheter to replace the needle or wire, allowing easy identification of the course of the tract down to the site of the biopsy.[36] Whatever technique of utilization is used, the specimen should be x-rayed following removal to assure that the abnormal tissue or calcifications have been removed.

At this institution, the needle/wire technique is used, employing a Kopan's wire. The operation is performed utilizing a combination of local anesthesia and intravenous sedation. This allows continuous monitoring by the anesthesiologists, allowing significant safe sedation that makes the surgery far easier for the patient. While local anesthesia alone may be sufficient, the anxiety provoked by the procedure itself and the discomfort associated with the use of only a local anesthetic prompts our use of intravenous sedation in virtually all cases. The surgical technique employed is similar to that described under the breast biopsy technique.

Biopsy in a patient with inflammatory carcinoma. Inflammatory breast cancer patients typically present with erythema and skin edema overlying a large carcinoma of the breast. The carcinoma is most often of a diffuse type and may not be appreciated easily by palpation. The biopsy site should be directly over the most central portion of the abnormality, and an incisional type biopsy only should be used, aimed at confirming diagnosis and obtaining appropriate hormone receptor analysis and other specialized information. The skin should be biopsied to document the presence of tumor emboli in the skin lymphatics. It should be emphasized that the underlying fat appears normal in most instances and may be fairly thick secondary to the edema and to the depth of the fatty layer itself. The underlying breast tissue is diffusely involved; a small incisional biopsy is usually sufficient for all of the studies that are required. The surgeon should carefully record the location and extent of skin edema and erythema so that the subsequent elliptical skin incision used for mastectomy will remove the area of maximal skin involvement. Currently, we treat these patients initially with chemotherapy, hormonal therapy, and radiation therapy, which usually gives excellent resolution of all gross abnormalities, leaving only microscopic disease if any. The planning of the mastectomy incision depends upon the initial findings. As much skin as possible should be removed consistent with a primary closure. The operation that has been used as the final stage of treatment has been a modified radical mastectomy.

Biopsy for nipple discharge. If a mass or mammographic abnormality is present, it must be removed by the usual techniques already described. In the absence of a mass, the entire duct is excised. This operation can be performed entirely through a circumareolar incision. The duct is identified by expressing the discharge at surgery and by clearly marking it at the time of that preincision physical examination. It is ligated at the undersurface of the nipple's skin. The breast is then dissected free from the surrounding fat to the periphery of the breast and the entire duct with surrounding parenchyma is excised. With these excisions the breast tissue usually can be approximated without any distortion. A combination of local anesthesia and intravenous sedation has sufficed for this surgery despite the significant amount of breast tissue being removed.

Other surgeons have advocated placement of a small probe or injection with vital dyes to help to isolate the ductal system involved. I have not found this helpful and have relied upon a complete excision of a wedge of tissue surrounding the identified duct. This does not create any significant cosmetic defect, again provided that the fat layer is well preserved by a meticulous dissection at the interface of breast and fat tissue.

SURGICAL MANAGEMENT OF PRIMARY BREAST CANCER

Mastectomy

Surgical attempts to treat breast carcinoma are traceable to the early periods of history. Descriptions are found as early as 1600 BC. Treatment consisted of either burning the lesion directly or removing it with sharp instruments. Throughout the nineteenth century, surgical treatment was aimed at providing local control of the disease and usually resulted in failure. Advanced bulky disease was the usual presentation and rates of local recurrence and death from the disease were inordinately high.

In 1894 Halsted published the description of his technique for radical mastectomy. This operation included excision of a margin of skin, development of flaps and en bloc removal of the breast, axillary nodes, and both pectoral muscles. Local control of the disease with a low local recurrence rate[30] established this procedure as the operation of choice for carcinoma of the breast. It became firmly entrenched in medical practice and for the ensuing 75 years was the measure against which all other proposed treatments for breast carcinoma were gauged.

Extensions of the radical mastectomy were described by Urban and Baker,[70] adding en bloc dissection of the internal mammary chain to the earlier procedure. This more radical extension of the original operation never gained popular acceptance. An international cooperative trial[38] did not show a difference in either overall survival rates or local-regional control. In a trial in the United States, there were no significant differences in 10-year survival rates but a statistical advantage in 10-year survival rates for extended mastectomy in patients with central or medial tumors was shown. Patients with lateral tumors did not benefit from this approach.[44]

Further analysis of the international cooperative trial by Lacour et al.[37] demonstrated improvements in survival when analyzed for the subset of patients with inner tumors and positive axillary nodes. The benefit of extended radical mastectomy was matched, however, by those patients treated by radical mastectomy and radiation therapy.

The extended radical mastectomy never gained great acceptance because of the doubts concerning its benefits and because of the additional morbidity that could be expected from the more radical surgery. The improvement in radiotherapy techniques and the demonstration that the radical mastectomy plus radiation therapy was equally beneficial, even in inner quadrant lesions, has led to the abandonment of the extended radical mastectomy. We have applied these concepts to our own practice by encouraging breast conservation radiation therapy in acceptable candidates with inner quadrant lesions and by the consideration of postoperative radiation therapy in those patients with inner quadrant lesions and positive axillary nodes treated by mastectomy.

During the same time period, other surgeons sought to diminish the extent of local resection in order to provide a better cosmetic and functional result without sacrificing local-regional control. This modified radical mastectomy was originally described by Patey to include total mastectomy, axillary dissection and excision of the pectoralis minor muscle. The pectoralis major muscle was preserved.[48] It was later modified by Auchincloss to include preservation of the pectoralis minor muscle as well.[2] The preservation of the pectoralis minor muscle does not appear important. I continue to remove the pectoralis minor muscle to provide optimal access to the highest lymph nodes in the parasternal area at the sternoclavicular junction. With this technique, combined with the use of muscle relaxants, the operative exposure of the complete axilla and all levels is equal to that of a radical mastectomy (Fig. 4-1).

Modified radical mastectomy has been the standard surgical approach since 1970. Multiple studies of long-term results have shown its effectiveness in both treatment of the breast and axilla.[74] When combined with a transverse incision that removes both the biopsy site and nipple/areolar complex, the operation can be performed with satisfactory cosmetic result and with excellent opportunity for prosthetic reconstruction without the need for tissue transfer techniques. Retrospective analysis of pa-

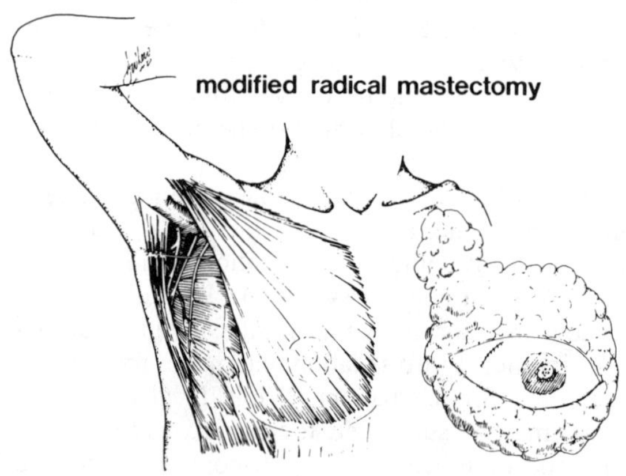

Fig. 4-1 A modified radical mastectomy removes the breast and axillary contents. Removal of the pectoralis minor muscle provides axillary exposure equal to that of a radical mastectomy. The finished dissection demonstrates the limits of dissection and the preservation of the intercostobrachial, long thoracic, and thoracodorsal nerves.

tients treated at Johns Hopkins Hospital[3] confirmed the similarity in 5-year survival and local recurrence rates in treatment of patients with stage I and stage II disease when treated by either radical mastectomy or modified radical mastectomy. In a 10-year follow-up of a trial in Manchester, U.K.,[69] modified radical mastectomy compared favorably with radical mastectomy in terms of survival, disease-free survival, and local recurrence rates and cases of distant metastases. The operation of modified radical mastectomy does not remove the interpectoral lymph nodes (Rotter's nodes). The possibility of unresected lymph nodes becoming the source of either recurrence or distant disseminators of future tumor concerns some that the modified mastectomy was conceptually inferior to radical mastectomy. In an extensive analysis of the interpectoral lymph nodes, Cody et al.[10] indicated that there were extremely few axillary node-negative patients with positive interpectoral node disease. Even patients with other positive axillary lymph nodes had a low incidence (8.2%) of positive interpectoral nodes. I routinely examine the interpectoral nodes and, if suspicious, biopsy these for confirmation. Should interpectoral nodes be positive, then postoperative radiation therapy is utilized.[10]

While there are retrospective studies showing that the local recurrence rate is not influenced by the proximity of the tumor to the pectoralis fascia, some authors recommend an excision of a portion of muscle beneath the tumor for a wider margin of resection. Analysis of close margins of 1 mm or less showed few local recurrences, suggesting that an intact pectoral fascia is an effective tumor barrier.[45] In our approach, close surgical margins in any direction are treated by subsequent radiation therapy. Therefore a posteriorly located tumor with a very narrow margin of resection would be aggressively treated not by conversion to radical mastectomy but by the use of postoperative radiation therapy. Obviously any direct involvement of the pectoralis major muscle, which is quite unusual in our patient population, would call for full resection of the pectoralis major muscle for treatment.

Total mastectomy removes the entire breast and includes the nipple/areolar complex. However, nodal dissection is not performed and the pectoral muscles are left intact. This operation generally has been reserved for patients with noninvasive ductal carcinoma. Even in extensive intraductal carcinoma, involvement of the lymph nodes with metastatic disease is extremely low.[65] In removing the tail of Spence area, a few small nodes can be removed as samples and the nodes can be clinically evaluated. Patients undergoing prophylactic mastectomy because of high-risk conditions for the development of carcinoma do not require nodal dissection, and total mastectomy is the operation of choice. Finally, total mastectomy has been generally employed for those patients who experience breast disease recurrence after partial mastectomy, axillary dissection, and radiation therapy. However, the upper axillary levels should be inspected and the axillary dissection completed if any suspicious nodes are found. Additionally, any nodes remaining in the previously dissected level I area should be removed, as this area will be exposed surgically in performing the total mastectomy.

Rationale for mastectomy. The rationale for mastectomy relates to the incidence of multicentric or multifocal breast cancer. When sections of breast tissue are taken from the quadrants excluding the primary tumor, multicentricity has been reported in a significant number of patients. Rosen et al.[56] carefully analyzed 203 mastectomy specimens after operations for unilateral invasive carcinoma. Following the removal by mastectomy, a bench dissection was performed to remove the primary tumor quadrant and to assess the disease remaining in the other three quadrants. When the primary lesion was >2 cm in diameter, 38% of patients had carcinoma remaining in the breast. When the lesion was <2 cm in size, 26% had carcinoma remaining in the breast. In analyzing subsets, residual carcinoma was found in 80% of patients with lesions in the subareolar area. None of nine patients with medullary or colloid-type carcinomas that measured <2 cm had carcinoma in the breast outside of the primary quadrant. The incidence of multifocal breast carcinoma increased with increasing primary tumor size so that 63% of patients with a tumor size >4 cm had residual carcinoma. Similarly, multicentricity is evident in patients who have had mastectomy for in situ carcinoma. These studies have been confirmed in other studies of mastectomy specimens, indicating that even the smallest lesions are associated with multicentricity, and that the incidence of multicentricity increases with increasing tumor size.[40,55] Therefore the possibility of multicentric disease dictates some continued caution in the application of partial mastectomy and radiation therapy. The question of whether these histologic findings, particularly when confined to noninvasive ductal carcinoma, will develop into invasive carcinoma of clinical importance remains unanswered.

Axillary node treatment

Axillary lymph node metastases occur in approximately 40% of patients with operable invasive breast cancer. There is a direct correlation between metastases and primary tumor size, with increased metastases noted as the tumor increases in size.[18]

However, in this study by Fisher et al., even the smallest tumors, measuring <1 cm, had a significant percentage of positive lymph nodes. Combined with the high incidence of both false-positive and false-negative detection of axillary involvement by physical examination, nodal dissection for accurate staging of the disease is essential. The importance of histologically negative axillary nodes as a prognostic indicator for improved survival has been documented clearly. Furthermore, the prognosis of these patients worsens as the number of involved lymph nodes increases.[19] The presence and the extent of metastases to the axilla remain an important prognostic factor and one of the most important indicators for additional therapy following treatment of the primary carcinoma.

The axilla is divided into three arbitrary levels. The level I lymph nodes are located lateral and inferior to the pectoralis minor muscle, the level II lymph nodes are located beneath the pectoralis minor muscle, and the level III lymph nodes are superior and medial to the pectoralis minor muscle. Involvement of these level III lymph nodes is unusual in the absence of involvement of the level I or level II lymph nodes. Involvement of the highest nodes at the apex of the axilla indicates a very poor prognosis. Multiple studies[57,72] have analyzed the distribution of node metastases. In patients with positive nodes, level I involvement was seen in approximately 60% of patients and involvement of the higher levels was seen in the additional 40%. Level II and level III lymph nodes were involved, in the absence of level I lymph node involvement, in only 4% of cases. These results demonstrate a largely sequential involvement of the axilla, making a level I dissection highly accurate in determining the presence of axillary lymph node involvement.

Present studies cast doubt about the importance of therapeutic axillary dissection in terms of improving overall survival. The removal of lymph nodes does, however, carry the benefit of therapy to prevent subsequent bulky nodal recurrence of disease that might lead to lymphedema of the extremity or painful involvement by direct extension to the neurovascular structures of the supraclavicular and axillary spaces. An axillary lymph node dissection will provide good local control of the axilla. Although axillary nodes were not specifically mentioned, the low rates of regional recurrence in all three arms of the NSABP B-06 study[17] suggested good local control of the axilla. In patients treated in the Milan trial,[71] no axillary nodal recurrences were seen. Patients in that series were treated by complete axillary dissection, demonstrating the good local control of the axilla that can be obtained by surgery alone.

In a study comparing the addition of radiation therapy to complete axillary dissection in node-positive patients with complete axillary dissection alone, Sarrazin et al.[59] did not demonstrate any difference in recurrence rates between the two groups, again demonstrating the therapeutic effectiveness of an axillary dissection. Patients with negative axillary sampling of the level I nodes did not receive additional radiation therapy, and only 2% developed recurrent disease in the axilla.

Conservative surgery and radiation for early-stage invasive breast cancer

A number of studies have reported that local tumor resection and radiation therapy have given survival and local regional control rates similar to those achieved with radical or modified radical mastectomy. Several of these individual protocols report results from more than 20 years observation.[1,29] Three large randomized trials have not shown any difference in either local-regional control or survival rates between the groups treated with conservative surgery plus radiation and those treated with more extensive surgery. Sarrazin et al.[59] treated patients with a primary tumor of ≤2 cm size and with positive or negative axillary lymph nodes. The patients were randomized to mastectomy with limited dissection or to local resection with a grossly negative margin combined with low axillary dissection and radiation therapy. At 10 years, no differences were demonstrated between the two groups in terms of overall survival rates, local recurrence rates or disease-free survival rates. Veronesi et al.[71] randomized patients with tumors ≤2 cm by pathologic measurement to either radical mastectomy or quadrantectomy, full axillary dissection, and radiation therapy. Overall survival and disease-free survival rates were similar. Node-positive patients treated by quadrantectomy and radiation therapy fared slightly better than those with radical mastectomy.

The largest study was the United States trial reported by Fisher.[17] This study treated patients with tumors ≤4 cm in size by modified radical mastectomy, local resection and axillary dissection without radiation therapy or local resection, and axillary dissection and radiation therapy. This trial required histologically negative surgical margins to qualify for the segmental mastectomy arms. At both 5 and 8 years, no difference in terms of survival or local-regional recurrence was found between the mastectomy group and the local resection/radiation therapy group. The group receiving local resection and axillary dissection without radiation therapy had a local recurrence rate of 28% at 5 years and 39% at 8 years. Despite these differences in local recurrence rates, overall survival rates were not different among the three arms. The analysis of 8-year data did not show any difference among the treatment arms when stratified for either node-positive or node-negative patients. As a result of these controlled trials, as well as many uncontrolled trials, conservative surgery and radiation therapy clearly have been demonstrated to be effective for early-stage breast cancer. Local recurrences have been extensively analyzed in an attempt to maximize the beneficial effects of the treatment.

Conservative breast surgery is designed to control local and regional disease with breast prevention. In our series, the surgery always has been combined with radiation therapy. We have not utilized resection alone for therapy even in patients with very small carcinomas or in patients with in situ ductal carcinoma that has been excised completely. Recommendations for adjuvant chemotherapy and hormonal therapy follow the same indications as for patients who have undergone a mastectomy. Integration of both radiation therapy and chemotherapy have not significantly adversely affected the cosmetic result.[12] In our experience, the combined use of radiation therapy and chemotherapy has not adversely affected the total dose obtainable with either modality.[27]

Eligibility criteria for conservative surgery and radiation therapy at this institution include a tumor size ≤5 cm, which is resectable with normal margins and with a cosmetically acceptable result. Analyses comparing primary tumor site size and treatment failure have not found differences in outcome with primary sizes of ≤5 cm.[5,20] While tumors ≤5 cm in size may be treated effectively, caution should be exercised as this tumor size in most normal-sized breasts will not allow for a cosmetically acceptable resection with normal surgical margins. Tumor location does not play a role in eligibility for radiation therapy except for those tumors that are close to the nipple/areolar complex. The presence of a subareolar primary tumor may require removal of the nipple/areolar complex in order to achieve total gross excision. This would impair the cosmetic benefit of the breast-conserving procedure. In analyzing involvement of the nipple and areola in carcinoma of the breast, Smith et al.[67] noted a 12% incidence of involvement of the nipple and areola by primary carcinomas of the breast. If the nipple appeared normal, involvement of the nipple and areola by carcinoma was rare if the primary tumor was <2 cm and was not situated behind the areola. Tumors within 2 cm of the nipple/areolar complex have been noted to involve the actual nipple in upwards of 40% of cases. Because tumor may extend along the ducts, achieving negative margins would be more difficult. In isolated incidences a small lesion in the region of the areola may be totally excised and its margins prove to be negative; for that specific patient breast conservation might be considered. However, in general patients with subareolar tumors should best be considered as candidates for mastectomy.

Other conditions that favor the use of mastectomy include very large, pendulous breasts that would present technical difficulties in obtaining appropriate radiation dosage. This is usually not a significant problem except in the very largest of breasts. Patients with extremely small breasts and larger tumors might not achieve a beneficial cosmetic result and might, at times, be better advised to have mastectomy with a reconstruction rather than breast conservation treatment with a poor cosmetic outcome. These are obviously highly subjective judgments and will depend in part upon the experience and expertise of both the surgical and radiation therapy teams. Patients with diffuse microcalcifications or multifocal gross malignant disease in the breast have been excluded from breast conservation therapy at the University of Pennsylvania. In an analysis of 40 such patients, 47% were found to have involvement of more than one quadrant of the breast and 40% had involved axillary lymph nodes, 70% of whom had four or more positive axillary nodes. Because these two features were associated with extensive disease in the breast and axilla, modified radical mastectomy was recommended. Depending on the extent of the disease in the axilla and the margins of resection, postoperative radiation therapy additionally may be required.

Surgical resection continues to be an important part of the treatment arm. Local control is less effective when either incision or needle biopsies are used as opposed to a complete excision of the tumor.[8,50] After accepting an excisional biopsy requirement, the question remains whether this should be a grossly negative margin or microscopically negative. Most of the major trials (except for the NSABP B-06 trial) required only grossly negative margins. Multiple series have demonstrated that residual tumor is left behind when only gross tumor excision is performed with no attempt at obtaining a surgically negative margin except by gross examination.[62,68] Despite this probable residual tumor burden, local recurrence and survival rates have not been affected adversely in those studies requiring only gross tumor excision. Unless unusual factors in selection in these prospective trials were operative, one could expect that similar rates of residual tumor were present in the breasts so treated. These results suggest that radiation therapy can control microscopic residual disease. Admitting this statistical possibility, we have formulated the policy that treatment by radiation therapy requires complete surgical excision with margins that are negative for both invasive ductal carcinoma and for extensive intraductal carcinoma. While a small focus of invasive or intraductal carcinoma may be acceptable for treatment, failure to obtain a margin that is free of significant disease is referred for mastectomy. The rationale for this also takes into account the high precedence of multicentric disease present with extensive in situ intraductal carcinoma.

Treatment with local resection and radiation therapy leaves the great majority of breast tissue at risk for either tumor recurrence or new tumor formation.[35] On this basis, patients must be followed faithfully by experienced clinicians for detection of recurrences both by clinical examination and by routine mammographic screening on a yearly basis. Kurtz et al.[35] has reported a favorable experience for breast disease recurrences following radiation therapy. Of 181 recurrences, only 10 had distant metastases and 93% of the local tumors were removable by either further local excision or mastectomy. He reported an overall survival rate of 57% at 10 years. Unlike chest wall metastases, recurrences in the breast can appear over a longer period.[61] Actuarial recurrence rates were 1.5% per year for the first 10 years and 1.1% per year for the subsequent 5 years. Similar results have been reported in many other series.[29] The more favorable results, compared to survival data following post-mastectomy chest wall recurrences, may reflect the fact that these local recurrences actually represent new primary tumor formation.

Partial mastectomy (lumpectomy). Lumpectomy is the term most commonly applied to conservative surgery, although it clearly is not an appropriate description. The aim of surgery is to excise the tumor totally and leave a normal margin of surrounding tissue. The term that we have used has been "partial mastectomy," which seems more appropriate in describing the procedure. If the diagnosis is uncertain, this partial mastectomy is performed as a first procedure utilizing local anesthesia with intravenous sedation. While general anesthesia may be used, it is not necessary and certainly adds to the expense of the procedure,[46] and probably to the chances of morbidity. Conversely, axillary dissection has been performed utilizing general anesthesia. If the patient confidently can be expected to be a good candidate for radiation therapy, then the initial procedure is carried out as a single procedure with general anesthesia. The partial mastectomy is performed first to document the diagnosis and the suitability of breast conservation therapy. The breast is then reprepared and redraped, all instruments and all personnel gown and gloves are changed, and the axillary dissection is performed as a second separate procedure. The partial mastectomy incision is covered with a small gauze bandage and a plastic occlusive dressing before repreparation of the axillary area.

The location of acceptable incisions is illustrated in Fig. 4-2. Almost all procedures in the upper breast can be performed with a crescent-shaped incision. Most authorities agree that a radial incision is preferable medially. I believe that radial incisions also can give better results inferiorly, and I frequently use these incisions instead of crescent-shaped incisions for tumors that are clearly malignant. When the lesion is more likely benign, a crescent-shaped incision can be used inferiorly as smaller amounts of tissue would be removed and the overall appearance might be somewhat better in terms of the scar. There have been no clear trials of the superiority of one incision over another, provided all are done with attention to cosmetic detail. If one chooses a radial incision, it is essential to provide several small cross marks to be certain that the skin is realigned in its normal position. Proper realignment may not be easily achieved in a radial incision once the underlying tissue has been dissected widely unless there are clear-cut lines of apposition to guide the surgeon. It should further be stressed that a radial incision always is used if skin is to be removed, because it produces the least cosmetic distortion. Closure of crescent-shaped incisions with skin removal would require complex plastic closures or a musculocutaneous interposition to prevent distortion and dislocation of the nipple. Therefore in superficial tumors where skin

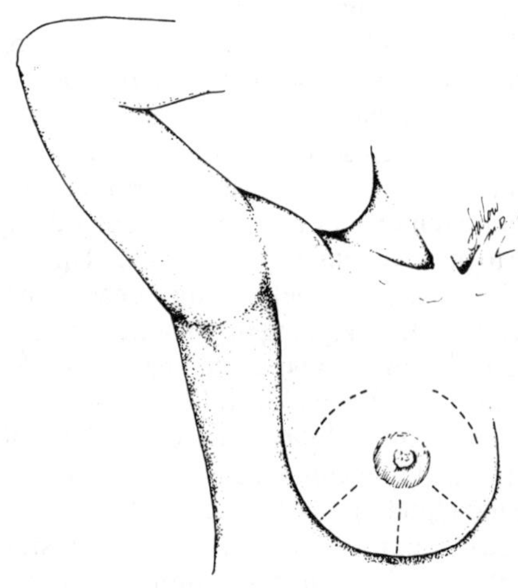

Fig. 4-2 Incisions for partial mastectomy are illustrated. The author favors radial incisions below the midplane of the breast. If skin removal is required, a radial incision is always used, regardless of the breast quadrant.

resection is necessary, a radial incision always should be used, whether the operation is in the upper or lower quadrants.

The key to a best cosmetic result is preservation of the fat in the subcutaneous area. Therefore the dissection is carried down to the interface between the fat and breast and the fat is widely dissected away from the underlying breast tissue (Fig. 4-3). Preservation of this fat layer allows very extensive breast tissue removal without any significant cosmetic sacrifice. A clear margin of breast tissue can therefore be excised easily around the tumor. This can be accomplished whether the operation is for primary removal or represents a reexcision for the removal of additional tissue following an initial biopsy. The margins of the specimen should be marked carefully by the pathologist in direct communication with the surgeon. The frozen section report should include an assessment of that margin. We aim for a negative margin of 1 or 2 cm in relation to the gross tumor, based upon the early data that tumor excision and radiation therapy produce lower local recurrence rates than radiotherapy alone, and that complete gross excision is superior to incomplete excision.[1,8] It is apparent from reviews of pathologic data that the line of resection can be reasonably small. I think that this is particularly true of the line of resection in reference to the subcutaneous tissue. If a breast tumor is located very superficially, then the dissection through the fatty tissue is performed through grossly normal tissue, but without an attempt to obtain a wide margin. Similarly, in tumors located posteriorly, removal of the pectoral fascia makes the widest margin possible and is acceptable. The pathologist

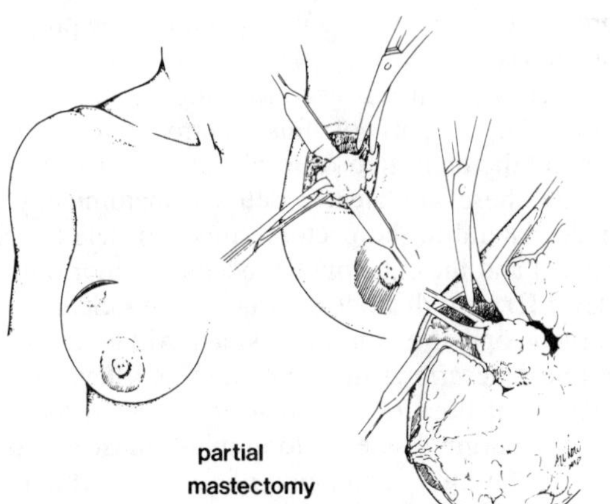

Fig. 4-3 A circumareolar incision overlying the mass, along with adequate superiorly and inferiorly applied traction, allows for dissection through normal tissue around the mass. The key to an excellent cosmetic result is the preservation of the subcutaneous fat layer.

may report these superficial or deep margins as positive or close to positive, but no further tissue can be realistically taken. Within the breast tissue itself, wider margins are taken because of the uncertainty of extensions of the tumor within the parenchyma of the breast. Radiation therapy can eradicate small foci of tumor, and it is on this basis that the margin in the subcutaneous tissue or at the fascial level is taken as a gross margin without the need to wait for the pathologist's final report. However, within the breast tissue itself we have insisted upon a negative margin, both grossly and microscopically. The rationale for the importance of the breast margin relates not only to residual microscopic tumor but to assessment of the risk of multicentricity based upon the extent of local disease.

The extension of our requirement to microscopically negative margins has been made despite the fact that only the NSABP trial required microscopically negative margins; the other major trials relied upon gross margins only. As the results of those trials are not significantly different, there is at present no controlled trial that addresses the issue of a microscopically positive margin. Multicentric disease occurring at distances up to 10 cm from the tumor is expected in a significant number of patients.[9,32] Even with reported pathologically clear margins, residual breast cancer can be found in 25% of the patients later subjected to mastectomy.[25] This correlates with the demonstrated local recurrence rates documented in the NSABP trial arm employing surgical resection without radiation therapy.[16] Negative margins may be especially important in minimizing the risk of breast recurrence in patients with an invasive cancer with an extensive intraductal component. When margins of resection were unknown in these patients, breast disease recurrence was 22% at 5 years.[47]

All agree that the margin of the gross tumor should be negative for carcinoma. We believe that microscopic examination should confirm that the tumor has been removed completely and that the tumor itself does not extend to the margin of resection. Failure to demonstrate this by a microscopic technique leaves us with the surgeon as the only witness that the tumor was grossly removed. Because some tumors infiltrate in an uneven fashion, this clearly would be unsatisfactory. Therefore, if the microscopic margins are not clearly negative by careful pathologic examination, we would recommend a reexcision to be certain that all of the gross tumor has been removed. Unfortunately, the strongest recommendation for reexcision comes from an inadequate description and documentation of the margins at the initial time of removal. In this situation, there is no clear information to allow for a confident prediction of gross removal of the tumor, leaving reexcision[25] the only alternative. More careful initial removal of the specimen as a single piece and more careful communication between surgeon and pathologist in preparation of the biopsy specimen would reduce the frequency of required reexcisions.

Foci of carcinoma present at the margin, representing probable multifocal disease, is a second problem. This often takes the form of an isolated focus of in situ intraductal carcinoma, although it may represent actual infiltrating carcinoma. In either instance, we routinely have recommended reexcision for positive margins, whether this represented ductal in situ carcinoma or infiltrating carcinoma. If a wider dissection still revealed infiltrating carcinoma at the margin, then mastectomy is advised because of the relatively diffuse nature of the infiltrating tumor. A small focus of invasive or intraductal carcinoma at the margin would not preclude radiation therapy, whereas a more diffuse multifocal in situ intraductal carcinoma also would not be acceptable for radiation therapy. Therefore, when either ductal in situ carcinoma or invasive cancer is present at the first resection margin, a further excision is obtained to seek a normal margin. Failure to achieve a microscopically negative margin at that time would lead to a recommendation for mastectomy.

Axillary node dissection. Axillary node dissection does not represent random sampling, but an anatomic dissection of the fat pad bearing the axillary lymph nodes. The prophylactic removal of lymph nodes probably does not affect overall survival.[16] The purpose of dissection in clinically node-negative patients is to provide information regarding prognosis and the possible use of adjuvant therapy. Small breast carcinomas[51] without clinical evidence of involved lymph nodes are being diagnosed more frequently. We continue to do axillary dissection for any invasive carcinoma, regardless of primary tumor size, because of the risk of significant node metastases, even with lesions <1 cm.[15] If specialized studies involving hormone receptors, flow cytometry, cathepsin-D, oncogenes, and the like, replace lymph node metastasis as an indicator for the need for additional therapy, then node-negative patients in the future might not have to undergo axillary dissection in certain circumstances. However, the data to allow for such discrimination is not yet available. We do not currently dissect nodes in patients with in situ intraductal carcinoma who are clinically node negative.

The incision for axillary dissection is placed in the lower hairline of the axilla and should be kept completely posterior to the pectoral muscle (Fig. 4-4). If increased incision length is required, it should be extended posteriorly. This incision will be completely within the hollow of the axilla and is a cosmetically excellent incision. If it extends at all onto the pectoral muscle, it will later be clearly visible and detract from the cosmetic appearance. I routinely use muscle relaxants, allowing easy retraction of the muscle for a satisfactory dissection of the lateral chest wall. This does remove a slight safety factor in dissecting the long thoracic and thoracodorsal nerves, but these are protected easily when a dissection is done properly under visual control.

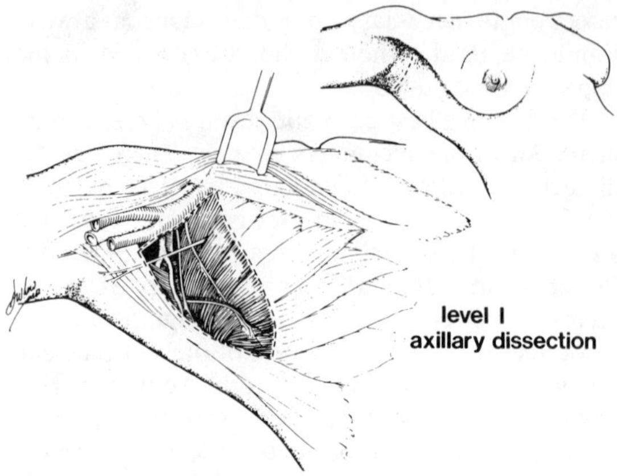

Fig. 4-4 The axillary dissection is carried out through a separate incision from that of the partial mastectomy. The incision *(upper right)* is within the confines of the axilla, kept posterior to the pectoralis major muscle. This incision will allow for adequate exposure of the axillary region. Dissection should be carried anterior to the long thoracic nerve and should spare the intercostobrachial nerve as well as the thoracodorsal neurovascular bundle. The extent of dissection is illustrated by the shaded area.

There is controversy concerning the nodes to be removed. A part of this controversy revolves around the definition of level I and level II nodes. While these are clearly defined anatomically as nodes lateral to the pectoral minor muscle (level I nodes) and those below the pectoral minor muscle (level II), that distinction is not always clear to the surgeon operating through a small axillary incision. While I described my dissection as a level I dissection, it does extend to some extent below the lateral margin of the pectoral minor muscle. However, a careful examination of the pectoral muscle would indicate that it extends almost to the sternal border and fans out quite broadly. Most surgeons do not dissect to the full medial extent of this muscle, although almost all do remove at least a portion of the level II nodes. The landmarks that I utilize are the axillary vein, the thoracodorsal nerve, and the long thoracic nerve. The axillary vein provides the border superiorly and the thoracodorsal nerve bundle supplies the resection laterally. On the chest wall, I clearly go well medial to the long thoracic nerve but do not make a definite attempt to go medial to the pectoral muscle. The intercostobrachial nerve should be identified and protected, because transection of this nerve leads to the need for anesthesia in the triceps area of the arm.

Information concerning skip areas has led to the practice of dissecting both level I and level II nodes. As I have indicated, I do not believe that most surgeons perform an actual complete level II dissection, although most do remove a portion of these nodes. The risk of positive nodes in the level II and level III areas when the level I nodes are negative is quite low.[7] The possibility of skip metastases should be evaluated by direct palpation of the remaining lymph nodes as well as by palpation of the interpectoral (Rotter's) nodes. This direct palpation, however, does not guarantee detection of small metastases.[24] Other authors have advocated a complete dissection of the level II nodes because of the possibility of skip metastases being present in a higher percentage of cases in their particular series.[11,63] Skip metastases to level III (when both level I and level II are negative) are quite unusual, and most practitioners agree that in the clinically negative axilla, level III nodes do not require dissection. As I have indicated, the dissection that I utilize is a full dissection of the level I nodes and a dissection of a portion of the level II nodes. Emphasis is placed upon the lateral chest wall dissection, clearly exposing the area medial to the long thoracic nerve and dissecting all of the tissue from the serratus muscle out to the lateral border of the latissimus dorsi muscle. Additionally, the area that is probably most difficult to dissect because of an uneasy cleavage plane is the axillary fat pad itself along the skin of the hair-bearing axilla. This should be included in the level I dissection. My personal belief is that the nodal areas that are least well dissected are the subcutaneous fat in the axillary skin area (see earlier discussion) and the nodal tissues along the serratus muscle in the inferior portion of the dissection. At completion, the axillary dissection should appear as illustrated in Fig. 4-4.

The operation is begun by developing the inferior skin flap at a 45-degree downward angle to the chest wall. The serratus muscle, latissimus dorsi, and pectoral muscles are all dissected free from this fat pad inferiorly. The axillary vein can then be identified by retraction of the pectoral muscles medially. As indicated above, muscle relaxants are used to facilitate an easy retraction of these muscles. The axillary vein is then dissected free of the vessels, nerves, and lymphatics except for the thoracodorsal, long thoracic, and intercostobrachial nerves. The latter can be seen emerging from the second interspace below the pectoralis minor muscle belly and should be directly visualized and protected. The axillary skin flap is created by dissecting the hair-bearing skin of the axilla down to the level of the axillary vein. This isolates the triangle of tissue to be removed and identifies the major neurovascular structures to be preserved. The dissection then proceeds downward from the axillary vein along the serratus muscle to completely remove all of the tissue except for the essential structures to be preserved. While this clearly includes a part of the level II nodes, it does not include a dissection past the medial border, which would involve an unnecessarily large axillary dissection in my opinion.

Treatment of in situ ductal carcinoma

Most patients historically have been treated with mastectomy when the diagnosis of in situ intraductal carcinoma was established. This was based upon studies that demonstrated progression to invasive carcinoma when these patients were treated by biopsy alone. Invasive carcinoma developed in 30% of patients followed for up to 10 years.[6] The tumor was noted to occur in the same quadrant and close to the original biopsy site. This demonstrated multicentricity of in situ ductal carcinoma, together with excellent local tumor control and excellent survival rates for total mastectomy has led to the adoption of mastectomy as the treatment of choice for all but very localized in situ ductal carcinomas.

However, new data and approaches to in situ ductal carcinoma have led to new treatment options in this disease. Lagios et al.[39] have characterized in situ ductal carcinoma by nuclear grade, growth pattern, and the presence or absence of necrosis. They found correlation with high nuclear grade and necrosis in terms of a higher risk of local recurrence in the breast and a shorter time from treatment to recurrence. They also noted that the tumor was likely to recur in the immediate vicinity of the biopsy site. In contrast, low-grade lesions had a lower risk of local recurrence.[39,41] Obviously, long-term follow-up will be necessary to determine the effectiveness of the staging by subtypes and the effect on prognosis for recurrence following therapy. Further attempts have been made to classify the ductal carcinoma on the basis of the extent of the lesion within the breast tissue.[28] In considering combinations of these different staging approaches, the major finding that appears to be associated with occult invasion in other parts of the breast is the comedo type of ductal carcinoma with high nuclear grade and necrosis combined with a size >4 cm. On the basis of these findings, prospective trials for conservative management of in situ ductal carcinoma without invasion have been formulated. These treatment options include excision combined with radiation therapy or excision alone. Both options provide breast preservation. Recurrence rates after irradiation range up to 10%. The results of the NSABP B-06 trial compare the two therapeutic modalities and suggest a benefit from radiation therapy.[22] Higher local recurrence rates have been demonstrated with centrally located in situ ductal carcinoma.[49]

This retrospective study from our institution and the Joint Center for Radiation Therapy has led to the policy of requiring negative margins for treatment by local resection and radiation therapy. Therefore, significant in situ ductal carcinoma at the original margin of resection requires a reexcision for further evaluation. If clear margins cannot be obtained, then mastectomy is recommended. A further important consideration in the use of radiation therapy for localized in situ ductal carcinoma is that a local recurrence is likely to be treatable despite the fact that invasive carcinoma is frequently present at the time of relapse. It has been estimated that approximately 50% of patients in whom disease recurs will develop invasive carcinoma even when the initial biopsy showed in situ carcinoma only.[49] Salvage for patients who have been treated previously with radiation therapy requires a mastectomy. The long-term outcome of a recurrence within the breast in terms of survival remains uncertain and therefore all attempts should be made to keep local recurrence rates as low as possible. This includes acceptance of strict criteria for applying breast conservation treatment programs combined with careful monitoring by physician follow-up and mammography during the postoperative period.

Occult carcinoma of the breast presenting as axillary metastases

Occasionally an axillary mass is the abnormality first noted, before the diagnosis of breast carcinoma.[23] While such a tumor may represent adenocarcinoma from a site other than the breast, extensive evaluations generally have not revealed another primary site. The breast is the source of such a carcinoma in most instances. Thorough examination and mammography obviously are indicated. Any breast abnormality uncovered would require biopsy. Kemeny et al.[33] recently examined the histories of 20 such patients. An exhaustive search for the primary tumor (outside of the breast) was largely unsuccessful. Of the 11 of 20 patients who underwent a mastectomy, five were confirmed to have breast carcinoma. Baron[4] reviewed the charts of 35 patients with adenocarcinoma of the axilla without a known primary tumor. While adenocarcinoma of other sites (lung, thyroid, colon, and the like) was searched for, these tumors were not found. A mastectomy was performed in 28 of the 35 patients, and in four of the 35 excision of a suspicious area in the breast was done. Twenty-two patients (67%) were found to have breast carcinoma. Of interest, both authors pointed out that those patients treated by less drastic techniques than mastectomy (axillary dissection, radiation therapy, chemotherapy) had similar survival curves.

Both of these series confirmed the presence of breast carcinoma in a significant percentage of these patients, confirming the wisdom of the usual recommendation for surgery that includes mastectomy. However, the absence of carcinoma in one half to one third of the resected specimens, together with the similar survival curves of those treated without mastectomy, argues somewhat in favor of axillary dissection combined with radiation therapy to the breast itself. Hormonal therapy and chemotherapy are obviously indicated in the presence of this nodal disease. This would, of course, be a more tenable approach in older patients where the breast has been largely replaced by fat and the mammographic examination is extremely accurate. In younger women with dense breasts, mastectomy clearly would be indicated because of the unreliability of diagnostic procedures.

Our present approach is to continue to perform mastectomy because of the significant number of breast carcinomas identified. Full axillary dissection is required to treat the axilla. Many of these patients will have bulky nodal disease, and in those instances postoperative radiation therapy is utilized as well to prevent local-regional recurrence.

REFERENCES

1. Almaric R, Santamaria F, Robert F, et al: Radiation therapy with or without limited surgery for operable breast cancer: a 20 year experience at the Marseilles Cancer Institute, Cancer 49:30, 1982.
2. Auchincloss H: Significance of location and number of axillary metastases in carcinoma of the breast, Ann Surg 158:37, 1963.
3. Baker RR, Montague ACW, and Childs NJ: A comparison of modified radical mastectomy to radical mastectomy in the treatment of operable breast cancer, Ann Surg 189:553, 1979.
4. Baron BL, Moore MP, and Kinne DW: Occult breast cancer presenting with axillary metastases, Arch Surg 125:210, 1990.
5. Bartelink H, Borger JH, Van Donzen JA, et al: The impact of tumor size and histology on local control after breast conserving therapy, Radiother Oncol 11:297, 1988.
6. Betsill WL, Rosen PP, Lieberman PH, and Robbins GF:

Intraductal carcinoma: long-term follow-up after treatment by biopsy alone, JAMA 239:1863, 1978.
7. Boova RS, Bonani R, and Rosato FE: Patterns of axillary and nodal involvement in breast cancer: predictability of level one dissection, Ann Surg 196:642, 1982.
8. Calle R, Pelleron JP, Schleinger P, et al: Conservative management of operable breast cancer: ten years' experience at the Foundation Curie, Cancer 42:2045, 1978.
9. Carter D: Margins of lumpectomy for breast cancer, Hum Pathol 17:330, 1986.
10. Cody HS, Egeli RA, and Urban JA: Rotter's nodes metastases: therapeutic and prognostic considerations in early breast carcinoma, Ann Surg 199:266, 1984.
11. Danforth DN, Findlay PA, McDonald HD, et al: Complete axillary node lymph dissection for stage I-II carcinoma of the breast, J Clin Oncol 4:655, 1986.
12. Danoff BF, Goodman BL, Glick JH, et al: The effect of adjuvant chemotherapy on cosmesis and complications in patients with breast cancer treated by definitive irradiation, Int J Radiat Oncol Biol Phys 9:1625, 1983.
13. Devitt JE: Management of nipple discharge by clinical findings, Am J Surg 149:789, 1985.
14. Egan JF, Sayler CB, and Goodman MJ: A technique for localizing occult breast lesions, CA 26:32, 1976.
15. Fisher B, Redmond C, Fisher ER, and Caplan R: Relative worth of estrogen or progesterone receptor and pathologic characteristics of differentiation as indicators of prognosis in node negative breast cancer patients: findings from National Surgical Adjuvant Breast and Bowel Project (Protocol B-06), J Clin Oncol 6(7):1076, 1988.
16. Fisher B, Redmond C, Poisson R, et al: Five year results of a randomized clinical trial comparing total mastectomy and lumpectomy with or without radiation, N Engl J Med 312:674, 1985.
17. Fisher B, Redmond C, Poisson R, et al: Eight year results of randomized clinical trial comparing total mastectomy and lumpectomy with or without radiation in the treatment of breast cancer, N Engl J Med 320:822, 1989.
18. Fisher B, Slack NH, and Bross IDJ: Cancer of the breast: size of neoplasm and prognosis, Cancer 33:1145, 1974.
19. Fisher B, Slack N, Katrych D, and Wolmark N: Ten year follow-up of results of patients with carcinoma of the breast in a co-operative clinical trial evaluating surgical adjuvant chemotherapy, Surg Gynecol Obstet 140:528, 1975.
20. Fisher B and Wolmark N: Limited surgical management for primary breast cancer: a commentary on the NSABP reports, World J Surg 9:682, 1985.
21. Fisher ER, Sass R, and Fisher B: Biologic consideration regarding the one and two step procedures and management of patients with invasive carcinoma of the breast, Surg Gynecol Obstet 161:245, 1985.
22. Fisher ER, Sass R, Fisher B, et al: Pathologic findings from the National Surgical Adjuvant Breast Project (Protocol 6). I. Intraductal carcinoma (DCIS), Cancer 57:197, 1986.
23. Fitts WT, Steiner GC, and Enterline HT: Prognosis of occult carcinoma of the breast, Am J Surg 106:460, 1963.
24. Forrest APM, Stewart JH, Roberts MM, et al: Simple mastectomy and axillary node sampling (pectoral node biopsy) in the management of primary breast cancer, Ann Surg 196:371, 1982.
25. Frazier TG, Wong RW, and Rose D: Implications of accurate pathologic margins in the treatment of breast cancer, Arch Surg 1224:37, 1989.
26. Glen PM and Dargulies D: Electrocautery and hormone receptor status in breast biopsy, Am J Surg 158:6, 1989.
27. Glick JH, Fowble BL, Haller DG, et al: Integration of full dose adjuvant chemotherapy with definitive radiotherapy for primary breast cancer: four year update, NCI Monogr 6:297, 1988.
28. Graverson HP, Blichert-Toft M, Dyreborg U, et al: In situ carcinoma of the female breast: incidence, clinical findings and DBCG proposals for management, Acta Oncol 27:679, 1988.
29. Haffty BG, Goldberg NB, Rose M, et al: Conservative surgery with radiation therapy in clinical stage I and II breast cancer: results of a 20 year experience, Arch Surg 124:1266, 1989.
30. Halsted WH: The results of operations for the cure of cancer of the breast performed at the Johns Hopkins Hospital from June, 1889 to January, 1894, Johns Hopkins Hosp Bull 4:497, 1984.
31. Hassan J, Luhan PA, and Kohl MW: Comparison of estrogen levels in breast cancer samples from mastectomy and frozen section specimens, Cancer 47:138, 1981.
32. Holland R, Veling SH, Mravunac M, et al: Histologic multifocality of TIS, T1-2 breast carcinomas: implications for clinical trials of breast conserving surgery, Cancer 56:979, 1985.
33. Kemeny MM, Rivera DE, Terz JJ, and Benfield JR: Occult primary adenocarcinoma with axillary metastases, Am J Surg 152:43, 1986.
34. Kopans DB and Meyer JE: Versatile spring hookwire breast lesion localizer, AJR 138:586, 1982.
35. Kurtz JM, Spitalier JM, Almaric R, et al: Results of wide excision for local recurrence after breast conserving therapy, Cancer 61:1969, 1989.
36. Kwasnik EM, Sadowsky NL, and Vollman RW: An improved system for surgical excision of needle-localized nonpalpable breast lesions, Am J Surg 154:476, 1987.
37. Lacour J, Le MG, Hill C, et al: Is it useful to remove internal mammary lymph nodes in operable breast cancer? Eur J Surg Oncol 13:309, 1987.
38. Lacour J, Monique L, Caceres E, et al: Radical mastectomy versus radical mastectomy plus internal mammary dissection, Cancer 51:1941, 1983.
39. Lagios MD, Margolin FR, Westdahl PR, et al: Mammographically detected duct carcinoma in situ: frequency of local recurrence following tylectomy and prognostic effect of nuclear grade on local recurrence, Cancer 63:618, 1989.
40. Lagios MD, Richards VE, Rose MR, and Yee E: Segmental mastectomy without radiotherapy: short-term follow-up, Cancer 52:2173, 1983.
41. Lagios MD, Westdahl PR, Margolin FR, et al: Duct carcinoma in situ: relationship of extent of noninvasive disease to the frequency of occult invasion, multicentricity, lymph node metastases and short term treatment failures, Cancer 59:1309, 1982.
42. Leis HP: Management of nipple discharge, World J Surg 13:736, 1989.
43. Martin HE and Ellis EB: Biopsy by needle procedure and aspiration, Ann Surg 92:169, 1930.
44. Meier P, Ferguson D, and Karrison T: A controlled trial of extended radical versus radical mastectomy: ten year results, Cancer 63:599, 1989.
45. Mentzer SJ, Osteen RT, and Wilson RE: Local recurrence and the deep resection margin in carcinoma of the breast, Surg Gynecol Obstet 16:513, 1986.
46. Norton LW, Zeligman BE, and Pearlman NW: Accuracy and cost of needle localization breast biopsy, Arch Surg 123:947, 1988.
47. Osteen RT, Connolly JL, Recht A, et al: Identification of patients at high risk for local recurrence after conservative surgery and radiation therapy for stages I and II breast cancer, Arch Surg 122:1248, 1987.
48. Patey DH and Dyson WH: The prognosis of carcinoma of the breast in relation to type of mastectomy performed, Br J Cancer 2:7, 1948.
49. Recht A, Danoff BS, Solin LJ, et al: Intraductal carcinoma of the breast: results of treatment with excisional biopsy and irradiation, J Clin Oncol 3:1339, 1985.

50. Recht A, Silver B, Schnitts S, et al: Breast relapse following primary radiation therapy for early breast cancer. I Classification frequency and salvage, Int J Radiat Oncol Biol Phys 9:339, 1983.
51. Reger V, Beito G, and Jolly P: Factors affecting the incidence of lymph node metastases in small cancers of the breast, Am J Surg 157:501, 1989.
52. Rosato FE, Thomas J, and Rosato EF: Operative management of nonpalpable lesions detected by mammography, Surg Gynecol Obstet 137:491, 1983.
53. Rosemund GP, Maier WP, and Brobyn TJ: Needle aspiration of breast cysts, Surg Gynecol Obstet 138:351, 1969.
54. Rosen PP: Frozen section diagnosis of breast lesions: recent experience with 556 consecutive biopsies, Ann Surg 187:17, 1978.
55. Rosen PP, Braun DW, and Kinne DW: The clinical significance of preinvasive breast carcinoma, Cancer 46:919, 1980.
56. Rosen PP, Fracchia AA, and Urban JA: "Residual" mammary carcinoma after simulated partial mastectomy, Cancer 35:739, 1975.
57. Rosen PP, Lesser ML, Kinne DW, and Beattie EJ: Discontinuous or "skip" metastases in breast carcinoma, Ann Surg 187:276, 1983.
58. Rosenthal LJ: Discrepant estrogen receptor protein levels according to surgical technique, Am J Surg 138:680, 1879.
59. Sarrazin D, Le M, Arriagada R, et al: Ten-year results of a randomized trial comparing a conservative treatment to mastectomy in early breast cancer, Radiother Oncol 14:177, 1989.
60. Sarrazin D, Le M, Rousse J, et al: Conservative treatment vs mastectomy in breast cancer tumors with macroscopic diameter of 20mm or less, Cancer 53:1209, 1984.
61. Schnitt S, Connolly J, Recht A, et al: Breast relapse following primary radiation therapy for early breast cancer. II. Detection, pathologic features, and prognostic significance, Int J Radiat Oncol Biol Phys 11:1277, 1985.
62. Schnitt SJ, Connolly JL, Khettry U, et al: Pathologic findings on re-excision of the primary site in breast cancer patients considered for treatment by primary radiation therapy, Cancer 59:675, 1987.
63. Schwartz GF, D'Ugo DM, and Rosenberg AL: Extent of axillary dissection preceding irradiation for carcinoma of the breast, Arch Surg 1231:1395, 1986.
64. Seltzer MH, Perloff LJ, Kelley RI, and Fitts WT: The significance of age in patients with nipple discharge, Surg Gynecol Obstet 131:519, 1970.
65. Silverstein MJ, Rosser RJ, Gierson ED, et al: Axillary lymph node dissection for intraductal breast carcinoma: is it indicated? Cancer 59:1819, 1987.
66. Smith C, Butler J, Cobb C, and State D: Fine needle aspiration cytology in the diagnosis of primary breast cancer, Surg 103:178, 1988.
67. Smith J, Payne WS, and Carney JA: Involvement of the nipple and areola in carcinoma of the breast, Surg Gynecol Obstet 153:546, 1976.
68. Solin LJ, Fowble B, Martz K, et al: Results of re-excisional biopsy of the primary tumor in preparation for definitive irradiation of patients with early stage breast cancer, Int J Radiat Oncol Biol Phys 12:721, 1986.
69. Turner L, Swindell R, Bell WG, et al: Radical versus modified radical mastectomy for breast cancer, Ann R Coll Surg 63:239, 1981.
70. Urban JA and Baker HW: Radical mastectomy in continuity with en bloc resection of the internal mammary lymph node chain, Cancer 5:992, 1952.
71. Veronesi U, Banfi A, Del Vecchio M, et al: Comparison of Halsted mastectomy with quadrantectomy, axillary dissection and radiotherapy in early breast cancer: long-term results, Eur J Cancer Clin Oncol 22:1085, 1986.
72. Veronesi U, Rilke F, and Luini A: Distribution of axillary node metastases by level, Cancer 59:682, 1987.
73. Wilkinson EJ, Schuettke CM, Ferrier CM, et al: Fine needle aspiration of breast masses: analysis of 276 aspirates, Acta Cytol 33:613, 1989.
74. Wilson RE, Donegan WL, Mettlin C, et al: The 1982 National Survey of carcinoma of the breast in the United States by the American College of Surgeons, Surg Gynecol Obstet 159:309, 1984.
75. Wolberg WH: Fine needle aspiration for breast mass diagnosis, Arch Surg 123:814, 1989.

5 Conservative Surgery and Radiation for Early Breast Cancer

Barbara Fowble, Lawrence J. Solin, and Delray J. Schultz

The results of prospective randomized trials comparing conservative surgery and radiation to either radical mastectomy or modified radical mastectomy were presented in Chapter 3. In summary, no difference between the two treatments has been demonstrated in terms of local-regional recurrence, distant metastases, long-term survival (i.e., ≥10 years), or the risk of contralateral breast cancer or a second malignancy not involving the breast. The results of multiple retrospective series also were presented in Chapter 3; these series continue to support the role of conservative surgery and radiation in the treatment of early breast cancer.

The goals of the conservative approach are to eradicate microscopic foci of multicentric cancer with moderate doses of radiation, to minimize local recurrence at the primary site, and to maximize benefit in terms of quality of life with a minimal risk of complications and second malignancy and with an acceptable cosmetic result. The success of the conservative approach, however, depends on the expertise and collaboration of the diagnostic radiologist, surgeon, pathologist, radiation oncologist, and medical oncologist. Each of these specialists plays a major role in determining which patients are candidates for conservative surgery and radiation with or without adjuvant systemic therapy, in assuring the delivery of an optimal treatment program, and in diligent follow-up once treatment has been completed.

PATIENT SELECTION

Conservative surgery and radiation represent an alternative equal to mastectomy when outcome for the two treatments is comparable in terms of long-term or disease-free survival and local-regional recurrence. Not all patients with early breast cancer are candidates for conservative surgery and radiation. Patients may not be considered acceptable candidates either because the risk of a breast recurrence following the conservative approach is significant enough to warrant mastectomy or because the likelihood of an unacceptable cosmetic result is high.

Cosmetic considerations

Factors relevant to the cosmetic outcome include the primary tumor size and its location, the overall breast size or total body weight, and a history of a preexisting collagen vascular disease. For the patient with a very small breast, a complete excision of the primary tumor may result in a significant cosmetic defect. This patient may be better treated by mastectomy and reconstruction. However, a recent report from the National Cancer Institute in Milan indicated that 20% of patients who undergo quadrantectomy experience a deformity that merits surgical correction.[60] The authors report successful reconstruction with reshaping of the breast and volume augmentation with a custom prosthesis. Therefore breast size relative to tumor size may become less of a consideration. Patients with large pendulous breasts or obese patients are less likely to achieve a good to excellent cosmetic result when treatment involves conservative surgery and radiation because of increased breast fibrosis and retraction.[25,106,132] Approximately 50% to 60% of obese women or women with large breasts will have a good to excellent cosmetic result, compared to 80% to 90% of women with small to moderate size breasts or a body weight <160 lb.[25,106,132] An additional cosmetic consideration is the patient with a subareolar primary tumor. Resection of the nipple areolar complex may be required to achieve complete excision of the primary tumor. This may result in an unacceptable cosmetic result for the patient, although, as noted by Recht and Harris,[137] the appearance of the remaining breast may be as good as that of a reconstructed breast following mastectomy. Patients with subareolar primary tumors, however, may not be candidates for the conservative approach because of extensive disease along the ducts of the breast as discussed in the following section. Patients with a preexisting history of collagen vascular disease such as scleroderma or lupus erythematosus have been reported to develop marked fibrosis and soft tissue and bone necrosis following conservative surgery and radiation for early-stage breast cancer.[48,108,131] The relatively high incidence of complications in this group of patients is considered an indication for mastectomy.

Factors affecting breast cancer recurrence in conservatively treated patients

Factors affecting breast recurrence can be divided into three categories: 1) clinical factors; 2) histopathologic factors; and 3) treatment-related factors. Clinical factors include patient age, tumor size, tumor location, gross multicentricity, mammographic evidence of diffuse microcalcifications, and the estrogen and progesterone receptor status. Histopathologic factors include histologic or nuclear grade, tumor necrosis, vascular or lymphatic invasion, inflammatory infiltrate, the presence of intraductal noninvasive cancer in association with an invasive ductal cancer, margins of resection, histology other than infiltrating ductal carcinoma, and the pathologic nodal status. Treatment-related factors include the extent of the surgical resection for the primary tumor, radiation technique, and the use of adjuvant systemic chemotherapy or hormonal therapy.

Multiple series have evaluated the impact of these factors on breast disease recurrence rates following conservative surgery and radiation. The results have been both confirmatory and conflicting. Varying results may be caused by subtle but important differences in treatment, patient selection, or chance. The interaction of various factors may have an impact on the relative importance of each factor. While no consensus exists as to which factors predispose the patient to a risk of breast recurrence that is significant enough to warrant mastectomy, there is general agreement in certain areas.

Recurrence following conservative surgery and radiation is related to the presence of a significant residual tumor burden following excisional biopsy that cannot be controlled with moderate doses of radiation. The likelihood of a significant residual tumor burden has been correlated with both clinical and pathologic factors, including tumor location, the presence of gross multicentric or multifocal disease, diffuse microcalcifications, the association of an extensive intraductal component with an invasive ductal carcinoma, and infiltrating lobular histology.

Tumor location. An increased incidence of multicentricity has been noted for central tumors when compared to inner or outer quadrant lesions[98] and for those involving the nipple.[46] Histopathologic studies[93,116,177] have demonstrated that tumors within 2 to 2½ cm of the nipple areolar complex involve the structure in 40% to 50% of cases. The most common mechanism for involvement is intraductal spread of the tumor.[116,177] Other mechanisms include stromal invasion and lymphatic emboli. The likelihood of nipple involvement also increases with an increase in primary tumor size.[93,116,195] Patients with subareolar tumors may have extensive tumor along the ducts that is not grossly appreciated. Fisher et al.[39] noted that central tumors were more likely to have positive margins of resection following an excisional biopsy. While breast disease recurrence following conservative surgery and radiation has not been correlated with tumor location (Table 5-1), caution must be applied to tumors in the subareolar region. These patients should be considered candidates for conservative surgery and radiation only if adequate excision can be accomplished with negative margins of resection and if the tumor is well localized.

Table 5-1 Breast recurrence following conservative surgery and radiation related to location of primary tumor

	Breast recurrence (%)	
Author	Central/Inner	Outer
Calle et al.[16]	9	7
Balawajder et al.[1]	14	10
Van Limbergen et al.[182]	9	9
Boyages et al.[13]	9	11

Gross multicentric or multifocal disease. The presence of gross multicentric disease demonstrated either clinically or mammographically has been correlated with extensive disease in the breast in studies at the University of Pennsylvania. An example of gross multicentric disease is demonstrated in Fig. 5-1. Fig. 5-2 demonstrates gross multifocal disease in which two discrete masses are identified in the same quadrant. A total of 17 patients with gross multicentric or multifocal disease underwent mastectomy at the University of Pennsylvania following an initial excisional biopsy. Detection was by mammogram only in two patients and by a combination of physical examination and mammography in 15 patients. Eight patients had two lesions demonstrated, eight patients had three, and one patient had five lesions. Clinical and/or mammographic evaluation revealed that in 16 of the 17 patients one or two quadrants of the breast were involved. Pathologic assessment of the mastectomy specimens, however, revealed three or four quadrants of the breast to be involved in nine patients, with one quadrant involved in one patient, and two quadrants involved in five patients. Two patients had no residual tumor at the time of mastectomy. These findings suggest that in this subset of patients with gross multicentric or multifocal

A B

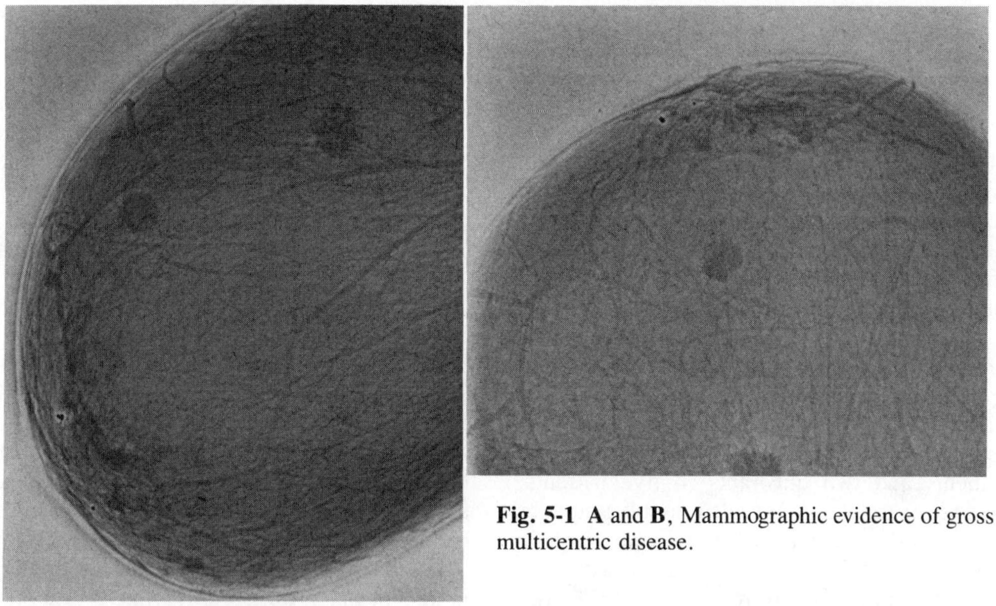

Fig. 5-1 **A** and **B**, Mammographic evidence of gross multicentric disease.

A B

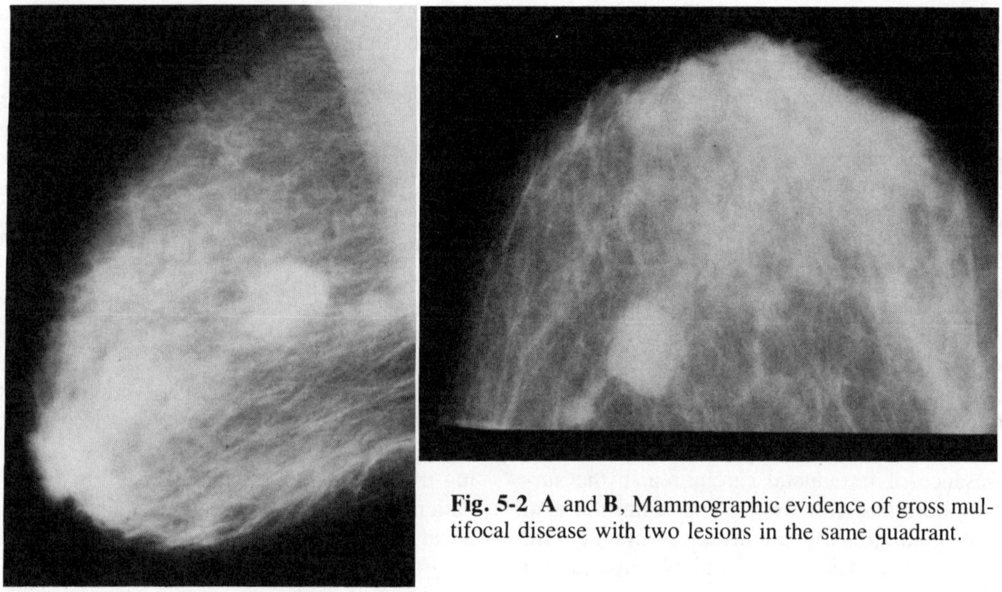

Fig. 5-2 **A** and **B**, Mammographic evidence of gross multifocal disease with two lesions in the same quadrant.

disease, the disease is more extensive in the breast than what is appreciated clinically.

The presence of gross multicentric or multifocal disease has been associated with a high risk of breast recurrence in patients undergoing conservative surgery and radiation. Leopold et al.[97] reported breast recurrence in four of ten patients with gross multicentric or multifocal disease who underwent conservative surgery and radiation at the Joint Center for Radiotherapy. The recurrence rate was 37% in patients who had clinical evidence of gross multicentric or multifocal disease and 50% for those in whom the gross multifocal and multicentric disease was an incidental finding by the pathologist. Kurtz et al.[85] and Clark et al.[24] also reported an increased risk for breast recurrence in patients with macroscopic multifocal tumors. This is in contrast to microscopic multifocal disease, which is not associated with an increased risk of breast recurrence in conservatively treated patients.

Singletary and McNeese[163] reported a breast recurrence rate to be 8% in patients with microscopic, multifocal invasive disease and 4% in patients with microscopic, multifocal noninvasive disease. Despite excisional biopsy in patients with gross multicentric or multifocal disease, a significant residual tumor burden appears to be responsible for the high risk of recurrence.

Diffuse microcalcifications. Similar pathologic findings have been reported in patients whose mammograms revealed diffuse microcalcifications.[33] Sixteen patients with diffuse microcalcifications on mammography and biopsy-proven invasive cancer underwent mastectomy at the University of Pennsylvania. Preoperatively the clinical extent was confined to a single quadrant in 11 patients and two quadrants in five patients. Pathologic examination revealed involvement of four quadrants in one patient and two quadrants in six patients. Of the seven of 16 patients with positive axillary nodes, six were found to have four or more positive nodes. These patients had extensive disease not only in the breast but also in the axilla. Patients with gross multicentric or multifocal disease or diffuse microcalcifications are not candidates for conservative surgery and radiation because of the presence of extensive disease in the breast, which has resulted in a high breast disease recurrence rate.

Extensive intraductal component with invasive ductal carcinoma. The presence of an extensive intraductal component (EIC) in association with an infiltrating ductal carcinoma also has been correlated with the likelihood of having a significant residual tumor burden following gross excision.[74] First described by Schnitt et al.[154] from the Joint Center for Radiation Therapy, the entity by definition consists of the simultaneous presence of an intraductal, noninvasive carcinoma comprising 25% or more of the primary invasive tumor and the presence of intraductal carcinoma in the surrounding normal breast tissue. The definition also includes predominantly noninvasive tumors with focal areas of invasion. The clinical presentation of EIC-positive tumors is most often one of mammographic microcalcifications without an associated mass.[70] Holland et al.[74] in a serial subgross and correlated mammographic examination of 217 mastectomy specimens, correlated the presence of an extensive intraductal component in an invasive ductal cancer with the incidence of residual tumor following excisional biopsy. EIC-positive tumors were significantly more likely to have residual tumor and tumor at greater distances from the primary than EIC-negative tumors. The residual tumor was predominantly noninvasive. At a distance of 2 cm from the edge of the primary tumor, 59% of EIC-positive tumors had residual tumor, as compared to 29% of EIC-negative tumors. At a distance of 6 cm from the edge of the primary tumor, 21% of EIC-positive tumors had residual carcinoma, compared to 8% of EIC-negative tumors. Fisher et al.[46] also correlated multicentricity with the presence of a noninvasive cancer in the vicinity of a dominant mass.

The risk of a breast recurrence following conservative surgery and radiation has been related to the presence of EIC. Recht et al.[138] report the 5-year actuarial recurrence rate to be 23% in patients in whom EIC was present, with a 10-year actuarial rate of 33%. An extensive intraductal component existed in 32% of the patient population. When EIC was absent this 5-year actuarial breast recurrence rate was 5%, and the 10-year actuarial rate was 8%. Both features must be present for the risk of a breast recurrence to be increased. With an extensive intraductal component in the primary tumor only, the 5-year actuarial breast recurrence rate was 5%, and in the presence of intraductal carcinoma in the adjacent breast tissue only, the 5-year actuarial breast recurrence rate was 6%.[13] The absence of both of these features resulted in a 5-year actuarial rate of 3%.[13] The mere presence of an intraductal component has not been associated with an increased risk of breast recurrence.[27,34,182] Osteen et al.[122] further subdivided the entity into macroscopic EIC, in which there is a clinically defined tumor mass with the intraductal component limited to the palpable abnormality, and microscopic EIC, in which the intraductal component is detected only on permanent histologic section and is not obvious to either the surgeon or the pathologist at the time of gross inspection or frozen section. Macroscopic EIC was associated with a 5-year actuarial risk of breast disease recurrence of 8%, whereas that for microscopic EIC was 27%. It must be emphasized that data regarding the risk of a breast recurrence in EIC-positive patients treated at the Joint Center was obtained during a period of time in which preoperative mammograms were not performed routinely and assessment of resection margins was not standard policy.

Multiple other series have assessed the impact of an extensive intraductal component on breast recurrence (Tables 5-2 and 5-3). Unfortunately, there has not been uniformity in adherence to the original definition, and changes in the definition have resulted in significant variations in the percentage of patients with this feature in the total patient population. The intraductal component has been assessed in terms of its mere presence or absence, its extent in the primary tumor only, its extent in the primary tumor and presence in adja-

Table 5-2 Breast recurrence related to the presence/extent of an intraductal noninvasive component (IC)

Author	Total no. pts.	Surgery	IC present (%)	Definition
Boyages et al.[13]	445	LE	32	>25% primary tumor + outside
Bartelink et al.[3]	495	LE, WE	16	>25% tumor area
Fourquet et al.[50]	424	WE	15	>25% primary tumor + >25% outside
Koper et al.[82]	566	WE	50	Primary tumor + adjacent area
Kurtz et al.[85]	496	WE	21	>25% primary tumor + outside
Lindley et al.[102]	265	LE	19	>25% primary tumor
Van Limbergen et al.[182]	233	WE, Q	9	Extensive involvement
Clarke et al.[27]	375	WE, Q	28	IC present
Maylin et al.[110]	340	LE	20	IC present
Delouche et al.[34]	372	LE	19	IC present

LE, local excision; WE, wide excision; Q, quadrantectomy.

cent tissue, or its extent in the primary tumor and its extent in adjacent tissue. Only one other series[85] has employed the criteria established by the Joint Center. Breast recurrence related to EIC is presented in Table 5-2. Differences in the magnitude of the recurrence in EIC-positive tumors are noted. The extent of the surgery for the primary tumor as well as the use of different definitions may be responsible for these variations. In series where margins of resection have been assessed and are negative,[3,47,197] EIC has not been a prognostic factor for recurrence. There is a single exception to this observation. Kurtz et al.[86] reported that negative margins of resection did not decrease the risk of a breast recurrence significantly in young women (<40 years of age) with either a major cellular reaction (moderate to marked lymphocytic or lymphoplasmocytic cell reaction within the tumor stroma), and/or more than 50% intraductal carcinoma within the tumor. The breast recurrence rate was 31% for patients with negative margins, 45% for those with indeterminate margins, and 67% for those with positive margins. Margin assessment was not performed by routine inking of the specimen but was assessed retrospectively by reviewing routine sections through the tumor as well as those taken at the periphery. It is difficult to know whether this method of margin assessment may be responsible for the finding that negative margins of resection did not decrease the risk of a breast recurrence in young women with EIC-positive tumors. The significance of EIC in predicting for a breast recurrence also appears to be age related. Kurtz et al.[85] found EIC to be a significant factor for breast recurrence only in premenopausal women. The risk was not influenced by the addition of single-agent chemotherapy. However, Rose et al.[142] also have reported a decrease in the risk of such recurrence in premenopausal patients with EIC-positive tumors who received multiagent adjuvant chemotherapy (30% vs. 13%).

Table 5-3 Breast recurrence related to intraductal component within and adjacent to primary tumor

	No. pts.	Breast recurrence (%) 5 yr.	10 yr.
EIC-negative			
Recht et al.[138]	302	5	8
Zafrani et al.[197]	361	6	5
Bartelink et al.[3]	208	2	
Koper et al.[82]	283	13	
Kurtz et al.[85]	390	8	
EIC-positive			
Recht et al.[138]	143	23	33
Zafrani et al.[197]	63	11	23
Bartelink et al.[3]	79	9	
Koper et al.[82]	283	10	
Kurtz et al.[85]	106	18	

EIC, extensive intraductal component.

It should be emphasized that EIC-positive tumors are not associated with an increased risk of distant metastases. Schnitt et al.[157] reported distant metastases in 20% of patients with EIC-positive tumors, compared to 21% of those with EIC-negative tumors. The presence of an intraductal component in an invasive ductal cancer has been associated with an overall better prognosis.[145,162]

Therefore the presence of an extensive intraductal component is a pathologic indicator that the disease in the breast may be more extensive than what is appreciated clinically. Assessment of resection margins in these patients is important in

Table 5-4 Breast recurrence related to histology

Histologic subtype	Breast recurrence at 5 yr (%)		
	Mate[107]	Schnitt[156]	Kurtz[87]
Infiltrating ductal carcinoma	13 [108]	11 [561]	9 [709]
Infiltrating lobular carcinoma	25 [12]	12 [49]	13.5 [67]
Medullary carcinoma			4 [27]
Colloid carcinoma			0 [11]

[ ], total no. pts.

determining treatment options. Patients with EIC-positive tumors in whom the initial margins of resection are positive should undergo reexcision. If the reexcision margins are negative, current information would suggest that they are appropriate candidates for conservative surgery and radiation,[3,47,197] although a single series[86] suggests that even the existence of negative margins of resection in premenopausal women with EIC-positive tumors does not reduce the risk of a breast recurrence. If the reexcision margins are positive, mastectomy is the preferred treatment.

Infiltrating lobular histology. Multicentricity for invasive breast cancer also has been associated with an infiltrating lobular histology. Approximately 50% of patients with an invasive lobular cancer will have residual tumor in the breast following an initial excisional biopsy, as demonstrated by mastectomy specimens,[61,98,144] compared to 15% to 30% of patients with an invasive ductal cancer.[61,98,144] Breast recurrence related to histologic subtype following conservative surgery and radiation is presented in Table 5-4. While Mate et al.[107] reported an increased risk of such recurrence in patients with infiltrating lobular carcinoma, their conclusion was based on 12 patients. Schnitt et al.[156] and Kurtz et al.,[87] reporting on larger number of patients, noted a minimal increase in risk for patients with infiltrating lobular carcinomas when compared to infiltrating ductal carcinomas. The risk appears small for patients with medullary or colloid carcinomas.

Tumor size. The likelihood of multicentric breast cancer or a significant residual tumor following excisional biopsy has not been correlated with a primary tumor size of <4 to 5 cm. The risk of multicentric breast cancer is not greater for T_2 tumors when compared to T_1 tumors.[46,61,75,145] Rosen et al.[144] found the risk of multicentricity to increase only for tumors >4 cm and Fisher et al.[46] found an increased risk of multicentricity only for tumors >5 cm. These findings correlate well with the observation that patients with T_2 tumors undergoing conservative surgery and radiation do not have an increased risk of breast disease recurrence when compared to patients with T_1 tumors provided that an excisional biopsy has been performed (Table 5-5).

Other factors studied following conservative surgery and radiation

Axillary node status. Multicentricity appears not to be related to the pathologic axillary nodal status. While Lesser et al.[98] noted an increased incidence of multicentricity with histologically positive axillary nodes when compared to those with negative axillary, Fisher et al.[46] and Lagios et al.[92] noted no correlation with histologic nodal status and the incidence of multicentricity. Table 5-6 presents the influence of pathologic axillary node status on breast recurrence in patients undergoing conservative surgery and radiation. Unlike a chest wall recurrence after mastectomy, there appears to be no increased risk of a breast recurrence in patients with histologically positive axillary nodes. This finding correlates with the fact that patients with positive axillary nodes do not have a greater risk of a significant residual tumor burden.[46,92]

Patient age. Patient age has not been correlated with a greater incidence of multicentricity.[46] However, an initial report from Vilcoq et al.[192] suggested that patients ≤30 years of age who underwent conservative surgery and radiation had a local-regional recurrence rate of 35% as compared to 4% in those >30 years of age. A subsequent update by Fourquet et al.[50] confirmed these initial findings. In patients ≤32 years of age at the time of diagnosis, the 10-year actuarial breast disease recurrence rate was 43%, compared to 15% for patients of age 33 to 45 years, 6% for age 46 to 55 years, and 3% for age >55 years. Subsequent reports with age divisions less than or greater than 50 years, less than or greater than 40 years, or less than or greater than 35 years have produced varying results (Tables 5-7, 5-8, and 5-9). Recht et al.[135] reported a 5-year actuarial breast recurrence rate of 26% in 47 women <35 years of age at the time of treatment. The University of Pennsylvania has demonstrated

Table 5-5 Breast recurrence related to clinical tumor size following excisional biopsy or quadrantectomy and radiation

Author	Breast recurrence (%)	
	T_1	T_2
NSABP B-06[43]	7	10
Veronesi et al.[184]	4	
Clarke et al.[27]	6	3
Calle et al.[16]	7	11
Delouche et al.[34]	6	14
Solin et al.[169]	5	8
Spitalier et al.[175]	13	15
Van Limbergen et al.[182]	5	15
Boyages et al.[13]	10	10
Nobler and Venet[118]	7	8

Table 5-6 Breast recurrence following conservative surgery and radiation related to pathologic nodal status

Author	Breast recurrence (%)	
	Node-negative	Node-positive
NSABP B-06[43]	12	6
Clarke et al.[27]	4	7
Solin et al.[169]	7	4
Durand et al.[38]	1	4
Van Limbergen et al.[182]	10	15
Recht et al.[138]	12	10
Bedwinek et al.[7]	8	6

Table 5-7 Breast recurrence related to age ≤35 years vs. >35 years

Author	Breast recurrence (%)		Follow-up
	≤35 yr age	>35 yr age	
Clarke et al.[27]	9 [32]	5 [424]	5-yr mean
Recht et al.[135]	26 [47]	10 [560]	5-yr actuarial
Muscolino et al.[117]	9 [95]	4 [1137]	—
Kurtz et al.[89]	16 [91]	10 [1291]	11-yr mean
Mathews et al.[109]	15 [72]	5 [306]	≥2 yr
Solin et al.[173]	9 [86]	8 [798]	5-yr actuarial

[ ], total no. pts.

Table 5-8 Breast recurrence related to age <40 yr vs. ≥40 yr

Author	Breast recurrence (%)		Follow-up
	<40 yr age	≥40 yr age	
Vilcoq et al.[192]	14 [70]	3 [235]	≥3 yr
Delouche et al.[34]	20 [71]	7 [339]	11-yr median
Van Limbergen et al.[182]	21	6-11	5-yr actuarial
Kurtz et al.[89]	12 [210]	6 [1172]	5-yr actuarial
	19 [210]	9 [1172]	11-yr median
Maylin et al.[110]	20 [82]	5 [328]	≥5 yr
Ryoo et al.[148]	16 [51]	5 [342]	3.5-yr median

[ ], total no. pts.

Table 5-9 Breast recurrence related to age ≤50 yr vs. >50 yr

Author	Breast recurrence (%)		Follow-up
	≤50 yr age	>50 yr age	
Delouche et al.[34]	13 [210]	6 [200]	11-yr median
Mate et al.[107]	12 [57]	12 [94]	5 yr
Nobler and Venet[118]	27 [15]	3 [128]	3.8-yr median
Fisher et al.[39]	9 [242]	6.5 [324]	5-yr actuarial
Recht et al.[135]	16 [298]	6 [309]	5-yr actuarial
Kurtz et al.[89]	13 [695]	8 [687]	11-yr median
Mathews et al.[109]	12 [205]	5 [173]	≥2 yr
Vilcoq et al.[192]	10 [183]	0 [131]	≥3 yr

[ ], total no. pts.

no increase in breast recurrence in young women.[173] While younger women tended to have an earlier pattern of failure, the difference between the actuarial percentage of failures at 5 years was not statistically significant. The 5-year actuarial risk of such recurrence was 9% in women ≤35 years of age, compared to 8% for those >35 years of age. Kurtz et al.[89] reported this rate to be 12% in women <40 years of age with a crude rate of 19% compared to 6% and 9% in women >40 years of age. In a multivariate analysis[85] age was not a predictor for breast recurrence.

Because age alone has not been correlated with an increased incidence of significant residual tumor burden,[46] attention has been drawn to the presence of additional factors in these young women that could account for an increased risk of breast recurrence. Three series have reported a greater prevalence of EIC-positive tumors in young women.[50,86,135] Because EIC-positive tumors are associated with an increased risk of a significant residual tumor burden,[74] the association of young age and EIC-positive tumors may account for the increased risk in young women. However, Recht et al.[135] noted that the presence of EIC was not entirely responsible for the increased risk of breast recurrence because the recurrence in young patients was 22% when EIC was absent compared to 3% in older women. Fourquet et al.[50] also noted a greater prevalence of inadequate surgery in young women. Inadequate surgery for the primary tumor clearly results in a greater incidence of breast recurrence[7,20,136,182] and may be an additional factor. Kurtz et al.[86] also noted that younger women more often had tumors exhibiting a major cellular reaction, and that this pathologic factor was found in a multivariate analysis to be a significant predictor for breast recurrence. The significance of young age as a predictor for breast recurrence in conservatively treated patients also may be influenced by treatment-related factors. As previously noted, inadequate surgery of the primary tumor may be responsible for an increased risk of a breast recurrence.[50] Several series have noted a decrease in the risk of breast recurrence in patients receiving multiagent chemotherapy and radiation.[11,43,142,169] Specifically for young women, Rose et al.[142] reported a breast recurrence rate of 9% in women <35 years of age who were treated with conservative surgery and radiotherapy with adjuvant chemotherapy, compared to 26% for those who did not receive adjuvant chemotherapy. Kurtz et al.[86] failed to note a significant decrease in breast recurrence in young women receiving adjuvant chemotherapy, although most of the patients received only perioperative single-agent treatment.[85] Similarly, the authors failed to note a decrease in breast recurrence rates in young women with negative margins of resection who had either EIC-positive tumors or a major cellular reaction.[86] In Table 5-10 the crude and actuarial breast recurrence rates for five major series are presented.[89,109,135,173,182] Variations exist in the use of reexcision of the primary tumor, evaluation of pathologic margins of

Table 5-10 Results of definitive irradiation and conservative surgery for early breast cancer in young women: summary of series reporting breast recurrence rates

	Recht[135]	Mathews[109]	Van Limbergen[182]	Kurtz[89]	Solin[173]
Age	≤34 yr	≤35 yr	≤39 yr	≤39 yr	≤35 yr
Treatment period	1968-1981	1955-1983	1966-1979	1963-1981	1977-1986
No. treated breasts	47	72	NS	210	88
T_1 lesions (%)	53	NS	24*	58	50
Reexcision of the primary tumor (%)	NS	NS	NS	NS	64
Evaluation of the pathology margins of the primary tumor (%)	NS	NS	NS	NS	53
Axillary lymph node dissection (%)	85	57*	60*	30	100
Pathologic N_1 axillae (%)	40	29*	NS	56	37
Chemotherapy (%)	32	NS	14*	16	40
Breast recurrence					
Actuarial at 5 years (%)	26	NS	21	12	9
Crude (%)	23	12	NS	20	7

NS, not stated.
*For younger and older women combined.
From Solin et al: Int J Radiat Oncol Biol Phys 12:721, 1986.

Table 5-11 Survival following conservative surgery and radiation for early-stage breast cancer related to age

Author		5-yr survival (%)		
		<35 yr		>35 yr	
Recht et al.[135]		89		85	
Solin et al.[173]		94 [78]		90 [81]	
Mathews et al.[109]		85 [70]		87 [82]	
Calle et al.[16]	≤32 [68]		33-50 [87]		≥51 [80]

[ ], disease-free survival.

resection, and the use of adjuvant systemic chemotherapy. It is possible that significant differences in treatment account for the variations in the breast recurrence rate as well as the relative significance of age as a predictor for breast recurrence. In the University of Pennsylvania series, where emphasis is placed on complete gross excision of the primary tumor with reexcision where indicated and assessment of resection margins as well as the use of adjuvant systemic chemotherapy in all premenopausal node-positive patients, there is no increased risk of breast recurrence associated with young age.

There is no evidence to suggest that younger women who undergo conservative surgery and radiation for the treatment of early breast cancer have a diminished 5-year survival when compared to older women (Table 5-11), although Mathews et al.[109] and Calle et al.[16] have reported a decreased disease-free survival rate in young women. Table 5-12 compares 5-year survival rates and disease-free survival rates in young women undergoing conservative surgery and radiation with those treated by mastectomy from retrospective series. There appears to be no survival benefit associated with mastectomy in this group of patients.

Histologic grade, vascular/lymphatic invasion, necrosis, and inflammatory infiltrate. The likelihood of multicentricity has not been correlated with various other histopathologic factors including histologic grade, the presence or absence of vascular or lymphatic invasion, tumor necrosis, or a prominent inflammatory infiltrate.[46] The relative significance of these factors in predicting for a breast recurrence in patients undergoing conservative surgery and radiation is presented in Tables 5-13 and 5-14. Again, there appears to be no universal agreement as to the significance of these factors. While there is a trend for an increased risk of breast recurrence in patients with histologic grade III tumors or those with vascular or lymphatic invasion, these findings are not always confirmed in a multivariate analysis (Table 5-15). Schnitt et al.[154] reported a higher breast recurrence rate in patients with nuclear grade III tumors (15%) when compared to nuclear grade I or grade II (3%). Two series have suggested that the presence of tumor necrosis is associated with an increased risk of recurrence,[102,107] however, in the Yale series the significance was associated with necrosis in the invasive component of the tumor[107] whereas in the Westminster series[102] it was associated with necro-

Table 5-12 Results of treatment of young women with early-stage breast cancer

Author	No. pts.	Age (yr)	5-yr survival (%) Conservative surgery and R	5-yr survival (%) Mastectomy
Calle et al.[16]	32	≤32	[68]	
Recht et al.[135]	47	<35	89	
Mathews et al.[109]	113	≤35	85 [70]	75 [70]
Clark et al.[27]	44	≤35	73	
Solin et al.[173]	86	≤35	94 [77]	
Rosen et al.[146]	166	≤35		75 [70]
Noyes et al.[119]	84	≤30		[51]
Hermann et al.[71]	64	≤35		64

R, radiation; [ ], disease-free survival.

Table 5-13 Breast recurrence related to histologic grade

Author	Breast recurrence (%)		
	I	II	III
Mate et al.[107]	4	13	16
Fisher et al.[47]	0	3	6
Calle et al.[16]	5	12	5
Clarke et al.[27]	1	6	4
Van Limbergen et al.[182]	5	10	16
Kurtz et al.[85]	3	9	17
Lindley et al.[102]	4	11	21
Pezner et al.[123]	3		18

Table 5-14 Breast recurrence related to vascular/lymphatic invasion

Author	Breast recurrence (%)	
	No	Yes
Singletary and McNeese[163]	—	11
Fisher et al.[47]	3	8
Mate et al.[107]	11	19
Fourquet et al.[50]	10	25
Lindley et al.[102]	—	19
Koper et al.[82]	7	22

Table 5-15 Significant pathologic discriminants for a breast recurrence: multivariate analysis

Author	Necrosis	Lymphatic/vascular invasion	Inflammatory infiltrate	Histologic grade
JCRT[13,154]	No	No	No	No
Marseille[85]	No	No	Yes	Yes
Curie[50]	—	Yes	—	No
Yale[107]	Yes	No	No	No
Westminster[102]	Yes	No	Yes	Yes
Rotterdam[82]	—	Yes	—	No
IGR[27]	—	—	—	Yes
NSABP B-06[47]	No	No	No	No

sis in the noninvasive component of the tumor. A prominent inflammatory infiltrate has been associated with an increased risk of breast recurrence in two series,[85,102] but not in one additional series.[107]

Estrogen and progesterone receptor status. The impact of estrogen and progesterone receptor status on breast recurrence in patients undergoing conservative surgery and radiation is uncertain. Kurtz et al.[89] demonstrated an increased risk of breast recurrence in women <40 years of age with estrogen receptor–negative tumors. Ryoo et al.[148] also reported a breast recurrence rate of 16% in patients with negative estrogen receptor status, as compared to a rate of 4% in patients with positive estrogen receptor status. In a multivariate analysis negative estrogen receptor status correlated significantly with breast recurrence. Others[47,82,110] have found no correlation between estrogen receptor status and breast recurrence. Similarly, a negative progesterone receptor status has been correlated with breast recurrence in one study[82] and not in three others.[47,89,110]

Risk factors for breast recurrence by institution

In summary, the identification of factors associated with a significant risk for recurrence of breast disease in patients undergoing conservative surgery and radiation is a complex issue. Table 5-16 summarizes the risk factors identified by various institutions, the recurrence rates associated with these factors, and the percentage of patients treated who presented with these factors. It is apparent that the simultaneous presence of several features enhances the risk for a breast recurrence and that the majority of patients treated are not in the high-risk group. However, the importance of each of these factors clearly can be modified by treatment including wider surgical resections, negative margins, and the use of adjuvant systemic chemotherapy or hormonal therapy. For example, the presence of an extensive intraductal component has not been found to be a significant factor for breast recurrence in patients with negative margins of resection,[3,47,197] although Kurtz et al.[86] noted no decrease in recur-

Table 5-16 Identification of patients with greatest risk for breast recurrence by institutional experience

	5-yr actuarial breast recurrence (%)	All pts. (%)
Joint Center[13,97,122,135,138]		
Gross multicentric	40 (crude)	1
Age <35	26	8
EIC+	23	32
EIC+, age <35	38	4
EIC+, Grade 3	37	24
EIC+, LVI	34	9
Micro EIC+	27	9
Micro EIC+, age <50	40	—
M.D. Anderson[163]		
Gr 3, lymphatic invasion	21 (crude)	—
Yale[107]		
Necrosis	20	30
Marseille[85]		
Premenopausal EIC+, MCR+	53	8 (pre)
Postmenopausal Gr 3, positive or unknown margin	33	13 (post)
Curie[50]		
Inadequate surgery	28 (10 yr)	14
Age <32 yr	43 (10 yr)	7
Vascular/lymphatic invasion	25 (10 yr)	6

EIC, extensive intraductal component; MCR, major mononuclear cell reaction.

rence rates in premenopausal women with EIC-positive tumors and negative margins of resection. While larger resections of the primary tumor such as quadrantectomy for reexcision may decrease breast recurrence in EIC-positive tumors, the use of large-volume implants with doses >7000 cGy does not decrease the recurrence rate in these patients. Boyages et al.[13] reported a 33% 5-year actuarial breast recurrence in EIC-positive patients who received >7000 cGy to the primary site or an implant whose volume was >75 seeds. This was compared to a 5-year actuarial breast recurrence rate of 23% in patients in whom the dose to the primary tumor site was <7000 cGy or the implant volume was <75 seeds. The addition of adjuvant chemotherapy to conservative surgery and radiation has resulted in a decreased breast recurrence rate both in EIC-positive patients and young women. Rose et al.[142] reported a decrease in breast recurrence rates from 30% to 13% with the addition of chemotherapy in EIC-positive premenopausal patients, and a decrease from 26% to 9% in women <35 years of age. Kurtz et al.[86] reported no significant decrease in breast recurrence with the addition of chemotherapy in premenopausal women, although the chemotherapy was often single agent and not multiagent. Tamoxifen also has resulted in a significant decrease in breast recurrence in node-negative, estrogen receptor (ER)–positive patients undergoing conservative surgery and radiation as reported in the NSABP B-14 study.[40] The NSABP B-06 study identified no significant clinical or histopathologic features that correlated with breast recurrence in patients undergoing conservative surgery and radiation whose margins of resection were histologically negative.[47] Kurtz et al.[85] also identified no histopathologic factors that could predict for a breast recurrence in postmenopausal women whose margins of resection were negative and in premenopausal women with negative margins of resection; only the presence of an extensive intraductal component or a major cellular reaction significantly correlated breast recurrence.

Status of resection margin

A final issue is whether patients with microscopically positive margins of resection are candidates for conservative surgery and radiation. In the NSABP B-06 protocol,[39] an arbitrary decision was made to treat patients with microscopically positive

Table 5-17 Incidence of microscopically positive margin(s) following initial excisional biopsy

Author	No. pts.	Primary tumor size (cm)	Surgery	Positive margin (%)
Volterrani et al.[193]	291	≤2.5	LE	16
Clarke et al.[27]	362	≤2.5	WE	24
Hunig et al.[77]	109	≤3	LE	14
Fisher et al.[39]	625	≤4	WE	7
Solin et al.[169]	218	<5	LE, WE	25
McCormick et al.[111]	75	≤5	WE	28
Bartelink et al.[3]	369	≤5	WE	9
Lagios et al.[94]	43	≤5	WE	23

LE, local excision; WE, wide excision.

margins of resection with mastectomy. Assessment of resection margins is a sampling tool that provides a guide for the extent of surgical resection, an estimate of the residual tumor burden, and information for treatment decisions. In general the margin is considered positive when tumor cells are noted at the resection margin, close when tumor cells are within 2 mm of the resection margin, or negative when the tumor margin is >2 mm. If margins are positive it must be determined whether they are grossly positive or microscopically positive, how many of the margins are positive, whether the involvement is focal or diffuse, and whether there is an invasive or a noninvasive tumor at the margin. The location of the margin involvement also should be stated. Involvement of the most superficial or anterior margin may have little significance because these more superficial tissues are removed. Similarly, a positive deep margin at the pectoral fascia without extension through the fascia may not be clinically important. Grossly positive margins of resection are associated with an increased risk of the breast recurrence. Zafrani et al.[197] reported a 10-year actuarial breast recurrence rate of 24% in patients with grossly positive margins, as compared to 9% in those with grossly negative margins. Therefore patients with grossly positive margins of resection must undergo reexcision before the initiation of radiation.

Microscopically positive margins of resection have been reported in 20% to 25% of patients undergoing an initial excisional biopsy (Table 5-17). The likelihood of obtaining negative margins of resection is related to the initial surgical procedure, the primary tumor size, and histology. Surgical resections such as a wide excision or quadrantectomy result in a lower incidence of microscopically positive margins (Table 5-18). Patients with T_2 primary tumors have a greater incidence of microscopically positive margins (Table 5-19). Fisher et al.[39] also noted a higher incidence of microscopically positive margins in patients with histologically positive nodes, although McCormick et al.[111] reported a higher incidence in histologically node-negative patients. Patients with an extensive intraductal component have a higher incidence of both initial margin positivity and reexcision margin positivity. Schnitt et al.[155] reported 95% initial margin positivity and 60% reexcision margin positivity in 25 patients with an extensive intraductal component. In 45 patients in whom an extensive intraductal component was absent the initial margin positivity rate was 65% and the reexcision margin was positive in 31%. Fisher et al.[39] also have reported an increased incidence of margin positivity in patients with central primary tumors.

Breast recurrence related to the status of the resection margin is presented in Table 5-20. In

Table 5-18 Incidence of microscopically positive margin related to surgical procedure

	Microscopically positive margin (%)		
Author	LE	WE	Q
Kantorowitz et al.[81]		6	0
Volterrani et al.[193]		16	3
Ghossein et al.[57]	37	15	6
Frazier et al.[55]	46		

LE, local excision; WE, wide excision; Q, quadrantectomy.

Table 5-19 Factors related to microscopically positive margin of resection

	Positive margin (%)		
Factor	Fisher[39]	Hunig[77]	McCormick[111]
T size			
T_1	7	6	23
T_2	13	26	38
Pathologic nodal status			
N_0	7		29
N_1	15		22

general for patients with microscopically positive margins of resection there is no evidence of an increased risk of breast recurrence, provided that boost doses of radiation are employed. At the University of Pennsylvania, the 5-year actuarial risk of a breast disease recurrence was 7% in patients with negative margins, 9% in those with unknown margins, 11% in those with close margins, and 2% in those with positive margins. It must be emphasized that for the most part these margins were focally and not diffusely positive. Patients with diffuse margin involvement underwent mastectomy. Kurtz et al.[85] reported a 5-year actuarial recurrence rate of 6% in patients with negative margins of resection, compared to 22.5% in patients with positive margins of resection. However, the status of the margins was not determined by inking of the pathologic specimen but by a retrospective review of sections taken from the tumor and peripheral tissue. Microscopically positive margins of resection are, therefore, not a contraindication to conservative surgery and radiation provided that a boost dose of radiation is employed and margin involvement is not diffuse. Omission of the boost in patients with microscopically positive margins has been correlated with an increased incidence of breast recurrence.[148] Patients with EIC-positive tumors are more likely to have a positive margin of reexcision, and in these patients negative margins of resection appear essential to minimize the risk of a breast recurrence. Microscopic involvement of a margin in patients who do not have EIC-positive tumors does not appear to be associated with an increased risk of recurrence.

Selection of candidates for conservative treatment

Of the various clinical and histopathologic factors that investigators have analyzed for their ability to predict breast disease recurrence in patients undergoing conservative surgery and radiation, at the present time only the following appear to have an impact on patient selection: the presence of gross multicentric or multifocal disease, diffuse microcalcifications, or the presence of an extensive intraductal component. Patients with gross multicentric or multifocal disease or diffuse microcalcifications on a mammogram have a significant residual tumor burden following excisional biopsy, and a breast recurrence rate high enough to warrant mastectomy. Patients with an extensive intraductal component must be evaluated thoroughly with preoperative mammograms to exclude the possibility of diffuse microcalcifications. Assessment of resection margins should be performed. EIC-positive patients with negative margins of resection appear to have an acceptably low risk of breast recurrence. Patients with multiple positive margins of resection after reexcision should be referred for mastectomy. Young age by itself is not a contraindication to conservative surgery and radiation. Careful assessment of tumors in the subareolar location also must be performed since these patients often have extensive disease along the ducts.

Patients who are considered good candidates for conservative surgery and radiation are those with

Table 5-20 Breast recurrence related to microscopic margin of resection

Author	Positive	Close	Negative	Unknown	Follow-up (yr)
University of Pennsylvania	2 [57]	11 [37]	7 [257]	9 [346]	5 (actuarial)
Hunig et al.[77]	7 [15]		6 [90]		2.3 (median)
Clarke et al.[27]	9 [88]		4 [274]		5 (mean)
Bartelink et al.[3]	7 [32]		2 [242]		6 (actuarial)
Schmidt-Ullrich et al.[153]	0 [46]		0 [61]		4.7 (median)
Fisher et al.[43]			10 [629]		8 (actuarial)
Zafrani et al.[197]			9		10 (actuarial)
Kurtz et al.[86]	24 [49]		8 [283]	16 [164]	5.9 (median)
Ryoo et al.[148]	13 [23]	8 [87]	6 [283]		3.5 (median)

[ ], total no. pts.

Table 5-21 Local recurrence following conservative surgery and radiation stage I and stage II breast cancer

Author	Local recurrence (%)		
	Excisional biopsy	Incisional biopsy	Follow-up (yr)
Van Limbergen et al.[182]	10	30	5 (actuarial)
Recht et al.[136]	7	31	5 (actuarial)
Bedwinek et al.[7]	5	20	3.4 (median)
Chu et al.[20]	10	39	4.2 (median)

Table 5-22 Local recurrence related to extent of breast surgery

Author	Local recurrence (%)	
	Excisional biopsy	Quadrantectomy
Clarke et al.[27]	5 [369]	9 [43]
Van Limbergen et al.[182]	15 [149]	7 [69]
Nobler and Venet[118]	7 [87]	6 [48]
Chu et al.[20]	10 [110]	11 [18]
NSABP B-06[43]	10 [629]	
Milan[185]		4 [352]

[ ], total no. pts.

a primary tumor size ≤4 to 5 cm and a single discrete tumor; if microcalcifications are present, they must be focal. In patients with focal microcalcifications, all microcalcifications should be removed before initiation of radiotherapy. Patients with a preexisting history of collagen vascular disease should not be offered conservative surgery and radiation because of the high risk of complications associated with this treatment. Radiation should not be employed in the treatment of a pregnant woman with early breast cancer; either it is delayed until the postpartum period or the pregnancy is terminated.

Table 5-23 Breast recurrence related to extent of primary surgery

Author	5-yr actuarial breast recurrence (%)		
	LE	WE	Q
Recht et al.[138]	10		
Kurtz et al.[84]		7	
Fourquet et al.[50]		7	
Veronesi et al.[185]			4
Kantorowitz et al.[81]	[16]	[12]	[3]
Van Limbergen et al.[182]		12	5
Ghossein et al.[57]	[12]	[6]	[6]

LE, local excision; WE, wide excision; Q, quadrantectomy; [ ], crude breast recurrence.

SURGICAL CONSIDERATIONS IN PATIENTS UNDERGOING CONSERVATIVE SURGERY AND RADIATION

Primary tumor

The extent of surgical resection of the primary tumor before radiation has ranged from simple excision without regard to surgical margins to wide resection, removing from 1 to 2 cm of normal surrounding breast tissue to performing quadrantectomy in which the entire quadrant with the overlying skin and underlying fascia is removed. Incisional biopsies are not appropriate as they result in a threefold to fourfold increase in breast recurrence rates when moderate doses of radiation are employed (Table 5-21). When compared with wide excision, quadrantectomy results in a less optimal cosmetic result, with obvious volume loss of the breast (Figs. 5-3 and 5-4). Tables 5-22 and 5-23 present breast recurrence rates related to the extent of surgery for the primary tumor. There appears to be no significant reduction in the recurrence rate with the use of quadrantectomy. A comparison of two prospective randomized trials reveals a 10% recurrence rate for patients undergoing wide excision with negative margins of resection in the NSABP B-06 study[43] compared to a 4% rate in the Milan trial[185] in which quadrantectomy was employed. While wider resection may be required for patients with an extensive intraductal component, there appears to be little advantage for more extensive resection on a routine basis. From 1985 to 1987 the National Cancer Institute in Milan conducted a prospective randomized trial comparing tumorectomy (removal of the primary tumor with <1.0 cm margin of normal tissue) and boost with a single-plane iridium-192 implant to quadrantec-

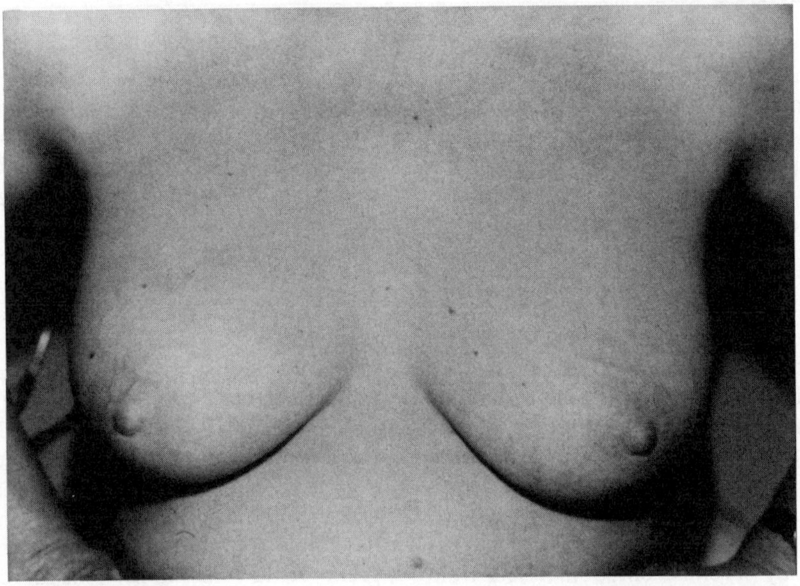

Fig. 5-3 Cosmetic appearance of the breast *(right)* in a patient who has undergone wide excision of the primary tumor.

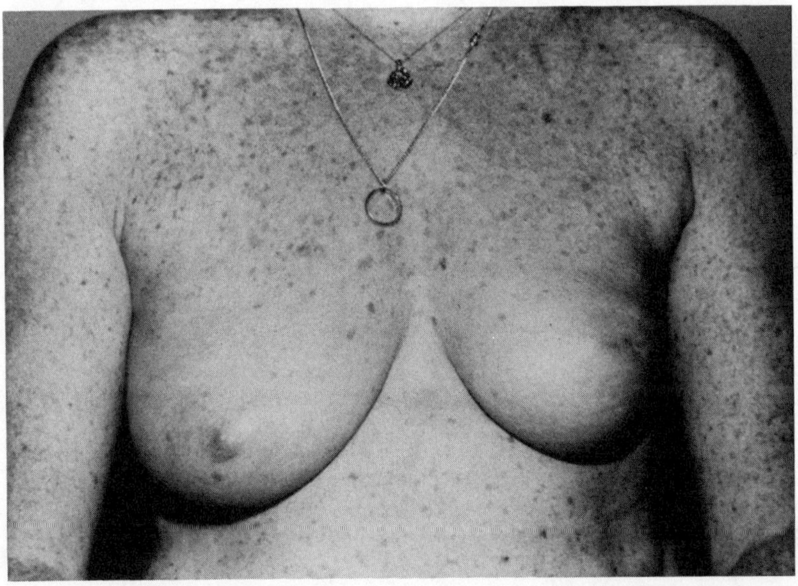

Fig. 5-4 Cosmetic appearance of the breast *(left)* in a patient who has undergone quadrantectomy. There is obvious volume loss of the breast. (From Danoff BF et al: Ann Intern Med 102:639, 1985.)

Table 5-24 Incidence of residual tumor at the time of reexcision

Author	No. pts.	Indication	Positive residual (%)
Montague[114]	67	Biopsy elsewhere	57
McCormick et al.[111]	22	Biopsy elsewhere, positive margin	50
Schwartz et al.[160]	—	Biopsy elsewhere	32
Solin et al.[171]	181	Unknown or positive margin	50
Schnitt et al.[155]	71	EIC or positive margin	62

tomy in patients with primary tumors ≤2.5 cm undergoing conservative surgery and radiation.[183] Seven hundred and five patients were randomized. While cosmesis was superior in the tumorectomy group, the breast recurrence rate was also higher (7% vs. 1%). The very limited surgical resection with a single-plane implant may be partly responsible for the increased recurrence rate in the tumorectomy patients. With a median follow-up of 4 years there were no differences in overall survival rates or the incidence of distant metastases. The long-term results of this trial will help to provide further information regarding the optimal surgical procedure for the primary tumor that best minimizes breast disease recurrence and produces optimal cosmesis.

The role of reexcision of the primary tumor has been evaluated by several institutions. Data from the M.D. Anderson Hospital[163] and Institut Gustave Roussy[27] suggest that patients undergoing a single biopsy outside of the parent institution have an increased risk of breast recurrence. A single biopsy elsewhere resulted in a recurrence rate of 13%, compared to 7% when the single biopsy was performed at the M.D. Anderson.[163] Similarly, the breast recurrence rate was 5% for a single biopsy at the Institut Gustave-Roussy, compared to 10% for a single biopsy elsewhere.[27] These observations resulted in a policy of reexcision of the primary tumor site at several institutions in patients in whom the completeness of the initial surgical resection could not be determined. The incidence of residual tumor in the reexcision specimen and the indications for reexcision are given in Table 5-24. Approximately 50% of patients who underwent reexcision in these series were found to have residual tumor at the primary tumor site. The likelihood of finding residual tumor was related to the initial margin of resection, the primary tumor size, the presence of an extensive intraductal component, and the finding of residual microcalcifications at the primary tumor site on a postbiopsy mammogram (Table 5-25). Indications for reexcision of the primary tumor, therefore, include an initial incisional biopsy, positive or unknown pathologic margins on an initial excisional biopsy specimen, the presence of an extensive intraductal component demonstrated on an initial excisional biopsy in which margins of resection are questionable or unknown, and residual microcalcifications on a post-

Table 5-25 Factors related to positive reexcision

	Positive reexcision (%)		
Factor	Solin[170]	Schnitt[155]	McCormick[111]
Margin of resection			
Negative		33	
Positive	60	69	55
Unknown	49		
T size			
T_1	45	63	
T_2	63	58	
Residual microcalcifications on mammogram	86		
EIC			
Yes		88	
No		48	

biopsy mammogram. Reexcision has not had an adverse impact on cosmesis at the University of Pennsylvania, where approximately 90% of patients achieve a good to excellent cosmetic result. Complete excision of all focal microcalcifications in the area of the primary tumor should be performed before the initiation of radiation therapy.

Axillary node dissection

An axillary staging procedure is recommended before initiating radiotherapy. The value of the procedure is both prognostic and therapeutic. It identifies a subgroup of patients with histologically positive nodes who may benefit from adjuvant chemotherapy, it reduces the axillary recurrence rate, it provides prognostic information in terms of the number of positive axillary nodes, and it identifies a group of patients in whom regional nodal irradiation may be omitted (i.e., those with pathologically negative axillary nodes). The benefit of an axillary staging procedure may be questioned in patients with a clinically negative axilla, as the indications for adjuvant systemic therapy have been expanded to include patients with histologically negative axillary nodes. However, clinical examination of the axilla is associated with a 25% to 40% incidence of false negativity as well as a 30% incidence of false positivity.[15,30,45,62,149,158,164] Adjuvant programs for node-negative patients may be different from those for node-positive patients, especially for those who have extensive nodal involvement. Therefore the axillary staging procedure is currently of value in identifying various prognostic subgroups for whom different adjuvant chemotherapy regimens are appropriate, and it continues to identify a subset of patients for whom no adjuvant therapy may be indicated.

Controversy exists concerning the optimal staging procedure. This has varied from an axillary sampling that involves a selective removal of only those nodes that appear suspicious, to a level I axillary dissection (formal node dissection removing nodes lateral to the pectoralis minor muscle), to a level I-II axillary dissection (removal of lymph nodes lateral and beneath the pectoralis minor muscle), to a complete axillary dissection (dissection of the nodes lateral, beneath, and medial to the pectoralis minor muscle). The merits of the various procedures can be evaluated in terms of their ability to detect positive nodes, to determine the extent of nodal positivity, and their associated morbidity (i.e., breast and arm edema). Table 5-26 presents the likelihood of finding positive nodes only in the level(s) above the one that was dissected. If a level I dissection is performed and is negative, the likelihood of finding positive nodes at level II or level III ranges from 1.5% to 29%. However, if a level I or level II node dissection is performed and is negative, the likelihood of finding positive nodes at level III is ≤10% and for the most part is <3%. Therefore, a level I or level II axillary node dissection will miss approximately 3% of patients with positive nodes. By definition, a complete axillary dissection is 100% accurate in assessing whether nodes are positive or negative. Danforth et al.[30] have demonstrated no significant benefit in evaluating the extent of nodal positivity (i.e., four or more positive nodes) with a complete axillary dissection when compared to a level I to level II dissection. Thirty-three percent of patients with a level I to level II dissection were found to have four or more positive nodes, compared to 35% of patients who had a complete axillary dissection. The incidence of arm edema related to the extent of axillary surgery and the addition of radiation is presented in Table 5-27. The incidence of arm edema is relatively low with either a limited axillary dissection or complete axillary dissection and no radiation. However, the incidence is markedly increased in patients who have undergone a complete axillary dissection and subsequently receive axillary radiation. Complete axillary dissection

Table 5-26 Axillary node dissection and the incidence of skip metastases in lymph node–positive patients

Author	No. pts.	Negative level I, positive level II-III (%)	Negative level I-II, positive level III (%)
Forrest et al.[49]	43	12	2
Danforth et al.[30]	65	29	3
Boova et al.[10]	80	9	1
Pigott et al.[128]	80	25	1
Schwartz et al.[159]	127	13	2
Smith et al.[165]	304	25	10
Ciatto et al.[23]	392	9	1
Rosen et al.[147]	508	—	3
Veronesi et al.[187]	539	1.5	0.4

Table 5-27 Incidence of arm edema (%) related to extent of axillary surgery and radiation

	No R		R		
Author	**LAD**	**CAD**	**None**	**LAD**	**CAD**
Veronesi et al.[188]		3			
Larson et al.[95]			4	8	43
Solin et al.[169]	3			10	
Durand et al.[38]	1			9	
Delouche et al.[34]			3	9	
Clarke et al.[26]			3		
Groupe European[127]	2		2	9	
Lichter et al.[101]					18

R, radiation; LAD, limited axillary dissection; CAD, complete axillary dissection.

also increases the incidence of breast edema (Table 5-28). Therefore a level I or level II axillary node dissection is the preferred procedure in the majority of patients, because it adequately determines nodal positivity as well as the extent of nodal positivity, and it is associated with a lower incidence of breast and arm edema when compared to a complete axillary dissection.

Fisher et al.[45] have correlated axillary recurrence with the number of axillary nodes removed at the time of the dissection. The axillary recurrence was 21% when no nodes were removed, 11% for fewer than five, 5% for six to 10 nodes, and <1% for more than 10 nodes. Similarly, the likelihood of skip metastases also has been correlated with the number of nodes removed at the time of a level I axillary node dissection. Boova et al.[10] reported 14 as the mean number of nodes removed at level I axillary dissection for patients without skip metastases; the mean number for patients with skip metastases was 3.4. Ciatto et al.[23] reported a 13% incidence of skip metastases with fewer than eight nodes removed at a level I dissection, compared to 6% when eight or more nodes were removed. A limited axillary dissection typically removes 10 to 15 axillary nodes. Ten or more nodes should be removed for pathologic examination to minimize axillary recurrence and for adequate assessment of the extent of nodal positivity.

TECHNICAL ASPECTS OF THE DELIVERY OF DEFINITIVE BREAST IRRADIATION

The technical delivery of definitive breast irradiation after breast-conserving surgery demands careful attention to detail with the integration of the clinical, mammographic, pathologic, and surgical findings in the breast and regional lymph nodes. The current treatment policies for definitive breast irradiation at the University of Pennsylvania are presented in this section.

For the majority of patients in whom axillary lymph node staging is performed, radiation therapy simulation is performed 2 to 4 weeks after surgery to allow for wound healing and adequate arm mobility. Prolonged delays in the initiation of definitive irradiation have been associated with increased local recurrence rates.[27,68] For the small number of patients who are treated without axillary staging (i.e., for patients with noninvasive ductal carcinoma or with medical contraindications to general anesthesia), simulation is performed 1 to 2 weeks after excisional biopsy.

All patients are casted to minimize daily varia-

Table 5-28 Incidence of breast edema related to the extent of the axillary surgery

	Axillary surgery			
Author	**None**	**Sampling**	**Level I**	**Level I-III**
Clarke et al.[16]	7	25		87
Beadle et al.[4]	6		17	
Pezner et al.[125]		18		39
Montague et al.[115]			13	100
Hayward et al.[69]				51

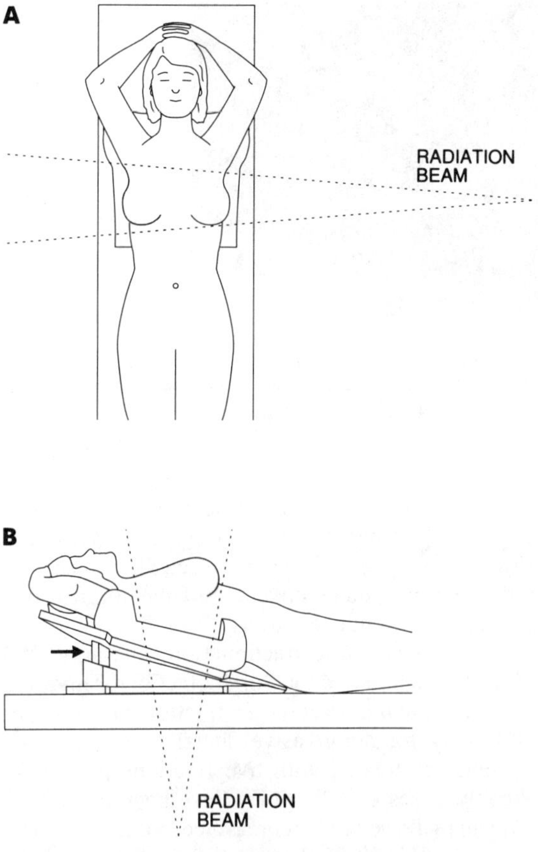

Fig. 5-5 The patient in the standard treatment position. The patient lies in a customized cast which has been placed on top of the breast board. **A,** Overhead view of the medial tangential field. **B,** Lateral view of the lateral tangential field. A plastic insert *(arrow)* of variable height is used to adjust the angle of the breast board to the desired position.

tion in patient setup. The treatment position (Fig. 5-5) is with the fingers interlocked on the top of the head and with the elbows out to the side of the body. The cast provides ipsilateral arm and shoulder support after axillary surgery.

Daily radiation treatments are delivered with the patient in a cast and on an angle board. The optimal angle of the angle board for the individual patient is determined clinically for the position of the breast and to align the chest wall in the horizontal plane.

Table 5-29 outlines the target volumes for definitive breast irradiation. Each of these volumes will be discussed in turn.

Whole breast radiotherapy

After breast-conserving surgery, all patients are treated initially with whole breast irradiation either with or without regional nodal irradiation. The whole breast irradiation is followed by a boost to the excisional biopsy site.

In patients with pathologically negative axillary lymph nodes or with noninvasive ductal carcinoma, conventional breast tangents alone are used without regional nodal irradiation. The clinical landmarks used to set up conventional breast tangents are as follows: (1) cephalad, the inferior border of the clavicular head; (2) caudad, 2 cm caudad to palpable breast tissue; (3) laterally, 2 cm lateral to palpable breast tissue; and (4) medially, midline. If extended breast tangents are used for treatment of the internal mammary lymph nodes, the medial border is placed 3 cm across midline to the contralateral side.

Fig. 5-6 shows a standard breast tangential field. The four radiographic borders of the field are: (1)

Table 5-29 Target volumes for definitive breast irradiation

Target volume	Technique	Dose (cGy)	Indication
Whole breast	Tangential fields	4500-5000	All pts.
Boost to the biopsy site	Electrons or iridium implant	1000-2000	All pts.
Total dose (whole breast plus boost to the biopsy site)	—	6000-6600	All pts.
Axilla	Anterior axillary/supraclavicular field plus posterior axillary boost	4500-4600	Pathologically node-positive axilla, no axillary staging, or inadequate axillary staging
Supraclavicular fossa	Anterior axillary/supraclavicular field	4500-4600	Pathologically node-positive axilla, no axillary staging, or inadequate axillary staging
Internal mammary lymph nodes	Extended tangential fields or en face field	4500-4600	Uncertain (possibly for inner quadrant or central lesion and node-positive axilla)

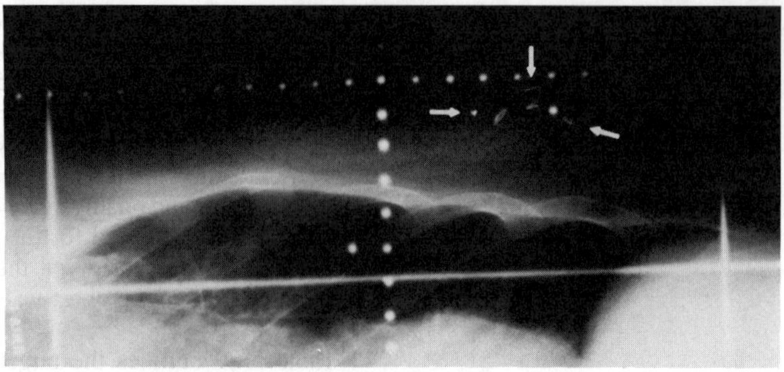

Fig. 5-6 Lateral breast tangential field. The surgical clips *(arrows)* are well encompassed within the field. (From Solin LJ et al: Int J Radiat Oncol Biol Phys 11:1215, 1985.)

cephalad, the inferior border of the clavicular head; (2) caudad, 2 cm caudad to the edge of the breast; (3) anteriorly, a minimum of 1.5 cm of flash in air beyond the edge of the breast; and (4) posteriorly, 2.0 to 3.0 cm of lung. In general a minimum of 2 cm of lung is necessary in order to assure adequate coverage of the breast because of the curvature of the breast around the chest wall. Because the amount of lung seen on the simulator film correlates with the volume of lung irradiated,[14,32] the amount of lung seen on the simulator film is restricted to ≤3 cm. A separate electron beam field may be required to treat the medial aspect of the breast to minimize the volume of lung and heart included within the tangential fields.

At the time of excisional biopsy or reexcision of the primary tumor, radiopaque surgical clips are placed to outline the primary tumor bed.[168] The tangential fields are checked at the time of simulation to confirm adequate coverage of the tumor bed as delineated by the surgical clips. Occasionally, breast tangent fields for patients with very medial or very lateral lesions close to the chest wall will have inadequate coverage of the surgical bed on the initial simulator films (Fig. 5-7).

The standard dose fractionation schema is 200 cGy per fraction to a total of 4600 cGy for invasive carcinoma and 200 cGy per fraction to a total of 5000 cGy for noninvasive ductal carcinoma. All patients are treated with five fractions per week. Weekly doses of <800 cGy have been associated with an increased risk of breast recurrence.[88,121] The energy used is 6 mV photons without bolus; cobalt-60 is not used. However, these guidelines may be adjusted for clinical considerations. For example, higher energy photons (e.g., 10 mV or 15 mV) or reduced daily fractions of 180 cGy are used occasionally for a patient with a large breast or a large separation where the dose inhomogeneity with 6 mV photons is excessive (>15%). When

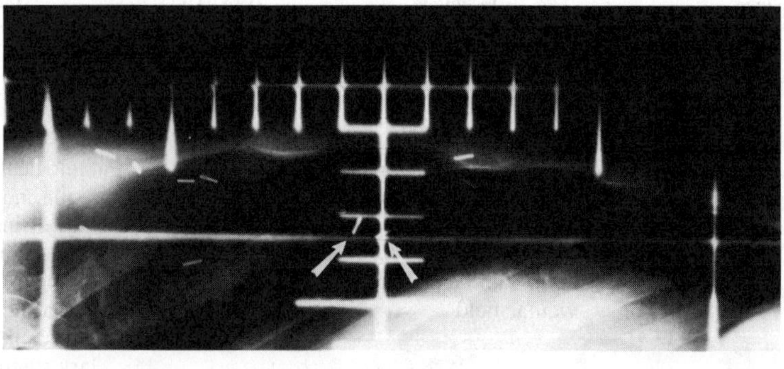

Fig. 5-7 Breast tangential field from the initial clinical setup. The posterior edge of the breast tangential fields is not adequate to cover the deepest clips *(arrows)* placed at the time of lumpectomy. Adequate coverage of the target volume was accomplished by symmetrically widening the width of the field without a change in the isocenter. (From Solin LJ et al: Int J Radiat Oncol Biol Phys 11:1215, 1985.)

Table 5-30 Guidelines for the total dose delivered from the whole breast irradiation plus the boost

Reexcision	Residual tumor present on reexcision	Final pathology margin	Dose (cGy)
No	—	Negative	6000-6400
No	—	Unknown	6400-6600
No	—	Close or positive	6500-6600
Yes	No	Negative	6000-6200
Yes	Yes	Negative	6000-6400
Yes	Yes	Unknown	6400-6600
Yes	Yes	Close or positive	6500-6600

higher energy photons are used, a beam spoiler is used to increase the dose within the build-up region.[37,179,196]

Boost to biopsy site

Following whole breast tangential irradiation, all patients are treated with a boost. The boost is delivered using either electrons of varying energy or an iridium implant. The rationale for the boost is based on the fact that the majority of breast recurrences occur in the vicinity of the original primary tumor and that the majority of residual tumors following an excisional biopsy are found adjacent to the primary tumor.[75]

The dose for the boost is based on the pathologic margins of the primary tumor excision, the use of a reexcisional biopsy, and the presence of residual tumor in the reexcision specimen (Table 5-30). The volume for the boost is determined by the clinical features of the primary tumor, including the clinical and pathologic tumor size, the pathologic evaluation of the margins of excision, and the use of a reexcision. For example, wider margins are utilized when the pathology margins of the tumor excision are close or positive. Larger volumes are also used for T_2 as opposed to T_1 lesions. Relatively tight margins are utilized when pathology margins are negative or when there is no residual tumor on reexcision of the primary tumor site.

When an electron beam boost is selected, individualized cutouts are utilized (Fig. 5-8). The target volume for the boost is considered to be the entire surgical bed.[168] A minimum of five surgical clips are placed to outline the primary tumor bed. These are placed by the surgeon medially, laterally, cephalad, caudad, and deep in the primary tumor bed. The surgical clips plus the biopsy incision on the skin surface delineate the surgical volume of the biopsy site, and this volume determines the target volume. However, problems may arise when the surgical incision is placed at a location distant from the primary tumor bed or when the surgical incision is unnecessarily long. Under such circumstances the target volume is adjusted in order to reduce the total body volume that receives the boost by focusing primarily on the primary tumor bed while minimizing or excluding the area of the surgical skin incision. The determination of the depth from the skin surface to the surgical marking clips can be accomplished using either computerized tomography (CT) scanning or surface contour mapping with orthogonal or stereo shift radiographs.[166,168]

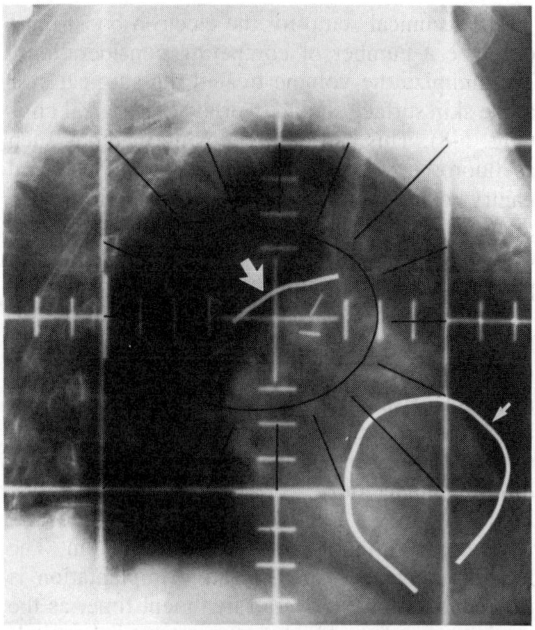

Fig. 5-8 Electron boost field. A customized electron cutout is utilized for each patient. A solder wire *(large arrow)* is placed on the surgical skin incision, and a second solder wire *(small arrow)* is placed to mark the areola. The surgical marking clips delineate the tumor bed. The surgical scar at the skin surface overlies the surgical marking clips. The external landmarks of the surgical skin incision and the areola are used clinically to verify the location of the electron boost field on the patient.

Table 5-31 Outcome related to type of boost treatment following excisional biopsy

	Breast recurrence (%)		
Author	**External**	**Iridium-192**	**Electrons**
Nobler and Venet[118]		8.5	0
Clark et al.[24]	7		
Triedman et al.[180]		9	8
Veronesi et al.[185]	4		
Ray et al.[132]			1
Gerard et al.[56]	10	4	
Fowble et al.[51]		4	2
Van Limbergen et al.[182]			10
Hunig et al.[77]			6
Sarrazin et al.[150]	5		
Hery et al.[73]	6		
Mate et al.[107]			8
Pezner et al.[123]		14	7

Table 5-32 Cosmetic outcome related to type of boost treatment following excisional biopsy

	Good-excellent cosmesis (%)		
Author	**External**	**Iridium-192**	**Electrons**
Veronesi[186]	70		
Ray et al.[132]			91
Fowble et al.[51]		88	96
Triedman et al.[180]		88	96
Gerard et al.[56]	70	70	
Hunig et al.[77]			80

The technical setup for the electron boost must optimize a number of competing considerations. To minimize the volume treated the surgical scar at the skin surface should overlay the surgical clips (Fig. 5-8). This can be done using methods such as fluoroscopy or CT planning.[166,168] Couch and gantry rotations may be indicated to optimize the relationship of the electron beam to the target volume. Another technique is to deliver the electrons perpendicular to the skin surface.

Implants have been used successfully for boosts.[10,20,66,67] Recent reports have described methods of optimizing the placement of iridium implants based on coverage of the surgical bed.[5,79,112] Perioperative implants have been described to position the catheters optimally at the time of lumpectomy.[79,112] However, perioperative implantation is a relatively recent technique that will require further follow-up for evaluation. The major advantage of perioperative implantation is the reduction of the overall treatment time, as the implant is performed while the patient is hospitalized for the excisional or reexcisional biopsy.

Both electrons and implants used as a boost are effective in local tumor control. At the present time, as demonstrated in Table 5-31, no difference has been shown in the relative effectiveness for local tumor control of electron vs. implant boosts, although cosmesis appears to be superior with the use of electrons. Table 5-32 presents cosmetic outcome related to the type of boost. In our own patients we have found no difference in the risk of a recurrence of breast disease or cosmetic outcome when comparing boost treatment with electrons vs. implant. Between 1977 and 1985, 659 patients received definitive radiation with a boost for stage I or stage II breast cancer. For 169 patients the boost was delivered by an iridium-192 implant and for 490 the boost was with electrons. The 5-year actuarial breast disease recurrence rate was 9% in the electron group vs. 6% in the implant group. For patients with negative margins of resection the 5-year actuarial rate of breast recurrence was 8% for both groups. For patients with microscopically positive margins of resection the 5-year actuarial recurrence rate was 3% for the electron boost and 0 for patients receiving the implant. For patients with unknown margins of resection the 5-year actuarial recurrence rate was 11% for electron boosts and 6% for implant boosts. Further information will be available from the prospective, randomized trial comparing electrons and implants that has been conducted by the Radiation Therapy Oncology Group (RTOG).

One major unresolved issue is the necessity for a boost in the presence of pathologically confirmed negative margins. Table 5-33 presents breast recurrence rates related to boost treatment following excisional biopsy. The addition of the boost has resulted in a decreased incidence of recurrence in series where margins of resection are unknown. In the NSABP B-06 study a boost dose was not employed and the whole breast received 5000 cGy. The 8-year actuarial breast recurrence rate was 10% with a 5-year actuarial rate of 8%.[43] The European Organization for Research and Treatment of Cancer (EORTC) has initiated a prospective randomized trial for patients with primary tumors $\leq$3 cm in diameter with either clinically positive or negative axillary nodes. All patients will undergo tumorectomy and axillary dissection and subsequently be randomized to receive a boost dose or not. The boost will employ either electrons (1000 cGy) or

Table 5-33 Breast recurrence related to boost treatment following excisional biopsy

Author	Surgery for primary tumor	Margins	Breast recurrence (%)	
			Boost	No boost
NSABP B-06[43]	WE	Negative		10
Cedermark et al.[17]	WE	Unknown		1
Veronesi et al.[185]	Q	Unknown	4	
Bedwinek et al.[7]	WE	Unknown	5	5
Nobler and Venet[118]	LE	Unknown	6	9
Harris et al.[65]	LE	Unknown	6	12
Clark et al.[24]	LE	Unknown	11	17
Chu et al.[20]	LE	Unknown	7	20

WE, wide excision; LE, local excision; Q, quadrantectomy.

iridium-192 (1500 cGy). Preliminary results from this trial[140] show no difference in terms of breast recurrence. The long-term results of this trial will provide further information regarding the role of the boost. Boost treatment is indicated clearly in patients with focally positive microscopic margins of resection. Ryoo et al.[148] reported a 30% breast recurrence rate in patients with positive or close margins who received no boost, compared to 7% in those who received a boost. However, increasing the volume or dose of the boost has not resulted in a decreased breast recurrence rate in patients with an extensive intraductal component at the Joint Center.[13] Therefore in certain patients who are deemed at high risk for a breast recurrence, the boost may not decrease this risk. Our current policy is to utilize a boost in all patients. Our results have documented excellent local control utilizing a modest volume-customized boost.[169] Further, cosmesis does not appear to be compromised through the use of a modest boost volume. Although both electrons and implants have been used in our department, our current policy is to employ electrons because we have demonstrated excellent cosmesis with this form of boost and the use of electrons avoids hospitalization.[51]

TREATMENT OF THE AXILLA

The management of the axillary region requires close cooperation between the surgeon and radiation oncologist. Our current surgical approach is to perform a limited axillary dissection of level I and level II. Axillary recurrence can be correlated to pathologic nodal status, the extent of the axillary dissection, and the addition of axillary radiation (Table 5-34). For patients with histologically negative axillary nodes there is no difference in the incidence of axillary recurrence when comparing a complete axillary dissection to a limited axillary dissection. The addition of axillary radiation to a

Table 5-34 Axillary recurrence related to pathologic nodal status, extent of axillary dissection, and radiation

Author	Total no. pts.	Follow-up	Axillary recurrence (%)						
			Pathologic N_0			Pathologic N_1			
			LAD	LAD and R	CAD	LAD	LAD and R	CAD	CAD and R
Dewar et al.[36]	592	5 (actuarial)	0.7	—	3	33	0	0	0
Cedermark et al.[17]	154	6 mo-5 yr	2.5						
Hery et al.[73]	92	5 yr (median)	4				0		
Gerard et al.[56]	165	5 yr (actuarial)	1.2		0				0
Veronesi et al.[190]	342	8 yr (median)			0			0	
University of Pennsylvania[52]	990	3.3 yr (median)	1.6	0	—	0	1.6	—	—

LAD, limited axillary dissection; R, radiation; CAD, complete axillary dissection.
From Fowble et al: Int J Radiat Oncol Biol Phys 17:703, 1989.

limited axillary dissection in patients with histologically negative axillary nodes does not reduce the axillary recurrence rate significantly. Therefore in patients with histologically negative axillary nodes who have undergone either a limited (level I to level II) or complete axillary dissection there appears to be no role for axillary radiation. In patients with positive axillary nodes, Dewar et al.[36] reported an axillary recurrence rate of 33% in patients who underwent a limited axillary dissection without radiation. In our own series, axillary radiation was omitted only in patients who had one to three positive nodes following a limited axillary dissection. The axillary recurrence rate in this group of patients was 0%. Veronesi et al.[187] have correlated the likelihood of positive level II to level III nodes with the number of nodes positive at level I. For patients with a single positive node at level I only 8% had positive level II to level III nodes. For patients with two or three positive nodes at level I, 25% to 30% had positive level II or level III nodes. For patients with four or more positive nodes at level I, 66% had positive nodes at level II to level III. Lloyd et al.[104] also correlated the incidence of positive nodes at level II and level III with the number of positive nodes at level I. The incidence of positive nodes at level II and level III was 20% for a single positive node at level I, 50% for two nodes positive at level I, 50% for three nodes positive at level I, and 58% for four or more nodes positive at level I. Therefore indications for axillary radiation in patients who have undergone a limited axillary dissection include the presence of four or more positive nodes, extracapsular nodal extension, or the highest axillary node positive. There is no role for axillary radiation in patients who have undergone a complete axillary dissection and are found to have positive nodes. The addition of axillary radiation to a complete axillary dissection increases the incidence of arm edema but does not significantly decrease the risk of an axillary recurrence.

The apical axillary nodes are treated within the supraclavicular field (Fig. 5-9). A posterior axillary boost field (Fig. 5-10) may be utilized to bring the midplane of the axilla to a total dose of approximately 4500 to 4600 cGy.[172] The posterior

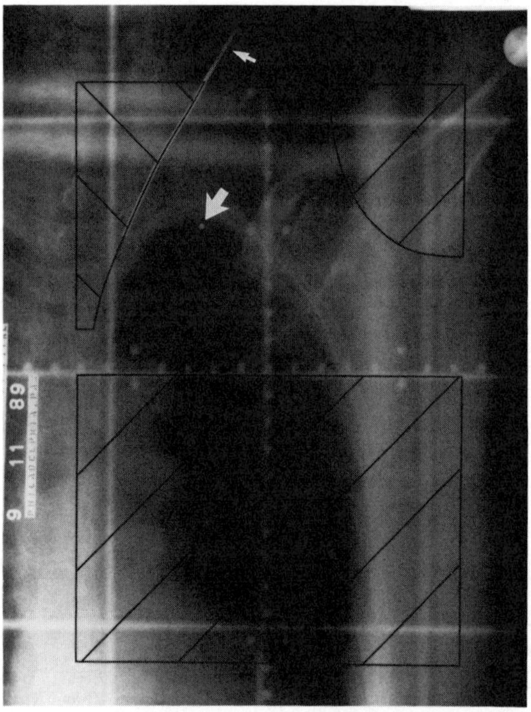

Fig. 5-9 Anterior axillary/supraclavicular field. The field is treated to a depth of 3 cm. The depth is measured at the supraclavicular fossa, marked by the BB *(large arrow)*. When the axillary apex is to be included within the supraclavicular field, the lateral border is placed as shown at the mid aspect of the humeral head. When only the supraclavicular fossa is to be treated, the lateral border is moved medially to the medial edge of the humeral head. A solder wire *(small arrow)* is placed 1 cm medially to the medial border of the sternocleidomastoid muscle and the area medial to the solder wire is blocked.

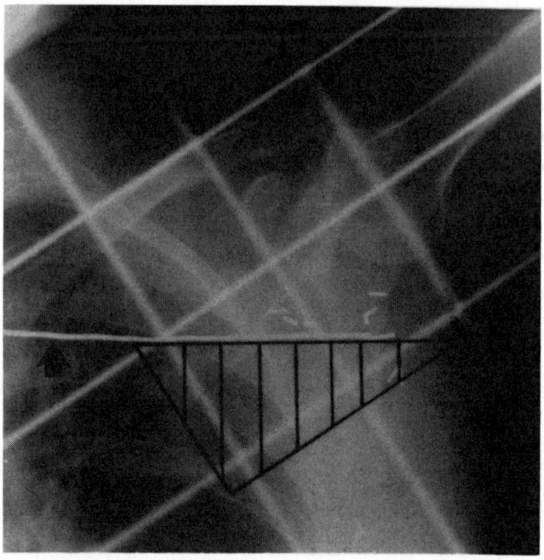

Fig. 5-10 Posterior axillary boost field. The wire *(arrow)* shows the match plane between the breast tangential fields and the supraclavicular fields. A block is used inferior to the match plane to block the area treated in the tangential fields. (Reproduced with permission from Solin LJ et al: Int J Radiat Oncol Biol Phys 12:2040, 1986.)

axillary boost field is delivered at 100 cGy per fraction with two or three fractions weekly as required. For the average patient the total posterior boost dose is approximately 800 to 1000 cGy. The radiographic borders of the posterior axillary boost field are as follows: 1) inferiorly at the match plane; 2) superiorly at the midclavicle; 3) medially 1 cm medial to the chest wall; and 4) laterally at the midhumeral head. Using fluoroscopy, a collimator angle is used such that the superior field border is parallel with the clavicle and the medial field border is parallel with the chest wall.

Treatment of the supraclavicular nodes

The incidence of supraclavicular recurrence is correlated with positive axillary nodes and ranges from 10% to 26%.[44,189] Prophylactic irradiation of the supraclavicular region has been shown to decrease supraclavicular recurrences significantly without a demonstrable survival benefit.[44] Therefore prophylactic irradiation of this region in axillary node-positive patients can be justified only on the basis of a decrease in the incidence of supraclavicular recurrences. Supraclavicular irradiation is not indicated in patients with histologically negative axillary nodes.

When a supraclavicular field is to be utilized, the initial step is to set up a match plane. A match plane is required rather than a matchline in order to minimize the inhomogeneity at the junction of the supraclavicular field and the tangential breast fields. Hunt et al.[78] and Lichter et al.[100] have evaluated the dosimetry across the match plane. The inhomogeneity across the match plane is minimized when techniques are utilized to obtain a match plane rather than a matchline.

The borders of the field for the supraclavicular field are as follows: 1) inferiorly, at the inferior aspect of the clavicular head; 2) superiorly, at the cricothyroid notch; 3) laterally, at the medial aspect of the humeral head; and 4) medially, 1 cm to the contralateral side of midline at the sternal notch. The lateral border is extended to the midhumeral head when the remaining axilla is to be treated (Fig. 5-9) (i.e., for patients with multiple positive nodes or extracapsular extension). A half-beam block is utilized to define the match plane. The supraclavicular field is angled 11 to 12 degrees in order to avoid the spinal cord. A solder wire is placed 1 cm medial to the medial border of the sternocleidomastoid muscle, and the area medial to the solder wire is blocked to shield the trachea and larynx. A number of techniques have been utilized to match the supraclavicular fields with the tangential fields.[28,96,100,129,161,178] Our current technique for matching has been described in detail by Chu et al.[21] and is a modification of the hanging block technique.[147,178] This technique utilizes a half-beam block for the supraclavicular field and a rod-chain combination to define the match plane for the tangential fields. The rod-chain technique is highly efficient and yields an exact geometric solution for the matching problem. Further, the rod-chain technique is sensitive to deviations from exact matching as small as ½ degree for the couch position (Fig. 5-11).

A

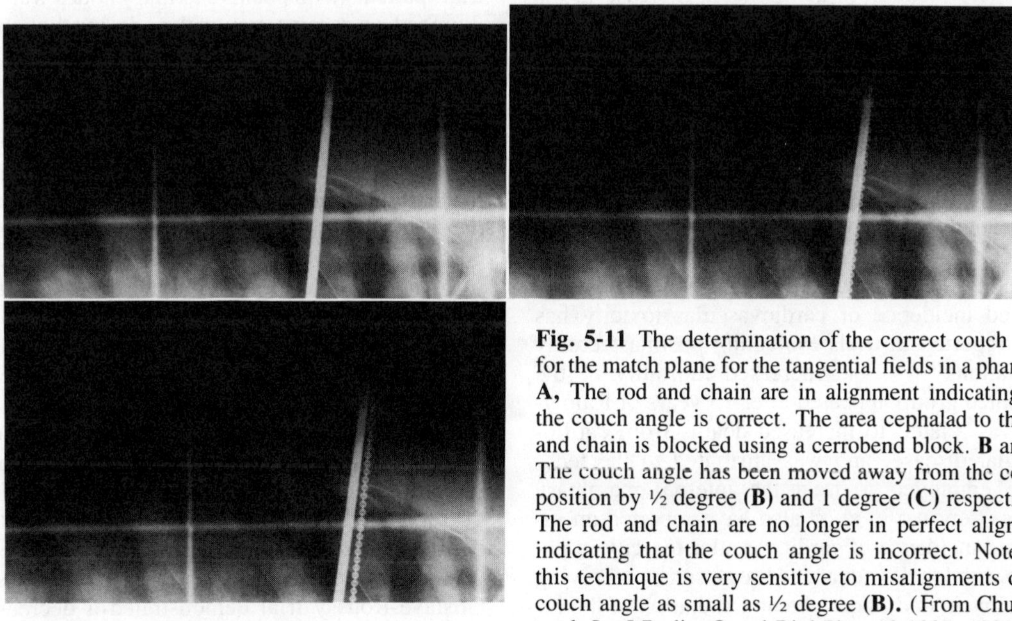

B

C

Fig. 5-11 The determination of the correct couch angle for the match plane for the tangential fields in a phantom. **A,** The rod and chain are in alignment indicating that the couch angle is correct. The area cephalad to the rod and chain is blocked using a cerrobend block. **B** and **C,** The couch angle has been moved away from the correct position by ½ degree **(B)** and 1 degree **(C)** respectively. The rod and chain are no longer in perfect alignment indicating that the couch angle is incorrect. Note that this technique is very sensitive to misalignments of the couch angle as small as ½ degree **(B).** (From Chu JCH et al: Int J Radiat Oncol Biol Phys 19:1037, 1990.)

Treatment of the internal mammary lymph nodes

Treatment of the internal mammary lymph nodes with radiation is controversial. Our current treatment policy is not to treat these nodes in patients with breast cancer in early stages. The rationale for this policy is the lack of clear evidence to support such treatment, the extraordinarily low risk of clinical internal mammary node failure in the untreated patient with early-stage breast cancer, and the increased volume of normal tissues treated when such treatment is utilized, as well as the possible need to treat the contralateral breast at some time in the future. A detailed discussion of the role of treatment of the internal mammary nodes is presented in Chapter 3.

Complications related to internal mammary node irradiation with photons include decreased hematologic tolerance to chemotherapy, an increased incidence of symptomatic pneumonitis, and an increased incidence of cardiovascular disease. It is postulated that the increased hematologic toxicity is related to either photon irradiation of the mediastinum and circulating blood pool or to the thoracic bone marrow.[6,99] Romsdahl et al.[141] reported a 9% incidence of symptomatic pneumonitis in patients in whom cobalt-60 was employed to treat the regional nodes, compared with a 2% incidence when the regional nodes were treated with a combination of photons and electrons. The area of lung treated with various techniques has been analyzed by Roberson et al.[139] When tangents and a direct photon beam internal mammary node field were used, 36% of the ipsilateral lung received ≥2000 cGy. Angling the photon beam internal mammary node field resulted in a significant increase in the area of lung treated (i.e., 60%). The combination of tangents with mixed electron-photon irradiation of the internal mammary nodes resulted in 20% of the ipsilateral lung receiving ≥2000 cGy. The use of deep tangents (i.e., extension of the medial entrance point 3 cm to the contralateral side) resulted in a 38% area of ipsilateral lung receiving ≥2000 cGy. Therefore the technique that best minimizes the area of lung treated is one employing electrons or a combination of electrons and photons. An increased incidence of cardiovascular toxicity has been reported in trials evaluating postmastectomy irradiation.[29,72,80] The increased mortality in the irradiated group appeared after 15 years of follow-up, was related to increased deaths from cardiovascular disease, and was attributed to the technique employed to treat the internal mammary nodes. Loprinzi et al.[105] also have reported an increased incidence of cardiovascular toxicity in patients with locally advanced breast cancer receiving Adriamycin and photon beam irradiation of the internal mammary nodes. CT scans performed in the treatment position have revealed that the standard hockey stick field encompasses approximately 50% of the volume of the heart for lesions on the left side and 20% for lesions on the right side.[32] Internal mammary irradiation in patients with breast cancer in the early stages does not decrease the incidence of regional recurrence in the internal mammary nodes significantly. At the University of Pennsylvania there have been no internal mammary node failures in 218 patients with positive axillary nodes who did not receive treatment to this region. There also appears to be no survival benefit for internal mammary node irradiation in patients with early breast cancer.[90,91,113,189] However, the potential for complications clearly exists in terms of an increased incidence of symptomatic pneumonitis, cardiovascular disease, or hematologic toxicity. If a decision is made to treat the internal mammary nodes, the nodal technique that best minimizes treatment to normal structures is one that employs electrons for the entire treatment or electrons mixed with photons. We continue to advocate omission of internal mammary node irradiation even in node-positive patients with early-stage breast cancer for the reasons stated above.

Prospective randomized trials evaluating regional node irradiation

Two prospective randomized trials have evaluated regional node irradiation in early breast cancer. These trials investigated the possibility of omitting regional node irradiation in patients with histologically positive axillary nodes following complete axillary dissection. In the first 2 years of the Milan trial, patients with positive axillary nodes were randomized to receive regional node irradiation (33 patients) or no regional node irradiation (23 patients). The 5-year relapse-free survival rate was 74% in patients who received no nodal radiation, compared to 49% in those who did. At 10 years the disease-free survival rate was 68% in the group that received no regional node irradiation, compared to 40% in the group that did.[191] In the Institut Gustave-Roussy trial[151] patients with positive axillary nodes underwent a complete axillary dissection and were randomized to regional node irradiation (41 patients) or no further treatment (31 patients). The 5-year relapse-free survival rate was 66% in the patients who received no nodal irradiation, as compared to 62% in the group that received nodal irradiation. Regional recurrences were decreased from 35% to 19% with the addition of regional node irradiation. While these trials demonstrate no benefit in terms of relapse-free survival for regional node irradiation, the Institut Gustave-Roussy trial demonstrated a decrease in the incidence of regional node recurrence. In the NSABP B-06 trial, treatment was directed to the breast only in both node-negative and node-positive patients. With a median follow-up of 81 months, the regional recurrence rate was 3.9% in the group of patients undergoing total mastectomy, compared to 5.4% in those undergoing conservative surgery and radiation.[43] Regional node recurrence was not reported separately for node-positive and node-negative patients. Similarly, in the Milan trial, regional node recurrence was 2.6% for patients undergoing radical mastectomy and 2.3% for patients undergoing quandrantectomy and axillary dissection and radiation.[190] The majority of patients in this latter group received no regional node irradiation.

These findings have led to the consideration of omission of regional node irradiation in patients with positive axillary nodes. Axillary irradiation is not indicated in patients who have undergone a complete axillary dissection and are found to have positive nodes; however, in patients undergoing a limited axillary dissection the likelihood of positive nodes at level II or level III increases with the number of positive nodes at level I. For patients with four or more positive nodes at level I, the likelihood of positive nodes at level II or level III is 66%.[187] Dewar et al.[36] have demonstrated a high risk of axillary recurrence in patients who have undergone a limited axillary dissection without radiation. Consideration should be given to axillary irradiation in patients with four or more positive nodes, extracapsular nodal extension, or the highest axillary node positive. Because the likelihood of a supraclavicular recurrence is related to positive axillary nodes and because supraclavicular recurrences have been decreased significantly with prophylactic irradiation of the supraclavicular region,[44] consideration also should be given to treatment of the supraclavicular region in patients with positive axillary nodes. In general all patients with positive axillary nodes at the University of Pennsylvania who have undergone a limited axillary node dissection receive radiation to the supraclavicular and apical axillary nodes. The only exception to this policy has been patients who have a single positive node at level I.

BILATERAL BREAST CANCER

With the growing popularity of definitive breast irradiation the number of patients requiring bilateral breast irradiation has been rising. The incidence of bilateral breast cancer in reported series of definitive breast irradiation ranges from 0.7% to 5.5%.[7,20,66,183] A recent study by Solin et al.[174] described the use of bilateral definitive irradiation for patients with bilateral early-stage breast cancer.

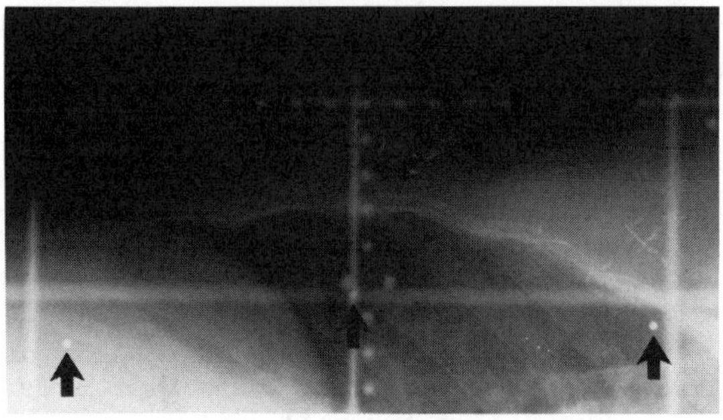

Fig. 5-12 The medial tangential field for the second *(right)* breast cancer from sequential, bilateral breast cancers treated bilaterally with definitive breast irradiation. The right breast was treated 20 months following left breast irradiation. The tattoos from the medial entrance of the first *(left)* tangential fields have been marked with BBs *(arrows)*. Because the breast tangents curve along the chest wall, there is a gap between the tangential fields in the area cephalad and caudad to the isocenter. Note that the second *(right)* breast cancer is matched in the transverse plane through the isocenter to the first *(left)* breast cancer without overlap.

This study showed that the delivery of definitive irradiation technically can be accomplished without undue morbidity.

Fig. 5-12 shows the medial breast tangential field from the second breast cancer in a patient treated sequentially with definitive breast irradiation. The medial entrance point for the second breast cancer is matched to the medial entrance point for the first breast cancer. Our current policy is to avoid overlapping tangential fields for patients with bilateral breast cancer, even if the first breast cancer had a medial entrance point across midline. For patients treated with concurrent bilateral breast carcinoma, the medial entrance point for both breasts is placed at the midline.

The technical delivery of bilateral breast irradiation differs between patients with concurrent vs. those with sequential cancers. For patients with concurrent bilateral breast cancer, the tangential fields are matched at the midline in the transverse plane through the isocenter. As the tangential fields curve slightly along the chest wall in the cephalad and caudad directions, there are no areas of overlap utilizing such a setup. The setup for patients with sequential bilateral breast cancer is limited by the technical delivery of treatment to the first breast. In cases in which the medial entrance point is across midline, our current approach is to avoid areas of overlap if at all possible because of the potential risk of late complications such as soft tissue fibrosis or sternal necrosis. The medial entrance point for

Table 5-35 Evaluation of calculations using inhomogeneity corrections for 6 mV photons

Author	Parameter evaluated	Off-axis planes included in calculations	Inhomogeneity corrections (%)	
			No	Yes
Chin et al.[18]	Irradiated volume receiving >105%	Yes	14*	20-29*
	Irradiated volume receiving >110%	Yes	4*	5-8*
Fraass et al.[53]	Maximum isodose for 2 cm^2 area in central axis	Yes	100-102	110-112
	Volume of breast tissue receiving dose >110%	Yes	0	20
Kuchnir et al.[83]	Target in central axis receiving >115%	Yes	0	2
	Volume of target receiving >115%	Yes	0	5
Solin et al.[167]	Maximum isodose covering 5% of target volume	Yes	110	114-115
	Maximum point dose	Yes	111-114	114-117
Webb et al.[194]	Central axis dose inhomogeneity	Yes	4-9	7-18

*Estimated from curves.

treatment of the second breast is also matched to the medial entrance point for the first breast (see Fig. 5-12).

THREE-DIMENSIONAL TREATMENT PLANNING

Dosimetry calculations for conventional breast tangential irradiation commonly are performed using a single transverse contour through the isocenter of the tangential fields with the calculations performed without inhomogeneity (e.g., lung density) corrections. Extensive clinical experience has been obtained using such treatment planning techniques in many centers, and long-term results are now available. These results generally show excellent rates of local control with low rates of complications.

A number of recent reports have evaluated the findings from three-dimensional treatment planning for intact breast irradiation. Such treatment planning requires the ability to outline the anatomic structures in three dimensions. This is done most commonly using CT scanning through the body with multiple transverse planes. CT scanning has the added benefit of allowing for density corrections for inhomogeneity calculations based on CT numbers. The two major advantages of three-dimensional treatment planning over conventional treatment planning are the integration of off-axis planes and the incorporation of inhomogeneity corrections for the dosimetry calculations. The most significant effect of inhomogeneity corrections is from the presence of significant volumes of lung within the treatment field.

Table 5-35 shows the results of five studies that have evaluated the use of plans calculated with inhomogeneity corrections vs. those without inhomogeneity corrections. All plans were studied using 6 mV photons, as this is one of the commonly used energy levels for breast irradiation. Although the end points measured in each study differ, all of the parameters evaluated in the studies showed an increase in the amount of dosimetric inhomogeneity regardless of the parameter evaluated. The magnitude of the increase in inhomogeneity varied depending upon the parameters studied.

Table 5-36 shows the results of five studies that have evaluated the degree of inhomogeneity in off-axis planes. All plans were calculated using 6 mV photons. There were significant differences in the

Table 5-36 Evaluation of calculations for inhomogeneity in off-axis planes for 6 mV photons

Author	No. pts.	No. CT slices	CT slice spacing	Inhomogeneity corrections included in calculations	Inhomogeneity in off-axis planes (%)
Chin et al.[19]	1*	3	7-8 cm	No	110
Chu et al.[22]	1	—	1 cm	Yes	110-115
Fraass et al.[53]	34	3	>3 cm	Yes	102-111
Solin et al.[167]	2	26-34	1 cm	Yes	110-118
Webb et al.[194]	30	3	—	Yes	+20

*Phantom.

number of patients studied, the number of CT slices utilized, the CT slice spacing and the use of inhomogeneity corrections in the dose calculations. Even though there were significant differences in the methodologies between the studies, all the studies showed significant inhomogeneities in off-axis planes, generally with a maximum of 10% to 20%. The inhomogeneities in the off-axis planes were caused by contour changes in the off-axis planes with decreasing separations as well as lung density corrections.

Fig. 5-13 shows isodose distributions from one patient treated with definitive breast irradiation. These isodose distributions show the increase in the magnitude and the volume of the hot spots in the central plane and in the off-axis planes when inhomogeneity corrections are utilized. These hot spots are seen both within the breast tissue as well as within the normal tissues of lung, chest wall, and soft tissue. The hot spots identified in the off-axis planes are secondary to the lung inhomogeneity corrections and the changing contours with decreasing separations.

Three studies have evaluated the effects of varying energies for breast tangential fields.[18,53,167] Fig. 5-14 shows a comparison of the use of cobalt-60 vs. 6 mV photons vs. 15 mV photons in one patient from the study by Solin et al.[167] Although 15 mV photons reduced the hot spots, there was less tumor coverage because of the extended build-up region. Cobalt-60 was found to have increased hot spots as compared to 6 mV photons with only minimal improvement in the build-up region. These results are similar to those found in two other studies.[18,53] Based on these three studies, a medium energy photon, such as 6 mV, would appear to be the energy of choice for the average patient. However, consideration should be given to the use of higher-

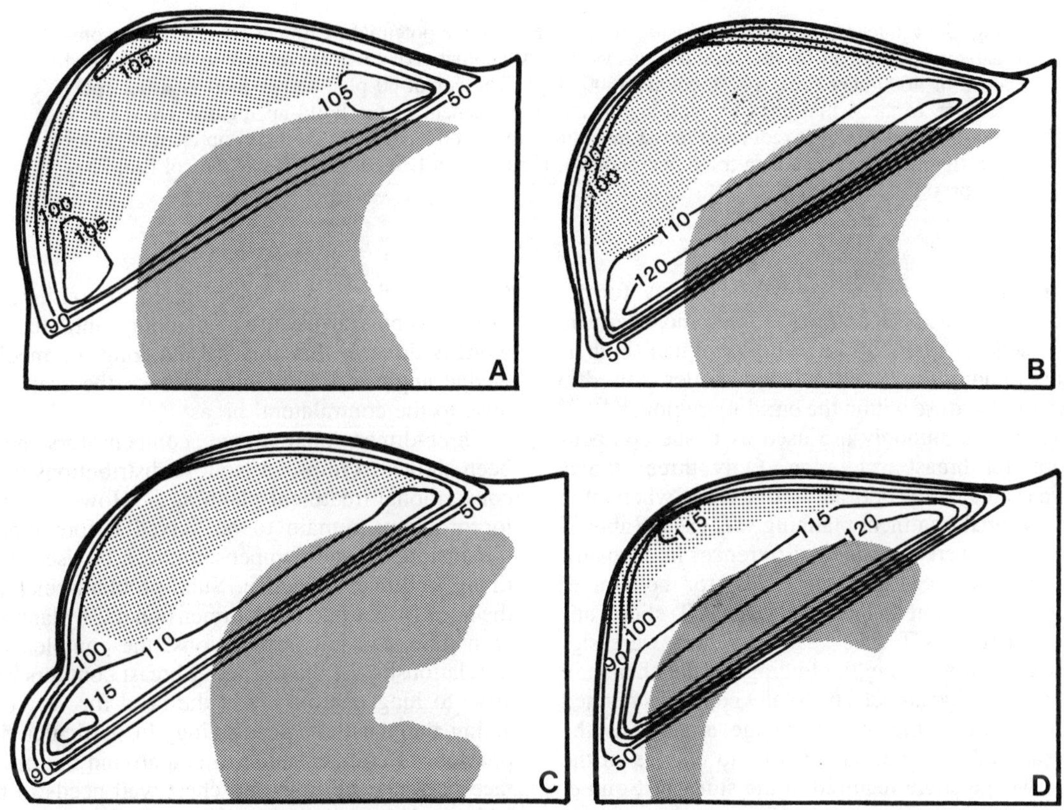

Fig. 5-13 Isodose distributions in the transverse plane for breast tangential irradiation calculated without and with inhomogeneity corrections. **A,** Isodose distribution through the isocenter calculated without inhomogeneity corrections. **B,** Isodose distribution through the isocenter calculated with inhomogeneity corrections. There is a significant increase in the hot spots seen because of the change in the lung density. **C,** Isodose distribution at a level 5 cm cephalad to the isocenter. The plan is calculated with inhomogeneity corrections. **D,** Isodose distribution at a level 5 cm caudad to the isocenter. The plan is calculated with inhomogeneity corrections. In all figures, the breast is indicated by *light shading,* and the right lung is indicated by *dark shading*. (Modified and redrawn from Solin LJ et al: Int J Radiat Oncol Biol Phys [in press].)

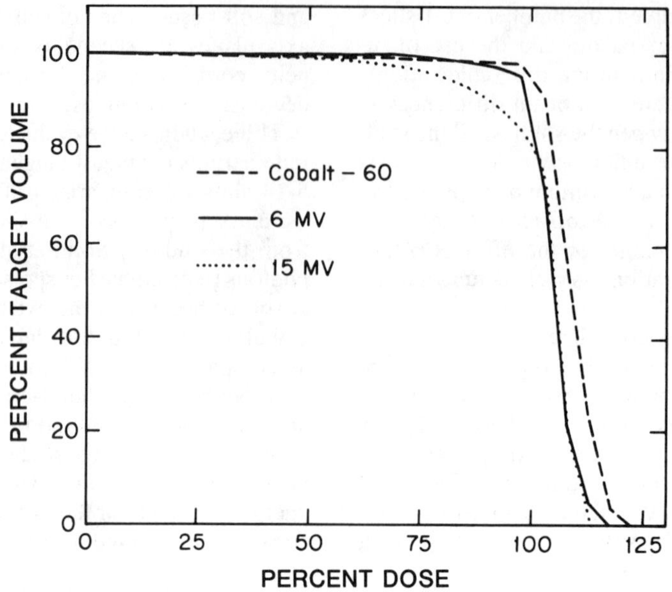

Fig. 5-14 Integral dose-volume histogram comparing three potential treatment energies. The comparison is for cobalt-60 vs. 6 mV photons vs. 15 mV photons. All doses are relative to the prescribed dose of 4600 cGy (i.e., 100% equals 4600 cGy). The cobalt-60 plan shows increased hot spots relative to the 6 mV photons with significant improvement in the build-up region. The 15 mV photons show a slight reduction in the magnitude of the hot spots, but the build-up characteristics are significantly worse than the 6 mV photons. (From Solin LJ et al: Int J Radiat Oncol Biol Phys [in press].)

energy photons such as 10 mV or 15 mV for patients with large separations or inhomogeneity in the isodose distribution >15%. When higher-energy photons are used, a beam spoiler is used to increase the dose within the build-up region.[37,179,196]

Wedges commonly are used as tissue compensation for breast irradiation. Only three studies have evaluated the optimal wedge angle when three dimensional treatment planning was used (Table 5-37). There were significant differences in the methodologies between the three studies for the number of patients studied, the number of CT slices utilized, and the CT slice spacing. There were significant differences in the findings in the change in the total wedge angle. The total wedge was defined as the sum of the medial wedge angle plus the lateral wedge angle. There was no change in the total wedge angle required in the study of Solin et al.[167] because of competing factors: the need to decrease the wedge angle in the central plane because of lung inhomogeneity corrections, and the need to increase the wedge in the off-axis planes because of contour separation changes. Based on the excellent local control rates and low complication rates in historic studies using conventional treatment planning and based on the conflicting results from three-dimensional treatment planning (see Table 5-37), we have elected to continue to use conventional treatment planning until further work is done in this area. Minimizing the medial wedge angle is important to reduce the scattered dose to the contralateral breast.[54,152]

Three-dimensional tissue compensators have been shown to improve isodose distributions over conventional treatment planning.[167] However, major problems remain to be solved before three-dimensional tissue compensators can be used routinely in clinical practice. Such problems include the need for routine three-dimensional CT planning with inhomogeneity corrections, the complex interrelationship of the changing breast contours relative to lung contours, and the need for very exacting daily patient positioning. In particular the problem of compensation in and around the interface between the lung and chest wall needs to be addressed carefully before tissue compensators can be used routinely.

INTEGRATION OF PRIMARY RADIOTHERAPY AND ADJUVANT SYSTEMIC CHEMOTHERAPY

The ability to integrate adjuvant systemic chemotherapy with conservative surgery and radiation has raised questions about the following: 1) the proper

Table 5-37 Evaluation of the use of wedges for tissue compensation for 6 mV photons

Author	No pts.	No. CT slices	CT slice spacing (cm)	Change in total wedge angle
Fraass et al.[53]	34	3	>3	Decrease 36 degrees
Kuchnir et al.[83]	4	6-9	2	Decrease 0-15 degrees
Solin et al.[167]	2	26-34	1	No change

sequencing of chemotherapy and radiotherapy; 2) the ability to deliver optimal doses of chemotherapy; and 3) the incidence of complications with chemotherapy, including cosmetic results.

Sequencing of chemotherapy and radiotherapy

Because the efficacy of adjuvant chemotherapy appears to be related to its prompt initiation following surgery and the ability to deliver optimal doses, emphasis has been placed on sequential regimens employing chemotherapy first. However, radiation in the conservation approach represents an integral part of the treatment of the primary tumor and should not be considered adjuvant therapy. The NSABP B-06 study has shown clearly that chemotherapy alone does not prevent breast recurrence.[43] In node-positive patients who underwent segmental mastectomy without radiation and who received adjuvant chemotherapy consisting of 5-fluorouracil and Alkeran, the recurrence rate was 43%, compared to 6% in the group that received radiation. Approximately 25% of these recurrences occurred during the first year. In contrast, it appears that the combination of adjuvant systemic chemotherapy and radiation results in a decreased incidence of breast recurrence (Table 5-38). The question arises as to whether a delay in the initiation of radiation is detrimental in terms of breast recurrence rates. There is minimal data that would suggest that a delay of 7 or 8 weeks may predispose the patient to a higher risk of recurrence of disease in the breast. Harter et al.[68] reported an 18% breast recurrence rate in 16 patients whose radiotherapy was delayed for two cycles of cyclophosphamide, methotrexate, and 5-fluorouracil (CMF). Clarke et al.[27] reported an increased risk of breast disease recurrence in patients whose radiotherapy was delayed >7 weeks. However, Boyages et al.[13] noted no increase in recurrence with a delay in the initiation of radiation of >7 weeks.

Gore et al.[59] reported a decrease incidence of local recurrence in 41 patients who received concurrent treatment with cyclosphosphamide, methotrexate, and 5-fluorouracil (CMF) and radiation compared to 41 patients who received sequential treatment with radiation given first. Although cosmesis was worse in the concurrent group, it most likely was related to the concurrent use of methotrexate. The University of Pennsylvania has routinely employed a concurrent regimen with cyclophosphamide and 5-fluorouracil given during radiation with methotrexate or adriamycin added after the completion of radiation. The 5-year actuarial recurrence rate was 3%.[169] The concurrent use of both modalities has the potential for minimizing breast recurrence as well as allowing for prompt initiation of systemic chemotherapy.

In the NSABP B-16[42] trial node-positive breast cancer patients ≥50 years of age were randomized to either tamoxifen for 5 years or tamoxifen and chemotherapy. All patients had "tamoxifen responsive" tumors (i.e., age 50 to 59 years and progesterone receptor ≥10 fmol/mg cytosol protein or age ≥60 years). Chemotherapy consisted of melphalan and 5-fluorouracil (PF) ± Adriamycin (PAF) or Adriamycin and cyclophosphamide (AC). Twenty-eight percent of patients had lumpectomy and radiation. Patients randomized to PFT and tamoxifen (PFT) or PAF and tamoxifen (PAFT) received breast irradiation following one cycle of chemotherapy, and patients randomized to AC and tamoxifen (ACT) received breast irradiation following four cycles of chemotherapy (approximately 12 weeks). All patients received tamoxifen following lumpectomy. At 3 years, there were no breast recurrences in the ACT group (106 patients)

Table 5-38 Breast recurrence following conservative surgery, radiation, and adjuvant chemotherapy for stage I and stage II breast cancer

	Breast recurrence (%)	
Author	Chemotherapy	No chemotherapy
Solin et al.[169]	3	8
NSABP B-06[43]	6	12
NSABP B-13[41]*	1	4
Borger and Keijser[11]	0	5
Rose et al.[142]†	5	17

*Node-negative, ER-negative patients.
†Premenopausal patients.

Table 5-39 Ability to deliver optimal adjuvant chemotherapy (level I) in patients undergoing conservative surgery and radiation

		Level I (%)	
Author	Agents	Radiation	Mastectomy
Glick et al.[58]	CMFP	71 [96]	87 [40]
Bonadonna et al.[9]	CMF	95 [157]	99 [171]
Lippman et al.[103]	AC	83 [17]	91 [20]
Botnick et al.[12]	CMF	85 [46]	
Bluming et al.[8]	AC or ACT CMF or CMFT	82 [50]	

[ ], no. pts.

and one each in the PFT group (20 patients) and PAFT group (86 patients). The delay in radiation in the ACT group appears not to have affected the recurrence rate adversely, although the addition of tamoxifen may contribute to this observation, because in the NSABP B-14[40] trial patients who received tamoxifen and radiation had a significantly decreased breast recurrence rate when compared to patients treated with radiation alone.

The Dana Farber Cancer Institute initiated a randomized trial in 1984 for patients with primary tumors ≤5 cm in diameter with negative margins of resection and histologically positive axillary nodes. Following surgery, patients were randomized to receive radiation first or chemotherapy first. The chemotherapy consisted of cyclophosphamide, Adriamycin, 5-fluorouracil, methotrexate, and prednisone (CAFMP) for four cycles given every 3 weeks. A concurrent regimen was not evaluated. The results of this trial will provide further data regarding breast recurrence related to a delay in the initiation of radiation as well as overall and disease-free survival for delays in the initiation of chemotherapy.

Most of the current national cooperative adjuvant trials employ sequential rather than concurrent regimens. However, a single trial in the Southwest Oncology Group (8313) employs a concurrent regimen of cyclosphosphamide and 5-fluorouracil during radiation followed by either cyclophosphamide, methotrexate, 5-fluorouracil, vincristine, and prednisone (CMFVP) or 5-fluorouracil, Adriamycin, cyclophosphamide, and methotrexate (FAC-M) for ER-negative stage II breast cancer patients. Information from these trials will help to determine the optimal sequencing. This issue is especially relevant in node-negative patients who receive adjuvant systemic chemotherapy where the risk of a breast recurrence without appropriate radiation may be equal to that of distant metastases.

Ability to deliver optimal doses of chemotherapy

The ability to deliver optimal doses of chemotherapy in patients receiving primary radiotherapy is demonstrated in Table 5-39. Radiotherapy technique can have a significant impact on hematologic tolerance, and the use of a direct photon beam to treat the internal mammary nodes has been associated with a decreased ability to deliver optimal doses.[2,76,99] This may be related to the dose of radiation delivered to the thoracic spine[99] or to radiation of the circulating blood in the mediastinum resulting in a decrease in the peripheral leukocyte count, especially the lymphocytes.[6] Studies that have not employed a direct photon beam field to treat the internal mammary nodes have demonstrated no significant compromise in the ability to deliver optimal doses of chemotherapy.[8,9,12,58,103]

Incidence of complications with adjuvant chemotherapy

The impact of adjuvant systemic chemotherapy on complications is presented in Table 5-40. The addition of adjuvant systemic chemotherapy has been associated with a somewhat increased incidence of rib fractures, arm edema, and symptomatic pneumonitis, although this has not been a uniform finding in all series. The concurrent use of methotrexate during radiation may be responsible for the increased incidence of symptomatic pneumonitis in some series.[12] Several series[4,58,101,134] have demonstrated an increased incidence of fair to poor cosmetic result with the addition of adjuvant systemic chemotherapy to radiation, although the magnitude of this effect has varied. At the University of Pennsylvania[58] the incidence of fair to poor cosmetic results was 16% in patients receiving adjuvant chemotherapy, compared to 10% in those who did not. Rose et al.[143] reported a 20% incidence of fair to poor cosmetic results at 5 years in 134

Table 5-40 Incidence of complications in patients undergoing conservative surgery and radiation with or without adjuvant systemic chemotherapy

Complication	Treatment	Palo Alto[134]	National Cancer Institute[101]	University of Pennsylvania[31]	Joint Center[12,95]	Instituut Limburg[11]
Rib fractures	Chemotherapy and R	12	20	4	—	0
	R	4	11	1	—	0
Arm edema	Chemotherapy and R	12	—	13	8	5
	R	5	—	4	6	5
Symptomatic pneumonitis	Chemotherapy and R	2	0	4	6	6
	R	1	0	5	0	0

R, radiation.

patients receiving adjuvant systemic chemotherapy, compared to 8% in 459 patients receiving radiation alone. Ray et al.[134] reported a 17% incidence of fair to poor cosmesis in patients receiving adjuvant chemotherapy compared to 5% with radiation alone, and Lichter et al.[101] reported a 30% incidence of fair to poor cosmesis in patients receiving chemotherapy and radiation compared to 22% in those receiving radiation alone. Borger and Keijser[11] reported a 64% incidence of good to excellent cosmesis in 17 patients receiving cyclophosphamide, Adriamycin, and 5-fluorouracil. The impact of Adriamycin-containing regimens on complications and cosmesis will require further evaluation.

COSMETIC RESULT

Assessment

The goal of conservative surgery and radiation is the preservation of an intact breast that is cosmetically acceptable. For the most part a physician assessment cosmetic scale as initially suggested by Harris et al.[64] has been employed. The overall cosmetic score is deemed excellent if the treated breast is almost identical to the untreated breast (Fig. 5-15). A score of good recognizes differences between the treated breast and untreated breast that are slight (Fig. 5-16). A fair cosmetic result indicates obvious differences between the treated breast and untreated breast (Fig. 5-17). A poor cosmetic result is associated with marked distortion

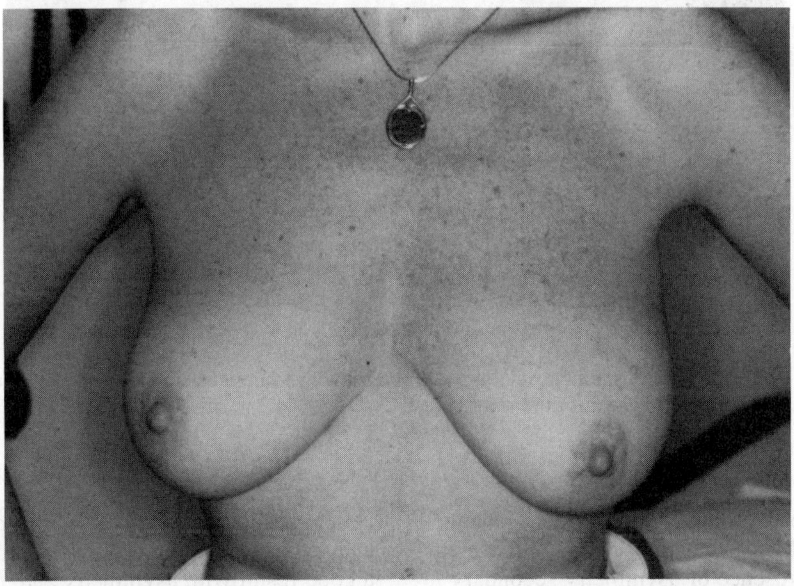

Fig. 5-15 Excellent cosmetic result following conservative surgery and radiation. Treated breast *(left)* is almost identical to the untreated. (From Danoff BF et al: Ann Intern Med 102:639, 1985.)

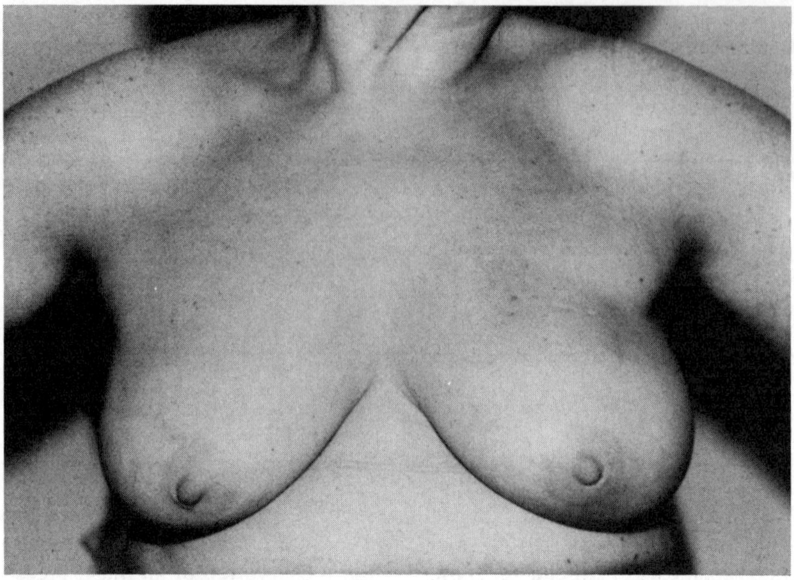

Fig. 5-16 Good cosmetic result following conservative surgery and radiation. Treated breast *(left)* reveals persistent edema and some volume loss and induration in the implant site *(upper central)*.

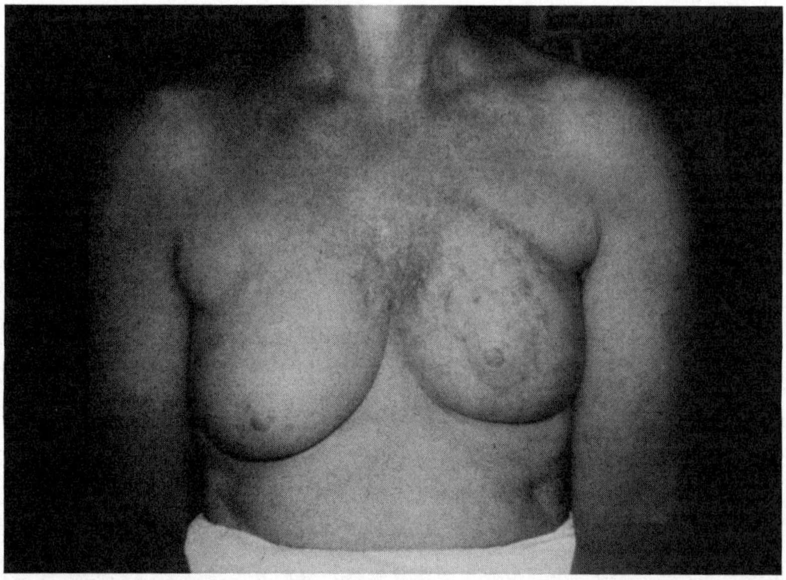

Fig. 5-17 Fair to poor cosmetic result in the left breast with telangiectasias, fibrosis, and retraction. Good cosmetic result is seen in the right breast.

of the treated breast (Fig. 5-18). Primary changes in the treated breast that impact on the cosmetic score are the presence of asymmetry secondary to a large surgical resection or significant breast fibrosis and retraction, or the presence of marked breast edema or telangiectasia. In general an excellent result is associated with no skin changes and either no asymmetry or minimal asymmetry, a good result with asymmetry and/or skin changes involving less than one quarter of the breast, a fair result with asymmetry and/or skin changes involving between 25% and 50% of the breast, and

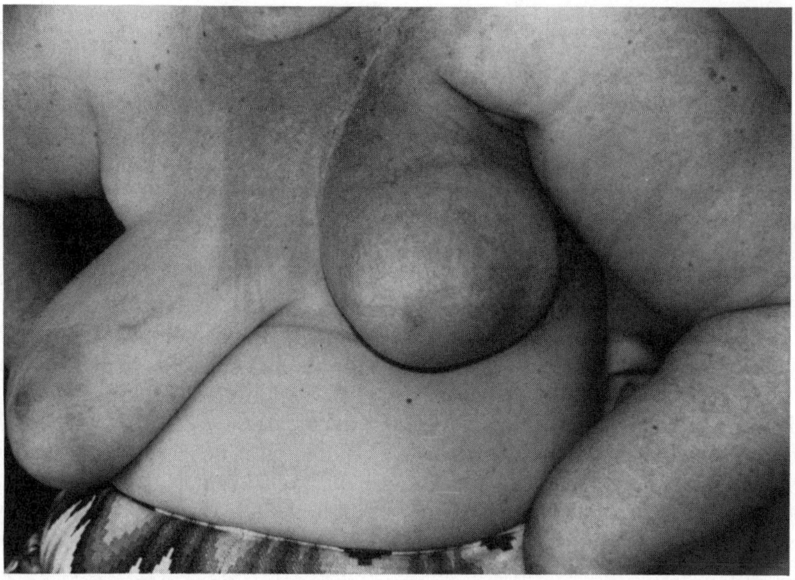

Fig. 5-18 Poor cosmetic result left breast with marked fibrosis and retraction in an obese patient with large pendulous breast. (From Danoff BF et al: Ann Intern Med 102:639, 1985.)

the poor result with deformity of greater than one half of the breast.[124] Table 5-41 presents cosmetic results from series employing conservative surgery and radiation for early breast cancer. As can be seen the majority of patients achieve a good to excellent cosmetic result. Factors that impact on cosmetic outcome can be divided into patient-related factors and treatment-related factors including surgery, radiotherapy, and chemotherapy.

Patient-related factors

Patient-related factors include breast size, body weight, the presence of a preexisting collagen vascular disease, and primary tumor size and location. Martinez et al.[106] reported good to excellent cosmetic results in 46% of patients whose weight was >161 lb, compared to 80% to 90% in patients <160 lb. Similarly, large breast size has been associated with good to excellent cosmetic results in 50% to 60% of patients.[106,132] Several authors have reported an increased incidence of marked fibrosis, telangiectasia, and soft tissue complications in patients with a preexisting history of collagen vascular disease.[48,108,131] Large primary tumor size also has been correlated with a decrease in the incidence of good to excellent cosmetic results.[35,132,143] Rose et al.[143] reported no effect of tumor location on ultimate cosmetic result; however, Van Limbergen et al.[181] noted a worse cosmetic result with tumors that were inferior or medial in location. While subareolar primary tumors may require sacrifice of the nipple areolar complex, the ultimate cosmetic result in these patients may be superior to mastectomy and reconstruction.[137]

Table 5-41 Cosmetic results conservative surgery and radiation for early breast cancer

Author	Good to excellent result (%)
Montague et al.[115]	75
Beadle et al.[4]	86
Solin et al.[169]	90
Bedwinek et al.[7]	84
Ray et al.[132]	81
Prosnitz et al.[130]	69
Bluming et al.[8]	81
Delouche et al.[34]	76
Spitalier et al.[175]	70
Pierquin et al.[126]	75
Calle et al.[16]	73
Veronesi et al.[186]	70
Hunig et al.[77]	83

Treatment-related factors

Choice and extent of surgery can affect the cosmetic outcomes. Extensive surgical resections of the primary tumor clearly result in increased deformity of the breast and a decreased incidence of good to excellent cosmetic results.[35,64,106,120,124,132,181] Veronesi et al.[186] reported satisfactory results in more than 70% of patients undergoing quadrantectomy for T_1 tumors. Grisotti et al.[60] reported that approximately 20% of patients undergoing quadrantectomy developed a deformity that was worthy of reconstruction. The extent of the axillary dissection has an impact not only on arm edema but also on breast edema. Patients undergoing a complete axillary dissection have a greater incidence of breast edema than those undergoing no dissection or a limited dissection.[26,69,115,125] Van Limbergen et al.[181] also noted a worse cosmetic result when the axillary dissection was performed in conjunction with the excision of the primary tumor, compared to a separate incision for the axillary dissection.

Radiotherapy factors that impact on the cosmetic result include delivery of the dose to the entire breast, the daily fraction, the type of boost, the volume of the boost as well as boost dose, and the matchline technique. Doses to the entire breast >5000 to 6000 cGy have been associated with increased fibrosis and retraction and a worse cosmetic result.[64,120,181] The use of an iridium-192 implant has been associated with a worse cosmetic result when compared to electrons or no boost at all.[51,120,132] The use of a large-volume boost with an implant also has been associated with impaired cosmetic results.[4] Daily fractions >250 cGy per day to the entire breast have been associated with a marked increase in fibrosis and ultimately a worse cosmetic result.[35,106,181] The overlap of adjacent radiotherapy fields results in matchline fibrosis and telangiectasia (Fig. 5-19). The use of regional node irradiation in conjunction with tangential breast irradiation has been associated with worse cosmetic results from matchline fibrosis.[64,120,133,181]

The addition of adjuvant systemic chemotherapy to conservative surgery and radiation has resulted in an increased incidence of fair to poor cosmetic results in several series,[4,58,101,134] although the magnitude of the impact has varied. It has been suggested by Gore et al.[59] that the use of concurrent regimens may result in a worse cosmetic result than sequential regimens. This has not been confirmed by the University of Pennsylvania, where concurrent regimens are employed routinely and where methotrexate is omitted during the radiation. Eighty-four percent of patients undergoing concurrent chemotherapy and radiation at the University of Pennsylvania experienced a good to excellent cosmetic result,[58] compared to 70% at the Joint Center.[59] It is uncertain as to whether there will be a difference in cosmetic outcome with the use of Adriamycin versus non–Adriamycin-containing regimens. The cosmetic result at 3 years and 5 years is fairly predictive of long-term results[120] and reflects the fact that progressive worsening is a relatively uncommon event. At the University of Pennsylvania 93% of patients had a good to excellent result at 10 years.

THE UNIVERSITY OF PENNSYLVANIA EXPERIENCE WITH CONSERVATIVE SURGERY AND RADIATION

Between 1977 and 1989, 1542 patients underwent conservative surgery and radiation at the University of Pennsylvania and Fox Chase Cancer Center for stage I and stage II breast cancer. A subgroup of 697 women treated between 1977 and 1986 have

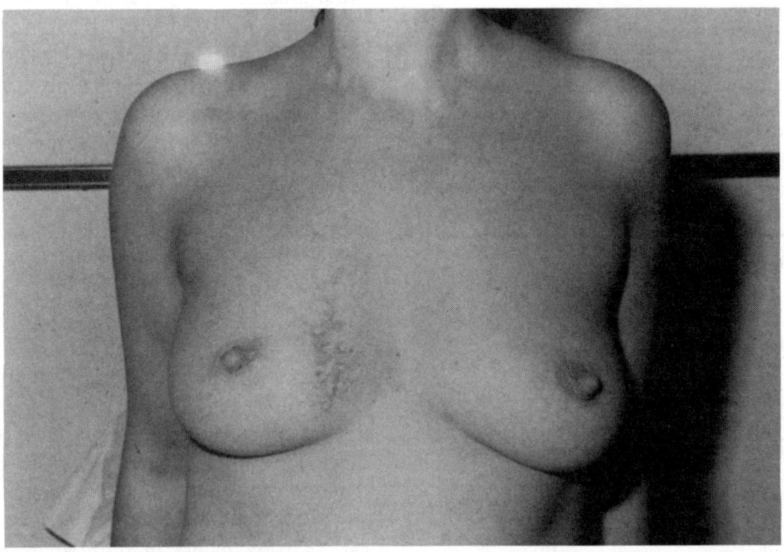

Fig. 5-19 Matchline fibrosis with linear telangiectasia in area of overlap of the medial breast tangential field and the direct photon beam internal mammary field.

been identified for long-term follow-up. All patients underwent excisional biopsy and axillary dissection and definitive radiation. The median followup was 58 months (range 2 to 37 months) with a mean of 61 months. The median age was 51 years with a range of 22 to 85 years. There were 411 patients with T_1 lesions and 286 patients with T_2 lesions. Reexcision of the primary tumor was performed in 330 and residual tumor was identified in 57% of these patients. Margins of resection were assessed in 50% and 250 patients had final margins of resection that were negative. In 408 patients axillary dissection was negative and in 217 nodes were histologically positive. Of the latter, 168 patients had one to three positive nodes and 49 patients had four or more positive nodes. The radiotherapy technique is described in the section on technical aspects of definitive radiotherapy. Adjuvant systemic chemotherapy consisting of CMF with or without prednisone or tamoxifen was given to 185 patients. Seventy-nine percent of node positive patients received chemotherapy. Of premenopausal node-positive patients 93% received adjuvant chemotherapy compared to 67% of postmenopausal women. Of the patients with histologically negative axillary nodes 3% received adjuvant systemic chemotherapy, and 20 patients received tamoxifen alone.

The results of treatment in terms of survival and breast disease recurrence are presented in Table 5-42. The 10-year actuarial survival rate for the entire group was 83% with a no evidence of disease (NED) survival of 73%. The 10-year actuarial survival rate was 87% for clinical stage I patterns and 77% for stage II patients. Patients with histologically negative axillary nodes had a 10-year survival rate of 86%, compared to 74% for those with positive nodes. Sixty-one patients developed a recurrence in the treated breast and in seven of these it was associated with simultaneous distant metastasis. The actuarial probability of an isolated breast recurrence was 6% at 5 years and 16% at 10 years. The overall breast recurrence rate (i.e., including those who present with simultaneous distant metastasis) was 8% at 5 years and 18% at 10 years. Breast recurrence was unrelated to T stage, clinical stage, or histologic nodal status. In patients with negative margins of resection, the 5- and 10-year actuarial overall breast recurrence rates were 8% and 14%. While chemotherapy decreased the breast recurrence rate at 5 years (9% vs. 5%), no impact was observed at 10 years (19% vs. 19%). Of the recurrences occurring within 5 years 78% were located in the vicinity of the original primary tumor and 62% involved initial T_1 lesions. Of the recurrences between 5 and 10 years 56% were true or marginal (i.e., in the vicinity of the original tumor) and 82% involved initial T_1 lesions. Complications of treatment included moderate arm edema in 5%, symptomatic pneumonitis in <1%, rib fractures in 1%, pericarditis in 0%, and brachial plexopathy in <1%. The incidence of symptomatic pneumonitis

Table 5-42 Results of conservative surgery and radiation in patients with stage I and stage II breast cancer at the University of Pennsylvania

	Overall survival		NED survival		Relapse-free survival		Breast recurrence ± distant metastases	
	5 yr	10 yr	5 yr	10 yr	5 yr	10 yr	5 yr	10 yr
All pts.	90	83	81	73	75	61	8	18
Clinical stage								
I	93	87	88	79	81	63	9	21
II	87	77	72	67	68	59	7	13
Pathologic nodal status								
Negative	92	86	84	78	78	65	8	18
Positive	87	74	74	66	70	51	7	21
Clinical tumor size								
T_1	93	87	88	79	81	64	8	20
T_2	86	77	70	65	67	58	8	14
Pathologic stage								
I	93	88	88	82	81	66	8	19
II	87	77	74	65	70	56	8	17

was 2% in patients receiving adjuvant chemotherapy and <1% in those who did not. There was no significant difference in the incidence of symptomatic pneumonitis when comparing sequential treatment (0 of 23 patients) with concurrent chemotherapy and radiation (2 of 158 patients). Methotrexate was not given during the radiation treatment period. Cosmesis was judged to be good to excellent in 91% of those treated at 5 years and 93% at 10 years, demonstrating the stability of the cosmetic result. Our 5-year results show no impact of young age on breast recurrence.[173] Patients with microscopic margins of resection that are focally positive have not experienced an increased risk of breast recurrence when a boost dose of radiation was employed, and we have found no correlation with primary tumor size or pathologic nodal status provided that an excisional biopsy was performed (see Tables 5-5, 5-6, and 5-20).

A detailed review of histopathologic factors re-

Table 5-43 Histopathologic factors correlated with breast recurrence—univariate and multivariate analysis at the University of Pennsylvania

Histopathologic factors	No. pts.	Actuarial breast recurrence (%) 5 yr	10 yr	p value (univariate)
Histologic grade				.0005
1	23	4	4	
2	51	7	16	
3	191	4	14	
4	10	47	—	
Necrosis of intraductal component*				.057
None	67	2	14	
Slight	71	1	9	
Moderate	54	18	23	
Marked	15	7	7	
Inflammatory response				.04
1+	121	4	15	
2+	78	6	9	
3+	30	3	3	
4+	11	20	20	
Absent	35	14	30	
Retrograde cancerization				.015
Present	74	15	18	
Absent	176	2	12	
Fibrocystic changes*				.015
Present	81	11	18	
Absent	140	2	7	
Epithelial hyperplasia				.04
Slight	19	6	6	
Moderate	17	6	17	
Atypical	11	19	46	
Absent	173	4	10	
Extensive intraductal component				.03
Positive	23	22	22	
Negative	252	4	11	
Progesterone receptor				.03
Negative	63	2	—	
Positive	83	12	—	

*Significant factors in a multivariate analysis.

lated to breast recurrence is presented in Chapter 7. Briefly, a retrospective pathologic review of 275 patients with infiltrating ductal carcinoma (stage I or stage II) who underwent conservative surgery and radiation between 1977 and 1986 was performed. The median follow-up time was 6.3 years. Reexcision was performed in 30% and residual tumor was identified in 68%. Margins were assessed in 40% and were positive in 24%, close in 16%, and negative in 60%. Axillary dissection was performed in 93% and 80 patients had positive nodes (31%). Seventy-three patients received chemotherapy consisting of CMF with or without prednisone and tamoxifen. For the entire group, the 5-year actuarial risk of a breast failure was 6% with a 10-year actuarial risk of 14%. The following factors were analyzed for their ability to predict for breast recurrence: primary tumor size, histologic type, histologic and nuclear grade, the presence or absence of an extensive intraductal component, nipple involvement, retrograde cancerization of the breast, fibrosis, the percentage of tumor per unit area, necrosis in either the noninvasive or invasive component of the tumor, inflammatory response, mitotic index, lymphatic or blood vessel invasion, growth pattern of the infiltrating carcinoma, tumor border, background breast changes (fibrocystic disease, atypical epithelial hyperplasia, atrophy), final pathologic margin, and estrogen and progesterone receptor status. In a univariate analysis, histologic grade, moderate to marked necrosis within the intraductal component, the absence of an inflammatory response, retrograde cancerization, fibrocystic changes, epithelial hyperplasia, an extensive intraductal component and progesterone receptor positivity significantly correlated with the 5- and 10-year actuarial risk of a breast recurrence (Table 5-43). In a multivariate analysis only the presence of moderate or marked necrosis in the intraductal component and the presence of fibrocystic changes were significant. Specifically for EIC, the definition employed was that used by the Joint Center.[154] Only 8% of patients were EIC positive, but this may be a reflection of our patient selection. Patients with diffuse or widespread microcalcifications were referred for mastectomy. As previously noted the most common clinical presentation of EIC-positive tumors is one of mammographic calcifications without an associated mass.[70] The 5- and 10-year actuarial risk for a breast disease recurrence was 22% for EIC-positive tumors compared to 4% and 11% for EIC-negative tumors. Five of 23 patients with EIC-positive tumors developed a recurrence. None of four patients with positive or close margins had a recurrence compared to one of five with negative margins and four of 14 with unknown margins. It is difficult to draw conclusions from these small numbers; however, the number of recurrences in the unknown margin group suggests inadequate evaluation of the tumor extent.

In summary, the series from the University of Pennsylvania is relatively contemporary in that all patients had an excisional biopsy, 47% underwent a reexcision, 50% had margin assessment, axillary dissection was performed in 100%, and 79% of all node-positive patients received adjuvant chemotherapy. It must be emphasized that criteria for patient selection were rather stringent and patients with gross multicentric disease, diffuse microcalcifications, or diffuse margin involvement were referred for mastectomy. Preoperative mammograms were assessed routinely and postbiopsy mammograms were obtained in patients who presented with focal microcalcifications to insure complete removal of the microcalcifications. The radiotherapy treatment policy during this time was consistent and a boost dose was given routinely to the biopsy site. The 10-year breast disease recurrence rate is quite comparable to that reported by others[24,63,84,138,176] and reflects the results in patients treated in the early part of the study in whom reexcision was not performed and in whom margins were not assessed routinely. Further follow-up in the group of patients with margin assessment will provide long-term information on breast recurrence rates in this group of patients.

REFERENCES

1. Balawajder I, Antich PP, and Boland J: The management of breast carcinoma by primary radiotherapy at Mount Sinai Hospital from 1962-1979, Cancer 49:1587, 1982.
2. Banerjee RK, Hoehn JL, Greenlaw RH, and Jacoby C: Chemotherapy drug dose alternative due to radiation therapy in an adjuvant situation in breast cancer, Am J Clin Oncol 7:437, 1984.
3. Bartelink H, Border JH, van Dongen JA, and Peterse JL: The impact of tumor size and histology on local control after breast-conserving therapy, Radiother Oncol 11:297, 1988.
4. Beadle GF, Harris JR, Silver B, et al: Cosmetic results following primary radiation therapy for early breast cancer, Cancer 54:2911, 1984.
5. Bedwinek J: Preoperative planning of breast implants using the breast implant planning device (BIPD), Int J Radiat Oncol Biol Phys 14:817, 1988.
6. Bedwinek J: Adjuvant irradiation for early breast cancer. An on-going controversy, Cancer 53:729, 1984.
7. Bedwinek JM, Perez CA, Kramer S, et al: Irradiation as the primary management of stage I and II adenocarcinoma of the breast, Cancer Clin Trials 3:11, 1980.
8. Bluming AZ, Dosik G, Lowiz B, et al: Treatment of primary breast cancer without mastectomy: the Los Angeles Community experience and review of the literature, Ann Surg 204:136, 1986.
9. Bonadonna G, Valagussa P, Zucali R, et al: Feasibility of adjuvant chemotherapy plus radiotherapy in operable breast cancer. In Harris J, Hellman S, and Silen W, editors: Conservative management of breast cancer, Philadelphia, 1983, JB Lippincott, pp 329-338.
10. Boova RS, Bonanni R, and Rosato FE: Patterns of axillary

nodal involvement in breast cancer: predictability of level one dissection, Ann Surg 196:642, 1982.
11. Borger JH and Keijser AH: Conservative breast cancer treatment: analysis of cosmetic results and the role of concomitant adjuvant chemotherapy, Int J Radiat Oncol Biol Phys 13:1173, 1987.
12. Botnick L, Come S, Rose C, et al: Primary breast irradiation and concomitant adjuvant chemotherapy. In Harris J, Hellman S, and Silen W, editors: Conservative management of breast cancer, Philadelphia, 1983, JB Lippincott, pp 321-328.
13. Boyages J, Recht A, Connolly J, et al: Factors associated with local recurrence as a first site of failure following conservative treatment of early breast cancer, Recent Results Cancer Res 115:92, 1989.
14. Bronstein BA, Cheng CW, Rhodes L, et al: Can measurements taken at simulation be used to predict the volume of lung within the radiation therapy treatment field in breast cancer patients? Int J Radiat Oncol Biol Phys 15(suppl):192, 1988 (abstract).
15. Butcher HR: Radical mastectomy for mammary carcinoma, Ann Surg 170:883, 1969.
16. Calle R, Vilcoq JR, Zafrani B, et al: Local control and survival of breast cancer treated by limited surgery followed by irradiation, Int J Radiat Oncol Biol Phys 12:873, 1986.
17. Cedermark B, Askergren J, Alveryd A, et al: Breast-conserving treatment for breast cancer in Stockholm, Sweden 1977 to 1981, Cancer 53:1253, 1984.
18. Chin LM, Chenk CW, Siddon RL, et al: Three-dimensional photon dose distributions with and without lung corrections for tangential breast intact treatments, Int J Radiat Oncol Biol Phys 17:1327, 1989.
19. Chin LM, Siddon RL, Svensson GK, and Rose C: Progress in 3-D treatment planning for photon beam therapy, Int J Radiat Oncol Biol Phys 11:2011, 1985.
20. Chu AM, Cope O, Russo R, and Lew R: Patterns of local-regional recurrence and results in stages I and II breast cancer treated by irradiation following limited surgery, Am J Clin Oncol 7:221, 1984.
21. Chu JCH, Solin LJ, Whang CC, et al: A nondivergent three field matching technique for breast irradiation, Int J Radiat Oncol Biol Phys 19:1037, 1990.
22. Chu JCH, Sontag MR, Danoff BF, and Goodman RL: Assessment of dose uniformity in the irradiation of the intact breast using three-dimensional dose calculations, Int J Radiat Oncol Biol Phys 11(suppl I):613, 1985 (abstract).
23. Ciatto S, Pacini P, DelTurco MR, et al: Patterns of axillary metastases in breast cancer, Radiother Oncol 5:91, 1986.
24. Clark RM, Wilkinson RH, Miceli PN, and MacDonald WD: Breast cancer: experiences with conservation therapy, Am J Clin Oncol 10:461, 1987.
25. Clarke D, Martinez A, and Cox RS: Analysis of cosmetic results and complications in patients with stage I and II breast cancer treated by biopsy and irradiation, Int J Radiat Oncol Biol Phys 9:1807, 1983.
26. Clarke D, Martinez A, Cox RS, and Goffinet DR: Breast edema following staging axillary node dissection in patients with breast carcinoma treated by radical radiotherapy, Cancer 49:2295, 1982.
27. Clarke DH, Le MG, Sarrazin D, Lacombe M, et al: Analysis of local-regional relapse in patients with early breast cancers treated by excision and radiotherapy: experience of the Institut Gustave-Roussy, Int J Radiat Oncol Biol Phys 11:137, 1985.
28. Conte G, Nascimben O, Turcato G, et al: Three-field isocentric technique for breast irradiation using individualized shielding blocks, Int J Radiat Oncol Biol Phys 14:1299, 1988.
29. Cuzick J, Stewart H, Peto H, et al: Overview of randomized trials of postoperative adjuvant radiotherapy in breast cancer, Cancer Treat Rep 71:15, 1987.
30. Danforth DM, Findlay PA, McDonald HD, et al: Complete axillary lymph node dissection for Stage I-II carcinoma of the breast, J Clin Oncol 4:655, 1986.
31. Danoff B, Goodman RL, and Glick JH: The effect of adjuvant chemotherapy on cosmesis and complications in patients with breast carcinoma treated by definitive irradiation, Int J Radiat Oncol Biol Phys 9:1625, 1983.
32. Danoff BF, Galvin JM, Cheng E, et al: The clinical application of CT scanning in the treatment of primary breast cancer. In Ames FC, Blumenschein GR, and Montague ED, editors: Current controversies in breast cancer, Austin, 1984, University of Texas Press, pp 391-397.
33. Danoff BF and Goodman RL: Identification of a subset of patients with early breast cancer in whom conservative surgery and radiation is contraindicated, Int J Radiat Oncol Biol Phys 11:104, 1985 (abstract).
34. Delouche G, Bachelot F, Premont M, and Kurtz JM: Conservation treatment of early breast cancer: long term results and complications, Int J Radiat Oncol Biol Phys 13:29, 1987.
35. Dewar JA, Benhamou S, Benhamou E, et al: Cosmetic results following lumpectomy, axillary dissection and radiotherapy for small breast cancers, Radiother Oncol 12:273, 1988.
36. Dewar JA, Sarrazin D, Benhamou E, et al: Management of the axilla in conservatively treated breast cancer: 592 patients treated at Institut Gustave-Roussey, Int J Radiat Oncol Biol Phys 13:475, 1987.
37. Doppke K, Novvack D, and Wang CC: Physical considerations in the treatment of advanced carcinomas of the larynx and pyriform sinuses using 10 MV X rays, Int J Radiat Oncol Biol Phys 6:1251, 1980.
38. Durand JC, Poljicak M, LeFranc JP, and Pilleron JP: Wide excision of the tumor, axillary dissection, and post-operative radiotherapy as treatment of small breast cancers, Cancer 53:2439, 1984.
39. Fisher B, Bauer M, Margolese R, et al: Five-year results of a randomized clinical trial comparing total mastectomy and segmental mastectomy with or without radiation in the treatment of breast cancer, N Engl J Med 312:665, 1985.
40. Fisher B, Costantino J, Redmond C, et al: A randomized clinical trial evaluating tamoxifen in the treatment of patients with node-negative breast cancer who have estrogen-receptor-positive tumors, N Engl J Med 320:479, 1989.
41. Fisher B, Redmond C, Dimitrov NV, et al: A randomized clinical trial evaluating sequential methotrexate and fluorouracil in the treatment of patients with node-negative breast cancer who have estrogen-receptor-negative tumors, N Engl J Med 320:473, 1989.
42. Fisher B, Redmond C, Legault-Poisson S, et al: Postoperative chemotherapy and tamoxifen compared with tamoxifen alone in the treatment of positive-node breast cancer patients aged 50 years and older with tumors responsive to tamoxifen: results from the National Surgical Breast and Bowel Project B-16, J Clin Oncol 8:1005, 1990.
43. Fisher B, Redmond C, Poisson R, et al: Eight-year results of a randomized clinical trial comparing total mastectomy and lumpectomy with or without irradiation in the treatment of breast cancer, N Engl J Med 320:822, 1989.
44. Fisher B, Slack NH, Cavanaugh PJ, et al: Postoperative radiotherapy in the treatment of breast cancer: results of the NSABP clinical trial, Ann Surg 172:711, 1970.
45. Fisher B, Wolmark N, Bauer M, et al: The accuracy of clinical nodal staging and of limited axillary dissection as

a determinant of histologic nodal status in carcinoma of the breast, Surg Gyn Obstet 152:765, 1981.
46. Fisher ER, Gregorio R, Redmond C, et al: Pathologic findings from the National Surgical Adjuvant Breast Project (Protocol 4): I. Observations concerning the multicentricity of mammary cancer, Cancer 35:247, 1975.
47. Fisher ER, Sass R, Fisher B, et al: Pathologic findings from the National Surgical Adjuvant Breast Project (Protocol 6) II. Relation of local breast recurrence to multicentricity, Cancer 57:1717, 1986.
48. Fleck RS, McNeese MD, Ellerbrock NA, et al: Consequences of breast irradiation in patients with pre-existing collagen vascular disease, Int J Radiat Oncol Biol Phys 17:829, 1989.
49. Forrest APM, Stewart HJ, Roberts MM, and Steele RJC: Simple mastectomy and axillary node sampling (pectoral node biopsy) in the management of primary breast cancer, Ann Surg 196:371, 1982.
50. Fourquet A, Campana F, Zafrani B, et al: Prognostic factors in the conservative management of early breast cancer: a 25 year follow-up at the Institut Curie, Int J Radiat Oncol Biol Phys 17:7199, 1989.
51. Fowble B, Solin LJ, Martz KL, et al: The influence of the type of boost (electrons vs. implant) on local control and cosmesis in patients with stages I and II breast cancer undergoing conservative surgery and radiation, Int J Radiat Oncol Biol Phys 12:150, 1986 (abstract).
52. Fowble B, Solin LJ, Schultz DJ, and Goodman RL: Frequency, sites of relapse and outcome of regional node failures following conservative surgery and radiation for early breast cancer, Int J Radiat Oncol Biol Phys 17:703, 1989.
53. Fraass BA, Lichter AS, McShan DL, et al: The influence of lung density corrections on treatment planning for primary breast cancer, Int J Radiat Oncol Biol Phys 14:179, 1988.
54. Fraass BA, Robertson PL, and Lichter AS: Dose to the contralateral breast due to primary breast irradiation, Int J Radiat Oncol Biol Phys 11:485, 1985.
55. Frazier TG, Wong RWY, and Rose D: Implications of accurate pathologic margins in the treatment of primary breast cancer, Arch Surg 124:37, 1989.
56. Gerard JP, Montbarbon JF, Chassard JL, et al: Conservative treatment of early carcinoma of the breast: significance of axillary dissection and iridium implant, Radiother Oncol 3:17, 1985.
57. Ghossein NA, Barba JP, Alpert S, et al: Importance of adequate surgical excision prior to radiotherapy in the local control of patients treated conservatively for breast cancer. Proceedings of the seventeenth International Congress of Radiation Oncology, Paris, 1989, p. 48 (abstract).
58. Glick JH, Fowble BL, Haller DG, et al: Integration of full dose adjuvant chemotherapy with definitive radiotherapy for primary breast cancer: a four year update. Interaction of radiation therapy and chemotherapy, NCI Monogr 6:297, 1988.
59. Gore SM, Come SE, Griem K, et al: Influence of the sequencing of chemotherapy and radiation therapy in node positive breast cancer patients treated by conservative surgery and radiation. In Salmon SE, editor: Adjuvant therapy of cancer V, Orlando, Fla, 1987, Grune & Stratton, Inc, pp 365-373.
60. Grisotti A, Luini A, Callegari M, et al: Reconstruction after conservative treatment for breast cancer, Breast Cancer Res Treat 12:117, 1988.
61. Gump FE, Shikora S, Habif DV, et al: The extent and distribution of cancer in breasts with palpable primary tumors, Ann Surg 204:384, 1986.
62. Haagensen CD: The natural history of breast carcinoma. In Haagensen CD, editor: Diseases of the breast, ed 3, Philadelphia, 1986, WB Saunders Co, pp 635-718.
63. Haffty BG, Goldberg NB, Fischer D, et al: Conservative surgery and radiation therapy in breast carcinoma: local recurrence and prognostic implications, Int J Radiat Oncol Biol Phys 17:727, 1989.
64. Harris JL, Levene MB, Svensson G, and Hellman S: Analysis of cosmetic results following primary radiation for stages I and II carcinoma of the breast, Int J Radiat Oncol Biol Phys 5:257, 1979.
65. Harris JR, Beadle GF, and Hellman S: Clinical studies on the use of radiation therapy as primary treatment of early breast cancer, Cancer 53:705, 1984.
66. Harris JR, Botnick L, Bloomer WD, et al: Primary radiation therapy for early breast cancer: the experience at the Joint Center for Radiation Therapy, Int J Radiat Biol Phys 7:1549, 1981.
67. Harris JR and Hellman S: The results of primary irradiation therapy for early breast cancer at the Joint Center for Radiation Therapy. In Harris JR, Hellman S, and Silen W, editors: Conservative management of breast cancer: new surgical and radiotherapeutic techniques, Philadelphia, 1983, JB Lippincott, pp 47-52.
68. Harter K, Goldberg R, Bryne P, et al: Local recurrence of breast cancer following lumpectomy in patients receiving adjuvant chemotherapy prior to definitive breast irradiation, Proc Am Soc Clin Oncol 3:125, 1984 (abstract).
69. Hayward JL, Winter PJ, Tong D, et al: A new combined approach to the conservative treatment of early breast cancer, Surgery 95:270, 1984.
70. Healey EA, Osteen RT, Schnitt SJ, et al: Can the initial clinical and mammographic features predict the presence of an extensive intraductal component in early stage breast cancer, Int J Radiat Oncol Biol Phys 17:1217, 1989.
71. Hermann RE, Esselstyn CB, Crile G, et al: Results of conservative operations for breast cancer, Arch Surg 120:746, 1985.
72. Hermann RE, Esselstyn CB, and Grundfest-Broniatowski S: The treatment of curable breast cancer—the Cleveland Clinic experience. In Grundfest-Broniatowski S and Esselstyn CB, editors: Controversies in breast disease: diagnosis and management, New York, 1988, Marcel Dekker Inc, pp 287-306.
73. Hery M, Namer M, Verschoore J, et al: Conservative treatment of breast cancer. A report of 108 patients, Int J Radiat Oncol Biol Phys 10:2185, 1984.
74. Holland R, Connolly J, Gelman R, et al: The presence of an extensive intraductal component following a limited excision correlates with prominent residual disease in the remainder of the breast, J Clin Oncol 8:113, 1990.
75. Holland R, Veling S, Mravunac M, and Hendriks J: Histologic multifocality of Tis T1-2 breast carcinomas. Implications for clinical trials of breast-conserving surgery, Cancer 56:979, 1985.
76. Holland TF and Glidewell O: Adverse effect of radiotherapy on adjuvant chemotherapy for carcinoma of the breast, Surg Gynecol Obstet 150:817, 1980.
77. Hunig R, Walther E, Harder F, et al: The Basel lumpectomy protocol: 5 year experience with a prospective study for conservative treatment of breast cancer. In Harris JR, Hellman S, and Silen W, editors: Conservative management of breast cancer, Philadelphia, 1983, JB Lippincott, pp 23-35.
78. Hunt MA, Kutcher GJ, and Martel MK: Matchline dosimetry of a three field technique for breast treatment using Cobalt or 6 MV x-rays, Int J Radiat Oncol Biol Phys 13:1099, 1987.
79. Jewell WR, Krishnan L, Reddy EK, et al: Intraoperative implantation radiation therapy plus lumpectomy for carcinoma of the breast, Arch Surg 122:687, 1987.
80. Jones JM and Ribeiro GG: Mortality patterns over 34 years

of breast cancer patients in a clinical trial of post-operative radiotherapy, Clin Radiol 40:204, 1989.
81. Kantorowitz DA, Poulter CA, Rubin P, et al: Treatment of breast cancer with segmental mastectomy alone or segmental mastectomy plus radiation, Radiother Oncol 15:141, 1989.
82. Koper PCM, van Putten WLJ, Wijnmaalen AJ, et al: Breast conserving surgery and radiotherapy in early stage breast cancer, Int J Radiat Oncol Biol Phys (in press).
83. Kuchnir FT, Chen GTY, Pelizzari CA, et al: Application of the Moire photography to multi-level treatment planning in radiation therapy the intact breast, Int J Radiat Oncol Biol Phys 13 (suppl 1):197, 1987 (abstract).
84. Kurtz JM, Amalric R, Brandone H, et al: Local recurrence after breast-conserving surgery and radiotherapy. Frequency, time course and prognosis, Cancer 63:1912, 1989.
85. Kurtz JM, Jacquemier J, Amalric R, et al: Risk factors of breast recurrence in pre- and postmenopausal patients with ductal cancers, Cancer 65:1867, 1990.
86. Kurtz JM, Jacquemier J, Amalric R, et al: Why are local recurrences after breast conserving therapy more frequent in young patients? J Clin Oncol 8:591, 1990.
87. Kurtz JM, Jacquemier J, Torhorst J, et al: Conservation therapy for breast cancers other than infiltrating ductal carcinoma, Cancer 63:1630, 1989.
88. Kurtz JM, Spitalier J, and Amalric R: Late breast recurrence after lumpectomy and irradiation, Int J Radiat Oncol Biol Phys 9:1191, 1983.
89. Kurtz JM, Spitalier JM, Brandone H, et al: Mammary recurrences in women younger than forty, Int J Radiat Oncol Biol Phys 15:271, 1988.
90. Lacour J, Bucalossi P, Cacers E, et al: Radical mastectomy vs. radical mastectomy plus internal mammary dissection. Five year results of an international cooperative study, Cancer 37:206, 1976.
91. Lacour J, Le M, Caceres E, et al: Radical mastectomy versus radical mastectomy plus internal mammary dissection. Ten year results of an international cooperative trial in breast cancer, Cancer 51:1941, 1983.
92. Lagios MD: Multicentricity of breast carcinoma demonstrated by routine correlated serial subgross and radiographic examination, Cancer 40:1726, 1977.
93. Lagios MD, Gates EA, Westdahl PR, et al: A guide to the frequency of nipple involvement in breast cancer: a study of 149 consecutive mastectomies using a serial subgross and correlated radiographic technique, Am J Surg 138:135, 1979.
94. Lagios MD, Richards UE, Rose MR, and Yee E: Segmental mastectomy without radiotherapy. Short-term follow-up, Cancer 52:2173, 1983.
95. Larson P, Weinstein M, Goldberg I, et al: Edema of the arm as a function of the extent of axillary surgery in patients with Stage I-II carcinoma of the breast treated with primary radiotherapy, Int J Radiat Oncol Biol Phys 12:1575, 1986.
96. Lepesque JV: Field matching in breast irradiation: an exact solution to a geometrical problem, Radiother Oncol 5:45, 1986.
97. Leopold KA, Recht A, Schnitt SJ, et al: Results of conservative surgery and radiation for multiple synchronous cancers of one breast, Int J Radiat Oncol Biol Phys 16:11, 1989.
98. Lesser ML, Rosen PP, and Kinne DW: Multicentricity and bilaterality in invasive breast carcinoma, Surgery 91:234, 1982.
99. Levine TF, Coleman CM, Cot RS, et al: The effect of post-operative and primary radiation therapy in delivered dose of adjuvant cyclophosphamide, methotrexate and 5-fluorouracil (CMF) chemotherapy in breast cancer, Cancer 53:237, 1984.
100. Lichter AS, Fraass BA, van de Geijn J, and Padikal TN: A technique for field matching and primary breast irradiation, Int J Radiat Oncol Biol Phys 9:263, 1983.
101. Lichter AS, Lippman ME, Gorrell CR, et al: Adjuvant chemotherapy in patients treated primarily with irradiation for localized breast cancer. In Harris J, Hellman S, and Silen W, editors: Conservative management of breast cancer, Philadelphia, 1983, JB Lippincott, pp 299-310.
102. Lindley R, Bulman A, Parsons P, et al: Histologic features predictive of an increased risk of early local recurrence after treatment of breast cancer by local tumor excision and radical radiotherapy, Surgery 105:13, 1989.
103. Lippman ME, Lichter AS, Edwards BK, et al: The impact of primary irradiation treatment of localized breast cancer on the ability to administer systemic adjuvant chemotherapy, J Clin Oncol 2:21, 1984.
104. Lloyd LR, Waits RK, Schroder P, et al: Axillary dissection for breast carcinoma: the myth of skip metastases, Am Surg 55:381, 1989.
105. Loprinzi CL, Carbone PP, Tormey DC, et al: Aggressive combined modality therapy for advanced local-regional breast carcinoma, J Clin Oncol 2:157, 1984.
106. Martinez AA and Clarke D: Treatment results, cosmesis and complications in stages I and II breast cancer patients treated by excisional biopsy and irradiation. In Ames FC, Blumenschein GR, and Montague ED, editors: Current controversies in breast cancer, Austin, 1984, University of Texas Press, pp 369-381.
107. Mate TP, Carter D, Fischer DB, et al: A clinical and histopathologic analysis of the results of conservation surgery and radiation therapy in Stage I and II breast carcinoma, Cancer 58:1995, 1986.
108. Mathews RH: Collagen vascular disease and irradiation, Int J Radiat Oncol Biol Phys 17:1123, 1989.
109. Mathews RH, McNeese M, Montague ED, and Oswald NJ: Prognostic implications of age in breast cancer patients treated with tumorectomy and irradiation or with mastectomy, Int J Radiat Oncol Biol Phys 14:659, 1988.
110. Maylin C, Socie G, Clot PH, et al: Five years local control after conservative treatment in breast cancer with intra-operative brachytherapy. Uni- and multivariate analysis of 410 cases stage I-II. UICC. St. Louis Hospital Experience—Paris. Proceedings of the seventeenth International Congress of Radiation Oncology, Paris, 1989, p 49 (abstract).
111. McCormick B, Kinne D, Petrek J, et al: Limited resection for breast cancer: a study of inked specimen margins before radiotherapy, Int J Radiat Oncol Biol Phys 13:1667, 1987.
112. McCormick B, Wesson MF, Cox L, et al: Iridium 92 implants for primary breast cancer: experience with placement at the time of wide local excision, Int J Radiat Oncol Biol Phys 15:745, 1988.
113. Meier P, Ferguson DJ, and Karrison T: A controlled trial of extended radical versus radical mastectomy. Ten-year results, Cancer 63:188, 1989.
114. Montague ED: Conservative surgery and radiation therapy in the treatment of operable breast cancer, Cancer 53:700, 1984.
115. Montague ED, Schell SR, Romsdahl MD, and Ames FS: Conservative surgery and irradiation in clinically favorable breast cancer—the M.D. Anderson experience. In Harris J, Hellman S, and Silen W, editors: Conservative management of breast cancer, Philadelphia, 1983, JB Lippincott, pp 53-60.
116. Morimoto T, Komaki K, Inui K, et al: Involvement of the nipple and areola in early breast cancer, Cancer 55:2459, 1985.

117. Muscolino G, Luini A, Bedini AV, et al: Impact of young age on local recurrence risk in patients with early breast cancer who have undergone Q.U.A.R.T. Paper presented at the Breast Conference, San Antonio, Texas, 1988 (abstract).
118. Nobler MP and Venet L: Prognostic factors in patients undergoing curative irradiation for breast cancer, Int J Radiol Oncol Biol Phys 11:123, 1985.
119. Noyes RD, Spanos WJ, and Montague ED: Breast cancer in women aged 30 and under, Cancer 39:1302, 1982.
120. Olivotto IA, Rose MA, Osteen RT, et al: Late cosmetic outcome after conservative surgery and radiotherapy: analysis of causes of cosmetic failure, Int J Radiat Oncol Biol Phys 17:747, 1989.
121. Osborne MP, Ormiston N, Harmer CL, et al: Breast conservation in the treatment of early breast cancer, Cancer 53:349, 1984.
122. Osteen RT, Connolly JL, Recht A, et al: Identification of patients at high risk for local recurrence after conservative surgery and radiation therapy for Stage I or II breast cancer, Arch Surg 122:1248, 1987.
123. Pezner RD, Lipsett JA, Desai K, et al: To boost or not to boost: decreasing radiation therapy in conservative breast cancer treatment when "inked" tumor resection margins are pathologically free of cancer, Int J Radiat Oncol Biol Phys 14:873, 1988.
124. Pezner RD, Lipsett JA, Vera NL, and Desai KR: Limited usefulness of observer-based cosmesis scales employed to evaluate patients treated conservatively for breast cancer, Int J Radiat Oncol Biol Phys 11:1117, 1985.
125. Pezner RD, Patterson MP, Hill LR, et al: Breast edema in patients treated conservatively for stage I and II breast cancer, Int J Radiat Oncol Biol Phys 11:1765, 1985.
126. Pierquin B: Conservative treatment for carcinoma of the breast: experience of Creteil—ten year results. In Harris J, Hellman S, and Silen W, editors: Conservative management of breast cancer, Philadelphia, 1983, JB Lippincott, pp 11-14.
127. Pierquin B, Mazeron J, and Glaubiger D: Conservative treatment of breast cancer in Europe: report of the Groupe Europeen du Curietherapie, Radiother Oncol 6:187, 1986.
128. Pigott J, Nichols R, Maddox WA, and Balch CM: Metastases to the upper levels of the axillary nodes in carcinoma of the breast and its implications for nodal sampling procedures, Surg Gyn Obstet 158:255, 1984.
129. Podgorsak EB, Gosselin M, Pla M, et al: A simple isocentric technique for irradiation of the breast, chest wall and peripheral lymphatics, Br J Radiol 57:57, 1984.
130. Prosnitz LR, Weshler Z, and Goldenberg IS: Primary radiotherapy for breast carcinoma instead of mastectomy: the Yale experience. In Harris J, Hellman S, and Silen W, editors: Conservative management of breast cancer, Philadelphia, 1983, JB Lippincott, pp 61-70.
131. Ransom DT and Cameron FG: Scleroderma: a possible contraindication to lumpectomy and radiotherapy in breast cancer, Australas Radiol 31:317, 1987.
132. Ray GR and Fish VJ: Biopsy and definitive radiation therapy in stage I and II adenocarcinoma of the female breast: analysis of cosmesis and the role of electron beam supplementation, Int J Radiat Oncol Biol Phys 9:813, 1983.
133. Ray GR, Fish VJ, Lee RH, et al: Biopsy and definitive radiation therapy in stages I and II carcinoma of the female breast, Int J Radiat Oncol Biol Phys 9:23, 1983.
134. Ray GR, Fish VJ, Marmor JB, et al: Impact of adjuvant chemotherapy on cosmesis and complications in stages I and II carcinoma of the breast treated by biopsy and radiation therapy, Int J Radiat Oncol Biol Phys 10:837, 1984.
135. Recht A, Connolly JL, Schnitt SJ, et al: The effect of young age on tumor recurrence in the treated breast after conservative surgery and radiotherapy, Int J Radiat Oncol Biol Phys 14:3, 1988.
136. Recht A, Connolly JL, Schnitt SJ, et al: Conservative surgery and radiation therapy for early breast cancer: results, controversies, and unsolved problems, Semin Oncol 13:434, 1986.
137. Recht A and Harris JR: Selection of patients with early-stage breast cancer for conservative surgery and radiation, Oncology 4:23, 1990.
138. Recht A, Silen W, Schnitt SJ, et al: Time course of local recurrence following conservative surgery and radiotherapy for early stage breast cancer, Int J Radiat Oncol Biol Phys 15:255, 1988.
139. Roberson PL, Lichter AS, Bodner A, et al: Dose to lung in primary breast irradiation, Int J Radiat Oncol Biol Phys 9:97, 1982.
140. Romestaing P, Carrie C, Ardiet JM, et al: Conservative treatment of small breast cancer. Relevance of a boost after 50 GY on the whole breast. Preliminary results of a randomized trial. Proceedings of the Seventeenth International Congress of Radiation Oncology, Paris, 1989, p 55 (abstract).
141. Romsdahl MM, Montague ED, Ames FC, et al: Conservation surgery and irradiation as treatment for early breast cancer, Arch Surg 118:521, 1983.
142. Rose MA, Henderson IC, Gelman R, et al: Premenopausal breast cancer patients treated with conservative surgery, radiotherapy and adjuvant chemotherapy have a low risk of local failure, Int J Radiat Oncol Biol Phys 17:711, 1989.
143. Rose MA, Olivotto I, Cady B, et al: Conservative surgery and radiation therapy for early breast cancer. Long term cosmetic results, Arch Surg 124:153, 1989.
144. Rosen PP, Fracchia AA, Urban JA, et al: "Residual" mammary carcinoma following simulated partial mastectomy, Cancer 35:739, 1975.
145. Rosen PP, Kinne DW, Lesser M, and Hellman S: Are prognostic factors for local control of breast cancer treated by primary radiotherapy significant for patients treated by mastectomy? Cancer 57:1415, 1986.
146. Rosen PP, Lesser ML, Kinne DW, and Beattie EJ: Breast carcinoma in women 35 years of age or younger, Ann Surg 199:133, 1984.
147. Rosen PP, Lesser ML, Kinne DW, and Beattie EJ: Discontinuous or "skip" metastasis in breast carcinoma, Ann Surg 197:276, 1983.
148. Ryoo ME, Kagan AR, Wollin M, et al: Prognostic factors for recurrence and cosmesis in 393 patients after radiation therapy for early mammary carcinoma, Radiology 172:555, 1989.
149. Sacre RA: Clinical evaluation of axillary lymph nodes compared to surgical and pathologic findings, Eur J Surg Oncol 12:169, 1986.
150. Sarrazin D, Dewar JA, Arriagada R, et al: Conservative management of breast cancer, Br J Surg 73:604, 1986.
151. Sarrazin D, Le MG, Fontaine MF, and Arriagada R: Conservative treatment versus mastectomy in T_1 or small T_2 breast cancer—a randomized clinical trial. In Harris J, Hellman S, and Silen W, editors: Conservative management of breast cancer, Philadelphia, 1983, JB Lippincott, pp 101-111.
152. Schell MC, Peksens R, Albright N, and Ling C: Dose to the opposite breast, Med Phys 13:599, 1986 (abstract).
153. Schmidt-Ullrich R, Wazer DE, Tercilla O, et al: Tumor margin assessment as a guide to optimal conservation surgery and irradiation in early stage breast cancer, Int J Radiat Oncol Biol Phys 17:733, 1989.

154. Schnitt SJ, Connolly JL, Harris JR, et al: Pathologic predictors of early local recurrence in Stage I and II breast cancer treated by primary radiation therapy, Cancer 53:1049, 1984.
155. Schnitt SJ, Connolly JL, Khettry U, et al: Pathologic findings on re-excision of the primary site in breast cancer patients considered for treatment by primary radiation therapy, Cancer 59:675, 1987.
156. Schnitt SJ, Connolly JL, Recht A, et al: Influence of infiltrating lobular histology on local tumor control in breast cancer patients treated with conservative surgery and radiotherapy, Cancer 64:448, 1989.
157. Schnitt SJ, Connolly JL, Silver B, et al: Updated results on the influence of pathologic features on treatment outcome in Stage I and II breast cancer patients treated by primary radiation therapy, Int J Radiol Oncol Biol Phys 11:104, 1985 (abstract).
158. Schottenfeld D, Nash AG, Robbins GF, and Beattie EJ: Ten-year results of the treatment of primary operable breast carcinoma, Cancer 38:1001, 1976.
159. Schwartz GF, D'ugo DM, and Rosenberg AL: Extent of axillary dissection preceding irradiation for carcinoma of the breast, Arch Surg 121:1395, 1986.
160. Schwartz GF, Rosenberg AL, Danoff BF, et al: Lumpectomy and level I axillary dissection prior to irradiation for "operable" breast cancer, Ann Surg 200:554, 1984.
161. Siddon RL, Buck BA, Harris JR, and Svensson GK: Three-field technique for breast irradiation using tangential field corner blocks, Int J Radiat Oncol Biol Phys 9:583, 1983.
162. Silverberg S and Chitale AR: Assessment of significance of porportions of intraductal and infiltrating tumor growth in ductal carcinoma of the breast, Cancer 32:830, 1973.
163. Singletary SE and McNeese M: Segmental mastectomy and irradiation in the treatment of breast cancer, Am J Clin Oncol 11:679, 1988.
164. Smart CR, Myers MH, and Gloecker LA: Implications from SEER data on breast cancer management, Cancer 41:787, 1978.
165. Smith JA, Gamez-Araujo J, Gallagher HS, et al: Carcinoma of the breast. Analysis of total lymph node involvement versus level of metastases, Cancer 39:527, 1977.
166. Solin LJ, Chu JCH, Larsen R, et al: Determination of depth for electron breast boosts, Int J Radiat Oncol Biol Phys 13:1915, 1987.
167. Solin LJ, Chu JCH, Sontag MR, et al: Three-dimensional photon treatment planning of the intact breast, Int J Radiat Oncol Biol Phys (in press).
168. Solin LJ, Danoff BF, Schwartz GF, et al: A practical technique for the localization of the tumor volume in definitive irradiation of the breast, Int J Radiat Oncol Biol Phys 11:1215, 1985.
169. Solin LJ, Fowble B, Martz KL, and Goodman RL: Definitive irradiation for early stage breast cancer: the University of Pennsylvania experience, Int J Radiat Oncol Biol Phys 14:235, 1988.
170. Solin LJ, Fowble B, Martz K, et al: Does residual tumor adversely impact on the outcome of patients undergoing definitive irradiation for early stage breast cancer? Int J Radiat Oncol Biol Phys 12:91, 1986 (abstract).
171. Solin LJ, Fowble B, Martz KL, et al: Results of reexcisional biopsy of the primary tumor in preparation for definitive irradiation of patients with early stage breast cancer, Int J Radiat Oncol Biol Phys 12:721, 1986.
172. Solin LJ, Fowble B, Miller-Wilson P, et al: A practical method of delivering the posterior axillary boost for the treatment of patients with breast cancer, Int J Radiat Oncol Biol Phys 12:2040, 1986.
173. Solin LJ, Fowble B, Schultz DJ, and Goodman RL: Age as a prognostic factor for patients treated with definitive irradiation for early stage breast cancer, Int J Radiat Oncol Biol Phys 16:373, 1989.
174. Solin LJ, Fowble B, Schultz DJ, and Goodman RL: Bilateral breast carcinoma treated with definitive radiation, Int J Radiat Oncol Biol Phys 17:263, 1989.
175. Spitalier JM, Gambarelli J, Brandone H, et al: Breast conserving surgery with radiation therapy for operable mammary carcinoma: a 25 year experience, World J Surg 10:1014, 1986.
176. Stotter AT, McNeese MD, Ames FC, et al: Predicting the rate and extent of locoregional failure after breast conservation therapy for early breast cancer, Cancer 64:2217, 1989.
177. Suehiro S, Inai K, Tokuoka S, et al: Involvement of the nipple in early carcinoma of the breast, Surg Gynecol Obstet 168:244, 1989.
178. Svensson GK, Chin LM, Siddon RL, and Harris JR: Breast treatment techniques at the Joint Center for Radiation Therapy. In Harris JR, Hellman S, and Silen W, editors: Conservative management of breast cancer, Philadelphia, 1983, JB Lippincott, pp 239-255.
179. Ten Haken RK, Lichter AS, and Fraass BA: The use of 10 MV photon beam for isocentric beam treatments: beam spoilers, bolus, and more, Med Phys 13:599, 1986 (abstract).
180. Triedman S, Boyages J, Silver B, et al: A comparison of local control and cosmetic outcome in patients boosted with electrons or implant in the conservative management of early breast cancer. Proceedings of the Seventeenth International Congress of Radiation Oncology, Paris, July, 1989, p 48 (abstract).
181. Van Limbergen E, Rijnders A, van der Schueren E, et al: Cosmetic evaluation of breast conserving treatment for mammary cancer. 2. A quantitative analysis of the influence of radiation dose, fractionation schedules and surgical treatment techniques on cosmetic results, Radiother Oncol 16:253, 1989.
182. Van Limbergen E, Van der Bogaert W, Van der Schueren E, and Rijnders A: Tumor excision and radiotherapy as primary treatment of breast cancer analysis of patient and treatment parameters and local control, Radiother Oncol 8:1, 1987.
183. Veronesi U: Breast conservation trials of the NCI-Milan. Proceedings of the NIH Consensus Development Conference on Early Stage Breast Cancer, June 1990, pp 19-22.
184. Veronesi U, Banfi A, DelVecchio M, et al: Comparison of Halsted mastectomy with quadrantectomy, axillary dissection and radiotherapy in early breast cancers: long-term results, Eur J Cancer Clin Oncol 22:1085, 1986.
185. Veronesi U, Cascinelli N, and Luini AL: The surgical treatment of curable breast cancer: the Milan experience. In Grundfest-Broniatowski S and Esselstyn CB, editors: Controversies in breast disease: diagnosis and management, New York, 1988, Marcel Dekker Inc, pp 307-318.
186. Veronesi U, DelVecchio M, and Greco M: Results of quadrantectomy, axillary dissection and radiotherapy (QUART) in T1 N0 patients. In Harris J, Hellman S, and Silen W, editors: Conservative management of breast cancer, Philadelphia, 1983, JB Lippincott, pp 91-99.
187. Veronesi U, Rilke F, Luini A, et al: Distribution of axillary node metastases by level of invasion, Cancer 59:682, 1987.
188. Veronesi U, Saccozzi R, DelVecchio M, et al: Comparing radical mastectomy with quadrantectomy, axillary dissection and radiotherapy in patients with small cancers of the breast, N Engl J Med 305:6, 1981.
189. Veronesi U and Valagussa P: Inefficacy of internal mammary nodes dissection in breast cancer surgery, Cancer 47:170, 1981.

190. Veronesi U, Zucali R, and DelVecchio M: Conservative treatment of breast cancer with the Q.U.A.R.T. technique, World J Surg 9:767, 1985.
191. Veronesi U, Zucali R, and Luini A: Local control and survival in early breast cancer: the Milan trial, Int J Radiat Oncol Biol Phys 12:717, 1986.
192. Vilcoq JR, Calle R, Stacey P, and Ghossein NA: The outcome of treatment by tumorectomy and radiotherapy of patients with operable breast cancer, Int J Radiat Oncol Biol Phys 7:1327, 1981.
193. Volterrani F, Veronesi U, Marubini E, et al: TART vs. QUART in the treatment of T1-2 (≤2.5 cm) N0 N1a,b M0 breast cancer. Proceedings of the Seventh Annual Meeting of the European Society for Therapeutic Radiology and Oncology, Den Haag, 1988, p 212.
194. Webb S, Leach MO, Bentley RE, et al: Clinical dosimetry for radiotherapy to the breast based on imaging with the prototype Royal Marsden Hospital CT simulator, Phys Med Biol 32:835, 1987.
195. Wertheim U and Ozzello L: Neoplastic involvement of nipple and skin flap in carcinoma of the breast, Am J Surg Pathol 4:543, 1980.
196. Wu A: Effects of an acrylic resin tray on relative surface doses for 10 MV X ray beams, Int J Radiat Oncol Biol Phys 6:1257, 1980.
197. Zafrani B, Vielh P, Fourquet A, et al: Conservative treatment of early breast cancer: prognostic value of ductal in situ component and other pathologic variables on local control and survival, Eur J Cancer Clin Oncol 25:1645, 1989.

6 Mammographic Evaluation of Patients Treated with Conservative Surgery and Radiation

Rosalind H. Troupin** and **Elizabeth A. Patterson

Mammography makes potentially significant contributions to the follow-up evaluation of patients treated by lumpectomy and radiation therapy. Its dual functions are to detect recurrent tumor at the lumpectomy site and to evaluate both breasts for new areas of suspicion. An appreciation of the major alterations that follow treatment is needed, because these changes may interfere with mammographic technique and interpretation in ways that can both mask and simulate recurrent disease.

The first part of this chapter describes and illustrates acceptable and suspicious posttreatment mammographic appearances; the second part focuses on a detailed analysis of a group of treated patients who required a subsequent biopsy.

DIFFUSE CHANGES

Skin thickening

Virtually all patients seen in our series and those described in the literature show skin thickening on their early posttreatment mammograms. In our experience this was observed and illustrated much more easily on broad-latitude xeromammograms, the modality used in the early years of the University of Pennsylvania study. In deliberately high contrast film mammography with good penetration, specific scrutiny of the skin may require "hot-light" illumination to show the thickening.

Skin thickening is generally not uniform and is invariably most intense in the treated quadrant. This is not unexpected in view of the surgical trauma and the local "boost dose" effects. Its severity is affected by other treatment modalities. Dershaw et al.[3] reported that severe skin thickening was present in 59% of treated patients who also had undergone axillary dissection, but in only 21% of patients who had not. The same study found an increase in the severity of skin thickening in those patients who also had been treated with chemotherapy. In addition, individual variations are quite striking in groups of identically treated patients.

The skin thickening evolves in a fairly predictable way, with gradual subsidence over the first 2 or 3 years and stabilization of changes after that time (Fig. 6-1). Again, considerable individual variation occurs and persistent thickening should not be regarded as evidence of residual or recurrent neoplasm. Nisce et al.,[7] reporting on skin changes following irradiation of advanced tumors, suggested that an initial diminution in skin thickness followed by a subsequent increase was suspicious for recurrence. In the instances in which we observed this phenomenon, there were other mammographic or clinical findings as well, negating any unique usefulness of this mammographic sign (Fig. 6-2).

Stromal edema and fibrosis

Fluid, inflammatory infiltrate, and progressive fibrosis are responsible for coarsening of the stromal trabecula and Cooper's ligaments, findings most easily visible in the subcutaneous fat (see Fig. 6-1, *B*). Again, these changes are most evident on early posttreatment mammograms and show variable rates of regression and ultimate stabilization. As part of the fibrosis pattern, some overall contraction of the breast occurs, often with an element of localized retraction at the lumpectomy site.

CHANGES IN THE LUMPECTOMY BED

The evolving scar

In the immediate postoperative period the lumpectomy bed is a pocket of serosanguineous fluid that gradually clots, organizes, and contracts over a period of months. This is particularly true in the Fisher[4] surgical lumpectomy technique in which, in an attempt to minimize cosmetic contour loss, the deep tissues are not approximated or drained, and only the skin is sutured. The report by Mendelson[6] described an imaging follow-up protocol wherein the evolving fluid collection was followed closely by ultrasound as well as by mam-

A

B

C

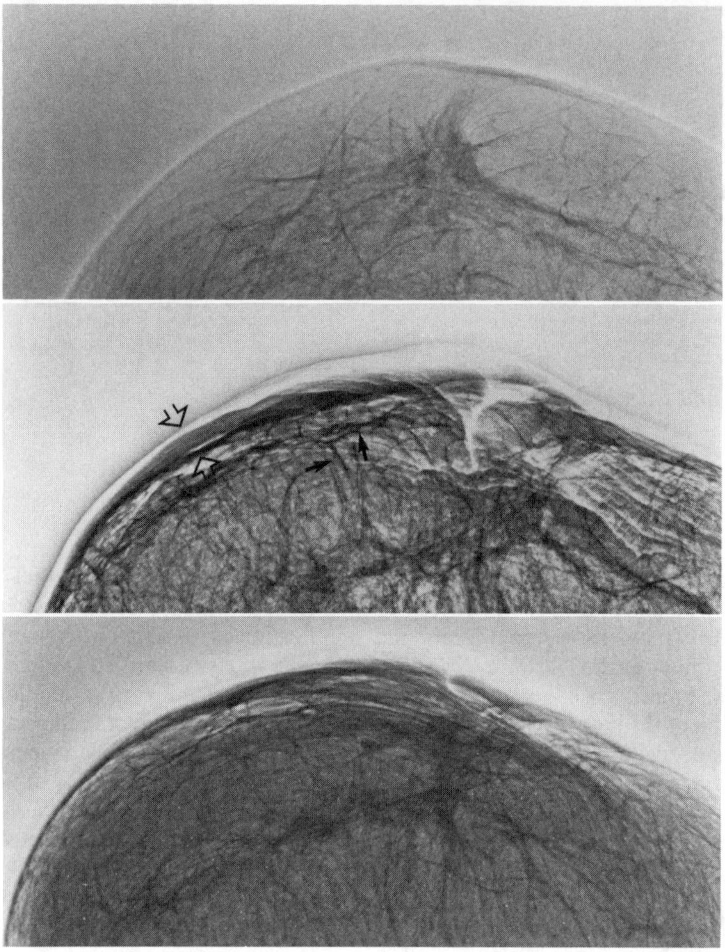

Fig. 6-1 Skin thickening and stromal fibrosis following lumpectomy and irradiation. **A**, Pretreatment; **B**, 1 year after treatment; and **C**, 4 years after treatment. Note in **B** and **C** the development and partial subsidence of skin thickening (*open arrows*) and trabecular coarsening (*solid arrows*).

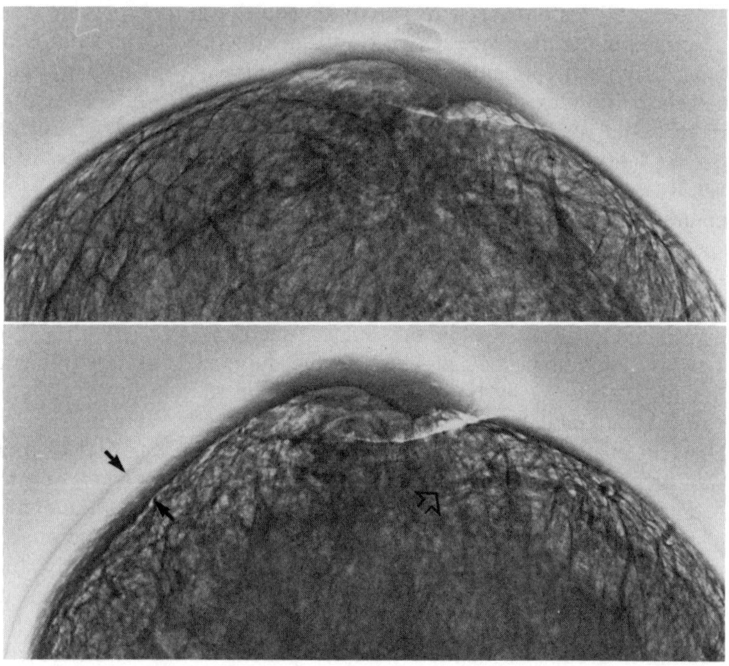

A

B

Fig. 6-2 Progressive skin thickening in patient with diffuse recurrence seen 12 **(A)** and 18 months **(B)** after treatment. In **B** thickened skin (*arrows*) was accompanied by diffuse parenchymal density, focal calcification (*open arrow*), and palpable induration.

mography. Sonographically, 50% of those collections remained cystic at 6 months and 20% were unresolved at 9 months. As expected, sonographic resolution of the hematoma was characterized by increasingly irregular margins and fibrosis-induced acoustic shadowing. The scars were ultimately indistinguishable from solid, irregular lesions; this informative basic research protocol is not a recommended follow-up method for detecting residual or recurrent neoplasm.

Initial mammography 6 to 12 months following lumpectomy and irradiation shows an excision site that varies from an unremarkable focus of linear distortion to an alarmingly stellate, slightly nodular density (Fig. 6-3, *A*). Surgical closure technique, breast parenchymal background, reaction to irradiation, and individual variation all contribute to the wide spectrum of appearances. In the absence of clinically worrisome features or mammographically suspect calcifications, mammography of an irregularly stellate focus seen on first examination should be repeated in 6 months to be certain that resolution, in the form of evolving contraction, is occurring. If this second examination suggests increasing nodularity, biopsy is advised. If the appearance is stable, another 6-month interval is in-

A

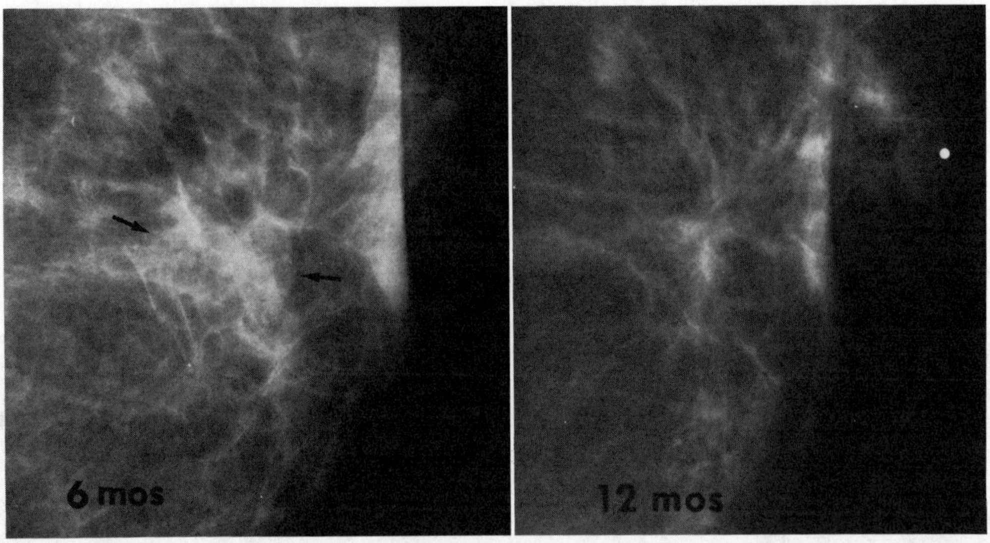

B

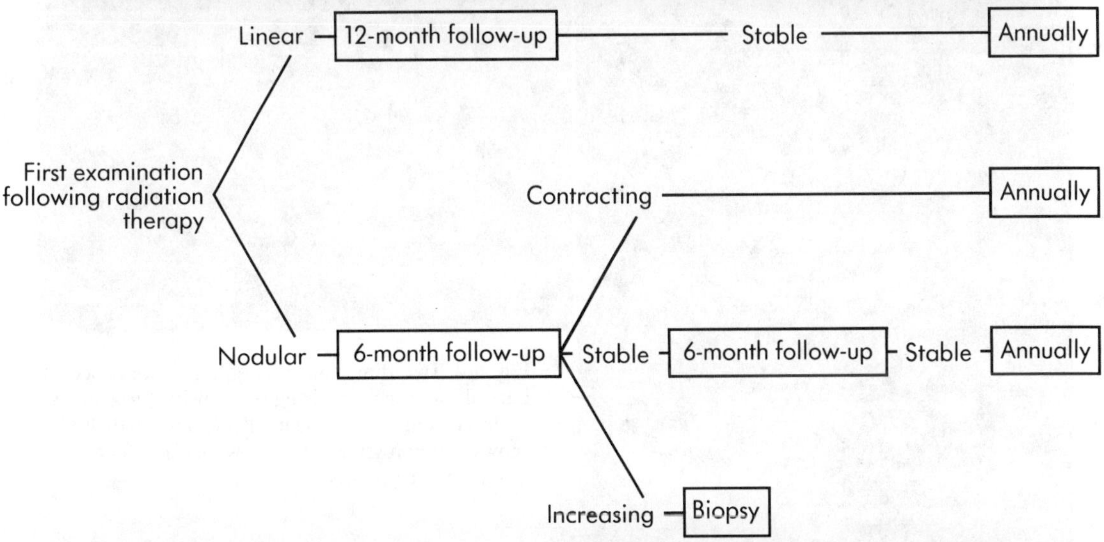

C

Fig. 6-3 Contracting scar following lumpectomy and irradiation seen 6 (**A**) and 12 months (**B**) after treatment. In **A** note irregular density (*arrows*) deep to distorted skin, with later image (**B**) showing a scar with less bulk and more stellate contraction. **C**, Algorithm for mammographic follow-up of a surgical scar.

dicated, and if it definitely is contracting (Fig. 6-3, *B*), the next follow-up interval can be lengthened to 12 months (Fig. 6-3, *C*).

While the only completely reassuring scenario is one in which a sequence of mammograms documents evolving contraction of the lumpectomy bed, decisions required at any given point early in the sequence are often very difficult. There are some guidelines and criteria that are helpful. A reasonably reliable feature of a benign scar is its tendency toward two-dimensionality. While very troubling in its stellate or slightly nodular appearance on one view, the right-angle projection often shows a more amorphous or wispy configuration (Fig. 6-4). Another reassuring feature is the presence of central radiolucency within the stellate focus characteristic of a lipid cyst[1] associated with fat necrosis (Fig. 6-5, *A* and *B*). If three-dimensional irregular nodularity is documented, biopsy rather than follow-up is recommended. Fig. 6-6 shows an example 1 year after lumpectomy; however, biopsy showed a persistent, organized hematoma. In a second instance of a false-positive mammogram, a nonpalpable smooth nodule that became visible 15 months after treatment was shown to be solid on ultrasound; on biopsy it was found to be a fibroadenoma (Fig. 6-7). A nodule with a similar appearance, developing between years 4 and 5 in another patient, however, was malignant (Fig. 6-8).

Developing calcifications

As discussed and illustrated in Chapter 2, calcifications are commonly the central issue in mammographic interpretation. In the other ipsilateral and contralateral quadrants of the patient who has undergone lumpectomy and irradiation, criteria for biopsy are the same as described previously. The thresholds must recognize both the high risk associated with this group of patients, and the realities of overlapping benign and malignant appearances, inevitably resulting in some level of false-positive calls. There is little information in the literature that specifically assesses the positive predictive yields for calcifications biopsied outside of the lumpectomy site in these patients. A previous publication from our group by Solin et al.[11] combined experiences from the University of Pennsylvania and Fox Chase Cancer Center in postlumpectomy patients undergoing biopsy based solely on detection of new calcifications. In 5 of the 19 patients, the calcifications were in a quadrant differ-

A

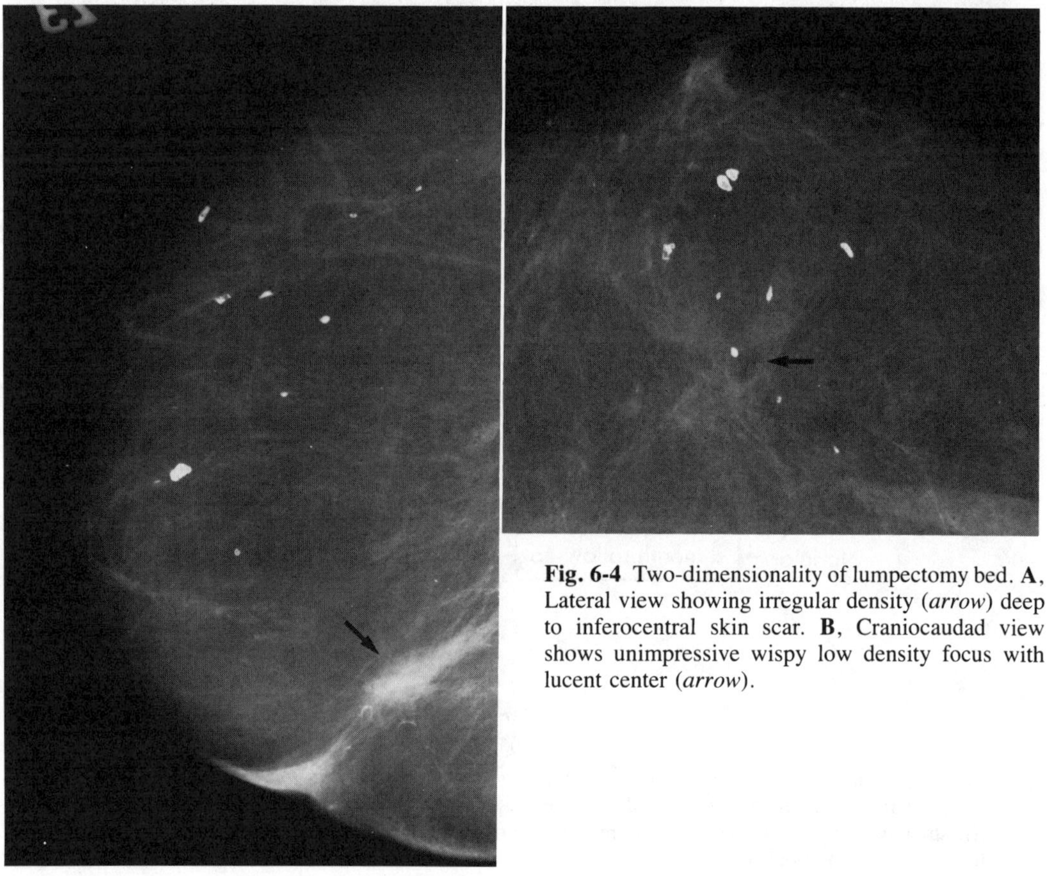

B

Fig. 6-4 Two-dimensionality of lumpectomy bed. **A**, Lateral view showing irregular density (*arrow*) deep to inferocentral skin scar. **B**, Craniocaudad view shows unimpressive wispy low density focus with lucent center (*arrow*).

A

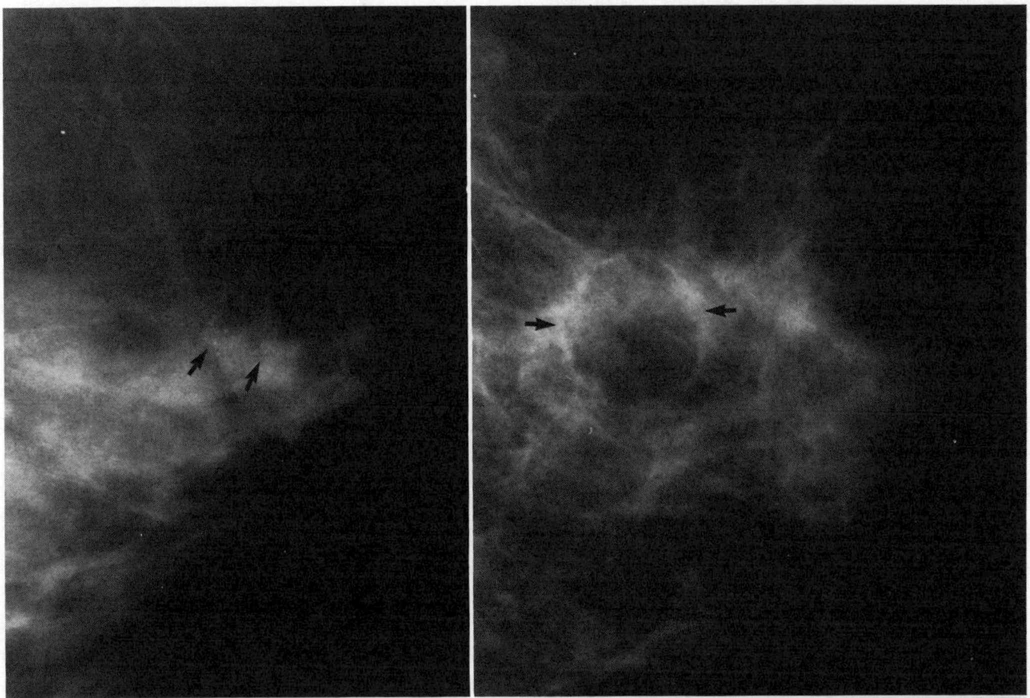

B

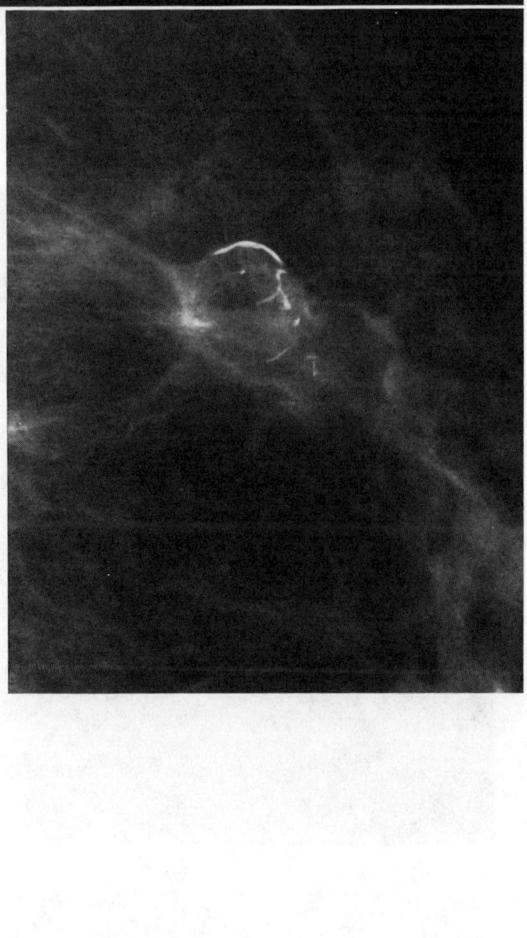

C

Fig. 6-5 Fat necrosis with lipid cyst. **A**, Preoperative focus of malignant calcification (*arrows*). **B**, Six months after treatment. Note lucent lipid cyst (*arrows*). **C**, Three years after treatment. Wall of lipid cyst shows benign calcific rim.

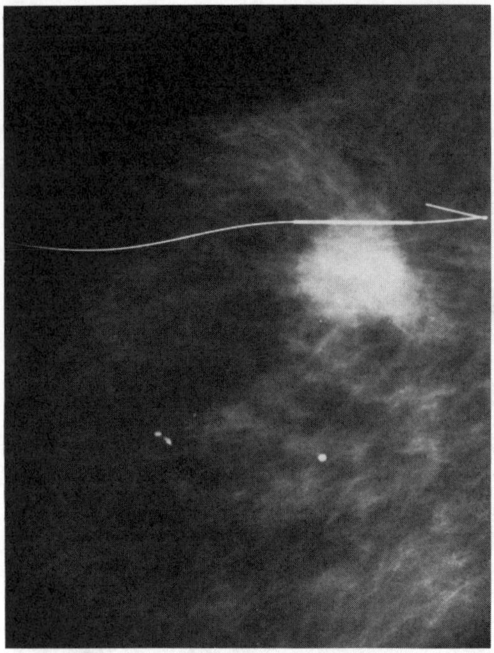

Fig. 6-6 Persistent nodule with irregular edges 1 year after treatment. It was not palpable and aspiration attempt under mammographic control yielded only a few drops of bloody fluid. Lesion was localized and excised. Diagnosis was organized hematoma.

ent from the initial tumor. Four of those five biopsies were positive for carcinoma.

Within the lumpectomized quadrant, traumatized by surgery and higher levels of radiation, analysis of calcifications is complicated by the frequent development of benign, dystrophic calcium deposits. Published series[3,5] report an approximately 25% incidence of benign calcifications developing during the follow-up of these patients. This contrasts strikingly with the 3% to 4% frequency of calcifications reported by Sickles[10] in 1049 biopsy sites to which radiation therapy had not been administered. After lumpectomy and irradiation, benign calcifications arise within areas of fat necrosis and stromal fibrosis. When allowed to develop fully, these benign calcifications tend to evolve toward coarse, so-called macrocalcifications. Curvilinear morphology generally correlates with mural calcification in the wall of a lipid cyst (see Figs. 6-5, *C*, and 6-15). Streaks, plaques, chunks, and smooth, round concretions are also characteristic of benign calcification (see Fig. 6-4). Occasionally, suture material also calcifies (Fig. 6-9).[2] Unfortunately, calcifications that are destined to become coarse start microscopically and evolve mammographically from invisible through barely discernible "microcalcifications," at which point they may be misinterpreted as malignant (Fig. 6-10).

Returning to the previously mentioned report by Solin et al.,[11] suspicious calcifications developed in the lumpectomized quadrant in 14 of the 19 biopsied cases; of those, 7 were malignant. It should be reemphasized that this group of 19 cases,

A

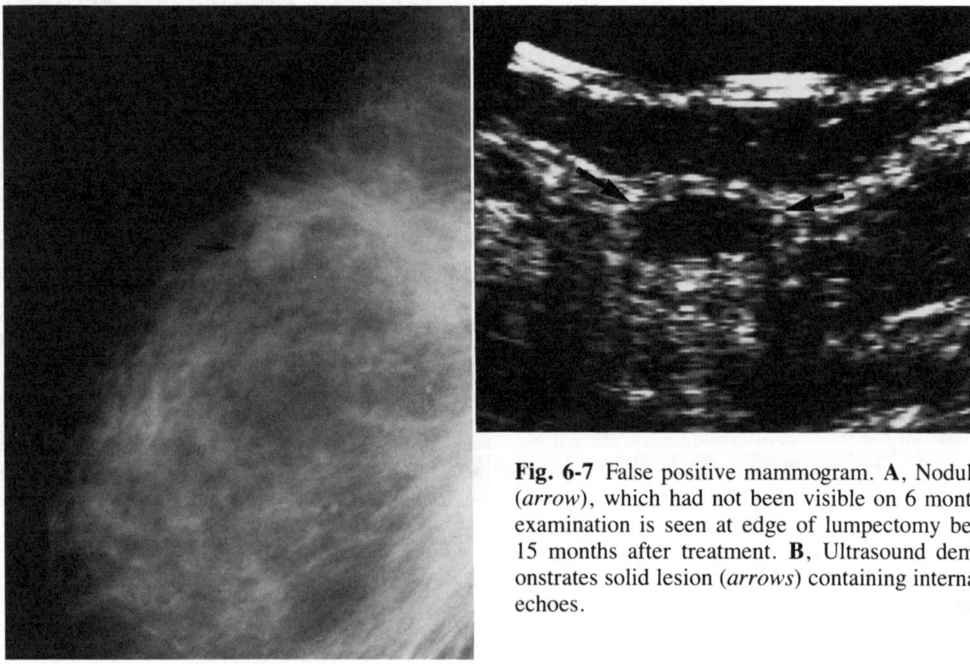

B

Fig. 6-7 False positive mammogram. **A**, Nodule (*arrow*), which had not been visible on 6 month examination is seen at edge of lumpectomy bed 15 months after treatment. **B**, Ultrasound demonstrates solid lesion (*arrows*) containing internal echoes.

A

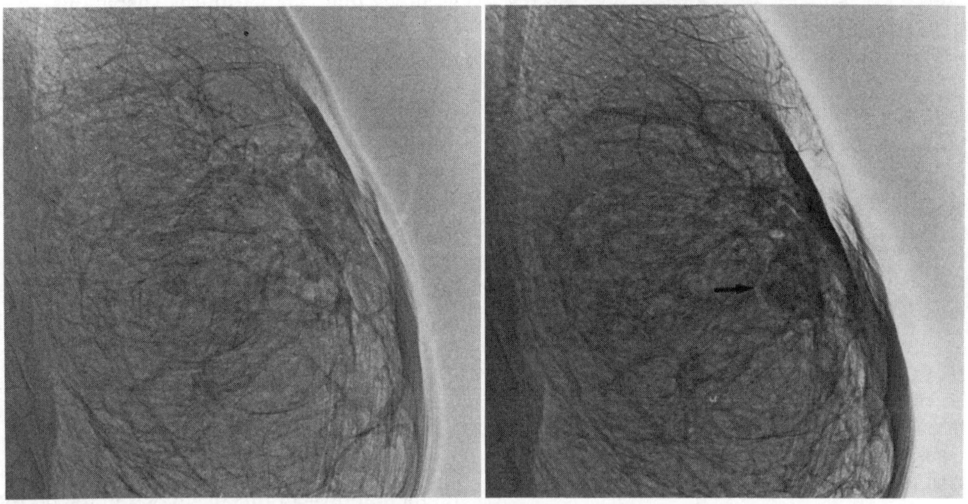

B

Fig. 6-8 True-positive mammogram. **A**, Lumpectomy site 4 years after treatment. **B**, One year later, nonpalpable nodule (*arrow*) has developed.

A

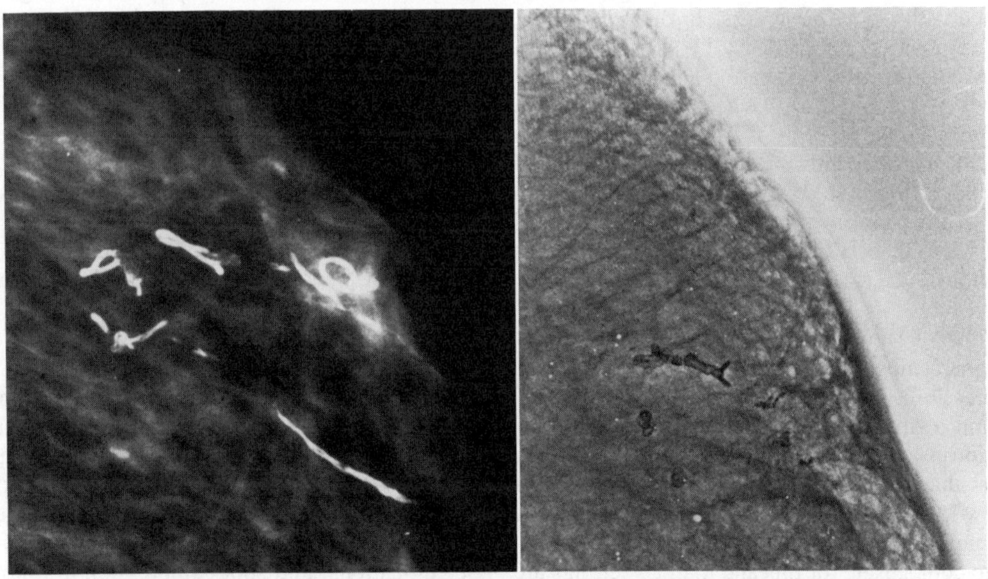

B

Fig. 6-9 Calcification of surgical sutures in two patients. **A**, Appearance using film-screen mammography. **B**, Second patient shown by xeromammography.

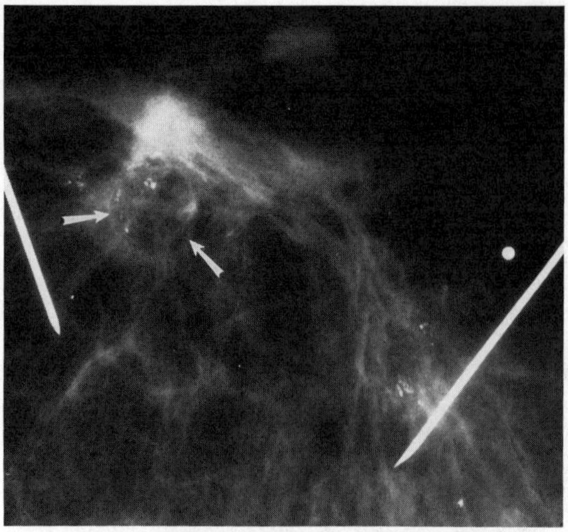

Fig. 6-10 False-positive mammogram for atypical calcifications of fat necrosis 2 years after treatment. Although lucency of a lipid cyst (*arrows*) indicated that fat necrosis was present, the associated calcifications were too atypical to justify follow-up without biopsy.

in which mammographic criteria were sufficiently suspicious to mandate biopsy, is a very small subset of posttreatment calcifications. Recurrences diagnosed on the basis of microcalcifications tend to be at an early stage, amenable to salvage, and associated with a good prognosis. In those 19 cases, 11 were positive and 7 of the 11 showed only in situ or microinvasive disease. This parallels the findings of Schnitt et al.,[9] who reported six cases of recurrence detected by microcalcifications that were all predominantly or exclusively intraductal carcinoma. In one study by Stomper et al.,[12] there were seven instances of noninvasive cancer, six of which were detected as mammographic microcalcifications.

SPECIAL IMAGING PROBLEMS

Skin thickening, stromal fibrosis, and decreased compressibility of the treated breast result in degradation of mammographic images. The breast is both intrinsically denser and artifactually thicker, factors that interfere with adequate penetration at the low kilovoltages needed to offer good contrast. In some instances the automatic phototimer is unable to compensate for this and manual settings are needed (Fig. 6-11). A technologist who is experienced in the special problems of this clinical group can sometimes, but not always, anticipate this difficulty, based on visual inspection and breast compressibility, thereby altering technique appropriately.[13] If there has been a previous posttreatment mammogram, reference obviously can be made to the technique recorded at that time. If not, a single test film should be taken, guiding technique selection for the other views. Doing the entire examination and then repeating a complete, corrected sequence causes anxiety in a patient who wrongly assumes that "something is suspicious."

A second technical problem occurs when xeromammography is used in a patient whose lumpectomy bed was marked by metallic surgical clips. In routine positive mode xerography, a halo caused by "powder depletion" artifact results in image loss adjacent to the dense metallic clips (Fig. 6-12). This can be prevented by reversing to negative mode or by using film mammography.

The final and major technical problem in posttreatment mammography is ensuring that the lumpectomy bed and the rest of the breast are imaged completely. Some of the original lesions were deep, or located far laterally and/or superiorly. With an element of posttreatment retraction and decreased overall pliability, coverage becomes even more difficult. The armamentarium of supplemental projections discussed in the pretreatment mammography chapter is even more valuable at this point. Our posttreatment examination routinely includes three views of each breast including the true mediolateral as well as the oblique mediolateral and cephalocaudad (CC) projections. In addition, technologists are instructed to be certain that the scar is included completely on the images, even if creative supplementary positioning is needed. Because such a large proportion of breast cancers occur in the outer quadrants, the most common supplemental view is the internally rotated CC projection, in which the patient and breast are rotated medially to emphasize coverage of the lateral quadrants (Fig. 6-13). This supplements, and is not a substitute for, the standard CC view, which is still needed for imaging of the medial half of the breast. Again, by including the extra view with the basic projections, the patient is not alarmed by being recalled into the mammography room after the radiologist has studied the films.

It is important to have the previous examinations and reports available at the time of the mammogram, so that tailored problem-solving of specific follow-up issues can be incorporated promptly into the filming sequence. Common examples of this include magnification for high-detail follow-up of calcifications, and spot compression to follow soft tissue density or distortion in the lumpectomy bed (Fig. 6-14). The old films are also critically important in interpreting the stability of findings (Fig. 6-15). Comparison judgments must take into account technical differences, including tissue contrast differences in xerography and film screen technique (Fig. 6-16).

A 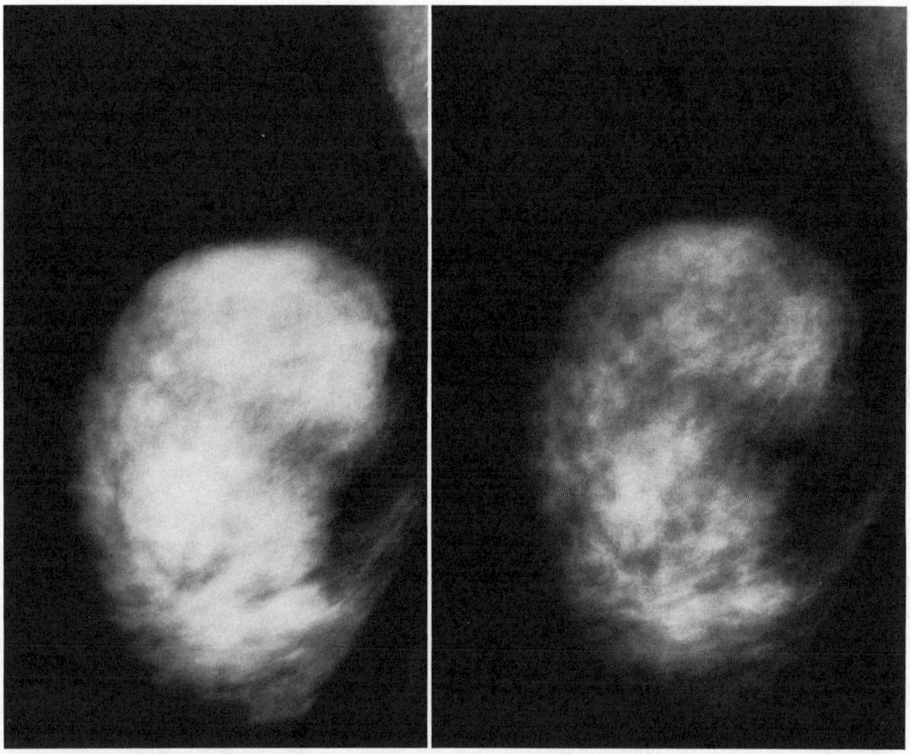 B

Fig. 6-11 Use of manual exposure factors when photo-timed automatic exposure fails. Very dense fibroglandular breast before treatment became even more impenetrable after lumpectomy and irradiation. **A**, Photo-timed exposure with regular molybdenum filtration using a modern General Electric CGR mammography unit. Penetration was insufficient to allow detection or exclusion of calcifications. **B**, Manual selection exposure at 120 mA and 36 kV using aluminum filtration. While soft tissue masses would be invisible against this fat-free background, calcification would be detectable.

A 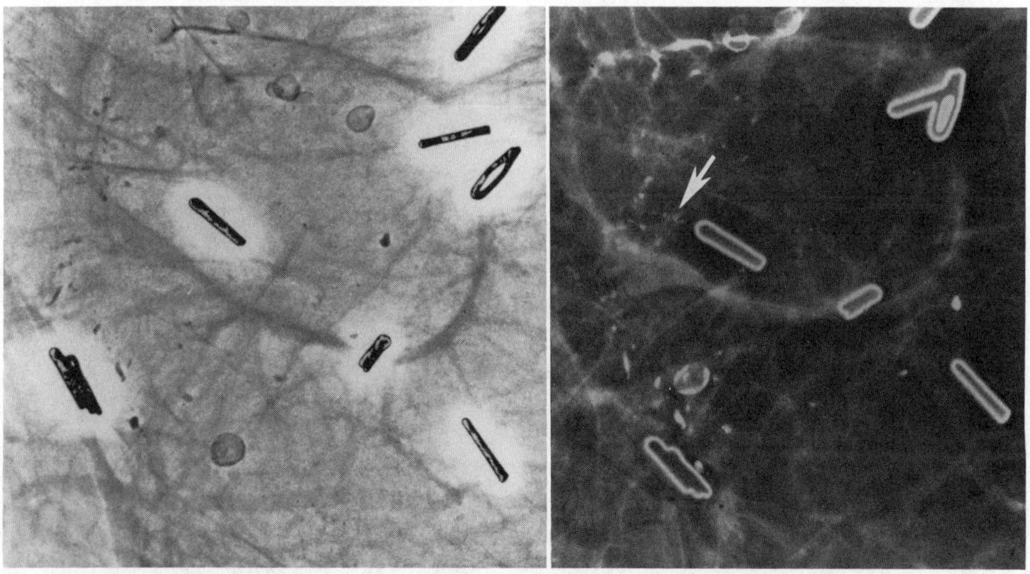 B

Fig. 6-12 "Powder depletion" artifact. In the electrostatic imaging of xeromammography, charged powder particles are attracted to very high density images such as metal clips, leaving a surrounding halo with no image. **A**, Positive mode xeromammogram showing halo around clips in treated patient with calcification. **B**, Polarity reversed to negative mode removing the halos, and showing additional calcifications (*arrow*). While this additional calcium was not decisive in this case, it could have been, had it been the only calcium.

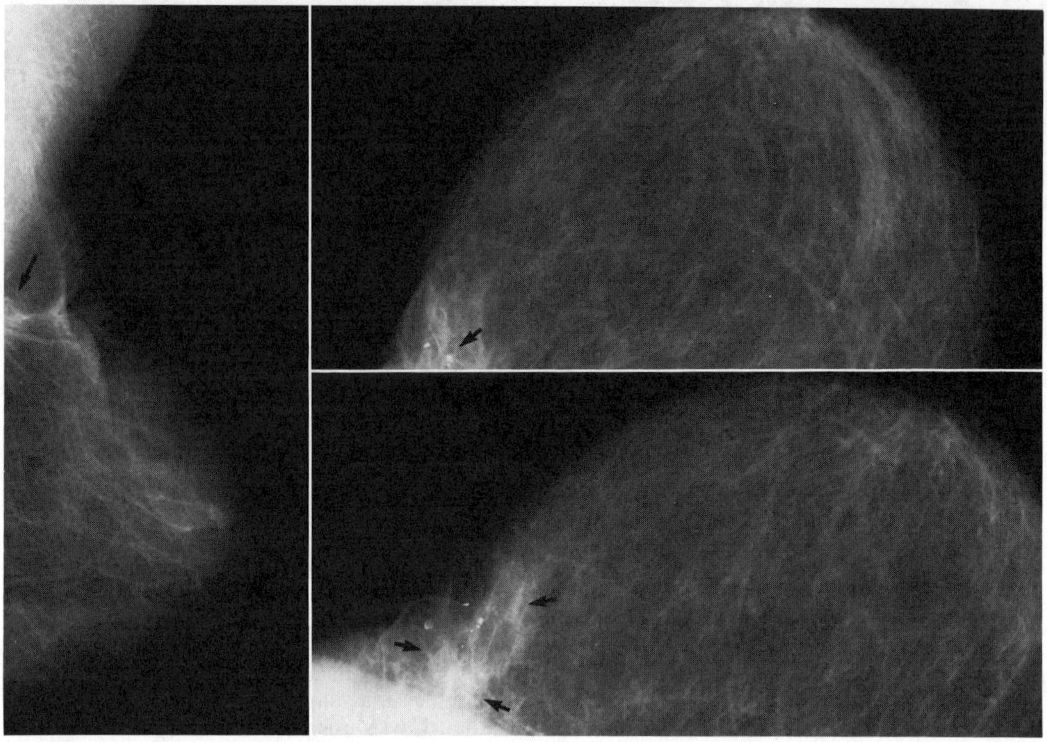

A B C

Fig. 6-13 Internally rotated craniocaudad (CC) view for lateral quadrant imaging. **A**, Oblique mediolateral view after lumpectomy and irradiation upper outer quadrant. Note focal retraction and incomplete visualization of lumpectomy bed (*arrow*). **B**, Regular CC view showing benign coarse calcification (*arrow*). **C**, Internally rotated CC view bringing remainder of benign calcium and scar into view. Oblique density is soft tissue fold.

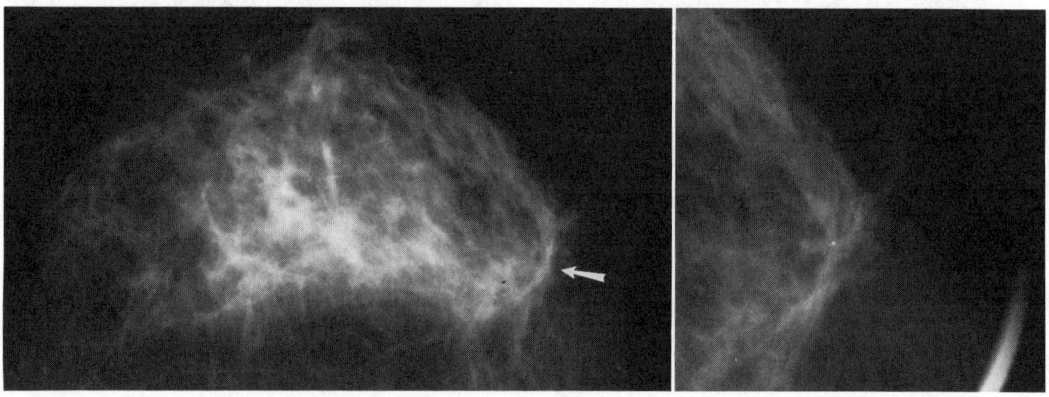

A B

Fig. 6-14 Spot compression and magnification of posttreatment scar. **A**, Craniocaudad view showing stellate retraction at lumpectomy site laterally (*arrow*). **B**, Focal compression and magnification show unremarkable linear stranding and a single benign calcific particle.

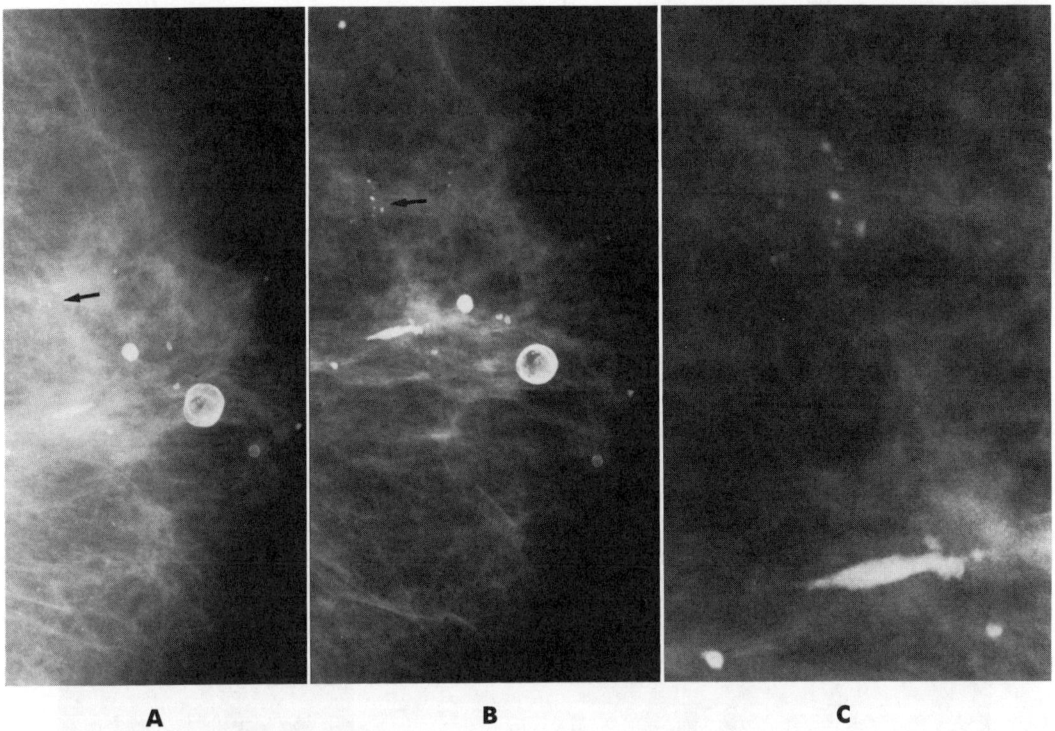

Fig. 6-15 Late follow-up films showing development of malignant calcifications. **A**, Seven years after treatment there are multiple benign, coarse calcifications in addition to three nonspecific flecks (*arrow*) that had not changed. **B**, One year later additional particles have developed in that area (*arrow*). **C**, Magnification of cluster shows their ambiguous morphology; however, they were biopsied because of their increasing number, and were found to be intraductal carcinoma.

MAMMOGRAPHIC ANALYSIS OF 58 PATIENTS REQUIRING SUBSEQUENT IPSILATERAL BIOPSY

Over 1500 breast cancer patients were evaluated and treated at the University of Pennsylvania by lumpectomy and irradiation between 1977 and 1989, 102 of whom required subsequent biopsy on the ipsilateral, treated side. We chose this group for a detailed analysis of the specific contributions, limitations, and diagnostic criteria of follow-up mammography. Because of the nature of our cancer center and its patient population, some of the follow-up mammograms were either performed at, or subsequently loaned out to, other cooperating hospitals. There were 58 patients in whom there were two mammographic examinations available for our review, one of which was performed within 3 months of the subsequent biopsy. In order to be certain that these 58 were representative of the total 102 and not an artifactually skewed subset, the relative numbers of positive biopsies in these groups were ascertained (Table 6-1). Positive biopsies were obtained in 69% of the total group and 65% of the group with films available for analysis.

Overall clinical and mammographic accuracy

Next examined were the relative, overall contributions of the clinical and mammographic examinations (Tables 6-2 and 6-3). The original mammographic interpretations were utilized in this and all subsequent analyses. In the 38 cases with positive biopsies, 34% were seen by mammography alone, with 45% detected on physical examination alone and the remainder evident by both modalities (see Table 6-2). Sixty percent of the benign biopsies were initiated by the physical findings, 30% by mammography, and 10% by both modalities. Combining the figures to encompass those cases in which both modalities were suspicious, a positive mammographic reading was correct 72% of the time, and a suspicious physical examination was confirmed by a positive biopsy in 64% of the instances (see Table 6-3). Significantly, in only 8 of the 38 positive biopsies did the two methods over-

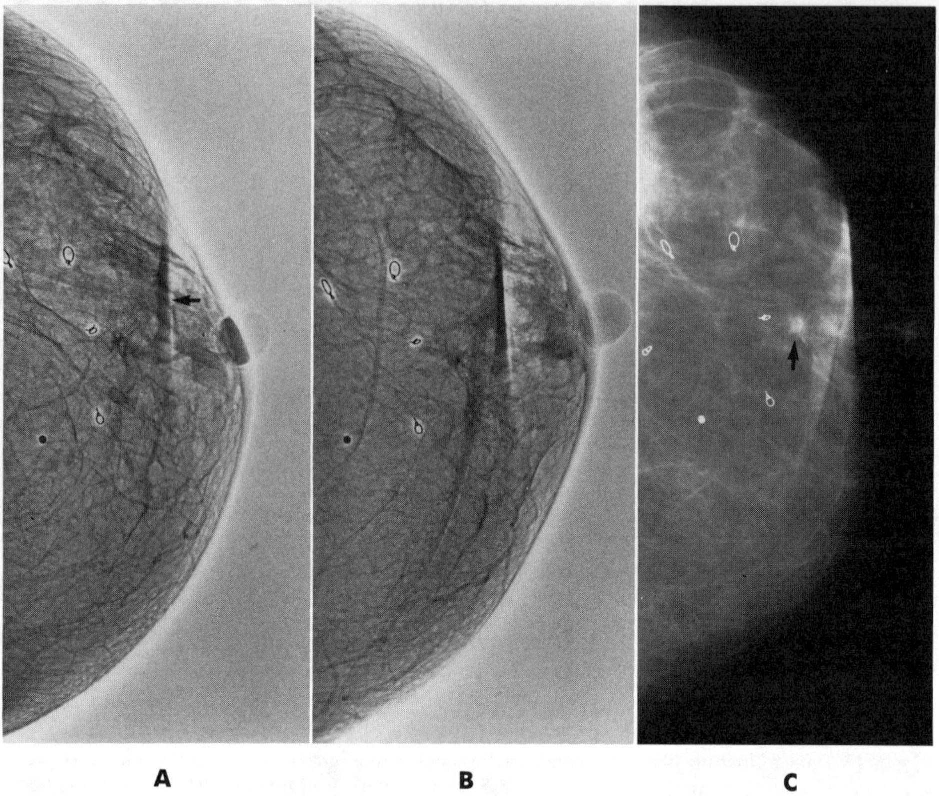

Fig. 6-16 Follow-up sequence with interval change from xeromammography to film screen mammography. **A**, Two years after lumpectomy and irradiation with bed marked by metal sutures. Note localized skin retraction (*arrow*). **B**, Four years after treatment, less contour deformity and deeper imaging coverage. **C**, Six years after treatment, film mammogram. Coverage now includes a deeper posterior suture and some posterior muscle. Tiny, stellate density anteriorly (*arrow*) is made prominently visible by high-contrast technique but is actually stable.

lap, indicating uniquely complementary roles for mammography and physical examination.

Comparison of these results to the 1987 study by Stomper et al.[12] from the Joint Center for Radiation Therapy in Boston shows some significant parallels and interesting differences. Their patient numbers were smaller (only 45 cases biopsied for suspected recurrence in the irradiated breast). Overall, cancer was found in 23 of 45 (51%) of the Boston patients and 38 of 58 (65%) of the University of Pennsylvania patients. Comparison initially focused on the positive predictive values (PPVs), defined as the percentage yield of positive biopsies resulting from a positive diagnostic finding. Biopsy PPVs for suspicious mammography (with or without clinical findings) was 72% in the University of Pennsylvania series and 61% for the Boston study group. Biopsy performed for suspicious clinical findings (with or without suspicious mammography) proved positive in 64% of our patients and 47% of the Boston group. Of note is that at each institution the mammographic and clinical thresholds were quite parallel, reflecting an appropriate compatibility of operational philosophies. As a result, the relative proportion of cancers detected by mammography alone might be expected to be similar at each institution. By a statistical coincidence it was identical: 8 of 23 (34.8%) in Boston and 13 of 38 (34.2%) at the University of Pennsylvania.

Selecting a threshold for biopsy involves weighing the risks of delayed detection against the negative physical and emotional consequences of a second biopsy for what proves to be benign disease. As criteria for biopsy are broadened, sensitivity improves, but PPVs must fall. This may be reflected in comparison of the mammographic results in these two study groups: sensitivities of 55% and 61% vs. PPVs of 72% and 61%, for the University of Pennsylvania and the Joint Center, respectively.

Table 6-1 Proportion of positive biopsies in total vs. analyzed groups

Biopsy results	No. all cases	No. analyzed cases
Malignant	71 [69]	38 [65]
Benign	31	20
TOTAL	102	58

[ ], percentage of cases.

Table 6-2 Relative contributions of mammography and palpation to detection of 38 cancers

Suspicious finding	No. malignant biopsies	No. benign biopsies
Mammogram only	13 [34.2]	6 [30.0]
Palpation only	17 [44.7]	12 [60.0]
Both	8 [21.1]	2 [10.0]
TOTAL	38 [100]	20 [100]

[ ], percentage of biopsies.

Table 6-3 Fifty-eight patients biopsied for suspicious findings: predictive values for mammography, palpation, and combined findings

Results	Findings on mammography only	Findings on palpation only	Findings on both	Mammography and both	Palpation and both
Malignant	13 [68.4]	17 [58.6]	8 [80]	21 [72.4]	25 [64.1]
Benign	6	12	2	8	14
TOTAL	19	29	10	29	39

[ ], percentage of total.

In selected cases, close clinical correlation and the liberal use of short-term mammographic follow-up can support the decision to defer biopsy in the presence of very low probability findings.

Accuracy related to quadrant

The analysis then investigated whether mammographic and clinical detection capabilities were altered within, and outside of, the lumpectomized quadrant. Of the 38 cancers detected in the 58 patients that underwent ipsilateral biopsy, 21 were clearly within the lumpectomized quadrant, the other 17 being distributed elsewhere in that breast. Within the lumpectomized quadrant, physical examination had substantially better sensitivity than mammography (Table 6-4). Operating at similar predictive values, palpation detected 71% of the 21 cancers, while mammography detected only 43%. These numbers total more than 100% because there were lesions detected with both modalities.

Detection sensitivities for the 17 cancers in the nonlumpectomized quadrants showed a very different pattern (Table 6-5). Of 14 cases called positive by mammography, 12 were positive for cancer on biopsy, for a PPV of 86% and a sensitivity of 71%. Ten of the 16 cases called positive on physical examination proved to be cancerous, for a PPV of 62% and sensitivity of 59%.

False negatives on physical examination did not appear to be affected by location. On palpation 13 cancers were missed—six within and seven outside of the lumpectomy quadrant—that were detected solely by mammography. Five of the seven were detected mammographically by calcium alone; two had associated nonpalpable mass (Fig. 6-17). Mammographic sensitivity was affected significantly by location. Twelve of the 17 cancers detected by palpation and missed by mammography were in the lumpectomy quadrant. None of these contained calcifications, emphasizing the poor detectability of soft tissue lesions in a dense or architecturally distorted background.

Analyzing the false positives displayed in Tables 6-4 and 6-5, physical examination performed uniformly in all quadrants; 35% and 37% false positive rates respectively within and outside of the lumpectomy quadrant. Contary to what might have been expected, the lumpectomy bed firmness and distortion did not result in any concentration of false positives by the clinical examiners. In contrast, mammographic false-positive rates were significantly influenced by location. Outside of the lumpectomy quadrant there was only a 14% overcall rate while within the treated quadrant the 40% mammographic false-positive rate was similar to the 35% clinical one. These mammographic in-

Table 6-4 Accuracy of mammography and palpation in the detection of 21 cancers within lumpectomy quadrant

Results	Mammography	Palpation
Cases called positive*	15	23
True positives	9	15
False positives	6 [40]	8 [34.8]
Sensitivity	9/21 [42.8]	15/21 [71.4]
Positive predictive value	9/15 [60]	15/23 [65.2]

[ ], percentage of cases.
*In three cases mammography and palpation agreed, therefore these are listed in both categories.

Table 6-5 Accuracy of mammography and palpation in the detection of 17 cancers outside lumpectomy quadrant

Results	Mammography	Palpation
Cases called positive*	14	16
True positives	12	10
False positives	2 [14]	6 [37.5]
Sensitivity	12/17 [70.6]	10/17 [58.8]
Positive predictive value	12/14 [85.7]	10/16 [62.5]

[ ], percentage of cases.
*In five cases mammography and palpation agreed, therefore these are listed in both columns.

quadrant overcalls comprise six cases, four of which were based on misinterpreted calcifications, showing our difficulty in confidently assigning a benign designation to certain developing calcifications (Fig. 6-18). A fifth in-quadrant overcall was the small fibroadenoma (see Fig. 6-7), detected 15 months after treatment when unmasked by the subsidence of surrounding treatment reaction. The sixth false positive in the lumpectomy quadrant proved to be a fibrotic density, visible and palpable 7 years following treatment. Interestingly, this error occurred during the University of Pennsylvania changeover from xeromammography to high contrast film mammography, a difficult year for documentation of scar stability.

Accuracy related to time elapsed

We began with an anecdotal hypothesis that follow-up mammographic cancer detection in the lumpectomy quadrant might be more impaired by reactive density early, but would improve after stabilization. As a dividing point, 2 years was arbitrarily selected; of the 21 recurrent malignancies in the treated quadrant five were diagnosed before, and 16 after, that point. Mammographic detection rates were no different (40% and 44% respectively) in the early and late follow-up groups. Selecting a different "stabilization point" at 3 years did not result in greater sensitivity. Parallel analysis of clinical accuracy in our early and late study groups similarly failed to show a trend toward improvement.

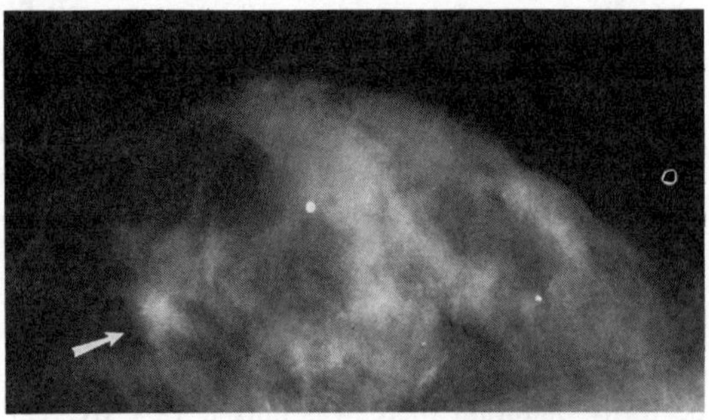

Fig. 6-17 Nonpalpable malignant stellate nodule (*arrow*) in medial breast, 4 years after lumpectomy and irradiation of the upper outer quadrant.

Accuracy related to background breast density

Another intuitive hypothesis that we investigated was the belief that in fatty breasts, mammography should be highly dependable. Indeed, in all five instances in which false positive benign biopsies were initiated by palpation in mammographically fatty breasts, mammography had been read as negative. All mammographers employ a working rule that a negative mammogram should never dissuade biopsy of a clinically suspicious focus. In a given case however, a very low level of clinical suspicion, coupled with a mammographically fatty background, might support consideration of a close-interval follow-up rather than biopsy. Judgment to defer biopsy in such an instance requires the close consultation of experienced radiologists and radiation oncologists, as well as an informed, reliable, patient. It cannot be overemphasized that in our study group there were three mammographic false negatives in fatty breasts, biopsied because of a significant clinical suspicion. In two, subtle induration and/or nodularity in the scar was palpable but mammographically invisible. In the third the pathologist found a microscopic focus of carcinoma adjacent to fat necrosis, the latter presumably responsible for the palpable firmness.

A 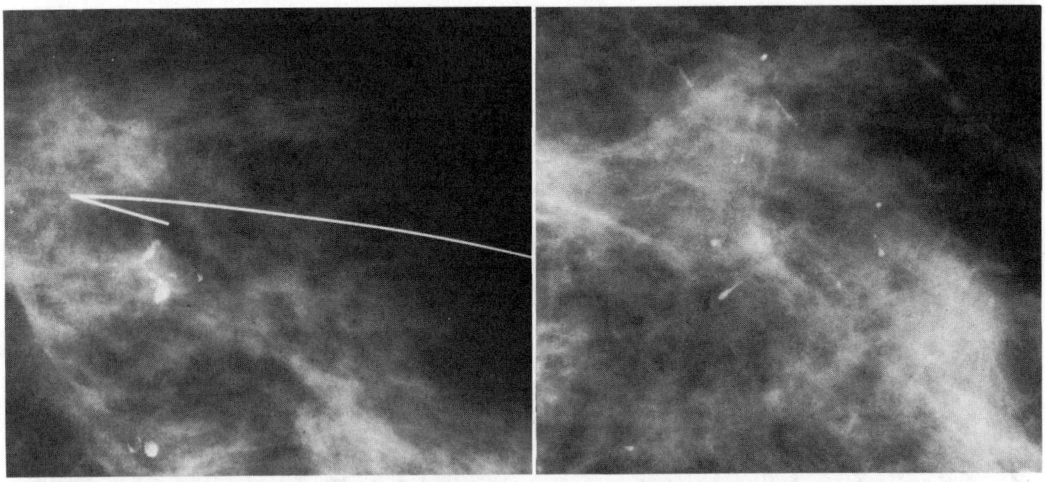 B

Fig. 6-18 False positive based on indeterminate calcifications. **A**, Bizarre calcification in screening mammogram prompted biopsy that showed carcinoma. **B**, One year after lumpectomy and irradiation atypical linear calcifications are present. Biopsy showed posttreatment changes, no malignancy.

Mammographic criteria for biopsy

Our study group included 29 patients in whom mammography was suspicious and biopsy was recommended. Table 6-6 lists the mammographic findings, the number of patients with each finding, and the biopsy results. We have combined our tabulation with the parallel data from the Boston study by Stomper et al.[12] Again, overall yields show some differences; 21 of 29 mammographically suspicious University of Pennsylvania cases had positive biopsies, for a PPV of 72%. Fourteen of 23 Boston cases were positive, for a PPV of 61%. There were identical predictive values for the lesions containing calcium, 16 of 21 University of Pennsylvania cases (76.2%) and 10 of 13 Boston cases (76.9%) showing malignancy. There was an apparent difference in uncalcified abnormalities, positive biopsies in 5 of 8 University of Pennsylvania (62.5%) and 4 of 10 Boston (40%) cases. Those numbers are small and of dubious significance. In all of the cases at both institutions (10 total) where both mass and calcifications were present, the biopsy was positive for malignancy.

The high yields related to calcifications are documented elsewhere in the literature. In the previous report from University of Pennsylvania/Fox Chase[11] describing results in 19 patients biopsied solely for calcifications (calcifications with associated mammographic or clinical masses having been excluded), 11 of 19 (58%) were positive. Rebner et al.,[8] reporting from University of Michigan, noted positive biopsies in 4 of 10 patients with calcifications developing in the treated quadrant after lumpectomy and irradiation. This was a subset from a total of 152 treated patients.

In order to see whether benign and malignant

Table 6-6 Results of suspicious mammograms: criteria and yield

	University of Pennsylvania (29 cases)		Boston Joint Center for Radiation Therapy (23 cases)	
Findings	**Malignant**	**Benign**	**Malignant**	**Benign**
Calcification alone	10 [47.6]	5	6 [42.8]	3
Calcification and mass	6 [28.6]	0	4 [28.6]	0
Mass or distortion	4 [19.0]	3	3 [21.4]	6
Inflammatory thickening	1 [4.8]	0	1 [7.1]	0
TOTAL	21 [100]	8	14 [100]	9

[ ], percentage of cases.

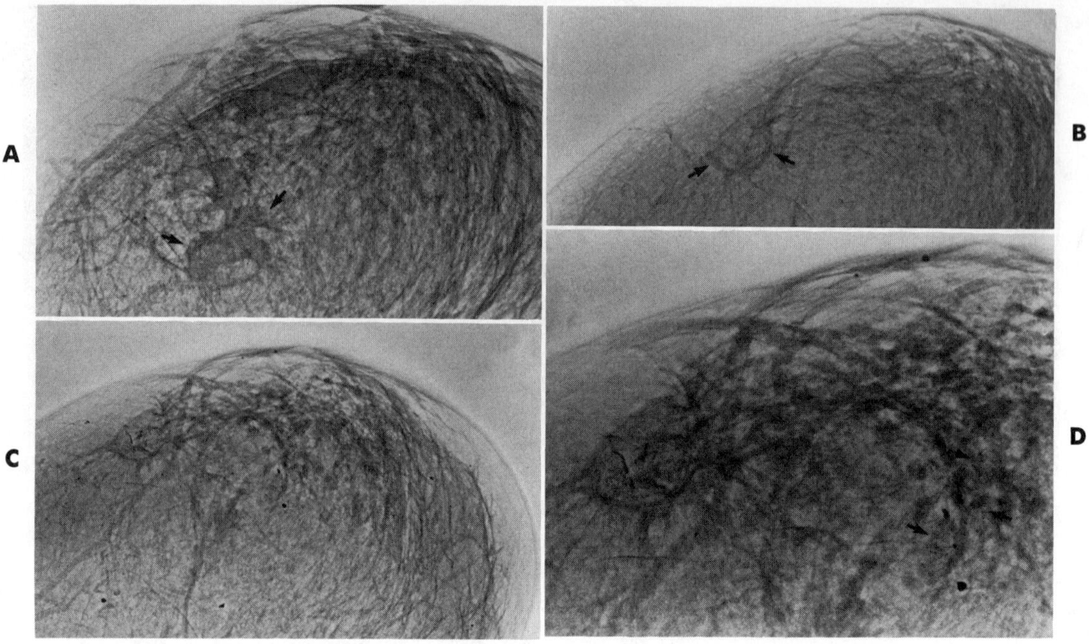

Fig. 6-19 Benign and malignant calcifications. **A**, Mammogram showing hematoma (*arrows*) at site of 2-week-old biopsy. **B**, Two years after treatment, lipid cyst with curvilinear wall (*arrows*) has developed. **C**, Three years after treatment there are benign-appearing calcifications at lipid cyst. **D**, Photographic enlargement confirms benign calcifications laterally but shows a linear array of malignant calcifications (*arrows*) in subareolar region.

calcifications differed in time of appearance, we studied the 21 cases with mammographically suspicious calcifications noting the time elapsed since treatment. All four cases that developed in the first 24 months were malignant, whereas only 12 of 17 (71%) developing afterwards were malignant. If "early" and "late" were split at 36 months, however, 9 of 12 (75%) early and 7 of 9 (78%) late were malignant. It should again be emphasized that all of these biopsies were done for mammographically suspicious calcifications; throughout all of the time course, dystrophic coarse or scattered calcifications developed, were noted, and were dismissed as benign. A pertinent example is shown in Fig. 6-19. Benign calcification at the treatment site and malignant calcification in the subareolar region developed simultaneously between the second and third posttreatment years.

REFERENCES

1. Bassett LW, Gold RH, and Mirra JM: Non-neoplastic breast calcifications in lipid cysts: development after excision and primary irradiation, AJR 138:335, 1982.
2. Davis SP, Stomper PC, Weidner N, and Meyer JE: Suture calcification mimicking recurrence in the irradiated breast: a potential pitfall in mammographic evaluation, Radiology 172:247, 1989.
3. Dershaw DD, Shank B, and Reisinger S: Mammographic findings after breast cancer treatment with local excision and definitive irradiation, Radiology 164:455, 1987.
4. Fisher B, Bauer M, Margolese R, et al: Five year results of a randomized clinical trial comparing total mastectomy and segmental mastectomy with or without radiation in the treatment of breast cancer, N Engl J Med 312:665, 1985.
5. Libshitz HI, Montague ED, and Paulus DD: Calcifications and the therapeutically irradiated breast, AJR 128:1021, 1977.
6. Mendelson EB: Imaging the post-surgical breast, Semin Ultrasound CT MR 10:154, 1989.
7. Nisce LZ, Snyder RE, and Chu FCH: The role of mammography in evaluating radiation response of inoperable primary breast cancer, Radiology 110:85, 1974.
8. Rebner M, Pennes DR, Adler DD, et al: Breast microcalcification after lumpectomy and radiation therapy, Radiology 170:691, 1989.
9. Schnitt SJ, Connolly JL, Recht A, et al: Breast relapse following primary radiation therapy for early breast cancer. II. Detection, pathologic features and prognostic significance, Int J Radiat Oncol Biol Phys 11:1277, 1985.
10. Sickles EA and Herzog KA: Mammography of the post-surgical breast, AJR 136:585, 1981.
11. Solin LJ, Fowble FL, Troupin RH, and Goodman RL: Biopsy results of new calcifications in the postirradiated breast, Cancer 63:1956, 1989.
12. Stomper PC, Recht A, Berenberg AL, et al: Mammographic detection of recurrent cancer in the irradiated breast, AJR 148:39, 1987.
13. Swann CA, Kopans DB, McCarthy KA, et al: Mammographic density and physical assessment of the breast, AJR 148:525, 1987.

7 Pathologic Assessment and Pathologic Prognostic Factors in Operable Breast Cancer

I'Tien Yeh, Barbara Fowble, Mary Jo Viglione, Virginia A. LiVolsi, and Delray J. Schultz

Breast carcinomas are heterogeneous neoplasms that manifest diverse biologic behavior. The ability to predict tumor behavior has major clinical implications in the selection of appropriate treatment for an individual patient. A number of pathologic findings have been correlated with clinical outcome. These factors can be divided into those that relate to tumor extent such as tumor size and axillary nodal metastases and those that relate to the inherent biologic aggressiveness of the tumor such as histologic subtype, histologic and nuclear grade, the presence or absence of lymphatic-vascular invasion, tumor necrosis, hormone receptor status, and measures of proliferative activity (i.e., thymidine labeling index, ploidy status, or S-phase fraction). The purpose of this chapter is to review the pathologic prognostic factors of tumor size, axillary nodal status, histologic subtype, the presence or absence of necrosis, lymphatic-vascular invasion, histologic and nuclear grade, multicentric disease, and margins of resection. These factors will be analyzed both in terms of their ability to predict for local-regional recurrence and overall and disease-free survival. The importance of each of these factors in determining treatment options also will be presented. The factors are reviewed for their relevance to operable invasive breast cancer. Prognostic factors for in situ breast cancer, i.e., in situ ductal and in situ lobular cancer, are presented in Chapter 13, and prognostic factors for locally advanced breast cancer are presented in Chapter 14. Biologic markers such as receptor status, measures of proliferative activity, oncogenes, cathepsin-D, and heat shock proteins are discussed in Chapter 8.

Accurate and complete pathologic examination is crucial to decisions regarding the appropriate management of the breast cancer patient. Because the manner in which specimens are handled at the time of initial surgery largely determines the quality and quantity of information that can later be derived from the excised tissues, a review of the appropriate processing of these specimens and a description of the information that should be derived from each is presented.

PATHOLOGIC SPECIMENS

Fine needle aspiration

For fine needle aspiration (FNA), microscopic fragments of tissue and individual cells are aspirated from tissue with the use of a syringe and a 22- to 25-gauge needle. The procedure is employed most commonly for palpable masses, although nonpalpable lesions visualized by mammography have been aspirated with mammographic guidance.[36] FNAs are a cytologic preparation and have the advantage of being less traumatic to the patient. They may be performed in the office or bedside setting with or without local anesthesia. Immediate feedback can be obtained as to the adequacy of the sample. In the event of an inadequate smear, the FNA can be repeated. A preliminary diagnosis can be established by the cytopathologist. In establishing a diagnosis of malignancy, the false-negative rate ranges from 5% to 20% depending on the technique employed to obtain the smear, the skill of the pathologist, and the strictness of the cytologic criteria applied.[42,93] In situations where an on-site pathologist is not available to assess the adequacy of the aspiration, the percentage of nondiagnostic samples may be higher. The fine needle aspiration is also limited in that noninvasive carcinomas cannot be distinguished from invasive carcinomas and histologic subtypes are more difficult to determine with this technique. False-positive diagnoses also have been made on fine needle aspiration (0 to 3%) and most cytopathologists generally prefer a frozen section confirmation of invasive malignancy before definitive treatment is initiated. Because a tissue diagnosis confirms greater information, many surgeons prefer to go directly to an excisional biopsy.

Core needle biopsy

This procedure involves the removal of a small cylinder or core of tissue, most often using a disposable Tru-Cut needle. The procedure requires local anesthesia and can be performed in the physician's office with relatively few complications. The tissue is submitted for histologic interpretation. With the Tru-Cut needle biopsy, noninvasive carcinomas can be distinguished from invasive carcinomas and the histologic subtype may be determined. However, the core biopsy may not provide a truly representative sample of the tumor.

Excisional biopsy

The most commonly employed initial surgical procedure for the diagnosis of a clinically suspicious lesion is the excisional biopsy (lumpectomy). Incisional biopsies may be performed on larger tumor masses. Submission of the unfixed, fresh biopsy specimen to the surgical pathology laboratory for an interoperative consultation is the procedure of choice. Tissue can then be put aside for special studies including estrogen and progesterone receptor assays and flow cytometry. Biochemical cytosolic assay for estrogen and progesterone receptor assays requires at least 500 mg of tissue. For very small lesions, immunohistochemical analysis for estrogen and progesterone receptors can be performed on frozen sections.[117] Formalin fixed paraffin sections also have been used recently for receptor assays, although the fixation and processing steps partially destroy receptor activity, making this assay less ideal.[37] Flow cytometry can be performed either from the scraping of the surface of the tumor or on tissue retrieved from the formalin fixed paraffin embedded blocks.[107] Because all patients potentially have breast cancer and may be candidates for breast conservation treatment, all excisional biopsies should be treated as lumpectomy specimens. The surgical margin of resection is painted with an indelible ink that survives the tissue processing procedure (generally India ink or varying colors of tattoo ink); thus, microscopic assessment of the margin can be definitely made. Painting the freshly inked specimen with Bouin's fixative aids in preventing ink diffusion and smearing. Orientation of this specimen may help determine the site of a positive margin to aid in reexcision strategy when necessary, although the entire biopsy cavity often is reexcised. Sutures placed at two margins are sufficient to orient the specimen in three dimensions (usually placed in the superior and lateral positions for superior-inferior, medial-lateral, and superficial-deep margins). The overall dimensions of the specimen as well as any gross lesions are recorded as well as the proximity of the gross tumor to the closest resection margin. Tumor circumscription, color, consistency, and the presence of necrosis also should be noted. A section of tumor nearest an inked resection margin is frozen to confirm malignancy microscopically and to assess the proximity to the margin. Tissue is then taken for hormone receptor assays and for flow cytometry. If a lesion seen on frozen section is purely in situ ductal carcinoma, the entire specimen should be blocked for permanent sections for evaluation of invasion. It is more important to document the presence of invasion than to obtain tissue for ancillary studies. However, extra frozen sections and a tissue scraping can be taken for immunohistochemical receptor studies and flow cytometry analysis.

Excisional biopsy specimens that are obtained with mammographic needle localization require special attention. Specimen radiography is performed on needle localization specimens for verification of excision of the abnormal area and to guide the pathologic examination. The specimen radiograph should be received in the pathology laboratory along with the specimen, with the area of calcifications or nodule clearly marked. The surgical margin is painted with an indelible ink and sutures are placed at two margins to orient the specimen in three dimensions. If there is no gross lesion present that corresponds to the mammographic abnormality, the area of interest is marked with eosin dye for complete processing later and the specimen is placed in formalin fixative to preserve the calcifications. If a gross lesion is evident, dimensions are recorded, including the size of the tumor and its proximity to the closest resection margin. The use of a dissecting microscope may aid in identifying an intraductal carcinoma or a very small lesion. The position of the calcifications or the mammographic mass relative to the edge of the specimen should be stated. A section of tumor nearest an inked resection margin is frozen to microscopically confirm malignancy and the status of the margin. Tissue is then taken for hormone receptor assays and flow cytometry.

Microscopic examination of an excisional biopsy specimen is usually carried out on the tissue in its entirety for lesions under 3 cm. In larger specimens, microscopic examination is performed on all parenchymal tissue with attention to grossly suspicious areas. Microscopic examination generally is not performed on grossly pure adipose tissue as this yields little additional diagnostic information. In a study by Owings et al.[167] the restriction of microscopic examination to areas of mammographic calcifications resulted in 37% fewer blocks being processed and a single case of ductal carcinoma in situ would have been missed. In a separate study by the same group,[202] limiting the number of blocks to 10 per case would have resulted in 18% fewer blocks processed and a single case of lobular carcinoma in situ would have been missed. Microscopic assessment of the excisional biopsy specimen should include tumor size, histologic subtype, the presence or absence of in situ component, the presence or absence of necrosis, lymphatic or vascular invasion, multifocal lesions, nuclear and histologic grade, and the status of the resection margins. Pathologic tumor size is defined by the invasive component of the primary tumor and does not include any noninvasive component. Margins generally are deemed positive if there are invasive or noninvasive cancers at the resection margin, close if there is tumor within 2 mm of the margin, and negative if the distance is >2 mm.

Mastectomy specimens

A gross description of the mastectomy specimen should include the extent of the tissues removed and record the overall size of the specimen as well as its dimension and should document the presence or absence of muscle and axillary tissue. Measurements of scars and incisions should be obtained, and the appearance of the skin, nipple, and areola also should be stated. If a gross lesion is identified, its size and its proximity to the deep margin should be indicated. The presence or absence of other lesions also should be recorded. The deep surface of the specimen should be inked.

The mastectomy specimen should be sectioned grossly at 1 cm intervals and representative sections of each quadrant, the deep margin, and the nipple should be taken. Each slice should be inspected visually and palpated for lesions. Adequate fixation is critical and over night fixation generally is recommended because of the high fat content and consequent slow fixation of breast tissue.

Microscopic assessment of the mastectomy specimen should include the pathologic tumor size, the histologic subtype, the presence or absence of an in situ component, nuclear and histologic grade, the presence or absence of necrosis, lymphatic or vascular invasion, the presence or absence of multicentric foci of invasive or noninvasive cancer, and assessment of the deep margin.

Axillary lymph nodes

Axillary node dissection specimens taken as part of a lumpectomy or mastectomy generally are examined by the pathologist while the tissue is unfixed. Gross involvement and a count of the number of nodes in the specimen can be recorded. For the reporting of the level of nodal involvement the specimen should be labeled appropriately by the surgeon in the operating room, because levels are determined relative to the pectoralis minor muscle, which is typically absent in an axillary node dissection performed for breast conservation therapy and may or may not be present in a modified radical mastectomy specimen.

Microscopic evaluation of the axillary nodes should include the total number of nodes removed, the number of positive nodes, the level(s) at which positive nodes are identified, and the presence of extracapsular nodal extension. Micrometastasis should be distinguished from macrometastasis. Micrometastasis, for definition, represents tumor infiltration <2 mm in diameter.

Various methods have been employed to detect early metastasis to lymph nodes. These include the clearing of axillary nodes with carnoy's solution, serial sectioning of axillary nodes, and immunohistochemical staining for keratin, which is very sensitive and specific for epithelial cells in lymph nodes.[209] The percentage of patients who ultimately are found to have positive nodes by any one of these methods after an initial report of negative nodes ranges from 0 to 24% (Table 7-1). Pickren[173] demonstrated no difference in 5-year survival rates for patients whose axillary nodes were reported initially as negative and were found subsequently to be positive by the clearing method. Fisher et al.[90] and Wilkinson et al.[238] also reported no significant difference in 5-year disease-free or overall survival rates when comparing patients whose axillary nodes were positive by serial sectioning to those whose axillary nodes were negative. However, a recent study by the International Breast Cancer Study Group[115] reported that serial sectioning of initially negative lymph nodes revealed positive nodes in 9% and that these patients had a significantly decreased disease-free and overall survival when compared to patients in whom no additional metastases were detected by serial sectioning. The significant difference in disease-free survival, however, was confined to patients with primary tumors >2 cm. In addition, two relatively recent studies have demonstrated that immuno-histochemical detection of lymph node metastases is associated with a worse prognosis.[210,226] However, in one study by Trojani et al.[226] the magnitude of the differences was not great (Table 7-1). It should be noted that when standard light microscopy is compared with immunohistochemistry there is no statistically significant difference in either sensitivity or specificity of detection.[209,210] Further studies will be required to demonstrate the role of immunohistochemical detection of axillary node metastasis. Because the overall incidence of nodal positivity with immu-

Table 7-1 Survival related to occult involvement of axillary nodes

Author	Method of detection	Positive node initially reported negative (%)	Survival (%)		
			Node-negative pts.	Node-positive pts.	Follow-up (yr)
Morrow et al.[159]	Clearing	0	—	—	—
Pickren[173]	Clearing	22	89	91	5
International Breast Cancer Study Group[115]	Serial sectioning	9	88 [74]	79 [58]	5
Fisher et al.[90]	Serial sectioning	24	73	67	5
Wilkinson et al.[238]	Serial sectioning	17	86 [80]	87 [79]	5
Apostolikas et al.[4]	Serial sectioning	14	—	—	—
Trojani et al.[226]	Immunohistochemical	14	98	93	5
			90	84	10

[ ], disease-free survival.

nohistochemical staining is small for axillary node-negative patients, standard light microscopy without serial sectioning or clearance remains the most commonly employed procedure. The presence of occult nodal metastasis also has been correlated with primary tumor size,[115] vascular or lymphatic invasion,[115,238] and the absence or minimal component of an in situ ductal carcinoma.[90] Therefore the presence of any of these factors in axillary node-negative patients may identify a poor prognostic subgroup without the need for immunohistochemical staining of the axillary nodes.

Differences in the number of axillary nodes recovered and examined are related to a combination of anatomic (patient) factors and surgical and pathologic dissection techniques. The complete axillary dissection results in the removal of more nodes than a level I or level I to level II axillary dissection. While clearing agents may increase the yield of lymph nodes,[61] careful manual dissection techniques have been reported to be the most cost effective.[159] The relative merits of the various axillary staging procedures employed in the breast conservation therapy are presented in Chapter 5.

PATHOLOGIC PROGNOSTIC FACTORS

Numerous pathologic factors have been evaluated for their ability to predict clinical outcome both in terms of local-regional recurrence and disease-free and overall survival. While early series tended to identify factors that would correlate with outcome in all patients with operable breast cancer, more recent studies have stressed the importance of distinguishing prognostic factors for patients with histologically positive axillary nodes and those with histologically negative axillary nodes. Most of the earlier studies evaluating prognostic factors were based on patients undergoing mastectomy. Recently, data have become available on patients undergoing conservative surgery and radiation. This section will review pathologic prognostic factors for survival and disease-free survival in patients undergoing mastectomy and breast conservation treatment. It also will identify pathologic factors that correlate with local-regional recurrence following either mastectomy or lumpectomy and radiation.

Tumor size

Pathologic tumor size is defined by the invasive component of the primary tumor. The American Joint Commission on Cancer (AJCC)/International Union against Cancer (UICC) staging system divides tumors into T_1 ($\leq$2 cm), T_2 ($>$2 cm but $\leq$5 cm), and T_3 ($>$5 cm).[14] Survival and disease-free survival rates as related to tumor size are demonstrated in Tables 7-2 through 7-7. Increasing tumor size has been associated with a decreased overall survival rate in a number of studies.[5,58,151,199,232] Tumor diameter was found to be an independent prognostic factor in a survey of 2740 breast cancer cases in the United States recorded by the Surveillance Epidemiology and End Results (SEER) Program.[33] The effect of tumor size was greater for node-positive patients than for node-negative patients, but was significant in both groups. Koscielny et al.[124] also have correlated the incidence of distant metastasis with increasing tumor size. Twenty-seven percent of patients with tumors 1 to 2.5 cm in diameter either presented with or developed distant metastasis over a period of 25 years. Distant metastasis occurred in 50% of patients with tumors 3.56 cm in diameter.

The impact of tumor size on outcome in histologically node-negative patients has been variable

Table 7-2 Outcome related to tumor size for operable breast cancer: all patients

		Survival (%) related to tumor size					
		≤2 cm		2-5 cm		>5 cm	
Author	Total no. pts.	5 yr	10 yr	5 yr	10 yr	5 yr	10 yr
Carter et al.[33]	24,740	91		80		63	
Schottenfeld et al.[207]	304	92	79	71	57	55	40
Nemoto et al.[161]	13,384	[62]		[49]		[34]	

[ ], disease-free survival.

(see Tables 7-3, 7-4, and 7-7). Clark et al.[38] reported no correlation between tumor size and overall or disease-free survival rates for node-negative patients. Courdi et al.,[45] in a univariate analysis, noted no significant correlation between tumor size and ralapse-free survival rates for node-negative patients. Bonadonna and Valagussa,[26] Silvestrini et al.,[217] and Sigurdsson et al.[214] noted tumor size to be a significant factor for relapse-free survival but not for overall survival. Fisher et al.[88] noted an increased 10-year treatment failure for tumors ≥2 cm in node-negative patients. Rosen et al.[186] noted a significant correlation for tumor size with relapse-free survival for T_1 histologically node-negative patients. Van de Velde et al.[228] noted a significant correlation between tumor size and disease-free survival rates for node-negative patients.

There appears to be some consistency in the finding that tumor size has an impact on relapse-free and overall survival in node-positive patients[26,39,88] (Tables 7-5 through 7-7). Increasing tumor size is associated with a worsening prognosis.

Tumor size has been correlated with the incidence of local-regional recurrence following mastectomy (Table 7-8). Increasing tumor size results in an increased incidence of local-regional recur-

Table 7-3 Outcome related to tumor size for operable breast cancer in T_1, axillary node-negative patients

	Survival (%)					
	Tumor size					
	<1 cm		1-2 cm		All T_1	
Author	5 yr	10 yr	5 yr	10 yr	5 yr	10 yr
Carter et al.[33]	98		86		96	
Fisher et al.[76]	76		85		—	
Payne et al[170]	89	67	87*	72*		
Rosen et al.[187-190]	98 [92]	95 [84]	96 [85]	93 [80]	95 [88]	[84]
Rosner and Lane[193]	96 [91]					
Wilkinson et al.[238]	91	74	87	75		
Donegan[58]	93	88	87	64		
Nemoto et al.[161]	[73]		[68]			
Moon et al.[156]	[88]	[85]	[82]	[74]	94 [84]	81 [77]
Milan	95 [90]		89 [83]			
Royal Marsden	91 [76]		80 [73]			
Bonadonna and Valagussa[26]					88 [80]	
Sigurdsson et al.[214]					88 [85]	
Say and Donegan[199]					87	83
Schottenfeld et al.[207]					91	82
Cutler et al.[47]					91†	87†

[ ], disease-free survival.
*1 to 3 cm.
†<2.5 cm.

Table 7-4 Outcome related to tumor size for operable breast cancer in T_2, axillary node-negative patients

	Survival (%)							
	Tumor size							
	2-2.9 cm		3-3.9 cm		4-4.9 cm		All T_2	
Author	5 yr	10 yr	5 yr	10 yr	5 yr	10 yr	5 yr	10 yr
Fisher et al.[76]	80		69		72			
Donegan[58]	78	55	94	71	80	—		
Carter et al.[33]							89	
Nemoto et al.[161]							[62]	
Valagussa et al.[227]							86	80
Cutler et al.[47]							82	70
Moon et al.[156]							87 [74]	76 [67]
Milan							86 [75]	
Royal Marsden							83 [64]	
Schottenfeld et al.[207]						87	65	

[ ], disease-free survival.

Table 7-5 Outcome related to tumor size and pathologic axillary nodal status in T_1, axillary node-positive patients

	Survival (%)					
	Tumor size					
	<1 cm		1-2 cm		T_1	
Author	5 yr	10 yr	5 yr	10 yr	5 yr	10 yr
Carter et al.[33]	94 (1-3)		87 (1-3)		87 (1-3)	
	54 (≥4)		67 (≥4)		66 (≥4)	
Fisher et al.[76]	100		67			
Payne et al.[170]	58	29	57*	43*		
Rosen et al.[187-190]	[81]	[65]	[73]	[60]	78 [60]	
					(1-3) [84]	[70]
					(≥4) [61]	[43]
Donegan[58]	80		73			
Nemoto et al.[161]	[54]		[39]			
Moon et al.[156]	—		—		[55]	[41]
Milan	74 [61]		66 [46]			
Royal Marsden	65 [59]		61 [50]			
M.D. Anderson	—		75 [61]			
Bonadonna and Valagussa[26]					74 [62]	
Say and Donegan[199]					46	27
Cutler et al.[47]					73†	52†
Valagussa et al.[227]					85	66

[ ], disease-free survival.
*1 to 3 cm.
†<2.5 cm.

Table 7-6 Outcome related to tumor size and pathologic axillary nodal status in T_2, axillary node-positive patients

	Survival (%)							
	Tumor size							
	2-2.9 cm		3-3.9 cm		4-4.9 cm		All T_2	
Author	5 yr	10 yr	5 yr	10 yr	5 yr	10 yr	5 yr	10 yr
Fisher et al.[76]	59		44		43			
Donegan[58]	63	31	54	—	43	43		
Carter et al.[33]							80 (1-3 positive nodes) 59 (≥4 positive nodes)	
Nemoto et al.[161]							[21]	
Valagussa et al[227]							56	41
Cutler et al.[47]							52	32
Moon et al.[156]							[41]	[28]
Milan							50 [36]	
Royal Marsden							54 [36]	
M.D. Anderson							58 [53]	

[ ], disease-free survival.

Table 7-7 Outcome related to tumor size and pathologic axillary in nodal status T_3 breast cancer patients

		Survival (%)			
		Node-negative		Node-positive	
Author	Total no. pts.	5 yr	10 yr	5 yr	10 yr
Carter et al.[33]	2698	82		73 (1-3 positive nodes) 46 (≥4 positive nodes)	
Valagussa et al.[227]	83	84	81	37	22
Cutler et al.[47]	112	78	63	0	0
Nemoto et al.[161]	1285	[57]		[21]	
Fisher et al.[76]	226	74		42 54 (1-3 positive nodes) 44 (≥4 positive nodes)	

[ ], disease-free survival.

Table 7-8 Incidence of postmastectomy local-regional recurrence related to primary tumor size

		Local-regional recurrence (%)			
Author	Treatment	T_1	T_2	T_3	Follow-up (yr)
Donegan et al.[78]	RM	7 [73]	16 [398]	30 [135]	5
Rosenman et al.[191]	RM/MRM	8 [51]	18 [87]	32 [44]	2-14
Dao and Nemoto[49]	RM	6 [36]	6 [70]	24 [29]	1.3-3+
Baker et al.[11]	MRM			39 [31]	5
	RM			9 [36]	5
Maddox et al.[146]	MRM			20 [20]	3-5
	RM			6 [16]	

RM, radical mastectomy; MRM, modified radical mastectomy; [ ], total no. pts.

Table 7-9 Breast recurrence related to clinical tumor size following excisional biopsy or quadrantectomy and radiation

Author	Breast disease recurrence (%) T_1	T_2
NSABP B-06[72]	7	10
Veronesi et al.[231]	4	
Clarke et al.[41]	6	3
Calle et al.[31]	7	11
Delouche et al.[53]	6	14
Solin et al.[221]	5	8
Spitalier et al.[222]	13	15
Van Limbergen et al.[229]	5	15
Boyages et al.[27]	10	10
Nobler and Venet[163]	7	8

rence, which approaches 30% for T_3 primary tumors. In contrast, there is no significant correlation between tumor size and breast recurrence rates following conservative surgery and radiation when comparing T_1 and T_2 tumors (Table 7-9).

Axillary node status

The axillary node status is the most important prognostic factor for operable breast cancer.[39,88,213] Survival and disease-free survival rates for axillary node-negative and axillary node-positive patients are presented in Tables 7-10, 7-11, and 7-12. The overall 5-year survival rate for axillary node negative patients is 80% to 90% with a 10-year survival rate of 70% to 80% (Table 7-10). More recently, several prospective randomized trials have evaluated the role of adjuvant chemotherapy or hormonal therapy in the treatment of node-negative breast cancer. Overall and disease-free survival rates for the observation arms in these trials are presented in Table 7-11. A comparison of the results in Tables 7-10 and 7-11 would suggest that the control arms in the prospective randomized trials have a worse prognosis than those reported in multiple retrospective series. However, it must be emphasized that there was significant patient selection for entry into these trials, some of which included only estrogen receptor negative patients.[70,73,243] Table 7-11 emphasizes the fact that within the node-negative patient population there can be significant variations in prognosis related to multiple factors that are addressed in the following sections and Chapters 8 and 9.

It is clear that patients with positive axillary nodes have a worse prognosis than those with negative axillary nodes (Table 7-10). The conventional nodal grouping of one to three vs. four or more positive axillary nodes was first suggested in 1968 by Fisher et al.[69] The lack of a significant difference

Table 7-10 Outcome related to pathologic axillary nodal status in node-negative patients with operable breast cancer, no adjuvant therapy used

Author	No. pts.	Survival (%) 5 yr	10 yr
Moon et al.[156]			
Milan	769	89 [81]	—
Royal Marsden	188	86 [69]	—
Winchester et al.[241]	257	91 [81]	—
Nemoto et al.[161]	12,299	72	—
Wilson et al.[240]	11,138	92	—
Carter et al.[33]	13,464	92	—
Martin et al.[151]	326	95	87
Finney et al.[65]	115	91	71
Madden et al.[145]	38	82	64
Fisher et al.[75]	219	78	65
Valagussa et al.[227]	335	88 [79]	83 [74]
Ariel[5]	596	81	63
Cutler et al.[47]	344	86	75
Donegan[58]	365	78 [70]	60 [52]
Payne et al.[170]	1,320	86	72
Ferguson et al.[64]	375	—	72
Schottenfeld et al.[207]	147	—	72
Haagensen[105]	562	—	77

[ ], disease-free survival.

Table 7-11 Outcome in prospective randomized trials comparing adjuvant therapy versus no adjuvant therapy node-negative breast cancer: survival in *observation only arm*

Trial	Patient selection	No. pts.	Survival (%)	Follow-up (yr)
NSABP B-13[70,73]	T_1-T_3 ER −	340	86 [71] T_1 [76] $T_{2\text{-}3}$ [63]	4
Intergroup[149,150]	ER −, ≥3 cm ER +	210	76 [61]	5
	<3 cm ER +	445	93	5
Ludwig Breast Cancer Group[144]	$T_{1\text{-}3}$	427	[69]	5
Milan[243]	$T_{1\text{-}3}$, ER −	45	66 [47]	5 (median)
Leningrad[211]	$T_{1\text{-}2}$	126	82	5
NSABP B-14[68,73]	$T_{1\text{-}3}$, ER +	1326	[77] T_1 [80] $T_{2\text{-}3}$ [73]	4
Scottish Cancer Trials[28]	$T_{1\text{-}3}$	374	82	5

ER −, estrogen receptor negative; ER +, estrogen receptor positive; [ ], disease-free survival.

in outcome for patients with one, two, or three positive nodes has been confirmed by additional studies.[26,67] The need to divide patients with four or more positive nodes into subgroups for greater prognostic relevance has resulted in various recommendations. Fisher et al.[67] and Ferguson et al.[64] have employed subdivisions of 4 to 6 positive nodes, 7 to 12 positive nodes, and ≥13 positive nodes. Nemoto et al.,[161] Bonadonna and Valagussa,[26] and Clark and McGuire[39] have employed subdivisions of 4 to 10 positive nodes vs. >10 positive nodes. Buzdar et al.[29] and Lee[140] have employed subdivisions of 4 to 9 positive nodes vs. 10 or more positive nodes. Each of these subdivisions identifies a high risk group of patients for whom the 5-year disease-free survival rate is less than 30% (Table 7-13). Fisher and Slack[74] demonstrated that only the number of positive nodes is important and not the percentage of positive nodes.

The size of the nodal metastasis also has been correlated with survival and disease-free survival. A micrometastasis is defined as tumor infiltration

Table 7-12 Outcome related to pathologic axillary nodal status in node-positive patients with operable breast cancer, no adjuvant therapy used

Author	Total no. pts.	All		1-3 nodes		≥4 nodes	
		5 yr	10 yr	5 yr	10 yr	5 yr	10 yr
Moon et al.[156]							
Milan	1,080	60 [44]		68 [53]		48 [31]	
Royal Marsden	516	59 [44]		70 [51]		42 [32]	
M.D. Anderson	432	62 [56]		71 [69]		53 [43]	
Nemoto et al.[161]	8,248	51					
Carter et al.[33]	11,276			81		57	
Valagussa et al.[227]	762	56 [36]	43 [26]	69 [46]	54 [33]	42 [26]	26 [15]
Ariel[5]	263			66	53	48	23
Cutler et al.[47]	512	53	35				
Haagensen[105]	746		48		63		28
Donegan[58]	287	45	22	[65]		[28]	
Payne et al.[170]	1,071	50	32				
Finney et al.[65]	112			83	61	46	31
Fisher et al.[75]	374	46	25	62	38	32	13
Schottenfeld et al.[207]	157		48				
Ferguson et al.[64]	240				52		

[ ], disease-free survival.

Table 7-13 Survival related to the number of positive nodes in patients with operable breast cancer

	Survival (%)					
	1-3 positive nodes		4-9 positive nodes		≥10 positive nodes	
Author	5 yr	10 yr	5 yr	10 yr	5 yr	10 yr
Moon et al.[156]	[57]	[43]	[46]	[36]	[28]	[15]
Nemoto et al.[161]	59-63		41-52		22-29	
Bonadonna and Valagussa[26]	78 [69]		60 [44][a]		54 [26]	
Smith et al.[219]		47		18		14
Clark and McGuire[39]	[72]		[59]		[44][b] [21][c]	
Fisher et al.[67]	73 [60]		54 [42][d] 50 [28][e]		28 [16][f]	
Ferguson et al.[64]		52		41[d] 25[e]		18[f]

[ ], disease-free survival.
[a]4 to 10 nodes.
[b]11 to 20 nodes.
[c]>20 nodes.
[d]4 to 6 nodes.
[e]7 to 12 nodes.
[f]≥13 nodes.

<2 mm in diameter. Micrometastases account for <10% of patients with positive nodes and are more frequent in patients with a primary tumor size <2 cm or with 1 to 3 positive nodes.[26] Macrometastasis is defined as tumor infiltration ≥2 mm in diameter. Survival related to microscopic vs. macroscopic nodal involvement is presented in Table 7-14. Patients with microscopic nodal involvement have a better prognosis than those with macroscopic nodal involvement.[8,86,189] Fisher et al.[86] noted no difference in overall survival rates when comparing patients with microscopic nodal involvement and those with negative axillary nodes. However, a significant decrease in relapse-free survival was noted for those with microscopic nodal involvement. Bonadonna and Valagussa[26] reported an improved 10-year relapse-free and overall survival rate for patients with T_1 lesions with a single micrometastasis when compared to those with negative axillary nodes. For patients with T_1 and T_2 lesions combined and a single micrometastasis, the 5-year relapse-free survival and overall

Table 7-14 Survival related to size of axillary nodal metastasis (macroscopic vs. microscopic) in patients with operable breast cancer

		Survival (%)			
			Node-positive		
Author	Tumor type	Node negative	Single microscopic	Single macroscopic	Follow-up (yr)
Bonadonna and Valagussa[26]	T_1	86 [80]	92 [91]	83 [72]	10
	T_{1-2}	83 [75]	78 [61]	73 [55]	5
Rosen et al.[189]	T_1	[88]	[84]	[76]	5
		[84]	[70]	[63]	10
	T_2	[87]	[89]	[65]	5
		[69]	[82]	[55]	10
Fisher et al.[86]*		90 [90]	91 [62]	61 [44]	4
Attiyeh et al.[8]*			82	62	5
			77	53	10

[ ], disease-free survival.
*Any no. positive nodes.

Table 7-15 Survival related to the highest level of involvement of axillary nodes in patients with operable breast cancer

Author	Survival (%) Highest level positive I	II	III	Follow-up (yr)
Berg[16]	87	75	36	3
Adair[1]	65	45	28	5
Donegan[58]	29	32	10	10
Schottenfeld et al.[207]	81	46		5
	65	31		10

survival rates were worse than those for patients with negative axillary nodes. Rosen et al.[189] reported an increased relapse rate at 10 years for patients with T_1 lesions with a single micrometastasis when compared to node-negative patients. This finding, however, was not observed for T_2 tumors. The number of positive nodes is more important than the size of the metastasis.[86]

Survival also has been related to the highest level of axillary nodal involvement (Table 7-15). Patients with positive nodes at level III have a decreased survival when compared to those with positive nodes only at level I or II. Smith et al.[219] reported that for a comparable number of positive nodes, the level involved did not affect survival. As the number of positive nodes increased, the number of levels involved also increased.

Extension of tumor beyond the lymph node capsule initially was associated with a greater short-term treatment failure in the NSABP B-04 study.[82] Patients with extranodal capsular extension had a 47% treatment failure compared to 29% treatment failure in those without extracapsular extension. However, in the 10-year analysis this factor lost significance as an independent indicator of prognosis and was associated more closely with nodal status.[88] Mambo and Gallagher[148] found extranodal extension to be an unfavorable prognostic factor in patients with one to three positive nodes. The 5-year survival rate was 74% for those patients without extracapsular extension, compared to 40% for those with extracapsular extension. For patients with four or more positive nodes, extracapsular node extension did not have a significant impact on survival rates (33% vs. 43%).

While the axillary nodal status is an independent prognostic factor for survival and disease-free survival in breast cancer,[33,87,213] it is related to tumor size. Koscielny et al.[123] developed a method for computing the distribution of tumor size at the time of development of the first, second, third, and so on, axillary metastasis based on a study population of 2408 women treated for invasive breast cancer at the Institut Gustave Roussy between 1954 and 1979. The authors found a progressive increase in both the incidence of axillary involvement and the number of positive nodes with tumor size. The mean tumor volume for the initiation of the first axillary node metastasis was 1.2 ml, corresponding to a tumor diameter of 1.32 cm. Table 7-16 dem-

Table 7-16 Incidence of positive axillary nodes related to primary tumor size

Author	Positive nodes (%) related to tumor size <1 cm	1-1.9 cm	2-2.9 cm	3-4.9 cm	≥5 cm
Haagensen[105]	28 [25]	27 [96]	28 [214]	45 [350]	52 [222]
Fisher et al.[76]	22 [52]	39 [375]	42 [611]	53 [996]	53 [665]
Nemoto et al.[161]	25 [1107]	34 [4044]	43 [3546]	52 [3052]	65 [1232]
Carter et al.[33]	21 [1335]	33 [6985]	45 [7282]	55 [6441]	70 [2698]
University of Pennsylvania	20 [81]	26 [284]	33 [298]	41 [196]	
Roger et al.[181]	8 [178]	27 [356]			
Say and Donegan[199]	33 [101]		51 [196]		

[ ], total no. pts.

Table 7-17 Incidence of local-regional recurrence after radical mastectomy (RM) or modified radical mastectomy (MRM) related to axillary nodal status

Author	Surgery	Local-regional recurrence (%)				Follow-up (yr)
		Negative nodes	Positive nodes			
			All	1-3	≥4	
Haagensen[105]	RM	3	—	4	22	10-37
Donegan et al.[59]	RM	6	27	12	38	5
Fisher et al.[77]	RM	8	24	24	31	5
Valagussa et al.[227]	RM/ERM	8	27	—	—	10
Rosenman et al.[191]	RM/MRM	4	—	17	22	2-14
Lee[138]	RM/MRM	6	—	11	37	4.4 (median)
Dao and Nemoto[49]	RM	0	16	—	—	1.3-3+
Deck and Kern[52]	RM/MRM	4	11	—	—	3+

onstrates the increasing incidence of axillary node metastasis with increasing tumor size. Increasing histologic grade also has been associated with a higher incidence of positive axillary nodes.[88,110,181] Additional pathologic factors that have been correlated with axillary node positivity include the presence of lymphatic or vascular invasion, high nuclear grade, and histologic subtype.[88] Therefore, while axillary nodal status is an independent prognostic factor, it is related to several additional pathologic factors. For further discussion see Chapters 3 and 8.

Local-regional recurrence has been correlated with axillary nodal status in patients undergoing mastectomy (Table 7-17). Patients with positive axillary nodes have a higher local-regional recurrence rate than those with negative axillary nodes, and the rate of recurrence increases with the number of positive nodes. Mambo and Gallagher,[148] however, found no correlation between the presence of extracapsular nodal extension and local recurrence in patients undergoing mastectomy. The level of positive nodes also has been correlated with local-regional recurrence in patients undergoing mastectomy. Smith et al.[219] reported an 8% local recurrence rate with a single level of nodal involvement vs. 24% for multilevel involvement. Donegan[58] reported a 28% local recurrence rate if only level I nodes were involved, a 33% local recurrence rate if level II nodes were involved, and a 45% local recurrence rate if level III nodes were involved. In contrast, the status of axillary nodes does not affect the breast recurrence rate in patients undergoing conservative surgery and radiation for stage I and stage II breast cancer (Table 7-18). This may be related to the fact that patients undergoing conservative surgery and radiation who also receive adjuvant systemic chemotherapy have a decreased risk of breast recurrence.[72,221]

Table 7-18 Breast recurrence following conservative surgery and radiation related to pathologic nodal status

Author	Breast recurrence (%)	
	Node negative	Node positive
NSABP B-06[72]	12	6
Clarke et al.[41]	4	7
Solin et al.[221]	7	4
Durand et al.[60]	1	4
Van Limbergen et al.[229]	10	15
Recht et al.[177]	12	10
Bedwinek et al.[15]	8	6

Histologic subtype

The vast majority of breast carcinomas are epithelial neoplasms that arise from the terminal ducts and are designated as invasive carcinoma not otherwise specified (NOS) or of no special type (NST) (Fig. 7-1). NST tumors have been defined as tumors in which >50% of the neoplasm lacks the histologic features of a specific type.[168] The presence of multiple histologic patterns in association with an invasive ductal carcinoma is categorized as an invasive ductal carcinoma. The relatively favorable prognosis associated with certain histologic subtype applies only to tumors composed entirely or mostly of that special type (see p. 179).

Special types of breast carcinoma associated with a more favorable prognosis include tubular carcinoma, mucinous or colloid carcinoma, and papillary carcinoma. For these tumors, 5-year sur-

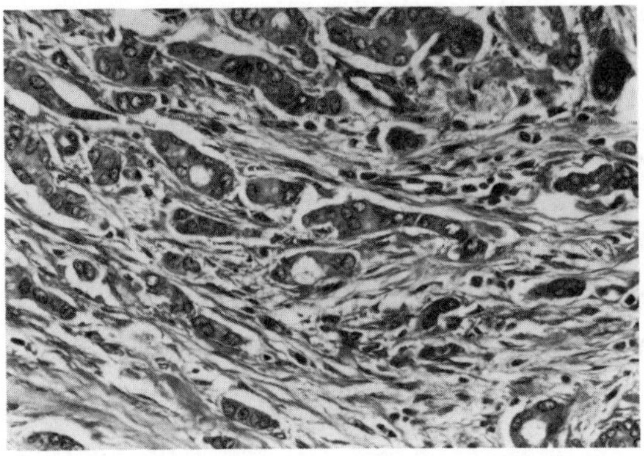

Fig. 7-1 Invasive ductal carcinoma of no special type. Some tubule formation is present (histologic grade II).

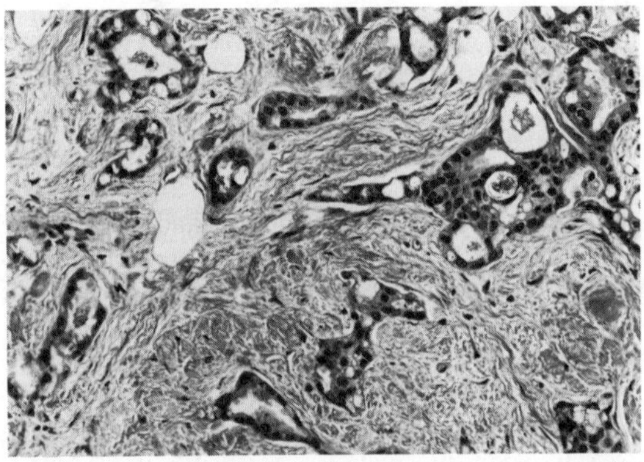

Fig. 7-2 Tubular carcinoma. Special form of invasive duct carcinoma composed almost exclusively of tubules.

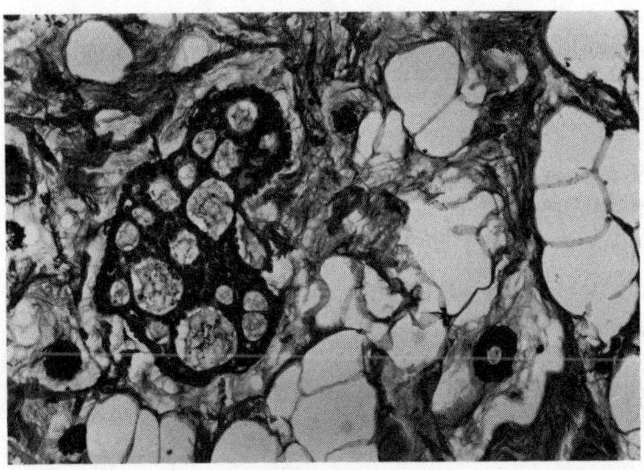

Fig. 7-3 Colloid carcinoma. Groups of relatively uniform cells within pools of mucin.

WORLD HEALTH ORGANIZATION HISTOLOGIC CLASSIFICATION OF MALIGNANT EPITHELIAL BREAST TUMORS[9]

1. Noninvasive
   a. Intraductal carcinoma
   b. Lobular carcinoma in situ
2. Invasive
   a. Invasive ductal carcinoma
   b. Invasive ductal carcinoma with a predominant intraductal component
   c. Invasive lobular carcinoma
   d. Mucinous carcinoma
   e. Medullary carcinoma
   f. Papillary carcinoma
   g. Tubular carcinoma
   h. Adenoid cystic carcinoma
   i. Secretory (juvenile) carcinoma
   j. Apocrine carcinoma
   k. Carcinoma with metaplasia
   l. Others
3. Paget's disease of the nipple

vival rates range from 85% to 90% or greater (Table 7-19). These three histologic subtypes comprise 3% to 6% of all breast cancers.[34,44,85,165,171,182] Tubular carcinoma is a variant of invasive ductal carcinoma characterized microscopically by a proliferation of small glands or tubules that resemble normal mammary ductals and are embedded in a moderately cellular stroma (Fig. 7-2). Mucinous or colloid carcinoma is distinguished by the abundant accumulation of extracellular mucinous secretion around tumor cells (Fig. 7-3). Papillary carcinomas are characterized by a frond-forming or papillary growth pattern. An additional histologic subtype that has been associated with a favorable prognosis is the cribiform carcinoma, which was first described by Page et al.[169] and is characterized by a complex architecture with extensive gland lumen formation and low nuclear grade. It often is associated with either tubular carcinoma or intraductal carcinoma of the cribriform type. A 5-year survival of 93% was reported by Venable et al.[230] for cribriform carcinoma.

The prognosis for patients with infiltrating lobular and medullary carcinomas is not as favorable as that for those with tubular, colloid, or papillary carcinomas but is better than that associated with infiltrating ductal carcinomas NOS, provided adherence to classical definitions is maintained (Table 7-20). Infiltrating lobular carcinoma is defined by a single filing of small regular epithelial cells with

Table 7-19 Survival related to histologic subtype in patients with operable breast cancer

Author	Survival (%)			
	Colloid carcinoma	Tubular carcinoma	Papillary carcinoma	Follow-up (yr)
Lee[140]	[92]			5
Ariel[5]	77			5
	64			10
Cutler et al.[47]	87		31	5
Robinson et al.[180]	88		86	5
Fisher et al.[85]	[98]	[85]	[85]	5
Silverberg et al.[216]	68			5
Norris and Taylor [164]	71			5
	55			10
Snyder and Tobon[220]	92			5
	77			10
Geschickter[97]	75			5
Lee et al.[137]	57			5
Kouchoukos et al.[125]	87		83	5
Carter et al.[34]			[40]	5
Cooper et al.[44]		100		5
Peters et al.[171]		100		—
Deos and Morris[54]		90		5
Oberman and Fidler[165]		100		7.5 mean

[ ], disease-free survival.

a targetoid pattern around benign ducts. It often has a diffuse multifocal distribution. Inclusion of variant patterns such as the pleomorphic lobular pattern and signet cell pattern have led to differences in the reported prognosis of infiltrating lobular carcinoma.[56] The histopathologic features that characterize medullary carcinoma (Fig. 7-4) include gross and microscopic circumscription, an intense lymphoplasmocytic reaction within and around the tumor, poorly differentiated nuclear grade, a syncytial growth pattern, and the absence of significant fibrosis or an in situ component, although intraductal carcinoma is frequently present at the periphery of the tumor.[157,179] Tumors that have some but not all of the features of medullary carcinoma have been termed atypical or medullary variants. The prognosis associated with atypical medullary carcinoma is not as good as that of medullary carcinoma but better than that of infiltrating ductal carcinoma NOS (Table 7-21).

Table 7-20 Survival related to histologic subtype in patients with operable breast cancer

Author	Survival (%)			
	Invasive ductal carcinoma	Invasive lobular carcinoma	Medullary carcinoma	Follow-up (yr)
Lee[140]	[62]	[65]	[54]	5
Ariel[5]	68	67	68	5
	53	50	62	10
Martin et al.[151]	76	89		8
Fisher et al.[85]	[58]	[65]	[73]	5
Ridolfi et al.[179]	72		88	5
	58		84	10
DiCostanzo et al.[56]	83 [67]	83 [76]		5
Ashikari et al.[6]		73		5
		58		10
Dixon et al.[57]	57	76		5
	42	58		10

[ ], disease-free survival.

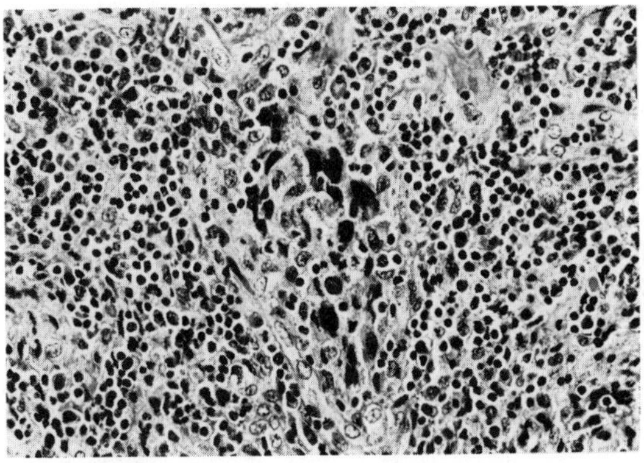

Fig. 7-4 Medullary carcinoma. Highly atypical nuclei in syncytial groups with background of lymphocytes and plasma cells.

It appears that the recognition of special histologic subtypes is most important in node-negative breast cancer.[87,185] Survival related to histologic subtype in axillary node-negative patients is presented in Table 7-22. The favorable histologic patterns of mucinous or colloid carcinoma and tubular or papillary carcinoma are associated with 5- and 10-year survival rates of 90%. Invasive lobular or medullary carcinoma has an intermediate survival of 80% to 90% with that of invasive ductal carcinoma ranging from 70% to 80%.

There has been no correlation with local-regional recurrence and histologic subtype for patients undergoing mastectomy. Recurrence related to histologic subtype in patients undergoing conservative surgery and radiation is presented in Table 7-23. There is no impact of histologic subtype on breast recurrence in these patients.

Table 7-21 Survival for medullary carcinoma in patients with operable breast cancer

	Survival (%)					
	Medullary carcinoma		Atypical medullary carcinoma		Nonmedullary carcinoma	
Author	5 yr	10 yr	5 yr	10 yr	5 yr	10 yr
Cutler et al.[47]	64	43				
Robinson et al.[180]	81					
Bloom and Field[24]	82	74				
Kouchoukos et al.[125]	68					
Maier et al.[147]	64	50				
Black et al.[20]	50	35				
Ridolfi et al.[179]	88	84	80	74	64	63
Richardson[178]	82 [78]	64 [64]				
Wargotz and Silverberg[234]	95		80		70	
Gorski et al.[103]		68				52
Rapin et al.[176]	96 [92]	92 [92]	76 [64]	62 [53]	67 [67]	61 [52]
Moore and Foote[157]	[83]					

[ ], disease-free survival.

Table 7-22 Survival related to histologic subtype in axillary node-negative patients

	Survival (%)			
Author	Invasive ductal carcinoma	Invasive lobular or medullary carcinoma	Mucinous (colloid) tubular papillary carcinoma	Follow-up (yr)
Rosen and Groshen[185]	[76]	[78]	[89]	10
Fisher et al.[87]	79	91	96	5
	66	82	92	8

[ ], disease-free survival.

Table 7-23 Breast recurrence related to histology in patients undergoing conservative surgery and radiation: 5-year follow-up

	Breast recurrence (%)			
Author	Infiltrating ductal carcinoma	Infiltrating lobular carcinoma	Medullary carcinoma	Colloid carcinoma
Mate et al.[152]	13 [108]	25 [12]		
Schnitt et al.[204]	11 [561]	12 [49]		
Kurtz et al.[128]	9 [709]	13.5 [67]	4 [27]	0 [11]

[ ], total no. pts.

Ductal carcinoma in situ (DCIS) in association with an invasive ductal cancer

Intraductal (noninvasive) carcinoma is frequently present within infiltrating ductal carcinomas (Fig. 7-5), although about half of breast tumors do not contain an in situ component.[214] The presence of an intraductal component has been associated with an overall decreased recurrence rate when compared to infiltrating ductal carcinomas without an intraductal component in patients undergoing mastectomy.[187,215] A similar finding has been observed in patients undergoing conservative surgery and radiation.[166] In an analysis of prognostic factors for histologically node-negative patients entered into the NSABP B-06 trial who underwent either lumpectomy with or without radiation or mastectomy, Fisher et al.[87] found the presence of an intraductal component to be associated with a significant improvement in overall survival in a univariate analysis but not in a multivariate analysis.

The presence of an intraductal component appears to have its greatest significance as a prognostic factor for breast disease recurrence in patients undergoing conservative surgery and radiation. While the mere presence of an intraductal component has not been associated with an increased risk of breast disease recurrence,[41,53,229] the presence of an extensive intraductal component (EIC) has been associated with an increased risk of such recurrence. EIC was first described by Schnitt et al.[202] By definition, it consists of the simultaneous presence of an intraductal noninvasive carcinoma comprising 25% or more the primary invasive tumor and the presence of intraductal carcinoma in the surrounding normal breast tissue (Fig. 7-6). The definition also includes predominantly noninvasive tumors with focal areas of invasion. Recht et al.[177] reported a 5-year actuarial breast recurrence rate of 23% in EIC-positive patients with a 10-year actuarial rate of 33%. An extensive intraductal component was present in 32% of the patient population. When EIC was absent, the 5-year actuarial breast recurrence rate was 5%, with a 10-year actuarial rate of 8%. It must be emphasized that both features must be present for the risk of a breast recurrence to be

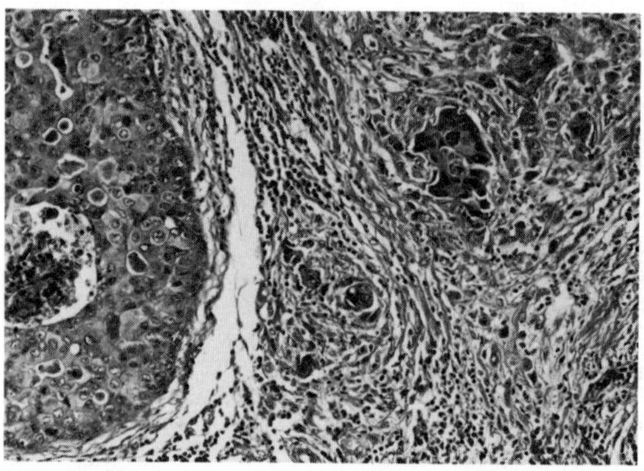

Fig. 7-5 Intraductal component, comedo subtype, within invasive duct carcinoma. Both intraductal and invasive components exhibit high nuclear grade.

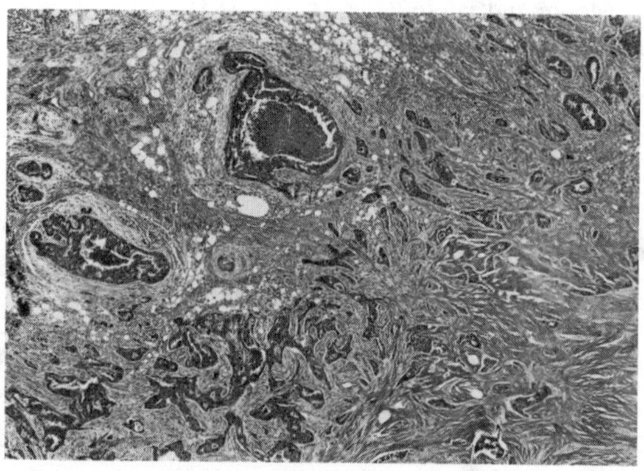

Fig. 7-6 Extensive intraductal component. Note intraductal carcinoma, comedo subtype, admixed with invasive duct carcinoma. Intraductal carcinoma comprises over 25% of the tumor area.

Table 7-24 Breast recurrence related to intraductal component within and adjacent to primary tumor in patients undergoing conservative surgery and radiation

	Author	No. pts.	Breast recurrence (%) 5 yr	10 yr
EIC negative	Recht et al.[177]	302	5	8
	Zafrani et al.[242]	361	6	5
	Bartelink et al.[12]	208	2	
	Koper et al.[122]	283	13	
	Kurtz et al.[126]	390	8	
EIC positive	Recht et al.[177]	143	23	33
	Zafrani et al.[242]	63	11	23
	Bartelink et al.[12]	79	9	
	Koper et al.[122]	283	10	
	Kurtz et al.[126]	106	18	

increased. An extensive intraductal component in the primary tumor only resulted in a 5-year actuarial breast recurrence rate of 5% and the presence of a intraductal carcinoma in the adjacent breast tissue only resulted in a 5-year actuarial breast recurrence rate of 6%.[27] The absence of both of these features resulted in a 5-year actuarial breast recurrence rate of 3%.[27] The risk of a breast recurrence in patients undergoing conservative surgery and radiation with EIC-positive tumors is presented in Table 7-24. While others have observed an increased risk of breast recurrence in EIC-positive patients, the magnitude of this risk is less than that reported by Recht et al.[177] It must be emphasized that data regarding the risk of a breast recurrence in EIC-positive patients treated at the Joint Center were obtained during a period of time in which preoperative mammograms were not performed routinely and assessment of resection margins was not standard policy. In series where margins of resection have been assessed and are negative,[12,89,242] EIC has not been a prognostic factor for breast recurrence. There is a single exception to this observation. Kurtz et al.[127] reported that negative margins of resection did not significantly decrease the risk of a breast recurrence in young women (<40 years of age) with either a major cellular reaction (moderate to marked lymphocytic or lymphoplasmocytic cell reaction within the tumor stroma) and/or more than 50% intraductal carcinoma within the tumor. The breast recurrence rate was 31% for patients with negative margins, 45% for those with indeterminate margins, and 67% with positive margins. However, margin assessment in this study was not performed by routine inking of the specimen. It was retrospectively assessed by reviewing routine sections from the tumor as well as those taken at the periphery. The increased risk of a breast recurrence in EIC-positive patients appears to be related to inadequate primary surgery with a resultant significant residual tumor burden that cannot be controlled by moderate doses of radiation. Holland et al.,[108] in serial subgross and correlated mammographic examination of 217 mastectomy specimens, correlated the presence of an extensive intraductal component in an invasive ductal cancer with the incidence of residual tumor following excisional biopsy. EIC-positive tumors were significantly more likely to have residual tumor and tumor at greater distances from the primary tumor than EIC-negative tumors. The residual tumor was predominantly noninvasive cancer. Ichihara et al.[114] reported that 33% of patients who had invasive ductal carcinoma with an intraductal component ≥1 cm had two or more separate invasive nodules in their mastectomy specimens. These nodules often were not recognized grossly and frequently were separated widely and located in fibrotic areas or adipose tissue around the intraductal component. It therefore appears that, in patients with EIC-positive tumors, negative margins of resection and wide excisions are required to decrease the increased risk of breast recurrence. An increased risk of local-regional recurrence with EIC-positive tumors has not been found in patients undergoing mastectomy.[187]

Multicentricity

Multicentricity in breast cancer has been defined variably with some authors accepting any amount of normal tissue between sites of carcinoma, whereas others require specific distances between tumor sites or the presence of tumor in multiple quadrants. The inclusion of lobular carcinoma in situ, atypical hyperplastic lesions, and lesions

Table 7-25 Incidence of residual carcinoma following excisional biopsy in patients undergoing mastectomy

Author	No. pts.	Margin	Positive residual carcinoma (%)	
			T_1	T_1 and T_2
Holland et al.[109]	282	>2 cm	42	43
		3 cm	17	18
		4 cm	10	11
Gump et al.[104]	657	>2 cm	18	27
Rosen et al.[187]	573	Separate quadrant	22	26
Lagios[130]	85	Separate quadrant		21
Lesser et al.[142]	687	Separate quadrant		27
Cahill et al.[30]	107	Separate quadrant		20
Fisher et al.[81]	904	Separate quadrant		13
Morgenstern et al.[158]	500	Separate quadrant		31

in the same vicinity as the main tumor mass yield a higher percentage. The incidence also depends upon the thoroughness of the pathologic sampling and examination of the mastectomy specimen. The random section technique provides less information than Eagan's technique of serial subgross and correlated mammographic examination that was employed by Holland et al.[109] and Lagios.[130] As noted in Table 7-25, the incidence of residual cancer in the breast following excisional biopsy in patients undergoing mastectomy ranges from 13% to 43%. Approximately one half to two thirds of the residual cancer is noninvasive, with one third being invasive cancer.[109,142] The incidence of multicentricity is unrelated to tumor size for T_1 and T_2 tumors but is related to histology (Table 7-26). Multicentricity is more common with invasive lobular carcinoma than invasive ductal carcinoma and also has been correlated with the presence of an extensive intraductal component. The incidence of multifocal disease has not been correlated with the presence of positive axillary nodes or patient age.[236] Multicentric carcinomas of varying histologic types have been associated with a poor prognosis when compared to unicentric single type carcinomas in patients undergoing mastectomy.[62]

The influence of multicentric disease on local-regional recurrence rates in patients undergoing mastectomy is unknown. However, patients with gross multicentric or multifocal disease have been reported to have an increased risk of breast recurrence when treated with conservative surgery and radiation.[40,126,141] Leopold et al.[141] reported a recurrence rate of 37% in patients who had clinical evidence of gross multicentric or multifocal disease and 50% for those in whom the gross multifocal and multicentric disease was an incidental finding by the pathologist. Kurtz et al.[126] and Clark et al.[40] also reported an increased risk for breast recurrence in patients with macroscopic multifocal tumor. This is in contrast to microscopic multifocal disease, which is not associated with an increased risk of

Table 7-26 Incidence of residual or multicentric carcinoma related to the histology of invasive cancer

Author	Residual or multicentric carcinoma (%)				
	Ductal	Ductal and EIC	Lobular	Medullary	Colloid
Holland et al.[108]	42 [151]	74 [66]			
Shah et al.[212]	55 [359]		77 [39]	42 [12]	55 [9]
Gump et al.[104]	19 [496]		50 [92]		
Rosen et al.[184]	33 [165]		50 [10]		
Lagios[130]	14 [56]		22 [9]		
Tinnemans et al.[225]	52 [44]		83 [6]		
Lesser et al.[142]	26 [635]		54 [70]	10 [58]	

[ ], total no. pts.

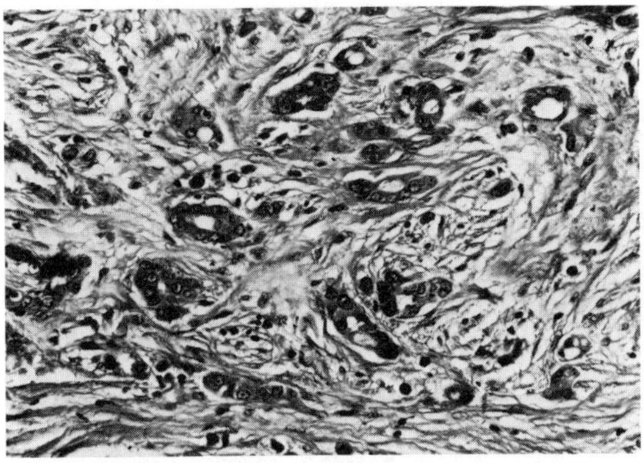

Fig. 7-7 Histologic differentiation, invasive duct carcinoma NST. Grade I: tubule formation is predominant.

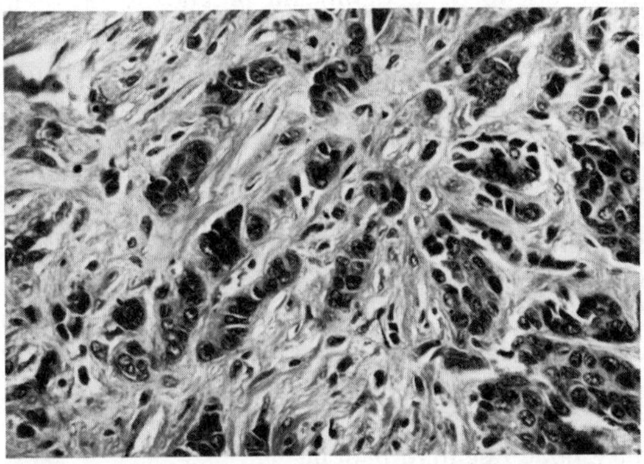

Fig. 7-8 Grade III: tumor is predominantly invading in cords and nests, without significant tubule formation.

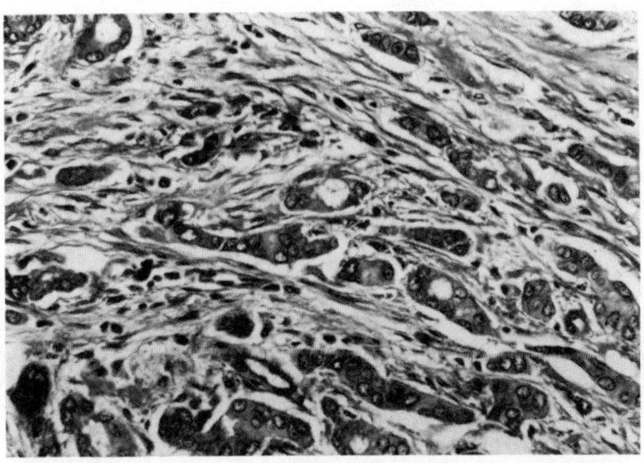

Fig. 7-9 Grade II: tubules are admixed with areas of invasive cancer in cords and nests.

breast recurrence in conservatively treated patients. Singletary and McNeese[218] reported a breast recurrence rate in patients with microscopic multifocal invasive disease to be 8% and in patients with microscopic multifocal noninvasive disease it was 4%. A significant residual tumor burden despite excisional biopsy in patients with gross multicentric and multifocal disease appears to be responsible for the high risk of breast recurrence. The presence of gross multicentric disease demonstrated either clinically or mammographically has been correlated with extensive disease in the breast in studies at the University of Pennsylvania. A total of 17 patients with gross multicentric or multifocal disease underwent mastectomy following an initial excisional biopsy. Detection was by mammogram only in 2 patients and by a combination of physical examination and mammography in 15 patients. Eight patients had two lesions demonstrated, 8 patients had three, and 1 patient had five. Preoperative evaluation revealed 16 of the 17 patients to have one or two quadrants of the breast involved. Pathologic assessment of the mastectomy specimens, however, revealed three or four quadrants of the breast to be involved in 9 patients with one quadrant involved in 1 patient, and two quadrants involved in 5 patients. Two patients had no residual disease at the time of mastectomy.

Histologic and nuclear grade

Histologic grading can be applied most easily to infiltrating ductal carcinomas NOS, which comprise over half of all breast malignancies. The commonly used scheme is derived from Bloom and Richardson[25] and Scarff and Handley[200] and divides infiltrating ductal carcinomas into three grades by evaluating the degree of tubular formation, nuclear morphology, and mitotic index. Grade I (well differentiated) tumors are characterized by well defined tubular formation, relatively uniform nuclei, and a low mitotic rate (Fig. 7-7). Grade III (poorly differentiated) tumors are characterized by little or no tubular formation, pleomorphic nuclei, and a high mitotic rate (Fig. 7-8). Grade II (moderately differentiated) tumors have intermediate characteristics (Fig. 7-9). Tubular formation and mitotic rate indirectly reflect differentiation and growth fraction, which recently have been measured by more complex techniques such as hormone receptor status, oncogenic expression, DNA index, and S-phase fraction.

Table 7-27 presents survival and disease-free survival rates related to histologic grade in all patients with operable breast cancer. Histologic grade has been shown to be an independent prognostic variable in several studies.[174,194] Survival related to histologic grade in patients with node-negative

Table 7-27 Survival related to histologic grade in patients with operable breast cancer

Author	Survival (%) related to histologic grade			Follow-up (yr)
	Low	Intermediate	High	
Martin et al.[151]	92	85	71	8
Contesso et al.[43]	91	74	61	5
Baak et al.[10]	97	78	55	5
Rosen et al.[187]	95 [85]	83 [76]	73 [60]	5
Bloom and Richardson[25]	75	53	31	5
	47	27	18	10

[ ], disease-free survival.

breast cancer is presented in Table 7-28. Fisher et al.[88] reported histologic grade to be a significant prognostic factor for a 10-year treatment failure in patients undergoing mastectomy in the NSABP B-04 protocol. Relapse-free survival has been significantly correlated with histologic grade in node-negative patients in several studies.[45,51,186,208,228] Roses et al.,[192] however, found no significant correlation with histologic grade and outcome in patients with T_1 node-negative breast cancer. Fisher et al.[87] identified histologic grade as a significant prognostic factor for overall survival in node-negative breast cancer patients entered into the NSABP B-06 protocol but did not find it to be significant in a multivariate analysis. Survival related to histologic grade in node-positive patients is presented in Table 7-29. Fisher et al.[88] correlated 10-year treatment failure with histologic grade in patients with four or more positive nodes. There was no correlation in patients with one to three positive nodes. Rosen et al.[186] found histologic grade not to be a significant prognostic factor in patients with T_1 node-positive breast cancer.

The incidence of local-regional recurrence following either mastectomy or conservative surgery and radiation has been correlated with histologic grade. Donegan et al.[59] reported a 0 and 11% risk of local-regional recurrence for grade I and grade II tumors vs. 18% and 34% for grade III and grade IV tumors in patients who underwent mastectomy. Hopton et al.[110] and Williams et al.[239] reported a local-regional recurrence rate of approximately

Table 7-28 Survival related to histologic grade in axillary node-negative patients

Author	Survival (%) related to histologic grade				Follow-up (yr)
		Intermediate			
	Low I-II	II	III	High III-IV	
Fisher et al.[88]	93			86	5
	87			73	10
Ariel[5]	87	73	62	29	5
	67	59	47	29	10
Payne et al.[170]	100	91	90	81	5
	100	85	74	66	10
Hopton et al.[110]	92			72	5
Courdi et al.[45]	[79]	[61]		[67]	8
International Breast Cancer Study Group[115]	[83]	[71]		[70]	5
Bloom and Richardson[25]	86	68		64	5
	61	47		42	10
Sarrazin et al.[198]	100 [93]	82 [75]		86 [70]	7
Wilkinson et al.[238]	90	83		73	5
	80	73		57	10
Rosen et al.[186]*	67	75		65	10

[ ], disease-free survival.
*T_1 only determinant survival.

Table 7-29 Survival related to histologic grade in axillary node-positive patients

	Survival (%) related to histologic grade			
Author	Low	Intermediate	High	Follow-up (yr)
Payne et al.[170]	90	65	43	5
	79	40	28	10
Hopton et al.[110]	80		46	5
Davis et al.[51]	86 [64]	70 [51]	57 [42]	5
Bloom and Richardson[25]	66	33	19	5
	51	14	9	10
Sarrazin et al.[198]	95 [84]*	75 [70]*	53 [48]*	7*
	93 [83]†	50 [41]†	41 [40]†	
Rosen et al.[186]‡	96	82	81	10

[ ], disease-free survival.
*1 to 3 positive nodes.
†≥4 positive nodes.
‡T_1 only determinant survival.

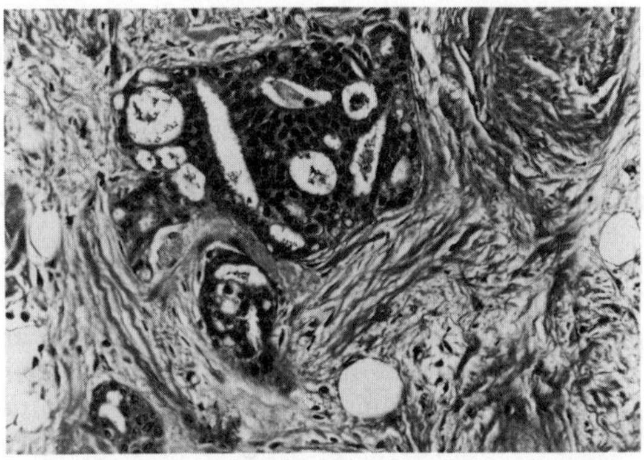

Fig. 7-10 Nuclear differentiation, invasive duct carcinoma NST. Grade I: nuclei are uniform in size and shape with fine chromatin and small nucleoli.

Table 7-30 Breast recurrence related to histologic grade in patients undergoing conservative surgery and radiation

	Breast disease recurrence (%)		
Author	I	II	III
Mate et al.[152]	4	13	16
Fisher et al.[89]	0	3	6
Calle et al.[31]	5	12	5
Clarke et al.[41]	1	6	4
Van Limbergen et al.[229]	5	10	16
Kurtz et al.[126]	3	9	17
Lindley et al.[143]	4	11	21
Pezner et al.[172]	3		18

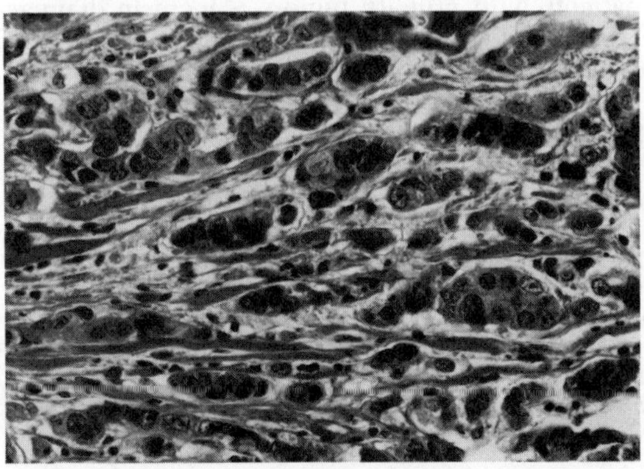

Fig. 7-11 Grade II: nuclei are more variable in size and shape, with prominent nucleoli.

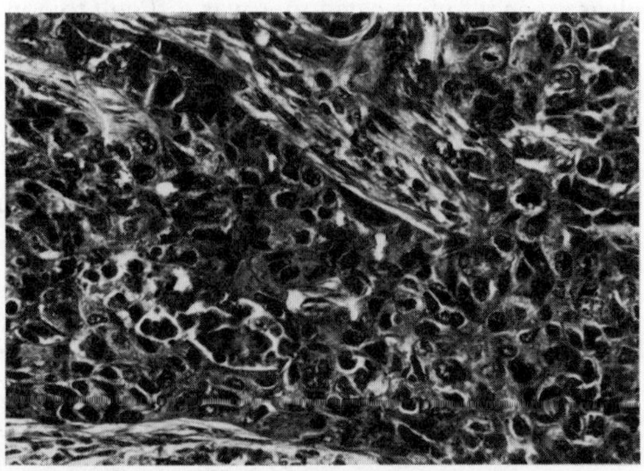

Fig. 7-12 Grade III: highly pleomorphic nuclei with coarse chromatin. Mitotic figures are identified easily and necrosis is also seen.

Table 7-31 Survival related to nuclear grade in axillary node-negative patients

Author	Survival (%) related to nuclear grade			Follow-up (yr)
	Good	Intermediate	Poor	
Cutler et al.[47]	95	87	81	5
	90	76	79	10
Fisher et al.[71,87]	93		79	5
	86		64	8
Rosner and Lane[193]	[91]		[91]	5
Black et al.[21]	88		69	5
Kister et al.[119]	95	74	75	10
Rosen et al.[186]*	91	87	78	10

[ ], disease-free survival.
*T_1 only determinant survival.

20% in patients with histologic grade III tumors and negative axillary nodes who underwent mastectomy, compared to a rate of <10% for grade I tumors. Breast recurrence related to histologic grade in patients undergoing conservative surgery and radiation is presented in Table 7-30. While patients with histologic grade III tumors appear to have an increased risk of breast recurrence, histologic grade was a significant predictor for breast recurrence in only three series.[41,126,143]

Nuclear grade has been considered to be more important than architectural grade.[22,175] Black et al.[22] proposed a separation of nuclear characteristics from tubule formation. Nuclear grade was thought to reflect the growth potential of tumors and included evaluation of nuclear pleomorphism, chromatin structure, nuclei, and mitosis. Five nuclear grades from 0 to 4 were used, 4 being the best differentiated and 0 being the most poorly differentiated (i.e., the reverse of the numerical convention used for histologic grading and for grading tumors in other sites). The division of nuclear grade into five categories was difficult to consistently follow,[46] and Black et al.[21] later utilized three grades. Most pathologists now use two (good and poor[87]) or three grades (1 equals best differentiated, 3 equals worst differentiated).[80,175] Figs. 7-10, 7-11, and 7-12 demonstrate nuclear differentiation for invasive ductal carcinoma.

Survival and disease-free survival rates related to nuclear grade for axillary node-negative and axillary positive patients are presented in Tables 7-31 and 7-32. In a multivariate analysis, Fisher et al.[87] identified nuclear grade as one of the most significant pathologic predictors for overall survival in axillary node-negative patients entered into the B-06 protocol. Bauer et al.[13] also correlated short-term recurrence (i.e., within 2 years) with high nuclear grade in node-negative, estrogen receptor–negative breast cancer patients. Van de Velde et al.[228] reported nuclear grade as a significant factor for disease-free survival in axillary node-negative patients. Rosen et al.[186] also reported nuclear grade as a significant factor for relapse-free survival in T_1 node-negative breast cancer patients. Rosner and Lane[193] showed no correlation between nuclear grade and relapse-free survival rates for patients with primary tumors ≤1 cm in diameter with histologically negative axillary nodes. Winchester et al.[241] reported nuclear grade to be a sig-

Table 7-32 Survival related to nuclear grade in axillary node-positive patients

Author	Survival (%) related to nuclear grade			Follow-up (yr)
	Good	Intermediate	Poor	
Cutler et al.[47]	80	59	44	5
	61	37	26	10
Black et al.[21]	54		39	5
Kister et al.[119]	57	67	51	10
Rosen et al.[186]*	83	72	67	10

*T_1 only determinant survival.

nificant prognostic factor for relapse-free survival in axillary node-negative patients. Prediction of survival in node-negative patients by nuclear grade appears to be at least equivocal to the newer techniques such as flow cytometry or examination of the C-erb B-2 (neu) protooncogene expression.[87,134]

The primary criticism of histologic and nuclear grading has been its subjectivity and lack of interobserver and even intraobserver consistency.[46] In an analysis of the "local" vs. "central" pathologist grading of breast tumors by the Ludwig Breast Cancer Study Group, there was exact agreement in only 54% of cases.[51] However, disagreement of more than one grade accounted for only 3% of cases and significant prognostic information about overall and disease-free survival rates was obtained using the "local" grading. Gilchrist et al.[101] noted complete agreement on nuclear grade by 11 pathologists in only 2% of cases, with agreement among six reviewers in 12% of cases. Hopton et al.[111] noted complete agreement for histologic grade among 11 pathologists in 78% of the 874 breast cancer mastectomy specimens that were reviewed. Numerous modifications of the criteria of Bloom and Richardson and Black have been proposed and have been employed by various breast cancer study groups. The variation in the proportions of tumors reported as grades I, II, and III reflects the different definitions employed. Nevertheless, pathologists who routinely work together and use a defined set of criteria for grading, such as those in the NSABP trials, report complete agreement in 90% of cases.[79] A recent modification of the Scarff-Bloom-Richardson scheme separates tumors by scoring ductoglandular differentiation, nuclear characteristics, and mitotic grade and stratifying patients into five distinct prognostic groups.[133] This modified scheme is said to be the most important factor for prediction of relapse in node-negative patients. The routine application among surgical pathologists of a scheme as complicated as this is unlikely unless it proves to be extremely useful in clinical decision making. A simplification of the grading scheme as recommended by Fisher et al.[87] should lead to greater interobserver agreement.

A more objective approach to grading recently has been attempted using computerized image analysis.[120,121,132] Parameters assessed by image analysis include nuclear area, area of condensed chromatin, nuclear shape, and degree of tubule formation. These techniques are promising and will require further investigation.

Vascular and lymphatic invasion

Lymphatic tumor emboli in the breast are found in approximately 25% of invasive ductal carcinomas and in 10% to 15% of patients with invasive ductal carcinomas who have histologically negative axillary nodes.[183] A major problem in the pathologic diagnosis of tumor emboli in lymphatics is that interpretation is subject to fixation artifact that may produce spaces around tumor cells (Fig. 7-13). These spaces simulate lymphatic spaces, and there is poor interobserver concurrence in the recognition of lymphatic involvement, which was reported as only 34% by a group of experts in an Eastern Cooperative Oncology Group (ECOG) study.[99] Rosen[183] proposed the following strict histologic criteria for the diagnosis of lymphatic space involvement: 1) evaluation of lymphatic invasion in tissue peripheral to the tumor; 2) the identification of coexistent blood vessels adjacent to the lymphatic space; 3) lining of the space by endothelial cells; 4) the contour of the suspicious embolus must be different from the space in which it lies (Fig. 7-14). Reevaluation of the ECOG data with Rosen's criteria would have lead to 77% concur-

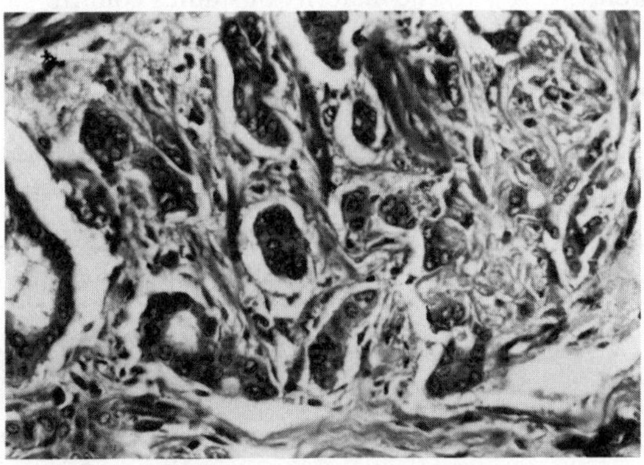

Fig. 7-13 Invasive duct carcinoma showing artifactual spaces around groups of tumor cells.

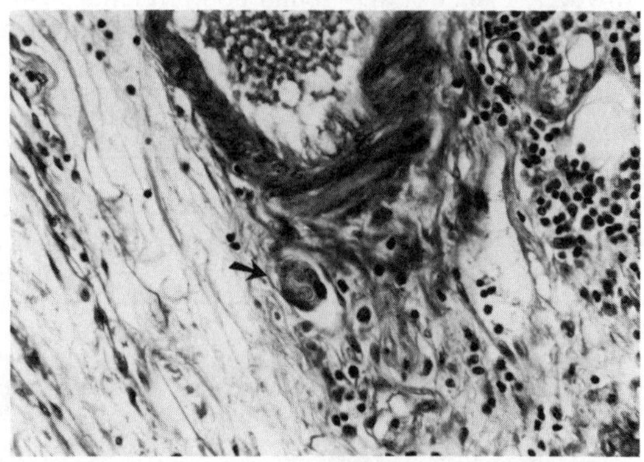

Fig. 7-14 Peritumoral lymphatic invasion (*arrow*). Note endothelial lined space containing carcinoma cells, adjacent to larger vein.

rence.[19] Immunohistochemical staining for specific endothelial cell constituents holds promise for definitive identification of lymphovascular channels; antibodies that have been used include those made against factor VIII–related antigen, blood group ABO antigens, and Ulex europeaeus I agglutinin. Elastic stains and basement membrane antigenic components such as laminin and type IV collagen can be used to distinguish between lymphatics and vascular channels. Special stains for evaluation of lymphatic invasion, however, have not yet been proven to be better than careful examination of hematoxylin-eosin–stained sections.[136,196,237] The majority of patients with lymphatic tumor emboli in the breast have positive axillary nodes. Lymphatic invasion also has been correlated with tumor size for T_1 tumors.[186] Rosen et al.[186] reported a significant decrease in 10-year determinant survival rates for patients with T_1 tumors with histologically negative or histologically positive axillary nodes and lymphatic invasion. The 10-year determinant survival rate was 87% without lymphatic invasion for T_1 node-negative patients, compared to 70% for those with lymphatic invasion. The 10-year determinant survival rate for T_1 histologically node-positive patients was 74% in the absence of lymphatic invasion and 59% with lymphatic invasion. Several additional studies have demonstrated the prognostic value of lymphatic invasion in histologically node-negative patients.[18,135,162,192] Lee et al.[135] demonstrated a significant decrease in overall and disease-free survival rates in 221 axillary node-negative patients with either lymphatic or vascular invasion detected by immunohistochemical techniques. The 5- and 10-year actuarial survival rates were 98% and 92% without lymphatic-vascular invasion, compared to 75% and 55% when this feature was present. Similar findings were noted at 10 years. In a multivariate analysis, lymphatic or vascular invasion was an independent prognostic factor. However, Fisher et al.[88] found no correlation with 10-year treatment failure in node-negative patients entered into the NSABP B-04 protocol who had lymphatic invasion. Bauer et al.[13] also found no correlation with short-term treatment failure (within 2 years) in axillary node-negative, estrogen receptor–negative patients who had lymphatic invasion.

There has been no correlation between the presence of lymphatic invasion in the breast and local-regional recurrence in patients undergoing mastectomy.[162] However, breast recurrence in patients undergoing conservative surgery and radiation has been correlated with the presence of vascular or lymphatic invasion (Table 7-33). Although the presence of vascular or lymphatic invasion is associated with an increased breast recurrence rate, it has been shown to be a significant pathologic prognostic factor for breast recurrence in only two series.[91,122]

Blood vessel invasion is demonstrated by the presence of tumor in the lumen of an artery or vein. These vessels are identified by the presence of a smooth muscle wall supported by elastic fibers. Special stains for elastic tissue often are required to demonstrate blood vessel invasion. The incidence of blood vessel invasion ranges from 10% to 49%.[7,19,95,186,197,235] The variation is related primarily to the method by which blood vessel invasion was identified. Blood vessel invasion has been correlated with increasing tumor size.[186]

The prognostic significance of blood vessel invasion has been variable. Survival and disease-free survival rates for axillary node-negative and axillary node-positive patients are presented in Tables 7-34 and 7-35. The presence of blood vessel invasion in patients with histologically negative axillary nodes has been correlated with a decreased survival[135,224] and disease-free survival rates.[115,135] However, several additional studies have found no correlation between survival and the presence of blood vessel invasion in axillary node-negative patients.[13,88,118,235] The majority of studies confirm the

Table 7-33 Breast recurrence related to vascular/lymphatic invasion in patients undergoing conservative surgery and radiation

	Breast recurrence (%)	
Author	Pts. without vascular/lymphatic invasion	Pts. with vascular/lymphatic invasion
Singletary and McNeese[218]	—	11
Fisher et al.[89]	3	8
Mate et al.[152]	11	19
Fourquet et al.[91]	10	25
Lindley et al.[143]	—	19
Koper et al.[122]	7	22

Table 7-34 Survival related to blood vessel invasion in axillary node-negative patients

Author	Survival (%) No blood vessel invasion	Survival (%) Blood vessel invasion	Follow-up (yr)
Rosen et al.[186]*	87	72	10
Bettelheim et al.[19]	[87]	[53]	5
Sampat et al.[197]	98	59	5
	94	40	10
Friedell et al.[95]	[70]	[36]	5
Atiba et al.[7]†	91 [79]	43 [28]	5
Kister et al.[118]	78	70	10
International Breast Cancer Study Group[115]	[79]	[66]	5
Lee et al.[135]†	98 [90]	75 [60]	5
	92 [88]	55 [44]	10

[ ], disease-free survival.
*T_1 only determinant survival.
†Lymphatic or vascular invasion.

presence of blood vessel invasion as a poor prognostic factor in axillary node-positive patients.[118,159,235] However, Teel[224] found no correlation between survival and the presence of blood vessel invasion in axillary node-positive patients.

Necrosis

Tumor necrosis is found in approximately 60% of patients with invasive breast cancer.[84] Fisher et al.[84] have divided tumor necrosis into two types. The comedo type represents necrosis that is found within the intraductal component of an invasive tumor (see Fig. 7-5). Necrosis also may be found within the invasive component of the tumor. The presence of the comedo type of necrosis has been associated significantly with multicentric foci of cancer remote from the dominant mass.[84] Tumor necrosis is related primarily to histologic and nuclear grade.[13,84] Tumor necrosis has been associated with an increased incidence of nodal metastasis in mastectomy patients in one series[35]; however, this finding was not confirmed by Fisher et al.[84]

The presence of necrosis within the invasive component of a tumor has been associated with early recurrence and death in patients with axillary node-positive breast cancer[100] and increased treatment failure[84] and decreased overall survival and recurrence-free survival rates[152] in all patients. Epstein et al.[63] reported the presence of marked necrosis to be correlated significantly with distant failure in patients undergoing conservative surgery and radiation. Bauer et al.[13] reported the presence of marked tumor necrosis to be associated significantly with short-term treatment failure in patient with node-negative, estrogen receptor–negative breast cancer. Roses et al.,[192] however, found no

Table 7-35 Survival related to blood vessel invasion in axillary node-positive patients

Author	Survival (%) No invasion	Survival (%) Invasion	Follow-up (yr)
Rosen et al.[186]*	76	59	10
Bettelheim et al.[19]	[63]	[44]	5
Sampat et al.[197]	81	12	5
	63	3	10
Friedell et al.[95]	[28]	[24]	5
Davis et al.[50]†	82 [65]	71 [50]	4
Kister et al.[118]	62	33	10

[ ], disease-free survival.
*T_1 only determinant survival.
†Lymphatic or vascular invasion.

correlation between recurrence and the presence of tumor necrosis for T_1 node-negative breast cancer patients.

Two series have suggested that the presence of tumor necrosis is associated with an increased risk of breast recurrence in patients undergoing conservative surgery and radiation.[143,152] In the Yale series, the significance was associated with necrosis in the invasive component of the tumor,[152] whereas in the Westminster series[143] it was associated with necrosis in the noninvasive component of the tumor. Three additional series have found no correlation between the presence of necrosis and breast recurrence in patients undergoing conservative surgery and radiation.[27,89,126,203]

Inflammatory response

The presence of lymphoplasmocytic infiltration in the stroma has had variable prognostic significance. The favorable prognosis associated with medullary carcinoma has been attributed to the intense lymphoplasmocytic reaction.[157] However, approximately 20% of nonmedullary carcinomas also will have a moderate to marked lymphoplasmocytic reaction.[80,188] The prognostic significance of this inflammatory response in nonmedullary carcinoma has been variable. Several studies have suggested a worse prognosis,[188,192] while others have suggested an improved prognosis.[17,21,47] An intense lymphoplasmocytic reaction has been associated with high histologic grade and therefore, a worse prognosis by some.[84,186] Rosen et al.[186] reported that the presence of an intense lymphoplasmocytic peritumoral infiltrate was a significant prognostic factor for relapse-free survival in patients with tumors 1.1 to 2 cm in diameter that were histologically node negative. The moderate to marked lymphoplasmocytic infiltrate was associated with a significantly increased risk of recurrence and death caused by breast cancer. Differing patterns of lymphoid infiltration have been analyzed for their relationship to survival, but no consistent association has been demonstrated.[83] Subtype studies have shown that most breast carcinoma infiltrating lymphocytes are T suppressor cells;[102] the presence of plasma cells and B lymphocytes are relatively uncommon. Specific cell-mediated immunity as measured by skin window reactivity[23] or mixed lymphocyte culture[32] has been said to be predictive of survival in breast carcinoma patients.

A prominent inflammatory infiltrate has been associated with an increased risk of breast recurrence in patients undergoing conservative surgery and radiation.[126,143] Kurtz et al.[126] reported a 5-year actuarial breast recurrence rate of 53% in premenopausal patients with an extensive intraductal component and a major mononuclear reaction. Two additional studies have found no correlation between breast recurrence and the presence of an inflammatory infiltrate.[27,89,203]

Margins of resection

Pathologic assessment of the deep margin of resection in patients undergoing mastectomy has been relatively standard. However, the correlation between the status of the margin of resection and local-regional recurrence is controversial. Ahlborn et al.[2] reported a slightly higher incidence of local-regional recurrence (5.7%) in patients with a close margin (i.e., $\leq$4 mm) who underwent modified radical mastectomy for T_1 or T_2 tumors with histologically negative axillary nodes. No adjuvant therapy was given to this group of patients. The incidence of local-regional recurrence was 3.4% for those whose margins were >4 mm. A close deep margin was present in 27% of the 322 patients. Mentzer et al.[155] were unable to correlate the incidence of local-regional recurrence with margin status in 100 patients with stage II breast cancer who underwent mastectomy. Positive axillary nodes were present in 59% of patients. The deep margin, however, was measured grossly in 67% of patients, and only 39 patients had microscopic assessment. In patients who received no postoperative radiotherapy, 0 of 4 with a positive margin had a local-regional recurrence, and 3 of 25 patients with a margin $\leq$2 mm had a local recurrence. Five of 45 patients with a margin $\leq$5 mm had a local-regional recurrence, compared to 1 of 33 with a margin >5 mm. Overall, 35% of patients had a $\leq$2 mm margin. Therefore patients with close margins but an intact pectoral fascia had a somewhat higher but not significantly increased risk of local-regional recurrence. Pectoral fascial involvement has been associated with a 28% to 29% risk of local-regional recurrence in patients undergoing mastectomy.[48,92]

The assessment of resection margins in patients undergoing conservative surgery and radiation was mandatory for entry of patients into the NSABP B-06 protocol.[66] This protocol established guidelines for the pathologic assessment of resection margins and defined positive margins as those with tumor at the resection edge. An arbitrary decision was made to treat patients with microscopically positive margins of resection with mastectomy. The assessment of resection margins has been adopted by many institutions and provides a guide for the extent of surgical resection, an estimate of the residual tumor burden, and information for treatment decisions. There are obvious limitations with the prospective evaluation of margins, including sampling error, the noncontiguous nature of tumor extension, the interference of surgical cautery artifact

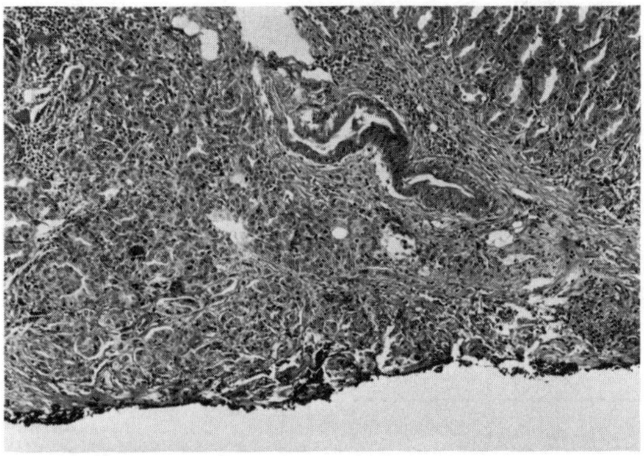

Fig. 7-15 Positive margin. Inked margin shows tumor to be transected. (Original magnification, ×10.)

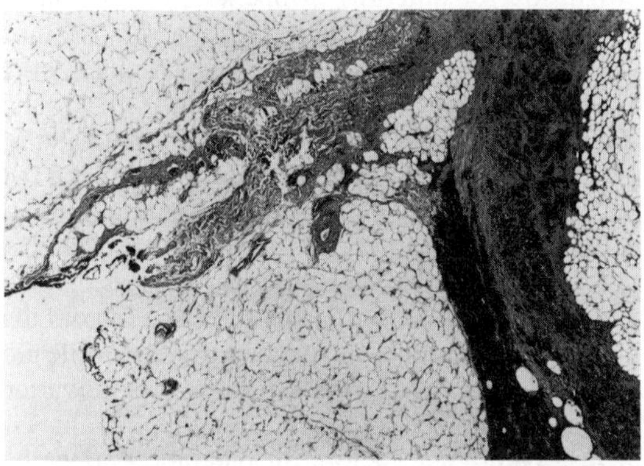

Fig. 7-16 Close margin. Tumor is within 2 mm of inked margin. (Original magnification, ×4.)

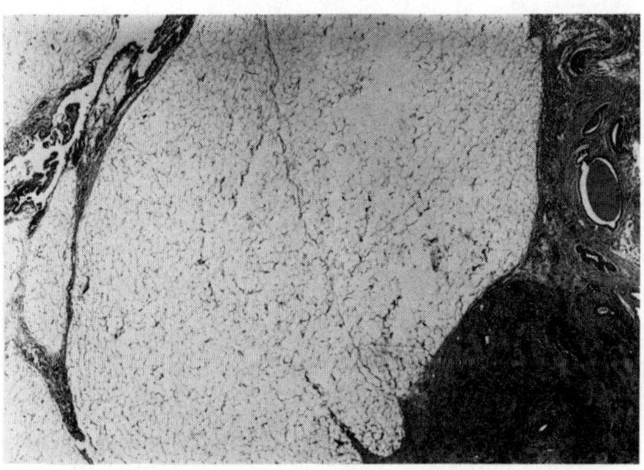

Fig. 7-17 Negative margin. Tumor is >2 mm from inked margin. (Original magnification, ×2.)

with histologic interpretation of margins, and the seeping of ink into the crevices making the true surgical margin difficult to define. Despite these limitations the assessment of margins provides significant clinical information for treatment decisions. In general the margin is considered positive when tumor cells are noted at the resection margin (Fig. 7-15), close when tumor cells are within 2 mm of the resection margin (Fig. 7-16), and negative when the tumor margin is >2 mm (Fig. 7-17). The nature of the positive margin should be stated (i.e., whether it is grossly or microscopically positive as well as the number of margins that are positive, whether the involvement is focal or diffuse, and whether there is invasive or noninvasive tumor at the margin). The location of the margin involvement also should be stated. Involvement of the most superficial and anterior margin may have little significance as these more superficial tissues are removed. Similarly, a positive, deep margin at the pectoral fascia without extension through the fascia may not be clinically important. Grossly positive margins of resection are associated with an increased risk of breast recurrence. Zafrani et al.[242] reported a 24% 10-year actuarial breast recurrence rate in patients with grossly positive margins, compared to 9% in those with grossly negative margins. Microscopically positive margins of resection have been reported in 20% to 25% of patients undergoing initial excisional biopsy (Table 7-36). The likelihood of obtaining negative margins of resection is related to the initial surgical procedure, the primary tumor size, and histology. Approximately 40% of patients who undergo a lumpectomy have positive margins of resection.[94,98] The incidence of microscopically positive margins for patients undergoing quadrantectomy ranges from 0 to 6%.[98,116,233] For patients undergoing wide excision, the incidence of a microscopically positive margin ranges from 6% to 16%.[116,206,233] Patients with T_2 primary tumors have a greater incidence of microscopically positive margins when compared to those with T_1 tumors.[66,112,154] Fisher et al.[66] also reported a higher incidence of microscopically positive margins in patients with histologically positive axillary nodes (15% vs. 7%). Patients with extensive intraductal component have both a higher incidence of initial margin positivity as well as reexcision margin positivity. Schnitt et al.[204] reported 95% initial margin positivity and 60% reexcision margin positivity in 25 patients with an extensive intraductal component. In 45 patients in whom an extensive intraductal component was absent, the initial margin positivity rate was 65% and the reexcision margin positive rate was 31%. The incidence of breast recurrence related to the status of the resection margin is presented in Table 7-37. In

Table 7-36 Incidence of microscopically positive margin(s) following initial excisional biopsy

Author	No. pts.	Primary tumor size (cm)	Surgery	Positive margin (%)
Volterrani et al.[233]	291	≤2.5	LE	16
Clarke et al.[41]	362	≤2.5	WE	24
Hunig et al.[112]	109	≤3	LE	14
Fisher et al.[66]	625	≤4	WE	7
Solin et al.[221]	218	<5	LE, WE	25
McCormick et al.[154]	75	≤5	WE	28
Bartelink et al.[12]	369	≤5	WE	9
Lagios et al.[131]	43	≤5	WE	23

LE, local excision; WE, wide excision.

general, for patients who have microscopically positive margins of resection, there is no evidence of an increased risk of breast recurrence provided that boost doses of radiation are employed. Therefore knowledge of the status of the resection margin provides a guide for the final radiation dose. Omission of the boost in patients with microscopically positive margins of resection has been correlated with an increased incidence of breast recurrence.[195] Patients with EIC-positive tumors are more likely to have a positive margin of excision, and in these patients negative margins of resection appear essential to minimize the risk of a breast recurrence. Therefore, in patients with EIC-positive tumors, knowledge of the resection margin is extremely important. Patients with EIC-positive tumors who have an initial positive margin of resection should undergo reexcision and, if the margin remains positive, mastectomy is the recommended treatment. Microscopic margin involvement in patients who do not have EIC-positive tumors is not associated with an increased risk of breast recurrence, and in these patients it is not a contraindication to conservative surgery and radiation.

Relative significance of histopathologic factors for outcome in the treatment of operable breast cancer

While multiple histopathologic factors have proven prognostic for outcome in operable breast cancer, it is important to determine which factors are most significant in predicting outcome. The interaction among factors such as tumor size and axillary nodal status or histologic grade and axillary nodal status may impact on the overall significance of each factor. Univariate analysis selects factors that individually impact on either recurrence, relapse-free, or overall survival rates. Multivariate regression techniques have the advantage of selecting factors that independently influence survival from multiple factors that are shown to be important in a univariate analysis. A review of series presenting an analysis of histopathologic factors for outcome in operable breast cancer appears in Table 7-38. Outcome has been measured either in terms of overall survival rates, relapse-free survival rates, or recurrence rates. For all series, axillary nodal status is the most important factor. Tumor size has been shown to be a significant factor in the majority of series, and

Table 7-37 Breast recurrence related to microscopic margin of resection

Author	Positive	Close	Negative	Unknown	Follow-up (yr)
University of Pennsylvania	2 [57]	11 [37]	7 [257]	9 [346]	5 (actuarial)
Hunig et al.[112]	7 [15]		6 [90]		2.3 (median)
Clarke et al.[41]	9 [88]		4 [274]		5 (mean)
Bartelink et al.[12]	7 [32]		2 [242]		6 (actuarial)
Schmidt-Ullrich et al.[201]	0 [46]		0 [61]		4.7 (median)
Fisher et al.[72]			10 [629]		8 (actuarial)
Zafrani et al.[241]			9		10 (actuarial)
Kurtz et al.[127]	24 [49]		8 [283]	16 [164]	5.9 (median)
Ryoo et al.[195]	13 [23]	8 [87]	6 [283]		3.5 (median)

[ ], total no. pts.

Table 7-38 Significant histopathologic factors correlating with outcome in patients with operable breast cancer

Author	Outcome	Tumor size	Nodal status	Histologic subtype	Histologic grade	Nuclear grade	Necrosis	Lymphatic/vascular invasion	Inflammatory response
Contesso et al.[43]	OS	No	Yes	No	Yes	—	—	—	—
Shek and Godolphin[213]	OS	Yes*	Yes*	No	No	No	Yes*	—	—
Russo et al.[194]	RFS	Yes	Yes	—	Yes	Yes	—	—	—
Stenkvist et al.[223]	Recurrence with 2.5 yr	Yes*	Yes*	No	Yes*	Yes*	No	No	Yes*
Alderson et al.[3]	OS	Yes*	Yes*	—	Yes*	—	—	—	Yes*
Carter et al.[33]	OS	Yes	Yes	—	—	—	—	—	—
Fisher et al.[88]	Recurrence	Yes	Yes	No	Yes	—	No	Yes	No
Friedell et al.[96]	Recurrence	No	Yes	—	—	No	—	Yes	—
Lee and Chan[139]	DFS	Yes	Yes	Yes	—	—	—	—	—
Breast Cancer Study Group[174]	Recurrence within 2 yr								
	Pre	Yes*	Yes*	—	Yes*	No	—	Yes*	—
	Post	Yes*	Yes*	—	No	No	—	No	—

OS, overall survival; DFS, disease-free survival; RFS, relapse-free survival; —, factor not analyzed.
*Significant in multivariate analysis.

Table 7-39 Significant histopathologic factors correlating with outcome in histologic node-negative breast cancer patients

Author	Outcome	Tumor size	Histologic subtype	Histologic grade	Nuclear grade	Necrosis	Lymphatic/ vascular invasion	Inflammatory response
Fisher et al.[88]	(B-04) recurrence	Yes	No	Yes	—	No	No	No
Fisher et al.[87]	(B-06) OS	No	Yes*	Yes	Yes*	Yes	No	No
Clark and McGuire[39]	DFS	Yes*						
Nealon et al.[160]	OS	—	—	Yes	—	—	Yes	—
Rosen et al.[186]	T_1 RFS	Yes	Yes	Yes	Yes	—	Yes	Yes
Van de Velde et al.[228]	Recurrence	Yes	Yes	Yes	Yes	No	Yes	No
Huseby et al.[113]	Recurrence							
	Premenopausal	Yes	—	No	No	—	—	—
	Postmenopausal	Yes	—	Yes	Yes	—	—	—
Bauer et al.[13]	ER-negative, recurrence within 2 yr	No	No	No	Yes*	Yes*	No	No
Sears et al.[208]	Recurrence	No	No	Yes	Yes	—	No	—
Bonadonna and Valagussa[26]	OS	No	—	—	—	—	—	—
	RFS	Yes	—	—	—	—	—	—
Roses et al.[192]	T_1, recurrence	—	Yes	No	—	No	Yes	No
Courdi et al.[45]	RFS	No	—	Yes	—	—	—	—
Winchester et al.[241]	Recurrence, OS	Yes	—	Yes	Yes	—	—	—
Rosner and Lane[193]	≤1 cm, RFS, OS	No	—	No	No	—	—	—
Lee et al.[135]		No	—	No	No	No	Yes*	—

RFS, relapse-free survival; DFS, disease-free survival; OS, overall survival.
*Significant factor in multivariate analysis.

Table 7-40 Significant histopathologic factors correlating with outcome in histologic node-positive patients with operable breast cancer

Author	Outcome	Tumor size	Histologic subtype	Histologic grade	Nuclear grade	Necrosis	Lymphatic/ vascular invasion	Inflammatory response
Clark and McGuire[39]	DFS	Yes*	—	—	—	—	—	—
Fisher et al.[88]	B-04, recurrence							
	1-3 positive nodes	No	No	No	—	No	No	No
	≥4 positive nodes	Yes	Yes	No	—	No	No	No
Rosen et al.[186]	T_1, RFS	No	No	No	No	—	Yes	Yes†
Davis et al.[50]	DFS, OS	No	—	Yes	—	—	No	—
Gilchrist et al.[100]	Recurrence, OS	No	—	—	—	Yes*	—	No
Bonadonna and Valagussa et al.[26]	RFS, OS	Yes	—	—	—	—	—	—

DFS, disease-free survival; OS, overall survival; RFS, relapse-free survival.
*Significant factor in multivariate analysis.
† 1 to 3 positive nodes only.

histologic grade appears to be a consistent factor in series where this feature was analyzed. Results relating to the presence of necrosis within the invasive component of a tumor, lymphatic or vascular invasion, or inflammatory response are variable.

Histopathologic factors correlating with outcome in axillary node-negative patients are presented in Table 7-39. Histologic and nuclear grade are significant in the majority of series. In two series, nuclear grade was a significant factor for either overall survival rates or recurrence rates within 2 years in a multivariate analysis.[87,159] Several series have identified various histologic subtypes as significantly improving prognosis.[87,186,192,228] The significance of necrosis within the invasive component of the tumor, vascular or lymphatic invasion, or inflammatory response has been variable. It must be emphasized that not all factors were analyzed in each series, and for the most part multivariate analyses were performed infrequently. Further studies employing multivariate analysis for node-negative patients will be important in determining the most significant histopathologic variables.

For patients with histologically positive axillary nodes the number of positive nodes remains the most significant prognostic factor (Table 7-40). Gilchrist et al.[100] identified necrosis within the invasive component of the tumor as a significant factor for recurrence and overall survival rates in node-positive patients entered into the ECOG surgical adjuvant chemotherapy trials. Davis et al.[50] identified histologic grade as a significant factor for disease-free and overall survival rates for node-positive patients entered into the Ludwig adjuvant trials.

Data obtained for Tables 7-38 to 7-40 for the most part have been collected from mastectomy series. The report of Fisher et al.[87] for patients entered into the NSABP B-06 trial includes patients who underwent lumpectomy with or without radiation. Several series have evaluated the influence of histopathologic features on disease-free survival in patients undergoing conservative surgery and radiation (Table 7-41). There appears to be little difference between these series and mastectomy series in terms of the identification of histopathologic factors that are prognostic for disease-free survival or distant relapse.

University of Pennsylvania experience

An analysis of histopathologic features that are prognostic for breast recurrence and disease-free and overall survival in patients undergoing conservative surgery and radiation at the University of Pennsylvania was performed and included 275 patients with clinical stages I and II infiltrating ductal carcinoma of the breast. All cases were examined by at least two pathologists for a consensus opinion. The median follow-up was 76 months with a range of 28 to 147 months. All patients

Table 7-41 Histopathologic factors correlated with disease-free survival in patients undergoing conservative surgery and radiation for early breast cancer: univariate and multivariate analysis

	Mate et al.[152]	Epstein et al.[63]*	Dewar et al.[55]*	Zafrani et al.[242]†	University of Pennsylvania
Tumor size	Yes‡	Yes	Yes	Yes	Yes‡
Nodal status	Yes‡	Yes‡	Yes	—	Yes‡
Histologic subtype	Yes‡	—	—	—	—
Histologic grade	No	Yes‡	Yes	Yes	No
Nuclear grade	—	No	—	—	No
Vascular-lymphatic invasion	No	Yes‡	—	Yes	No
Necrosis	Yes‡	Yes‡	—	—	No
Presence of in situ ductal carcinoma	No	No	—	Yes	—
Inflammatory response	No	—	—	—	No

*Factors significant for distant relapse.
†Factors significant for overall survival.
‡Significant in a multivariate analysis.

underwent an excisional biopsy. Reexcision was performed in 82 patients; in 26 it was negative and in 56 it was positive. One hundred fifty-six patients had T_1 tumors and 119 had T_2 tumors. The final margin of resection was assessed in 109 patients. In 66 patients the final margin was negative and in 26 the final margin was positive, and 17 had a close final margin. Two hundred fifty-five patients underwent an axillary node dissection. One hundred seventy-five had negative nodes, 80 had positive nodes with 59 patients having one to three positive nodes and 21 had four or more positive nodes. Seventy-three patients received adjuvant chemotherapy consisting of cyclophosphamide, methotrexate, and 5-fluorouracil. Breast recurrence was defined as any first treatment failure in the breast with or without simultaneous distant metastases. For the entire group the 5-year actuarial breast recurrence rate was 6% with a 10-year actuarial breast recurrence rate of 14%.

Pathologic features that were examined in the primary tumor included tumor size, histologic grade, nuclear grade, necrosis, inflammatory response, mitotic index, amount of fibrosis, lymphatic invasion, and the percentage of intraductal carcinoma within and beyond the confines of the main tumor mass. In addition, the presence of retrograde cancerization, Paget's disease, background breast tissue, pathology, tumor growth pattern, tumor border, and the presence of tumor at the margin of resection were all recorded. Three grades were used for evaluation of histologic and nuclear characteristics using modified criteria of Bloom and Richardson. Necrosis and inflammatory response were evaluated as none, slight, moderate, or marked, with distinctions made between the intraductal and invasive portions of the tumor. The predominant cell type in the inflammatory response was recorded. Lymphatic invasion was evaluated outside the main tumor mass using Rosen's criteria. The percentage of intraductal carcinoma was estimated by screening all available histologic sections. An extensive intraductal component was identified if >25% of the main tumor mass was composed of intraductal carcinoma and there was intraductal carcinoma outside the main tumor mass. Background breast tissue was examined for the presence of fibrocystic changes with notation of the degree of proliferation of epithelial elements. The margin of resection was evaluated only if indelible ink was used during processing. The final margin was judged to be positive if tumor was present at the inked margin of the primary resection or the reexcision specimen if further breast tissue was removed. The margin was judged to be close if tumor was seen within 2 mm of the inked resection margin and negative if the margin was >2 mm.

Overall breast recurrence rates at 5 and 10 years for the various histopathologic features are presented in Tables 7-42 and 7-43. In a univariate analysis, factors that significantly correlated with breast recurrence included histologic grade, moderate to marked necrosis in the intraductal component of the tumor, the absence of inflammatory response, retrograde cancerization, other fibrocystic changes, positive progesterone receptors, the presence of epithelial hyperplasia, and an extensive intraductal component. Histologic grade has been identified by three other series as an important prognostic factor for a breast recurrence.[41,126,143] Lindley et al.[143] also identified the presence of marked necrosis within the intraductal component of a tumor

Table 7-42 Histopathologic factors related to breast recurrence: University of Pennsylvania

	No. pts.	Actuarial breast recurrence (%) 5 yr	10 yr	p value
Tumor size (cm)				
≤1	27	8	19	.76
1-2	69	2	18	
>2-3	67	6	6	
>3-4	24	9	9	
>4-5	9	0	0	
Unknown	81	9	17	
Histologic nodal status				
Negative	175	8	14	.47
1-3	59	2	15	
≥4	21	5	—	
Histologic grade				
1	23	4	4	.0005
2	51	7	16	
3	191	4	14	
4	10	47	—	
Nuclear grade				
1	32	3	7	.82
2	98	6	14	
3	139	6	15	
Lymphatic invasion				
No	213	5	14	.44
Yes	54	10	16	
Inflammation				
1+	121	4	15	.04
2+	78	6	9	
3+	30	3	3	
4+	11	20	20	
Absent	35	14	30	
Lymphocyte: plasma cell ratio				
L > P	221	5	13	.51
P > L	9	0	—	
P = L	4	0	—	
Absent	14	7	—	
EIC positive (≥25% of primary tumor and in surrounding breast)	23	22	22	.03
EIC negative	252	4	11	
Necrosis intraductal				
None	67	2	14	.057
Slight	71	1	9	
Moderate	54	18	23	
Marked	15	7	7	
Necrosis invasive				
None	148	4	17	.82
Slight	82	8	13	
Moderate	24	5	5	
Marked	16	7	7	
Retrograde cancerization				
Present	74	15	18	.015
Absent	176	2	12	

as a significant factor for breast recurrence. The presence of an inflammatory infiltrate was identified by Kurtz et al.[126] as a significant factor for breast recurrence in premenopausal patients undergoing conservative surgery and radiation. In the present series the absence of an inflammatory response was associated with the highest risk of breast disease recurrence. In the present series EIC-positive tumors had a 22% 5-year and 10-year actuarial risk of breast recurrence. However, only 8% of the patients had EIC-positive tumors, and this is in contrast to the Joint Center series in which approximately one third of patients were found to have EIC-positive tumors.[27] This difference may be related to the patient selection policy at the University of Pennsylvania, where patients with diffuse or widespread microcalcifications were referred for mastectomy. As previously noted, the

Table 7-43 Histopathologic factors related to breast recurrence: University of Pennsylvania

		Actuarial breast recurrence (%)		
	No. pts.	5 yr	10 yr	p value
Growth pattern of infiltrating cancer				
Single mass	204	4	11	.11
Discontiguous nodules	56	8	19	
Gross tumor border				
Pushing	34	7	7	.52
Infiltrative	59	6	—	
Not available	181	6	17	
Microscopic tumor border				
Pushing	57	13	23	.18
Infiltrative	129	1	13	
Pushing-mixed	52	8	8	
Infiltrative-mixed	25	8	8	
Fibrosis				
Slight	29	4	10	.99
Moderate	149	8	12	
Marked	95	3	17	
Absent	1	—	—	
Background breast				
Atrophic	148	2	9	.10
Premenopausal	77	11	17	
Secretory	1	0	0	
Other fibrocystic changes				
Present	81	11	18	.015
Absent	140	2	7	
Epithelial hyperplasia				
Slight	19	6	6	.04
Moderate	17	6	17	
Atypical	11	19	46	
Absent	173	4	10	
Estrogen receptor				
Negative	55	5	13	.68
Borderline positive	133	6	11	
Progesterone receptor				
Negative	63	2	—	.03
Borderline positive	83	12	—	

most common clinical presentation of EIC-positive tumors is one of mammographic calcifications without an associated mass.[106] Five of the 23 patients with EIC-positive tumors developed a recurrence. None of the tumors in 4 patients with positive or close margins recurred, compared to 1 of 5 in patients with negative margins and 4 of 14 in patients with unknown margins. It is difficult to draw conclusions from these small numbers, but the number of recurrences in the one unknown margin group suggest inadequate evaluation of the tumor extent. In the present study a positive progesterone receptor was associated with an increased risk of breast disease recurrence. This finding has

Table 7-44 Histopathologic prognostic factors for disease-free survival—univariate analysis at the University of Pennsylvania

	No. pts.	5-yr actuarial disease-free survival (%)	p value
Tumor size (cm)			
≤1	27	96	.004
>1-2	69	88	
>2-3	65	71	
>3-4	24	87	
>4-5	9	52	
Unknown	81	87	
Histologic nodal status			
Negative	175	86	.0001
Positive			
1-3 nodes	59	90	
≥4 nodes	21	53	
Lymphatic invasion			
Present	54	75	.08
Absent	213	85	
Inflammation			
1+	121	85	.98
2+	78	83	
3+	30	80	
4+	11	82	
Absent	35	85	
Histologic grade			
1	23	100	.33
2	51	83	
3	191	82	
4	10	80	
Nuclear grade			
1	32	100	.12
2	98	84	
3	139	79	
Necrosis intraductal			
None	67	76	.52
Slight	71	90	
Moderate	54	83	
Marked	15	87	
Necrosis invasive			
None	148	85	.72
Slight	82	81	
Moderate	24	79	
Marked	16	88	

not been documented by other studies. A single study has reported an increased recurrence rate in progesterone receptor negative patients,[122] while others found no impact on progesterone receptor status and breast recurrence.[89,129,153] The association of an increased rate of breast recurrence with retrograde cancerization, other fibrocystic changes, and epithelial hyperplasia has not been reported by other groups. Of the univariate factors analyzed, only intraductal necrosis (moderate and marked) and the presence of other fibrocystic changes were significant in a multivariate analysis.

Table 7-45 Histopathologic prognostic factors for overall survival: univariate analysis at the University of Pennsylvania

	5-yr survival (%)	p value
Tumor size (cm)		
≤1 cm	100	.32
>1-2	95	
>2-3	91	
>3-4	100	
>4-5	100	
Unknown	92	
Histologic nodal status		
Negative	96	.09
Positive		
1-3 nodes	96	
≥4 nodes	88	
Lymphatic invasion		
Present	92	.22
Absent	95	
Inflammation		
1+	94	.96
2+	96	
3+	93	
4+	100	
Absent	93	
Histologic grade		
1	100	.35
2	93	
3	94	
4	89	
Nuclear grade		
1	100	.04
2	95	
3	94	
Necrosis intraductal		
None	92	.81
Slight	97	
Moderate	94	
Marked	100	
Necrosis invasive		
None	96	.25
Slight	92	
Moderate	96	
Marked	93	

Tables 7-44 and 7-45 present histopathologic factors correlating with disease-free and overall survival rates at 5 years. A significant correlation with 5-year actuarial disease-free survival was found for tumor size and histologic nodal status. The only factor that correlated with overall survival was nuclear grade. The findings are compared with others in the literature in Table 7-42 and again confirm the importance of tumor size and histologic nodal status.

SUMMARY

Analysis of histopathologic factors plays a major role in establishing significant prognostic factors for local-regional recurrence (either postmastectomy or following conservative surgery and radiation) as well as overall, relapse-free, and disease-free survival. The identification of these factors may impact on treatment recommendations as well as the identification of subsets of patients for whom the results of current treatment warrant improvement. At present the two most important factors for relapse-free and overall survival are tumor size and histologic nodal status. Increasing attention has been focused on the identification of prognostic factors in node-negative breast cancer patients and of the various histopathologic features, nuclear grade, or histologic grade and histologic subtype appear to be the most important. Further studies, however, are required to establish the relative importance of each of these factors in a multivariate analysis.

REFERENCES

1. Adair FE: Surgical problems involved in breast cancer, Ann R Coll Surg Engl 4:360, 1949.
2. Ahlborn TN, Gump FE, Bodian C, et al: Tumor to fascia margin as a factor in local recurrence after modified radical mastectomy, Surg Gynecol Obstet 166:523, 1988.
3. Alderson MR, Hamlin I, and Staunton MD: The relative significance of prognostic factors in breast carcinoma, Br J Cancer 25:646, 1971.
4. Apostolikas N, Petraki C, and Agnantis NJ: The reliability of histologically negative axillary lymph nodes in breast cancer. Preliminary report, Pathol Res Pract 184:35, 1989.
5. Ariel JM: Results of treating 1178 patients with breast cancer by radical mastectomy and postoperative irradiation where metastases to axillary lymph nodes occurred, J Surg Oncol 12:137, 1989.
6. Ashikari R, Huvos AG, Urban JA, and Robbins GF: Infiltrating lobular carcinoma of the breast, Cancer 31:110, 1973.
7. Atiba J, Coppin C, Ragaz J, et al: Clinical significance

of lymphatic, vascular or neural invasion in node-negative breast cancer, Proc Am Soc Clin Oncol 7:12, 1988.
8. Attiyeh FF, Jensen M, Huvos AG, and Fracchia A: Axillary micrometastasis and macrometastasis in carcinoma of the breast, Surg Gynecol Obstet 144:839, 1977.
9. Azzopardi JG, Chepick OF, Hartmann WH, et al: The World Health Organization histological typing of breast tumors—second edition, Am J Clin Pathol 78(6):806, 1982.
10. Baak JPA, Van Dop H, Kurver PHJ, and Herman SJ: The value of morphometry to classic prognosticators in breast cancer, Cancer 56:374, 1985.
11. Baker RR, Montague ACW, and Childs JN: A comparison of modified radical mastectomy to radical mastectomy in the treatment of operable breast cancer, Ann Surg 189:553, 1979.
12. Bartelink H, Border JH, van Dongen JA, and Peterse JL: The impact of tumor size and histology on local control after breast-conserving therapy, Radiother Oncol 11:297, 1988.
13. Bauer TW, O'Ceallaigh D, Eggelston JC, et al: Prognostic factors in patients with stage I, estrogen receptor-negative carcinoma of the breast. A clinicopathologic study, Cancer 52:1423, 1983.
14. Beahrs OH, Henson DE, Hutter RVP, and Myers MH, editors: Manual for staging of cancer: American Joint Committee on Cancer, ed 3, Philadelphia, 1988, JB Lippincott Co, pp 145-150.
15. Bedwinek JM, Perez CA, Kramer S, et al: Irradiation as the primary management of stage I and II adenocarcinoma of the breast, Cancer Clin Trials 3:11, 1980.
16. Berg JW: The significance of axillary node levels in the study of breast carcinoma, Cancer 8:776, 1955.
17. Berg JW: Morphological evidence for immune response to breast cancer. A historical review, Cancer 28:1453, 1971.
18. Bettelheim R and Neville AM: Lymphatic and vascular channel involvement within infiltrative breast carcinomas as a guide to prognosis at the time of primary surgical treatment, Lancet ii:631, 1981.
19. Bettelheim R, Penman HG, Thornton-Jones H, and Neville AM: Prognostic significance of peritumoral vascular invasion in breast cancer, Br J Cancer 50:771, 1984.
20. Black CL, Morris DM, Goldman LI, and McDonald JC: The significance of lymph node involvement in patients with medullary carcinoma of the breast, Surg Gynecol Obstet 157:497, 1983.
21. Black MM, Barclay THC, and Hankey BF: Prognosis in breast cancer utilizing histologic characteristics of the primary tumor, Cancer 36:2048, 1975.
22. Black MM, Opler SR, and Speer FD: Survival in breast cancer cases in relation to the structure of the primary tumor and regional lymph nodes, Surg Gynecol Obstet 100:543, 1955.
23. Black MM, Zachrau RE, Hankey BF, and Wesley M: Skin window reactivity to autologous breast cancer. An index of prognostically significant cell-mediated immunity, Cancer 62:72, 1988.
24. Bloom HJG and Field JR: Impact of tumor grade and host resistance on survival of women with breast cancer, Cancer 28:1580, 1971.
25. Bloom HJG and Richardson WW: Histological grading and prognosis in breast cancer. A study of 1409 cases of which 359 have been followed for 15 years, Br J Cancer 11:359, 1957.
26. Bonadonna G and Valagussa P: Contribution of prognostic factors to adjuvant chemotherapy in breast cancer, Recent Results Cancer Res 96:34, 1984.
27. Boyages J, Recht A, Connolly J, et al: Factors associated with local recurrence as a first site of failure following conservative treatment of early breast cancer, Recent Results Cancer Res 115:92, 1989.
28. Breast Cancer Trials Committee: Adjuvant tamoxifen in the management of operable breast cancer: the Scottish trial, Lancet ii:171, 1987.
29. Buzdar A, Smith T, Blumenschein G, et al: Adjuvant chemotherapy with fluorouracil, doxorubicin, and cyclophosphamide (FAC) for stage II or III breast cancer: 5 year results. In Salmon SE and Jones SE, editors: Adjuvant therapy for cancer III, New York, 1981, Grune & Stratton, pp 419-426.
30. Cahill CJ, Gibbs NM, Boulter PS, et al: Invasive breast cancer—the tip of an iceberg, Ann R Coll Surg Engl 65:356, 1983.
31. Calle R, Vilcoq JR, Zafrani B, et al: Local control and survival of breast cancer treated by limited surgery followed by irradiation, Int J Radiat Oncol Biol Phys 12:873, 1986.
32. Cannon GB and Pomerantz R: Cell-mediated immune responses—prognostic indicators of survival from breast cancer, Int J Cancer 44:995, 1989.
33. Carter CL, Allen C, and Henson DE: Relation of tumor size, lymph node status, and survival in 24,740 breast cancer cases, Cancer 63:181, 1989.
34. Carter D, Orr SL, and Merino MJ: Intracystic papillary carcinoma of the breast after mastectomy, radiotherapy or excisional biopsy alone, Cancer 52:14, 1983.
35. Carter D, Pipkin RD, Shepard RH, et al: Relationship of necrosis and tumor border to lymph node metastases and 10-year survival in carcinoma of the breast, Am J Surg Pathol 2:39, 1978.
36. Chen HH, Bernstein JR, Paige ML, and Crampton AR: Needle localization of nonpalpable breast lesions with a portable dual-grid compression system, Radiology 170:687, 1989.
37. Cheng L, Binder SW, Fu YS, and Lewin KH: Demonstration of estrogen receptors by monoclonal antibody in formalin-fixed breast tumors, Lab Invest 58(3):346, 1988.
38. Clark GM, Dressler LG, Owens MA, et al: Prediction of relapse or survival in patients with node-negative breast by DNA flow cytometry, N Engl J Med 320:627, 1989.
39. Clark EM and McGuire WL: New biologic prognostic factors in breast cancer, Oncology 3:49, 1989.
40. Clark RM, Wilkinson RH, Miceli PN, and MacDonald WD: Breast cancer: experiences with conservation therapy, Am J Clin Oncol 10:461, 1987.
41. Clarke DH, Le MG, Sarrazin D, et al: Analysis of local-regional relapse in patients with early breast cancers treated by excision and radiotherapy. Experience of the Institute Gustave-Roussy, Int J Radiat Oncol Biol Phys 11:137, 1985.
42. Cohen MB, Channing D, Rodgers RPC, et al: Influence of training and experience in fine-needle aspiration biopsy of breast. Receiver operating characteristics curve analysis, Arch Pathol Lab Med 111:418, 1987.
43. Contesso G, Mouriesse H, Friedman S, et al: The importance of histologic grade in long-term prognosis of breast cancer: a study of 1,010 patients, uniformly treated at the Institut Gustave-Roussy, J Clin Oncol 5:1378, 1987.
44. Cooper HS, Patchefsky AS, and Krall RA: Tubular carcinoma of the breast, Cancer 42:2334, 1978.
45. Courdi A, Hery M, Dahan E, et al: Factors affecting relapse in node-negative breast cancer. A multivariate analysis including the labeling index, Eur J Clin Oncol 25:351, 1989.
46. Cutler SJ, Black MM, Friedell GH, et al: Prognostic factors in cancer of the female breast. II. Reproducibility of histopathologic classification, Cancer 15(1):75, 1966.

47. Cutler SJ, Black MM, Mork T, et al: Further observations on prognostic factors in cancer of the female breast, Cancer 24:653, 1969.
48. Danforth DM, Findlay PA, McDonald HD, et al: Complete axillary lymph node dissection for Stage I-II carcinoma of the breast, J Clin Oncol 4:655, 1986.
49. Dao TL and Nemoto T: The clinical significance of skin recurrence after radical mastectomy in women with cancer of the breast, Surg Gynecol Obstet 117:447, 1963.
50. Davis BW, Gelber R, Goldhirsch A, et al: Prognostic significance of peritumoral vessel invasion in clinical trials of adjuvant therapy for breast cancer with axillary lymph node metastasis, Hum Pathol 16:1212, 1985.
51. Davis BW, Gelber RD, Goldhirsch A, et al: Prognostic significance of tumor grade in clinical trials of adjuvant therapy for breast cancer with axillary lymph node metastasis, Cancer 58:2662, 1986.
52. Deck KB and Kern WH: Local recurrence of breast cancer, Arch Surg 111:323, 1976.
53. Delouche G, Bachelot F, Premont M, and Kurtz JM: Conservation treatment of early breast cancer: long term results and complications, Int J Radiat Oncol Biol Phys 13:29, 1987.
54. Deos PH and Morris HJ: Well-differentiated (tubular) carcinoma of the breast. A clinicopathologic study of 145 pure and mixed cases, Am J Clin Pathol 78:1, 1982.
55. Dewar JA, Benhamou E, Benhamou S, et al: Predictors of distant metastatic relapse in conservatively treated breast cancer, Proc ESTRO, 1987 (abstract).
56. DiCostanzo D, Rosen PP, Gareen I, et al: Prognosis in infiltrating lobular carcinoma. An analysis of "classical" and variant tumors, Am J Surg Pathol 14:12, 1990.
57. Dixon JM, Anderson JT, Page DL, et al: Infiltrating lobular carcinoma of the breast: an evaluation of the incidence and consequence of bilateral disease, Br J Surg 70:513, 1983.
58. Donegan WL: Staging and primary treatment. In Donegan WL and Spratt JS, editors: Cancer of the breast, ed 3, Philadelphia, 1988, WB Saunders Co, pp 336-402.
59. Donegan WL, Perez-Mesa CM, and Watson FR: A biostatistical study of locally recurrent breast carcinoma, Surg Gynecol Obstet 122:529, 1966.
60. Durand JC, Poljicak M, LeFranc JP, and Pilleron JP: Wide excision of the tumor, axillary dissection, and postoperative radiotherapy as treatment of small breast cancers, Cancer 53:2439, 1984.
61. Durkin K and Haagensen CD: An improved technique for the study of lymph nodes in surgical specimens, Ann Surg 191:419, 1980.
62. Egan RL and McSweeney MB: Multicentric breast carcinoma, Recent Results Cancer Res 90:28, 1984.
63. Epstein AH, Connolly JL, Gelman R, et al: The predictors of distant relapse following conservative surgery and radiotherapy for early breast cancer are similar to those following mastectomy, Int J Radiat Oncol Biol Phys 17:755, 1989.
64. Ferguson DJ, Meier P, Karrison T, et al: Staging of breast cancer and survival rates. An assessment based on 50 years of experience with radical mastectomy, JAMA 248:1337, 1982.
65. Finney GG Sr, Finney GG Jr, and Diamond EL: A rational approach to the treatment of carcinoma of the breast, Ann Surg 71:859, 1970.
66. Fisher B, Bauer M, Margolese R, et al: Five-year results of a randomized clinical trial comparing total mastectomy and segmental mastectomy with or without radiation in the treatment of breast cancer, N Engl J Med 312:665, 1985.
67. Fisher B, Bauer M, Wickerham L, et al: Relation of number of positive axillary nodes to prognosis of patients with primary breast cancer. An NSABP update, Cancer 52:1551, 1983.
68. Fisher B, Costantino J, Redmond C, et al: A randomized clinical trial evaluating tamoxifen in the treatment of patients with node-negative breast cancer who have estrogen-receptor-positive tumors, N Engl J Med 320:479, 1989.
69. Fisher B, Ravdin RG, Ausman RK, et al: Surgical adjuvant chemotherapy in cancer of the breast: results of a decade of cooperative investigation, Ann Surg 168:337, 1968.
70. Fisher B, Redmond C, Dimitrov NV, et al: A randomized clinical trial evaluating sequential methotrexate and fluorouracil in the treatment of patients with node-negative breast cancer who have estrogen-receptor-negative tumors, N Engl J Med 320:473, 1989.
71. Fisher B, Redmond C, Fisher ER, and Caplan R: Relative worth of estrogen or progesterone receptor and pathologic characteristics of differentiation as indicators of prognosis in node negative breast cancer patients: findings from National Surgical Adjuvant Breast and Bowel protocol B-06, J Clin Oncol 7:1076, 1988.
72. Fisher B, Redmond C, Poisson R, et al: Eight-year results of a randomized clinical trial comparing total mastectomy and lumpectomy with or without irradiation in the treatment of breast cancer, N Engl J Med 320:822, 1989.
73. Fisher B, Redmond C, Wickerham L, et al: Systemic therapy in patients with node-negative breast cancer, Ann Intern Med 111:703, 1989.
74. Fisher B and Slack NH: Number of lymph nodes examined and the prognosis of breast carcinoma, Surg Gynecol Obstet 131:79, 1970.
75. Fisher B, Slack N, Katrych D, and Wolmark N: Ten year follow-up of patients with carcinoma of the breast in a cooperative clinical trial evaluating surgical adjuvant chemotherapy, Surg Gynecol Obstet 140:528, 1975.
76. Fisher B, Slack NH, and Bross ID: I. Cancer of the breast: size of neoplasm and prognosis, Cancer 24:1071, 1969.
77. Fisher B, Slack NH, Cavanaugh PJ, et al: Post-operative radiotherapy in the treatment of breast cancer: results of the NSABP clinical trial, Ann Surg 172:711, 1970.
78. Fisher B, Wolmark N, Bauer M, et al: The accuracy of clinical nodal staging and of limited axillary dissection as a determinant of histological nodal status in carcinoma of the breast, Surg Gynecol Obstet 152:765, 1981.
79. Fisher ER: Comment on "Interobserver reproducibility of histopathologic features in stage II breast cancer" by Gilchrist KW et al, Breast Cancer Res Treat 5:11, 1985.
80. Fisher ER, Gregorio RM, Fisher B, et al: The pathology of invasive breast cancer. A syllabus derived from findings of the National Surgical Adjuvant Breast Project (protocol no. 4), Cancer 36(1):1, 1975.
81. Fisher ER, Gregorio RM, Redmond C, et al: Pathologic findings from the National Surgical Adjuvant Breast Project (protocol 4): I. Observations concerning the multicentricity of mammary cancer, Cancer 35:247, 1975.
82. Fisher ER, Gregorio RM, Redmond C, et al: Pathologic findings from the National Surgical Adjuvant Breast Project (protocol no. 4). III. The significant of extranodal extension of axillary metastases, Am J Clin Pathol 65:439, 1976.
83. Fisher ER, Kotwal N, Hermann C, et al: Types of tumor lymphoid response and sinus histiocytosis. Relationship to five-year, disease-free survival in patients with breast cancer, Arch Pathol Lab Med 107:222, 1983.
84. Fisher ER, Palekar AS, Gregorio RM, et al: Pathological findings from the National Surgical Adjuvant Breast Project (protocol no. 4): IV. Significance of tumor necrosis, Hum Pathol 9:523, 1978.

85. Fisher ER, Palekar AS, Redmond C, et al: Pathologic findings from the National Surgical Adjuvant Breast Project (protocol no. 4): VI. Invasive papillary cancer, Amer J Clin Pathol 73:313, 1980.
86. Fisher ER, Palekar AS, Rockette H, et al: Pathologic findings from the National Surgical Adjuvant Breast Project (protocol 4): V. Significance of axillary nodal micro- and macrometastases, Cancer 42:2032, 1978.
87. Fisher ER, Redmond C, Fisher B, and Bass G: Pathologic findings from the National Surgical Adjuvant Breast and Bowel Projects (NSABP) prognostic discriminants for 8 year survival for node-negative invasive breast cancer patients, Cancer 65:2121, 1990.
88. Fisher ER, Sass R, and Fisher B: Pathologic findings from the National Surgical Adjuvant Project for Breast Cancers (protocol no. 4): X. Discriminants for the tenth year treatment failure, Cancer 53:712, 1984.
89. Fisher ER, Sass R, Fisher B, et al: Pathologic findings from the National Surgical Adjuvant Breast Project (protocol 6): II. Relation of local breast recurrence to multicentricity, Cancer 57:1717, 1986.
90. Fisher ER, Swamidoss S, Lee CH, et al: Detection and significance of occult axillary node metastases in patients with invasive breast cancer, Cancer 43:2025, 1978.
91. Fourquet A, Campana F, Zafrani B, et al: Prognostic factors in the conservative management of early breast cancer. A 25 year follow-up at the Institut Curie, Int J Radiat Oncol Biol Phys 17:7199, 1989.
92. Fowble B, Gray R, Gilchrist K, et al: Identification of a subgroup of patients with breast cancer and histologically positive nodes receiving adjuvant chemotherapy who may benefit from postoperative radiotherapy, J Clin Oncol 6:1107, 1988.
93. Frable WJ: Needle aspiration biopsy: past, present, and future, Hum Pathol 20(6):504, 1989.
94. Frazier TG, Wong RWY, and Rose D: Implication of accurate pathologic margins in the treatment of primary breast cancer, Arch Surg 124:37, 1989.
95. Friedell GH, Betts A, and Sommers SC: The prognostic value of blood vessel invasion and lymphocytic infiltrates in breast carcinoma, Cancer 18:164, 1965.
96. Friedell GH, Goldenberg IS, Masnyk IJ, et al: Identification of breast cancer patients with high risk of early recurrence after radical mastectomy. I. Description of study, J Natl Cancer Inst 53:603, 1974.
97. Geschickter CF: Gelatinous mammary carcinoma, Ann Surg 108:321, 1938.
98. Ghossein NA, Barba JP, Alpert S, et al: Importance of adequate surgical excision prior to radiotherapy in the local control of patients treated conservatively for breast cancer. Proceedings of the seventeenth International Congress of Radiation Oncology, Paris, 1989, p 48 (abstract).
99. Gilchrist KW, Gould VE, Hirschl S, et al: Interobserver variation in the identification of breast carcinoma in intramammary lymphatics, Hum Pathol 13:179, 1982.
100. Gilchrist KW, Gray R, Fowble B, et al: Tumor necrosis is a histoprognosticator for early recurrence and death in stage II breast cancer, Lab Invest 58:34A, 1988 (abstract).
101. Gilchrist KW, Kalish L, Gould VE, et al: Interobserver reproducibility of histopathologic features in stage II breast cancer. An ECOG study, Breast Cancer Res Treat 5:3, 1985.
102. Giorno R; Mononuclear cells in malignant and benign human breast tissue, Arch Pathol Lab Med 107:415, 1983.
103. Gorski CM, Niepolomska W, Nowak K, et al: Clinical evaluation and pathologic grading in relation to other prognostic factors. In Forrest APM and Kunkler PB, editors: Prognostic factors in breast cancer, Baltimore, 1968, Williams & Wilkins, pp 309-317.
104. Gump FE, Shikora S, Habif DV, et al: The extent and distribution of cancer in breasts with palpable primary tumors, Ann Surg 204:384, 1986.
105. Haagensen CD: Results with Halsted's radical mastectomy. In Haagensen CD, editor: Disease of the breast, Philadelphia, 1986, WB Saunders Co, pp 903-932.
106. Healey EA, Osteen RT, Schnitt SJ, et al: Can the initial clinical and mammographic features predict the presence of an extensive intraductal component in early stage breast cancer? Int J Radiat Oncol Biol Phys 17:1217, 1989.
107. Hedley DW, Friedlander ML, Taylor IW, et al: Method of analysis of cellular DNA content of paraffin-embedded pathological material using flow cytometry, J Histochem Cytochem 31:1333, 1983.
108. Holland R, Connolly J, Gelman R, et al: The presence of an extensive intraductal component following a limited excision correlates with prominent residual disease in the remainder of the breast, J Clin Oncol 8:113, 1990.
109. Holland R, Veling S, Mravunac M, and Hendriks J: Histologic multifocality of Tis T1-2 breast carcinomas. Implications for clinical trials of breast-conserving surgery, Cancer 56:979, 1985.
110. Hopton DS, Thorogood J, Clayden AD, and Mackinnon D: Histologic grading of breast cancer: significance of grade on recurrence and mortality, Eur J Surg Oncol 15:25, 1989.
111. Hopton DS, Thorogood J, Clayden AD, and Mackinnon D: Observer variation in histologic grading of breast cancer, Eur J Surg Oncol 15:21, 1989.
112. Hunig R, Walther E, Harder F, et al: The Basel lumpectomy protocol: 5 year experience with a prospective study for conservative treatment of breast cancer. In Harris JR, Hellman S, and Silen W, editors: Conservative management of breast cancer, Philadelphia, 1983, JB Lippincott, pp 23-35.
113. Huseby RA, Ownby HE, Frederick J, et al: Node-negative breast cancer treated by modified radical mastectomy without adjuvant therapies: variables associated with disease recurrence and survivorship, J Clin Oncol 6:83, 1988.
114. Ichihara S, Aoyama H, Matsuyama T, et al: Relationship between the extent of intraductal component and that of invasive component in ductal carcinomas of the breast, Acta Pathol Jpn 39:786, 1989.
115. International (Ludwig) Breast Cancer Study Group: Prognostic importance of occult axillary lymph node micrometastases from breast cancer, Lancet i:1565, 1990.
116. Kantorowitz DA, Poulter CA, Rubin P, et al: Treatment of breast cancer with segmental mastectomy alone or segmental mastectomy plus radiation, Radiother Oncol 15:141, 1989.
117. King WJ, DeSombre ER, Jensen EV, and Greene GL: Comparison of immunocytochemical and steroid-binding assays for estrogen receptor in human breast tumors, Cancer Res 45:293, 1985.
118. Kister SJ, Sommers SC, Haagensen CD, and Cooley E: Reevaluation of blood-vessel invasion as a prognostic factor in carcinoma of the breast, Cancer 19:1213, 1966.
119. Kister SJ, Sommers SC, Haagensen CD, et al: Nuclear grade and sinus histiocytosis in cancer of the breast, Cancer 23:570, 1969.
120. Komitowski D and Janson C: Quantitative features of chromatin structure in the prognosis of breast cancer, Cancer 65:2725, 1990.
121. Komitowski D, Kett P, Janson C, and Jarasch ED: Quantitative aspects in defining prognostic factors in breast cancer, Pathol Res Pract 185:621, 1989.
122. Koper PCM, van Putten WLJ, Wijnmaalen AJ, et al: Breast conserving surgery and radiotherapy in early stage breast cancer, Int J Radiat Oncol Biol Phys (in press).

123. Koscielny S, Le MG, and Tubiana M: The natural history of human breast cancer. The relationship between involvement of axillary lymph nodes and the initiation of distant metastases, Br J Cancer 59:775, 1989.
124. Koscielny S, Tubiana M, Le MG, et al: Breast cancer: relationship between size of the primary tumor and probability of metastatic dissemination, Br J Cancer 49:709, 1984.
125. Kouchoukos NT, Ackerman LV, and Butcher HR: Prediction of axillary nodal metastases from the morphology of primary mammary carcinomas. Guide of operative therapy, Cancer 20:948, 1967.
126. Kurtz JM, Jacquemier J, Amalric R, et al: Risk factors of breast recurrence in pre- and postmenopausal patients with ductal cancers, Cancer 65:1867, 1990.
127. Kurtz JM, Jacquemier J, Amalric R, et al: Why are local recurrences after breast conserving therapy more frequent in young patients? J Clin Oncol 8:591, 1990.
128. Kurtz JM, Jacquemier J, Torherst J, et al: Conservation therapy for breast cancers other than infiltrating ductal carcinoma, Cancer 63:1630, 1989.
129. Kurtz JM, Spitalier JM, Brandone H, et al: Mammary recurrences in women younger than forty, Int J Radiat Oncol Biol Phys 15:271, 1988.
130. Lagios MD: Multicentricity of breast carcinoma demonstrated by routine correlated serial subgross and radiographic examination, Cancer 40:1726, 1977.
131. Lagios MD, Richards UE, Rose MR, and Yee E: Segmental mastectomy without radiotherapy. Short-term follow-up, Cancer 52:2173, 1983.
132. Larsimont D, Kiss R, d'Olne D, et al: Relationship between computerized morphonuclear image analysis and histopathologic grading of breast cancer, Anal Quant Cytol Histol 11:433, 1989.
133. Le Doussal V, Tubiana-Hulin M, Friedman S, et al: Prognostic value of histologic grade nuclear components of Scarff-Bloom-Richardson (SBR), Cancer 64:1914, 1989.
134. Le Doussal V, Tubiana-Hulin M, Hacene K, et al: Nuclear characteristics as indicators of prognosis in node negative breast cancer patients, Breast Cancer Res Treat 14:207, 1989.
135. Lee AKC, DeLellis RA, Silverman ML, et al: Prognostic significance of peritumoral lymphatic and blood vessel invasion in node negative carcinoma of the breast, J Clin Oncol 8:1457, 1990.
136. Lee AKC, DeLellis RA, Silverman ML, and Wolfe HJ: Lymphatic and blood vessel invasion in breast carcinoma: a useful prognostic indicator? Hum Pathol 17(10):984, 1986.
137. Lee BJ, Hauser H, and Pack GT: Gelatinous carcinoma of the breast, Surg Gynecol Obstet 59:841, 1934.
138. Lee YN: Breast carcinoma: pattern of recurrence and metastasis after mastectomy, Am J Clin Oncol 7:443, 1984.
139. Lee YN and Chan LS: Surgical treatment of carcinoma of the breast: II. Prognostic factors influencing relapse rate, J Surg Oncol 25:102, 1984.
140. Lee Y-T N: Surgical treatment of carcinoma of the breast: III. Pathological finding and probability of relapse, J Surg Oncol 25:109, 1984.
141. Leopold KA, Recht A, Schnitt SJ, et al: Results of conservative surgery and radiation for multiple synchronous cancers of one breast, Int J Radiat Oncol Biol Phys 16:11, 1989.
142. Lesser ML, Rosen PP, and Kinne DW: Multicentricity and bilaterality in invasive breast carcinoma, Surgery 91:234, 1982.
143. Lindley R, Bulman A, Parsons P, et al: Histologic features predictive of an increased risk of early local recurrence after treatment of breast cancer by local tumor excision and radical radiotherapy, Surgery 105:13, 1989.
144. Ludwig Breast Cancer Group: Prolonged disease-free survival after one course of preoperative adjuvant chemotherapy for node-negative breast cancer, N Engl J Med 320:491, 1989.
145. Madden JL, Kanadalaft S, and Bourque R-A: Modified radical mastectomy, Ann Surg 175:724, 1972.
146. Maddox WA, Carpenter JT, Laws HL, et al: A randomized perspective trial of radical mastectomy versus modified radical mastectomy in 311 breast cancer patients, Ann Surg 198:207, 1983.
147. Maier WP, Goldman LI, and Tyson RR: A ten year study of medullary carcinoma of the breast, Surg Gynecol Obstet 144:695, 1977.
148. Mambo NC and Gallagher HS: Carcinoma of the breast. The prognostic significance of extranodal extension of axillary disease, Cancer 39:2280, 1977.
149. Mansour E, Eudey L, Shatile A, et al: Adjuvant therapy in node-negative breast cancer. Is it necessary for all patients? An intergroup study. In Salmon SE, editor: Adjuvant therapy of cancer VI, Philadelphia, 1990, WB Saunders Co, pp 174-189.
150. Mansour EG, Gray R, Shatile AH, et al: Efficacy of adjuvant chemotherapy in high-risk node-negative breast cancer. An Intergroup Study, N Engl J Med 320:485, 1989.
151. Martin JK, Van Heerden JA, Taylor WF, and Gaffey TA: Is modified radical mastectomy really equivalent to radical mastectomy in treatment of carcinoma of the breast, Cancer 57:510, 1986.
152. Mate TP, Cater D, Fischer DB, et al: A clinical and histopathologic analysis of the results of conservation surgery and radiation therapy in stage I and II breast carcinoma, Cancer 58:1994, 1986.
153. Maylin C, Socie G, Clot PH, et al: Five years local control after conservative treatment in breast cancer with intraoperative brachytherapy. Uni- and multivariate analysis of 410 cases stage I-II. UICC, St. Louis Hospital Experience—Paris. Proceedings of the Seventeenth International Congress of Radiation Oncology, Paris, 1989, p 49 (abstract).
154. McCormick B, Kinne D, Petrek J, et al: Limited resection for breast cancer: a study of inked specimen margins before radiotherapy, Int J Radiat Oncol Biol Phys 13:1667, 1987.
155. Mentzer SJ, Osteen RT, and Wilson RE: Local recurrence and the deep resection margin in carcinoma of the breast, Surg Gynecol Obstet 163:513, 1986.
156. Moon TE, Jones SE, Bonadonna G, et al: Development and use of a natural history data base of breast cancer studies, Am J Clin Oncol 10:396, 1987.
157. Moore OS and Foote FW: The relatively favorable prognosis of medullary carcinoma of the breast, Cancer 2:635, 1949.
158. Morgenstern L, Kaufman PA, and Friedman NB: The case against tylectomy for carcinoma of the breast. The factor of multicentricity, Am J Surg 130:251, 1975.
159. Morrow M, Evans J, Rosen PP, and Kinne DW: Does clearing of axillary lymph nodes contribute to accurate staging of breast carcinoma, Cancer 53:1329, 1984.
160. Nealon TF Jr, Nkongho A, Grossi CE, et al: Treatment of early cancer of the breast ($T_1N_0M_0$ and $T_2N_0M_0$) on the basis of histologic characteristics, Surgery 89:279, 1981.
161. Nemoto T, Vana J, Bedwani RN, et al: Results of a national survey by the American College of Surgeons, Cancer 45:2917, 1980.
162. Nime FA, Rosen PP, Thaler HT, et al: Prognostic significance of tumor emboli in intramammary lymphatics in patients with mammary carcinoma, Am J Surg Pathol 1:25, 1977.

163. Nobler MP and Venet L: Prognostic factors in patients undergoing curative irradiation for breast cancer, Int J Radiat Oncol Biol Phys 11:123, 1985.
164. Norris HJ and Taylor HB: Prognosis of mucinous (gelatinous) carcinoma of the breast, Cancer 18:879, 1965.
165. Oberman HA and Fidler WJ: Tubular carcinoma of the breast, Am J Surg Pathol 13:387, 1979.
166. Osteen RT, Connolly JL, Recht A, et al: Identification of patients at high risk for local recurrence after conservative surgery and radiation therapy for stage I or II breast cancer, Arch Surg 122:1248, 1987.
167. Owings D, Hann L and Schnitt S: How thoroughly should needle localization breast biopsies (NLBB) be sampled for microscopic examination? A prospective mammographic-pathologic correlative study, Mod Pathol 2:69A, 1989.
168. Page DL and Anderson TJ: Diagnostic histopathology of the breast, New York 1987, Churchill Livingstone.
169. Page DL, Dixon JM, Anderson TJ, et al: Invasive cribiform carcinoma of the breast, Histopathology 7:525, 1983.
170. Payne WS, Taylor WF, Khonsari S, et al: Surgical treatment of breast cancer. Trends and factors affecting survival, Arch Surg 101:105, 1970.
171. Peters GM, Wolff M, and Haagensen CD: Tubular carcinoma of the breast. Clinical pathologic correlations based on 100 cases, Ann Surg 193:138, 1981.
172. Pezner RD, Lipsett JA, Desai K, et al: To boost or not to boost: decreasing radiation therapy in conservative breast cancer treatment when "inked" tumor resection margins are pathologically free of cancer, Int J Radiat Oncol Biol Phys 14:873, 1988.
173. Pickren JW: Significance of occult metastases. A study of breast cancer, Cancer 14:1266, 1961.
174. Primary Therapy of Breast Cancer Study Group: Identification of patients with high risk of early recurrence after radical mastectomy: II. Clinical and pathologic correlations: a report of the Primary Therapy of Breast Cancer Study Group, Cancer 42:2808, 1978.
175. Rank F, Dombernowsky P, Jespersen NCB, et al: Histologic malignancy grading of invasive ductal breast carcinoma. A regression analysis of prognostic factors in low-risk carcinomas from a multicenter trial, Cancer 60:1299, 1987.
176. Rapin V, Contesso G, Mouriesse H, et al: Medullary breast carcinoma. A reevaluation of 95 cases of breast cancer with inflammatory stroma, Cancer 61:2503, 1988.
177. Recht A, Silen W, Schnitt SJ, et al: Time course of local recurrence following conservative surgery and radiotherapy for early stage breast cancer, Int J Radiat Oncol Biol Phys 15:255, 1988.
178. Richardson WW: Medullary carcinoma of the breast. A distinctive tumor type with a relatively good prognosis following radical mastectomy, Br J Cancer 10:415, 1956.
179. Ridolfi RL, Rosen PP, Port A, et al: Medullary carcinoma of the breast. A clinicopathologic study with 10 year follow-up, Cancer 40:1365, 1977.
180. Robinson GN, Van Heerden JA, Payne WS, et al: The primary surgical treatment of carcinoma of the breast. A changing trend toward modified radical mastectomy, Mayo Clin Proc 51:433, 1976.
181. Roger V, Beito G, and Jolly PC: Factors affecting the incidence of lymph node metastases in small cancers of the breast, Am J Surg 157:501, 1989.
182. Rosen PP: The pathologic classification of human mammary carcinoma: past, present and future. Ann Clin Lab Sci 9:144, 1979.
183. Rosen PP: Tumor emboli in intramammary lymphatics in breast carcinoma: pathologic criteria for diagnosis and clinical significance, Pathol Annu 18(Part 2):215, 1983.
184. Rosen PP, Fracchia AA, Urban JA, et al: "Residual" mammary carcinoma following simulated partial mastectomy, Cancer 35:739, 1975.
185. Rosen PP and Groshen S: Survival and prognostic factors in node negative breast cancer: results of long-term follow-up studies. Presented at the NIH Consensus Conference Treatment of Early Stage Breast Cancer, Bethesda, Md, June 1990.
186. Rosen PP, Groshen S, Saigo PE, et al: Pathologic prognostic factors in stage I ($T_1N_0M_0$) and stage II ($T_1N_1M_0$) breast carcinoma: a study of 644 patients with medial follow-up of 18 years, J Clin Oncol 7:1239, 1989.
187. Rosen PP, Kinne DW, Lesser M, and Hellman S: Are prognostic factors for local control of breast cancer treated by primary radiotherapy significant for patients treated by mastectomy? Cancer 57:1415, 1986.
188. Rosen PP, Saigo PE, Braun DW, et al: Predictors of recurrence in stage I ($T_1N_0M_0$) breast carcinoma, Ann Surg 193:15, 1981.
189. Rosen PP, Saigo PE, Braun DW, et al: Axillary micro and macrometastases in breast cancer. Prognostic significance of tumor size, Ann Surg 194:585, 1981.
190. Rosen PP, Saigo PE, Braun DW, et al: Prognosis in stage II ($T_1N_1M_0$) breast cancer, Ann Surg 194:576, 1981.
191. Rosenman J, Bernard S, Kober C, et al: Local recurrences in patients with breast cancer treated at the North Carolina Memorial Hospital, Cancer 57:1421, 1986.
192. Roses DF, Bell DA, Fiotte TJ, et al: Pathologic predictors of recurrence in stage I ($T_1N_0M_0$) breast cancer, Am J Clin Pathol 78:817, 1982.
193. Rosner D and Lane WW: Node-negative minimal invasive breast cancer patients are not candidates for routine systemic adjuvant therapy, Cancer 66:199, 1990.
194. Russo J, Frederick J, Ownby HE, et al: Predictors of recurrence and survival of patients with breast cancer, Am J Clin Pathol 88:123, 1987.
195. Ryoo ME, Kagan AR, Wollin M, et al: Prognostic factors for recurrence and cosmesis in 393 patients after radiation therapy for early mammary carcinoma, Radiology 172:555, 1989.
196. Saigo PE and Rosen PP: The application of immunohistochemical stains to identify endothelial-lined channels in mammary carcinoma, Cancer 59:51, 1987.
197. Sampat MB, Sirsat MV, and Gangadharan P: Prognostic significance of blood vessel invasion in carcinoma of the breast in women, J Surg Oncol 9:623, 1977.
198. Sarrazin D, Le M, Mouriesse H, et al: Radiotherapeutic studies in breast cancer at Villejuif, Cancer Bull 34:242, 1982.
199. Say CC and Donegan WL: Invasive carcinoma of the breast: prognostic significance of tumor size and involved axillary lymph nodes, Cancer 34:468, 1984.
200. Scarff RW and Handley RS: Prognosis in carcinoma of the breast, Lancet ii:582, 1938.
201. Schmidt-Ullrich R, Wazer DE, Tercilla O, et al: Tumor margin assessment as a guide to optimal conservation surgery and irradiation in early stage breast cancer, Int J Radiat Oncol Biol Phys 17:733, 1989.
202. Schnitt SJ and Wang H: Histologic sampling of grossly benign breast biopsies. How much is enough? Am J Surg Pathol 13(6):505, 1989.
203. Schnitt SJ, Connolly JL, Harris JR, et al: Pathologic predictors of early local recurrence in Stage I and II breast cancer treated by primary radiation therapy, Cancer 53:1049, 1984.
204. Schnitt SJ, Connolly JL, Khettry U, et al: Pathologic findings on re-excision of the primary site in breast cancer patients considered for treatment by primary radiation therapy, Cancer 59:675, 1987.
205. Schnitt SJ, Connolly JL, Recht A, et al: Influence of

infiltrating lobular histology on local tumor control in breast cancer patients treated with conservative surgery and radiotherapy, Cancer 64:448, 1989.
206. Schnitt SJ, Connolly JL, Silver B, et al: Updated results on the influence of pathologic features on treatment outcome in Stage I and II breast cancer patients treated by primary radiation therapy, Int J Radiat Oncol Biol Phys 11:104, 1985 (abstract).
207. Schottenfeld D, Nash AG, Robbins GF, and Beattie EJ: Ten-year results of the treatment of primary operable breast carcinoma. A summary of 304 patients evaluated in the TNM system, Cancer 38:1001, 1976.
208. Sears HG, Janus C, Levy W, et al: Breast cancer without axillary metastases. Are there high risk biologic subpopulations? Cancer 50:1820, 1982.
209. Sedmak DD, Meineke TA, and Knechtges DS: Detection of metastatic breast carcinoma with monoclonal antibodies to cytokeratins, Arch Pathol Lab Med 113:786, 1989.
210. Sedmak DD, Meineke TA, Knechtges DS, and Anderson J: Prognostic significance of cytokeratin-positive breast cancer metastases, Mod Pathol 2(5):516, 1989.
211. Semiglazov VF, Bavli JL, Moiseyenko VM, et al: Clinical trials on adjuvant chemotherapy for breast cancer, Cancer 57:1957, 1985.
212. Shah JA, Rosen PP, and Robbins GF: Pitfalls of local excision in the treatment of carcinoma of the breast, Surg Gynecol Obstet 136:721, 1973.
213. Shek LLM and Godolphin W: Model for breast cancer survival: Relative prognostic roles of axillary nodal status, TNM stage, estrogen receptor concentration, and tumor necrosis, Cancer Res 48:5565, 1988.
214. Sigurdsson H, Baldetorp B, Borg A, et al: Indicators of prognosis in node-negative breast cancer, N Engl J Med 322:1045, 1990.
215. Silverberg SG and Chitale AR: Assessment of significance of proportions of intraductal and infiltrating tumor growth in ductal carcinoma of the breast, Cancer 32:830, 1973.
216. Silverberg SG, Kay S, Chitale AR, and Levitt SH: Colloid carcinoma of the breast, Am J Clin Pathol 55:355, 1971.
217. Silvestrini R, Daidone MG, DiFronzo G, et al: Prognostic implication of labeling index versus estrogen receptors and tumor size in node negative breast cancer, Breast Cancer Res Treat 7:161, 1986.
218. Singletary SE and McNeese M: Segmental mastectomy and irradiation in the treatment of breast cancer, Am J Clin Oncol 11:679, 1988.
219. Smith JA, Gamez-Araujo JJ, Gallagher HS, et al: Carcinoma of the breast. Analysis of total lymph node involvement versus level of metastasis, Cancer 39:527, 1977.
220. Snyder M and Tobon H: Primary mucinous carcinoma of the breast. Breast, Diseases of the Breast 3:17, 1977.
221. Solin LJ, Fowble B, Martz KL, and Goodman RL: Definitive irradiation for early stage breast cancer: the University of Pennsylvania Experience, Int J Radiat Oncol Biol Phys 14:235, 1988.
222. Spitalier JM, Gambarelli J, Brandone H, et al: Breast conserving surgery with radiation therapy for operable mammary carcinoma: a 25 year experience, World J Surg 10:1014, 1986.
223. Stenkvist B, Bengtsson E, Dahlqvist B, et al: Predicting breast cancer recurrence, Cancer 50:2884, 1982.
224. Teel P: Vascular invasion as a prognostic factor in breast carcinoma, Surg Gynecol Obstet 118:1006, 1964.
225. Tinnemans JGM, Wobbes T, Van der Sluis RF, et al: Multicentricity in nonpalpable breast carcinoma and its implications for treatment, Am J Surg 151:334, 1986.
226. Trojani M, de Mascarel I, Bonichon F, et al: Micrometastases to axillary lymph nodes from carcinoma of breast: detection of immunohistochemistry and prognostic significance, Br J Cancer 55:303, 1987.
227. Valagussa P, Bonadonna G, and Veronesi U: Patterns of relapse and survival following radical mastectomy: analysis of 716 consecutive patients, Cancer 41:1170, 1978.
228. Van de Velde CJH, Gallagher S, and Giacco GG: Prognosis in node-negative breast cancer, Breast Cancer Res Treat 8:189, 1986.
229. Van Limbergen E, Van der Bogaert W, Van der Schueren E, et al: Tumor excision and radiotherapy as primary treatment of breast cancer analysis of patient and treatment parameters and local control, Radiother Oncol 8:1, 1987.
230. Venable JG, Schwartz AM, and Silverberg SG: Infiltrating cribiform carcinoma of the breast: a distinctive clinicopathologic entity, Hum Pathol 21:333, 1990.
231. Veronesi U, Banfi A, DelVecchio M, et al: Comparison of Halsted mastectomy with quadrantectomy, axillary dissection and radiotherapy in early breast cancer: long-term results, Eur J Cancer Clin Oncol 22:1085, 1986.
232. Veronesi U, Salvadori B, Luini A, et al: Conservative treatment of early breast cancer. Long-term results of 1232 cases treated with quadrantectomy axillary dissection and radiotherapy, Ann Surg 211:250, 1990.
233. Volterrani F, Veronesi U, Marubini E, et al: TART vs. QUART in the treatment of T1-2 (≤2.5 cm) N0 N1a,b M0 breast cancer. Proceedings of the seventh annual meeting of the European Society for Therapeutic Radiology and Oncology, Den Haag, 1988, p 212.
234. Wargotz ES and Silverberg SG: Medullary carcinoma of the breast: a clinicopathologic study with appraisal of current diagnostic criteria, Hum Pathol 11:1340, 1988.
235. Weigan RA, Isenberg WM, Russo J, et al: Blood vessel invasion and axillary lymph node involvement as prognostic indicators for human breast cancer, Cancer 50:962, 1982.
236. Westman-Naeser S, Bengtsson E, Eriksson O, et al: Multifocal breast cancer, Am J Surg 142:255, 1981.
237. Wetzels RHW, Holland R, Van Haelstr UJGM, et al: Detection of basement membrane components and basal cell keratin 14 in noninvasive and invasive carcinomas of the breast, Am J Pathol 134(3):571, 1989.
238. Wilkinson EJ, Hause LL, Hoffman RG, et al: Occult axillary lymph node metastases in invasive breast carcinoma: characteristics of the primary tumor and significance of the metastases, Pathol Annu 17:67, 1982.
239. Williams MR, Hinton CP, Toddy JH, et al: The prediction of local or regional recurrence after simple mastectomy for operable breast cancer, Br J Surg 72:721, 1985.
240. Wilson RE, Donegan WL, Mettlin C, et al: The 1982 national survey of carcinoma of the breast in the United States by the American College of Surgeons, Surg Gynecol Obstet 159:309, 1984.
241. Winchester DJ, Duda RB, August CZ, et al: The importance of DNA flow cytometry in node-negative breast cancer, Arch Surg 125:886, 1990.
242. Zafrani B, Vielh P, Fourquet A, et al: Conservative treatment of early breast cancer: prognostic value of ductal in situ component and other pathologic variables on local control and survival. Long term results, Eur J Cancer Clin Oncol 11:1645, 1989.
243. Zambetti M, Valagussa P, Brambilla C, et al: Adjuvant CMF in node-negative and estrogen receptor negative breast cancer: updated results, Proc Am Soc Clin Oncol 8:21, 1989.

8 Biologic Markers of Breast Cancer Prognosis

Marisa C. Weiss and Martin L. Kelsten

The investigative efforts of a great many scientists in both basic and clinical research have been devoted to understanding the biology of breast cancer. From laboratory studies of the pathogenesis and metastatic potential of breast cancer, several protein products and genetic factors have been identified that may play important roles in the etiology and progression of breast cancer. Some of these molecular factors also have proved to be valuable predictors of clinical outcome in large series of patients. These "biologic markers" have been incorporated into treatment protocols as prognostic factors used to make important therapeutic decisions, such as the need for adjuvant chemotherapy in otherwise low-risk patients, or the need for more intensive chemotherapy with bone marrow rescue for high-risk patients. This chapter discusses estrogen and progesterone receptors, cathepsin D, heat shock proteins, DNA ploidy and proliferative indices, the HER-2/neu oncogene, and the epithelial growth factor receptor, all of which appear to have prognostic value in women with operable breast cancer.

Of all the clinicopathologic features of breast cancer that have been evaluated as prognostic factors, the presence of metastasis to axillary lymph nodes is clearly the most powerful predictor of outcome. However, there is a need for additional independent prognostic factors because the predictive power of lymph node status alone or in combination with other clinical factors is insufficient. For example, several studies of node-negative breast cancer patients demonstrated that 30% failed and 70% did well without adjuvant therapy.[55,63,104] This result implies that 70% of node-negative patients who received adjuvant therapy were treated unnecessarily. Similar problems apply in the operable node-positive patient group, where clinicopathologic factors fail to predict individual patient outcomes with sufficient certainty to base treatment on those factors alone. The 1990 National Institutes of Health (NIH) Consensus Conference concluded that "at present there is no reliable system for estimating an individual's risk of recurrence and death using available prognostic factors."[124a] Using the new prognostic parameters based on the molecular markers mentioned above, we will try to develop reasonable guidelines to address the two major clinical questions in the modern treatment of breast cancer: (1) which node-negative patients may benefit from adjuvant chemotherapy? and (2) which node-positive patients may benefit from intensified chemotherapy?

HORMONAL RECEPTORS

Both progesterone and estrogen play a role in the regulation of cell growth and differentiation in normal breast tissue. Their effects are mediated by specific receptors that bind their respective ligands and transport them to the nucleus. Estrogen is thought to stimulate the growth of estrogen-positive breast cancers through the same ligand-receptor mechanism that mediates its effect in normal tissue. The expression of progesterone receptors, in both normal breast and in human breast cancer cell lines, depends on estrogen stimulation.[79,110] Progesterone receptor (PR) positivity therefore signifies an intact estrogen receptor (ER)–dependent signal transduction pathway in the cell.[83] Because estrogen and progesterone appear to mediate some of the same growth regulatory functions in breast cancer cell lines in vitro as they do in normal tissues, it is reasonable to hypothesize that the presence and number of both hormone receptors in breast cancer correlates with the clinical behavior of the disease.

Methodology

There are many biochemical methods for steroid receptor analysis, but the most widely used technique, the dextran-coated charcoal assay, is based on the biochemical measurements of classic ligand binding interactions.[95,117] In short, radiolabeled hormones in competition with radioinert hormones are added in varying amounts to disrupted cells. Dextran-coated charcoal is added to adsorb nonspecific and unbound ligands, and the resultant radioactivity is quantitated. Although this assay is relatively simple and can be performed on a large number of samples, a radioactive probe is required and relatively large amounts of tissue are needed. Other biochemical methods include measurement of sucrose density gradients, chromatography, isoelectric focusing, and the like, which are laborious and, often, more expensive.

Morphologic methods have the advantage of permitting direct correlation of histology with receptor status, especially in specimens too small for biochemical assay. Reliable commercial antibodies have made these methods widely available. The estrogen receptor immunocytochemical assay (ER-ICA) is the most commonly used technique. It is a chromogen-conjugated antireceptor antibody technique (Fig. 8-1), which stains the nucleus predominantly, in contrast to the mostly cytosol identification of receptors in biochemical methods.[125,129] ER-ICA correlates in the 80% range with the dextran-coated charcoal assay and enzyme immunoassays.[44,71] This technique allows testing of small, paraffin-embedded tumors[148] and cytologic samples[58,103] originally too small for analysis. It overcomes the effect of stromal dilution, reveals receptor heterogeneity within samples, and allows confirmation that the receptor measured is within tumor cells. Similar biochemical and immunohistochemical methods have been developed for progesterone receptors.[21,136] Also available are immunoradiometric assays[21,66] and enzyme-linked immunoassays.[54,71] However, these methods have problems similar to those of other biochemical ligand-receptor interaction assays.[66] A promising antiestradiol immunoperoxidase assay has been recently reported.[125]

Quantitation is difficult to achieve with immunocytochemical methods. Image cytometric analysis does offer quantitation. Correlation with the dextran-coated charcoal assay is good and objective scores of heterogeneity and density also can be obtained.[30,38] Flow cytometric analysis[34,65,172] is not yet widely used.

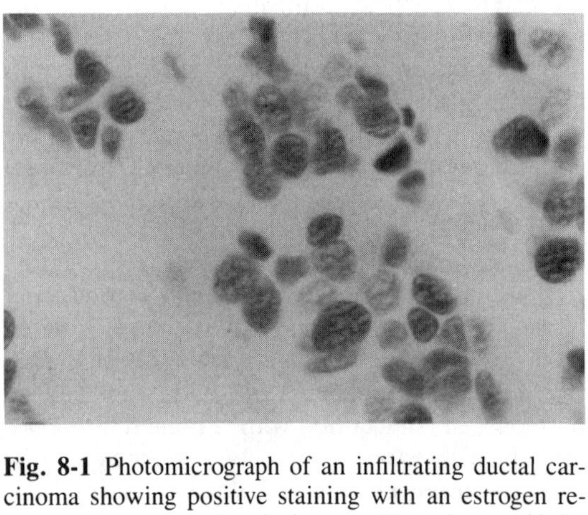

Fig. 8-1 Photomicrograph of an infiltrating ductal carcinoma showing positive staining with an estrogen receptor immunocytochemical assay. Note the specificity of staining for tumor nuclei and the heterogeneity of staining demonstrated throughout the field (400×).

Difficulty interpreting hormone receptor status. There is considerable variation in the cut-off point used to define hormone receptor positivity, and the basis for determining the cut-off value is not usually stated. Values range from 3 fmol/mg protein,[32] to 8[70,105,151,185] up to 10.[5,23,56,90,92,149] The cut-off point was not stated in two of the studies.[91,145]

This variability may not be important in determining prognosis as there does not appear to be a dose-response relationship between level of receptor positivity and prognosis. In fact, the actual level of ER positivity did not seem to affect the outcome in two large series: the prognostic power of ER did not improve as values increased from 3 to 10 fmol/mg protein[23] and from 10 to ≥100 fmol/mg protein.[56] Further, one study showed that increasing levels of progesterone receptors above 10 fmol/mg protein did not improve outcome.[56] But in another large study, patient outcome was directly proportional to the level of progesterone receptor positivity.[34] The variation in criteria for receptor positivity may compromise one's ability to predict a woman's response to hormonal therapy, however, because response to hormonal therapy clearly depends on the level of estrogen receptor positivity[16,110,129,132,141]: 40% to 80% of ER-positive tumors respond to hormone therapy (depending on the concentration of receptors), whereas <10% of ER-negative tumors respond. The highest response to hormonal therapy is seen in tumors that are both ER and PR positive.

In addition to the lack of consistent definition of ER positivity, one's difficulty in interpreting the literature is compounded by the substantial variability of ER measurements within the same tumor resulting from sampling variation. Intrinsic tumor heterogeneity is associated with variable levels of ER positivity; in some cases, some parts of the tumor are ER positive and other parts are ER negative. There is also the dilutional effect of nontumorous tissue within the sample analyzed.

The correlation between hormone receptor status and other prognostic variables

Sixty-four percent of premenopausal women and 75% of postmenopausal women had ER-positive tumors ($p < .05$), and 58% and 53% of these groups, respectively, were PR-positive ($p = .07$) in an analysis of 2800 women.[35] Hormone receptor status is dependent on histologic subtype: estrogen receptors are identified most commonly in lobular

Table 8-1 The correlation between EGFR and classic prognostic variables

Author	Tumor size	Stage	Age	Menopausal status	Histologic/ Nuclear grade	Lymph node status	ER/PR
Battaglia et al.[14]	—	—	—	—	—	Yes	Yes
Bolla et al.[18]	—	No	—	—	Yes	No	Yes
Reubi and Torhorst[139]	—	—	—	—	—	—	Yes
Sainsbury et al.[142]	Yes	—	—	—	Yes	No	Yes
Sainsbury et al.[143]	—	—	No	—	Yes	Yes	Yes
Toi et al.[168]	No	No	—	No	Yes	No	Yes

Yes, statistically significant ($p \leq .05$); No, not statistically significant.

carcinoma, tubular carcinoma, and mucinous carcinoma. They are common in medullary carcinoma and of intermediate prevalence in ductal carcinoma.[75] An inverse correlation has been demonstrated between receptor status and histologic grade (well-differentiated cancers are more often ER positive than poorly differentiated cancers),[75,103] pathologic stage (early-stage cancers are more often ER positive than advanced-stage lesions),[16,165] and epithelial growth factor receptor (EGFR) oncogene expression (EGFR positivity is more common in ER-negative than ER-positive cancers) (Table 8-1).

THE PROGNOSTIC VALUE OF HORMONE RECEPTOR STATUS

Operable breast cancer

Many studies have examined the prognostic value of ER status on disease-free survival and overall survival in operable breast cancer. Most were able to demonstrate a statistically significant disease-free and overall survival advantage for ER-positive patients in the range of 7% to 17%.

In an early study by Knight et al.,[92] ER status was shown as an independent predictor of disease-free survival, a finding confirmed by other investigators. Clark and McGuire[32] showed that ER positivity predicted a longer disease-free and overall survival regardless of axillary nodal status. Allegra et al.[5] showed that ER status had independent prognostic value, but were unable to show (in a small number of patients) an association between progesterone receptor status and disease-free survival. In a review by Hahnel et al.[70] there was a significant difference in disease-free survival at 3 years, but not at 5 years. A 3-year disease-free survival advantage for ER-positive patients, seen primarily in node-negative individuals, also was demonstrated by Cooke et al.[40] In contrast, Williams et al.[185] could not demonstrate an association between ER status and the length of the disease-free interval.

An overall survival advantage to patients with ER-positive tumors was reported by Hahnel et al.[70] ER-positive patients had an 173-month interval between mastectomy and death, compared to 87 months for patients with ER-negative cancers ($p < .05$). Two other studies confirmed this survival advantage, but were unable to demonstrate a definite disease-free survival advantage.[90,105] Progesterone receptors predicted both disease-free and overall survival in the study by Mason et al.[105] (Table 8-2). Multivariate analysis revealed a significant association between ER or PR status and overall survival, but the relationship between ER or PR status and disease-free survival was not significant. When the two hormone receptors were analyzed as a combined parameter, however, a significant difference in overall and disease-free survival occurred between ER-positive/PR-positive and ER-negative/PR-negative patients, in both node-positive and node-negative patients.

In addition to survival outcome, several investigators have correlated the presence of estrogen receptors with the pattern of metastatic failure. ER-negative bony metastases.[16,24,36,138]

Node-negative patients

The association of hormone receptor status and patient outcome in node-negative women has been evaluated in many studies in an attempt to identify a group of high-risk patients who may benefit from adjuvant chemotherapy. Some of the above studies examined the value of hormone receptor status in this subset of women, and additional studies focused exclusively on this group of women.

A statistically significant correlation between ER positivity and disease-free and/or overall survival has been demonstrated by many studies (Tables 8-2 and 8-3). Knight et al. was one of the first to show a difference in recurrence between ER-positive and ER-negative cancers,[92] an association confirmed by Cooke et al.[40] They showed that ER-negative patients had a lower 3-year disease-free

Table 8-2 Correlation between progesterone receptor status and patient outcome in axillary node-negative patients

Author	No. pts.	Follow-up (yr)	Disease-free survival (%)		Distant disease-free survival (%)		Overall survival (%)		Statistical significance of the differences between PR-positive and PR-negative pts.		
			PR-positive	PR-negative	PR-positive	PR-negative	PR-positive	PR-negative	Disease-free survival	Distant disease-free survival	Overall survival
Fisher et al.[56]*	1157	5	72	68	79	74	91	83	No	No	Yes
Mason et al.[105]†	224	2.6	82	80	—	—	94	89	No	—	No
Sigurdsson et al.[149]*	325	4	85	75	89	77	92	79	Yes	Yes	Yes

*PR positivity = 10 fmol/mg protein.
†PR positivity = 1 fmol/mg protein.

Table 8-3 Correlation between estrogen receptor status and patient outcome in axillary node-negative patients

Author	No. pts.	Follow-up (yr)	Disease-free survival (%)		Distant disease-free survival (%)		Overall survival (%)		Patient outcome		
			ER-positive	ER-negative	ER-positive	ER-negative	ER-positive	ER-negative	Disease-free survival	Distant disease-free survival	Overall survival
Allegra et al.[5]	82	2	90	73	—	—	—	—	Yes	—	—
Butler et al.[23]	556	6.3	83	86	—	—	94	91	No	—	No
Clark and McGuire[32]	2840	3.3	59	52	—	—	—	—	Yes	—	—
Cooke et al.[40]	245	3	94	30	—	—	—	—	Yes	—	—
Fisher et al.[56]	1157	5	74	66	80	72	92	82	Yes	Yes	Yes
Hahnel et al.[70]	161	3 for OS 5 for DFS	71	71	—	—	57	40	No	—	Yes
Kinne et al.[90]	553	1.2	[96]	95	—	—	99	99	[No]	—	No
Klintenberg et al.[91]	90	5	[82]	80	—	—	—	—	[No]	—	—
Knight et al.[92]	71	1.5	94	88	—	—	—	—	—	—	—
Mason et al.[105]	224	2.6	84	81	—	—	95	87	No	—	Yes
Sears et al.[145]	155	6	88	78	—	—	72	68	Yes	—	—
Sigurdsson et al.[149]	367	4	83	76	89	76	91	78	No	Yes	Yes
Silvestrini et al.[151]	215	5	[79]	62	—	—	—	—	[Yes]	—	—
Valagussa et al.[171]	422	3	82	45	—	—	—	—	Yes	—	—
Williams et al.[185]	401	7	60	60	—	—	70	70	No	—	No

[ ], relapse-free survival; DFS, disease-free survival; OS, overall survival; Yes, statistically significant ($p \leq .05$); No, not statistically significant.

survival rate than ER-positive patients. In fact, node-negative/ER-negative patients had a recurrence rate similar to all node-positive patients. Allegra et al.[5] showed a 17% difference in recurrence rates between ER-positive and ER-negative patients. Clark and McGuire[32] from San Antonio demonstrated a 9% reduction in 12-year disease-free survival in ER-negative patients, compared to patients with ER-positive tumors. Multivariate analysis of the San Antonio patients by Benner et al.[16] in the same year revealed that ER status and tumor size were the most important prognostic variables in 1461 node-negative patients. Patients with ER-positive tumors had a range of disease-free and overall survival of 83% to 64% and 88% to 83%, respectively, as tumor size increased from <2 to >5 cm. The range of disease-free and overall survival rates was 70% to 66% and 83% to 60% for patients with ER-negative tumors, depending on tumor size. The latest update on this patient population[33] showed a strong association between ER status and the rates of disease-free survival in 2264 node-negative women, but with only a 1.49 relative risk of recurrence. PR status did not correlate with disease-free survival.

Valagussa et al.[171] found a 37% difference in 5-year disease-free survival between ER-positive and ER-negative patients. Later, Silvestrini et al.,[151] from the same institution showed that ER status was only significant with respect to relapse-free and overall survival on univariate analysis. In a review by Mason et al.,[105] ER status affected overall survival, but not disease-free survival. PR status by itself did not chart patient outcome, but when combined with ER status, node-negative ER-negative/PR-negative patients showed a significant reduction in survival rate compared to node-positive ER-positive/PR-positive patients. Sigurdsson et al.[149] analyzed patient outcome in 346 Swedish women with ER determinations and 325 with PR determinations. Multivariate analysis revealed that S-phase fraction (SPF) had the most prognostic power, followed by PR and tumor size. They devised a prognostic model consisting of three co-variables: SPF, PR status, and tumor size. The combined parameters identified a high risk group (37% of node-negative patients) having a fourfold increased risk of distant recurrence, compared to the low-risk group of women (63%) with only a 3% incidence of distant metastases. Survival in the favorable group was similar to the expected survival of an age-matched group of normal Swedish women. Hahnel et al.[70] reported a 17% survival advantage of ER-positive patients compared to ER-negative patients.

Finally, Fisher et al. evaluated the prognostic importance of both ER and PR status in node-negative patients treated on the NSABP B-06 trial.[56] The 5-year disease-free, distant disease-free, and overall survival rates were significantly greater in ER-postive patients, than in ER-negative patients, but the difference was only 8% for both disease-free and distant disease-free survival, and 10% for overall survival. The difference in distant and disease-free survival, however, was only found to be significant in women ≥50 years of age. Multivariate analysis showed that ER status was significant with respect to survival only. Patients with PR-positive tumors had an 8% better 5-year overall survival than those with PR-negative tumors (seen mostly in women ≤49 years of age) on univariate analysis only. There was no significant difference in 5-year disease-free or distant disease-free survival between PR-positive and PR-negative patients. Three hundred and thirty-two patients, had an unknown ER or PR status, and these patients had outcomes similar to those of patients with ER-positive or PR-positive tumors, respectively. This is probably because unknown hormone status usually involves small tumors insufficient in size for the assay.

No prognostic value for ER could be demonstrated by Williams et al.,[185] Sears et al.,[145] Klintenberg et al.,[91] or Kinne et al.[90] These studies showed the same disease-free and overall survival rates for both the ER-positive and ER-negative patients. Furthermore, Butler et al.[23] could not demonstrate a statistically significant difference in disease-free or overall survival rates between ER-positive and ER-negative patients, even when the criteria for receptor positivity was increased from 3 to 10 fmol/mg protein.

Node-positive patients

Hormone receptor status predicts overall survival but has not consistently predicted disease-free survival in node-positive breast cancer patients by univariate analysis (Table 8-4).

Mason et al.[105] found a survival advantage for patients with ER-positive as well as PR-positive tumors. A 26% difference in overall survival rates between ER-positive and ER-negative patients was reported by Hahnel et al.[70] Although Williams et al.[185] also demonstrated an association between ER status and overall survival, this was not independent of histologic grade.

A disease-free survival difference of 13% and 33% was observed by Williams et al.[185] and Klintenberg et al.,[91] respectively. Mason et al.[105] demonstrated an overall survival-rate improvement in ER-positive (94% vs. 77%) and PR-positive (96% vs. 81%) patients and a disease-free survival improvement in PR-positive patients (68% vs. 53%). Allegra et al.[5] showed no difference in re-

Table 8-4 Correlation between estrogen receptor status and patient outcome in axillary node-positive patients

			Disease-free survival (%)		Overall survival (%)		Statistical significance of the difference between ER-positive and ER-negative pts.	
	No. pts.	Median follow-up (yr)	ER-positive	ER-negative	ER-positive	ER-negative	Disease-free survival	Overall survival
Allegra et al.[5]	41*	2	90	67	—	—	—	—
Clark and McGuire[32]	670	3.3	40	38	—	—	No	—
Hahnel et al.[70]	161	3 (length)	—	—	32	6	—	Yes
Kinne et al.[90]	450	1.2	89†	83†	95	87	(Yes)*	Yes*
Klintenberg et al.[91]	107	5	64†	31†	—	—	(Yes)	—
Mason et al.[105]	150	2.6	61	55	94	77	No	Yes
Williams et al.[185]	303	12	28	15	48	25	—	—

*Limited to pts. with four or more positive lymph nodes.
†Recurrence-free survival.

currence between ER-positive and ER-negative patients with one to three positive lymph nodes; however, in patients with four or more positive lymph nodes, ER-positive patients had a 10% failure rate (2/20) compared to 33% (7/21) in ER-negative patients. Similarly, Kinne et al.[90] could only demonstrate a difference in relapse-free and overall survival in patients with four or more positive lymph nodes. Hormone receptor status did not predict recurrence rate in a report by Cooke et al.[40]

Clark et al.[34] correlated hormone receptor status and disease-free survival in 318 node-positive patients. PR and ER status were significantly associated with disease-free survival by univariate analysis. But by multivariate analysis (including the following factors: number of involved lymph nodes, tumor size, age, ER status, PR status, menopausal status), only the number of positive lymph nodes and the level of PR had independent prognostic significance. With increasing levels of progesterone receptors, disease-free survival rates improved. A decreasing disease-free survival for ER-positive/PR-positive, ER-positive/PR-negative, and ER-negative/PR-negative patients was demonstrated, with a significant difference between the first two groups, but only a marginal difference in disease-free survival advantage between the second and third groups. In this small number of patients, these results suggest that PR status may be more significant than ER status with regard to disease-free survival. ER status did not offer any prognostic information beyond what the other factors provided. The population studied, however, was not representative of the whole population of women treated on the trial because only 60% of the patients had PR status determined, and these patients had a shorter overall disease-free survival compared to the patients with unknown PR status. Therefore the association of progesterone receptor status and outcome cannot be generalized to the rest of the women in the trial. Later, in 1988, Clark reported only a 5% difference in disease-free survival rates at 12 years between patients with ER-positive and ER-negative tumors.[32] Finally, in a 1989 update, PR status had a strong influence on disease-free survival in 1885 patients from the San Antonio Tumor Bank; ER status had none.[33]

Summary

In node-negative patients with primary breast cancer, there is a strong association between estrogen receptor positivity and improved disease-free and overall survival on multivariate analysis; however, the magnitude of the survival improvement in most studies is only 8% to 10%. These small differences in survival rates indicate that estrogen receptor status alone is an insufficient criterion for the selection of women who may benefit from adjuvant therapy.[56,111,113] When estrogen receptor status is combined with other prognostic parameters such as tumor size, ploidy, and S-phase fraction, much stronger criteria for the selection of patients for adjuvant chemotherapy emerge.

Essentially all studies show a limited prognostic role for progesterone receptor status in node-negative breast cancer patients.

In node-positive patients, ER status predicts 7% to 26% differences in rates of overall survival. When these differences are statistically significant, it is by univariate, not multivariate analysis. The role of ER status in predicting disease- or relapse-free survival is even less clear. In the poor prognostic group of patients with four or more positive lymph nodes, ER negativity may confer an even worse outcome. PR status may have greater prognostic power than ER status in node-positive patients, primarily with respect to disease-free survival.

The main value of both hormone receptors is predicting a response to hormonal manipulation in early and advanced breast cancer patients.[16,110,129,132,141] Level of receptor positivity is also important in predicting hormone treatment response.

DNA CONTENT ANALYSIS

General

There is a rapidly growing experience in the use of the DNA index (aneuploidy vs. diploidy) and the proliferative index (% S, % G_2/M, or % S + % G_2/M) to assess the prognosis of breast cancer patients and to select women for adjuvant systemic therapy.

Two measurements of DNA content within tumors routinely are reported: relative DNA content (ploidy analysis) and cell proliferation. Relative DNA content is expressed as the DNA index (DI), the ratio of the modal DNA content of the G_0/G_1 population of the abnormal population to that of the normal population (Fig. 8-2). A diploid population has a normal DNA content, an aneuploid population an abnormal DNA content. Most aneuploid tumors contain excess DNA (hyperdiploid, tetraploid, hypertetraploid, and multiploid). Only about 5% contain less than the normal amount of DNA (hypodiploid). Cell proliferative indices include the parameters % S, % G_2/M, or % S + % G_2/M; however, % S, otherwise called S-phase fraction, is used most commonly.

Of all breast carcinomas, 55% to 90% are aneuploid; of ductal carcinomas alone, 60% to 70%.[31,42,51] In the largest analysis available, of 21,480 specimens examined for both ploidy and S-phase fraction, 10,000 were aneuploid, and 68%

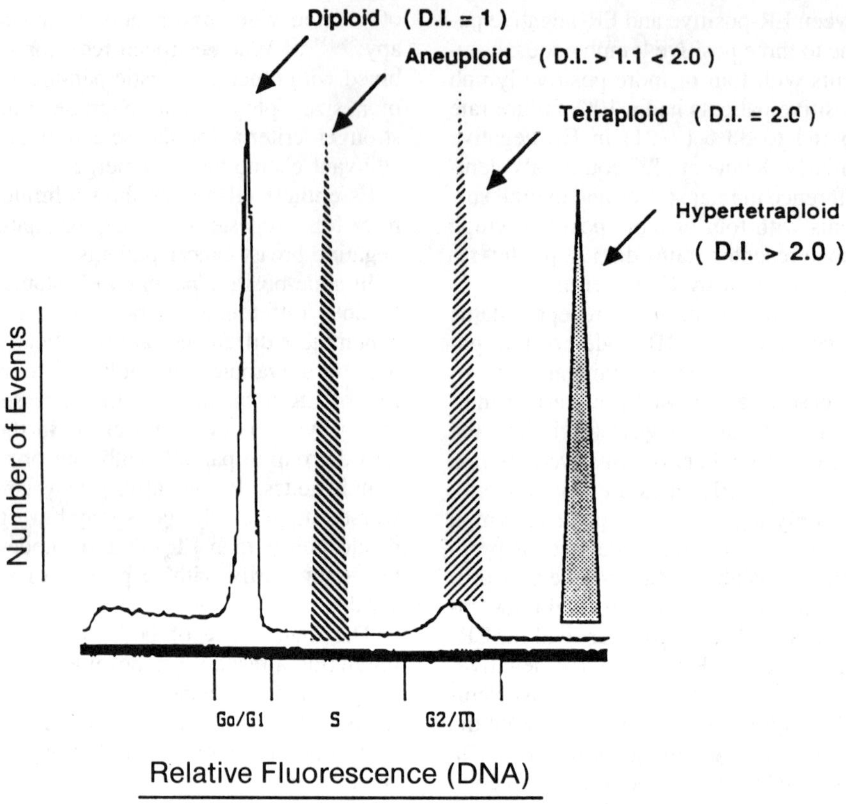

Fig. 8-2 Single-parameter DNA histogram (relative DNA fluorescence *vs.* number of events) with superimposed G_0/G_1 peaks of abnormal DNA content demonstrating aneuploid, tetraploid, and hypertetraploid patterns. DNA index (DI) is a measure of relative DNA content compared to the standard diploid population (i.e., DI = [mean DNA content of tumor G_0/G_1 population] / [mean DNA content of standard diploid G_0/G_1 population]).

of these had high S-phase fractions. Of the 12,000 patients with diploid tumors, 18% had high S-phase fractions.[133]

Methodology

Flow cytometry detects intrinsic features, such as cell size and cell granularity, by light scatter, and extrinsic features, including DNA and/or RNA content and antigens on the surface of the cell, in its cytoplasm or in the nucleus, by fluorescence. Whether one starts with fresh, frozen, or fixed tissue, cytologic specimens or paraffin blocks, the goal of processing is to obtain a single cell suspension that can be stained and analyzed. The analysis entails streaming the cells past a focused light source (e.g., a laser), which results in scattered light and stimulated fluorochromes (e.g., FITC-conjugated antibodies for antigen detection, propidium iodide for DNA). The signals emitted are collected by detectors and analyzed by a computer program.

Image analysis uses similar principles based on the measurement of individual cellular characteristics. However, this technology involves the transfer of a few hundred microscope slide–based images to a statistical database that must be further processed to yield interpretable data. The major advantage of this approach is its ability to quantitate small cell samples in cytologic smears and in the context of intact morphology (e.g., quantitation of estrogen receptor immunocytochemistry, analysis of DNA content, etc.). Both flow cytometry and image analysis yield comparable results in DNA analysis. Although image systems have a higher specificity in detecting aneuploidy,[170,184] flow cytometry has the further advantage of being able to analyze larger populations of cells and to analyze proliferative index. The agreement between these two methods is as high as 90%.[91] There are many reviews of these methods.[41,76,102,147,181]

These techniques can resolve the equivalent of two entire chromosomes. Normal cycling human

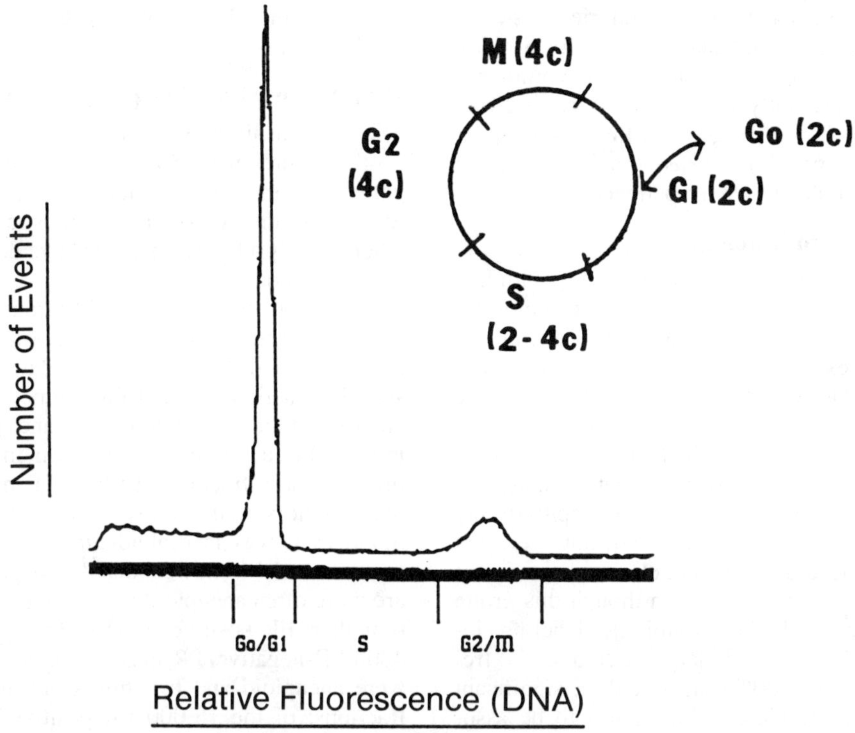

Fig. 8-3 Single-parameter DNA histogram (relative DNA fluorescence *vs*. number of events) showing a normal diploid cell population distribution and its relationship with the cell cycle.

cells have two sets of 23 chromosomes with a normal diploid DNA histogram (Fig. 8-3). The subpopulations defined relate to the phases of the cell cycle: G_0/G_1 (2C), S (2-4C), G_2/M (4C). The quality of the histogram and the heterogeneity of the sample are described by the coefficient of variation (CV), a measure of the width of the G_0/G_1 peak. In normal peripheral blood lymphocytes this should be $<2\%$ and in tumors $<8\%$.

Ploidy and S-phase fraction determinations depend on which part of the tumor is sampled because of inherent tumor heterogeneity.[137,150] There was a 90% concordance between ploidy measurements and a 77% concordance of S-phase fraction determinations when two adjacent parts of the same tumor were analyzed.[150] When adjoining samples of breast tissue had discordant S-phase fraction determinations, the relative risk of distant recurrence was determined by the less favorable reading. Tumors of mixed ploidy had an intermediate risk of distant recurrence between pure diploid and pure aneuploid tumors.

Several of the studies cited in this chapter assess cell cycle kinetics using the thymidine labeling index (TLI), an autoradiographic method of detecting cells that are synthesizing DNA. The concordance of flow cytometric measurements and thymidine labeling studies has been relatively good.[109] TLI has many disadvantages: it requires fresh tissue; the exposure time to radioactive thymidine is relatively long; it is time-consuming; and it is limited by the number of cells it can count (~3000 to 10,000); and a skilled pathologist is often required to interpret the results. In addition, the results are dependent on conditions such as temperature and background noise.[51,109] TLI tends to overestimate S-phase fraction (SPF), especially in tumors with overlapping populations of DNA content. But this can be improved substantially with proper procedures and correction for debris.[107,109,116] Flow cytometry has the advantage of being able to evaluate large numbers of cells and is therefore more accurate. It is capable of assessing several parameters simultaneously, for example, S-phase fraction, DNA ploidy, and neu oncogene expression.[86] One disadvantage of flow cytometry is the dilutional effect of normal surrounding breast tissue and inflammatory cells on the measurements of a cancer. A second disadvantage is the effect of nuclear debris on the distribution. Software that allows for debris subtraction and population overlap is available and provides more accurate determinations. The methods used to derive these numbers have not been systematically applied, however, resulting in great variability between laboratories. As a result, an ideal universal "cut-off point" for S-phase determination, the parameter most commonly used, is not presently achievable. A further disadvantage of flow cytometry is that, even under optimal conditions, the S-phase fraction cannot be determined in about 20% of patients.[130]

Correlation with histology

Numerous studies have correlated ploidy with histologic type.[78,108,118,126,128] Of all breast carcinomas, 55% to 90% are aneuploid; however, if ductal carcinomas are examined alone, 60% to 70% exhibit an abnormal DNA content.[42,51] An analysis of cycle distribution in various histologic types,[126] found that medullary carcinoma had the highest proliferative index, followed by ductal carcinomas, and then low-grade histologies, such as papillary and tubular carcinomas. Meyer showed, however, that TLI did not accurately predict clinical behavior of medullary cancer patients, even though this group had consistently higher thymidine labeling indices.[116] Although medullary carcinoma is frequently (85% to 100%) aneuploid, a significant proportion is tetraploid, which tends to be associated with a more favorable outcome than other aneuploid subtypes.[9,53,85]

Intraductal carcinoma only has been investigated rarely in this manner, with one study showing 58% aneuploidy.[108] Ductal variants, such as tubular, papillary, and colloid carcinomas almost uniformly show a diploid pattern. Lobular carcinoma tends to have normal DNA content in approximately 65% to 80% of cases.

Correlation with other prognostic variables

The relationship between DNA content and prognostic features has been studied by many investigators. The majority of studies have correlated ploidy with the classical prognostic indicators, whereas only a limited number have done the same with proliferative index.

In general, ploidy (Table 8-5) consistently correlates with tumor grade, lymph node status, and ER status, and it frequently correlates with tumor size, histologic type, and PR status. There is also an association between ploidy and proliferative index. In a study by Kallioniemi et al.,[84] mean S-phase fraction was twice as high in aneuploid tumors (particularly in hypertetraploid tumors) as it was in diploid tumors. Furthermore, Owens et al.[133] showed that ER-negative tumors are more often aneuploid with a high S-phase fraction than ER-positive tumors. Of approximately 4000 ER-negative/PR-negative tumors, two thirds were aneuploid and two thirds had high S-phase fractions; of the 15,000 ER-positive/PR-positive tumors, half were aneuploid and one third had high S-phase fractions.

No correlation between ploidy and stage has been shown, and association with age or menopausal status is unusual. Measures of cell proliferation (Table 8-6) consistently correlate with tumor grade and are inversely proportional to ER and

Table 8-5 The correlation between DNA content and classical prognostic variables

Author	No. specimens	Age	Menopause	Tumor size	Grade	ER/PR	Lymph node status
University of Pennsylvania*	327	Yes	No	No	—	No	No
Muss et al.[122]†	101	No	—	No	No	No	N/A
Hatschek et al.[73]*	430	—	—	Yes	Yes	No	Yes
Dressler et al.[51]*	1184	No	Yes	—	—	Yes	Yes
Moran et al.[118]‡	76	—	—	—	Yes	Yes	No
Kallioniemi et al.[84]‡	308	No	No	No	Yes	Yes	Yes
Fallenius et al.[53]‡	227	—	—	Yes	Yes	—	No
Kallioniemi et al.[85]*	308	Yes	No	No	Yes	Yes	Yes
Cornelisse et al.[42]*	565	—	No	Yes	—	Yes	Yes
Hedley[74]‡	473	—	Yes	No	Yes	Yes	Yes
McDivitt et al.[108]‡	168	—	—	No	No	No	No
Thorud et al.[166]†	59	—	Yes	Yes	Yes	No	—
Olszewski et al.[126, 127]§	92	—	—	—	Yes	Yes	—
Von Rosen et al.[178, 179]	?	Yes	—	Yes	—	Yes	No

Yes, statistically significant ($p \leq .05$); No, not statistically significant.
*All stages.
†Stage I.
‡Up to stage III.
§Stage not specified.

Table 8-6 The correlation between proliferative index and classical prognostic variables

Author	No. pts.	Age	Menopause	Tumor size	Grade	ER	Lymph node status
Muss et al.[122]*	101	Yes	—	No	Yes	Yes	N/A
Kallioniemi et al.[85]†	308	No	No	No	Yes	No	No
Hedley et al.[74]†	473	—	No	No	Yes	No	No
McDivitt et al.[108]†	168	—	—	—	Yes	Yes	No
Gentili et al.[62]‡	541	—	Yes	No	—	—	No
Sigurdsson et al.[149]*	367	Yes	—	Yes	—	Yes	N/A

Yes, statistically significant ($p \leq .05$); No, not statistically significant.
*Stage I.
†Stage I to stage III.
‡All stages.

PR status. No correlation of proliferative index with tumor size or lymph node status has been seen, and rarely has it been associated with age, menopausal status, or histology.

The prognostic value of DNA ploidy and proliferative index in breast cancer

As a univariate indicator, aneuploidy has frequently been a marker of decreased disease-free and overall survival, a correlation not always sustained by multivariate analysis. But an elevated proliferative index consistently carries a negative prognosis with respect to both disease-free and overall survival, a finding usually supported by multivariate analysis.

It is difficult to make generalizations on the prognostic value of ploidy and proliferative index in breast cancer because of the lack of standardization and systematic analyses in the literature. Most studies refer to breast cancer as a single disease without reference to its histologic variants. Variation among studies with regard to stage, number of patients, therapeutic manipulations, statistical methods, and definition of analytic variables greatly weakens conclusions. Further, the population of tumors analyzed with ploidy and proliferative index is biased to tumors large enough to allow measurements of these nonclassical parameters, in addition to the more conventional ones. For example, Klintenberg et al.[91] demonstrated that patients whose tumors were not analyzed for proliferative index had a 5-year relapse-free survival rate similar to that of patients with a low proliferative index. There have been some multivariate analyses of the various prognostic parameters, including tumor size, in an attempt to elucidate the independent value of ploidy and proliferative index.

Operable breast cancer. Proliferative index and ploidy studies in women with operable breast cancer (node-positive and node-negative combined) give strong independent prognostic significance to proliferative index for disease-free and overall survival and inconsistent prognostic significance to ploidy (Tables 8-7 and 8-8).

Ploidy alone has been analyzed in stage I to stage III breast cancer patients (Table 8-8). Fallenius et al.[52] reported significant differences in survival associated with diploid, triploid, and hypertetraploid tumors at 5 years and 10 years (Table 8-9). The relative risk of recurrence for aneuploid tumors was about four times higher than for diploid tumors. Ploidy was an independent prognostic factor only in postmenopausal patients with operable breast cancer in a review by Cornelisse et al.[42] In a multivariate analysis Von Rosen showed that ploidy had prognostic value only in node-negative patients.[179]

Proliferative index has been shown to be an independent predictor of overall and disease-free survival in studies of stage I to stage III breast cancer patients (see Tables 8-10 and 8-11). Meyer and Province[116] showed that thymidine labeling index was a strong independent predictor for relapse-free and overall survival in all women. Its strongest predictive value was in node-negative patients with small tumors, but it also had predictive value for node-positive patients with large tumors. They divided the population of women into three groups: patients had high, mid, or low levels of TLI, with about a 30% difference in overall and relapse-free survival between the high and the low values. Ten-year results reported by Tubiana et al.[169] revealed that TLI was the most powerful independent predictor of survival, followed by tumor size, histologic grade, and number of positive lymph nodes. For relapse-free survival, histologic grading was the most important predictor, followed by TLI, tumor size, and inflammatory reaction. In 1988 Silvestrini et al.[153] confirmed the prognostic significance of TLI in 971 operable breast cancer patients and suggested a role for TLI in identifying those patients who may benefit from chemotherapy.

Table 8-7 The prognostic value of proliferative index (PI) in stage I to stage III breast cancer

Author	No. pts.	PI	Disease-free survival (%)	Overall survival (%)	Outcome based on PI: Disease-free survival	Outcome based on PI: Overall survival	Follow-up (yr)
Kallioniemi et al.[84,85]	308				—	Yes (U)	8
Klintenberg et al.[91]	210	Low	71*	—	Yes (M)*†	—	5 (minimum)
		High	54*	—			
Meyer and Province[116]	718	Low		79	Yes (M)‡	Yes (M)‡	5
		Mid	49	61			
		High	41	51			
Tubiana et al.[169]	125	Low	75*	70	Yes (M)*§	Yes (M)*§	10
		Mid	47*	48			
		High	38*	38			

(U), univariate anaylsis; (M), multivariate analysis; Yes, statistically significant ($p \leq .05$); No, not statistically significant.
*Relapse-free survival.
†Independent of lymph node status, number of positive lymph nodes, and ER status.
‡Independent of stage and ER/PR status.
§Independent of tumor size, histologic grade, and inflammatory reaction.

Table 8-8 The prognostic value of ploidy in stage I to stage III breast cancer patients

Author	No. pts.	Ploidy	Outcome: Disease-free survival (%)	Outcome: Overall survival (%)	Outcome based on ploidy: diploid vs. aneuploid: Disease-free survival	Outcome based on ploidy: diploid vs. aneuploid: Overall survival	Follow-up (yr)
Cornelisse et al.[42]*	565	Diploid	78†	80	BS (U)†	Yes (U)	3 (disease-free survival), 5 (overall survival)
		Aneuploid	67†	69			
Fallenius et al.[53]	409	Diploid	76†	—	Yes (U)†	—	—
		Aneuploid	45†	—			
Kallioniemi et al.[84,85]	308	Diploid	—	74	—	Yes (M)§	8
		Aneuploid	—	51			
Klintenberg et al.[91]	210	Diploid	60‡	—	No (U)‡	—	5 (minimum)
		Aneuploid	64‡	—			
Von Rosen et al.[179]	464	Diploid	90‡	—	Yes (M)‡	—	3.5
		Aneuploid	82‡	—			

BS, borderline significance; (U), univariate analysis; (M), multivariate analysis; Yes, statistically significant ($p \leq .05$); No, not statistically significant.
*Stage I to stage IV; only includes 12 stage IV patients.
†Distant relapse-free survival.
‡Relapse-free survival.
§Independent of tumor size, nodal status, ER/PR, or age.

Table 8-9 The association between ploidy subtype and overall survival

Ploidy subtype	Overall survival (%) 5 yr	10 yr
Diploid	78	64
Triploid	67	59
Hypertetraploid	49	42

Adapted from Fallenius A, Aver G, and Carstensen J: Cancer 62:331, 1988.

A recent update by Sigurdsson et al.[150] on 584 women revealed significant prognostic value for S-phase fraction in both node-negative and node-positive women.

Several studies examined both cell cycle kinetics and ploidy in the same stage I to stage III breast cancer patients. Kallioniemi et al.[84] showed a 23% difference in 8-year survival rates and an approximately threefold risk of death for patients with aneuploid tumors as compared to these with diploid tumors. Within the group of patients with aneuploid tumors, those with tetraploid tumors had a relatively good prognosis compared to those with hypertetraploid tumors (statistically significant on multivariate analysis). In a later report by the same author, S-phase fraction had more independent prognostic importance than ploidy.[85] By combining these two prognostic variables, an even stronger parameter emerged. Women with diploid/low S-phase fraction cancers had a very favorable outcome, an 8-year cumulative survival of 90%; women with aneuploid/high S-phase fraction tumors were at high risk for failure, with an 8-year cumulative survival of 50%. The risk of death in the high-risk group was eight times that observed in the favorable group. These combined factors had significant prognostic value in both node-negative and node-positive patient groups. The combined parameters had independent prognostic significance stronger than tumor size, lymph node status, or estrogen or progesterone status on multivariate analysis. Klintenberg et al.[91] showed independent prognostic value for S-phase fraction with respect to 5-year relapse-free survival rates, but could not demonstrate a difference in rates of overall or relapse free survival between patients with aneuploid and diploid tumors.

Node-negative breast cancer. Many studies have examined the prognostic value of proliferative index in node-negative women (Table 8-10). Hery et al.[77] found that thymidine labeling index predicted relapse-free and overall survival outcome in a prospective study of 76 stage I patients treated with radical mastectomy or lumpectomy and radiation at a mean follow-up of 6 years. Patients with a high TLI had an 84% and a 36% overall survival rate at 5 and 8 years, respectively, compared to a 100% survival rate for low TLI tumors at similar follow-up. High TLI also was associated with early relapse: 29% of patients with high TLI relapsed within the first 2 years, compared to none of the low TLI patients. Although Gentili et al.[62] demonstrated a significant overall association between high TLI and relapse by univariate analysis, by multivariate analysis they showed an improvement in relapse-free survival only in premenopausal patients (no relapses were observed in low TLI patients (0/37) compared to a 67% (22/33) recurrence rate in high TLI patients). In an early report, Meyer et al.[115] showed that TLI predicts for early recurrence and overall survival. Later they showed that TLI could identify a subgroup of patients with a 40% risk of relapse and a 50% survival rate at 5 years within a group of surgically treated node-negative women (268 women).[116] TLI had predictive power within different categories of vascular invasion and nuclear grade. Further, it could predict overall survival rates (differences of 25% to 50%) and relapse-free survival rates (differences of 31% to 38%) in stage I patients within subgroups of ER-positive and ER-negative patients, and for PR-positive patients. This prognostic value was confirmed on multivariate analysis. The low-risk group determined by TLI represents about one third of the population analyzed (a subset only, of course, of the total number of patients seen in that hospital during the study period).

Silvestrini et al.[152] showed a statistically significant difference in 6-year relapse-free and overall survival rates based on TLI. These results were statistically significant for postmenopausal women, and highly significant for premenopausal and perimenopausal women. In a second report by Silvestrini et al.[151] TLI was the only independent predictor of early relapse, being more important than ER/PR status on multivariate analysis. In addition, TLI could identify those patients with ER-negative and ER-positive borderline tumors who were at highest risk of relapse (Table 8-11). In an updated report in 1988,[153] a highly statistically significant difference in 5-year relapse-free and overall survival rates was again confirmed between patients with high and low TLI.

Proliferative index and ploidy. Several studies that analyzed both ploidy and S-phase fraction in node-negative patients showed prognostic value for S-phase fraction but not for ploidy (Tables 8-10, 8-12, and 8-13). Ploidy was not of prognostic value

Table 8-10 The prognostic value of proliferative index in axillary node-negative patients

			Survival (%)		Outcome based on PI: low vs. high		
Author	No. pts.	Proliferative index	Disease-free survival	Overall survival	Disease-free survival	Overall survival	Follow-up (yr)
Gentilli et al.[62]	145	Low	88	—	Yes (U)	—	4
		High	72	—			
Hery et al.[77]	76	High	71	84	—	—	2 (disease-free survival), 5 (overall survival)
		Low	100	100			
Meyer and Province[116]	268	High	61	64	Yes (U)	Yes (U)	5
		Mid	59	66			
		Low	80	89			
Silvestrini et al.[151]	215	—	—		Yes	Yes	5
		—	—				
Silvestrini et al.[152]	258	High	60	75	—	—	6
		Low	81	91			
Silvestrini et al.[153]	414	High	60	86	Yes	Yes	5
		Low	83	96			
Clark et al.[31]*	253	Low	90	—	Yes (M)†	—	5 (median)
		High	70	—			
Dressler et al.[50]*	409				Yes	—	4 (median)
Muss et al.[122]	101	Low	78‡	87	No	Yes (M)	4.3 (median)
		High	67‡	70			
Sigurdsson et al.[149]	367	Low	89	93	Yes (U)	Yes (M)	4 (median)
		High	69	71	No (M)		

Yes, statistically significant ($p<.05$); No, not statistically significant; (U), univariate analysis; (M), multivariate analysis. When the type of analysis is not specified by the author, no (U) or (M) appears after "Yes" or "No."
*Reporting from same institution, San Antonio.
†In diploid tumors only, but independent of tumor size, ER/PR status, age.
‡Relapse-free survival.

in node-negative patients treated on EST 1180 protocol.[50] An elevated S-phase fraction, however, significantly predicted decreased relapse-free survival rates compared to those patients with a normal S-phase fraction. The lack of prognostic significance of ploidy also was demonstrated by Cornelisse et al.[42] Muss et al.[122] found that neither ploidy nor proliferative index correlated with time to relapse on multivariate analysis. With respect to survival,

Table 8-11 Five-year relapse-free survival rate based on combined thymidine labeling index (TLI) and ER status

	TLI status	
Hormone receptor status	Low	High
ER-positive/borderline	86	67
ER-negative	81	52

Adapted from Silvestrini R, Daidone M, Di Fronzo G, et al: Breast Cancer Res Treat 7:161, 1986.

the full parameter $S/G_2/M$ was a significant independent predictor of survival; %S was borderline, and ploidy was not significant. In a paper by Sigurdsson et al.,[149] S-phase fraction had the most prognostic power, followed by PR and tumor size, in a multivariate analysis (including age, tumor size, ER/PR status, ploidy, and S-phase fraction). The risk of death in patients with high S-phase fraction was twice as high as that for patients with low S-phase fraction. Ploidy did not provide any additional prognostic information; patients with low S-phase fraction and either diploid or aneuploid tumors had similar 4-year overall survival rates. The mortality from breast cancer was higher in patients with diploid/high S-phase fraction tumors, compared to those with aneuploid/low S-phase fraction tumors. They devised a prognostic model consisting of three covariables: S-phase fraction, PR status, and tumor size. In a multivariate analysis, no other prognostic variable was significant. Sixty-three percent of the women had a low-risk combined parameter, and only 3% of them

Table 8-12 The prognostic value of ploidy in axillary node-negative patients

Author	No. pts.	Survival (%)		Outcome based on ploidy: diploid vs. aneuploid			
		Disease-free survival	Overall survival	Disease-free survival	Overall survival	Ploidy	Follow-up (yr)
Clark et al.[31]*	345	88	—	Yes (M)†	No (U)‡	Diploid	5 (median)
		74	—			Aneuploid	
Cornelisse et al.[42]	263	88§	93	Yes (U)§	No (U)	Diploid	3 (distant disease-free survival), 5 (overall survival)
		82§	85			Aneupolid	
Dressler et al.[50]*	563	—	—	No	—	—	4 (median)
Muss et al.[122]	101	80‖	83	No	No‖	Diploid	4.3 (median)
		72‖	80			Aneuploid	
Sigurdsson et al.[149]	367	88	95	Yes (U)	Yes (U)	Diploid	4 (median), 5 (overall survival)
		78	80	No (M)	No (M)	Aneuploid	

Yes, statistically significant ($p<.05$); No, not significant; (U), significant only on univariate analysis; (M), significant on multivariate analysis.
*Reporting from same institution, San Antonio.
†Independent of tumor size, ER/PR status, age.
‡Borderline significance.
§Distant relapse-free survival.
‖Relapse-free survival.

developed distant metastases. Survival rates in this favorable group were similar to the expected survival rates of an age-matched group of normal Swedish women. The combined parameter identified a high-risk group consisting of 37% of the patients as having a four-fold increase in the risk of distant recurrence compared to the low-risk group.

High S-phase fraction and aneuploidy were associated with early relapse independent of tumor size and ER status in an analysis by Clark et al.[31] Multivariate analysis showed that ploidy was the only significant variable in predicting time of recurrence. S-phase fraction was then determined and found to be important in identifying which patients with diploid tumors were most likely to fail; patients with low S-phase fraction had a 5-year probable disease-free survival rate of 90% compared to 70% in those patients with high S-phase fraction. Similar differences reportedly were obtained for rates of overall survival, although these data were not provided. Multivariate analysis of diploid tumors using S-phase fraction, tumor size, ER and PR status, and age as variables demonstrated that S-phase fraction was the only significant variable in predicting disease-free or overall survival. Pa-

Table 8-13 The prognostic value of ploidy in axillary node-positive patients

Author	No. pts.	Outcome based on ploidy: diploid vs. aneuploid			Survival (%)		
		Disease-free survival	Overall survival	Ploidy	Disease-free survival	Overall survival	Follow-up (yr)
Hedley et al.[74]	428	Yes (U)	Yes (U)	Diploid	64	81	5
		No (M)*	No (M)*	Aneuploid	53	63-70	
Kute et al.[96]	197	No (U)	No (U)	Diploid	61	66	5
				Aneuploid	48	64	

Yes, statistically significant ($p<.05$); No, not significant; (U), significant only on univariate analysis; (M), significant on multivariate analysis.
*Independent only of number of positive lymph nodes and menopausal status.

tients with high S-phase fractions had a fourfold greater risk of recurrence than those with low S-phase fraction. S-phase fraction had no prognostic value in aneuploid tumors. Progesterone receptor status was the only significant factor with respect to overall survival in aneuploid tumors; patients with diploid/low S-phase fraction tumors had survival rates similar to those of patients with aneuploid/PR-positive tumors; patients with diploid/high S-phase fraction tumors had rates similar to those of patients with aneuploid/PR-negative tumors. In this study population, while patients with diploid/high S-phase fraction and aneuploid tumors were at relatively high risk for failure, this group included most patients, and therefore these two parameters alone would be inadequate criteria on which to base the selection of chemotherapy.

Node-positive breast cancer. Limited data on ploidy and S-phase fraction are available for women with node-positive breast cancer. The following studies show that when proliferative index predicts disease-free or relapse-free survival, it is only able to do so by univariate analysis or limited multivariate analysis[74,116,152] (Table 8-14). Similarly, significant differences in overall survival rates were seen only in subgroups of node-positive women and by limited multivariate analysis.[74,152] The prognostic value of ploidy was also limited to subgroups of node-positive women and by univariate analysis only.[42,74,96]

Meyer and Province[116] found TLI to be an independent prognostic variable on multivariate analysis in 246 operable node-positive patients. Silvestrini et al. analyzed 557 patients of whom 306 had less than three positive lymph nodes.[152] In this group, there was a statistically significant overall difference in relapse-free survival rates; however the relapse-free survival rate was similar for patients with both high and low TLI tumors treated with full-dose chemotherapy, compared to a significant difference in rates of relapse-free survival for similar patients who received less than full-dose therapy. There was no difference in rates of overall survival. In the 251 patients with three or more positive lymph nodes, there was a 15% to 20% significant difference in both relapse-free and overall survival. In a review by Cornelisse et al.,[42] aneuploidy was associated with a difference in overall survival by univariate analysis; however, this difference was observed only in postmenopausal patients on multivariate analysis. In patients with three or more positive lymph nodes, those with diploid tumors had better distant relapse-free survival and overall survival rates than those with aneuploid tumors by univariate analysis. Hedley et al.[74] retrospectively measured ploidy in 428 node-positive patients and S-phase fraction in 285 of 490 consecutive node-positive patients treated on randomized trials (premenopausal patients received mastectomy followed by various chemotherapeutic regimens; postmenopausal patients were randomized between chemotherapy, hormonal manipulation, and observation) (see Table 8-13). There was

Table 8-14 The prognostic value of proliferative index (PI) in axillary node-positive patients

			Outcome (%)		Outcome based on PI (low vs. high)		
Author	**No. pts.**	**PI**	**Disease-free survival**	**Overall survival**	**Disease-free survival**	**Overall survival**	**Follow-up (yr)**
Hedley et al.[74]	285	Low	66	—	Yes (M)*	Yes (M)*	5
		High	49	—			
Kute et al.[96]	197	Low	59	67	No (U)	No (U)	5
		High	56	60			
Meyer and Province[116]	256	Low	65†	79	Yes (M)†‡	Yes (M)†‡	5
		Mid	53†	73			
		High	40†	52			
Silvestrini et al.[153]	306§	Low	78†	87	Yes (U)†	No (U)	5
		High	61†	82			
	251‖	Low	52†	81	Yes (U)†	Yes (U)	
		High	37†	60			

(M), significant on multivariate analysis; (U), significant on univariate analysis only.
*Independent of number of positive lymph nodes and menopausal status only.
†Relapse-free survival.
‡Independent of tumor size, age, number of positive lymph nodes, ER/PR status, and thymidine labeling index.
§Three or fewer positive lymph nodes.
‖More than three positive lymph nodes.

a statistically significant correlation between ploidy, and disease-free and overall survival rates by univariate analysis. Ploidy had no significance, however, independent of lymph node status, menopausal status, ER/PR status, or grade. Low S-phase fraction had a very significant association with increased rate of disease-free survival by univariate analysis. In a multivariate analysis, S-phase fraction was a prognosticator of disease-free and overall survival rates independent of lymph node and menopausal status, but not independent of tumor grade, ER/PR status, and tumor size. The combined prognostic parameter of S-phase fraction and ploidy could not be assessed satisfactorily because in many cases both factors could not be determined reliably. These findings are in disagreement with Kute et al., who showed no independent prognostic significance for S-phase fraction, but did prove significance for ploidy in hormone receptor-negative patients (see Table 8-13).[96]

Summary. The prognostic value of DNA ploidy and proliferative indices is weakened by the lack of standardization in the techniques used to measure the parameters and the criteria used to determine a positive test, both within and between institutions. Despite these limitations in the literature, it is possible to make some conclusions.

Overall, studies of operable breast cancer patients demonstrate that proliferative index can independently predict disease-free and overall survival. The prognostic value of DNA ploidy is restricted almost entirely to univariate analysis. In the occasional study that demonstrates its independent prognostic significance, ploidy is less powerful than S-phase fraction as a predictor.

The prognostic role of proliferative index and ploidy is weak in women with node-positive breast cancer. The role of DNA ploidy and proliferative index in assessing the prognosis of node-negative women with breast cancer has been evaluated by many studies with the hope of discovering better criteria for the selection of women who may benefit from adjuvant chemotherapy. S-phase fraction is a stronger determinant of patient outcome than ploidy. Disease-free and overall survival rates have differences of 10% to 30% (most range between 20% and 30%) for patients with low and high S-phase fractions; this may justify the use of S-phase fraction alone as an indicator for chemotherapy. The ideal cutoff value used to define an elevated S-phase fraction needs to be determined and then standardized to facilitate comparison of data between institutions. Certainly, the combination of S-phase fraction with other prognostic variables such as ploidy, hormone receptor status, tumor size, and/or nuclear grade is a sufficiently powerful criteria on which to base the recommendation of adjuvant chemotherapy. The best combination of prognostic parameters will be better defined by current randomized studies.

CATHEPSIN D

Cathepsin D is a lysosomal hydrolase with at least two biologic properties: estrogen and/or growth factor–dependent mitogenic activity and enzymatic activity on proteoglycans, extracellular matrix, and basement membrane.[22,140,177] These properties suggest a potential role for cathepsin D in the invasion and metastasis of cancer cells.[99]

Cathepsin D exists in three forms: it is secreted as a proenzyme, which is then activated by an acidic pH to its intermediate 48 kd and mature 34 kd forms.[25,119] Located on chromosome 11, the difference between procathepsin D in the breast cancer cell line MCF-7 and normal human kidney procathepsin D is one amino acid substitution.[8]

There is a significant interaction between hormones, growth factors, and cathepsin D. Estrogens can stimulate both the growth of breast cancer cells and the production of several growth regulatory factors: cathepsin D[28,177,183] and growth factors such as TGF-alpha and IGF-1.[100] In ER-positive tumors, estrogen can increase cathepsin D levels significantly; and in ER-negative tumors, cathepsin D is usually constitutive and responds minimally to estrogen.[61] In addition, the growth factors IGF-I and epithelial growth factor (EGF) have been shown to increase cathepsin D mRNA levels.[28] Furthermore, cathepsin D itself has autocrine growth stimulation properties on human breast cancer cell lines.[177] Thus estrogens and growth factors may mediate tumor proliferation, invasion, and metastasis through the agency of cathepsin D.

In breast cancer cell lines in vitro, there is a substantial increase (two- to 30-fold) in the amount of cathepsin D produced by malignant cells compared to normal breast tissue growing at the same rate[26]; in addition, the processing of the various forms of cathepsin D is delayed.[140] Ex vivo, cathepsin D levels are slightly higher than normal in benign mastopathies and substantially higher still (three to four times) in primary and metastatic breast cancers.[15]

Correlation between cathepsin D and other prognostic variables

There appears to be a correlation between very high levels and low levels of cathepsin D (but not the actual concentration of cathepsin D) and estrogen receptor status in nonmetastatic breast cancer patients.[106] Thorpe et al.[164] could only demonstrate an association between high cathepsin D levels and

Table 8-15 The prognostic value of cathepsin D in operable breast cancer

Author	No. pts.	Level	Survival (%)			Outcome based on high vs. low levels of cathepsin D			Level
			Disease-free survival	Distant disease-free survival	Overall survival	Disease-free survival	Distant disease-free survival	Overall survival	
Namer et al.[123]	141 node-negative	Low	—[a]	—[a]	—[a]	—	—	No	6
	96 node-positive	High	—[a]	—[a]	—[a]	—	—	Yes (U)	
Spyratos et al.[157]	122	Low	—[a]	67	—[a]		Yes (M)	Yes (U)[c]	7, 4.6 (median)
		High	—[a]	22	—[a]				
Tandon et al.[162]	199 node-negative	Low	70	—	80	Yes (M)[d]	—	Yes (M)[d]	5.3
		High	48	—	51				
	98 node-positive	Low	—[a]	—[e]	—[a]	No	—	No	4.7
		High	—[a]	—[e]	—[a]				
Thorpe et al.[164]	242 pre/peri-menopausal	Low	64[f]	—[e]	—[a]	BS	—[e]	No	7
		Mid	48[f]	—[e]	—[a]				
		High	32[f]	—[e]	—[a]				
	150 post-menopausal	Low	61[f]	—[e]	—[a]	Yes	—[e]	No	7
		Mid	42[f]	—[e]	—[a]				
		High	18[f]	—[e]	—[a]				

Yes, statistically significant ($p \leq .05$); No, not significant ($p > .05$); BS, borderline significant ($p = .06$); (U), univariate analysis; (M), multivariate analysis.
[a]Authors did not provide actual values.
[b]Independent only of lymph node status.
[c]Seen only in patients with cathepsin D levels 70 pmol/mg.
[d]Independent of age, ploidy, tumor size, ER/PR status.
[e]Not done by authors.
[f]Relapse free survival.

ER-positive tumors in premenopausal and perimenopausal patients. Additional reports were unable to show an association between ER status and levels of cathepsin D,[46,123] even when the cut-off point used to define a positive cathepsin D level was varied.[46]

No significant association between cathepsin D and age, lymph node status, tumor size, progesterone status, histologic grade,[106,123,164] epithelial growth factor receptors (EGFRs), ploidy, or S-phase fraction[46] was observed. Aneuploidy was associated with cathepsin D levels only in node-negative patients.[162]

The prognostic value of cathepsin D in patients with operable breast cancer

Cathepsin D has been found to be an independent prognostic factor, having a greater impact on disease-free and distant disease-free survival rates than lymph node status[157] (Table 8-15). In an analysis of women treated in Danish Breast Cancer Cooperative Group trials,[164] cathepsin D was found to be an independent prognostic factor for relapse-free survival rates, approaching the significance of lymph node status. The prognostic significance of cathepsin D depended on menopausal status: the shorter relapse-free survival is observed in a small fraction of premenopausal and perimenopausal patients with the highest cathepsin D levels (borderline significant, $p=.06$), whereas decreased relapse-free survival rates observed in the majority of postmenopausal patients with similarly high levels of cathepsin D (statistically significant). There was a trend for shorter overall survival only in the postmenopausal patient group. A potential bias exists in this analysis, however, because the tumors analyzed were not representative of those in the general population of patients. The tumors analyzed were generally larger, of higher grade, and were more commonly ER-negative, and patients were more often premenopausal or perimenopausal, when compared to the group that was not analyzed.

In a separate analysis of node-negative patients, two studies demonstrated prognostic value for cathepsin D and a third study did not. A high level of cathepsin D was the most important independent prognostic factor with respect to disease-free and overall survival rates in node-negative women in a study by Tandon et al.[162] Node-negative patients with high cathepsin D levels had 2.6 relative risk of tumor recurrence and a 3.9 relative risk of death compared to node-negative patients with low cathepsin D levels.[162] In a low-risk group of node-negative patients (ER-positive/PR-positive, diploid, small tumors), Spyratos et al. showed that high levels of cathepsin D predicted for decreased rates of distant disease-free survival.[157] Cathepsin D had no impact on survival rates in an analysis of 141 node-negative patients by Namer et al.[123]

The two studies that analyzed the prognostic importance of cathepsin D in node-positive patients found conflicting results. Although Tandon et al.[162] were unable to demonstrate a significant impact on patient outcome, Namer et al.[123] reported that measurement of cathepsin D levels effectively split node-positive patients into low- and high-risk groups. Node-positive/low cathepsin D patients had similar overall survival rates to node-negative patients.

HER-2/neu ONCOGENE

The neu oncogene was discovered in ethylnitrosourea-induced neuroblastomas in rats.[144] Neuroblastoma cell DNA transfected into NIH3T3 cells causes transformation. Human homologues are HER-2/neu, c-erbB-2, and MAC 117.[43,88,146] The neu oncogene, located on chromosone 17q21,[43,60] is activated by mutation in the transmembrane domain.[11] Because neu is highly homologous to epithelial growth factor receptor,[10,88,187,188] it is probably a growth factor receptor, although its ligand is not yet identified. The oncogene encodes a 180-190 kd protein, depending on its source, human or rat.[2,69,144] Neu and the mutated neu have tyrosine kinase activity,[12,144,158] which is involved in the transforming properties of neu.[182] Furthermore, EGF can stimulate the phosphorylation of neu, mutated neu, and the neu gene products resulting in increased tyrosine kinase activity.[1,87,93,159]

The transforming, tumorigenic properties of neu have been extensively studied. In vitro transformation of NIH3T3 cells occurs by overexpression of the protooncogene[45,80] or by transfection with oncogenic (mutated) neu alone.[94] Monoclonal antibodies against neu oncoprotein partially revert the transformed phenotype.[49] Transformation of NIH3T3 cells also occurs by cotransfection of protooncogenic neu and epithelial growth factor receptor.[94] This synergy suggests important interactions between neu and epithelial growth factor receptor genes. Intermolecular association of these receptors by heterodimerization can be induced by cross-linking reagents or EGF.[180]

In vitro results have been extrapolated to in vivo models. Cell lines transformed by both neu and epithelial growth factor receptor are tumorigenic in animals, and tumor growth can be arrested by antireceptor antibodies as demonstrated in studies at the University of Pennsylvania by Mark Greene. When neu is introduced into male or female transgenic mice, mammary adenocarcinomas occur in 100% of recipients.[120] Protooncogenic neu amplification in vivo occurs in glandular tissue and adenocarcinomas.[88,188,189] Its presence in both intraductal and infiltrating ductal carcinoma suggests a carcinogenic role.[13]

Amplification of the HER-2/neu oncogene is detected by Southern blot of DNA extracted from the specimen. Overexpression via mRNA is measured by Northern blot; and the presence of the oncoprotein can be determined by Western blot or immunohistochemistry. The HER-2/neu oncogene and/or oncoprotein can be detected in fresh, frozen, or paraffin-embedded tissue,[154] and ethanol or Bouin fixed tissue.[86]

Variable results of HER-2/neu oncogene amplification or expression result from difficulties in assessing these parameters. Patients studied for the presence of HER-2/neu amplification or overexpression are a subset of those treated at a given institution. They are not representative of the general patient population as only the larger tumors allow the full battery of conventional analyses as well as those for the nonclassical parameters such as the HER-2/neu oncogene. Some studies have performed multivariate analyses to clarify any selection bias.

There are many pitfalls in tumor analysis that can produce variable results within and between studies. There is inherent heterogeneity within most tumor specimens,[3,97,154] which lowers the reproducibility of results within the same tumor. Technical difficulties occur with all methods used to assess amplification and overexpression,[3,4,17,20,69,89,97,154,156,176] There was 90% overall concordance of results obtained by Southern, Northern, and Western blots and immunohistochemistry (IHC),[154] in which at least two of the three methods were used to detect expression. Western blot was least reliable method, with discordance in 6% of cases, followed by Southern and Northern blot analyses (2%) and IHC (1%). This discordance is most likely on the basis of the dilutional effect[3,89,154,156] that can occur if normal surrounding tissue is mixed in with the tumor, diluting the level of DNA, RNA, or the protein of interest. Because normal tissue is relatively acellular with a protein content greater than the RNA or DNA content, dilution affects Western more than Southern and Northern blot measurements. Underestimation of gene copy number secondary to the dilutional effect or disruption of DNA integrity while processing the tissue (particularly in archival specimens), is more common than overestimating the number of copies present. Furthermore, amplification is real and not a result of chromosome duplication.[3,154]

Immunohistochemistry is unaffected by the dilutional effect because one can see if the antibody is reacting with normal vs. malignant tissue (Fig. 8-4); however, this technique is somewhat subjective and thus more dependent on its interpreter.[69,176] Specimens with extensive amplification usually show overexpression, but it is not uncommon for IHC to be positive with a Southern blot showing only one to three copies of neu[17,20,176] (Table 8-16). The quality of IHC depends upon the quality of the substrate. Tumor fixed in formalin and then embedded in paraffin has less antigen reactivity than fresh tissue. Reactivity is also dependent on the duration of fixation. Slamon and Clark[154] found that formalin fixation depressed reactivity when compared to freshly frozen tissue. High levels of protein were detected in all formalin-fixed and frozen preparations, but moderate levels of protein were not always detected in the formalin-fixed tissue. Most of these cases had only two-fold to five-fold amplification. Ten percent of overexpressed cases had only a single copy of DNA. Studies (Table 8-17) that examined both amplification and overexpression in the same tumors demonstrate a 9% to 23% discrepancy, in overexpression more than amplification. The mechanism for overexpression without amplification (beyond the technical considerations discussed above), is not well understood.

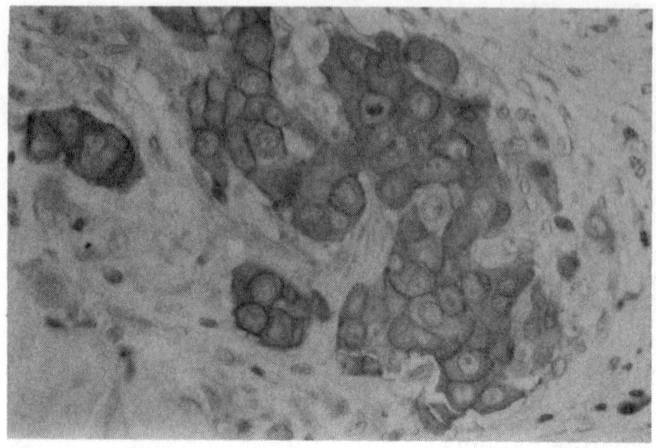

Fig. 8-4 Photomicrograph of an infiltrating ductal carcinoma showing delicate membrane staining with a polyclonal antibody to the c-erbB-2 oncoprotein.[53] Note that immunoreactivity is localized to tumor cells and that stroma is negative (400×).

Many studies measure only gene amplification and not gene expression. It is likely that expression of the gene determines its effect, rather than merely the presence of the amplified gene. But occasionally gene amplification, not overexpression, is of prognostic value.[156]

The definition of amplification and overexpression is not standardized. This further confounds one's ability to interpret the literature.

Finally, it is possible that the number of patients

Table 8-16 Incidence of HER-2/neu amplification and/or overexpression in patients with operable breast cancer

Author	Amplification		Overexpression	
	No. pts.	Incidence (%)	No. pts.	Incidence (%)
Ali et al.[4]	122	10	—	—
Allred et al.[7] *	727	14	—	—
Barnes et al.[13]	—	—	195	9
Berger et al.[17]	51	25	47	21
Borg et al.[20]	310	17	—	—
Cline et al.[37]	49	16	—	—
Fontaine et al.[59]	15	46	—	—
Guerin et al.[67]	92	20	92	36
King et al.[89]	61	6	61	19
O'Reilly et al.[126]	—	—	172	16
Paik et al.[134]	—	—	272	21
Slamon et al.[155,156]	181*	25*	—	—
	345†	27†	181†	25†
Varley et al.[174]	41	17	—	—
Ventner et al.[176]	36	33	12	66

*Node-negative patients only.
†Node-positive patients only.

studied in some series has insufficient statistical power to demonstrate significant differences between subgroups. We have therefore limited our discussion to larger studies.

Correlation between HER-2/neu oncogene amplification and/or overexpression and classic prognostic variables

There is no consistent relationship between HER-2/neu oncogene amplification and/or overexpression. Three of nine studies showed a correlation with increasing stage; six of 14 with positive nodal status, five of eight with higher histologic or nuclear grade, and five of 11 showed an inverse relationship with hormone receptor status (Table 8-18). HER-2/neu amplification and/or overexpression were proportional to the degree of nodal involvement.[20,155,163,172] Age association in two of six studies was inconclusive as one study showed a relationship to women >50 years of age[97] and the other with young women.[20] Similarly, the association between HER-2/neu and S-phase fraction and ploidy has been inconsistent; a significant association was demonstrated in one review[19] and no association was found in another.[126] Tumor size was proportional to the level of HER-2/neu amplification and overexpression.[20]

Table 8-17 Incidence of neu amplification vs. overexpression in patients with operable breast cancer

Author	Total no. pts.	Amplification (%)	Overexpression (%)
Berger et al.[17]	47	26	49
Guerin et al.[67]	92	20	36
King et al.[89]	61	10	19

The prognostic value of HER-2/neu amplification and/or overexpression

Noninvasive breast cancer. Several studies have examined the presence of the HER-2/neu oncoprotein with immunohistochemistry in different evolutionary stages of breast cancer, ranging from atypical ductal hyperplasia (ADH), to ductal carcinoma in situ (DCIS) with and without invasive ductal carcinoma (IDC), as well as IDC alone[6,64,101,172] (Table 8-19). ADH alone had HER-2/neu expression in 0 to 10% of cases analyzed. The neu oncogene is most likely found in in situ ductal carcinoma, specifically the comedo variant (60% to 100% for comedo vs. 8% to 11% for other subtypes of DCIS) and is less common in mixed DCIS and IDC (21%). Minimally invasive ductal carcinoma had an incidence of 38%, compared to 11% in frank IDC alone. These results suggest that HER-2/neu may be involved in the early development of breast cancer. In addition, HER-2/neu overexpression may serve as a marker for a rela-

Table 8-18 Correlations between HER-2/neu and classic prognostic parameters

Author	Stage	Lymph node status	Age	Hormone status	Histologic grade/ nuclear grade
Ali et al.[4]	No	No	—	No	—
Barnes et al.[13]	—	No	—	No	Yes
Berger et al.[17]	—	Yes	No	Yes	Yes
Borg et al.[20]	Yes	Yes	Yes	Yes	—
Cline et al.[37]	Yes	Yes	—	—	—
Slamon et al.[156] *	—	Yes	—	—	—
Fontaine et al.[59]	—	No	No	No	Yes
Guerin et al.[67]	—	Yes	No	Yes	No
King et al.[89]	No	No	—	—	—
Lacroix et al.[97]	No	No	Yes	No	—
O'Reilly et al.[126]	No	No	No	Yes	No
Paik et al.[134]	No	No	No	No	Yes
Van de Vijver et al.[172]	—	—	—	—	Yes
Varley et al.[174]	No	No	—	No	No
Zhou et al.[189]	Yes	No	No	No	No

Yes, statistically significant ($p \leq .05$); No, not significant.
*Node-positive patients.

tively aggressive variant of DCIS, the comedo variant, which is associated with increased thymidine labeling index,[114] a higher incidence of microinvasion,[135] and a higher recurrence rate following lumpectomy alone[98] compared to other subtypes of DCIS. The prognostic value of HER-2/neu in predicting tumor recurrence and the type of recurrence (DCIS vs. IDC), is not known.

Operable breast cancer. The ability of HER-2/neu to predict disease-free and overall survival rates in operable breast cancer patients as a whole is not well defined (Table 8-20). Two studies showed a significant relationship between HER-2/neu and disease-free survival,[37,186] one showed only borderline significance,[189] and four studies failed to demonstrate any association.[4,13,134,172] The relationship between HER-2/neu amplification and/or overexpression and rates of overall survival is similarly unclear. Three of the five studies showed a significant association with HER-2/neu and overall survival rates by univariate analysis,[134,172,186] but only one confirmed its prognostic significance by multivariate analysis.[134]

Separate analyses of node-negative and node-positive patients are presented in the following sections.

Node-negative breast cancer. Essentially all studies that analyzed node-negative breast cancer patients as a whole group failed to demonstrate a prognostic value for HER-2/neu amplification and/or overexpression with respect to disease-free survival[20,126,156,163] and overall survival rates [20,156,163] (Table 8-21). Only a small review of 14 patients by Cline et al.[37] showed a significant reduction in rates of relapse-free survival in women with amplification of HER-2/neu.

The prognostic value of HER-2/neu within subgroups of node-negative patients was evaluated by several authors. In patients with good nuclear grade treated on the NSABP B-06 trial,[134] HER-2/neu overexpression was able to predict independently a fivefold increase in the mortality rate. There was also a significant decrease in mortality in patients with HER-2/neu overexpression within the ER-positive, PR-positive, and PR-negative patient subgroups. Harris[72] showed that HER-2/neu predicted a decrease in overall survival rates and an increase in the rate of early recurrences within a relatively good prognostic group of ER-positive/EGFR-negative/lymph node–negative patients. There was progressive decline in rates of survival in patients who were EGFR-negative/HER-2/neu–negative to EGFR-positive/HER-2/neu–negative to EGFR-negative/HER-2/neu–positive to EGFR-positive/HER-2/neu–positive. Thus both EGFR and HER-2/neu provide important, independent information. Allred et al.[7] retrospectively determined the level of HER-2/neu expression in "good risk" (tumor <3 cm, ER-positive) and "poor risk" (tumor >3 cm or ER-negative) node-negative patients treated in the ECOG-E1180 protocol. In the good-risk patients, HER-2/neu overexpression predicted for a significantly higher recurrence rate at 3 years; 31% compared to 14% for patients without HER-2/neu overexpression. When patients with an in situ tumor component were excluded

Table 8-19 The correlation between breast disease and HER-2/neu overexpression

	Van de Vijver et al.[172]		Allred et al.[6]		Lodato et al.[101]		Goldschmidt et al.[64]	
Pathologic subtype	**No. pts.**	**Overexpression (%)**	**No. pts.**	**Overexpression (%)**	**No. pts.**	**Overexpression (%)**	**No. pts.**	**Overexpression (%)**
ADH	—	—	15	0	21	10	—	—
DCIS alone								
Comedo variant	29	66	40	78	10	100	29	59
Not otherwise specified	16	0	19	11	23	35	39	8
Combined DCIS and IDC								
DCIS	*	—	230	22	—	—	—	—
IDC	*	—	230	21	—	—	—	—
IDC alone	139	15	412	11.2	—	—	—	—

ADH, atypical ductal hyperplasia; IDC, infiltrating ductal carcinoma; DCIS, in situ ductal carcinoma.
*Three of 8 cases (38%) of DCIS with minimal invasive ductal carcinoma showed overexpression, however the authors did not indicate which component stained positive.

Table 8-20 Prognostic significance of HER-2/neu oncogene amplication or overexpression in stage I to stage III breast cancer

			Survival (%)		Outcome based on HER-2/neu status		
Author	**No. pts.**	**Amplification or overexpression**	**Disease-free survival**	**Overall survival**	**Disease-free survival**	**Overall survival**	**Follow-up (yr)**
Ali et al.[4]	122	Absent	—	—	No	No	4.4 (median)
		Present	—	—			
Barnes et al.[13,a]	195	Absent	54	64	No	No	10
		Present	39	50			
		Unknown	40	54			
Cline et al.[37,b]	48	Absent	34	—[d]	Yes[c]	—[d]	2
		Present	50	—[d]			
Paik et al.[134,a]	292	Absent	50	67	No	Yes[e]	8.3
		Present	47	47			
Van de Vijver et al.[172,a]	189	Absent	79	85	No[f]	Yes[c]	6, 4.3 (median)
		Present	74	70			
Wright et al.[186]	185	Absent	42	70	Yes[c]	Yes[c]	3.5, 2 (median)
		Present	21	37			
Zhou et al.[189]	51	Absent	67	—[d]	No	—[d]	3
		Present	33	—[d]			

Yes, statistically significant ($p \leq .05$); No, not significant ($p > .05$).
[a]Immunohistochemistry for overexpression.
[b]Southern blot for amplification.
[c]Significant on univariate analysis only.
[d]Analysis not done by author.
[e]Significant on multivariate analysis.
[f]Relapse-free survival.

Table 8-21 The prognostic value of HER-2/neu oncogene amplification or overexpression patients with node-negative breast cancer

		Outcome based on HER-2/neu status			
Author	No. pts.	Disease-free survival	Distant disease-free survival	Overall survival	Follow-up (yr)
Allred et al.[7]*	727 Low risk	Yes†	—	—	3.8 (median)
	High risk	No	—	—	
Borg et al.[20]‡	159/192§	No	No	No	3.8 (median)
Slamon et al.[156]‡	181	No	—	No	5
Tandon et al.[163]‖	378	No	—	No	6

*Immunohistochemistry analysis for overexpression.
†Significant on univariate analysis only.
‡Southern blot analysis for amplification.
§159 patients analyzed for amplification; 192 for overexpression.
‖Western blot analysis for overexpression.

from analysis, HER-2/neu expression became a stronger predictor of relapse, 57% vs. 15%. Thus HER-2/neu expression identified a group of women with a significant risk of failure within a group of women considered to be at low risk.

Node-positive breast cancer. HER-2/neu has prognostic importance in node-positive breast cancer patients (Table 8-22). Univariate and multivariate analyses revealed that HER-2/neu was an independent predictor of disease-free survival[126,155,156,163] and overall survival.[155,156,163] In a large review by Slamon et al.,[156] HER-2/neu was revealed as a stronger prognosticator than hormone receptor status, tumor size, and patient age. Borg et al.[20] demonstrated a significant reduction in disease-free, distant disease-free, and overall survival rates in patients with HER-2/neu amplification on univariate analysis, and found only a trend for overexpression. While multivariate analysis of these relationships failed to reach statistical significance, the combined parameter of negative progesterone receptor and HER-2/neu amplification offered significant prognostic value, being more important than the number of positive lymph nodes. O'Reilly et al.[126] showed that overexpression of HER-2/neu independently predicted for relapse-free survival on multivariate analysis of several variables including S-phase fraction. Further, Tandon et al.[136] showed that patient outcome was directly proportional to the number of involved axillary lymph nodes (Table 8-23).

Studies of breast cancer primary tumors and involved lymph nodes within the same patient showed similar patterns of HER-2/neu amplification and overexpression, suggesting that the oncogenic alterations occurred before metastasis.[13,97]

Inflammatory carcinoma. Two studies have assessed HER-2/neu and/or epithelial growth factor receptor amplification and overexpression in inflammatory breast cancer patients.[97] In a study by Lacroix et al.[97] overexpression of HER-2/neu was present in five of six patients, and three of those five also had amplification. In a second French study the same year, 41% (33/80) of inflammatory breast cancer patients had HER-2/neu amplification and 61% (46/75) had overexpression. In addition, overexpression of the EGFR was detected in 58% (31/53) of patients. When HER-2/neu and epithelial growth factor receptor analyses were performed in the same specimens, 91% had HER-2/neu and/or epithelial growth factor receptor overexpression. These oncogenic abnormalities were significantly higher in inflammatory breast cancer patients than in noninflammatory breast cancer patients at the same institution.

Summary

The biologic importance of HER-2/neu in breast cancer is under intense investigation. The high level of HER-2/neu amplification and/or overexpression in both noninvasive comedo-variant breast cancer and in inflammatory breast cancer is puzzling because the clinical behavior of these two disease presentations is antithetical. It is unlikely that HER-2/neu *alone* is critical in the pathogenesis of breast cancer; rather, its effect is probably dependent on interactions with other agents such as EGFR. Rodent cell lines that contain high levels of both EGFR and HER-2/neu demonstrate aggressive behavior in vitro and in vivo. Further, preliminary studies indicate that high levels of EGFR accompany HER-2/neu overexpression in most inflammatory breast cancer patients.

HER-2/neu provides independent prognostic information in node-positive patients for both disease-free and overall survival. In the overall

Table 8-22 The prognostic value of HER-2/neu overexpression in axillary node-positive breast cancer patients

			Survival (%)			Statistical significance of outcome based on presence or absence of the HER-2/neu oncogene			
Author	**No. pts.**	**Amplification and/or overexpression**	**Disease-free survival**	**Distant disease-free survival**	**Overall survival**	**Disease-free survival**	**Distant disease-free survival**	**Overall survival**	**Follow-up (yr)**
Borg et al.[20,1,b]	99	Absent	—[d]	47	—[d]	Yes[c]	Yes[c]	Yes[c]	6, 3.4 (median)
		Present	—[d]	30	—[d]				
Slamon et al.[155,a]	86	Absent	57	—[f]	54	Yes[e]	—[f]	Yes[e]	7
		Present	57	—[f]	41				
		Present/>5 copies	37	—[f]	40				
Slamon et al.[156,a]	345					4.8 (median)			
Tandon et al.[163,g]	350	Absent	45	—[f]	61	6, 4.2 (median)			
		Present	32	—[f]	40				

[a]Southern blot analysis for amplification.
[b]Significant with respect to amplification only; only a trend with overexpression.
[c]Significant on univariate analysis only.
[d]Authors did not provide actual values.
[e]Significant on multivariate analysis.
[f]Analysis not done.
[g]Western blot analysis for overexpression.

Table 8-23 HER-2/neu protein vs. positive nodes—effects on 5-year survival rates

No. positive nodes	HER-2/neu protein	No. pts.	Disease-free survival ± SD (%)	Overall survival ± SD (%)
1-3	Low	136	60 ± 5	81 ± 4
	High	19	37 ± 13	46 ± 14
4-10	Low	89	48 ± 6	66 ± 6
	High	23	34 ± 10	39 ± 12
>10	Low	66	20 ± 6	44 ± 7
	High	17	24 ± 12	36 ± 13

From Tandon A et al: J Clin Oncol 7(8):1120, 1989.

group of node-negative patients, however, HER-2/neu does not independently predict patient outcome. HER-2/neu amplification and/or overexpression, together with other more classic prognostic parameters, such as hormone receptor status, nuclear grade, and tumor size, does identify subgroups of node-negative breast cancer patients at high risk for failure.

Determinations of both HER-2/neu gene amplification and overexpression will better elucidate the mechanism by which this genetic abnormality has its effect and, in addition, will improve the ability to compare studies. Prospective analyses of HER-2/neu together with other prognostic variables (for example, EST 1189) will better define the independent prognostic significance of HER-2/neu and its role in selecting node-negative patients who are likely to benefit from adjuvant chemotherapy and node-positive patients who might benefit from more aggressive therapies.

EPITHELIAL GROWTH FACTOR RECEPTOR

Epithelial growth factor influences murine mammary carcinogenesis and may be important in human breast cancer. EGF induces mitosis in human breast cancer cells in vitro,[82,131] and its overexpression has been demonstrated in human breast cancer cells. The structural and functional relationship between the neu oncogene and EGFR is discussed in the previous section on the neu oncogene.

The epithelial growth factor receptor has an external domain, a transmembrane component, and a cytoplasmic component containing a tyrosine-specific protein kinase.[48] It is usually measured by a competitive binding assay using the radioligand iodine-125 EGF, but can also be detected by Northern blot and immunohistochemistry.[167] EGF and transforming growth factor alpha (TGF alpha) are the ligands for EGFR.[48,57] EGF binds to the external domain of EGFR, resulting in autophosphorylation leading to phosphorylation of cellular substrates and activation of tyrosine kinase.[27,81,180] Antibodies against TGF alpha or EGFR produce partial reversion of the transformed phenotype of the human breast cancer cell line MCF-7 in vitro.[112] Other agents can modulate EGFR function: estrogens can increase and antiestrogen can decrease certain growth factor activities.[100,121]

Increased EGFR expression is associated with aggressive tumor behavior in nonmammary epithelial tumors, such as those in the bladder,[124] lung,[175] and stomach.[160] EGFR rarely is seen in normal breast tissue,[68,139] and is uncommon in benign processes such as fibroadenomas.[68] EGFR elevation occurs in 25% to 57% of primary operable breast cancer patients (Table 8-24). A study of primary tumors and lymph node metastases in the same patients showed significantly higher levels of EGFR in the patients with metastases.[14]

Correlation with other prognostic variables

The association between EGFR and the classic prognostic variables such as tumor size, stage, age, menopausal status, histologic grade, lymph node status, and hormone receptor status is presented in Table 8-1.

Essentially, all studies demonstrate a strong inverse correlation between EGFR levels and hormone receptor status. But EGF expression may be more common in human breast tumors that express estrogen and progesterone mRNA than tumors that

Table 8-24 Incidence of EGFR positivity in operable breast cancer patients

Author	No. pts.	Incidence of elevation (%)
Battaglia et al.[14]	89	57
Bolla et al.[18]	177	25
Sainsbury et al.[142]	108	42
Toi et al.[167]	91	43

do not.[47] There is a consistent inverse relationship between EGFR expression and histologic grade, and a variable association between EGFR levels and lymph node status or tumor size. There is a significant association between EGFR expression and high proliferative index.[168]

The prognostic value of EGFR in operable breast cancer

Few studies have analyzed the prognostic value of EGFR expression in operable breast cancer (Table 8-25). The definition of positive EGFR used in these few studies ranged from 1 fmol/mg protein in one study[168] to 10 fmol/mg protein in the other two studies.[72,143] EGFR was an important predictor of relapse-free and overall survival rates by both univariate and multivariate (when available) analysis. EGFR was the most important prognosticator for predicting relapse-free survival (independent of tumor size, histologic grade, ER and lymph node status) and overall survival (only univariate analysis was available) in 135 operable breast cancer patients at 3 years.[143] By univariate analysis (multivariate analysis was unavailable), EGFR expression was the most significant prognosticator in node-negative patients and the second most important prognosticator in node-positive patients. In an analysis of 231 women with operable breast cancer at a median follow-up of 3 years, Harris demonstrated an association between elevated EGFR levels and decreased relapse-free and overall survival rates, independent of tumor size, histologic grade, and ER status.[72] EGFR expression also affected the pattern of metastatic disease: EGFR-positive patients had a pattern of visceral rather than bony metastases, the converse of EGFR-negative patients.[143,168]

When subsets of operable breast cancer patients were analyzed, EGFR expression was able to identify poor-risk patients within a relatively good-risk group, as well as good-risk patients within a relatively poor-risk group. For example, all EGFR-positive/ER-positive patients (four patients) died within 2 years; EGFR-negative/ER-negative patients had similar relapse-free survival rates and early overall survival rates compared to the general group of ER-positive patients.[143] Harris showed a significant reduction in the rate of relapse-free survival in EGFR-positive/ER-negative patients.[72] In node-negative patients, EGFR expression also had strong prognostic value with respect to rates of relapse-free survival[72,143] and overall survival.[72]

HEAT SHOCK STRESS PROTEINS

The level of heat shock or stress response proteins in breast cancer may be a measure of the biologic stress between patient and cancer and may predict the behavior of the cancer.

The prognostic value of this class of proteins was investigated by the San Antonio group in two separate reports. First, Chamness et al.[29] used Western blot to measure the estrogen-induced heat shock protein, hsp27, in 385 node-negative breast cancer specimens with a median follow-up of 53 months. A high level of hsp27, above 13.5 U, was associated with estrogen and progesterone positivity and aneuploidy, but not tumor size or age. Those patients with high hsp27 levels (23% of the group) had a 1.93 relative risk of recurrence, confirmed on multivariate analysis. ER-positive/low-hsp27 patients had a 15% actuarial 5-year recurrence rate, in contrast to 29% for ER-negative/low-hsp27 patients, and 39% for any high-hsp27 (ER-positive or ER-negative patients). Later, Tandon et al.[161] determined the levels of three heat shock proteins and one glucose regulatory protein in 400 breast cancer patients with Western blot analysis. While all four proteins were associated with increased levels of cathepsin D, only hsp70 was associated with ER/PR receptors, and hsp90 and grp94 were associated

Table 8-25 The correlation between EGFR status and patient outcome in patients with operable cancer

Author	No. pts.	EGFR status	Survival (%) Relapse-free survival	Survival (%) Overall survival	Follow-up (yr)
Toi et al.[168]	52	Negative	94	—	3.3, 2 (median)
		Positive	77	—	
Sainsbury et al.[143]	135	Negative	61	85	3
		Positive	33	38	
Harris[72]	Node-negative 30	Negative	75	88	4.6, 3 (median)
	20	Positive	37	58	
	Node-positive 44	Negative	37	47	
	35	Positive	31	31	

with aneuploidy and high nuclear grade. The median levels of all four proteins were significantly higher in node-positive patients than in node-negative patients; however, the level of protein had no prognostic value in node-positive patients. In the 200 node-negative patients, high levels of one or more of these proteins was associated with a significantly shorter relapse-free survival than those without detectable stress response protein. As the number of high-level stress response proteins increased from one to four, the actuarial recurrence rate increased from 24% to 80%.

Thus the class of heat shock or stress proteins may constitute yet another indicator of aggressive disease behavior within the group of node-negative patients. The association with other prognostic parameters and its independent prognostic value with respect to both disease-free and overall survival will be investigated further in women with node-negative breast cancer by the Southwest Oncology Group Protocol 9037, a companion protocol to EST-2188, CALGB-8897, and Intergroup 0102.

CONCLUSIONS

This chapter demonstrates the independent prognostic value of the newer biologic markers, particularly hormone receptors and proliferative index, on repeated clinical testing in node-negative breast cancer patients. By itself, each of these two parameters is insufficient criteria on which to base the administration of adjuvant chemotherapy. Together, they provide strong criteria. Ploidy is without consistent independent prognostic value in node-negative patients, but complements other factors. The combination of aneuploidy and a high proliferative index provides sufficiently strong criteria for the administration of adjuvant chemotherapy.

Cathepsin D possesses independent prognostic value in most of the limited number of clinical studies available. Its prognostic power may improve when combined with ploidy. Heat shock proteins demonstrated prognostic significance on preliminary univariate analyses.

The role of HER-2/neu in node-negative patients is unclear. Its predictive value is now limited to subgroups of patients already characterized by other prognostic factors such as hormone receptor status, nuclear grade, and tumor size. Early studies on the independent prognostic value of epithelial growth factor receptor are promising; however, the results of these studies must be substantiated by further investigation. Perhaps more exciting is the possible role of HER-2/neu and EGFR expression in the molecular mechanism of breast cancer carcinogenesis and progression, with its implications for future therapies.

HER-2/neu has independent predictive value in node-positive patients, although it has not yet served as a criterion for more intensive treatment of very high-risk patients in randomized studies. Hormone receptor status is an important predictor of a patient's response to hormonal manipulation. The other prognosticators—DNA ploidy and proliferative index, EGFR expression, heat shock proteins, and cathepsin D—are not clinically significant in node-positive patients at this time.

These new biologic markers need to be studied further. Standardization of the techniques for measuring the parameters, and the definition of a positive test would make the determinations much more useful and facilitate the comparison of studies. As laboratory assays improve and require less tissue, a greater number of tests can be performed on each tumor specimen. The population studied will become less biased towards larger tumors. Our goal is to devise strong, reliable, and widely available criteria to guide the clinician in delivering optimal therapy, observation or systemic intervention, to each patient. Current clinical trials, such as the Southwest Oncology Group Protocol 9037 (a companion protocol to EST-2188, CALGB-8897, and Intergroup 0102), are prospectively analyzing all of the biologic markers discussed in this chapter. The parameters that prove to have independent prognostic value will be important in selecting node-negative patients likely to benefit from adjuvant chemotherapy, and node-positive patients likely to benefit from autologous bone marrow transplantation and other more aggressive therapies.

REFERENCES

1. Akiyama T, Saito T, Ogawara H, et al: Tumor promoter and epidermal growth factor stimulate phosphorylation of the c-erbB-2 gene product in MKN-7 human adenocarcinoma cells, Mol Cell Biol 8:1019, 1988.
2. Akiyama T, Sudo C, Ogawara H, et al: The product of the human c-erbB-2 gene: a 185 kilodalton glycoprotein with tyrosine kinase activity, Science 232:1644, 1986.
3. Ali I, Campbell G, Lidereau R and Callahan R: Amplification of c-erbB-2 and aggressive human breast tumors? Science 240:1795, 1988.
4. Ali I, Campbell G, Lidereau R, and Callahan R: Lack of evidence for the prognostic significance of c-erbB-2 amplification in human breast carcinoma, Oncol Res 3(2):139, 1988.
5. Allegra J, Lippman M, Simon R, et al: Association between steroid hormone receptor status and disease-free interval in breast cancer, Cancer Treat Rep 63:1271, 1979.
6. Allred D, Clark G, Molina R, et al: Immunocytochemical evaluation of HER-2/neu oncogene expression in different evolutionary stages of breast carcinoma and correlation with clinical-pathological characteristics, Proc Am Soc Clin Oncol 9:23, 1990.
7. Allred D, Clark G, Tandon R, et al: HER-2/neu expression identified a group of node-negative breast cancer

patients at high risk for recurrence, Proc Am Soc Clin Oncol 9:23, 1990.
8. Augereau P, Garcia M, Mattei M, et al: Cloning and sequencing of the 52K cathepsin D complementary deoxyribonucleic acid of MCF7 breast cancer cells and mapping on chromosome 11, Mol Endocrinol 2:186, 1988.
9. Baildam A, Zaloudik J, Howell A, et al: DNA analysis by flow cytometry, response to endocrine treatment and prognosis in advanced carcinoma of the breast, Br J Cancer 55:553, 1987.
10. Bargmann C, Hung M-C, and Weinberg R: The neu oncogene encodes an epidermal growth factor receptor-related protein, Nature 319:226, 1986.
11. Bargmann C, Hung M-C, and Weinberg R: Multiple independent activation of the neu oncogene by point mutation altering the transmembrane domain of p185, Cell 45:649, 1986.
12. Bargmann C and Weinberg R: Increased tyrosine kinase activity with the protein encoded by the activated neu oncogene, Proc Natl Acad Sci USA 85:5394, 1988.
13. Barnes D, Lammie G, Millis R, et al: An immunohistochemical evaluation of c-erbB-2 expression in human breast carcinoma, Br J Cancer 58:448, 1988.
14. Battaglia F, Scambia G, Rossi S, et al: Epidermal growth factor receptor in human breast cancer: correlation with steroids hormone receptors and axillary lymph node involvement, Eur J Cancer Clin Oncol 24(11):1685, 1988.
15. Beaune J, Bagnard G, Rymer J, et al: Determination of 52k cathepsin D levels in normal tissues, benign mastopathies, breast cancers and metastatic cells, Breast Cancer Res Treat 16(2):181, 1990.
16. Benner S, Clark G, and McGuire W: Review: steroid receptors, cellular kinetics and lymph node status as prognostic factors in breast cancer, Am J Med Sci 1:59, 1988.
17. Berger M, Locher G, Saurer S, et al: Correlation of c-erbB-2 gene amplification and protein expression in human breast carcinoma with nodal status and nuclear grading, Cancer Res 48:1238, 1988.
18. Bolla M, Chedin M, Souvignet C, et al: Estimation of epidermal growth factor receptor in 177 breast cancers: correlation with prognostic factors, Breast Cancer Res Treat 16:97, 1990.
19. Borg A, Baldetorp B, Ferno M, et al: Oncogene amplification and breast cancer prognosis, Breast Cancer Res Treat 16(2):180, 1990.
20. Borg A, Tandon A, Sigurdsson H, et al: HER-2/neu amplification predicts poor survival in node-positive breast cancer, Cancer Res 50:4332, 1990.
21. Brailly S, Lorenzo F, Jolivet A, et al: Radioimmunoassay of progesterone receptor in human tissues: application to breast cancer, J Endocrinol 116:427, 1988.
22. Briozzo P, Morisset M, Capony F, et al: In vitro degradation of extracellular matrix with Mr 52,000 cathepsin D secreted by breast cancer cells, Cancer Res 48:3688, 1988.
23. Butler J, Bretsky S, Menendez-Botet C, and Kinne D: Estrogen receptor protein of breast cancer as a predictor of recurrence, Cancer 55:1178, 1985.
24. Campbell F, Blamey R, Elston C, et al: Oestrogen-receptor status and sites of metastasis in breast cancer, Br J Cancer 44:456, 1981.
25. Capony F, Garcia M, Capdevielle J, et al: Purification and first characterization of the secreted and cellular 52-kDa proteins regulated by estrogens in human breast cancer cells, Eur J Biochem 161:505, 1986.
26. Capony F, Rougeot C, Montcourrier P, et al: Increased secretion, altered processing and glycosylation of pro-cathepsin D in human mammary cancer cells, Cancer Res 49:3904, 1989.
27. Carpenter G: Receptors for epithelial growth factor and other polypeptide mitogens, Ann Rev Biochem 56:881, 1987.
28. Cavailles V, Augereau P, Garcia M, and Rochefort H: Estrogens and growth factors induce the mRNS of the 52K-pro-cathepsin-D secreted by breast cancer cells, Nucleic Acids Res 16(5):1903, 1988.
29. Chamness G, Ruiz A, Fulcher L, et al: Estrogen-inducible heat shock protein hsp27 predicts recurrence in node negative breast cancer, Proc Am Assoc Cancer Res 30:252, 1989.
30. Charpin C, Jacquemier J, Andrac L, et al: Multiparametric analysis (SAMBA 200) of the progesterone receptor immunocytochemical assay in nonmalignant and malignant breast disorders, Am J Pathol 132(2):199, 1988.
31. Clark G, Dressler L, Owens M, et al: Prediction of relapse or survival in patients with node-negative breast cancer by DNA flow cytometry, N Eng J Med 320(10):627, 1989.
32. Clark G and McGuire W: Steroid receptors and other prognostic factors in primary breast cancer, Semin Oncol 15 (2):20, 1988.
33. Clark G and McGuire W: New biologic prognostic factors in breast cancer, Oncology 3(5):49, 1989.
34. Clark G, McGuire W, and Hubay CA: Progesterone receptors as a prognostic factor in stage II breast cancer, N Engl J Med 309:1343, 1983.
35. Clark G, Osborne C, and McGuire W: Correlations between estrogen receptor, progesterone receptor, and patient characteristics in human breast cancer, J Clin Oncol 2:1102, 1984.
36. Clark G, Sledge G, Osborne C, and McGuire W: Survival from first recurrence: relative importance of prognostic factors in 1015 breast cancer patients, J Clin Oncol 5:55, 1987.
37. Cline M, Battifora H, and Yokota J: Proto-oncogene abnormalities in human breast cancer: correlations with anatomic features and clinical course of disease, J Clin Oncol 5(7):999, 1987.
38. Cohen O, Brugal G, Seigneurin D, and Demongeot J: Image cytometry of estrogen receptors in breast carcinomas, Cytometry 9:579, 1988.
39. Reference deleted.
40. Cooke T, George W, and Griffiths K: Possible tests for selection of adjuvant systemic therapy in early cancer of the breast, Br J Surg 67:747, 1980.
41. Coon J, Landau A, and Weinstein R: Advances in flow cytometry for diagnostic pathology, Lab Invest 57:453, 1988.
42. Cornelisse C, van de Velde C, Caspers R, et al: DNA ploidy and survival in breast cancer patients, Cytometry 8:225, 1987.
43. Coussens L, Yang-Feng T, Liao Y-C, et al: Tyrosine kinase receptor with extensive homology to EGF receptor shares chromosomal location with neu oncogene, Science 1132, 1985.
44. Cudany T, Boeryd B, Franlund B, and Nordenskjoeld B: A comparison of three different methods for the determination of estrogen receptors in human breast cancer, Am J Clin Pathol 90:583, 1988.
45. Di Fiore P, Pierce J, Kraus M, et al: erbB-2 is a potent oncogene when overexpressed in NIH/3T3 cells, Science 237:178, 1987.
46. Dollbaum C, Sylvester S, Howlett T, and Zava D: Cathepsin-D: relationship to other breast cancer prognostic indicators, Breast Cancer Res Treat 16(2):181, 1990.
47. Dotzlaw H, Miller T, Karvelas J, and Murphy L: Epidermal growth factor gene expression in human breast cancer biopsy samples: relationship to estrogen and progesterone receptor gene expression, Cancer Res 50:4204, 1990.

48. Downward J, Parker P, and Waterfield M: Autophosphorylation sites on the epidermal growth factor receptor, Nature 311:483, 1984.
49. Drebin J, Link V, Weinberg R, and Greene M: Inhibition of tumor growth by a monoclonal antibody reactive with an oncogene-encoded tumor antigen, Proc Natl Sci USA 83:9129, 1986.
50. Dressler L, Eudey L, Gray R, et al: DNA flow cytometry measurements are prognostic for time to recurrence in node negative breast cancer patients: an Eastern Cooperative Group (ECOG) intergroup study, Proc Am Soc Clin Oncol 9:22, 1990.
51. Dressler L, Seamer LC; Owens M, et al: DNA Flow cytometry and prognostic factors in 1331 frozen breast cancer specimens, Cancer 61:420, 1988.
52. Fallenius A, Auer G, and Carstensen J: Prognostic significance of DNA measurements in 409 consecutive breast cancer patients, Cancer 62:331, 1988.
53. Fallenius A, Franzen S, and Auer G: Predictive value of nuclear DNA content in breast cancer in relation to clinical and morphologic factors, Cancer 62:521, 1988.
54. Ferno M, Borg A, and Johansson U: Enzyme immunoassay of progesterone receptor in breast cancer biopsy samples, Acta Oncol 28:19, 1989.
55. Fisher B, Redmond C, Dimitrov N, et al: A randomized clinical trial evaluating sequential methotrexate and fluorouracil in the treatment of patients with node-negative breast cancer who have estrogen-receptor-negative tumors, N Engl J Med 320:473, 1989.
56. Fisher B, Redmond C, Fisher E, and Caplan R: Relative worth of estrogen or progesterone receptor and pathologic characteristics of differentiation as indicators of prognosis in node negative breast cancer patients: findings from National Surgical Adjuvant Breast and Bowel Project Protocol B-06, J Clin Oncol 6:1076, 1988.
57. Fitzpatrick S, Brightwell J, Wittliff J, et al: Epidermal growth factor binding by breast tumor biopsies and relationship to estrogen receptor and progestin receptor levels, Cancer Res 44:3448, 1984.
58. Flowers J, Burton G, Cox E, et al: Use of monoclonal anti-estrogen receptor antibody to evaluate estrogen receptor content in fine needle aspiration breast biopsies, Ann Surg 203:250, 1986.
59. Fontaine J, Tesseraux M, Klein V, et al: Gene amplification and expression of the neu (c-erbB-2) sequence in human mammary carcinoma, Oncology 45:360, 1988.
60. Fukushige S, Matsubara K, Yoshida M, et al: Localization of a novel v-erbB-related gene, c-erbB-2, on human chromosome-17 and its amplification in a gastric cancer cell line, Mol Cell Biol 6:955, 1986.
61. Garcia M, Lacombe M, Duplay H, et al: Immunohistochemical distribution of the 52-IDa protein in mammary tumors: a marker associated with cell proliferation rather than with hormone responsiveness, J Steroid Biochem 27:439, 1987.
62. Gentili C, Sanfilippo O, and Silvestrini R: Cell proliferation and its relationship to clinical features and relapse in breast cancers, Cancer 48:974, 1981.
63. Goldhirsch EA: Prolonged disease-free survival after one course of perioperative adjuvant chemotherapy for node-negative breast cancer, N Engl J Med 320:491, 1989.
64. Goldschmidt R, Prindiville S, Merkel D, et al: Comparison of HER-2 expression, histology, and flow cytometry in ductal carcinoma-in-situ, Breast Cancer Res Treat 16(2):191, 1990.
65. Graham M II, Bunn P Jr, Jewett P, et al: Simultaneous measurement of progesterone receptors and DNA indices by flow cytometry: characterization of an assay in breast cancer cell lines, Cancer Res 49:3934, 1989.
66. Greene G, Sobel N, King W, et al: Immunochemical studies of estrogen receptors, J Steroid Biochem 20:51, 1984.
67. Guerin M, Barrois M, Terrier M-J, et al: Overexpression of either c-myc or c-erbB-2/neu proto-oncogenes in human breast carcinomas: correlation with poor prognosis, Oncol Res 3(1):21, 1988.
68. Guerin M, Gabillot M, Mathieu M-C, et al: Structure and expression of C-erbB-2 and EGF receptor genes in inflammatory and non-inflammatory breast cancer: prognostic significance, Int J Cancer 43:201, 1989.
69. Gullick W, Berger M, Bennett P, et al: Expression of the c-erbB-2 protein in normal and transformed cells, Int J Cancer 40(2):236, 1987.
70. Hahnel R, Woodings T, and Vivian A: Prognostic value of estrogen receptors in primary breast cancer, Cancer 44:671, 1979.
71. Hanna W and Mobbs B: Comparative evaluation of ER-ICA and enzyme immunoassay for the quantitation of estrogen receptors in breast cancer, Am J Clin Pathol 91:182, 1989.
72. Harris A: Epidermal growth factor receptor and the HER-2/neu oncogene. Proceedings of the NIH Consensus Development Conference—Early Stage Breast Cancer, 1990, pp 107-110.
73. Hatschek Y, Fagerberg G, Stal O, et al: Cytometric characterization and clinical course of breast cancer diagnosed in a population-based screening program, Cancer 64:1074, 1989.
74. Hedley D, Rugg C, and Gelber R: Association of DNA index and S-phase fraction with prognosis of nodes positive early breast cancer, Cancer Res 47:4729, 1987.
75. Helin H, Helle M, Kallioniemi O, and Isola J: Immunohistochemical determination of estrogen and progesterone receptors in human breast carcinoma, Cancer 63:1761, 1989.
76. Herman C, McGraw T, Marder R, and Bauer K: Recent progress in clinical quantitative cytology, Arch Pathol Lab Med 111:505, 1987.
77. Hery M, Gioanni J, LaLanne C, et al: The DNA labelling index: a prognostic factor in node negative breast cancer, Breast Cancer Res Treat 9(3):207, 1987.
78. Horsfall D, Tilley W, Orell S, et al: Relationship between ploidy and steroid hormone receptors in primary invasive breast cancer, Br J Cancer 53:23, 1986.
79. Horwitz K, McGuire W, Pearson O, and Segaloff A: Predicting response to endocrine therapy in human breast cancer: a hypothesis, Science 189:726, 1975.
80. Hudziak R, Schlessinger J, and Ullrich A: Increased expression of the putative growth factor receptor p185HER2 causes transformation and tumorigenesis of NIH 3T3 cells, Proc Natl Acad Sci USA 84:7159, 1987.
81. Hunter T and Cooper J: Protein-tyrosine kinases, Ann Rev Biochem 54:897, 1985.
82. Imai Y, Leung C, Friesen H, and Shiu R: Epidermal growth factor receptors and effect of epidermal growth factor on growth of human breast cancer cells in long term tissue culture, Cancer Res 42:4394, 1982.
83. Jordon V: The control of hormone dependent breast cancer growth—are we talking about estrogen alone? Eur J Cancer Clin Oncol 24:1245, 1988.
84. Kallioniemi O-P, Blanco G, Alavaikko M, et al: Tumour DNA ploidy as an independent prognostic factor in breast cancer, Br J Cancer 56:637, 1987.
85. Kallioniemi O-P, Blanco G, Alavaikko M, et al: Improving the prognostic value of DNA flow cytometry in breast cancer by combining DNA index and S-phase fraction, Cancer 62:2183, 1988.
86. Kelsten M, Berger M, Maguire H Jr, et al: Analysis of c-erB-2 protein expression in conjunction with DNA con-

tent using multiparameter flow cytometry, Cytometry 11:522, 1990.
87. King C, Borrello I, Bellot F, et al: Egf binding to its receptor triggers a rapid tyrosine phosphorylation of the erB-2 protein in the mammary tumor cell line SK-BR-3, EMBO J 7(6):1647, 1988.
88. King C, Kraus M, and Aaronson S: Amplification of a novel v-erbB-related gene in a human mammary carcinoma, Science 229:974, 1985.
89. King C, Swain S, Porteer L, et al: Heterogeneous expression of erbB-2 messenger RNA in human breast cancer, Cancer Res 49:4185, 1989.
90. Kinne D, Ashikari R, Butler A, et al: Estrogen receptor protein in breast cancer as a predictor of recurrence, Cancer 47:2364, 1981.
91. Klintenberg C, Stal O, Nordenskjold B, et al: Proliferative index, cystosol estrogen receptor and axillary node status as prognostic predictors in human mammary carcinoma, Breast Cancer Res Treat 7(suppl):99, 1986.
92. Knight W, Livingston R, Gregory E, et al: Estrogen receptor as an independent prognostic factor for early recurrence in breast cancer, Cancer Res 37:4669, 1977.
93. Kokai Y, Dobashi K, Weiner D, et al: Phosphorylation process induced by epidermal growth factor receptor alters the oncogenic and cellular neu (NGL) gene products, Proc Natl Acad Sci USA 85:5389, 1988.
94. Kokai Y, Myers J, Wada T, et al: Synergistic interaction of p185c-neu and the EGF receptor leads to transformation of rodent fibroblasts, Cell 58:287, 1989.
95. Korenman S: Radio-ligand binding assay of specific estrogens using a soluble uterine macromolecule, J Clin Endocrinol Metabol 28:127, 1968.
96. Kute T, Muss H, Cooper M, et al: The use of flow cytometry for the prognosis of stage II adjuvant treated breast cancer patients, Cancer 66:1810, 1990.
97. Lacroix H, Iglehard J, Skinner M, and Kraus M: Overexpression of erbB-2 or EGF receptor proteins present in early stage mammary carcinoma is detected simultaneously in matched primary tumors and regional metastases, Oncogene 4:145, 1989.
98. Lagios M, Margolin F, Westdahl P, and Rose M: Mammographically detected duct carcinoma in situ: frequency of local recurrence following tylectomy and prognostic effect of nuclear grade on local recurrence, Cancer 63:6188, 1989.
99. Liotta L: Gene products which may play a role in cancer invasion and metastasis, Breast Cancer Res Treat 11:113, 1988.
100. Lippman M, Dickson R, Bates S, et al: Autocrine and paracrine growth regulation of human breast cancer, Breast Cancer Res Treat 7:59, 1986.
101. Lodato R, Maguire H Jr, Greene M, et al: Immunohistochemical evaluation of c-erbB-2 oncogene expression in ductal carcinoma in situ and atypical ductal hyperplasia of the breast, Mod Pathol 3(4):449, 1990.
102. Lovett E, Schnitzer B, Karen D, et al: Application of flow cytometry to diagnostic pathology, Lab Invest 50:115, 1984.
103. Lozowski M, Mishriki Y, Chao S, et al: Estrogen receptor determination in fine needle aspirates of the breast, Cancer 31:557, 1987.
104. Mansour E, Gray R, Shatila A, et al: Efficacy of adjuvant chemotherapy in high risk node negative breast cancer, N Engl J Med 320:485, 1989.
105. Mason B, Holdaway I, Mullins P, et al: Progesterone and estrogen receptors as prognostic variables in breast cancer, Cancer Res 43:2985, 1983.
106. Maudelonde T, Khalaf S, Garcia M, et al: Immunoenzymatic assay of Mr52,000 cathepsin D in 182 breast cancer cytosols: low correlation with other prognostic parameters, Cancer Res 48:462, 1988.
107. McDivitt R, Stone K, Craig R, and Meyer J: A comparison of human breast cancer cell kinetics measured by flow cytometry and thymidine labeling, Lab Invest 52(3):287, 1985.
108. McDivitt R, Stone K, Craig R, et al: A proposed classification of breast cancer based on kinetic information, Cancer 57:269, 1986.
109. McDivitt R, Stone K, and Meyer J: A method for dissociation of viable human breast cancer cells that produces flow cytometric kinetic information similar to that obtained by thymidine labeling, Cancer Res 44:2628, 1984.
110. McGuire W: Hormone receptors: their role in predicting prognosis and response to endocrine therapy, Semin Oncol 5:428, 1978.
111. McGuire W: Estrogen receptor versus nuclear grade as prognostic factors in axillary node negative breast cancer, J Clin Oncol 6:1071, 1988.
112. McGuire W, Dickson R, Osborne C, and Salomon D: The role of growth factors in breast cancer, Breast Cancer Res Treat 12:159, 1988.
113. McGuire W, Tandon A, Allred D, et al: How to use prognostic factors in axillary node-negative breast cancer patients, J Natl Cancer Inst 82(12):1006, 1990.
114. Meyer J: Cell kinetics of histologic variants of in situ breast carcinoma, Breast Cancer Res Treat 7:171, 1986.
115. Meyer J, Friedman E, McCrate M, and Bauer W: Prediction of early course of breast cancer by thymidine labelling, Cancer 51(10):1879, 1983.
116. Meyer J and Province M: Proliferative index of breast carcinoma by thymidine labeling: prognostic power independent of stage, estrogen and progesterone receptors, Cancer Res Treat 12:191, 1988.
117. Meyer J, Stevens S, White W, and Hixon B: Estrogen receptor assay of carcinomas of the breast by a simplified dextran-charcoal method, Am J Clin Pathol 70:655, 1978.
118. Moran R, Black M, Alpert L, and Straus M: Correlation of cell-cycle kinetics, hormone receptors, histopathology and nodal status in human breast cancer, Cancer 54(8):1586, 1984.
119. Morisset M, Capony F, and Rochefort H: Processing and estrogen regulation of the 52 kDa protein inside MCF-7 breast cancer cell, Endocrinology 110:2773, 1986.
120. Mueller WJ, Sinn E, Pattengale PK, et al: Single-step induction of mammary adenocarcinoma in transgenic mice bearing the activated c-neu oncogene, Cell 54(1):105, 1988.
121. Murphy LC, Murphy LJ, Dubik D, et al: Epidermal growth factor gene expression in human breast cancer cells: regulation of expression by progestins, Cancer Res 48:4555, 1988.
122. Muss H, Kute T, Case D, et al: The relation of flow cytometry to clinical and biologic characteristics in women with node negative primary breast cancer, Cancer 64:1894, 1989.
123. Namer M, Etienne M, Fontana X, et al: Prognostic value of total cathepsine D in breast cancer, Breast Cancer Res Treat 14:135, 1989.
124. Neal D, Marsh C, Bennett M, et al: Epidermal-growth-factor receptors in human bladder cancer: comparison of invasive and superficial tumours, Lancet i:366, 1985.
124a. NIH Conference: Treatment of early stage breast cancer, JAMA 265:391, 1991.
125. O'Keane J, Okon E, Moroz K, et al: Anti-estradiol immunoperoxidase labelling of nuclei, not cytoplasm, in paraffin sections, determines estrogen receptor status of breast cancer, Am J Surg Pathol 14:121, 1990.
126. Olszewski W, Darzynkiewicz Z, Rosen P, et al: Flow

cytometry of breast carcinoma. II. Relation of tumor cell cycle distribution to histology and estrogen receptor, Cancer 48:985, 1981.

127. Olszewski W, Darzynkiewicz Z, Rosen P, et al: Flow cytometry of breast carcinoma. I. Relation of DNA ploidy level to histology and estrogen receptor, Cancer 48:980, 1981.

128. O'Reilly S, Barnes D, Camplejohn R, and Richards M: C-erbB-2 expression and S-phase fraction are independent prognostic factors in node positive cancer, Breast Cancer Res Treat 16(2):182, 1990.

129. Osborne C: Heterogeneity in hormone receptor status in primary and metastatic breast cancer, Semin Oncol 12(3):317, 1985.

130. Osborne C: DNA flow cytometry in early breast cancer: a step in the right direction, J Natl Cancer Inst 81(18):1344, 1989 (editorial).

131. Osborne C, Hamilton B, Titus G, and Livingston R: Epidermal growth factor stimulation of human breast cancer cells in culture, Cancer Res 40:2361, 1980.

132. Osborne C, Yochmowitz M, Knight W III, and McGuire W: The value of estrogen and progesterone receptors in the treatment of breast cancer, Cancer 46:2884, 1980.

133. Owens M, Beardslee S, Wenger C, et al: DNA flow cytometry correlates with other prognostic factors for breast cancer, Breast Cancer Res Treat 14:134, 1989.

134. Paik S, Hazan R, Fisher E, et al: Pathologic findings from the National Surgical Adjuvant Breast and Bowel Project: prognostic significance of cerbB-2 protein overexpression in primary breast cancer, J Clin Oncol 8(1):103, 1990.

135. Patchefsky A, Schwartz G, Finkelstein S, et al: Heterogeneity of intraductal carcinoma of the breast, Cancer 63(4):731, 1979.

136. Pertschuk L, Tobin E, Brigati D, and Gaetjens E: Morphologic assay of steroid hormone receptors in human neoplasia, Pathol Ann 15 (part 2):143, 1980.

137. Prey M, Meyer J, Stone K, and McDivitt R: Heterogeneity of breast carcinomas determined by flow cytometric analysis, J Surg Oncol 29:35, 1985.

138. Qazi R, Chuang J, and Drobyski W: Estrogen receptors and the pattern of relapse in breast cancer, Arch Intern Med 144:2365, 1984.

139. Reubi J-C and Torhorst J: The relationship between somatostatin, epidermal growth factor and steroid hormone receptors in breast cancer, Cancer 64:124, 1989.

140. Rochefort H: Cathepsin D in breast cancer, Breast Cancer Res Treat 16:3, 1990.

141. Rutqvist L, Cedermark B, Fornander T, et al: The relationship between hormone receptor content and the effect of adjuvant tamoxifen in operable breast cancer, J Clin Oncol 17(10):1474, 1989.

142. Sainsbury J, Malcolm A, Appleton D, et al: Presence of epidermal growth factor receptor as an indicator of poor prognosis in patients with breast cancer, J Clin Pathol 38:1225, 1985.

143. Sainsbury J, Farndon J, Needham G, et al: Epidermal-growth-factor receptor status as predictor of early recurrence of and death from breast cancer, Lancet i:1398, 1987.

144. Schechter A, Stern D, Vaidyanathan L, et al: The neu oncogene: erb-B-related gene encoding a 185,000-M tumour antigen, Nature 312:513, 1984.

145. Sears H, Janus C, Levy W, et al: Breast cancer without axillary metastases, Cancer 50:1820, 1982.

146. Semba K, Kamata N, Toyoshima K, and Yamamoto T: A v-erbB-related proto-oncogene, c-erbB-2, is distinct from the c-erbB-i/epithelial growth factor-receptor gene and is amplified in human salivary gland adenocarcinoma, Proc Natl Acad Sci USA 82:6497, 1985.

147. Shapiro H: Practical flow cytometry, ed 2, New York, 1988, Liss.

148. Shintaku P and Said J: Detection of estrogen receptors with monoclonal antibodies in routinely processed formalin-fixed paraffin sections of breast carcinoma, Am J Clin Pathol 87:161, 1987.

149. Sigurdsson H, Baldetorp B, Borg A, et al: Indicators of prognosis in node-negative breast cancer, N Engl J Med 322(15):2046, 1990.

150. Sigurdsson H, Baldetorp B, Borg A, et al: Correspondence, N Engl J Med 323(19):1349, 1990.

151. Silvestrini R, Daidone M, Di Fronzo G, et al: Prognostic implication of labeling index versus estrogen receptors and tumor size in node-negative breast cancer, Breast Cancer Res Treat 7:161, 1986.

152. Silvestrini R, Daidone M, and Gasparini G: Cell kinetics as a prognostic marker in node-negative breast cancer, Cancer 56:1982, 1985.

153. Silvestrini R, Daidone M, Selvi C, et al: Cell kinetics as a prognostic indicator in operable breast cancers: updated report, Proc Am Soc Clin Oncol 7:24, 1988.

154. Slamon D and Clark G: Amplification of c-erbB-2 and aggressive human breast tumors? Science 240:1796, 1988.

155. Slamon D, Clark G, Wong S, et al: Human breast cancer: correlation of relapse and survival with amplification of the HER-2/neu oncogene, Science 235:177, 1987.

156. Slamon D, Godolphin W, Lovell A, et al: Studies of the HER-2/neu proto-oncogene in human breast and ovarian cancer, Science 244:708, 1989.

157. Spyratos F, Brouillet J-P, Defrenne A, et al: Cathepsin D: an independent prognostic factor for metastasis of breast cancer, Lancet ii:1115, 1989.

158. Stern D, Heffernan P, and Weinberg R: p185, a product of the neu proto-oncogene, is a receptorlike protein associated with tyrosine kinase activity, Mol Cell Biol 6(5):1729, 1986.

159. Stern D, Kamps M, and Cao H: Oncogenic activation of p185-neu stimulates tyrosine phosphorylation in vivo, Mol Cell Biol 9:3969, 1988.

160. Tahara E, Sumiyoshi H, Hata J, et al: Human epidermal growth factor in gastric cancer as a biological marker of high malignancy, Jpn J Cancer Res 77:145, 1986.

161. Tandon A, Clark G, Chamness G, et al: Heat shock/stress proteins: biological and clinical significance in breast cancer, Proc Am Soc Clin Oncol 9:23, 1990.

162. Tandon A, Clark G, Chamness G, et al: Cathepsin D and prognosis in breast cancer, N Engl J Med 322(5):297, 1990.

163. Tandon A, Clark G, Chamness G, et al: HER-2/neu oncogene protein and prognosis in breast cancer, J Clin Oncol 7(8):1120, 1989.

164. Thorpe A, Rochefort H, Garcia M, et al: Association between high concentrations of Mr52,000 cathepsin D and poor prognosis in primary human breast cancer, Cancer Res 49:6008, 1989.

165. Thorpe S: Estrogen and progesterone receptor determinations in breast cancer, Acta Oncol 27:1, 1988.

166. Thorud E, Fossa S, Vaage S, et al: Primary breast cancer: flow cytometric DNA pattern in relation to clinical and histopathologic characteristics, Cancer 57:808, 1986.

167. Toi M, Hamada T, Nakamura H, et al: Immunocytochemical and biochemical analysis of epidermal growth factor receptor expression in human breast cancer tissues: relationship to estrogen receptor and lymphatic invasion, Int J Cancer 43:220, 1989.

168. Toi M, Nakamura T, Mukaida H, et al: Relationship between epidermal growth factor, receptor status and various prognostic factors in human breast cancer, Cancer 65:1980, 1990.

169. Tubiani M, Pejovic M, Chavaudra N, et al: The long-term prognostic significance of the thymidine labelling index in breast cancer, Int J Cancer 33:441, 1984.
170. Uyterlinde A, Schipper N, and Baak J: Comparison of extent of disease and morphometric and DNA flow cytometric prognostic factors in invasive ductal breast cancer, J Clin Pathol 40:1432, 1987.
171. Valagussa P, Di Fronzo G, Bignami P, et al: Prognostic importance of estrogen receptors to select node negative patients for adjuvant chemotherapy. In Salmon SE and Jones SE, editors: Adjuvant therapy of cancer III: proceedings of the Third International Conference on the Adjuvant Therapy of Cancer, Tucson, Arizona, March 18-21, 1981, New York, 1981, Grune & Stratton.
172. Van N, Raber M, Barrows G, and Barlogie B: Estrogen receptor analysis by flow cytometry, Science 224:876, 1984.
173. van de Vijver M, Peterse J, Mooi W, et al: Neu-protein overexpression in breast cancer: association with comedo-type ductal carcinoma in situ and limited prognostic value in stage II breast cancer, N Engl J Med 319(19):1239, 1988.
174. Varley J, Swalow J, Brammar W, et al: Alterations to either c-erbB-2 (neu) or c-myc proto-oncogenes in breast carcinomas correlate with poor short-term prognosis, Oncogene 1:423, 1987.
175. Veale D, Marsh C, Ashcroft T, and Harris A: Epidermal growth factor receptors in non-small cell lung cancer, Br J Cancer 52:441, 1985.
176. Venter D, Tuzi N, Kumar S, and Gullick W: Overexpression of the c-erbB-2 oncoprotein in human breast carcinomas: immunohistological assessment correlates with gene amplification, Lancet ii:69, 1987.
177. Vignon F, Capony F, Chambon M, et al: Autocrine growth stimulation of the MCF 7 breast cancer cells by the estrogen-regulated 52 K protein, Endocrinology 118(4):1537, 1986.
178. Von Rosen A, Fallenius A, Sundelin B, and Auer G: Nuclear DNA content in mammary carcinomas in women aged 35 or younger, Am J Clin Oncol 9(5):382, 1986.
179. Von Rosen A, Rutqvist L, Carstensen J, et al: Prognostic value of nuclear DNA content in breast cancer in relation to tumor size, nodal status and estrogen receptor content, Breast Cancer Res Treat 13:23, 1989.
180. Wada T, Qian X, and Greene M: Intermolecular association of the p185neu protein and EGF receptor modulates EGF receptor function, Cell 61:1339, 1990.
181. Weid G, Bartels P, Bibbo M, and Dytch H: Image analysis in quantitative cytopathology and histopathology, Hum Pathol 20:549, 1989.
182. Weiner D, Kokai Y, Wada T, et al: Linkage of tyrosine kinase activity with transforming ability of the p185neu oncoprotein, Oncogene 4:1175, 1989.
183. Westley B and Rochefort H: A secreted glycoprotein induced by estrogen in human breast cancer cell lines, Cell 20:353, 1980.
184. Wilbur D, Zakowski M, Kosciol C, et al: DNA ploidy in breast lesions: a comparison study using two commercial image analysis systems and flow cytometry, Anal Quant Cytol Histol 12:28, 1990.
185. Williams M, Todd J, Ellis I, et al: Oestrogen receptors in primary and advanced breast cancer: an eight year review of 704 cases, Br J Cancer 55:67, 1987.
186. Wright C, Angus B, Nicholson S, et al: Expression of c-erbB-2 oncoprotein: a prognostic indicator in human breast cancer, Cancer Res 49:2087, 1989.
187. Yamamoto T, Ikawa S, Akiyama T, et al: Similarity of protein encoded by the human c-erb-B-2 gene to epidermal growth factor receptor, Nature 319:230, 1986.
188. Yokota J, Toyoshima K, Sugimura T, et al: Amplification of c-erb B-2 oncogene in human adenocarcinomas in vivo, Lancet 5:765, 1986.
189. Zhou D, Battifora H, Yokota J, et al: Association of multiple copies of the c-erbB-2 oncogene with spread of breast cancer, Cancer Res 47:6123, 1987.

9 Adjuvant Therapy for Node-Negative Breast Cancer

John H. Glick

In 1991, 175,000 new patients will be diagnosed with invasive breast carcinoma. Of these patients, 75% to 80% had clinical stage I or stage II disease, and approximately two thirds of these patients had histologically negative axillary lymph nodes. Increasing numbers of cases of breast cancer in the early stages are being reported, and this is partially attributable to early detection following the wider use of screening mammography. The majority of the cancers detected by mammography are in patients with smaller primary breast tumors that will have no axillary lymph node involvement. Despite advances in early diagnosis and primary treatment of breast cancer with surgery, radiation therapy, or both modalities, approximately 30% of the 70,000 newly diagnosed women with node-negative breast cancer will develop metastatic disease and ultimately die each year. If none of these women receive adjuvant therapy, in the United States alone approximately 20,000 of these women will eventually die. Thus node-negative breast cancer is not a uniformly favorable diagnosis, but represents a heterogeneous group of patients for whom adjuvant systemic therapy is indicated in subsets of patients with unfavorable prognostic factors.

In 1985 the NIH Consensus Conference on the Adjuvant Therapy of Breast Cancer reviewed the data available at that time and concluded that the administration of adjuvant therapy in node-negative patients could not be routinely recommended.[9] The Consensus Panel recommended that further research be conducted to determine which node-negative patients might benefit from adjuvant therapy. Even in 1985 the Consensus Panel did identify certain groups of high-risk node-negative patients who had a significantly greater chance of recurrence (large tumor size, negative hormone receptors, younger age, and higher degree of cellular proliferation). In these high-risk patients, the Panel concluded that adjuvant chemotherapy should be considered outside the context of a clinical trial.[9] Although this distinguished Panel recommended adjuvant therapy for selected groups of high-risk patients, this cautious recommendation was not utilized widely in clinical practice.

In 1988 the National Cancer Institute issued a Clinical Alert describing the preliminary results from three major randomized node-negative adjuvant studies. The Clinical Alert concluded that "adjuvant hormonal or cytotoxic chemotherapy can have a meaningful impact on the natural history of stage I breast cancer patients."[8] Many physicians interpreted the Clinical Alert as strongly recommending adjuvant therapy for all node-negative breast cancer patients. The publication of the Clinical Alert generated great controversy at that time over whether all node-negative patients benefit from some form of adjuvant therapy. This controversy persists to the present time.

Although all patients with node-negative breast cancer are at risk for disease recurrence, the majority of these patients are cured with local-regional therapy. During the past decade, intensive research efforts to define potentially important prognostic factors have made it possible to define subsets of node-negative patients with a very low risk of recurrence, as well as a high-risk group that clearly would benefit from adjuvant therapy. The challenge remains: with currently available knowledge, which node-negative patients should receive adjuvant therapy outside the context of a clinical trial, and which subsets have a favorable enough prognosis to be observed without adjuvant therapy?

GOALS OF ADJUVANT THERAPY

The primary goal of adjuvant therapy for node-negative breast cancer is to prolong survival significantly while maintaining a high quality of life. The major end-point is overall survival. However, disease-free survival, defined as the length of time free of recurrence, is also an important goal. Prolonged periods of disease-free survival are of benefit to patients because the quality of survival generally is better before relapse than after it. Once breast cancer recurs the patient cannot be salvaged or cured with secondary therapy, and the patient will ultimately die of their metastatic disease. In any trial of adjuvant therapy with short follow-up the first expected benefit of the experimental treatment will be a significant prolongation of disease-free survival. In general one does not expect to see a significant improvement in overall survival rates without first observing prolonged periods of disease-free survival.[23] Physicians and their patients frequently must make decisions based on disease-free survival data, as significant improvements in overall survival may not be detected for 5 to 10 years because palliative therapy for metastatic disease is frequently effective in prolonging survival.

Thus individual physicians and their patients must grapple with two questions: What probability of tumor recurrence is acceptable in order to simply observe the patient without adjuvant therapy? What improvement in disease-free survival or proportional reduction in the risk of relapse is necessary in order to treat an entire subset of patients? If currently available prognostic factors can identify a subset of node-negative patients with an excellent prognosis (e.g., 90% 5-year disease-free survival), then it is logical to observe this group without adjuvant therapy. However, if prognostic factors identify a group of node-negative patients with only a 50% chance of disease-free survival at 5 years, then it is appropriate to offer adjuvant therapy to this subset of patients outside the context of a clinical trial.[23] The clinical decision process becomes more difficult when a large subset of patients is identified with an estimated disease-free survival rate of 70% at 5 years. This situation is analogous to the control or untreated arms of the recently reported node-negative clinical trials. However, it is well recognized that these untreated patients still have short follow-up, and that by 10 years substantially more of the control patients will have experienced a recurrence of disease and will have died. Thus a paucity of 10-year data is available, and individual physicians and their patients must cope with this uncertainty in the decision-making process.

The second question presented above is an even more difficult challenge: What improvement in disease-free survival or reduction in the risk of relapse will you accept in order to treat an entire subset of patients? Does an improvement of 15% in the absolute risk of disease-free survival argue for the administration of systemic adjuvant therapy to an entire cohort of patients, when 70% will survive free of disease without treatment and 20% will relapse despite adjuvant therapy? There are no rigidly defined criteria for deciding how great the reduction in the risk of relapse must be before adjuvant therapy is prescribed. Therefore this decision is usually made through a discussion of the risks and the benefits of adjuvant therapy between an individual patient and his or her physician. However, the knowledgeable clinician must be able to interpret the data from controlled trials not only in terms of differences in absolute risk of disease-free or overall survival, but he or she must also consider relative risk (reduction in treatment failure) or relative odds ratio (greater chance of remaining disease-free) methodologies.[23] All these statistical measures are valid and provide clinicians and their patients with the data to make an intelligent decision.

Although estimates of the proportional reduction in the risk of relapse can be estimated from a knowledge of current clinical data, the clinician also must balance any potential benefits against both the short- and long-term side effects of adjuvant therapy. Therefore quality of life is an important measure for the evaluation of any adjuvant treatment program. However, there is little agreement among either clinicians or investigators pertaining to the evaluation of quality of life. Gelber and Goldhirsch[21] and Goldhirsch et al.[25] have commented that the evaluation of quality of life in patients undergoing adjuvant therapy for breast cancer is complex and is related to the specific methods used, including recording and grading acute toxic effects of treatment with a special emphasis on those subjectively experienced by the patients. These authors also noted that methods for measuring patients' perceptions of toxic side effects of treatment, including personal psychosocial and economical costs, must be factored into the equation. Methods for measuring the impact of relapse, its symptoms, and the treatment required for advanced metastatic disease, with its attendant toxic effects on the quality of life of those patients who relapse, must be weighed carefully in the decision to use adjuvant therapy at the time of diagnosis. Comparison of the quality of time with or without the burden of toxicity related to the adjuvant therapy program and quality of life as related to relapse are critically important.[21,22,25]

Assessing quality of life for cancer patients has become increasingly focused on the development of quality of life measurement instruments. Scales measuring different dimensions of well-being, mood, activity, pain, and appetite include the linear analogue self-assessment scale, and the Baum and Priestman scale, among others. Performance status, which relates the capacity to perform daily activities, is estimated by medical personnel frequently using the Karnofsky or Eastern Cooperative Oncology Group (ECOG) scales. In addition, a variety of measures have been developed using scales that rate feelings of well-being, providing a more complex evaluation of ability and disability. Gelber and Goldhirsch developed an approach known as the quality-adjusted TWiST (time without symptoms of disease and toxic effects of treatment).[22,25] The Q-TWiST methodology is a novel attempt to quantify the benefits of adjuvant therapy by considering the balance in reduction of symptoms of recurrent disease, as compared with the toxic effects of either adjuvant therapy or treatment at the time of relapse.

A more conventional method of weighing the risks and benefits of adjuvant therapy is to evaluate both the short- and long-term side effects of a specific adjuvant therapy regimen. One must balance the expected and potentially desirable side effects such as granulocytopenia, which indicates that appropriate full doses of chemotherapy were administered, against unexpected and life-threatening side effects such as pulmonary embolism, severe systemic infections, and rarely, second malignancies. However, recently completed and ongoing trials make us acutely aware of the short-term side effects, of the need to eliminate mortality in this prognostically favorable group of patients, and of the importance of not ignoring the ultimate endpoint of improving the therapeutic outcome for the patients being evaluated. Although long-term side effects of adjuvant therapy for node-negative patients are not yet known with certainty, data are available from node-positive trials with >10 years of follow-up. In these trials, long-term side effects of adjuvant chemotherapy or tamoxifen are rare. Nonetheless, physicians must inform their patients of the potential short- and long-term side effects of any adjuvant therapy regimen; they also must be able to place these side effects in perspective when compared to the potential benefit of the treatment program under consideration. The challenge remains: which patients with node-negative breast cancer should receive adjuvant therapy outside the context of a clinical trial?

PROGNOSTIC FACTORS

The majority of women with axillary node-negative breast cancer are cured following surgery and/or radiotherapy. Although there are now data from prospective, randomized clinical trials indicating that adjuvant chemotherapy or tamoxifen prolongs disease-free survival, it is not appropriate to recommend adjuvant therapy for all node-negative patients. Thus current and proposed prognostic factors are used to separate node-negative patients into low- and high-risk groups. The goal is to use a battery of prognostic assays to help the physician and patient make an intelligent decision as to whether adjuvant therapy is indicated, or to determine whether the patient has a good enough prognosis to be observed without systemic therapy. Unfortunately, no one prognostic feature or group of prognostic factors completely fills this objective. Therefore physicians must use their clinical judgment and the multiple prognostic factors now available to identify patients with a higher likelihood of recurrence.

PROGNOSTIC FACTORS

- Tumor size
- Estrogen and progesterone receptors
- Nuclear and histologic grade
- Ploidy
- Proliferative rate (S-phase fraction)
- HER-2 oncogene
- Cathepsin D

The 1990 NIH Consensus Panel[44] noted that a useful prognostic factor had the following characteristics: (1) it had significant and independent predictive value that has been validated by clinical testing; (2) its determination must be feasible, reproducible, and widely available with good quality control; and (3) it must be readily interpretable by the clinician and have therapeutic implications. The major prognostic factors available in clinical practice are listed above.

Tumor size

Primary tumor size has been shown to be an important prognostic factor in node-negative patients.[18,40,43,52,53,64] Tumors <2 cm in diameter demonstrate an excellent prognosis, with a 5-year relapse rate of approximately 11%. Multiple studies have noted that for patients with primary tumors measuring 2 to 5 cm, the 5-year relapse rate is approximately 22%, more than double the relapse rate for T_1 tumors. Rosen et al.[53] recently reported that patients with T_1N_0 tumors $\leq$1.0 cm in size had a significantly better 20-year disease-free survival rate (86%) than did T_1N_0 patients with tumors measuring 1.1 to 2.0 cm (74%).

Using 5-year overall survival data is not an optimal method for evaluating prognosis in breast cancer, because many recurrences occur beyond 5 years, and even if disease recurs within 5 years, the affected patient may live for a long time with currently available palliative chemotherapy or hormonal regimens. The data from the Surveillance, Epidemiology, and End Results (SEER) Program of the National Cancer Institute reported 5-year survival rates in relation to tumor size in node-negative breast cancer patients: patients with tumor size $\leq$1.0 cm had a 98% 5-year survival, compared to 92% for tumors measuring 1.0 to 1.9 cm, 91% for tumors 2.0 to 2.9 cm, 86% for tumors 3.0 to 3.9 cm, and 85% for tumors in the 4.0 to 4.9 cm range.[5] Thus it is clear that primary tumor size is an important prognostic variable, because there is a strong correlation between tumor size and the risk of recurrence. Patients with tumors measuring ≤1.0 cm have an excellent prognosis (<10% recurrence at 10 years), and thus generally do not require systemic adjuvant therapy outside of clinical trials. In contrast, patients with tumors measuring ≥2.0 cm should be considered for adjuvant therapy regardless of other prognostic factors. For patients with tumors measuring 1.1 to 2.0 cm, other major prognostic factors (to be discussed below) must be taken into consideration when deciding which patients should receive adjuvant therapy outside of a clinical trial. Tumor size should be determined by the pathologist, who must perform a careful gross examination with precise documentation of tumor size in order to give the clinician and the patient important prognostic information. Approximately 40% of node-negative patients have tumors <2.0 cm in size.[5] Thus tumor size alone remains an extremely important variable in deciding which patients should receive adjuvant therapy.

Estrogen and progesterone receptor determinations

Knight et al.[30] from the San Antonio Group were the first to demonstrate that estrogen receptor (ER) assays could identify both node-positive and node-negative patients at high risk for recurrent disease. This group recently updated their data on more than 2000 women with node-negative breast cancer, and again observed that estrogen receptor status remained an important factor in predicting recurrence.[37] For estrogen receptor–positive patients the 5-year disease-free survival rate was 76%, compared to 67% for estrogen receptor–negative patients (p = .001). Parallel figures for 5-year overall survival were 84% for the ER-positive patients, compared to 75% for the ER-negative patients (p = <.001).[37] These data have been confirmed by the National Surgical Adjuvant Breast and Bowel Project (NSABP), which also noted a highly significant improvement in disease-free and overall survival rates in patients with ER-positive tumors.[17] Although it is clear that patients with ER-positive tumors have a better prognosis than those with ER-negative tumors, the difference in recurrence rates at 5 years is only 8% to 10%. McGuire et al.[38] has argued that estrogen receptor status alone is not a sufficiently strong prognostic factor on which to base the decision to use adjuvant therapy. Although progesterone receptor determinations are an important prognostic variable in node-positive patients, controversy persists concerning the prognostic significance of progesterone receptors in node-negative patients. Recently, Clark et al.[6] reported the importance of progesterone receptor status when combined with ploidy in a multivariate analysis.

Nuclear grade and histologic factors

B. Fisher et al.[17] and E.R. Fisher et al.[19] from the NSABP were the first to document that nuclear grade was an important prognostic factor using a large series of patients. They grouped nuclear grade I and grade II together in a category that they labeled "nuclear grade good" and compared this with "nuclear grade poor" tumors. An 80% 5-year disease-free survival for nuclear grade good was reported, compared to 64% for nuclear grade poor.[17] The 5-year overall survival rate for patients labeled nuclear grade good was 93%, compared to 79% for those labeled nuclear grade poor. This study was performed by one very experienced pathologist, and questions have been raised as to whether these data can be replicated by other pathologists in normal clinical conditions in a multitude of hospitals. Recently, McGuire et al.[38] of the San Antonio group reported their experience using nuclear grade, which they divided into three categories according to the Scarff-Bloom-Richardson (SBR) system. They observed that SBR nuclear grade I or its equivalent identified a small set of node-negative patients at very low risk of tumor recurrence (<10% at 5 years). Thus the 1990 NIH Consensus Panel concluded that nuclear grade was a well-documented prognostic factor, and when determined by experienced pathologists, it discriminates favorable and unfavorable prognostic subgroups.[44] The Panel report observed that high nuclear grade clearly is associated with an increased rate of recurrence, and places a patient into the high-risk category. However, nuclear grade is not currently part of the routine pathologic review of breast cancer tumor specimens in many institutions. The Panel urged the pathology community to adopt a uniform grading system and to use nuclear grade routinely in clinical practice. Rosen et al.[51] also reported that nuclear grade was significantly related to disease-free survival (p = .02), and a similar trend was observed for histologic grade as well.

In Rosen's analysis of 474 T_1N_0 node-negative patients, those with infiltrating duct carcinoma and infiltrating lobular carcinoma did not differ significantly with respect to recurrence or overall survival rates.[51,53] However, recurrences were significantly less common in the category labelled "other" tumor types (tubular, medullary, papillary, and colloid) than in patients with invasive duct and lobular carcinomas. The projected 20-year recurrence rate was only 6% in the group labelled "other" carcinomas (p = .008). None of the patients in this category had peritumoral lymphatic tumor emboli or intratumoral blood vessel invasion. Although the "other" tumor types are a distinct minority of all breast cancer cases, the tubular, colloid (mucinous), and papillary histologies represent a very favorable prognostic subgroup and should be included in the low-risk or good prognostic category.

The prognostic significance of peritumoral lymphatic tumor emboli (LI) and blood vessel invasion (BVI) is controversial. These histologic factors have been questioned because of the low reproducibility and inconsistency of the methods used in assessing vessel involvement in routine histologic sections. Rosen et al.[51] reported that LI was detected in only 8% of cases but was associated with a significantly increased risk of recurrence. The impact of LI on disease-free survival was most pronounced among women with tumors measuring 1.1 to 2.0 cm. This group of investigators also noted that BVI was detected in elastic tissue stained sections of only 14% of breast tumors, all of which were invasive, ductal, or lobular carcinomas.[51] Patients with BVI involvement had a significantly higher recurrence rate, compared with patients in whom this factor was absent.

Recently, Lee et al.,[31] applied monoclonal antibodies to ABH isoantigens of endothelial cells to identify peritumoral lymphatic and blood vessel invasion. With their technique they were able to identify these factors more objectively, thereby reducing the proportion of false-positive cases, as well as identifying additional patients who would not have been identified in routinely stained sections. They observed that patients with both peritumoral lymphatic and blood vessel invasion had a significantly higher risk of death, as compared to patients with absence of these factors. However, their data showed that nearly half of the recurrences in this series were not predicted by this test, whereas half of the patients with both factors present were assigned incorrectly to a high-risk group.[31] Thus it remains to be determined whether the technique of Lee et al. will retain its prognostic effect, as compared with other prognostic factors when they are evaluated by multivariate statistical analysis.

Ploidy and proliferative rate

Quantitative measurements of cellular proliferation in breast cancer specimens using either the technique of thymidine-labeling index or flow cytometry have demonstrated a strong correlation with disease-free survival.[38] These studies indicate that both ploidy and proliferative rate are important prognostic features independent of tumor size, estrogen receptor content, and stage. The important retrospective study of Clark et al.[6] utilized DNA flow cytometric measurements of ploidy and S-phase fraction (the percentage of cells in the synthesis phase of the cell cycle) in 345 evaluable specimens from node-negative breast cancer patients. The median duration of follow-up for patients still alive was 59 months. Thirty-two percent of the specimens were diploid and 68% were aneuploid. The probability of 5-year disease-free survival was 88% for patients with diploid tumors, as compared to 74% for those with aneuploid tumors ($p = .02$). In patients with aneuploid tumors there were no differences in disease-free survival rates between high S-phase fraction tumors and those with low S-phase fraction tumors. However, for patients with diploid tumors the probability of disease-free survival with low S-phase fraction tumors was 95% at 5 years as compared to only 70% for those with diploid tumors and high S-phase fractions ($p = .007$). Similar differences in overall survival rates were noted. However, only 13% of diploid patients fell into the high S-phase group. Thus Clark et al.[6] identified only 28% of all node-negative patients with both diploid and low S-phase tumors. These patients are considered to be part of a good prognosis subgroup and might not require adjuvant systemic therapy. In contrast, approximately 72% of the patients had either aneuploid tumors or diploid tumors with high S-phase. These groups are clearly at an increased risk of recurrence and might well benefit from adjuvant therapy. Similar data have been reported by Kallioniemi et al.[29] from Finland, who also used DNA flow cytometry by combining DNA index and the S-phase fraction.

Dressler et al.[11] recently reported the preliminary results of an ancillary study to the Intergroup node-negative clinical trial. Flow cytometry measurements of ploidy and proliferative capacity were evaluated retrospectively for their ability to predict patient prognosis. Of the 563 specimens, 64% were aneuploid. Proliferative capacity was estimated by the percentage of cells in the S-phase of the cell cycle. The median S-phase value cut-off for the entire group was 6.9%. This median value defined the cut-off for interpretation of "high" or "low" S-phase values. At a median follow-up of 4.2 years they observed that S-phase fraction but not ploidy status was a significant prognostic factor in node-negative patients randomized to either the chemotherapy or observation arms.[11] These investigators also reported that the median S-phase values were higher in patients in the randomized portion of the study (ER-negative or ER-positive with tumor size >3.0 cm) compared with the group of patients registered only to observation (ER-positive with tumors ≤ 3.0 cm). This relationship was largely explained by the inverse correlation of S-phase fraction and ER receptor status and the strong correlation of S-phase fraction and tumor size. Dressler et al.[11] also noted that S-phase fraction was a significant predictor for disease-free survival as well as overall survival. Patients with a low S-phase fraction had a significantly longer time to recurrence and longer survival compared with patients with high S-phase fraction. Clark et al.[7] used the tumor specimens from the same population of patients and employed improved S-phase modeling techniques. The early results from this investigation and other studies demonstrated that S-phase can discriminate between a high or low probability of relapse in the aneuploid population as well.[7,39,47]

The 1990 NIH Consensus Panel concluded that DNA flow cytometry should be widely available for the determination of S-phase fraction as well as ploidy status.[44] However, the Panel noted that up to 25% of specimens were not evaluable by flow cytometry because of methodologic problems, and that because of the complexity of the technology, quality control was particularly important. The Panel concluded that although S-phase action has been shown to be an independent prognostic factor in some studies, its clinical value was still being defined.[44] This recommendation is too conservative, as S-phase fraction determination should be used routinely as an important prognostic factor in clinical practice. Ploidy status alone is not yet of clearly proven prognostic value, but it does appear that patients with aneuploid tumors, especially those with a high S-phase fraction, do have a significantly higher rate of recurrence.

In the current Intergroup protocol, patients with node-negative breast cancer in the "intermediate" risk group (i.e., ER and/or PgR-positive tumors <2 cm in diameter) are required to have paraffin blocks of tumor sent to a reference laboratory for flow cytometry. Patients with tumors <2 cm in size with S-phase <4.4% for diploid tumors or <7.0% for aneuploid tumors are placed in a low-risk group and simply are observed without adjuvant therapy. Patients with an S-phase fraction ≥4.4% for diploid tumors or ≥7.0% for aneuploid tumors are placed in a high-risk group and are randomized to one of two chemotherapy regimens followed by a secondary randomization at the conclusion of chemotherapy to tamoxifen or observation. Thus data from flow cytometry determinations are being used in current clinical trials as well as in clinical practice to determine prognosis and the need for systemic adjuvant therapy.

HER-2 oncogene

Recently, Slamon et al.[56] reported their studies of the HER-2 oncogene in early-stage breast cancer. HER-2 is identified in approximately 25% to 30% of human breast cancers. Slamon reported that HER-2 oncogene application is an independent predictor of both disease-free and overall survival in node-positive breast cancer. However, in node-negative tumors, neither univariate or multivariate analysis demonstrated an association between HER-2 amplification and disease outcome.[57] Other investigators also failed to demonstrate any value for measuring HER-2 oncogene amplification in node-negative patients.[30] However, the more recent data of Paik et al.[48] found that HER-2 overexpression was associated with decreased survival among women with tumors of good nuclear grade. In their retrospective study of 292 node-negative patients, HER-2 overexpression in tumors of good nuclear grade was associated with an approximately five-fold increase in mortality ($p = .00001$).[48] Allred et al.[1] from San Antonio also retrospectively evaluated HER-2 in a group of 235 node-negative patients who were followed on the observation arm of the Intergroup study (estrogen receptor–positive tumors that were <3.0 cm in tumor size). In patients with pure invasive ductal carcinomas (without any ductal carcinoma in situ component), they demonstrated that HER-2 overexpression was associated with a high rate of early recurrence. Thus McGuire[38] has suggested that there may be a role for HER-2 oncogene studies in selected subsets of node-negative patients. These would include patients with pure invasive ductal carcinoma (without any ductal carcinoma in situ component) who fall into the otherwise good-risk category of estrogen receptor–positive tumors with primary size <2.0 cm and nuclear grade I. However, this observation needs to be confirmed before being used commonly as a prognostic factor. At the present time, routine measurements for HER-2 oncogene overexpression in node-negative patients do not appear to be required in clinical practice outside of a clinical trial.

Cathepsin D

Rochefort's group from France first reported on the prognostic significance of measuring the lysosomal enzyme cathepsin D in breast cancer patients.[50] They noted that high levels of cathepsin D correlated with decreased disease-free and overall survival. Tandon et al.[60] from San Antonio performed a larger analysis of cathepsin D in node-negative breast cancer, and their initial data also revealed a high correlation between decreased disease-free survival and high levels of cathepsin D. The actuarial 5-year recurrence rate of node-negative aneuploid tumors with high levels of cathepsin D was 60%, as compared to 29% in aneuploid patients with low levels of cathepsin D.[60] These data also were confirmed by a Danish group of investigators.[61] Although three independent series of patients reported that overexpression of cathepsin D is an independent prognostic factor in node-negative breast cancer, the 1990 Consensus Panel was reluctant to make a definitive statement on the value of routine measurements of cathepsin D levels.[44] Although confirmatory large-scale data clearly need to be reported, high levels of cathepsin D are associated with an unfavorable prognosis, particularly in aneuploid patients, and should be considered as an independent prognostic factor.

Stress response proteins

Tandon et al.[59] recently reported that several families of heat shock/stress response proteins could be utilized as prognostic factors in a retrospective study of 200 node-negative patients. The presence of all four heat shock/stress proteins (hsp27, hsp70, hsp90, and grp94) was also associated with high levels of cathepsin D. Hsp70 was associated with estrogen and progesterone receptors, while hsp90 and the related grp94 were associated with aneuploidy and high nuclear grade. Higher levels of all the hsp except grp94 were associated with shortened disease-free survival. The 5-year actuarial recurrence rate increased from 24% to 80% as the number of high level hsp increased from zero to four.[39,59] Although these data are provocative, they clearly need to be confirmed and expanded before being accepted in routine practice. The current ancillary study to the Intergroup protocol will prospectively evaluate the role of stress response proteins and their correlation with disease-free and overall survival.

Estimating individual risks using prognostic factors

From the above discussion, it is apparent that currently available prognostic factors are associated with a broad range of recurrence rates in node-negative breast cancer patients. In 1990 the NIH Consensus Panel concluded that "there are extremes of high and low risk where it is possible to make recommendations about adjuvant systemic therapy."[44] However, this distinguished panel did not define what they meant by high- and low-risk subsets, other than to comment that patients with tumors $\leq$1 cm in diameter have less than a 10% recurrence rate at 10 years and should not be treated. The Panel concluded that a major future goal was the development of risk profile systems with sufficient accuracy and reproducibility to estimate prognosis in the individual patient.

However, the data are available today to allow individual physicians and their patients to use currently available prognostic factors to make rational treatment decisions outside the context of a clinical trial. Estimates of the 5-year probability of recurrence can be made using tumor size, estrogen receptor status, histologic factors such as nuclear grade, determination of ploidy, and S-phase fraction. These prognostic factors should be determined for every patient with node-negative breast cancer. Measurements of cathepsin D also may be important, but are not yet as widely available as is flow cytometry. Because a computer model has not yet been developed to predict accurately the probability of recurrence utilizing the known prognostic factors in node-negative patients, the clinician must use currently available prognostic factors to estimate a patient's individual risk of recurrence. McGuire[39] has developed a chart (Fig. 9-1) as a guide to estimate the 5-year probability of recurrence according to a patient's prognostic factors. Although patients frequently do not fit neatly into a particular prognostic category, using this chart to provide a reasonable estimate of the risk of relapse ($\pm$5% to 10%) is justified. In the case where the patient has both favorable and unfavorable risk factors, emphasis should be based on the most adverse prognostic factor. The value of using prognostic factors and a chart such as that of McGuire is to identify patients with such a low probability of recurrence (<15%) that they could be observed without adjuvant therapy. Although the ultimate decision regarding the administration of adjuvant therapy remains with the patient, it is the responsibility of the individual oncologist to make a recommendation regarding the benefits and risks of adjuvant therapy based not only on the patient's known prognostic factors, but also on the interpretation of the results of controlled clinical trials.

ADJUVANT CHEMOTHERAPY TRIALS

The importance of adjuvant chemotherapy in the treatment of node-positive breast cancer patients has been clearly established for more than a decade, particularly for premenopausal patients. Until recently the indications for administering adjuvant chemotherapy in node-negative breast cancer patients were controversial. The data base from which to make decisions was either incomplete, or large-scale randomized clinical trials had not yet matured to the point where firm conclusions could be made.

Early studies using adjuvant chemotherapy in node-negative patients were started more than three decades ago.[45] However, updated reports of the long-term effects of adjuvant therapy from these early studies have not been published. In 1974 the Swiss Cooperative Oncology Group (OSAKO) initiated a randomized prospective trial in which 122 node-negative patients were stratified separately from node-positive patients.[54] All patients underwent a modified radical mastectomy and were randomized either to surgery alone or adjuvant chemotherapy with chlorambucil, methotrexate, and

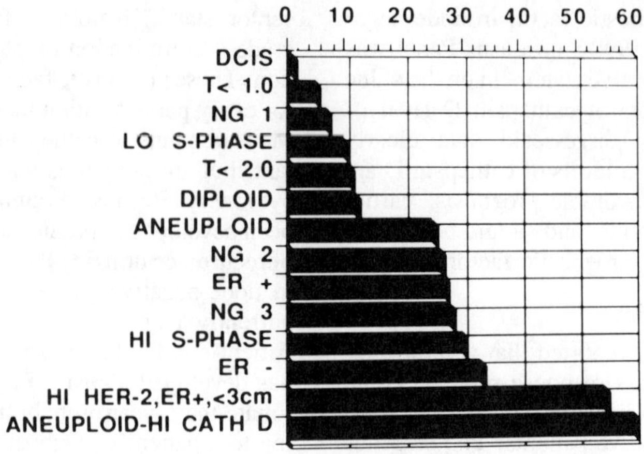

Fig. 9-1 Probability (%) of recurrence at 5 years on the basis of tumor characteristics in node-negative breast cancer patients. Values were derived from published references or estimated. *DCIS*, ductal carcinoma in situ; *T*, tumor size; *NG*, nuclear grade; *LO*, low level; *ER*, estrogen receptor; *HI*, high level; *CATH D*, cathepsin D. (Reprinted with permission from McGuire WL et al: How to use prognostic factors in axillary node-negative breast cancer patients, J Natl Cancer Inst 82:1011, 1990).

fluorouracil (LMF) for 6 months, followed by Calmette-Guerin bacillus (BCG) immunotherapy for 2 years or to the time of relapse. This study accrued patients between 1975 and 1977. Significant differences in relapse-free and overall survival initially were described only in the first 5 years (relapse-free survival) and 8 years (overall survival), respectively. Subsequent reports described a consistent trend towards better and longer survival of the LMF-treated patients.[55] The small actual differences in relapse-free and overall survival probably would have reached statistical significance if more patients had been included in this study. At the recent 1990 NIH Consensus Conference, Jungi and Senn[28] updated the results of the OSAKO trial at 14 years. There was no longer a significant difference in relapse-free survival. However, there now appeared to be a significant benefit in overall survival favoring the LMF-treated patients, 79% of whom were alive as compared to 62% of the controls (p = .019). This overall survival benefit was seen in both premenopausal and postmenopausal women.[28] It is difficult to understand how a benefit in overall survival was observed when there was no longer a difference in relapse-free survival. Interestingly, the number of second malignancies was lower in the chemotherapy group than in the control group. However, little is to be gained from further long-term follow-up of these patients, because the sample size was small and was unselected for hormone receptor status. In addition, the low doses of chemotherapy administered in this study have little resemblance to the doses of chemotherapy used in the modern era.

The West Midlands Oncology Association used virtually the same LMF regimen as the OSAKO group, and randomized 574 patients after simple mastectomy with axillary node sampling to either no further treatment or adjuvant chemotherapy.[41] Randomization was stratified by menopausal status and tumor size. Postoperative radiotherapy was not given. Patients were accrued to the study between 1976 and 1984. With a median follow-up of 7 years for disease-free survival and 10 years for overall survival, there remains no evidence for any overall treatment effect.[42] There are no significant differences between the chemotherapy and the control arms in disease-free or overall survival. Although local-regional relapse was decreased significantly in the LMF-treated patients, this group had an increased incidence of distant metastases. No subgroup of patients benefited from LMF chemotherapy. The authors concluded that LMF was not an effective combination for node-negative patients.

In 1980 the Milan Cancer Institute initiated a prospective randomized trial in node-negative, ER-negative patients.[3] Patient accural was terminated in mid-1985 after only 90 patients had been entered. Patients were randomized to receive either cyclophosphamide-methotrexate-fluorouracil (CMF) IV every 3 weeks for a total of 12 courses over 9 months or to a control group. The doses of CMF used in this study included cyclophosphamide

600 mg/m², methotrexate 40 mg/m², and fluorouracil 600 mg/m² all IV on day one of a 21-day cycle. Patients were entered on this trial after primary therapy either with a total mastectomy or breast conservation therapy. Table 9-1 summarizes the results of this trial.[2] The 7-year disease-free survival rate was significantly better for patients given CMF (85%) compared to the untreated controls (46%) (p = .0001). This benefit was seen for both premenopausal and postmenopausal patients, for those undergoing a total mastectomy as compared to a quadrantectomy and radiotherapy, as well as for those with T_1 and T_2 lesions. The 7-year overall survival rate also significantly favored CMF-treated patients (86% alive) compared to only 58% of the control group (p = .012). Patients with a high thymidine-labeling index appeared to benefit most from CMF adjuvant chemotherapy. In both arms of this study, new disease manifestations were first noted in sites of distant visceral metastases. Although IV CMF did not produce severe toxicity, 11 of 45 women refused to complete this adjuvant chemotherapy program, primarily for psychologic reasons.[2] This trial demonstrates the most dramatic benefit of adjuvant chemotherapy reported to date for node-negative patients. The small patient sample in the Milan trial and the significantly inferior disease-free survival of the control group may indicate differences in the patient population between the Milan trial and those entered into the NSABP and Intergroup trials discussed below. However, the 7-year data from the Milan group, demonstrating that 86% of CMF-treated, estrogen receptor–negative patients are alive and free of disease, are important results requiring confirmation.

Perioperative adjuvant chemotherapy is not a new concept. In the mid-1960s the Scandinavian Group, under the leadership of Nissen-Meyer, initiated a trial comparing 6 days of perioperative adjuvant cyclophosphamide to a control group of untreated node-negative patients. An overall advantage in terms of survival for all subgroups of patients treated with this perioperative chemotherapy in that trial was reported in 1987.[45]

Table 9-1 Milan estrogen receptor–negative, node-negative trial

7-year disease-free survival	CMF	Control	p value
All patients	85%	42%	.0001
7-year survival	**CMF**	**Control**	**p value**
All patients	86%	58%	.012

CMF, cyclophosphamide, methotrexate, fluorouracil.
Modified from Bonadonna G: In Program of the NIH Consensus Development Conference on Early Stage Breast Cancer, 1990, pp 49-50.

However, it was not until 1981 that a large-scale, well-controlled trial of perioperative chemotherapy was initiated. The International Breast Cancer Study Group recently updated the 5-year results of their study, which randomized 1275 patients to a single perioperative cycle of adjuvant CMF chemotherapy compared to a control group.[35] All patients underwent either total mastectomy with axillary clearance or modified radical mastectomy. The original chemotherapy regimen included 400 mg/m² of cyclophosphamide, 40 mg/m² of methotrexate, and 600 mg/m² of fluorouracil, all administered IV on days 1 and 8 with chemotherapy scheduled to begin within 36 hours after mastectomy. Unexpected severe early toxicity was observed, resulting in the addition of calcium leucovorin on days 2 and 9 (i.e., 24 hours after chemotherapy). The 5-year disease-free survival rate in the group receiving perioperative chemotherapy was 74%, as compared with 68% for those patients who received no adjuvant treatment (p = .003) (Table 9-2). This translated into a 22% reduction of the risk of relapse at 5 years favoring the chemotherapy arm.[24] For all patients entered onto this trial, the 5-year overall survival rate was similar for the chemotherapy group (88%), as compared to 85% for the control population (p = .31). However, the subset of postmenopausal patients with estrogen receptor–negative tumors demonstrated significantly improved disease-free survival rates with adjuvant chemotherapy (79% vs. 56%, p = .0003), as well as an advantage in terms of overall survival (91% vs. 70%, p = .0008).[24] This significant improvement in disease-free and overall survival in postmenopausal, estrogen receptor–negative patients with a single course of perioperative chemotherapy is an important observation, and is similar to the significant benefit noted by the NSABP for a different chemotherapy regimen in the same subset of patients.[15] Analysis of the patterns of relapse in the International trial demonstrated a significant reduction of relapses in regional sites, as compared to local recurrences or distant metastases. However, in the postmenopausal estrogen receptor–negative cohort, perioperative chemotherapy decreased the rate of recurrences in local, regional, and distant sites. The effect of a single course of perioperative CMF in premenopausal patients was less dramatic, but, extrapolating from the results of the node-positive portion of this trial, it seems that prolonged maintenance treatment after perioperative chemotherapy would probably be a more effective treatment strategy in this subset of patients.

Table 9-2 International breast cancer study group: perioperative adjuvant chemotherapy—single perioperative course of CMF + leucovorin vs. control in 1275 patients

	5-year DFS (%)			5-year survival (%)		
	CMF	Control	p	CMF	Control	p
All patients	74	68	.003	88	85	.31
Post, ER negative	79	56	.0003	91	70	.0008

CMF, cyclophosphamide, methotrexate, fluorouracil; ER, estrogen receptors; DFS, disease-free survival; Post, post-menopausal.
From Goldhirsch A et al: In Program of the NIH Consensus Development Conference on Early Stage Breast Cancer, 1990, pp 57-60.

One unexpected finding of the International trial was the observation that the prognosis of node-negative patients was worse than expected.[24] An investigation of prognostic factors was performed to identify why there was an increased risk of relapse. Following serial sectioning of ipsilateral axillary lymph nodes considered to be negative after routine histologic examination, micrometastases were detected in 83 (9%) of 921 breast cancer subjects for whom material was available for central pathologic review.[27] These patients had significantly inferior 5-year disease-free survival rates (56% vs. 74%; p = .003) and 5-year overall survival rates (79% vs. 88%; p = .002) than patients whose nodes remained negative after serial sectioning. Although the information gained from such a careful pathologic search for occult micrometastases of ipsilateral lymph nodes is potentially significant and might be used to identify a high-risk node-negative population, this technique would be costly and labor intensive, and would be difficult to perform in routine surgical pathology laboratories.

Severe toxicity was rare in the International trial but did include three deaths (0.2%) secondary to perioperative chemotherapy early in the study before leucovorin was added.[35] After modification of the protocol to include leucovorin, further deaths did not occur, and infectious complications were reduced significantly. Thrombophlebitis and embolism were seen in 0.5% of patients, while amenorrhea was observed in 31% of patients who received a single course of perioperative chemotherapy as compared to 21% in the control group.[27,35]

Follow-up is significantly shorter for a different perioperative chemotherapy trial initiated by the Cancer Research Campaign (CRC). This trial was intended to repeat the Scandinavian Chemotherapy Study Group's perioperative cyclophosphamide trial. The CRC trial administered cyclophosphamide at a dose of 30 mg/kg (maximum 2400 mg) IV for 6 days postoperatively. With a median follow-up of <4 years, the data have been reported in terms of observed O/E (ratios) for first events. In premenopausal node-negative patients, the O/E ratio for cyclophosphamide was 0.93 compared to 1.08 for the control group.[10] As noted in other trials, postmenopausal patients appeared to have a greater benefit with chemotherapy, as this trial reported an O/E ratio of 0.81 for the cyclophosphamide-treated group as compared to 1.21 for the controls. As yet, no advantage in terms of survival has been observed and further follow-up is required.

By 1980 the benefits of a 6-month course of adjuvant CMF chemotherapy for premenopausal node-positive women were accepted widely as demonstrating a significant improvement in rates of both disease-free and overall survival. Thus, in 1981, the Eastern Cooperative Oncology Group initiated a randomized trial for node-negative patients (see Fig. 9-2 for schema). Eligibility for this trial included patients with tumors of any size with negative estrogen receptors, or tumors measuring ≥3 cm with positive estrogen receptors. Patients with positive estrogen receptors whose tumors measured <3 cm in diameter were registered and observed without adjuvant therapy. Subsequently, the Southwest Oncology Group and the Cancer and Leukemia Group B joined this study, which became known as the Intergroup Trial.[36] Patients on the randomized portion of this trial received either CMFP chemotherapy for six monthly cycles or were observed without treatment. The CMFP regimen included cyclophosphamide 100 mg/m^2 PO on days 1 to 14, methotrexate 40 mg/m^2 and fluorouracil 600 mg/m^2 IV on days 1 and 8, and prednisone 40 mg/m^2 po on days 1 to 14. Randomization was stratified by type of surgical procedure, menopausal status, tumor size, and ER status. Treatment arms for the randomized patients were balanced for important pretreatment characteristics. The initial 3-year results of this trial were

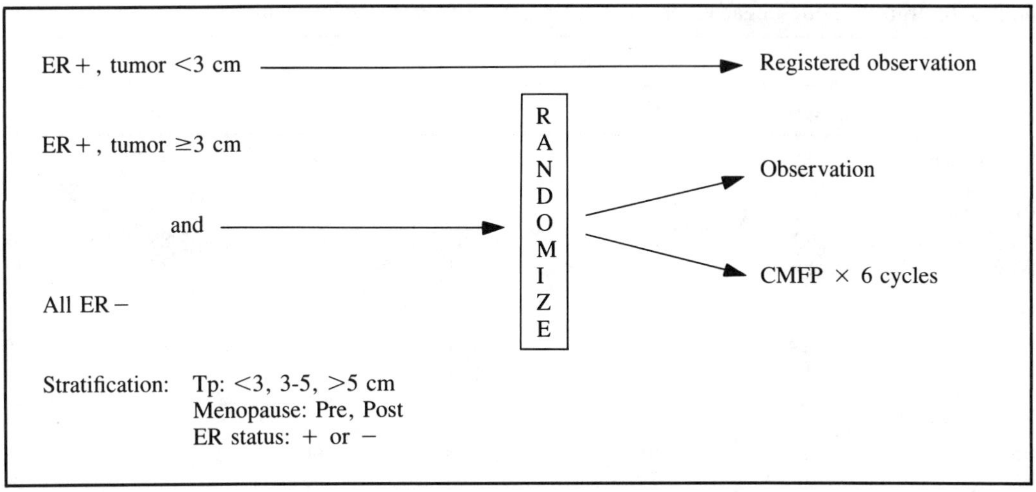

Fig. 9-2 Intergroup node-negative breast cancer trial.

published in 1989 by Mansour et al.[36] Recently, Tormey et al.[62] updated the 5-year actuarial results of this trial for the 425 eligible patients entered into the randomized portion of this study. The median followup of the randomized cohort is 4.5 years. The results of this trial are summarized in Table 9-3. The overall 5-year disease-free survival among the randomized patients was 83% with CMFP compared to 61% on the observation arm (p = .0001). Significant improvement in disease-free survival was observed in both premenopausal and postmenopausal patients, in women with ER-positive or ER-negative tumors, as well as in patients with tumors <3 cm or ≥3 cm. Five-year survival rates for the randomized treatments and the log rank p-values for the randomized comparisons also are shown in Table 9-3. Although the overall 5-year survival among the randomized patients was 86% with CMFP, compared with 80% on the observation arm (p = .31), this translated into a relative reduction in the risk of mortality of 26%. A statistically significant benefit in overall survival was observed for postmenopausal patients on CMFP (p= .04), as well as for patients with ER-positive tumors (p = .03).[62] With further follow-up the large differences in disease-free survival in other subgroups may also translate into overall survival differences.

Hematologic toxicity was observed in 33% of the CMFP patients, defined primarily as leukopenia with a WBC less than 4000/mm^3.[36] However, nadir counts were not reported and this degree of leukopenia should be expected with the CMFP combination. One treatment-related death occurred in association with a WBC of 200/mm^3, complicated by pulmonary embolism and secondary pneumonia.

In addition to the randomized portion of the trial, patients with ER-positive tumors <3 cm in diameter were entered into a separate registration arm of the protocol that observed these patients without treatment. The 5-year disease-free survival rate for the 445 eligible registered patients was 78%, with no differences noted for premenopausal and postmenopausal patients. The 5-year disease-free survival of 81% in the ER-positive patients with tumor size <2.0 cm was significantly higher than the disease-free survival of 74% for patients with 2.0 to 2.9 cm tumors (p = .04). The 5-year overall survival of all registered patients was 93% for ER-positive patients. With a tumor size of <2.0 cm, the 5-year survival rate was 94% as compared to 91% for patients with tumor size 2.0 to 2.9 cm (p = .39).[62] Although the disease-free and overall survival rates of the registered patients are better than those reported on the observation arm of the randomized portion of the study, the registered group of patients does not have a uniformly favorable prognosis.

An ancillary study to the Intergroup node-negative trial was performed by Dressler et al.[11] to retrospectively evaluate DNA flow cytometry measurements of ploidy and proliferative complicity for their ability to predict patient prognosis. The preliminary report from this ancillary study noted that S-phase fraction, but not ploidy status, was a significant predictor of time to recurrence. Overall, patients with a high S-phase fraction had a shorter time to recurrence as compared with patients who had a low S-phase fraction (p = .02). Among ran-

Table 9-3 Intergroup node-negative breast cancer trial: 5-year actuarial results

	% disease-free survival			% overall survival		
	Observ	**CMFP**	**p**	**Observ**	**CMFP**	**p**
All patients	61	83	<.0001	80	86	.31
Tumor size						
<3 cm	72	85	.05	90	88	.67
≥3 cm	54	81	.0001	74	84	.15
ER status						
Negative	68	82	.01	85	84	.90
Positive	42	86	.0001	68	92	.03
Menopause						
Pre	82	85	.0003	84	84	.78
Post	60	79	.03	74	89	.04

From Tormey DC et al: In Program of the NIH Consensus Development Conference on Early Stage Breast Cancer, 1990, pp 61-62.

domized patients whose tumors demonstrated a high S-phase, CMFP treatment was associated with a significantly lower recurrence rate compared to the observation arm.[11]

In 1981 the NSABP also initiated a large-scale randomized trial evaluating chemotherapy compared to a no treatment control group for patients with node-negative, estrogen receptor–negative tumors.[15] Following either a total mastectomy or lumpectomy and radiation therapy, 737 eligible patients were randomized to receive either no treatment or IV methotrexate (100 mg/m^2) followed 1 hour later by fluorouracil (600 mg/m^2) administered on days 1 and 8 of an every four week cycle. Calcium leucovorin (10 mg/m^2) was given orally every 6 hours for six consecutive doses 24 hours after methotrexate. These two antimetabolites were chosen despite the lack of adequate data demonstrating activity for this combination in metastatic disease. Alkylating agents were not added to the NSABP regimen because of the potential risk of inducing leukemia or second tumors. With a median time on study of 54 months, updated findings from this trial presented at the 1990 Consensus Conference failed to identify subgroups of patients who did not achieve significant disease-free survival benefit from the methotrexate-fluorouracil regimen.[15] Table 9-4 summarizes the absolute differences in disease-free survival favoring the chemotherapy arm, as well as the reduction in risk of relapse and the p values. As noted, patients ≤49 years of age, as well as those ≥50, had a significant benefit in disease-free survival with chemotherapy. Patients with tumor size ≤2 cm as well as those with larger tumor size had a significant improvement in disease-free survival rates with the methotrexate-fluorouracil regimen. There was a reduction in both local-regional and distant sites of treatment failure with chemotherapy. Ipsilateral breast tumor recurrence in the lumpectomy and radiation patients was reduced following methotrexate-fluorouracil therapy. Multivariate analysis for potential interactions failed to identify any subset of patients who did not benefit from adjuvant chemotherapy.

Only a borderline difference in statistical sig-

Table 9-4 NSABP B-13 estrogen receptor–negative, node-negative trial at 5 years: benefit of sequential methotrexate → fluorouracil + leucovorin × 12 courses vs. control in 737 patients

	Absolute difference in DFS (%)	**Reduction in risk of relapse (%)**	**p value**
All patients	9	27	<.0007
≤49 y.o.	6	16	<.05
≥50 y.o.	14	50	<.0007

From Fisher B et al: In Program on the NIH Consensus Development Conference on Early Stage Breast Cancer, 1990, p 63.

nificance for overall survival was observed in favor of this adjuvant chemotherapy regimen in this NSABP trial (p = .09). However, using hazard ratios, a 26% relative reduction in the risk of mortality for all patients was reported. Moreover, for patients ≥50 years, the methotrexate-fluorouracil combination significantly improved overall survival (p = .004), while the relative reduction in the risk of mortality in this age group was 65% on the chemotherapy arm.[15] The significant benefit in overall survival for patients ≥50 with estrogen receptor–negative tumors treated with chemotherapy on the NSABP trial is similar to the significant improvement in overall survival rate for perioperative CMF in postmenopausal, estrogen receptor–negative patients reported by the International Breast Cancer Study, as well as for all postmenopausal patients treated with CMFP in the Intergroup Trial. In the NSABP methotrexate-fluorouracil trial, no difference in overall survival for patients ≤49 years of age has been reported to date, despite a significant improvement in rates of disease-free survival.[15]

Toxicity from the methotrexate-fluorouracil regimen was mild, with only four patients having a WBC below 2500/mm^3; thrombocytopenia below 75,000/mm^3 was similarly rare. No patient died as a result of this chemotherapy program, and none have developed leukemia. The conclusions of the NSABP investigators remain as stated in their original publication in that all subgroups of node-negative estrogen receptor–negative patients benefited from adjuvant methotrexate-fluorouracil.[15,16] Because women with tumors too small for conventional analysis of ER are not included in this study, the NSABP does not recommend systemic adjuvant treatment for this subgroup of patients outside a clinical trial.

Thus the current results from four major trials using different adjuvant chemotherapy regimens for node-negative, estrogen receptor–negative patients all indicate a significant improvement in disease-free survival on the chemotherapy arm. The relative reduction in the risk of relapse ranges from 22% to 40%, and the relative reduction in the risk of mortality ranges from 15% to 25% for all the patients entered into these studies. The four major trials are also consistent in their observation that postmenopausal patients, particularly those with estrogen receptor-negative tumors, also achieve significantly improved overall survival rates with adjuvant chemotherapy. Premenopausal patients in these trials also demonstrate a significant benefit in disease-free survival rates with adjuvant chemotherapy, but this has not yet translated into an overall survival benefit, although the follow-up remains short. Thus, outside the context of a clinical trial, for the subgroup of node-negative patients who are also estrogen receptor negative, and particularly for postmenopausal patients with this prognostic feature, it is appropriate to administer adjuvant chemotherapy as standard treatment for this population. For the node-negative, estrogen receptor–negative patient, a no treatment control arm is no longer justified in patients with tumor size >1.0 cm. The choice of an optimal chemotherapy regimen for these patients is currently under investigation. In clinical practice the oncologist can reasonably use either the CMF or methotrexate-fluorouracil regimen for node-negative, estrogen receptor–negative patients.

ADJUVANT TAMOXIFEN TRIALS

Multiple trials of adjuvant tamoxifen in node-negative breast cancer patients have been conducted since the late 1970s, but it is only recently that the efficacy of adjuvant tamoxifen has emerged with the publication of major large-scale controlled clinical trials.

Riberio and Swindell[49] recently updated the Christie Hospital trial after 10 years of follow-up in a study begun in 1976. This small trial randomized 112 node-negative premenopausal patients following surgery to either irradiation-induced menopause or tamoxifen 20 mg daily for 1 year. Estrogen receptor data was not generally available at the start of this trial. The 10-year survival rate of the tamoxifen-treated patients was 93% compared to 82% in the irradiation-induced menopause group. The survival difference is not statistically significant (p = .09), primarily because of the small numbers of patients in each subgroup. The lack of a no treatment control arm also confounds interpretation of these results. However, the overall survival rate of the tamoxifen-treated patients must be regarded as excellent with long-term follow-up.

The Nolvadex Adjuvant Trial Organization (NATO) randomized 605 postmenopausal node-negative patients to a control group or to a group given tamoxifen (10 mg po) twice daily for 2 years following local-regional therapy. Only one half of patients had estrogen receptor analyses performed on their primary tumor specimens. With a median follow-up of 66 months, O/E ratios were calculated for the tamoxifen and control groups. The O/E risk for experiencing an event was 0.8 for tamoxifen compared to 1.17 for the control group.[46] Similar O/E ratios for survival were observed. The investigators concluded that 2 years of treatment with tamoxifen significantly reduced both disease recurrences and deaths. There did not appear to be evidence of a rebound increase in the number of recurrences or deaths following withdrawal of tamoxifen after 2 years. The NATO trial failed to demonstrate any correlation between estrogen receptor status and the effect of tamoxifen on either disease-free or overall survival rates.

Stewart[58] recently updated the results from the Scottish Adjuvant Tamoxifen Trial, which differed from most other studies by randomizing patients to 5 years of therapy with tamoxifen (20 mg po per day) or to a no treatment control group. After 5 years of tamoxifen, patients were rerandomized to either continue tamoxifen to relapse or to stop this hormonal agent. Patients on the control arm received tamoxifen at first relapse.[4] The authors reported that 751 patients (212 premenopausal and 539 postmenopausal patients) were entered into this study with median follow-up ranging from 5 to 10 years. Of premenopausal patients, 21% on the tamoxifen arm and 35% on the observation arm relapsed ($p = .018$). Of postmenopausal patients, 23% treated with tamoxifen and 34% on the observation arm relapsed ($p = .00026$). Tamoxifen-treated patients achieved a 38% relative reduction in the risk of recurrence.[58] When one considers the first site of recurrence, the effect of adjuvant tamoxifen was fairly consistent in all sites in premenopausal patients, but in postmenopausal women tamoxifen's major effect was to decrease local-regional recurrences and contralateral breast disease. Although there was a trend towards significantly improved overall survival rates on the tamoxifen arm ($p = .07$ for all node-negative patients), this translated into a 23% relative reduction in the risk of mortality for patients initially randomized to tamoxifen. Thus the results from the Scottish trial indicate a pronounced advantage for adjuvant tamoxifen administered for at least 5 years compared to a control group who received tamoxifen only at the time of first recurrence.

Subgroup analysis from the Scottish trial did not identify any group of patients for whom the benefit of tamoxifen was not apparent. Although estrogen receptor data was available in only 59% of patients, tamoxifen appeared to benefit estrogen receptor–negative patients as well.[4,58] However, the investigators defined estrogen receptor–rich or positive patients as having an ER value of ≥20 fmol, while ER-poor was defined as either absent ER or levels ≤20 fmol. In the ER-rich group, 19% of patients randomized to adjuvant tamoxifen have relapsed as compared with 34% on the observation arm ($p = .003$). In ER-poor patients, 32% of the tamoxifen group have relapsed, compared to 37% of patients on the observation arm. Thus, the greatest benefit for tamoxifen was demonstrated in those patients with the highest positive ER levels, a finding that is not unexpected. The investigators noted that the toxicity from adjuvant tamoxifen given for 5 years appeared no greater than in their earlier experience, when tamoxifen was given for shorter intervals of time.[4,58] Deaths from causes other than breast cancer have not increased in the tamoxifen-treated patients. In postmenopausal patients there appeared to be a reduction in deaths from acute myocardial infarction on the tamoxifen arm. No increase was found in the incidence of endometrial carcinoma in the tamoxifen-treated patients. This well-designed and important study clearly demonstrates a significant benefit for adjuvant tamoxifen irrespective of menopausal status.

The Cancer Research Campaign (CRC) initiated an adjuvant trial in 1980 aimed at repeating the Scandinavian Chemotherapy Study Group's cyclophosphamide perioperative trial as well as NATO's tamoxifen study. The CRC trial utilized a 2×2 factorial design, allowing two separate questions to be investigated simultaneously.[10] In the tamoxifen portion of the trial, 800 premenopausal, node-negative patients were entered and randomized to tamoxifen (10 mg po) twice daily for 2 years or to a control arm. At a medium follow-up of slightly more than 3 years, an event-free survival analysis has been performed. The investigators defined an event as not only a relapse, but also the development of a second primary breast cancer, and death from any cause. Of the 316 premenopausal patients, the O/E analysis for all events demonstrates a ratio of 0.74 for tamoxifen and 1.30 for the control group. For postmenopausal patients, the O/E ratio was 0.69 for tamoxifen and 1.27 for the control group. Although the follow-up is short, this trial already has shown that 2 years of adjuvant tamoxifen significantly improves the event-free survival for premenopausal and postmenopausal patients.[10] At 5 years, 90% of the tamoxifen-treated patients remain disease-free, compared to 76% on the control arm. As yet, a survival advantage for adjuvant tamoxifen has not emerged within the trial, but insufficient deaths have occurred to detect a 20% to 30% reduction in the 5-year mortality rates. An important initial observation in this trial is that adjuvant tamoxifen reduced the number of new contralateral breast carcinomas. The observation that tamoxifen-treated patients have a decreased frequency of second contralateral breast cancers has also been reported by Fornander et al.,[20] and by Stewart[58] for the Scottish Group.

NSABP investigators recently updated the results of their B-14 trial, which was initiated in 1981.[13,14] This study randomized both premenopausal and postmenopausal patients with estrogen receptor–positive tumors to either tamoxifen (10 mg po twice a day) for 5 years or to a placebo group. In 1987 the study was modified so that all patients who had completed the initial 5 years of tamoxifen were assigned randomly to receive either tamoxifen or placebo for an additional 5 years. In this study, ER-positive tumors were defined as having an ER value of ≥10 fmol. The 2644 eligible patients were stratified according to age, tumor size on clinical evaluation, and level of estrogen receptor concentration. Thirty-one per cent of patients entered onto this trial were ≤49 years of age. With an average time on study of 54 months, tamoxifen conferred a highly significant prolongation of disease-free survival compared with those receiving placebo (Table 9-5). Although the absolute difference in disease-free survival for all patients was only 10%, there was a 36% reduction in the risk of relapse in the tamoxifen-treated patients.[14] This benefit was observed in patients ≤49 years of age as well as in those ≥50 years of age. It is interesting to note that the benefit of tamoxifen appeared more pronounced in younger patients. Multivariate analysis indicated that all subgroups of patients benefited. Interestingly, patients with tumors measuring ≤1.0 cm had an 85% disease-free survival rate at 5 years with tamoxifen. Tamoxifen significantly reduced the rate of treatment failure at both local and distant sites, the incidence of tumors in the contralateral breast, and the incidence of recurrent or new tumors in the ipsilateral breast after lumpectomy and irradiation. Despite statistically significant differences in disease-free survival rates, no evidence of an overall survival benefit was observed in the tamoxifen-treated patients for any subset ($p = .3$). However, using the proportional hazard ratio model, there was an 18% reduction in the relative risk of mortality in patients treated with adjuvant tamoxifen.[14] The benefits achieved with tamoxifen were obtained with a low incidence of side effects. However, 1.3% of patients on the tamoxifen arm had thromboembolic events, and two deaths from pulmonary emboli were observed.

Athough there is no survival advantage for tamoxifen as yet in the NSABP trial, one would not expect to see such a survival advantage with <5 years of follow-up.[14] In the NSABP trials for node-positive patients evaluating adjuvant tamoxifen and/or chemotherapy, survival differences only became apparent 5 to 7 years after randomization. Because patients with ER-positive tumors who relapse are frequently treated with palliative secondary hormonal therapy and then chemotherapy, they may survive for many years with metastatic disease. Thus, small but significant advantages in terms of survival gained from the use of adjuvant tamoxifen in node-negative, ER-positive patients on NSABP protocol B-14 may not be observed for another 2 to 4 years.

When one evaluates the sum of data from these and other tamoxifen trials, there is a consistent effect of tamoxifen on reducing the risk of recurrence for women with node-negative breast cancer. The relative reduction in the risk of recurrence is in the range of 36% to 38%, and significant improvement in the disease-free survival rate of women receiving tamoxifen is reported in all studies. This benefit is seen irrespective of age or menopausal status, duration of tamoxifen therapy, and, in some trials, a significant benefit was seen in estrogen receptor–negative as well as estrogen receptor–positive patients. The relative reduction in the risk of mortality favoring tamoxifen ranges from 18% on the NSABP trial to 23% on the Scottish study.[14,58] This proportional reduction in the risk of death is remarkably similar to that reported by Peto in the overview analysis, which reported an 18% reduction in the relative risk of death in 16,000 node-negative women treated with tamoxifen.[12]

The potential benefit from adjuvant tamoxifen will depend on the predicted recurrence rate for patients with a specific profile of prognostic factors. In addition, potential benefits from tamoxifen must be balanced against an assessment of the potential toxicity of this hormonal agent. The effect of tamoxifen on inducing deep vein thrombophlebitis or pulmonary embolism is controversial. The NSABP observed an increased incidence of thromboembolism in patients receiving tamoxifen, while this has not been confirmed either by the NATO or Scottish investigators.[13,16,58] Although tamoxifen is an antiestrogen, this hormonal agent is known to have agonistic estrogenic properties. This has raised the concern that tamoxifen might cause the

Table 9-5 NSABP B-14 estrogen receptor–positive, node-negative trial at 5 years: benefit of tamoxifen vs. control in 2644 patients

	Absolute difference in DFS (%)	Reduction in risk of relapse (%)	p value
All patients	10	36	<.000005
≤49 y.o.	15	44	<.0001
≥50 y.o.	8	31	<.000005

From Fisher B et al: In Program of the NIH Consensus Development Conference on Early Stage Breast Cancer, 1990, p 64.

acceleration of osteoporosis. Prospective clinical data investigating the effect of long-term tamoxifen therapy on bone metabolism is limited. However, in the few studies reported to date, no differences in bone mineral density between tamoxifen and a control group of patients have been observed.[26,32,33]

Although hot flashes are the most common side effect of tamoxifen (reported by 62% of patients in the NSABP trial), they are rarely debilitating.[14] The number of patients who discontinued treatment in the NSABP trial was virtually identical for the tamoxifen group as compared to the placebo-treated patients. A recent concern that tamoxifen may induce uterine cancer has been raised by Fornander et al.[20] Utilizing data from the Cancer Registry in Sweden, these investigators examined the accumulated frequency of uterine cancer in patients who received tamoxifen at a dose of 20 mg twice daily for 5 years as compared to those who received tamoxifen for only 2 years or to those in no treatment control groups. They noted that uterine cancers were significantly more prevalent in the tamoxifen group than in the no treatment controls. Moreover, the accumulated frequency of uterine cancer was greater in patients who took tamoxifen for 5 years than those who received it for a shorter duration. The dose of tamoxifen used in this trial was twice that used by the NSABP, Scottish, and NATO investigators. To date, an increased risk of endometrial carcinoma has not been reported by other investigators including the large-scale Scottish, NATO, and NSABP trials.[14,46,58]

In addition to the controversy over the risk to benefit ratio of adjuvant tamoxifen, uncertainty exists concerning the use of adjuvant tamoxifen in premenopausal patients, the optimal duration of tamoxifen administration, the use of tamoxifen in estrogen receptor–negative patients, and the use of tamoxifen combined with chemotherapy. Further controversies also include whether tamoxifen reduces the incidence of new contralateral breast cancers and/or reduces the risk of recurrence in the ipsilateral breast treated with lumpectomy and radiation. In addition, tamoxifen therapy in the United States is expensive. Prolonged therapy for 5 years or even on an indefinite basis may prove to be an economic hardship for many patients. Thus questions pertaining to the optimal duration of tamoxifen administration are extremely important. The recently completed trials discussed above used adjuvant tamoxifen for different durations of time ranging from 1 to 2 years to 5 years or longer. Animal data indicates that tamoxifen is usually a cytostatic agent.[32] Thus prolonged durations of tamoxifen therapy theoretically should produce significantly improved disease-free survival rates. The Scottish trial, which administered tamoxifen for 5 years or longer, clearly supports this observation.[4] The NSABP B-14 protocol, which randomized patients to 5 years of tamoxifen or a control group, with the patients receiving tamoxifen subsequently randomized at the end of 5 years to receiving this drug for a further 5 years vs. stopping this agent, will be important in ultimately defining the optimal duration of tamoxifen administration. In addition, cooperative group results from trials involving node-positive patients who were randomized to 1 vs. 5 years of tamoxifen therapy should soon be available and will be important in defining guidelines for the duration of tamoxifen therapy in node-negative patients as well. At the present time, outside of a clinical trial setting, long-term administration of tamoxifen for at least 5 years appears indicated when this agent is used as adjuvant therapy for node-negative patients.

The role of tamoxifen in estrogen receptor–negative, node-negative patients also remains controversial. The NATO trial failed to demonstrate any correlation between estrogen receptor status and the effect of tamoxifen on either disease-free or overall survival rates, but estrogen receptor data were available in only approximately half the patients entered on this study.[46] Although the Scottish trial reported a disease-free survival benefit of tamoxifen in estrogen receptor–poor tumors, this difference was not statistically significant.[58] However, in the Scottish trial patients with high levels of positive estrogen receptors given tamoxifen clearly had improved disease-free survival rates as compared to tamoxifen-treated patients whose tumors were estrogen receptor poor. At the present time, the potential value of adjuvant tamoxifen alone in estrogen receptor–negative patients is unproven. Current evidence is not adequate to recommend adjuvant tamoxifen for the treatment of estrogen receptor–negative patients outside of a clinical trial. This is particularly true because the benefits of adjuvant chemotherapy in estrogen receptor–negative patients now show a significant survival benefit, leading to the recommendation that adjuvant chemotherapy should be administered for this subgroup of patients. However, the use of tamoxifen in estrogen receptor–negative patients, particularly after they have received initial adjuvant chemotherapy, is an important question that is now being addressed in the most recent Intergroup contolled clinical trial.

The role of tamoxifen given concurrently with adjuvant chemotherapy in the treatment of patients with node-negative breast cancer is now also under investigation. Recently completed large-scale studies did not investigate the role of tamoxifen combined with chemotherapy compared to tamoxifen alone. It is difficult to extrapolate from node-positive trials, particularly in postmenopausal patients, comparing chemotherapy plus tamoxifen to tamoxifen alone since the results are contradictory. Numerous studies have failed to demonstrate either a disease-free survival or overall survival advantage of tamoxifen combined with chemotherapy in postmenopausal, estrogen receptor–positive, node-positive patients, as compared to tamoxifen alone. New clinical trials in node-negative, ER-positive patients have been activated investigating the question of tamoxifen alone as compared to chemotherapy plus tamoxifen as compared to chemotherapy followed by tamoxifen. The results of these trials may not be available for many years. At the present time, we do not know the optimal way to combine chemotherapy and tamoxifen, and it remains uncertain if both modalities are indicated in certain subgroups of node-negative, estrogen receptor–positive patients.

Thus, although controversy continues to exist and many important questions remain unresolved, the benefits of adjuvant tamoxifen for many patients with estrogen receptor–positive, node-negative breast cancer appear to be established. The challenge remains as to which of these patients can be spared the use of adjuvant tamoxifen because of very favorable prognostic factors. In addition, we must recognize that estrogen receptor–positive patients treated with tamoxifen alone still have a considerable recurrence rate at 5 years. The next generation of clinical trials will search for an improvement in therapeutic efficacy by comparing tamoxifen alone to either chemotherapy plus concurrent tamoxifen or chemotherapy followed by tamoxifen.

1990 NIH CONSENSUS CONFERENCE

In June 1990 the NIH held the Consensus Development Conference on Early Stage Breast Cancer. The data presented at that conference on prognostic factors, chemotherapy, and adjuvant tamoxifen is summarized in previous sections of this chapter. After extensive deliberations, the Panel presented and published their conclusions and recommendations as follows[44]:

- The majority of patients with node-negative breast cancer are cured by breast-conserving treatment or total mastectomy and axillary dissection.
- There is clear evidence that the rate of local and distant recurrence is decreased by both adjuvant combination cytotoxic therapy and adjuvant tamoxifen. Adjuvant systemic therapy reduces the rate of recurrence by approximately one third.
- At the present time, reduced mortality is seen in nearly all trials but is not statistically significant in most. However, the rate of death in node-negative patients is low, so a clinically important reduction of mortality may require a long follow-up to achieve statistical significance.
- The many unanswered questions in the adjuvant systemic treatment of node-negative breast cancer make it imperative that all patients who are candidates for clinical trials be offered the opportunity to participate.

The Panel then issued following recommendations for patients who are not candidates for clinical trials or who refuse participation:

- All node-negative patients should be made aware of the benefits and risks of adjuvant systemic therapy. The decision to use adjuvant treatment should follow a thorough discussion with a patient regarding the likely risk of recurrence without adjuvant therapy, the expected reduction in risk with adjuvant therapy, toxicities of therapy, and its impact on the quality of life. Some degrees of improvement may be so small that they are outweighed by the disadvantages of therapy.
- Adjuvant therapy should consist of either combination chemotherapy or tamoxifen.
- While all node-negative patients are at some risk for recurrence, patients with tumors ≤ 1 cm have an excellent prognosis and do not require adjuvant systemic therapy outside of clinical trials.

The Panel went on to comment that they had reviewed the data from 10 randomized trials (summarized earlier in this chapter), but noted that the completed studies were not large enough nor was follow-up long enough to estimate with accurate precision the interactions between menopausal status and hormone receptor positivity and the effects of adjuvant therapy.[44] Although the Panel observed that the overall benefits from tamoxifen in postmenopausal patients clearly outweighed any toxicities currently described, they did not specify which subsets of patients should actually receive tamoxifen. The conservative, and almost defensive, tone of the Consensus Statement was echoed by the Panel's warnings that the administration of tamoxifen in premenopausal patients may cause endocrine abnormalities with uncertain long-term consequences. Little data were presented to support this conclusion. The Panel noted that, although there did not appear to be an excess number of cases of endometrial carcinoma in tamoxifen-treated premenopausal patients, the follow-up was too short to predict whether this will be observed or not.

It is unfortunate that the Panel did not define more precisely subsets of node-negative patients with either a high or low risk of recurrence, and therefore did not provide clinical practice guidelines for the use of adjuvant therapy in node-negative patients. The Panel concluded that a major goal for the future was the development of risk profile systems with sufficient accuracy and reproducibility to estimate prognosis in the individual patient. Other than stating that it would be reasonable not to treat patients with tumors ≤1 cm in diameter because their chance of recurrence is less than 10% at 10 years, the Panel did not provide treatment recommendations for any other subgroups of patients.[44] Instead the Panel left the individual patient and practicing physician in a quandary by abandoning their responsibility to provide treatment guidelines for specific subsets of node-negative patients.

TREATMENT RECOMMENDATIONS

Although the 1990 Consensus Panel strongly recommended that all node-negative patients who are candidates for clinical trials be offered the opportunity to participate, <5% of all such patients in the United States actually are entered into a clinical trial of adjuvant therapy. Thus practicing oncologists and their patients are faced with a therapeutic dilemma as to which node-negative patients should be observed and which should be treated with adjuvant therapy ouside the setting of a clinical trial. My treatment recommendations for node-negative breast cancer patients are summarized at right.

The minimal/low risk category includes patients with noninvasive tumors (ductal carcinoma in situ) and those with incidentally discovered small invasive tumors detected by mammography or by microscopic examination of tissue removed because of benign breast disease or in situ breast cancer. In addition, patients with tubular, colloid (mucinous), and papillary tumor subtypes are included in this subgroup because of their low risk of recurrence. Finally, I concur with the Consensus Panel that, in general, patients with tumors ≤1 cm in diameter have an excellent prognosis. Patients in the minimal/low risk subgroup usually have a very favorable prognosis. Overall, patients in this category have a <10% recurrence rate at 10 years. Moreover, patients in this category were not eligible and were not entered into the major clinical trials of adjuvant therapy discussed in this chapter. For almost all of the patients in the minimal/low risk category adjuvant systemic therapy is not indicated. However, there may be infrequent exceptions to this recommendation. For example, a patient may have a 0.8-cm tumor that is estrogen receptor negative with high nuclear grade and in which flow cytometry demonstrates a high S-phase. In this hypothetical patient, the administration of adjuvant chemotherapy would be indicated.

A good risk subgroup can be defined as those patients with approximately a 90% chance of remaining disease-free at 5 years. This category includes patients who meet all the following criteria: estrogen receptor–positive tumors <2 cm, which are nuclear grade good, and which are diploid with a low S-phase. Observation without adjuvant therapy for the good risk category remains the most appropriate recommendation at the present time. It is this subgroup of patients that will be registered

SUMMARY OF TREATMENT RECOMMENDATIONS FOR NODE-NEGATIVE BREAST CANCER

Minimal risk

Noninvasive tumors
Small invasive tumors discovered by mammography or at time of surgery for benign or in situ disease

Treatment recommendation

Observation

Good risk

ER-positive
Diploid and low S-phase
Tumor ≤2 cm size

Treatment recommendation

Observation

Intermediate risk

Tumor size 1 to 2 cm
ER-positive/negative
Nuclear grade II
Aneuploid with low S-phase
Low cathepsin D level

Treatment recommendation

Discuss risks and benefits with patients:
- Observation
- Tamoxifen
- Chemotherapy

High risk

Tumor size >2 cm
ER-negative
Nuclear grade III (poor)
High S-phase: diploid or aneuploid
High cathepsin D level

Treatment recommendation

Adjuvant therapy:
- Tamoxifen
- Chemotherapy

and followed without adjuvant therapy in the recently activated Intergroup protocol. However, it is important to note that approximately one half of patients entered into the NSABP B-14 protocol had tumors measuring ≤2.0 cm in size that were ER positive. These patients apparently gain a disease-free survival benefit with tamoxifen, but as yet no advantage in terms of overall survival has been observed. In the good risk group of patients, the ultimate benefit of tamoxifen remains to be determined. At the present time, there is clearly no role for adjuvant chemotherapy in this prognostically favorable category of patients.

Conversely, a high risk subgroup has been defined on the basis of well-known and accepted prognostic factors. This group includes patients with unequivocally estrogen receptor–negative tumors ≥1 cm in size, estrogen receptor–positive tumors ≥2 cm in diameter, and tumors that are either aneuploid or diploid with a high S-phase. The presence of any one of these unfavorable prognostic parameters justifies the use of adjuvant therapy outside the setting of a clinical trial. Additional prognostic factors such as poor nuclear grade, high cathepsin D level (especially in aneuploid tumors), and negative progesterone receptors can be added to the prognostic profile to guide the clinician and the individual patient. In addition to the consideration of these well-known prognostic factors, the physician must evaluate the patient's general medical condition and psychosocial status before deciding on a therapeutic recommendation.

Therefore patients in the high risk group should receive some form of adjuvant systemic therapy. All of the recent major clinical trials demonstrate significant prolongation of disease-free survival with either tamoxifen or chemotherapy for this subgroup of patients. In addition, evidence of a significant prolongation of overall survival is beginning to emerge from these trials as well. For example, the Intergroup trial demonstrated a significant improvement in survival for all postmenopausal patients and for the subgroup of patients with tumors ≥3 cm. Similar conclusions were obtained by the NSABP and International Breast Cancer Study Group, which demonstrated significant prolongation of overall survival with adjuvant chemotherapy in postmenopausal ER-negative patients.

Thus for the node-negative, estrogen receptor–negative patient, administration of adjuvant systemic chemotherapy is appropriate as standard treatment. A no treatment control arm in current and future clinical trials is no longer justified in patients with tumor size >1.0 cm. The choice of an optimal chemotherapy regimen for these patients currently is under investigation. In clinical practice the oncologist can reasonably administer the CMF or methotrexate-fluouracil regimen for node-negative, estrogen receptor–negative patients. No conclusion can be made at this time as to the superiority of CMF, sequential methotrexate-fluouracil, or an Adriamycin-containing regimen such as CAF (cyclophosphamide–Adriamycin–5-fluorouracil). The current Intergroup trial is directly comparing 6 months of CAF to CMF in high risk, node-negative patients (see Chapter 24). The role of perioperative chemotherapy is intriguing, but studies of node-positive patients demonstrate the superiority of perioperative chemotherapy combined with maintenance chemotherapy over perioperative chemotherapy alone.[34] Thus a single course of perioperative chemotherapy by itself cannot be recommended for node-negative patients. In all patients receiving chemotherapy, arbitrary dose modifications to reduce moderate and expected toxicity are not indicated.

For patients with estrogen receptor–positive tumors ≥2 cm, adjuvant systemic therapy also is indicated. The options for these patients include tamoxifen alone, adjuvant chemotherapy with CMF, or chemotherapy plus concurrent or sequential tamoxifen. In the absence of direct comparative data from the recently activated trials, this difficult choice also must be made on the basis of prognostic information for an individual patient, as well as the general medical condition of the patient. For example, an elderly patient with an estrogen receptor–positive tumor measuring 3 cm may not be able to tolerate full doses of chemotherapy. In this case, tamoxifen would be recommended. For other patients (e.g., one with a 4-cm ER-positive tumor with a high S-phase), combination chemotherapy plus tamoxifen (administered either concurrently or sequentially) is a reasonable alternative.

All the tamoxifen trials show a significant improvement in disease-free survival rates in patients with estrogen receptor–positive tumors who received tamoxifen. A trend toward significant improvement in overall survival in favor of tamoxifen is now beginning to emerge from the Scottish trial as well.[58] Moreover, Peto's overview analysis also demonstrates a significant survival benefit in favor of tamoxifen.[12] The recently completed large-scale adjuvant studies did not investigate the role of tamoxifen alone compared with the combination of tamoxifen plus chemotherapy in estrogen receptor–positive patients. Current clinical trials in node-negative, ER-positive patients are investigating the relative benefits of tamoxifen alone as compared to tamoxifen plus chemotherapy as compared to chemotherapy followed by tamoxifen. The results of these trials will not be available for many years. At the present time we do not know the optimal way to combine chemotherapy and tamoxifen, and it remains uncertain if both modalities are indicated in specific subgroups of node-negative, estrogen receptor–positive patients. Thus the clinical judgment of the oncologist remains critically important in recommending an appropriate adjuvant regimen for a specific patient. However, it is clear that all patients in the high risk category should receive some form of adjuvant therapy outside the context of a clinical trial. It is also important to recognize that a no treatment control arm for these ER-positive patients is no longer justified in a randomized clinical trial.

The practice of medicine would be much easier if patients fell neatly into good and high risk categories. However, many patients fall into an intermediate risk category, in which the risk of relapse at 5 years is betweeen 15% and 25%. Patients in the intermediate risk group frequently have an admixture of prognostic factors, including tumors measuring between 1 and 2 cm, estrogen receptors that may be positive but at a borderline level of positivity, nuclear grade II histology, and aneuploid tumors with low S-phase fractions. In this subgroup of intermediate risk patients, the decision to use adjuvant treatment should follow a thorough discussion with the patient regarding the likely risk of recurrence without adjuvant therapy, the expected reduction in risk with adjuvant treatment, the toxicities of therapy, and their impact on the patient's quality of life. While it might be appropriate to observe some patients in this category (e.g., an elderly patient with a history of other serious medical conditions), it is my recommendation that the majority of intermediate risk patients should be treated with adjuvant therapy even if not entered into a clinical trial. For example, in a patient with an estrogen receptor–positive, nuclear grade II, 1.5-cm tumor, which is aneuploid and low S-phase, a physician could recommend tamoxifen and/or adjuvant chemotherapy as appropriate systemic treatment. In the future, data from recently completed and currently active clinical trials should be able to answer the question definitively as to whether patients in the intermediate risk category will benefit from some form of adjuvant systemic treatment.

It is now apparent that all patients with node-negative breast cancer should have an oncologic consultation at the time of diagnosis, so that the patient and his or her physician can enter into a discussion of the patient's prognostic profile and the available therapeutic options for that patient, as well as the risk vs. benefit ratio. The first priority is to deliver excellent medical care, and the patient should be urged to participate in one of the available national clinical trials. However, given the extremely common situation in which most patients are treated outside a clinical trial, the physician should recommend adjuvant therapy for all high risk patients and for the majority of patients in the intermediate risk category. Treatment recommendations for intermediate and high risk node-negative breast cancer patients by estrogen receptor and menopausal status are summarized above. These recommendations are not fixed in stone, but must be regarded as dynamic. Longer follow-up of the recently completed adjuvant therapy trials and evaluations of the data that will emerge from newly activated clinical studies may well modify these guidelines in the future.

TREATMENT RECOMMENDATIONS FOR INTERMEDIATE OR HIGH-RISK, NODE-NEGATIVE PATIENTS OUTSIDE A CLINICAL TRIAL

	Premenopausal	Postmenopausal
ER-negative	Chemotherapy	Chemotherapy
ER-positive	Tamoxifen Chemotherapy Chemotherapy plus tamoxifen	Tamoxifen Chemotherapy Chemotherapy plus tamoxifen

It is now apparent that significant progress has been made using adjuvant therapy for node-negative breast cancer. The majority of node-negative patients, regardless of age or menopausal or receptor status, will benefit from some form of adjuvant chemotherapy and/or tamoxifen administration. Further clinical investigation is imperative, but it is now incumbent upon each physician to apply the known therapeutic regimens broadly, so as not to deny patients the specific benefits of adjuvant therapy that already have been demonstrated.

REFERENCES

1. Allred D, Clark G, Tandon A, et al: HER-2/neu expression identified a group of node-negative breast cancer patients at high-risk for recurrence, Proc Am Soc Clin Oncol 9:23, 1990.
2. Bonadonna G: Milan adjuvant chemotherapy trial for node negative breast cancer patients. Program of the NIH Consensus Development Conference on Early Stage Breast Cancer, 1990, pp 49-50.
3. Bonadonna G, Valagussa P, Zambetti M, et al: Milan adjuvant trials for stage I-II breast cancer. In Salmon SE, editor: Adjuvant therapy of cancer V, Orlando, 1987, Grune & Stratton, pp 211-221.
4. Breast Cancer Trials Committee: Adjuvant tamoxifen in the management of operable breast cancer: the Scottish trial, Lancet ii:171, 1987.

5. Carter CL, Allen C, and Henson DE: Relation of tumor size, lymph node status, and survival in 24,740 breast cancer cases, Cancer 63:181, 1989.
6. Clark GM, Dressler LG, Owens MA, et al: Prediction of relapse or survival in patients with node-negative breast cancer by DNA flow cytometry, N Engl J Med 320:627, 1989.
7. Clark GM, Owens MA, Dressler LG, et al: A new model for estimating S-phase fraction in node-negative breast cancer patients, Proc Am Assoc Cancer Res 31:184, 1990.
8. Clinical Alert, National Cancer Institute, Bethesda, May, 1988.
9. Consensus Development Conference Report: Adjuvant chemotherapy for breast cancer, JAMA 254:3461, 1985.
10. CRC Adjuvant Breast Trial Working Party: Cyclophosphamide and tamoxifen as adjuvant therapies in the management of breast cancer, Br J Cancer 57:604, 1988.
11. Dressler LG, Eudey L, Gray R, et al: DNA flow cytometry measurements are prognostic for time to recurrence in node-negative breast cancer: an Eastern Cooperative Group Intergroup study, Proc Am Soc Clin Oncol 9:22, 1990.
12. Early Breast Cancer Trialists, Collaborative Group: Effects of adjuvant tamoxifen and cytotoxic therapy on mortality in early breast cancer, N Engl J Med 319:1681, 1988.
13. Fisher B, Constantino J, Redmond C, et al: A randomized clinical trial evaluating tamoxifen in the treatment of patients with node-negative breast cancer who have estrogen-receptor-positive tumors, N Engl J Med 320:479, 1989.
14. Fisher B, Constantino J, et al: NSABP B-14: tamoxifen versus placebo in women with estrogen receptor positive, node negative breast cancer. Program of the NIH Consensus Development Conference on Early Stage Breast Cancer, 1990, p 64.
15. Fisher B, Redmond C, et al: NSABP B-13: methotrexate + 5 FU in women with estrogen receptor negative node negative breast cancer. Program of the NIH Consensus Development Conference on Early Stage Breast Cancer, 1990, p 63.
16. Fisher B, Redmond C, Dimitrov N, et al: A randomized clinical trial evaluating sequential methotrexate and fluorouracil in the treatment of patients with node-negative breast cancer who have estrogen-receptor-negative tumors, N Engl J Med 320:473, 1989.
17. Fisher B, Redmond C, Fisher ER, et al: Relative worth of estrogen or progesterone receptor and pathologic characteristics of differentiation as indicators of prognosis in node negative breast cancer patients: findings from National Surgical Adjuvant Breast and Bowel Project Protocol B-06, J Clin Oncol 6:1076, 1988.
18. Fisher B, Slack NH, Bross IDJ, et al: Cancer of the breast: size of neoplasm and prognosis, Cancer 24:1071, 1969.
19. Fisher ER, Redmond C, and Fisher B: Histologic grading of breast cancer. In Sommers SC and Rosen PP, editors: Pathology annual, Norwalk, CT, 1980, Appleton-Century-Crofts, pp 239-251.
20. Fornander T, Cedermark B, Mattsson A, et al: Adjuvant tamoxifen in early breast cancer: occurrence of new primary cancers, Lancet i:117, 1989.
21. Gelber R and Goldhirsch A: A new endpoint for the assessment of adjuvant therapy in postmenopausal women with operable breast cancer, J Clin Oncol 4:1772, 1986.
22. Gelber RD and Goldhirsch A: Quality of life in patients receiving adjuvant therapy. Program of the NIH Consensus Development Conference on Early Stage Breast Cancer, 1990, pp 71-73.
23. Glick JH: Adjuvant therapy for node negative breast cancer: a proactive view. In DeVita V, Hellman S, and Rosenberg S, editors: Advances in oncology, 1990, Philadelphia, JB Lippincott, pp 183-197.
24. Goldhirsch A, Castiglione M, and Gelber RD: International Breast Cancer Study Group trial of perioperative chemotherapy. Program of the NIH Consensus Development Conference on Early Stage Breast Cancer, 1990, pp 57-60.
25. Goldhirsch A, Gelber RD, Simes RJ, et al: Costs and benefits of adjuvant therapy in breast cancer: a quality-adjusted survival analysis, J Clin Oncol 7:36, 1989.
26. Gotfredsen A, Christiansen C, and Palshof T: The effect of tamoxifen on bone mineral content in premenopausal women with breast cancer, Cancer 53:853, 1984.
27. International (Ludwig) Breast Cancer Study Group: Prognostic importance of occult axillary lymph node micrometastases from breast cancer, Lancet 335:1565, 1990.
28. Jungi WF and Senn HJ: Swiss adjuvant trials in women with node negative breast cancer: 14-year results. Program of the NIH Consensus Development Conference on Early Stage Breast Cancer, 1990, pp 47-48.
29. Kallioniemi OP, Blanco G, Alavaikko M, et al: Improving the prognostic value of DNA flow cytometry in breast cancer by combining DNA index and S-phase fraction: a proposed classification of DNA histograms in breast cancer, Cancer 62:2183, 1988.
30. Knight WA, Livingston RB, Gregory EDJ, et al: Estrogen receptor as an independent prognostic factor for early recurrence in breast cancer, Cancer Res 37:4669, 1977.
31. Lee AKC, DeLellis RA, and Silverman ML: Prognostic significance of peritumoral lymphatic and blood vessel invasion in node negative carcinoma of the breast, J Clin Oncol 8:1457, 1990.
32. Love R: Tamoxifen therapy in primary breast cancer: biology, efficacy, and side effects, J Clin Oncol 7:803, 1989.
33. Love R, Mazess R, Tormey D, et al: Bone mineral density in woman with breast cancer treated for at least two years with tamoxifen, Breast Cancer Res Treat 12:297, 1988.
34. The Ludwig Breast Cancer Group: Combination adjuvant chemotherapy for node-positive breast cancer: inadequacy of a single perioperative cycle, N Engl J Med 319:1681, 1988.
35. The Ludwig Breast Cancer Study Group: Prolonged disease-free survival after one course of perioperative adjuvant chemotherapy for node-negative breast cancer, N Engl J Med 320:491, 1989.
36. Mansour E, Gray R, Shatila A, et al: Efficacy of adjuvant chemotherapy in high-risk node-negative breast cancer: an Intergroup study, N Engl J Med 320:485, 1989.
37. McGuire WL, Clark GM, Dressler LG, et al: Role of steroid hormone receptors as prognostic factors in primary breast cancer, NCI Monograph 1:19, 1986.
38. McGuire WL, Tandon AK, Allred DG, et al: How to use prognostic factors in axillary node-negative breast cancer, J Natl Cancer Inst 82:1006, 1990.
39. McGuire WL, Tandon A, Allred DC, et al: The relative value of tumor size, hormone receptors, flow cytometry, HER-2/neu oncogene, cathespin D, and stress response proteins in predicting patient outcome in axillary node negative breast cancer. Program of the NIH Consensus Development Conference on Early Stage Breast Cancer, 1990, pp 102-105.
40. Moon TE, Jones SE, Bonadonna G, et al: Development and use of a natural history data base of breast cancer studies, Am J Clin Oncol 10:396, 1987.
41. Morrison JM, Howell A, Grieve RJ, et al: The West Midlands Oncology Association trials of adjuvant chemotherapy for operable breast cancer. In Salmon SE, editor: Adjuvant therapy of cancer V, Orlando, 1987, Grune & Stratton, pp 311-318.
42. Morrison JM, Kelley KA, Howell A, et al: The West Midlands Oncology Association Trial of adjuvant chemotherapy for patients with node negative breast cancer. Program of the NIH Consensus Development Conference on Early Stage Breast Cancer, 1990, pp 51-56.

43. Nemoto T, Vana J, Bedwani RN, et al: Management and survival of female breast cancer: results of a national survey by the American College of Surgeons, Cancer 45:2917, 1980.
44. NIH Consensus Development Conference Statement: Treatment of early stage breast cancer. JAMA 265:391, 1991.
45. Nissen-Meyer R: Neoadjuvant chemotherapy in breast cancer: as single perioperative treatment and with supplementary long-term chemotherapy. In Salmon SE, editor: Adjuvant therapy of cancer V, Orlando, 1987, Grune & Stratton, pp 253-261.
46. Nolvadex Adjuvant Trial Organization: Controlled trial of tamoxifen as a single adjuvant agent in the management of early breast cancer: analysis at eight years, Br J Cancer 57:608, 1988.
47. Owens MA, Beardslee S, Wenger CR, et al: DNA ploidy and S-phase fractions by flow cytometry in a large breast cancer data base, Proc Am Assoc Cancer Res 31:184, 1990.
48. Paik S, Hazan R, Fisher ER, et al: Pathologic findings from the National Surgical Adjuvant Breast and Bowel Project: prognostic significance of erbB-2 protein overexpression in primary breast cancer, J Clin Oncol 8:103, 1990.
49. Riberio G and Swindell R: The Christie Hospital adjuvant tamoxifen trial-status at 10 years, Br J Cancer 57:601, 1988.
50. Rochefort H, Augereau P, Capony F, et al: The 52K cathespin-D of breast cancer: structure, regulation, function and clinical value. In Lippman ME and Dickson RB, editors: Breast cancer: cellular and molecular biology, Boston, 1988, Kluwer Acad, pp 207-221.
51. Rosen PP and Groshen S: Survival and prognostic factors in node-negative breast cancer: results of long-term followup studies. Program of the NIH Consensus Development Conference on Early Stage Breast Cancer, 1990, pp 86-91.
52. Rosen PP, Groshen S, Saigo PE, et al: A long-term follow-up study of survival in stage I ($T_1N_0M_0$) and stage II ($T_1N_1M_0$) breast carcinoma, J Clin Oncol 7:355, 1989.
53. Rosen PP, Groshen S, Saigo PE, et al: Pathological prognostic factors in stage I ($T_1N_0M_0$) and stage II ($T_1N_1M_0$) breast carcinoma: a study of 644 patients with median follow-up of 187 years, J Clin Oncol 7:1239, 1989.
54. Senn HJ and Mayr AC: Adjuvant chemotherapy in breast cancer: Swiss co-operative studies, Cancer Treat Rev 6:79, 1979.
55. Senn HJ and Barett-Mahler R: Update of Swiss adjuvant trials with LMF and CMF in operable breast cancer. In Salmon SE, editor: Adjuvant therapy of cancer V, Orlando, 1987, Grune & Stratton, pp 319-326.
56. Slamon DJ, Clark GM, Wong SG, et al: Human breast cancer: correlation of relapse and survival with amplification of the HER-2/neu oncogene, Science 235:177, 1987.
57. Slamon DJ, Godolphin W, Jones LA, et al: Studies of the HER-2/neu protooncogene in human breast and ovarian cancer, Science 244:707, 1989.
58. Stewart HJ: The Scottish adjuvant tamoxifen trials. Program of the NIH Consensus Development Conference on Early Stage Breast Cancer, 1990, pp 65-70.
59. Tandon AK, Clark GM, and Chamness GC: Heat shock/stress response proteins: biological and clinical significance in breast cancer, Proc Am Soc Clin Oncol 9:23, 1990.
60. Tandon AK, Clark GM, Chamness GC, et al: Cathepsin D and prognosis in breast cancer, N Engl J Med 322:297, 1990.
61. Thorpe SM, Rochefort H, Garcia M, et al: Association between high concentration of M_r 52,000 cathepsin D and poor prognosis in primary human breast cancer, Cancer Res 49:6008, 1989.
62. Tormey DC, Eudey L, Mansour EG, et al: CMFP versus observation in high-risk node negative breast cancer patients. Program of the NIH Consensus Development Conference on Early Stage Breast Cancer, 1990, pp 61-62.
63. Tsuda H, Hirohashi S, Shimosato Y, et al: Correlation between long-term survival in breast cancer patients and amplification of two putative oncogene-coamplification units: hst-1/int-2 and c-erbB-2/ear-1, Cancer Res 49:3104, 1989.
64. Valagussa P, Bonadonna G, and Veronesi U: Patterns of relapse and survival following radical mastectomy, Analysis of 716 consecutive patients, Cancer 41:1170, 1978.

10 Adjuvant Therapy of Node-Positive Operable Breast Cancer

Kevin R. Fox

Of the approximately 130,000 women in whom carcinoma of the breast is diagnosed each year in the United States, 40% to 50% have pathologic involvement of the axillary lymph nodes at the time of surgery. The risk of developing metastatic disease is altered dramatically by the presence of nodal involvement, as evidenced by the 10-year follow-up of patients treated with radical mastectomy alone[20,92] (Table 10-1). This increased risk of relapse translates directly into a marked reduction in overall survival, with 72% to 76% of node-negative patients surviving for 10 years and 35% to 48% of node-positive patients surviving for 10 years.[37,76,84]

The principle of adjuvant therapy of breast cancer is simple and is based on the assumption that a given percentage of patients with disease confined to the breast and axilla will be cured by local measures alone. The remainder, however, will remain at risk for systemic relapse because of the presence of micrometastatic disease in distant areas. Adjuvant therapy attempts to eradicate this subclinical disease and thus to improve overall patient survival.

HISTORY

The marked reduction in disease-free and overall survival rates associated with nodal involvement led to the first generation of adjuvant chemotherapy trials in the early 1970s, in which node-positive patients of all ages were randomized to receive some form of chemotherapy vs. local therapy (surgery) alone.

The National Surgical Adjuvant Breast Project (NSABP)[17,18] conducted the first trial, randomizing 349 patients between L-phenylalanine mustard (L-PAM) (0.15 mg/kg by mouth for 5 days, every 6 weeks for 2 years) vs. no chemotherapy. Shortly thereafter the National Cancer Institute of Milan[5] began a trial randomizing patients between no therapy and a combination of Cytoxan, methotrexate, and 5-fluorouracil (CMF) for 1 year (see below). Patients were stratified by true menstrual status (Milan) or by age (NSABP, age <50 years = premenopausal).

Table 10-2 illustrates the remarkable similarity in the results of these two trials. Data for disease-free survival are excluded for the sake of simplicity. In both trials, adjuvant chemotherapy improved survival rates at 10 years for premenopausal patients, with a 24% improvement in overall survival in the NSABP trial and a 12% improvement in the Milan trial. This survival benefit primarily applied to the premenopausal group with three or fewer lymph nodes involved. Premenopausal patients with four or more involved nodes enjoyed an improvement in survival that did not achieve statistical significance, while no survival benefit was noted for the entire postmenopausal group.

Bonadonna[3] has updated the original CMF trial with 14-year follow-up data. The data continues to show a significant improvement in the median duration of disease-free and overall survival in the chemotherapy treatment group, with the bulk of

Table 10-1 Percentage of disease-free survival in patients at 10 years according to degree of nodal involvement

Nodal involvement	Valagussa et al.[92]	Fisher et al.[20]
Node negative	72	76
1 to 3 positive nodes	34	36
≥4 positive nodes	16	14

THE CMF REGIMEN

Cytoxan: 100 mg/m² po on days to 1 to 14
Methotrexate: 40 mg/m² IV on days 1 and 8
5-Fluorouracil: 600 mg/m² IV on days 1 and 8

Cycle repeated every 28 days.

Table 10-2 Overall survival at 10 years in the NCI Milan[5] and NSABP[18] trials of adjuvant chemotherapy in node-positive breast cancer

	Overall survival (%)			
Pts.	L-PAM–treated pts.	Controls	CMF-treated pts.	Controls
Premenopausal	61	37*	59	45*
Premenopausal 1 to 3 nodes	81	48*	68	51*
Premenopausal ≥4 nodes	35	26	42	30
Postmenopausal	41	43	52	50

*p<.05.

this benefit still confined to the premenopausal patient (Table 10-3). This benefit continues to apply primarily to the group with three or fewer positive nodes (data not shown).

In 1975, after the accrual goals of the first CMF trial were met, a second trial was designed in which patients were randomized to receive either 12 months of CMF, as in the initial trial, or 6 months of identical chemotherapy. Both early and recent reports[3,86] indicate that there is no significant difference between the two treatment arms in terms of disease-free or overall survival rates. From this second Milan trial has emerged what most clinical oncologists consider the standard approach to the premenopausal, node-positive patient: 6 months of postoperative CMF chemotherapy.

Following these early, crucial clinical trials, clinical research in this area has been voluminous, the questions many and the answers relatively few and rarely clear-cut. Large-scale trials of endocrine therapy followed the early chemotherapeutic studies by only a few years, and their impact on the adjuvant therapy of breast cancer has been no less significant. The chapter discusses this treatment approach separately. The value of combining chemotherapeutic and hormonal interventions remains an unsolved research question.

Table 10-3 Median survival in months for patients treated in the first CMF trial at NCI Milan: 14-year follow-up[3]

Survival	Controls	CMF-treated pts.
Relapse-free survival (months)		
Premenopausal	32	141
Postmenopausal	59	64
Overall survival		
Premenopausal	96	NR
Postmenopausal	128	113

NR, median not reached.

INTERPRETING THE CLINICAL DATA

In his eloquent and exhaustive review of the subject, Henderson[38] warns of the many biases inherent in the literature on adjuvant therapy. The reader must remain circumspect with regard to the numbers of patients enrolled in such trials, the process of randomization, and the confidence limits imposed on the data. The reader's bias will be underscored by his or her personal requirement for a real "treatment benefit." The nihilist will interpret a 12% improvement in 10-year survival rates as seen in the Milan trial (43% vs. 31%) as a minor increment in the national history of breast cancer achieved only at great expense and with substantial toxicity and compromise of quality of life, while the activist will interpret this data as suggestive of a "cure" for thousands of patients per year, with only 6 months of effort and non–life-threatening toxicity.

"Publications bias" refers to the tendency for negative trials, which show no advantage to adjuvant therapy, to go unpublished. Furthermore, the statistical conventions applied to randomized trials ensure that 5% of "positive" trials actually are "false positives." This implies that more than 5% of the *published* "positive" trials actually are false positives.

Many adjuvant trials include subpopulations of patients that may be stratified prospectively or retrospectively by menopausal status, hormone receptor status, number of positive lymph nodes, histologic tumor grade, and flow cytometric analysis of tumor specimens. This enables the author to define subsets that may exceed 20 or 30 within a given clinical trial. Again, statistical convention allows 1 in 20 (or 5%) of these subgroups to display a positive result by chance alone, adding further to the false-positive bias of some clinical trials.

Finally, the reader must ask himself or herself which endpoints are most meaningful. It would seem most logical to observe overall survival as that endpoint that most closely approximates that percentage of patients actually cured by adjuvant therapy. This conclusion overlooks an important effect of adjuvant therapy which, while not implying cure, may imply a meaningful prolongation of life without evidence of metastatic cancer. In interpreting survival curves, one must be mindful of the fact that time is represented on the horizontal axis, and that a horizontal interpretation of data may predict a quantifiable prolongation of life for a given percentage (e.g., median number) of patients. For example, the median duration of disease-free survival in the initial Milan trial was 32 months for controls and 141 months for CMF-treated patients in the premenopausal group. Such a prolongation in time free of disease could be construed as worthy of 6 months (or 12 months) of treatment with unpleasant and occasionally toxic therapies.

ADJUVANT CHEMOTHERAPY

Overview analyses of randomized trials

It is generally accepted that adjuvant chemotherapy, in some form, will produce a benefit in disease-free and overall survival in premenopausal, node-positive patients with breast cancer. Given the relatively large number of clinical trials randomizing between some form of systemic chemotherapy and no therapy, this broad statement is best supported by two overview analyses that encompass all of these trials.

Himel et al.[44] reviewed trials published before December 1984. At this time, 14 published trials were referenced, 9 of which contained data sufficient for analysis, and 6 of which used combination chemotherapy rather than single agents. Whereas the 9 trials as a whole did not show an improvement in overall survival rates, those trials using multiagent chemotherapy did (Table 10-4). The overall survival benefit for premenopausal vs. postmenopausal patients could not be evaluated. However, when all 14 trials are examined individually for beneficial effect in the postmenopausal age group, none show significant improvement in overall or disease-free survival rates.[38]

The Early Breast Cancer Trialists Collaborative Group[14] analyzed all randomized adjuvant trials, published and unpublished and started before 1985, with respect to the reduction in the "odds of death" in treated vs. untreated groups. The report cited 31 clinical trials of adjuvant chemotherapy, involving over 7000 patients, with 27 trials randomizing between multiagent chemotherapy and no chemotherapy. Table 10-5 presents the overall results, which suggest an overall reduction in mortality in patients under 50 years of age treated with multiagent chemotherapy. The fact that CMF was the most commonly used regimen in these trials underscores the general acceptance of this regimen as standard in the premenopausal age group. Of additional interest, however, is the small but significant reduction in odds of death for patients over 50 years of age as well. This demonstrates the possibility of a subtle but real benefit to postmenopausal, node-positive patients with combination chemotherapy.

Despite the overwhelming evidence that the premenopausal, node-positive patient will enjoy an improved chance of survival with adjuvant chemotherapy, many outstanding questions remain and deserve individual discussion.

The reduced impact on the postmenopausal group

Why do postmenopausal patients derive less overall benefit, if any, from adjuvant chemotherapy? Several explanations have been set forth. First, there may be an inherent difference in the biology of breast cancer in older patients, which would render them inherently resistant to chemotherapy. This concept is only inferred from available clinical data and has not been proven conclusively in adjuvant

Table 10-4 Improvement in overall survival rates in patients receiving multiagent chemotherapy vs. control, or any chemotherapy vs. control, as analyzed by Himel et al.[44]

Treatment	Improvement in overall survival rates (% ± SD) 3-yr follow-up	5-yr follow-up
Multiagent chemotherapy	4.4 ± 3.5*	7 ± 6.5*
All chemotherapy	2 ± 3	4 ± 5

*Statistically significant.

Table 10-5 Reduction in annual odds of death in overview analysis[14] of all randomized trials prior to 1985

Treatment	Reduction in annual odds of death (% ± SD) Age ≤50	Age >50
Multiagent chemotherapy vs. no chemotherapy	26 ± 7	8 ± 6
Single-agent chemotherapy vs. no chemotherapy	11 ± 10	−4 ± 10
Multiagent chemotherapy vs. single-agent chemotherapy	21 ± 9	17 ± 8

trials. Second, the intensity of chemotherapy dosing in older patients may be compromised by their greater susceptibility to the toxicity of cytotoxic drugs. The benefit of sustained, full-dose or near full-dose chemotherapy in maximizing disease-free survival was first demonstrated in a retrospective analysis of the original Milan trial.[4] This benefit appeared to apply equally to both premenopausal and postmenopausal age groups. Nearly one half of the postmenopausal group received <65% of intended doses, while only 22% of the premenopausal group was so restricted (Table 10-6). In a more exhaustive analysis of 16 separate randomized trials, Hyriniuk and Levine[48] demonstrated a consistent improvement in relapse-free survival in studies using higher dose-intensity measured as total amount of drug administered per time unit. Again, this benefit applied both to premenopausal and postmenopausal groups; a tendency to reduce doses to a greater degree in older patients was not addressed in this analysis. Other studies analyzing dosing with respect to improvement in disease-free or overall survival have yielded conflicting results.[41]

Third, the benefit of adjuvant chemotherapy in overall survival of older, postmenopausal patients may be diluted by the many competing causes of death in these patients.[97] Finally, the most controversial issue regarding the postmenopausal group is the actual mechanism of action of adjuvant chemotherapy. It has been postulated that adjuvant cytotoxic chemotherapy works by inducing a "chemical oophorectomy" and that the postmenopausal group theoretically will derive no benefit because of preexisting ovarian nonfunction.[75] In a review of the experience in adjuvant trials in the Eastern Cooperative Oncology Group (ECOG), an improvement in disease-free and overall survival was seen in premenopausal patients who developed amenorrhea during chemotherapy compared to those who retained menses,[88] while a review of the Milan CMF trial detected no such difference.[6] The benefit of chemotherapy in postmenopausal, node-positive patients is marginal at best. The significant value of endocrine therapy in this group of patients (discussed later) leaves this issue to be resolved in further clinical trials. At the present time, if a postmenopausal patient is deemed to be a candidate for adjuvant chemotherapy in the absence of a clinical trial, good clinical sense requires maintenance of optimum, maximum chemotherapy dosing.

Table 10-6 Percentage of patients receiving different dose intensities in the original Milan CMF trial[4]

Percentage of full dose	Pt. group: Premenopausal	Pt. group: Postmenopausal
≥85%	58/262 (22%)	20/187 (11%)
<65%	58/262 (22%)	91/187 (48%)

Multidrug combinations vs. single agents

Despite the similarity in results obtained in the initial NSABP and Milan trials—the former trial utilizing the single agent L-PAM—the combination CMF regimen gradually secured a foothold as the standard adjuvant regimen. It may be that the increased leukemogenic risk of L-PAM, estimated at 1.1% ± 0.3% in patients treated with L-PAM alone (representing an elevenfold increase in leukemia risk compared to untreated controls) at 10 years, caused this drug to fall out of favor; however, the mortality from leukemia did not outweigh the survival benefit of adjuvant therapy.[24]

Henderson[38] has tabulated the clinical trials comparing single agents to multidrug combinations, and the results are conflicting. In the recent overview analysis,[14] results of trials utilizing single-agent chemotherapy vs. no chemotherapy (8 trials), and trials comparing polychemotherapy regimens vs. single agents (10 trials) were analyzed (see Table 10-5). These results favor the use of multidrug regimens. It is doubtful that the use of any single chemotherapeutic agent will reemerge in the adjuvant treatment of node-positive patients.

Optimum timing of initiation of therapy

The logic of adjuvant therapy suggests that treatment should be initiated at the earliest possible moment, when the burden of tumor is smallest and the chance of cure with cytotoxic therapy is therefore greatest. This logic would imply that therapy should commence in the immediate postoperative period or within several days to weeks of surgery after an appropriate convalescence. The in vivo biology of breast cancer suggests an observable clinical doubling time for macroscopic disease of 23 to 940 days, with averages of between approximately 3 months and 1 year.[43,63,64] This relatively slow growth suggests that the burden of tumor cells would not increase substantially in the first few postoperative weeks. The conventional clinical practice of initiating adjuvant chemotherapy within weeks, rather than days, of breast surgery seems appropriate.

The question of the optimal timing of drug therapy is of historical as well as practical interest. Two of the oldest and largest chemotherapeutic trials used chemotherapy in the perioperative and immediate postoperative period. In the NSABP B-01 trial, patients were randomized to receive ei-

Table 10-7 Treatment scheme* of the Ludwig V trial[62]

Treatment timing	Drugs	Schedule
Perioperative: <36 hr postoperative	Cytoxan	Days 1 and 8
	Methotrexate	Days 1 and 8
	5-Fluorouracil	Days 1 and 8
	Leucovorin	Days 2 and 9
Postoperative: commenced 25-32 days postoperative repeated q 28 days for 6 cycles	Cytoxan	Days 1-14
	Methotrexate	Days 1 and 8
	5-Fluorouracil	Days 1 and 8
	Prednisone	Daily
	Tamoxifen†	Daily

*Treatment group: I, perioperative; II, perioperative plus postoperative; III, postoperative only.
†Postmenopausal only.

ther no therapy or 3 consecutive days of intravenous thiotepa beginning on the day of surgery. A statistically significant advantage in survival at 5 years for premenopausal patients receiving chemotherapy was not maintained at 10 years of follow-up.[20] In an early Scandinavian trial[73] patients received either no perioperative therapy or 6 consecutive days of intravenous cyclophosphamide in the perioperative period. An advantage in overall survival for treated patients did not emerge until after 10 years of follow-up; it has been maintained to the present time. In a retrospective analysis of each contributing hospital, however, it was noted that one of the hospitals failed to show an overall survival benefit for its patients. It was discovered that this hospital's particular patients experienced a 2- to 4-week postoperative delay in initiation of chemotherapy, whereas other hospitals typically treated patients within the first postoperative week. The potentially detrimental effect of even a short delay in initiation of therapy became a reasonable hypothesis. Retrospective analysis of the timing of chemotherapy initiation in other studies have failed to confirm the harmful effects of such a delay.[9,30]

The question of optimal timing of chemotherapy has been addressed in a prospective, randomized fashion in only one study.[62] Between 1981 and 1985, 2628 patients were randomized preoperatively to receive one of three treatments (Table 10-7). Of the randomized patients, 1229 were classified as node positive. Patients received either a single perioperative cycle of a CMF regimen within 36 hours of surgery with no further treatment (group I), a single perioperative cycle plus six additional cycles of chemotherapy (group II), or no perioperative chemotherapy followed by a conventional 6 months of chemotherapy after a 25 to 32 day postoperative delay (group III). Table 10-8 presents 4 years of follow-up results.

The group receiving only a single cycle of postoperative chemotherapy had a poorer disease-free survival rate at 4 years than did group II and group III. This effect applied to both premenopausal and postmenopausal age groups (the postmenopausal

Table 10-8 Four-year disease-free survival by menopausal and nodal status in the Ludwig V trial[62]

Pt. group	Perioperative (I)	Combined (II)	Postoperative (III)
Premenopausal pts. (n = 715)			
All	40 ± 4	63 ± 4*	62 ± 4*
1-3 nodes	53 ± 5	77 ± 4*	76 ± 4*
4-9 nodes	26 ± 8	60 ± 8*	49 ± 8*
≥10 nodes	16 ± 6	19 ± 8	34 ± 10
Postmenopausal pts. (n = 514)			
All	40 ± 4	55 ± 5*	63 ± 4†
1-3 nodes	51 ± 6	60 ± 7*	70 ± 5*
4-9 nodes	28 ± 7	69 ± 8*	63 ± 7*
≥10 nodes	24 ± 9	15 ± 9	36 ± 11*

*p<.01.
†p=.06.

groups II and III also received 6 months of tamoxifen) and to all nodal subgroups in the premenopausal age group. Overall survival has not been improved upon, but mean follow-up of 42 months at publication may not be adequate to demonstrate a survival advantage.

A comparison of groups II and III shows no significant difference in disease-free survival for the entire groups of premenopausal and postmenopausal patients. This implies that a perioperative cycle of therapy confers no advantage on the node-positive patient and that the conventional approach, permitting a several-week delay before commencement of chemotherapy, is entirely acceptable and will remain the standard approach.

Optimum duration of chemotherapy

The first and second Milan CMF studies,[5,86] as discussed above, established both the efficacy of the CMF regimen and the fact that 6 months of therapy appeared to be as effective as a 12-month regimen. The efficacy of the 6-month treatment course has withstood the test of time, with 12-year follow-up reported recently.[3] Henderson[38] cites seven studies in which patients were randomized to two different durations of therapy. No survival advantage was demonstrated in any of the studies in which survival data was provided. However, two recent studies have reemphasized the apparent efficacy of relatively short durations of therapy. The Eastern Cooperative Oncology Group[16] randomized over 600 postmenopausal patients to receive either 4 or 12 months of CMF plus prednisone and tamoxifen (CMFPT). No significant difference in survival or freedom from relapse was noted between the two durations of therapy at over 4 years median follow-up. More recently, the NSABP has published the preliminary results of trial B-15,[95] in which patients were randomized to receive 12 weeks of an Adriamycin-Cytoxan combination, 6 months of conventional CMF, or a reinduction regimen of Adriamycin-Cytoxan of similar duration (12 weeks) followed 6 months later by 3 months of CMF. No differences among treatment groups have been noted at 3 years of median follow-up. Finally, investigators at the Dana Farber Cancer Institute performed a study with longer follow-up, in which high-risk patients (more than four positive nodes) received either 15 or 30 weeks of a Cytoxan-Adriamycin combination.[42] No survival advantage or disease-free advantage could be attributed to the longer course of therapy.

There seems to be no justification, therefore, for extending adjuvant therapy beyond a 4- to 6-month period. Obviously, minimizing toxicity is of paramount importance in the optimum application of adjuvant chemotherapy. Unfortunately, the use of a single perioperative cycle of treatment, while an appealing alternative, appears to be inadequate based on the results of the Ludwig V trial (see Table 10-8).[62]

Short-term and long-term toxicity of chemotherapy

The short-term toxicities of standard courses of chemotherapy are reproducible across multiple trials and are well understood. Most patients suffer some degree of nausea and/or vomiting and myelosuppression. Table 10-9 lists other side effects.[90] Most of these effects are short term in nature and consequence, with the possible exception of weight gain and amenorrhea. More serious and potentially life-threatening toxicities, such as systemic infection and deep venous thrombosis, may be increased with the concurrent use of prednisone; however, prednisone may reduce nausea and vomiting and

Table 10-9 Incidence of common acute toxicities in chemotherapy regimens[90]

	Incidence premenopausal (%)		Incidence postmenopausal (%)
Toxicity	CMF	CMF and prednisone	CMF and prednisone
WBC <2000	13.5	21.5	28
Platelets <50,000	3	1	10
Systemic infection	1	5	5
Nausea/vomiting*	19	5	4
Stomatitis*			11
Neurologic complications	7	17	17
Edema*	3	8	13
Weight gain >20%*	2	10	3
Deep venous thrombosis	0.5	1.5	3
Hot flashes	57	58	3
Amenorrhea	40	46	

*Severe enough to warrant chemotherapy dose reduction.

permit the use of higher doses of cytotoxic drugs.[57,90] Despite these toxicities a compelling statistic derived from patients treated in the United States suggested that 74% of those patients interviewed following adjuvant chemotherapy would recommend a course of adjuvant chemotherapy to a friend.[68]

Longer-term toxicities, particularly with respect to second malignancies, are less well understood and will require years of follow-up to be fully appreciated. The incidence of acute leukemia in melphalan-treated patients of 1.1% ± 0.3% at 10 years represents an elevenfold increase in comparison to controls treated with surgery alone.[24] Acute myelogenous leukemia occurred with a twenty-fourfold increase in likelihood in these patients. An increase in leukemia was also noted in patients receiving only radiotherapy in addition to surgery in this trial. The quantitative impact of radiation alone in the development of acute leukemia in breast cancer patients is not well understood. Because Cytoxan-containing regimens have proliferated in the adjuvant treatment of breast cancer, the leukemogenic effect of this particular alkylating agent must be evaluated. Cytoxan is a putative leukemogen in the laboratory and in other human malignancies, particularly the hematologic malignancies. However, retrospective analyses of CMF-treated patients have failed to show either an increased risk of leukemia or second malignancies in these patients.[45,93]

Qualitatively, for premenopausal, node-positive patients, toxicities of conventional adjuvant chemotherapy do not appear to outweigh the benefits. The Ludwig Breast Cancer Study Group has attempted to quantitate the benefit of adjuvant chemotherapy through the concept of "TWiST" (time without symptoms of disease and toxicity).[27,34] This analysis has thus far been confined to postmenopausal, node-positive patients treated in the Ludwig III trial.[25] In this trial, postmenopausal patients were randomized to adjuvant chemohormonal therapy, hormonal therapy, or no adjuvant therapy (see bottom left of this page).

The concept of TWiST, as initially defined, subtracted time spent with subjective symptoms relative to treatment, or time spent with distant or local recurrence, from the patient's overall survival. This yielded a net TWiST in months for each study arm. An abbreviated summary over 6 years of follow-up is shown in Table 10-10. This demonstrates a clear reduction in TWiST, as expected, for the chemotherapy-treated group in the first year relative to patients receiving less toxic hormonal therapy or no therapy, but by 6 years of follow-up the chemotherapy group was enjoying a significantly greater number of months of TWiST relative to untreated controls. If these data are examined after dividing the treatment groups into estrogen receptor–positive vs. estrogen receptor–negative groups, this statistical significance is lost (data not shown).

The TWiST construct is an honorable concept that attempts to quantitate the quality of life in these patients. The simplicity of the TWiST concept also may be considered its undoing, as it assumes that the relative quality of life is zero for women experiencing any toxicity and zero for any women with systemic relapse. Such an approach would inherently devalue quality survival for treated and untreated patients alike, but would be biased against patients receiving therapy in some form. With this in mind, Goldhirsch et al.[34] have reexamined the Ludwig III trial data and formulated a modification of TWiST, called "Q-TWiST," which deducts amounts of time with toxicity or relapse proportionately rather than absolutely from TWiST (see p. 272). The utility coefficients u_1 and u_2 are quite arbitrary and weight the relative quality of life from 0 ($u = 0$) to 100% ($u = 1$) during pe-

THE LUDWIG III TRIAL IN WHICH TWiST WAS EVALUATED[27]

Randomization
- No adjuvant therapy
- Tamoxifen and prednisone
- CMF, tamoxifen, prednisone

TWiST = OS − (A + B + C)

where OS = overall survival
A = time spent with subjective toxicity (nausea, vomiting, mucositis)
B = 3 months subtracted for weight gain, edema, or local recurrence
C = all months from systemic relapse until death

Table 10-10 Net months spent without toxicity (TWiST) in Ludwig III trial[26]

	Months postrandomization		
Treatment group	12	36	72
Untreated controls	11	25	38
Tamoxifen and prednisone	9	25	42
CMF, tamoxifen, and prednisone	3	21	44*

*Statistically significant relative to control.

Q-TWiST: A MODIFICATION OF TWiST

Q-TWiST = (u_1 × TOX) + TWiST + (u_2 × REL)

where TWiST = time without symptoms or toxicity

TOX = any reversible subjective toxicity during any treatment month, plus 3 months for alopecia and weight gain

REL = time spent with second malignancy or systemic relapse, and/or 3 months for local recurrence or contralateral breast cancer

u_1, u_2 = "utility coefficients" ranging from 0 to 1

Modified from Goldhirsch A et al: J Clin Oncol 7:36, 1989.

Table 10-11 Total time in Q-TWiST at median 7 years of follow-up in the Ludwig III trial

Treatment group	Months of Q-TWiST
Untreated control	51.9 ± 2.2
Tamoxifen and prednisone	54.6 ± 2.3
CMF, tamoxifen, and prednisone	58.7 ± 2.2*

*p = .05 relative to control.
Adapted from Goldhirsch A et al: J Clin Oncol 7:36, 1989.

riods of toxicity or relapse. Arbitrarily assigning a coefficient of 0.5 to these periods of time ($u_1 = u_2 = 0.5$), Table 10-11 shows the total amount of time spent in Q-TWiST for each treatment group at median 7 years of follow-up. This value approaches statistical significance for the chemotherapy-treated group relative to untreated patients.

The variations in calculating Q-TWiST are limitless. Perhaps this construct may be criticized on the grounds of being excessively arbitrary.[7] However, quantitating quality survival seems of paramount importance in assessing chemotherapy in postmenopausal patients, in whom the overall value of chemotherapy seems small, at best, at the present time.

The optimum chemotherapeutic regimen

If CMF chemotherapy today remains the standard regimen for treatment of premenopausal patients,[39] one must view the long-term survival data in the Milan trial with a critical eye (see Table 10-2). As the bulk of benefit in survival appears confined to the group with three or fewer positive nodes, this regimen could be construed as inadequate in the treatment of high-risk patients with extensive nodal involvement. Furthermore, can the 17% improvement in survival at 10 years in the patient with one to three positive nodes be improved upon with a better chemotherapeutic regimen? These issues remain the most critical ones as the present generation of adjuvant trials matures.

Efforts to improve on CMF have included randomized trials comparing standard CMF with regimens using CMF with prednisone (CMFP), or with vincristine and prednisone (CMFVP).[1,33,89] In a trial comparing CMF to CMFVP, Aisner et al. reported an advantage in disease-free survival in patients with 10 or more positive nodes.[1] However, the additional toxicities of vincristine and the inherent weakness of this drug as an agent in the treatment of breast cancer weigh against its inclusion in standard CMF regimens. Prednisone, on the other hand, seems to permit administration of higher doses of CMF by reducing the degree of neutropenia and thrombocytopenia.[89] This has not been translated into an improvement in disease-free or overall survival in the trials of CMFP vs. CMF cited in Table 10-12. The additional toxicities of prednisone in the CMFP regimen (see Table 10-9) are well known, and would rule against its routine inclusion in adjuvant chemotherapy.

For the moment, the most significant advance in the use of adjuvant chemotherapy seems to be the inclusion of doxorubicin (Adriamycin) in treatment regimens. Doxorubicin is one of the most active single agents in the treatment of metastatic breast carcinoma, and when Adriamycin-containing regimens (CAF) have been compared with CMF in metastatic cancer, both response rates and overall survival rates are superior.[1] Several trials have compared the results of doxorubicin-containing regimens with the results of more conventional treatments (Table 10-13). The NSABP randomized estrogen receptor–negative patients to receive either fluorouracil (5-FU) with melphalan, or 5-FU, melphalan, and doxorubicin.[19] Postmenopausal patients have shown an improvement in overall survival when receiving the doxorubicin-containing regimen when compared to patients who received 5-FU and melphalan alone. In a more compelling study, a French group has reported 7-year follow-up of a trial randomizing between CMF and a regimen of doxorubicin, vincristine, Cytoxan, and 5-fluorouracil (AVCF).[65,69] Both disease-free and overall survival rates were significantly improved for premenopausal patients only in the AVCF group.

The emerging evidence that doxorubicin-containing regimens should replace CMF as the standard of adjuvant therapy includes the elimination of CMF in the control arms of many ongoing

Table 10-12 Trials comparing CMF with regimens adding prednisone or vincristine and prednisone

Author	Randomization	Pts. menopausal status
CALGB[1]	CMF vs. CMFVP	Premenopausal and postmenopausal
Ludwig[33]	CMF vs. CMFP	Premenopausal only
ECOG[89]	CMF vs. CMFP	Premenopausal only

CALGB, Cancer and Leukemia Group B.

cooperative group studies. In the absence of an available clinical trial, the medical oncologist is forced to make a choice that remains somewhat empiric: should he or she accept the wealth of data supporting the use of CMF in the premenopausal patient? Or should he or she opt for a regimen of drugs that includes doxorubicin and accept the greater risk of alopecia and small risk of cardiotoxicity? Follow-up of present trials probably will resolve this issue in the next several years.

ADJUVANT ENDOCRINE THERAPY

The foregoing section purposely excluded a discussion of endocrine manipulations, particularly with respect to chemotherapy/endocrine therapy combinations. As discussed later in this chapter, the combination of chemotherapy and endocrine therapy in the adjuvant treatment of breast cancer is an unresolved issue. The history of endocrine therapy alone as adjuvant therapy deserves a separate discussion, as modern adjuvant endocrine therapy evolved parallel to early chemotherapy trials. Whereas the latter trials have affected the treatment of premenopausal, node-positive patients, the endocrine trials have had their greatest effects in the postmenopausal group. The respective roles of adjuvant chemotherapy and endocrine therapy may be mutually exclusive at the present time.

History and background

The responsiveness of metastatic breast cancer to endocrine manipulation is well known. Approximately one third of patients with metastatic disease will respond to endocrine manipulations of all types.[40] Surgical ablative procedures, such as oophorectomy, hypophysectomy, and adrenalectomy, and medical interventions, including the administration of estrogens, progesterones, aminoglutethimide, androgens, and tamoxifen, seem to be equally effective in treating metastatic disease. Some interventions, such as oophorectomy, are primarily effective in premenopausal patients and rarely produce significant responses in postmenopausal patients.

The effectiveness of endocrine therapies in the treatment of metastatic disease makes them appealing adjuvant interventions. The earliest adjuvant trials in the medical literature were trials of adjuvant oophorectomy. Henderson[38] has cited eight randomized trials of adjuvant oophorectomy or ovarian radioablation vs. surgical controls, all of which were started by 1965 and completed around the time of initiation of modern chemotherapy trials. These trials of ovarian ablation provide an interesting, although confusing, backdrop to modern endocrine therapy trials. All of the trials are limited by the fact that (1) estrogen receptor information on tumor tissue was unavailable at that time, (2) every trial included patients with *no* involved lymph nodes, and (3) many trials included postmenopausal patients, in whom adjuvant oophorectomy should have no logical role.

Indeed, only one trial suggested improvement in disease-free survival for postmenopausal patients, while overall survival rates have shown no significant improvement in any trial that included those patients. The benefits of oophorectomy or ovarian

Table 10-13 Trials comparing doxorubicin-containing regimens with non–doxorubicin-containing regimens

Author	Randomization	Pts. menopausal status
Misset et al.[69]	CMF vs. AVCF	Premenopausal and postmenopausal
Fisher et al.[19]	PamF vs. PamAF	Premenopausal and postmenopausal
Perloff et al.[77]	CMFVP vs. CMFVP/VATH	Premenopausal and postmenopausal

PamF, phenylalanine mustard; PamAF, phenylalanine mustard, Adriamycin (doxorubicin), and 5-fluorouracil; VATH, vinblastine, Adriamycin, tamoxifen, halostetin.

radioablation appear to be restricted, therefore, to the premenopausal population. Of the eight trials cited by Henderson,[38] only one has failed to show a trend in favor of improved overall survival. This improvement in overall survival reaches statistical significance in only two of these trials. In one of these two trials,[8] oophorectomy provided an 11% improvement in overall survival rates; while in the other[67] the benefit was confined to premenopausal women over the age of 45 who received small daily doses of prednisone in addition to ablative ovarian radiotherapy.

It is tantalizing to ponder the results of these trials of ovarian ablation had they been confined to premenopausal women with tumors positive for estrogen receptor. If one considers that perhaps only half of the premenopausal patients would have been receptor positive, the benefits of oophorectomy in the patients in these trials might be diluted by the substantial number of receptor-negative patients included, in whom endocrine manipulations are destined to fail under most circumstances. Unfortunately, other trials of endocrine manipulation in node-positive premenopausal patients have been less compelling (see discussion later in the chapter). The exact role of adjuvant ovarian ablation in the premenopausal patient remains uncertain.

Adjuvant tamoxifen

The minimal toxicity of tamoxifen makes it an attractive option for adjuvant endocrine therapy for breast cancer. Large-scale trials of adjuvant tamoxifen commenced in Europe in the mid-1970s and were directed largely at postmenopausal patients, as these patients were deemed to benefit little, if at all, from adjuvant chemotherapy. Henderson[38] cites 10 published trials of adjuvant tamoxifen. All of these trials have demonstrated an improvement in disease-free survival in the tamoxifen-treated patients. However, only two have demonstrated an overall survival benefit at this time and deserve separate mention.

The Nolvadex Adjuvant Therapy Organization (NATO) initiated its trials in Britain in 1977.[74] In this trial, over 1000 patients were randomized to receive either 2 years of tamoxifen or no adjuvant therapy regardless of menopausal status; both node-negative and node-positive patients were included. Nearly 90% of the patients were postmenopausal in this trial. The advantage in terms of survival at 8 years of follow-up was >10% for the treated group. A reduction in mortality was noted in both premenopausal and postmenopausal groups and in both node-positive and node-negative groups.

The Scottish National Trial Group study[80] began in 1978, randomizing over 1300 patients to receive 5 years of adjuvant tamoxifen or no therapy. Important differences in this trial included the fact that only node-negative premenopausal patients were included (19% of total patients), while both node-positive and node-negative postmenopausal patients were included, and that control patients were assigned to receive tamoxifen at the first sign of recurrence. At 8 years of follow-up the overall survival rate in the treated group was improved by 15% (82% vs. 67%). An overall reduction in the number of deaths was seen in all subgroups of patients regardless of menopausal or nodal status, but this was statistically significant only among postmenopausal and node-positive patients (Table 10-14).

How does the practicing physician distill this information into a clinically applicable treatment paradigm? Evidence of a survival benefit in premenopausal node-positive patients with adjuvant chemotherapy is irrefutable, while evidence that chemotherapy benefits the postmenopausal population is limited. Choosing among therapies can be simplified to a great degree by an understanding of the estrogen receptor (ER) and progesterone receptor (PR) status of the patients in these trials. The benefits of endocrine therapy in metastatic breast cancer has been shown to correlate well with estrogen receptor status (Table 10-15).[10,66] This would suggest the greater usefulness of adjuvant endocrine therapy in the treatment of patients with ER-positive tumors. In the NATO trial a reduction in deaths was described for *all* treatment groups

Table 10-14 The Scottish Trial: disease-free and overall survival for patients receiving 5 years of tamoxifen vs. no therapy[80]

	Disease-free survival (months)		Overall survival (months)	
Patient group	**Tamoxifen group**	**Controls**	**Tamoxifen group**	**Controls**
All pts.	*	73	*	95
Node-negative pts.	*	*	*	*
Node-positive pts.	84	31	85	63

*Median survival not reached at 8 years follow-up.

Table 10-15 Responses to endocrine therapy in metastatic cancer based on estrogen receptor (and progesterone receptor) status[10,66]

ER level (fm/mg)	Response (%)	ER/PR status	Response (%)
<3	6	ER−/PR−	9
>3, <100	46	ER+/PR−	32
>100	81	ER+/PR+	71

Table 10-16 Disease-free survival in patients in the Scottish Trial based on ER status[80]

		Disease-free survival at 3 years (%)	
ER level (fm/mg)	n	Tamoxifen group	Controls
0-4	218	65.6	55.1
5-19	89	71.7	60.5
20-99	214	85.6	73.8
>100	221	86.3	61.0
Not measured	570	79.7	65.3
Total no pts.	1312	78.9	64.1

Table 10-17 Reduction in mortality and estimated overall survival rates in patients treated with tamoxifen in overview analysis of all randomized trials of tamoxifen vs. no therapy[14]

	Overall survival (%)		
Patient age (yr)	Tamoxifen	Control	Reduction in annual odds of death (%)
<50	71.1	70.6	−1 ± 8
>50	73.4	67.6	20 ± 3

regardless of ER status. In the Scottish Trial, significant improvement in disease-free survival was seen only in the group with the highest ER level (Table 10-16), although a trend was noted in all ER-positive groups. Other trials, however, clearly have shown an advantage in terms of disease-free survival in estrogen receptor–positive patients, with only one exception. The value of adjuvant tamoxifen in estrogen receptor–negative patients has been mixed. No other trials have shown a statistically significant improvement or statistically significant decrement in disease-free or overall survival in these patients; trends have been seen in both directions.[38]

The overall value of adjuvant tamoxifen in all patients (node-negative and node-positive, premenopausal and postmenopausal) has been assessed in a recent overview analysis.[14] In this analysis, a clear reduction in mortality was seen in patients over age 50 treated with adjuvant tamoxifen vs. untreated controls. Such a benefit was not seen in patients below age 50 (Table 10-17).

Outstanding questions regarding adjuvant endocrine therapy

The toxicity of adjuvant endocrine therapy. As tamoxifen has been firmly established as the preferred adjuvant therapy in those patients deemed to derive benefit from an endocrine manipulation (i.e., ER-positive, postmenopausal patients), a critical appraisal of toxicity is mandatory. Fortunately, the toxicity of this drug in short-term usage (most adjuvant trials employed 1 to 2 years of therapy) appears minimal and acceptable. When tamoxifen is used in the treatment of metastatic disease, approximately 10% of patients experience transient nausea. A minority of patients experience a transient vaginal discharge, and rarely clinically insignificant thrombocytopenia is seen. Hot flashes occasionally occur, particularly in premenopausal patients.

The toxicity in adjuvant trials should not be considerably different, and the available toxicity data bear this out. In a study using tamoxifen or an actual placebo as adjuvant therapy for 2 years in postmenopausal patients, overall toxicities did not differ between the tamoxifen and placebo groups, except for a higher incidence of "hot flashes" in the tamoxifen group.[12] In one British trial, over 1000 patients were randomized to receive tamoxifen or a control treatment (*no* treatment if postmenopausal; ablative ovarian irradiation if premenopausal). The incidence of dose-reduction for toxicity in tamoxifen-treated patients was 2% and the overall incidence of premature cessation of therapy was 4% in the first year of treatment. In 199 premenopausal patients treated with tamoxifen, 28% developed menstrual irregularities or transient amenorrhea, and 19% developed permanent menopause.[81] In the NATO trial, when patients who died were evaluated for cause of death, causes "not due to breast cancer" were *not* increased in the tamoxifen group, implying a lack of toxic mortality for the drug.[74]

Most of the adjuvant tamoxifen trials have used relatively short durations of treatment (1, 2, or 5 years). The optimum duration of therapy is an unsettled issue (see below), and many investigators are advocating longer, perhaps indefinite, courses of therapy. The more serious potential toxicities of tamoxifen should be addressed in light of these emerging recommendations. When tamoxifen is used in metastatic disease, one study noted an increased incidence (1% to 3%) of thrombophlebitis,[60] while another reported an increase in the incidence of endometrial carcinoma.[55] In the latter study, the dose of tamoxifen used was higher than the standard dose of 20 mg per day. These studies require confirmation.

The "antiestrogenic" effects of tamoxifen have raised concern over an acceleration of the normal age-dependent loss of bone mineral density in women. Such an acceleration of bone mineral loss would place tamoxifen-treated patients at a theoretically increased risk of fracture over time. Several studies, using the technique of single or dual photon absorptiometry, have addressed these issues. Thus far, retrospective studies of postmenopausal women[25,61] and prospective studies of premenopausal[36] or postmenopausal women[91,96] or both[78] have shown *no* difference in measured bone density when compared to controls. One of these studies[91] actually has suggested an increase in bone density in tamoxifen-treated patients. These studies are limited in value because of small numbers of patients studied, short follow-up, and the fact that most of these patients received relatively short courses of tamoxifen therapy (maximum 5 years). The question of bone density loss with tamoxifen therapy remains open and will be resolved with larger studies and longer follow-up.

The optimum duration of tamoxifen therapy. All of the studies demonstrating an improvement in disease-free and overall survival benefit with adjuvant tamoxifen therapy have utilized finite periods of treatment of 1, 2, or 5 years. In animal models of adjuvant endocrine therapy, continuous treatment with tamoxifen is required to prevent regrowth of mammary tumors.[53] These laboratory findings suggest a suppressive or cytostatic effect, rather than a cytocidal effect, of tamoxifen in breast cancer and invite the hypothesis that longer (and perhaps indefinite) durations of treatment may produce greater disease-free and overall survival rates. The overview analysis[14] of adjuvant tamoxifen did not show a statistical advantage to more than 1 year of tamoxifen therapy, however (Table 10-18). Randomized trials comparing varying lengths of tamoxifen therapy are not yet published; the optimum duration of tamoxifen therapy remains an unresolved issue.

COMPARING AND COMBINING CHEMOTHERAPY AND ENDOCRINE THERAPY

The value of combination chemotherapy and endocrine therapy in the premenopausal and postmenopausal patients with node-positive stage II breast cancer is well established. Efforts to improve efficacy while limiting toxicity to an acceptable

Table 10-18 Overview analysis of adjuvant tamoxifen trials based upon duration of tamoxifen therapy[14]

		Reduction in annual odds of death (% ± SD)	
Duration of treatment	No. of trials	Age < 50 yr	Age > 50 yr
≤1 yr vs. control	9 (n = 5006)	−7 ± 15	15 ± 6
≥2 yr vs. control	19 (n = 11507)	1 ± 9	23 ± 4

Table 10-19 Assignment of risk by nodal status and receptor status in the GABG trial[52,54]

Nodal status	ER or PR positive	ER or PR negative
1-3 nodes	Low risk	High risk
≥4 nodes	High risk	High risk

ASSIGNMENT OF RANDOMIZATION BY RISK STATUS IN THE GABG TRIAL[52,54]

Low risk

Tamoxifen 30 mg per day for 2 years or CMF chemotherapy for 6 months.

High risk

Chemotherapy with Cytoxan and Adriamycin for 6 months or same chemotherapy plus tamoxifen 30 mg per day for 2 years.

level form the foundation for the present generation of clinical trials. In this vein, it has been postulated by some[75] that the value of chemotherapy in premenopausal women is attributable solely or partly to its endocrine effects. That is to say, the induction of a "chemical oophorectomy" confers a distinct relapse-free and overall survival benefit on the premenopausal patient,[65,88] and this effect may occur regardless of estrogen receptor status.

Although this endocrine hypothesis is refuted strongly by others,[5] it remains an inviting hypothesis. In light of the older oophorectomy trials from Canada, in which older (age >45 years) premenopausal patients seemed to derive benefit from adjuvant ovarian radioablation, a randomized comparison of chemotherapy and endocrine therapy seems in order. Such information was not available until recently, when 6 year follow-up results of such a trial were published. The Gynecological Adjuvant Breast Cancer Group (GABG) initiated the trial in 1981 and completed enrollment in May 1986. In this trial[52,54] node-positive patients were stratified into low-risk or high-risk groups based on nodal and/or estrogen receptor status (Table 10-19). Low-risk patients (ER- or PR-positive patients with one to three positive nodes) were randomized to receive 6 months of CMF chemotherapy or 2 years of tamoxifen. High-risk patients (any ER- or PR-negative patient, or any patient with more than four positive nodes) were randomized to receive a combination of chemotherapy (Cytoxan plus doxorubicin) or chemohormonal therapy (Cytoxan, doxorubicin, and tamoxifen, the latter for 2 years) (see above). Patients were treated only according to risk, regardless of age or menopausal status.

The results in the *low-risk* population will be considered here, as only this population of women serves to compare a purely endocrine vs. a purely chemotherapeutic maneuver. The 6-year results are shown in Table 10-20. In this relatively small study, survival for premenopausal patients was decidedly superior in the chemotherapy arm, while no significant difference existed in overall survival rates among postmenopausal patients. A *greater* risk of relapse was noted in the postmenopausal group treated with chemotherapy. This provocative study demonstrates a benefit of chemotherapy over tamoxifen therapy in a defined subpopulation of premenopausal women. Does it provide definitive proof that chemotherapy is unquestionably superior to endocrine therapy in younger women? Endocrine therapy with tamoxifen cannot be equated with oophorectomy, as most premenopausal patients will retain menses after a 1-year period of tamoxifen therapy.[81] Until trials randomizing between chemotherapy and oophorectomy are completed, chemotherapy alone will remain the mainstay of treatment in the premenopausal, node-positive patient. The 6-year follow-up data in the postmenopausal patient group reinforces the notion that chemotherapy *alone* offers no advantage over

Table 10-20 Six-year relapse and survival results for low-risk patients in GABG trial 1[52,54]

	Premenopausal pts. (%) (n = 119)		Postmenopausal pts. (%) (n = 157)	
Outcome	Tamoxifen	CMF	Tamoxifen	CMF
Relapse	51.1	15.7*	14.6†	38.3
Death	20.4	4.3‡	5.6	8.8

*p = .01.
†p = .003.
‡p = .002.

Table 10-21 The Ludwig III trial randomizing postmenopausal, node-positive patients to receive hormonal therapy, chemohormonal therapy, or no therapy[32]

Treatment group	Treatment	Evaluable pts.
Control	No treatment	156
Hormonal therapy	Tamoxifen + prednisone for 1 year	153
Chemohormonal therapy	CMF + prednisone + tamoxifen for 1 year	154

tamoxifen alone in the treatment of the node-positive, ER-positive patient.

Combining chemotherapy and endocrine therapy

The relative paucity of data comparing purely endocrine to purely chemotherapeutic interventions (as above) stands in sharp contrast to the wealth of data in clinical trials in which chemotherapy and endocrine therapy have been combined. The combination of modalities would seem inherently logical, as a given breast cancer might contain multiple clones of cells that may be endocrine-sensitive or chemotherapy-sensitive but not both, allowing for a superior tumor cell kill if both modalities are combined. Preclinical studies cast doubt on this hypothesis. In these in vitro experiments, low concentrations of tamoxifen inhibited the cytotoxic actions of doxorubicin and 5-fluorouracil on breast carcinoma lines.[47] In other systems, tamoxifen inhibited the cytotoxicity of melphalan[31] by inhibiting the uptake of melphalan into the tumor cell. In general it has been postulated that tamoxifen may indeed inhibit the cytotoxic effects of chemotherapy by prolonging the G_0 phase of cell growth, thus slowing cell growth in general and reducing the inherent action of cytotoxic drugs on actively dividing cells.[28] These laboratory data warn against the simultaneous applications of chemotherapeutic and hormonal treatments in adjuvant therapy. The clinical data are reviewed below.

Comparing chemohormonal therapy to endocrine therapy alone

Given the clear-cut role for adjuvant tamoxifen in the postmenopausal, node-positive, ER-positive patient, the pivotal question remains whether the combination of chemohormonal therapy might be beneficial to such patients, or to ER-negative patients.[46] The Ludwig III trial (Table 10-21)[32] is the most mature trial designed to address this question. Between 1978 and 1981 over 450 evaluable postmenopausal patients were randomized to receive no therapy, endocrine therapy with prednisone and tamoxifen for 12 months, or a 12-month course of CMF, prednisone, and tamoxifen. All patients were under 65 years of age. The disease-free and overall survival results at 7 years of median follow-up are shown in Table 10-22. Combination chemohormonal therapy produces improved disease-free survival rates when compared to hormonal therapy or observation, while overall survival rates compared to hormonal therapy approaches but does not quite reach statistical significance ($p = .08$). Estrogen receptor–negative patients also enjoy an improvement in disease-free survival, but not overall survival, when analyzed separately. A critical appraisal of the data in ER-negative patients is limited by the relatively small number of patients randomized in this study (n = 83, or 18% of total population).

More recently, two pivotal clinical trials limited to postmenopausal, ER-positive patients were eval-

Table 10-22 The Ludwig III trial: 7-year disease-free and overall survival results for postmenopausal patients[32]

	Disease-free survival (%)			Overall survival (%)		
	Pts. given CMF, prednisone and tamoxifen	Pts. given prednisone and tamoxifen	Observation group	Pts. given CMF, prednisone and tamoxifen	Pts. given prednisone and tamoxifen	Observation group
All pts.	51*	36	24	57	51	47
ER-positive pts.	52	39	26	61	57	59
ER-negative pts.	52*	20	21	55	37	38

*p<.01.

uated with short follow-up. The Intergroup[82] trial randomized 966 patients to receive either chemotherapy (CMFVP), hormonal therapy (tamoxifen), or a combination of chemohormonal therapy. This trial, unlike others, compares all three fundamental chemotherapeutic-hormonal interventions in this age group. Preliminary results at median follow-up of 4.3 years show no difference in overall survival rates in these treatment groups. Although the median follow-up is relatively short, the study suggests that tamoxifen remains the standard of care in this patient group and that the utility of chemohormonal combinations in the receptor-positive group requires further clinical trial with superior chemotherapy regimens. To this end, NSABP B-16 trial[21] compares tamoxifen alone to Adriamycin-Cytoxan-tamoxifen or L-PAM-5-FU-tamoxifen (with or without Adriamycin). Three-year results conflict with those of the above Intergroup study and suggest that the group receiving Adriamycin-Cytoxan-tamoxifen produces superior disease-free and overall survival rates when compared to the tamoxifen alone group. As data from this trial continue to mature, tamoxifen alone shall remain the preferred treatment in the postmenopausal, ER-positive group.

Comparing chemohormonal therapy to chemotherapy alone and/or no therapy

A relative wealth of clinical data addresses the value of chemohormonal therapy vs. that of chemotherapy alone and/or no therapy. In premenopausal patients, in whom the value of chemotherapy alone is unquestioned, the coadministration of hormonal therapy has yielded disappointing results. NSABP B-09 trial randomized over 1800 node-positive patients to receive either melphalan-5-FU or concurrent melphalan-5-FU-tamoxifen for 2 years. Patients under 50 years of age derived no benefit from the addition of tamoxifen therapy.[23] In the GABG trial discussed above, premenopausal patients determined to be high risk (any ER-negative patient, or one with four or more nodes) were randomized to receive a Cytoxan-Adriamycin combination for 6 months or the same chemotherapy plus tamoxifen concurrently for 2 years (see Table 10-19 and p. 277, top right). The 6-year results in the high-risk premenopausal group show no advantage to the addition of tamoxifen (Table 10-23). Other studies comparing chemotherapy with chemohormonal therapy,[49] or chemotherapy with chemotherapy plus oophorectomy[15,83] in premenopausal patients, have shown no significant improvements in survival rates, although trends have been observed.

Several mature trials have compared chemohormonal therapy to chemotherapy (or no therapy) in postmenopausal patients. The aforementioned NSABP B-09 trial compared melphalan-5-FU to melphalan-5-FU-concurrent tamoxifen in all node-positive patients. An improvement in disease-free and overall survival was seen in patients >50 years of age with more than four involved nodes in the combination therapy group. Improvement in disease-free survival rates was also dependent on estrogen and progesterone receptor content, with the advantage confined to those patients with positive receptors. These results contrast with those of the Eastern Cooperative Oncology Group,[87] whose trial randomized postmenopausal patients to receive no therapy, 1 year of chemotherapy with CMF plus prednisone (CMFP), or chemohormonal therapy with CMFP plus 1 year of tamoxifen (CMFPT). This study evaluated a total of 265 patients. Results at 5 years are summarized in Table 10-24. A disease-free survival benefit was noted in the *ER-negative* group only, with no improvement in overall survival in any group. A trend in favor of disease-free survival for the whole group was seen for CMFPT compared to CMFP or control, but this did not reach statistical significance.

In a similar three-arm trial conducted by the North Central Treatment Group (randomizing postmenopausal patients to receive CFP, CFP plus approximately 1 year of concurrent tamoxifen, or no therapy),[50] a disease-free survival benefit was seen for both the chemotherapy *and* chemohormonal groups relative to control, with no substantial difference noted between chemotherapy and chemohormonal therapy arms, even in hormone receptor

Table 10-23 Six-year relapse and survival results for high-risk patients in GABG trial 1[52]

	Premenopausal pts. (n = 212)		Postmenopausal pts. (n = 259)	
Outcome	Cytoxan and Adriamycin	Cytoxan, Adriamycin, and tamoxifen	Cytoxan and Adriamycin	Cytoxan, Adriamycin, and tamoxifen
Relapsed (%)	56.9	51.1	73.6	52.2*
Dead (%)	30.2	31.3	38.8	29.0

*$p<.01$.

Table 10-24 Five-year relapse-free and survival results in the randomized trial of chemohormonal therapy, chemotherapy, and observation in postmenopausal patients as shown by the Eastern Cooperative Oncology Group[87]

	Disease-free survival (%)			Overall survival (%)		
	Pts. given CMFPT	Pts. given CMFP	Observation group	Pts. given CMFPT	Pts. given CMFP	Observation group
All pts.	44	37	37	67	60	60
ER-positive pts.	43	39	50	72	66	76
ER-negative pts.	45*	34	15	57	51	58

*p = .002.

positive patients. In the GABG trial of Cytoxan-Adriamycin vs. Cytoxan-Adriamycin-tamoxifen in high-risk postmenopausal patients (see Tables 10-19 and 10-23 and p. 277, top right), the investigators observed a disease-free survival benefit and a beneficial trend in overall survival for the chemohormonal therapy group relative to the group treated with chemotherapy alone.

Both a superficial and an in-depth review of these trials is frustrating for the practicing physician in light of the occasionally conflicting results, the variability in the choices of chemotherapy, and the limited statistical power of the trials themselves. However, several conclusions can be drawn. First, *most* trials comparing chemohormonal therapy to chemotherapy alone have suggested improvements in disease-free survival only for the combined modality groups, but they have not shown improvements in overall survival. Unfortunately, it is not possible to define a subgroup of patients that is most likely to benefit from a combined modality effort. Second, these trials do not support the use of chemohormonal therapy in premenopausal patients.[71] Finally, virtually all of these clinical studies used cytotoxic therapy and hormone therapy concurrently; the preclinical data noted above do not support this mode of treatment, but rather suggest that these therapies are best applied sequentially, rather than concurrently, and that longer durations of tamoxifen therapy may be indicated.

To this end, the Eastern Cooperative Oncology Group conducted a large clinical trial comparing CMFPT for 4 months, CMFPT for 12 months, and CMFPT for 12 months followed by continuous tamoxifen for 5 years or more.[16] This recent study stands as the first published trial in which duration of tamoxifen therapy was examined and was restricted to postmenopausal patients. At 4 years of median follow-up, the Group noted an improvement in disease-free survival in the long-term tamoxifen group (Table 10-25). Patients received this hormone therapy both concurrently and sequentially in this group, and it may be agreed that the therapeutic benefit was entirely caused by tamoxifen. Nonetheless, this study illustrates the potential of tamoxifen applied as a long-term adjunct to chemotherapy in the postmenopausal patient. The true role of combined modality therapy remains an outstanding research question.

Table 10-25 Relapse-free survival results in a randomized trial comparing CMFPT for 4 months or 12 months, or 12 months followed by long-term tamoxifen[16]

Treatment	Disease-free survival at 4-yr median follow-up (%)
CMFPT for 4 months	52
CMFPT for 12 months	51
CMFPT for 12 months plus tamoxifen for 5 years or more	61

INTEGRATING PRIMARY BREAST RADIOTHERAPY AND ADJUVANT CHEMOTHERAPY

The primary management of breast carcinoma has evolved dramatically over the last 20 years. Breast conservation by lumpectomy and primary breast radiotherapy now is accepted widely as therapeutically equivalent and cosmetically superior to other techniques in the local management of breast cancer.[13,22,94] The application of adjuvant chemotherapy in most studies has been restricted, however, to patients receiving the more traditional mastectomy as primary management. Given the appropriateness of adjuvant chemotherapy for all node-positive premenopausal patients and many node-negative patients and the emerging use of chemotherapy in the node-positive postmenopausal group, development of programs combining the two modalities is essential.

The delivery of maximal chemotherapy dosing

appears to be critical to the effectiveness of adjuvant therapy.[4,46] The most important questions pertaining to combining modalities, then, appear to be:

1. Does primary breast radiotherapy compromise the ability to deliver adequate adjuvant chemotherapy?
2. What is the proper sequence of administration of these modalities?
3. Will breast cosmesis with radiotherapy be compromised by the concurrent administration of chemotherapy?

Several early, retrospective studies suggested that chemotherapy dosing would indeed be compromised by the combined administration of radiotherapy.[11,56] Since that time several centers have examined these issues with greater scrutiny.

In a prospective, randomized trial conducted at the National Cancer Institute, patients with small (<5 cm) breast cancers were randomized to receive either modified radical mastectomy or excisional biopsy/axillary dissection followed by primary breast radiotherapy.[59] Node-positive patients were assigned to receive adjuvant chemotherapy using a regimen of Cytoxan and Adriamycin for nine cycles. Patients undergoing primary breast radiotherapy first received two cycles of adjuvant chemotherapy, then received breast radiotherapy during the third cycle, with Adriamycin omitted only during this cycle. Scheduling of chemotherapy and dose modifications was identical for both mastectomy and radiation-treated patients. All patients were treated until equivalent bone marrow toxicity (granulocytopenia) was attained, with doses escalated until the nadir WBC was 2500 to 3000/mm^3 or total granulocyte count was no less than 1200/mm^3. In general total WBC, granulocyte, and platelet counts were lower in the radiation-treated group. This effect, however, did not prohibit the administration of intended drug doses, as 85% of irradiated patients received 85% or more of intended doses, compared to 90% of mastectomy patients. Further, patients who ultimately relapsed did *not* have significantly less chemotherapy dosing than patients who remained disease-free. These investigators concluded that radiotherapy did not prohibit the effective delivery of chemotherapy.

Investigators at the Joint Center for Radiation Therapy compared, in a nonrandomized fashion, the clinical outcomes for patients treated with either concurrent chemotherapy and primary breast radiation therapy or sequential radiation followed by chemotherapy.[35] In this analysis, 41 patients received primary breast radiotherapy while receiving a minimum of six cycles of standard CMF chemotherapy. Chemotherapy was not interrupted for delivery of radiation therapy in this concurrent group. The sequential group consisted of 41 patients receiving primary breast radiotherapy alone, followed by a minimum of six cycles of CMF chemotherapy after radiation therapy was complete. A summary of features and outcomes in this study is shown in Table 10-26. In this relatively small series of patients, the time to initiation of chemotherapy was considerably greater in the sequential group (median 97 vs. 15 days), as would be expected, because these patients awaited the completion of radiation therapy before the initiation of chemotherapy. This delay did not seem to compromise overall outcome (survival and freedom from distant relapse) in this relatively short period of follow-up. The total delivered dose of chemotherapy was not compromised by the concurrent administration of radiation therapy. Most striking, however, is the reduction in the number of patients enjoying an "excellent" clinical cosmetic response in the group receiving concurrent therapy. Such an adverse effect on cosmesis has been reported by others.[2,79]

Table 10-26 Comparison of groups receiving concurrent or sequential chemotherapy and radiation therapy in patients with stage II breast cancer[35]

Criteria	Concurrent group (n = 41)	Sequential group (n = 41)
Median time from axillary dissection to initiation of chemotherapy in weeks	15 (3-77)	97 (40-150)
Patients receiving ≥85% of prescribed chemotherapy dose	82%	72%
Actuarial overall survival at 5 years	85%	86%
Actuarial freedom from relapse at 5 years	80%	80%
Cosmetic outcome		
Excellent	12%	52%*
Good	58%	38%
Fair	19%	10%
Poor	11%	0%

*p = .004.

The reason for this compromise in cosmesis is unclear. Conceivably, the concurrent use of radiosensitizing drugs such as methotrexate or Adriamycin could enhance radiotherapeutic skin toxicity and thus jeopardize preservation of breast architecture. At the University of Pennsylvania, a clinical paradigm for combined modality therapy has been created that allows for the concurrent administration of chemotherapy and radiotherapy, circumventing the risk of chemotherapy-related skin toxicity and avoiding delays in the institution of chemotherapy while completing the radiotherapy. Representing the standard of management for node-positive patients undergoing lumpectomy and axillary dissection at the University of Pennsylvania since 1978, patients received primary breast radiotherapy while receiving two concurrent cycles of Cytoxan and 5-fluorouracil. Following completion of radiotherapy, a standard 6-month course of CMF or CMFP is administered.[13,29] The ability to administer appreciable doses of chemotherapy has been well documented,[29] wherein patients received an average of 95% of the optimal chemotherapy dose during the initial two cycles of CF, while receiving an average of 89% of optimum dose of CMFP in the 6 months that followed.

Two points deserve emphasis. First, the radiotherapeutic technique employed at the University of Pennsylvania avoids the use of a direct or angled beam to treat the internal mammary nodes, thus avoiding appreciable exposure to the thoracic spine and marrow. Second, the known lympholytic effects of radiation therapy alter the manner by which dose modifications are made. Radiotherapy-induced lymphopenia may produce an overall suppression of white blood cell count while leaving granulocytes relatively intact. Dose modifications of chemotherapy should therefore be based on the total granulocyte count rather than the total white blood cell count, thus avoiding unnecessary drug dosage reductions.

At the University of Pennsylvania, a total of 285 node-positive patients have been treated with lumpectomy and primary radiotherapy. One hundred and ninety-eight node-positive patients have received CMF chemotherapy (with or without prednisone or tamoxifen). Of patients receiving chemotherapy 88% (n = 176) received it by the conventional concurrent method, methotrexate being omitted during breast radiotherapy. The remaining patients (n = 22) received chemotherapy only after radiation therapy was completed.

Table 10-27 outlines survival data in the entire radiotherapy group, illustrating comparable survival rates at 5 years in the CMF-treated patients regardless of the method of chemotherapy/radiotherapy sequencing used. This data is not conclusive in a nonrandomized setting with unbalanced sample sizes, but it implies that survival is by no means jeopardized by the concurrent administration of radiation therapy and Cytoxan/5-FU.

Cosmetic results in the chemotherapy-treated groups are shown in Table 10-28. The concurrent use of CF chemotherapy with primary breast radiotherapy permits nearly 90% of patients to achieve and maintain "good to excellent" cosmesis at 5 years of follow-up. This result was comparable to patients receiving radiotherapy alone (data not shown) or to patients who subsequently received adjuvant CMF. Patients receiving concurrent therapy do not appear to be at an increased risk of a "poor" cosmetic result; in fact, the number of "poor" outcomes was greater at 5 years in the group receiving sequential therapy.

These data demonstrate the acceptable therapeutic and cosmetic outcomes with the concurrent use

Table 10-27 Primary breast radiotherapy in node-positive breast cancer: 5-year survival data at the University of Pennsylvania

Patient group	n	Relapse-free survival (%)	Overall survival (%)
Entire group	285	69	86
Nodal status			
1-3 nodes	214	75*	88
≥4 nodes	71	51*	81
Receptor status			
ER−	63	65	74*
ER+	153	72	91*
CMF chemotherapy			
Concurrently	176	70	89
Sequentially	22	79	95

*p = .002.

Table 10-28 Cosmetic results at 3 years and 5 years in patients treated with primary breast radiotherapy and concurrent or sequential chemotherapy at the University of Pennsylvania

	Concurrent group (%) (n = 176)		Sequential group (%) (n = 22)	
Result	3 yr	5 yr	3 yr	5 yr
Good/excellent	88	88	80	86
Fair	9	10	20	0
Poor	3	2	0	14

of systemic adjuvant chemotherapy with primary breast radiotherapy, with the omission of methotrexate during the radiotherapeutic course. It is unlikely that large-scale, randomized trials will be undertaken to address the optimum sequencing of both modalities. However, as the optimum timing of chemotherapy initiation has not been determined, the use of concurrent therapy will remain the standard approach at the University of Pennsylvania. This approach will not delay the timing of initiation of chemotherapy, nor will it compromise chemotherapy dose-intensity or cosmetic outcome.

NEOADJUVANT THERAPY

Virtually all clinical data of value in the field of adjuvant therapy of breast cancer follow the conventional sequence of local therapy (surgery or surgery-radiotherapy) followed by systemic therapy (adjuvant chemotherapy, hormonal therapy, or both). Such sequencing is entirely logical but is in essence empirical, and there is nothing to refute the notion that systemic therapy might be applied first, followed by local treatment.

Such a sequence has been employed in the preoperative management of inflammatory breast cancers and in noninflammatory, locally advanced breast cancers in which surgery is technically impossible or considered unsafe as the first therapeutic step. In these circumstances, initial application of systemic chemotherapy may render the disease operable or, under the best circumstances, clinically undetectable, allowing surgical or radiotherapeutic intervention and ultimately improving disease-free and overall survival. Such preoperative chemotherapy has not been emphasized in breast cancers that are deemed operable at the outset, but it has received increasing attention in some European centers. The advantages to a preoperative approach are both practical and theoretical. Presurgical therapy would allow an excellent in vivo test of drug sensitivity, allowing for manipulation of the drug regimen to maximize clinical response, using the same regimen in the postoperative setting in a true "adjuvant" fashion. Reduction in tumor mass might also render the patient treatable by lesser surgical means; the patient with a relatively large breast mass who is considered an unacceptable candidate for lumpectomy may be rendered acceptable by reduction of mass size. In the extreme, the need for local therapy might be obviated by eradication of all clinical evidence of malignancy, although this would represent a relatively uncommon and theoretically unsafe event. The potential disadvantages of a neoadjuvant approach are equally compelling. If the diagnosis of cancer is rendered by a minimally invasive technique, such as fine needle aspiration, then critical hormone receptor information would remain inaccessible, obligating all patients to receive systemic chemotherapy regardless of receptor status. If the diagnosis is rendered by incisional (or excisional) biopsy or by needle aspiration, no knowledge of the patient's nodal status will be obtained, and patients will receive systemic therapy even if node negative. The expanding use of tamoxifen and systemic chemotherapy in the node-negative population possibly makes this liability of neoadjuvant therapy decreasingly relevant.

Data in operable patients receiving neoadjuvant therapy is sparse, and there are no published, randomized trials to compare classical adjuvant therapy to neoadjuvant therapy in operable patients; however, two French trials deserve mention.

First, in a study of 252 patients, 130 of whom would be considered operable (stage I or stage II) by conventional criteria, patients received chemotherapy first, followed by external beam and iridium implant radiotherapy and maintenance chemotherapy (with or without tamoxifen) in a schedule that was escalated in intensity according to increasing clinical stage.[51] Patients were diagnosed exclusively by fine needle aspiration or drill biopsy. No surgery was performed in any of these patients. Chemotherapy consisted of thiotepa, vincristine, methotrexate, and 5-fluorouracil for the patients with the equivalent of stage I and stage II disease. Substantial tumor regression (over 75%) occurred in 63% of all cases. At 4 years median follow-up, the disease-free survival rate for "operable" patients (equivalent of clinical stage I or stage II) was 76%, with a local recurrence rate of only 4%.

In a second trial[85] restricted exclusively to operable patients with breast tumors of >3 cm, 119 women received preoperative chemotherapy (Adriamycin, vincristine, Cytoxan, methotrexate, 5-fluorouracil) for 3 months, followed by clinical reassessment and surgery. Patients whose tumors were reduced <3 cm in size underwent conservative surgery (lumpectomy); all others underwent mastectomy. Postoperative chemotherapy with 5-FU, Cytoxan, and Adriamycin was given for three courses along with primary breast radiotherapy for lumpectomy patients. The study reported an overall response rate to chemotherapy of 70%, with 11 patients enjoying a complete clinical response. Follow-up is extremely short in this trial, but the natural history of these patients who successfully underwent lumpectomy as a result of neoadjuvant cytoreduction will be most compelling.

CONCLUSIONS

In 1985 the National Institutes of Health convened the Consensus Development Conference on the Ad-

Table 10-29 Recommendations of the NIH Consensus Conference on the Adjuvant Therapy, 1985, for node-positive patients treated outside the context of a clinical trial

Pt. group	Treatment
Premenopausal	Combination chemotherapy
Postmenopausal, hormone receptor positive	Tamoxifen
Postmenopausal, hormone receptor negative	Combination chemotherapy should be considered but cannot be recommended as standard practice

juvant Chemotherapy and Endocrine Therapy for Breast Cancer. The conclusions of this panel with respect to the node-positive patient may be summarized as in Table 10-29. The Panel emphasized that (1) these conclusions were recommended outside of the context of a clinical trial, (2) optimum therapy had not been defined for any patient subgroup, and (3) participation in controlled clinical trials was recommended to all physicians.[58,72]

Five years later these conclusions may be both reinforced and modified. The lack of an *optimum* therapeutic regimen for any subgroup remains, as does the need for large-scale randomized trials to answer the remaining, critical therapeutic questions. In the absence of a clinical trial, however, the following recommendations are made based upon the patient's menopausal and hormone receptor status.

Premenopausal patients

Adjuvant cytotoxic chemotherapy remains the standard of care for premenopausal, node-positive patients regardless of hormone receptor status. The foregoing data suggest that this therapy should be applied for a period of approximately 6 months, and that maximum benefit will be derived with maintenance of maximum dose-intensity. The optimum regimen has not been defined. CMF remains the standard adjuvant regimen and, based on available data, should be recommended in the absence of a clinical trial. However, the use of Adriamycin-containing regimens may prove superior based on early data from some randomized trials.

Adjuvant tamoxifen therapy alone cannot be recommended for any subgroup of premenopausal, node-positive patients at this time. Further, clinical data presented herein do not support the use of concurrent combinations of chemotherapy and hormonal therapy in this patient group. The crucial clinical trials in premenopausal, node-positive patients will be those that define the optimum chemotherapeutic regimen, those that compare chemotherapy with chemotherapy followed by hormonal therapy (either tamoxifen or oophorectomy), and those that address the use of oophorectomy alone vs. chemotherapy, particularly in hormone-receptor positive patients. Effective therapies need to be defined for the very high-risk groups (>10 nodes) in whom conventional chemotherapies appear to be of little value. The use of autologous marrow transplantation is under investigation in some centers and will become part of randomized trials comparing conventional chemotherapy to transplantation in the next several years.

Postmenopausal, hormone receptor–positive patients

Based on the results of many, large-scale clinical trials and on the recent overview analysis,[14] tamoxifen therapy remains the standard approach in this patient group. Adjuvant tamoxifen improves relapse-free survival in virtually all trials, and overall survival in some. The optimum duration of therapy remains undefined, with 5 years of therapy representing the longest duration of treatment in any large randomized trial. Some authorities recommend longer, and perhaps indefinite, therapy with tamoxifen.[29] The role of chemotherapy alone in this group of patients appears to be marginal and cannot be recommended in lieu of tamoxifen therapy based on the results of GABG Trial I (see Table 10-20 and p. 277, top right). This statement does not presume that chemotherapy is of no value in this age group, and the maturity of NSABP B-16 trial may serve to alter the standard of care to chemohormonal therapy in this group. The Ludwig III Trial (see Table 10-22) demonstrates a significant improvement in disease-free survival rates for the postmenopausal patients treated with chemohormonal therapy vs. those treated with hormonal therapy, or no therapy, but this significance is lost when hormone receptor–positive patients are considered separately. Many trials have demonstrated the superiority of combined chemohormonal therapy vs. no therapy. Trials that define the optimum duration of tamoxifen therapy and trials that examine the difference between hormonal therapy alone vs. combined (or sequential) chemohormonal therapy are of the greatest importance in this patient group.

Postmenopausal, hormone receptor–negative patients

Therapeutic recommendations remain the most difficult in this group of patients. Popular prejudice assumes that tamoxifen therapy alone should have no effect on the hormone receptor–negative patient, although several large adjuvant trials[74,80] do demonstrate prolongation of disease-free and overall survival. This remains a point of controversy, as results lack consistency across all trials comparing tamoxifen therapy to no therapy in hormone receptor–negative patients. Given this uncertainty, the value of combining chemotherapy and hormonal therapy remains the outstanding issue in treating these patients.[70] Again, data from the Ludwig III trial suggest a benefit of combination therapy relative to hormones alone that is most pronounced in the receptor negative–patients. Maturity of data from ongoing clinical trials, as well as trials employing sequential chemohormonal therapy, will resolve the issue of "standard" therapy in the hormone receptor–negative patient.

Many issues remain to be resolved in the evolving clinical science of the adjuvant therapy of node-positive breast cancer. The optimum chemotherapeutic regimen, the optimum juxtaposition of chemotherapy and radiotherapy, and the optimum combination of chemotherapy and hormonal therapy pose continuing challenges to clinical investigators. As these issues approach resolution, the continued use of adjuvant therapies will cure thousands of patients per year, while providing additional thousands of patient-years of freedom from metastatic disease to others.

REFERENCES

1. Aisner J, Weinberg V, Perloff M, et al: Chemotherapy versus chemoimmunotherapy (CAF vs. CAFVP vs. CMF each plus/minus MER) for metastatic carcinoma of the breast. A CALGB study, J Clin Oncol 5:1523, 1987.
2. Beadle GF, Come SE, Henderson IC, et al: The effect of adjuvant chemotherapy on the cosmetic results after primary radiation treatment for early stage breast cancer: a preliminary analysis, Int J Radiat Oncol Biol Phys 10:2131, 1984.
3. Bonadonna G: Karnofsky memorial lecture: conceptual and practical advances in the management of breast cancer, J Clin Oncol 7:1380, 1989.
4. Bonadonna G and Valagussa P: Dose-response effect of adjuvant chemotherapy in breast cancer, N Engl J Med 304:10, 1981.
5. Bonadonna G, Valagussa P, Rossi A, et al: Ten-year experience with CMF-based adjuvant chemotherapy in resectable breast cancer, Breast Cancer Res Treat 5:95, 1985.
6. Bonadonna G, Valagussa P, Zambetti M, et al: The Milan experience with adjuvant chemotherapy in premenopausal women. In Senn HJ, Goldhirsch A, Gelber RD, et al, editors: Recent results in cancer research. Adjuvant therapy of primary breast cancer, Berlin Heidelberg, 1989, Springer-Verlag Berlin Heidelberg, pp 106-112.
7. Brunner KW: Adjuvant therapies in breast cancer and quality of life: a critical review of the TWiST concept. In Senn HJ, Goldhirsch A, Gelber RD, et al, editors: Recent results in cancer research. Adjuvant therapy of primary breast cancer, Berlin Heidelberg, 1989, Springer-Verlag Berlin Heidelberg, pp 239-243.
8. Bryant AJ and Weir JA: Prophylactic oophorectomy in operable instances of carcinoma of the breast, Surg Gynecol Obstet 153:660, 1981.
9. Buzdar AV, Smith TL, Powell KD, et al: Effect of timing of initiation of adjuvant chemotherapy in disease-free survival in breast cancer, Breast Cancer Res Treat 2:163, 1982.
10. Clark GM and McQuire WL: Progesterone receptors and human breast cancer, Breast Cancer Res Treat 3:157, 1983.
11. Cooper MR, Rhyne AL, Muss HB, et al: A randomized comparative trial of chemotherapy and irradiation therapy for stage II breast cancer, Cancer 47:2833, 1981.
12. Cummings FJ, Gray R, Davis TE, et al: Adjuvant tamoxifen treatment of elderly women with Stage II breast cancer: a double-blind comparison with placebo, Ann Intern Med 103:324, 1985.
13. Danoff B, Haller DG, Glick JH, et al: Conservative surgery and irradiation in the treatment of early breast cancer, Ann Intern Med 102:634, 1985.
14. Early Breast Cancer Trialists' Collaborative Group: Effects of adjuvant tamoxifen and of cytotoxic therapy on mortality in early breast cancer, N Engl J Med 319:1681, 1988.
15. Everson LK, Ingle JN, Wieand HS, et al: Randomized trial of adjuvant therapy with cyclophosphamide (C), 5-fluorouracil (F), prednisone (P) with or without tamoxifen (T) following mastectomy in premenopausal women with node-positive breast cancer, Proc Am Soc Clin Oncol 5:63, 1986.
16. Falkson HE, Gray RG, Wolberg WH, et al: Adjuvant trial of 12 cycles of CMFPT followed by observation or continuous tamoxifen versus 4 cycles of CMFPT in postmenopausal women with breast cancer: an Eastern Cooperative Oncology Group Phase III study, J Clin Oncol 8:599, 1990.
17. Fisher B: Adjuvant chemotherapy in breast cancer, Int J Radiat Oncol Biol Phys 4:295, 1978.
18. Fisher B, Fisher ER, and Redmond C: Ten-year results from the NSABP clinical trial evaluating the use of L-phenylalanine mustard (L-PAM) in the management of primary breast cancer, J Clin Oncol 4:929, 1986.
19. Fisher B, Redmond CK, and Wolmark N: Long term results from NSABP trials of adjuvant therapy for breast cancer. In Salmon SE, editor: Adjuvant therapy of cancer V, Orlando, 1987, Grune & Stratton, pp 283-295.
20. Fisher B, Slack N, and Katrych D: Ten year follow-up results of patients with carcinoma of the breast in a co-operative clinical trial evaluating surgical adjuvant chemotherapy, Surg Gynecol Obstet 140:528, 1975.
21. Fisher B, Redmond C, Brown A, et al: Adjuvant chemotherapy with and without tamoxifen in the treatment of primary breast cancer: 5-year results from the National Surgical Adjuvant Breast and Bowel Project Trial, J Clin Oncol 4:459, 1986.
22. Fisher B, Redmond C, Poisson R, et al: Eight-year results of a randomized clinical trial comparing total mastectomy and lumpectomy with or without irradiation in the treatment of breast cancer, N Engl J Med 320:822, 1989.
23. Fisher B, Redmond C, Poisson S, et al: Increased benefit from addition of adriamycin and cyclophosphamide (AC) to tamoxifen (TAM,T) for node-positive TAM-responsive postmenopausal breast cancer patients: results from NSABP B-16, Proc Am Soc Clin Oncol 9:20, 1990.
24. Fisher B, Rockette H, Fisher ER, et al: Leukemia in breast cancer patients following adjuvant chemotherapy or post-operative radiation: the NSABP experience, J Clin Oncol 3:1640, 1985.
25. Fornander T, Rutqvist LE, and Sjoberg HE: Long-term adjuvant tamoxifen in early breast cancer: risk of accelerated bone loss? Proc Am Soc Clin Oncol 8:21, 1989.
26. Gelber RD and Goldhirsch A for the Ludwig Breast Cancer Study Group: A new endpoint for the assessment of adjuvant therapy in postmenopausal women with operable breast cancer, J Clin Oncol 4:1772, 1986.

27. Gelber RD, Goldhirsch A, Castiglione M, et al: Time without symptoms and toxicity (TWiST): a quality-of-life-oriented endpoint to evaluate adjuvant therapy. In Salmon SE, editor: Adjuvant therapy of cancer V, Orlando, 1987, Grune & Stratton, pp 455-465.
28. Glick JH: Closing summary and outlook. In Senn HJ, Goldhirsch A, Gelber RD, et al, editors: Recent results in cancer research. Adjuvant therapy of primary breast cancer, Berlin Heidelberg, 1989, Springer-Verlag Heidelberg Berlin, pp 283-292.
29. Glick JH, Fowble BL, Haller DG, et al: Integration of full-dose adjuvant chemotherapy with definitive radiotherapy for primary breast cancer: four-year update, NCI Monogr 6:297, 1988.
30. Glucksberg H, Rivkin SE, Rasmussen S, et al: Combination chemotherapy (CMFVP) versus, L-phenylalanine mustard (L-PAM) for operable breast cancer with positive axillary nodes. A Southwest Oncology Group study, Cancer 50:423, 1982.
31. Goldenberg GJ: The effect of diethylstilbestrol (DES) and tamoxifen (T) on the cytocidal activity and uptake of melphalan (M) in human breast cancer cells *in vitro*, Proc Am Soc Clin Oncol 2:22, 1983.
32. Goldhirsch A and Gelber R: Adjuvant chemo-endocrine therapy or endocrine therapy alone for postmenopausal patients: Ludwig studies III and IV. In Senn HJ, Goldhirsch A, Gelber RD, et al, editors: Recent results in cancer research. Adjuvant therapy of primary breast cancer, Berlin Heidelberg, 1989, Springer-Verlag Berlin Heidelberg, pp 153-162.
33. Goldhirsch A and Gelber R: Adjuvant treatment for early breast cancer: the Ludwig Breast Cancer studies, NCI Monogr 1:55, 1986.
34. Goldhirsch A, Gelber RD, Simes JR, et al for the Ludwig Breast Cancer Study Group: Costs and benefits of adjuvant therapy in breast cancer: a quality-adjusted survival analysis, J Clin Oncol 7:36, 1989.
35. Gore SM, Come SE, Griem K, et al: Influence of the sequencing of chemotherapy and radiation therapy in node-negative breast cancer patients treated by conservative surgery and radiation therapy. In Salmon SE, editor: Adjuvant therapy of cancer V, Orlando, 1987, Grune & Stratton, pp 365-373.
36. Gotsfreden A, Christiansen C, and Palshof T: The effect of tamoxifen on bone mineral content in women with breast cancer, Cancer 53:853, 1984.
37. Haagensen CD: Treatment of curable carcinoma of the breast, Int J Radiat Oncol Biol Phys 2:975, 1977.
38. Henderson IC: Adjuvant systemic therapy for early breast cancer. Curr Probl Cancer 11:127, 1987.
39. Henderson IC: Adjuvant chemotherapy and endocrine therapy in patients with operable breast cancer, PPD Updates 1(3):1, 1987.
40. Henderson IC: Endocrine therapy in metastatic breast cancer. In Harris JR, Hellman S, Henderson IC, and Kinne DW, editors: Breast diseases, Philadelphia, 1987, JB Lippincott, pp 398-428.
41. Henderson IC, Hayes D, and Gelman R: Dose-response in the treatment of breast cancer: a critical review, J Clin Oncol 6:1501, 1988.
42. Henderson IC, Gelman RS, Harris JR, et al: Duration of therapy in adjuvant chemotherapy trials, NCI Monogr 1:95, 1986.
43. Heuser L, Spratt JS, and Polk HC: Growth rates of primary breast cancers, Cancer 43:1888, 1979.
44. Himel MN, Liberati A, Gelber RD, et al: Adjuvant chemotherapy for breast cancer: a pooled estimate based on published randomized control trials, JAMA 256:1148, 1986.
45. Holdener EE, Nissen-Meyer R, Bonadonna G, et al: Remaining problems of adjuvant chemotherapy in breast cancer. In Senn HJ, editor: Recent results in cancer research. Adjuvant chemotherapy of breast cancer, New York, 1984, Springer-Verlag, pp 188-196.
46. Hubay CA, Pearson OH, Gordon NH, et al: Randomized trial of endocrine versus endocrine plus cytotoxic chemotherapy in women with Stage II, estrogen-receptor positive breast cancer, Proc; Am Soc Clin Oncol 5:63, 1986.
47. Hug V, Hortobagyi GN, Drewinko R, et al: Tamoxifen-citrate counteracts the antitumor effects of cytotoxic drugs *in vitro*, J Clin Oncol 3:1672, 1985.
48. Hyriniuk W and Levine M: Analysis of dose intensity for adjuvant chemotherapy trials in Stage II breast cancer, J Clin Oncol 4:1162, 1986.
49. Ingle J, Everson LK, Wieand HS, et al: Randomized trial to evaluate the addition of tamoxifen to cyclophosphamide, 5-fluorouracil, prednisone adjuvant therapy in premenopausal women with node-positive breast cancer, Cancer 63:1257, 1989.
50. Ingle JN, Everson LK, Wieand HS, et al: Randomized trial of observation versus adjuvant therapy with cyclophosphamide, fluorouracil, prednisone with or without tamoxifen following mastectomy in postmenopausal women with node-positive breast cancer, J Clin Oncol 6:1388, 1988.
51. Jacquillat C, Weil M, Auclerc G, et al: Neoadjuvant chemotherapy in the conservative management of breast cancer: a study of 252 patients. In Senn HJ, Goldhirsch A, Gelber RD, et al, editors: Recent results in cancer research: adjuvant therapy of primary breast cancer, Berlin Heidelberg, 1989, Springer-Verlag Berlin Heidelberg, pp 36-42.
52. Jonat W, Kaufmann M, and Abel U: Chemo- or endocrine adjuvant therapy alone or combined in postmenopausal patients (GABG Trial I). In Senn HJ, Goldhirsch A, Gelber RD, et al, editors: Recent results in cancer research: adjuvant therapy of primary breast cancer, Berlin Heidelberg, 1989, Springer-Verlag Heidelberg Berlin, pp 163-169.
53. Jordan VC, Mirecki DM, and Gottardis MM: Continuous tamoxifen treatment prevents the appearance of mammary tumors in a model of adjuvant therapy. In Jones SE and Salmon SE, editors: Adjuvant therapy of cancer IV, Orlando, 1984, Grune & Stratton, pp 27-33.
54. Kaufman M, Jonat W, and Abel U: Adjuvant chemo- and endocrine therapy alone or in combination in premenopausal women (GABG Trial I). In Senn HJ, Goldhirsch A, Gelber RD, et al, editors: Recent results in cancer research: adjuvant therapy of primary breast cancer, Berlin Heidelberg, 1989, Springer-Verlag Heidelberg Berlin, pp 118-125.
55. Killacky MA, Hakes TB, and Pierce VK: Endometrial adenocarcinoma in breast cancer patients receiving antiestrogens, Cancer Treat Rep 69:237, 1985.
56. Levine JF, Coleman CN, Cot RS, et al: The effect of postoperative and primary radiation therapy on delivered dose of adjuvant cyclophosphamide, methotrexate, and 5-fluorouracil (CMF) chemotherapy in breast cancer, Cancer 53:237, 1984.
57. Levine MN, Gent M, Hirsch J, et al: The thrombogenic effect of anticancer drug therapy in women with Stage II breast cancer, N Engl J Med 318:404, 1988.
58. Lippman ME and Chabner BA: Editorial overview, NCI Monogr 1:5, 1986.
59. Lippman ME, Edwards BK, Findlay P, et al: Influence of definitive radiation therapy for primary breast cancer on ability to deliver adjuvant chemotherapy, NCI Monogr 1:99, 1986.
60. Lipton A, Harvey HA, and Hamilton RW: Venous thrombosis as a side-effect of tamoxifen treatment, Cancer Treat Rep 68:887, 1984.
61. Love RR, Mazess RB, Tormey DC, et al: Bone mineral density in women with breast cancer treated with adjuvant

tamoxifen for at least two years, Breast Cancer Res Treat 12:297, 1988.

62. The Ludwig Breast Cancer Study Group: Combination adjuvant chemotherapy for node-positive breast cancer: inadequacy of a single perioperative cycle, N Engl J Med 319:677, 1988.
63. Lundgren B: Observations on growth rate of breast carcinomas and its possible implications for lead time, Cancer 40:1722, 1977.
64. Malaise EP, Chauandra N, and Tublana M: The relationship between growth rate, labelling index, and histological type of human solid tumors, Eur J Cancer 9:305, 1973.
65. Mathe G, Plagne R, Morice V, et al: Consistencies and variations during serial analyses of a trial of adjuvant chemotherapy in breast cancer. In Salmon SE, editor: Adjuvant chemotherapy for cancer V, Orlando, 1987, Grune & Stratton, pp 271-280.
66. McGuire WL, Horwitz KB, Zava DT, et al: Progress in endocrinology and metabolism: hormones in breast cancer, Metabolism 27:487, 1978.
67. Meaken JW, Allt WEC, Beale FA, et al: Ovarian irradiation and prednisone following surgery and radiotherapy for carcinoma of the breast, Breast Cancer Res Treat 3(suppl):45, 1983.
68. Meyerowitz BE, Sparks FC, and Spears IK: Adjuvant chemotherapy for breast carcinoma: psychosocial implications, Cancer 43:1614, 1979.
69. Misset JL, DeVassal F, Delgado M, et al: Five-year results of the French adjuvant trial for breast cancer comparing CMF to a combination of adriamycin (ADM), vincristine (VCR), cyclophosphamide (CPM), and 5-fluorouracil. In Jones SE and Salmon SE, editors: Adjuvant therapy of cancer IV, Orlando, 1984, Grune & Stratton, pp 243-251.
70. Mouridsen HT: How to improve adjuvant treatment results in postmenopausal patients. In Senn HJ, Goldhirsch A, Gelber RD, et al, editors: Recent results in cancer research: adjuvant therapy of primary breast cancer, Berlin Heidelberg, 1989, Springer-Verlag Berlin Heidelberg, pp 144-152.
71. Mouridsen HT: Critical review of therapy in premenopausal patients. In Senn HJ, Goldhirsch A, Gelber RD, et al, editors: Recent results in cancer research: adjuvant therapy of primary breast cancer, Berlin Heidelberg, 1989, Springer-Verlag Heidelberg Berlin, pp 132-135.
72. NIH Consensus Conference: Adjuvant therapy for breast cancer, JAMA 254:3461, 1985.
73. Nissen-Meyer R, Kjellgren K, and Mansson B: Adjuvant chemotherapy in breast cancer, Cancer Res 80:142, 1982.
74. The Nolvadex Adjuvant Trial Organization: Controlled trial of tamoxifen as a single adjuvant agent in the management of early breast cancer, Br J Cancer 57:608, 1988.
75. Padmanabhan N, Howell A, and Rubens RD: Mechanism of action of adjuvant chemotherapy in early breast cancer, Lancet ii:411, 1986.
76. Payne WS, Taylor WF, and Khonjari S: Surgical treatment of breast cancer: trends and factors affecting survival, Arch Surg 101:105, 1970.
77. Perloff M, Norton L, Korzun A, et al: Advantage of an adriamycin (A) combination plus halotestin (H) after initial cyclophosphamide, methotrexate, 5-fluorouracil, vincristine, and prednisone (CMFVP) for adjuvant therapy of node-positive Stage II breast cancer, Proc Am Soc Clin Oncol 5:70, 1986.
78. Powles TJ, Hardy JR, Ashley SE, et al: A pilot trial to evaluate the acute toxicity and feasibility of tamoxifen for prevention of breast cancer, Br J Cancer 60:126, 1989.
79. Ray GR, Fish VJ, Lee RH, et al: Impact of adjuvant chemotherapy on cosmesis and complication in Stages I and II carcinoma of the breast treated by biopsy and radiation therapy, Int J Radiat Oncol Biol Phys 10:837, 1984.
80. Report from the Breast Cancer Trials Committee; Scottish Cancer Trials Office (MRC), Edinburgh: Adjuvant tamoxifen in the management of operable breast cancer: the Scottish Trial, Lancet ii:171, 1987.
81. Ribeiro G and Swindell R: The Christie Hospital adjuvant tamoxifen trial—status at 10 years, Br J Cancer 57:601, 1988.
82. Rivkin SE, Green S, Metch B, et al: Adjuvant combination chemotherapy (CMFVP) vs. tamoxifen vs. CMFVP + TAM for postmenopausal women with ER + operable breast cancer and positive axillary lymph nodes, Proc Am Soc Clin Oncol 9:24(87), 1990.
83. Rivkin SE, Knight WA, Cruz A, et al: Adjuvant chemotherapy and hormonal therapy for operable breast cancer with positive axillary nodes, Proc Am Assoc Cancer Res 25:181, 1984.
84. Schottenfeld D, Nash A, Robbins G, et al: Ten-year results of the treatment of primary operable breast carcinoma, Cancer 38:1001, 1976.
85. Spielmann M, Mathieu MC, Le Chevalier T, et al: Preliminary results of preoperative chemotherapy in patients (pts) with non-metastatic operable breast cancer of more than 3 cms, Proc Am Soc Clin Oncol 9:39, 1990.
86. Tancini G, Bonadonna G, Valagussa P, et al: Adjuvant CMF in breast cancer: comparative 5-year results of 12 versus 6 cycles, J Clin Oncol 1:2, 1983.
87. Taylor SG, Knuiman MW, Sleeper LA, et al: Six-year results of the Eastern Cooperative Oncology Group trial of observation versus CMFP versus CMFPT in postmenopausal patients with node-positive breast cancer, J Clin Oncol 7:879, 1989.
88. Tormey DC: Adjuvant therapy for premenopausal women: cytotoxic and endocrine mechanisms. In Senn HJ, Goldhirsch A, Gelber RD, et al, editors: Recent results in cancer research. Adjuvant therapy of primary breast cancer, Berlin Heidelberg, 1989, Springer-Verlag Berlin Heidelberg, pp 113-117.
89. Tormey DC: Clinical results III: experience of randomized trials without surgical controls. In Senn HJ, editor: Recent results in cancer research. Adjuvant chemotherapy of breast cancer, New York, 1984, Springer-Verlag, pp 155-165.
90. Tormey DC, Gray R, Taylor SG, et al: Postoperative chemotherapy and chemohormonal therapy in women with node-positive breast cancer, NCI Monogr 1:75, 1986.
91. Turken S, Siris E, Seldin D, et al: Effects of tamoxifen on spinal bone density in women with breast cancer, J Natl Cancer Inst 81:1086, 1989.
92. Valagussa P, Bonadonna G, and Veronesi U: Patterns of relapse and survival following radical mastectomy, Cancer 41:1170, 1978.
93. Valagussa P, Tancini G, and Bonadonna G: Second malignancies after CMF for resectable breast cancer. J Clin Oncol 5:1138, 1987.
94. Veronesi U, Saccozzi R, DelVecchio M, et al: Comparing radical mastectomy with quadrantectomy, axillary dissection, and radiotherapy in patients with small cancers of the breast, N Engl J Med 305:6, 1981.
95. Wickerham D, Fisher B, Brown A, et al: Two months of Adriamycin-cyclophosphamide with and without interval reinduction therapy vs. 6 months of conventional CMF in node-positive breast cancer patients non-responsive to tamoxifen: results of NSABP B-15, Proc Am Soc Clin Oncol 9:20, 1990.
96. Wolter J, Ryan WG, Subbaiah V, et al: Apparent beneficial effects of tamoxifen on serum lipoprotein subfractions and bone mineral content in patients with breast cancer, Proc Am Soc Clin Oncol 7:10, 1988.
97. Zelen M and Gelman R: Assessment of adjuvant trials in breast cancer, NCI Monogr 1:11, 1986.

11 The Role of Postmastectomy Adjuvant Radiotherapy for Operable Breast Cancer

Barbara Fowble

The rationale for postmastectomy adjuvant radiotherapy is the prevention of the local-regional recurrence of breast cancer. Theoretically, clinically occult persistent disease in the operative site or regional nodes could act as a source of distant metastases, and eradication of this disease may result in an enhanced disease-free and overall survival. The prevention of local-regional recurrence with adjuvant radiotherapy appears preferable to delaying treatment until the time of recurrence. At the time of recurrence, 30% to 40% of these patients will have associated distant metastases. Local-regional control is achieved in 50% to 60% of patients at best, and 5-year survival rates following recurrence range from 30% to 50%.[1,11,59,73] The morbidity of uncontrolled local-regional disease can be significant.

Some of the earliest prospective randomized trials evaluated the role of postmastectomy irradiation. These trials can be grouped into those that compared radical mastectomy to radical mastectomy and postoperative radiation, and those that compared simple mastectomy to simple mastectomy and postoperative radiation. Trials that compared lesser surgical procedures such as simple mastectomy with radiation to radical mastectomy are addressed in Chapter 3. Because these trials employed different surgical procedures as the primary treatment, their sole purpose was not to evaluate postoperative radiotherapy. Therefore they will not be considered in this section.

RANDOMIZED TRIALS EVALUATING POSTMASTECTOMY RADIATION

Radical or modified radical mastectomy with or without postoperative radiotherapy

Four prospective randomized trials have evaluated the addition of radiation to radical or modified mastectomy: the Manchester trial (I and II),[32,85] the National Surgical Adjuvant Breast Project (NSABP) B-02 trial,[41] the Stockholm trial,[93,103] and the Oslo trial (I and II).[55] The results of these trials are presented in Table 11-1. For the NSABP B-02 trial, comparisons are to the control patients who did not receive thiotepa. The trials were conducted over a wide range of time periods, from the late 1940s to the 1970s. Patient selection in the trials also varied. The NSABP B-02 and Stockholm trials included patients with operable stage III breast cancer, whereas the Manchester and Oslo trials included only stage I and stage II patients. Similarly, in the Manchester and NSABP B-02 trials, approximately 40% of patients had negative axillary nodes, whereas in the Stockholm and Oslo trials almost two thirds of the patients had negative axillary nodes. Surgery consisted of radical mastectomy in the Manchester and NSABP B-02 trials and modified radical mastectomy in the Stockholm and Oslo trials.

It is appropriate to review the radiotherapy technique employed in the trials, as their goal was to assess the role of postmastectomy radiotherapy. The use of inadequate radiotherapy has a definite potential for adversely affecting results. The radiotherapy dose was below current standards in the Manchester I trial,[32,85] the NSABP B-02 trial,[41] and the Oslo I trial.[55] Variations in the region(s) treated also may affect the results. The most common location for a local-regional recurrence following either radical or modified radical mastectomy is the chest wall.[6,34,41,50,51,66] Failure to include the chest wall in a course of postoperative radiotherapy has resulted in decreased survival rates[99] and increased incidence of local recurrence.[42] It is of note that the chest wall was omitted in the Manchester II trial, the NSABP B-02 trial, and the Oslo II trial.

The trials also have been criticized for lack of a consistent randomization process and inadequate stratification,[32,41,85] unequal patient distribution among the treatment arms,[41] and the use of confounding adjuvant therapy including oophorectomy[41,55] and chemotherapy.[41]

Despite these criticisms and the variations in patient population and radiotherapy technique, the results achieved have been quite similar. In all of the trials, the addition of radiation to either radical mastectomy or modified radical mastectomy has resulted in a decrease in the incidence of local-

Table 11-1 Prospective randomized trials comparing radical (RM) or modified radical mastectomy (MRM) with or without adjuvant radiation

	Manchester[32,85]								Oslo[55]			
	I		II		NSABP B-02[41]		Stockholm[93,103]		I		II	
Treatment period	1948-1952		1953-1955		1961-1968		1971-1976		1964-1967		1968-1972	
No. pts.	720		741		787		644		546		542	
Stage	I-II		I-II		I-III		I-III		I-II		I-II	
Node negative (%)	34		38		41		63		63		66	
≥4 positive nodes (%)	NS		NS		32		NS		9		8	
T_3 (%)	0		0		NS		12		0		0	
Surgery	RM		RM		RM		MRM		MRM		MRM	
Radiation												
Dose	Low		Adequate		Low		Adequate		Low		Adequate	
Region	CW and axilla		RN		RN		CW and RN		CW and RN		RN	
	RM	**RM and R**	**RM**	**RM and R**	**RM**	**RM and R**	**MRM**	**MRM and R**	**MRM**	**MRM and R**	**MRM**	**MRM and R**
Survival												
Overall N_0	24	12	25	16	62	56	65	70	I 69	70	76	63
	[.05]		[.13]				[>.05]		[>.05]		[.12]	
N_1	9	9	10	10					II 35	36	45	48
	[.9]		[.7]						[>.05]		[>.05]	
Disease-free	—	—	—	—	50	50	46	60	I 65	68	70	60
							[<.001]		[>.05]		[>.05]	
									II 36	38	39	47
									[>.05]		[.04]	
Follow-up (yr)	30		30		5		8-14		14		14	
Distant metastases						40						
(%)	—	—	—	—	32		40	33	II 56	46	50	33
									[>.05]		[>.05]	
Local-regional recurrence (%)	RM 32	RM and R 19			19	8	33	9	15	7	13	5
							[<.001]					

NS, not stated; CW, chest wall; RN, regional nodes; [ ], p value for comparison (adjacent columns).

regional recurrence. None of the trials demonstrated a survival benefit for the overall group of patients treated with follow-up periods ranging from 5 to 30 years. A significant decrease in distant metastases was noted in the Stockholm trial[93,103] only in node-positive patients. An update that combined both the Stockholm and Oslo trials[5] confirmed a significant decrease in distant metastases in node-positive patients with a follow-up of 13 to 16 years. A significant improvement in disease-free survival rates was noted in the Stockholm trial[93,103] and in the Oslo II trial,[55] but only for patients with stage II disease. While the NSABP B-02 trial[41] reported an improvement in 5-year disease-free survival rates for all node-positive patients with the addition of radiotherapy (38% vs. 32%), this difference was not statistically significant. A survival benefit of 22% was noted with radiation in the combined results of the Stockholm and Oslo trials for node-positive patients (p= .06).[5] There was no survival benefit for node-negative patients.

Simple mastectomy with or without postoperative radiotherapy

Results of prospective randomized trials comparing simple mastectomy with or without postoperative radiotherapy are presented in Tables 11-2 and 11-3. Five trials have evaluated the role of radiotherapy following simple mastectomy: the Cancer Research Campaign (CRC) trial,[12,23] the Southampton trial,[101] the Manchester regional trial,[71] the Edinburgh I trial,[43] and the NSABP B-04 trial.[38] In the NSABP B-04 trial, patients with clinically negative axillary nodes were randomized to radical mastectomy, total mastectomy, or total mastectomy and radiation. The NSABP B-04 was also the only trial that included operable T_3 lesions. Because the patients in the surgical arms of these trials were given either a simple or total mastectomy, pathologic assessment of the axillary nodes status was not performed routinely. However, pectoral lymph node biopsy was performed both in the Southampton trials and in the Edinburgh I trial. In the Cancer Research Campaign trial, axillary nodes were identified in 15% of the mastectomy specimens and 45% of these were negative.[12,23] Patients undergoing radical mastectomy in the NSABP B-04 trial had a complete axillary node resection. All of the trials employed radiotherapy directed to the chest wall and regional nodes. The radiotherapy dose delivered to these regions was low in the CRC trial[16] and the Manchester regional trial.[70] It was adequate in the remaining three trials. Of patients

Table 11-2 Results of randomized trials comparing simple mastectomy (SM) with simple mastectomy and radiation (SM and R)

	Cancer Research Campaign[12,23]	Southampton[101]	Manchester[71] regional	Edinburgh I[43]
Treatment period	1970-1975	1973-1976	1970-1975	1974-1979
No. pts.	2800	150	714	342
Stage	I and II	I and II	I	I and II
Node negative (%)	45	55	—	100
≥4 positive nodes (%)	NS	NS	—	0
T_3%				
Radiation	0	0	0	0
Dose				
Region	Low	Adequate	Low	Adequate
	CW and RN	CW and RN	CW and RN	CW and RN

	SM		SM and R	SM		SM and R	SM		SM and R	SM		SM and R
Survival (%)												
5-yr overall	70		73	78*	[>.05]	81*	69		74	80†		73†
5-yr DFS							49		65			
10-yr overall	55	[.88]	55				55	[.20]	62			
10-yr DFS							36	[<.0001]	52			
Distant metastases (%)	35		33	—		—	—		—	—		—
Local-regional recurrence (%)	39	[<.001]	17	28	[<.05]	9	42	[<.0001]	22	24		14
Follow-up (yr)	10			4			10			4		

*3-yr survival.
†4-yr survival.
DFS, disease-free survival; CW, chest wall; RN, regional nodes; NS, not stated; [ ], p value for comparison.

Table 11-3 Results of the NSABP B-04 randomized trial in clinically axillary node–negative patients[38]

Treatment period	Results 1971-1974		
No. pts.	1079		
Stage	T_{1-3} clinical N_0		
Node negative (%)	—		
≥4 positive nodes (%)	—		
T_3 (%)	NS		
Radiation			
Dose	Adequate		
Region	CW and RN		
	RM	TM	TM and R
5-year survival (%)			
Overall	75	74	75
Disease-free*	60	56	65
10-year survival (%)			
Overall	58	54	59 [.2]
Disease-free*	47	42	48 [.05]
Distant metastases (%)	30	34	32
Local-regional recurrence (%)*	9	14	5

CW, chest wall; RN, regional nodes; RM, radical mastectomy; TM, total mastectomy; R, radiation; [ ], p value for comparisons.
*Excludes patients with operable axillary recurrences.

with clinically negative nodes in the NSABP B-04 trial receiving radiotherapy, 82% had no significant variations in the treatment protocol.[36] Overall these trials demonstrated a greater uniformity in the patient population and in the radiotherapy technique and dosage.

The results of the trials again revealed no overall survival benefit with the addition of radiotherapy with follow-up ranging from 4 to 10 years. Analysis of the incidence of distant metastases was performed in the NSABP B-04 trial[36] and the Cancer Research Campaign trial[16]; neither of these produced a significant reduction in distant metastases with the addition of radiation. Local-regional recurrence was decreased in all of the trials except for the NSABP B-04 trial. It must be emphasized, however, that in this trial patients who developed an operable axillary recurrence were excluded from the statistical analysis of local-regional recurrence. Overall, 17.8% of patients who were clinically node-negative developed an axillary recurrence.[36] In the Cancer Research Campaign trial,[33] the rate of local-regional recurrence was significantly decreased with the addition of radiation only in node-positive patients and those with grade II or grade III tumors. A statistically significant improvement in disease-free survival at 10 years was noted in the Manchester regional study[70] as well as in the NSABP B-04 study[36] with the addition of radiation. Disease-free survival results were not reported in the Southampton trial,[101] the Cancer Research Campaign trial,[12,23] or the Edinburgh I trial.[43]

SURVIVAL OF PATIENTS WITH OR WITHOUT POSTOPERATIVE RADIOTHERAPY

In summary, prospective randomized trials evaluating the addition of radiation after either simple mastectomy, total mastectomy, or radical or modified radical mastectomy have demonstrated a benefit with a decrease in local-regional recurrence rates but no benefit in overall survival rates. Four studies have demonstrated a significant benefit in terms of disease-free survival.[38,55,71,93] While some of the studies have been flawed by the lack of a consistent randomization process, inadequate radiotherapy in terms of dose and region(s) treated, and the use of extraneous procedures including ovarian oblation, oophorectomy, or chemotherapy, the findings are fairly consistent.

It has been suggested that postmastectomy radiation may exert a detrimental effect on survival.[27,96] Stjernsward,[96] using the Mantel-Haenszel technique, combined the differences in individual survival results from four trials (Manchester,[32,85] Copenhagen,[61] Southeast Scotland,[65] and NSABP B-02[41]) and concluded that the differences in survival rates between irradiated and nonirradiated patients significantly favored the latter. However, in two of the trials (Copenhagen and Southeast Scotland) surgery in the two treatment arms was not identical; therefore these trials are not a strict comparison of surgery with or without postoperative radiotherapy. Levitt et al.[69] have reviewed Stjernsward's analysis and have found it to be invalid. It is also of note that with further follow-up the differences in favor of no radiotherapy have been eliminated. Cuzick et al.,[27] in an overview of mortality results of postmastectomy radiotherapy, analyzed results from the trials in Tables 11-2 and 11-3 (except for the NSABP B-02 trial), as well as those from an unpublished trial from Heidelberg comparing radical mastectomy to radical mastectomy and radiation. The authors noted no differences in survival for the first 10 years following treatment; however, follow-up after 15 years revealed a significant increase in mortality rates ($p<.001$) in patients who received radiotherapy. This increase in mortality was noted in the Manchester trial, the Oslo trial, the Cancer Research Campaign trial, and the Heidelberg trial, but not in the Stockholm trial. The mortality data was primarily drawn from the Manchester and Oslo trials. In the overview the causes of death were not known. However, further information is available from the Manchester trial, the Oslo trial, and Cancer Research Campaign trial. Jones and Ribeiro,[60] in a review of the Manchester trials I and II, noted no difference in survival rates for the first 15 years. After 15 years, a significant increase in mortality was noted in the radiotherapy group ($p = .0025$) and was related to increased deaths from cardiovascular disease. There was no difference in mortality from breast cancer or other causes between the two groups. There was no difference in the increased mortality from cardiovascular disease between patients with left- or right-sided primary tumors. The authors concluded that the technique and equipment (orthovoltage) employed in these trials were no longer used and most likely contributed to these deaths. In the Oslo trial[55] an increase in cardiovascular deaths primarily related to myocardial infarction was observed in stage I patients who received cobalt-60 irradiation to the regional nodes. The authors suggested that this phenomenon may be related to the radiotherapy technique employed to treat the internal mammary chain. A recent report from the Cancer Research Campaign trial[52] noted a slight but not significant increase in mortality rate in patients receiving postmastectomy radiation. The increase in mortality was related to an increase in nonbreast cancer deaths that occurred primarily in patients with left-sided tumors who received orthovoltage treatment. These studies demonstrate the effect of radiotherapy on patients with long-term cardiac complications. Modifications in technique that avoid irradiation of the heart virtually can eliminate increased mortality in these patients. Therefore there is little evidence to support a deleterious effect on survival with the use of postmastectomy adjuvant radiation except in these earlier studies where the radiotherapy technique contributed to an increased incidence of cardiovascular deaths.

SELECTING PATIENTS AT RISK FOR LOCAL-REGIONAL RECURRENCE

The question arises as to whether any benefit in terms of survival would have been expected from these adjuvant radiotherapy trials. The effect of adjuvant radiotherapy is to diminish the incidence of local-regional recurrence. This is obviously most important in patients in whom the risk of local-regional recurrence is significant. Data regarding patients at risk for local-regional recurrence following radical or modified radical mastectomy can be obtained from surgical series and are presented in Tables 11-4 through 11-7. It can be seen that the risk of a local-regional recurrence is related to the primary tumor size and the status of the axillary nodes. Patients with primary tumors $\geq$5 cm in diameter as well as those with four or more positive axillary nodes have a 25% to 30% incidence of local-regional recurrence. The risk is relatively low, i.e., $\leq$10%, for patients with T_1 lesions or negative axillary nodes. The risk is intermediate, i.e., approximately 15%, for patients with T_2 lesions or one to three positive axillary nodes. There is some evidence that patients with negative axillary nodes who have high-grade tumors have a risk of local-regional recurrence that approaches 20%.[54,104] The presence of tumor in intramammary lymphatics in patients with negative axillary nodes does not increase the risk for a local-regional recurrence.[81] There is also evidence that younger women have a higher incidence of local-regional recurrence. Donegan et al.[31] noted a 46% incidence of local-regional recurrence at 5 years (19/41) in women under the age of 40, compared to 12% (79/663) in women greater than 40 years of age. Mathews et al.[76] and Bartelink et al.[8] also have noted a higher incidence of local-regional recurrence following mastectomy in young women.

In summary, patients at greatest risk for a local-regional recurrence following mastectomy are

Table 11-4 Incidence of postmastectomy local-regional recurrence related to primary tumor size

Author	Surgery	Local-regional recurrence (%) T_1	T_2	T_3	Follow-up (yr)
Donegan et al.[31]	RM	7 [73]	16 [398]	30 [135]	5
Rosenman et al.[89]	RM/MRM	8 [51]	18 [87]	32 [44]	2-14
Dao and Nemoto[28]	RM	6 [36]	6 [70]	24 [29]	1.3-3+
Baker et al.[6]	MRM			39 [31]	5
	RM			9 [36]	5
Maddox et al.[72]	MRM			20 [20]	3-5
	RM			6 [16]	

RM, radical mastectomy; MRM, modified radical mastectomy; [ ], total no. pts.

Table 11-5 Incidence of postmastectomy local-regional recurrence in pathologic axillary node–negative patients

Author	No. pts.	Surgery	Local-regional recurrence (%)	Follow-up (yr)
Donegan et al.[31]	308	RM	6	5
Valagussa et al.[102]	335	RM/ERM	8	10
Haagensen[49]	562	RM	3	10-37
Rosenman et al.[89]	216	RM/MRM	4	2-14
Fisher et al.[41]	84	RM	8	5
Ahlborn et al.[2]	322	MRM	4	4 (mean)
Overgaard et al.[84]	3126	TM and AD	21	9
Williams et al.[104]	439	SM	19	4-10
Hopton et al.[54]	463	RM/SM	13	5
Deck and Kern[29]	617	RM/MRM/SM	4	3+
Dao and Nemoto[28]	55	RM	0	1.3-3+
Lee[67]	182	RM/MRM	6	4.4 (median)
Crowe et al.[26]	917	MRM	9	—

RM, radical mastectomy; ERM, extended radical mastectomy; TM, total mastectomy; AD, axillary dissection; MRM, modified radical mastectomy; SM, simple mastectomy.

Table 11-6 Incidence of postmastectomy local-regional recurrence in pathologic axillary node–positive patients

Author	No. pts.	Surgery	Local-regional recurrence (%)	Follow-up (yr)
Valagussa et al.[102]	381	RM/ERM	27	10
Donegan et al.[31]	395	RM	26	5
Fisher et al.[41]	185	RM	24	5
Hopton et al.[54]	366	RM/SM	29	5
Deck and Kern[29]	410	RM/MRM/SM	11	3+
Dao and Nemoto[28]	80	RM	16	1.3-3+

RM, radical mastectomy; ERM, extended radical mastectomy; SM, simple mastectomy; MRM, modified radical mastectomy.

Table 11-7 Incidence of postmastectomy local-regional recurrence related to the number of positive axillary nodes

Author	No. pts.	Surgery	Local-regional recurrence (%)		Follow-up (yr)
			1-3	≥4	
Haagensen[49]	373	RM	4	22	10-37
Donegan et al.[31]	395	RM	12	38	5
Fisher et al.[41]	185	RM	24	31	5
Rosenman et al.[89]	188	RM/MRM	17	22	2-14
Lee[67]	138	RM/MRM	11	37	4.4 (median)

RM, radical mastectomy; MRM, modified radical mastectomy.

those with a primary tumor ≥5 cm and four or more positive axillary nodes. Young age or histologic grade also may have an impact on the likelihood of local-regional recurrence. It is in this subgroup of patients that adjuvant radiotherapy would have its greatest impact and offer the potential for a survival benefit. It is highly unlikely that a reduction in local-regional recurrence in patients who are at low risk initially would translate into a survival benefit. A review of Table 11-1, which presents the trials of adjuvant radiotherapy in patients who had undergone either radical or modified radical mastectomy, reveals that in two of the trials (Stockholm[93,103] and Oslo[55]) approximately two thirds of the patients had negative axillary nodes. In the Manchester[32,85] and NSABP B-02[41] trials, approximately 40% of patients had negative axillary nodes and in the NSABP B-02 trial[41] 32% of the patients had four or more positive nodes. Patients with T_3 tumors were included in the NSABP B-02 trial but the percentage of patients in this category was not stated. T_3 tumors comprised 12% of the patients in the Stockholm trial.[93,103] Therefore patients entered into these trials were primarily in a low-risk category for local-regional recurrence. A review of Tables 11-2 and 11-3, presenting the results of adjuvant radiotherapy following simple mastectomy from randomized trials, reveals that only the NSABP B-04 trial[38] included patients with T_3 lesions. Again the percentage of patients in this category was not stated. Information regarding histologic nodal status is not available from the Manchester Regional trial or the NSABP B-04 trial, as axillary node dissection was not performed in patients undergoing simple or total mastectomy. In the Southampton trial[101] patients underwent a pectoral lymph node biopsy, and 55% of the patients entered into this trial had histologically negative axillary nodes. Similarly, in the Edinburgh I trial[43] all patients underwent pectoral node biopsy; they were eligible for this trial only if the nodes were negative or could not be identified. In the Cancer Research Campaign trial[33] 15% of patients had axillary nodes identified in the mastectomy specimen and 45% of these were negative. In these trials a survival benefit would not be expected for two reasons. First, many low-risk patients were included in the trials. Radiotherapy has little effect on reducing local-regional recurrence in low-risk patients. In the Cancer Research Campaign trial[33] there was no significant decrease in local-regional recurrence with radiation in patients with grade I tumors or negative axillary nodes. Second, unlike the radical or modified radical mastectomy trials, the primary site of local-regional recurrence was in the undissected axilla. The salvage rate for axillary failures in the clinically negative undissected axilla is relatively good,[22,25,38] and therefore this pattern of failure is unlikely to affect survival adversely.

In summary, the failure of randomized trials evaluating the role of adjuvant radiotherapy following either radical or modified radical mastectomy or simple or total mastectomy to demonstrate a survival benefit is not unexpected. The findings are consistent with the fact that in many of the trials the majority of patients entered were at low risk for local-regional recurrence, and in some inadequate radiotherapy (dose or region treated) was employed. While the trials also have been criticized for their lack of a consistent randomization process or the use of extraneous procedures, their findings are explained most readily by patient selection and, in some cases, inadequate radiotherapy.

THE ROLE OF ADJUVANT CHEMOTHERAPY IN PREVENTING LOCAL-REGIONAL RECURRENCE FOLLOWING MASTECTOMY

The role of postmastectomy radiation has been further challenged in the era of adjuvant chemotherapy. Can adjuvant chemotherapy, in addition to eradicating micrometastatic disease, prevent local-regional recurrence and thereby obviate the need for adjuvant radiation? Table 11-8 presents data regarding local-regional recurrence rates in prospective randomized trials comparing postmastectomy adjuvant chemotherapy to observation. Several of these studies[14,45,64,90] suggest that adjuvant chemotherapy does not alter the incidence of local-regional recurrence significantly when compared to an untreated group. The remainder of the studies, however, suggest that adjuvant chemotherapy reduces the incidence of local-regional recurrence. The overall incidence of local-regional recurrence in node-positive patients receiving various postmastectomy adjuvant chemotherapy regimens is presented in Table 11-9. The incidence of local-regional recurrence ranges from 8% to 29% and is highest for melphalan (L-PAM). Fisher et al.[40] reported a decrease in the incidence of local-regional recurrence with the addition of Adriamycin to L-PAM and 5-fluorouracil (27% vs. 16%). In general it is not established that Adriamycin-containing regimens are significantly more effective than non–Adriamycin-containing regimens in preventing postmastectomy local-regional recurrence. The dose of chemotherapy also does not appear to affect the incidence of local-regional recurrence in that patients who receive ≥85% of the prescribed dose do not have a lower incidence of local-regional recurrence when compared to those who receive <85%.[45,95] Table 11-10 presents the incidence of local-regional recurrence in node-positive patients

Table 11-8 Incidence of postmastectomy local-regional recurrence in randomized trials of adjuvant chemotherapy versus observation in node-positive patients

Author	Chemotherapy	No. pts.	Local-regional recurrence (%)		Follow-up (yr)
			Control	Chemotherapy	
Bonadonna et al.[14]	CMF	386	14	12	10
Howell et al.[56]	CMF	327	21	9	1-5
Fisher et al.[35]	L-PAM	380	24	14	10
Rubens et al.[90]	L-PAM	370	29	21	5
Koyama et al.[64]	MMC, C	229	4	16	7
Goldhirsh and Gelber[46]*	CMFPT	310	29	8	4 (median)
Ingle et al.[58]*	CFP	163	22	11	5 (median)
Fowble et al.[45]*	CMFP (T)	208	14	13	3

C, cyclophosphamide; M, methotrexate; F, 5-fluorouracil; P, prednisone; T, tamoxifen; MMC, mitomycin C.
*Postmenopausal pts. only.

receiving postmastectomy adjuvant chemotherapy related to the extent of nodal positivity and primary tumor size. The incidence of local-regional recurrence is ≤10% in patients with one to three positive nodes, 14% to 36% for patients with four or more positive nodes, and 18% to 31% for patients with T_3 primary tumors. The incidence of local-regional recurrence in high-risk patients, i.e., those with T_3 primary tumors or four or more positive nodes, is not significantly different from reports from surgical series alone (Tables 11-4 and 11-7). Therefore in this subset of patients chemotherapy does not appear to alter the local-regional recurrence rate when compared to surgery alone.

Young women receiving adjuvant chemotherapy also appear to have a higher risk of postmastectomy local-regional recurrence than older women. Rao et al.[87] reported a 19.3% incidence for women <50 years of age compared to 9.6% for those >50 years of age. Ingle et al.[57,58] reported a 17% incidence for premenopausal patients compared to 11% for postmenopausal patients. However, an analysis of the Eastern Cooperative Oncology Group (ECOG) adjuvant chemotherapy trials revealed no increased incidence for younger women (<40 years of age).[45] Sykes et al.[98] also identified patients who were node positive and estrogen receptor (ER) negative who received Adriamycin and Cytoxan as having a high risk of local-regional recurrence. The risk of a local-regional recurrence was 23% at 20 months in patients with ER-negative tumors and one to three positive nodes and 31% for patients with ER-negative tumors and four or more positive nodes. The incidence in this latter group increased to 41% at 30 months. Rutqvist et al.[92] noted no correlation with ER status and local-regional recurrence in postmenopausal patients receiving adjuvant chemotherapy. Node-negative patients

Table 11-9 Incidence of local-regional recurrence in node-positive patients receiving adjuvant chemotherapy

Regimen	Author	No. pts.	Local-regional recurrence (%)	Follow-up (yr)
L-PAM ± F	Rivkin et al.[88]	190	29	10
	Fisher et al.[40]	353	27	6
CMF	Wood et al.[105]	270	11	5
	Rutqvist et al.[93]	395	22	6.5 (mean)
CMFVP	Wood et al.[105]	258	8	5
	Rivkin et al.[88]	173	25	10
CFP	Ingle et al.[57,58]	202	17 premenopausal	5.3 (median)
		75	11 postmenopausal	
Adriamycin regimens				
L-PAM, A, F	Fisher et al.[40]	344	16	6
FAC	Buzdar et al.[19]	321	12	5

C, cyclophosphamide; M, methotrexate; F, 5-fluorouracil; V, vincristine; P, prednisone; A, Adriamycin.

Table 11-10 Incidence of local-regional recurrence in node-positive patients receiving postmastectomy adjuvant chemotherapy

		Local-regional recurrence (%)				
			Positive nodes			
Author	Chemotherapy	All pts.	1-3	≥4	T_3 tumors	Follow-up (yr)
Bonadonna et al.[14]	CMF	9	5	14* [21]	—	8
Stefanik et al.[95]	CMF	19	9	36	27	5
Tormey et al.[100]	CMF	—	—	18	—	2.8 (median)
	CMFVP	—	—	10	—	
Fowble et al.[45]	CMF (PT)	11	7	15	19	3
Rao et al.[87]	CMF or L-PAMFT	18	6	24	31	5.2 (median)
Lee[67]	CMF, L-PAM	20	9	27	—	4.4 (median)
Goldhirsch and Gelber[46]†	CMFP	11	8	15	—	4 (median)
Griem et al.[47]	CMF/MF	14	5	—	—	4.4 (median)
	CA			20	—	
Sykes et al.[98]	AC	—	10	10	28	2.9
Buzdar et al.[19]	FAC	12	7	14* [21]	18	5

C, cyclophosphamide; M, methotrexate; F, 5-fluorouracil; V, vincristine; P, prednisone; A, Adriamycin; T, tamoxifen; [ ], >10 positive nodes.
*4-10 positive nodes.
†Premenopausal pts. only.

receiving adjuvant chemotherapy have a predictably low risk for local-regional recurrence (Table 11-11).

EFFECTIVENESS OF ADJUVANT CHEMOTHERAPY VERSUS ADJUVANT RADIATION IN PREVENTING LOCAL-REGIONAL RECURRENCE

The majority of randomized trials evaluating adjuvant radiotherapy following radical or modified radical mastectomy (see Table 11-1) have demonstrated a local-regional recurrence rate of 5% to 9% with the addition of radiation; these trials have follow-up periods of 5 to 14 years. Beadle and Harris,[9] in a retrospective review, reported local-regional recurrence in 6% of 352 patients who received postmastectomy irradiation. Seventy-one percent of these patients had histologically positive axillary nodes. Fletcher et al.[42] reported local-regional recurrence rates in 412 patients who received radiation to the chest wall and regional nodes with a minimum follow-up of 10 years. The incidence of local-regional recurrence was 4% in patients with negative axillary nodes, 9% in those with one to three positive nodes, and 14% in those with four or more positive nodes. Therefore postmastectomy irradiation results in local-regional recurrence rates of approximately 10%.

A direct comparison of the effectiveness of radiation vs. chemotherapy in the prevention of post-

Table 11-11 Incidence of local-regional recurrence in node-negative patients receiving adjuvant chemotherapy postmastectomy

Author	Chemotherapy	Total no. pts.		Local-regional recurrence (%)	Follow-up (yr)
Sykes et al.[98]	AC	149	T_1	0	2.9
			T_2	5	
Caffier et al.[21]	CMF	73		10	3-7
Fisher et al.[37]*	M→F	339		4	4

C, cyclophosphamide; A, Adriamycin; M, methotrexate; F, 5-fluorouracil.
*Includes 31% of patients who underwent lumpectomy and radiation.

mastectomy local-regional recurrence was performed by the Stockholm Breast Cancer Group.[93] A randomized trial with more than 900 women entered was initiated in 1976. Premenopausal and postmenopausal patients <71 years of age with unilateral operable breast cancer were randomized following a modified radical mastectomy to postoperative radiotherapy or cyclophosphamide, methotrexate, and 5-fluorouracil (CMF) for a total of 12 courses. Patients included in the trial were those with histologically positive axillary nodes or primary tumor size >3 cm. With a 6½ year mean follow-up, local-regional recurrence was 12% in the group that received radiation vs. 22% in the group that received CMF ($p = .001$).[93] These findings suggest that radiotherapy is more effective than chemotherapy alone in preventing local-regional recurrence following mastectomy. However, the most effective treatment appears to be the combination of adjuvant systemic chemotherapy and radiation. Buzdar et al.[19] reported a 5-year local-regional recurrence rate of 10% with an historical control of 175 patients who received postmastectomy adjuvant radiation, compared to 5% in a group of patients who received postmastectomy irradiation and 5-fluorouracil, Adriamycin, and cyclophosphamide (FAC) chemotherapy. In the Danish Breast Cancer Cooperative Group (DBCG) trial 77B, premenopausal and perimenopausal women with positive nodes or T_3 primary tumors were randomized to postoperative radiotherapy alone, radiotherapy plus CMF, radiotherapy plus Cytoxan, or radiotherapy plus levamisole.[84] The actuarial risk of local-regional recurrence at 9 years was 12% in a group of patients who received radiotherapy alone, 6% in a group of patients who received radiotherapy and cyclophosphamide, and 8% in a group of patients who received radiotherapy and CMF. Similarly, in the Glasgow randomized trial[77,94] comparing postmastectomy radiation, CMF, and radiation and CMF, local-regional recurrence was lowest (12%) in the group of patients receiving both modalities. These three studies suggest that the risk of local-regional recurrence is lowest in the group of patients who receive both radiation and adjuvant systemic chemotherapy.

PATIENTS RECEIVING ADJUVANT CHEMOTHERAPY WHO MAY HAVE A SURVIVAL BENEFIT FROM POSTMASTECTOMY RADIATION

A subgroup of patients with histologically positive axillary nodes receiving adjuvant chemotherapy who may benefit from postoperative radiotherapy has been identified by Fowble et al.[45] In a review of 627 women entered into Eastern Cooperative Oncology Group adjuvant chemotherapy trials between 1978 and 1982, an overall local-regional recurrence of 11% was reported. None of these patients received adjuvant radiotherapy. The analysis was directed toward identifying prognostic factors that could predict the risk of an isolated local-regional recurrence as well as identifying factors that could discriminate between an isolated local-regional recurrence and distant metastases. In a multivariate analysis, the risk of an isolated local-regional recurrence significantly correlated with the number of positive axillary nodes, the primary tumor size, the presence of tumor necrosis, and the number of axillary nodes examined. Factors that significantly could determine the type of recurrence, i.e., isolated local-regional recurrence vs. distant metastases, were the number of positive nodes and primary tumor size. Patients with four to seven positive nodes or tumor size ≥5 cm had an almost equal chance of developing an isolated local-regional recurrence or distant metastases. It is of note that the majority of recurrences in patients with primary tumor size ≥5 cm and four to seven positive nodes were isolated local-regional recurrences and not distant metastases. The authors suggested that the group of patients in whom a potential for improved survival existed with the addition of adjuvant radiation were those with primary tumors ≥5 cm and four to seven positive axillary nodes. In this study, 29% of patients had four to seven positive nodes and 22% had primary tumors ≥5 cm. Therefore the subset of patients for whom a survival benefit may exist was not insignificant. While postmastectomy irradiation may be of benefit in terms of decreasing local-regional control in patients with eight or more positive nodes, a survival benefit could not be expected in this subgroup because distant metastases were the predominant form of recurrence.

RETROSPECTIVE REVIEWS COMPARING ADJUVANT SYSTEMIC CHEMOTHERAPY WITH ADJUVANT CHEMOTHERAPY AND POSTMASTECTOMY RADIATION

Several retrospective reviews have compared the results of postmastectomy adjuvant chemotherapy with postmastectomy adjuvant chemotherapy and radiation (Table 11-12). Sykes et al.[98] reported the results of adjuvant chemotherapy consisting of Adriamycin and cyclophosphamide with or without postmastectomy radiation in 400 women with stage II or stage III breast cancer. Patients were entered into the Arizona Adjuvant Chemotherapy trial; however, radiotherapy was not randomized. There

Table 11-12 Retrospective reviews comparing postmastectomy chemotherapy (C) with or without radiation (R)

	University of Arizona[98]			M.D. Anderson[19]				Southwestern Oncology Group[88]		Massachusetts General Hospital[24]			Mt. Sinai[53]	
No. pts.	400			768				363		101			100	
Treatment	1974-1985			1974-1982				1975-1978		1973-1974			NS	
≥4 positive nodes (%)	38			58				60		NS			100	
T_3 (%)	20			28				12		17			NS	
Chemotherapy	AC			FAC				CMFVP L-PAM		CMFVP			VPCMF	
	Disease Status	**C**	**C and R**	**Disease status**	**C**		**C and R**	**C**	**C and R**	**C**		**C and R**	**C**	**C and R**
Survival (%)														
Overall		—	—		—		—	—	—	58	[.40]	72	80	37
Disease-free		—	—		—		—	—	—					
Distant metastases (%)		—	—		—		—	—	—	34		46		
Local-regional recurrence (%)	T_2N_0	5	0		12	[<.01]	5	31	9	21		12		
	$T_{1\text{-}2}$, 1-3 positive nodes	10	0	II	11	[.04]	3							
	$T_{1\text{-}2}$, ≥4 positive nodes	10	8	T_3	18	[.04]	8							
	$T_3T_4N_2N_3$	28	15	1-3 positive nodes	7	[.04]	2							
				4-10 positive nodes	14	[.02]	5							
				>10 positive nodes	21	[.08]	8							
Follow-up (yr)		2.9			5			10		4			5	

A, Adriamycin; C, cyclophosphamide; F, 5-fluorouracil; V, vincristine; P, prednisone; [ ], p numbers for comparison between adjacent columns.

appeared to be no benefit for adjuvant radiotherapy in terms of local-regional control with an analysis at 35 months in patients with T_2 pathologically negative axillary nodes or in patients with $T_{1\text{-}2}$ tumors and four or more positive nodes. Patients who appeared to benefit from adjuvant radiotherapy in terms of local-regional control were those with $T_{1\text{-}2}$ primary tumors and three or fewer positive nodes, or T_3, T_4, N_2, or N_3 disease. The finding that local-regional recurrence was decreased significantly in patients with one to three positive nodes and not those with four or more positive nodes is contrary to what would be expected. It must be emphasized that 61% of the radiotherapy patients received <5000 rad. Overall, the radiotherapy patients were more advanced in stage, tumor size, and extent of nodal involvement. Of the patients who received chemotherapy and radiation, 29% had T_3 primary tumors, compared to 14% who received chemotherapy alone; 52% of the patients who received chemotherapy and radiation had four or more positive nodes as compared to 29% who received chemotherapy alone. Buzdar et al.,[19] in a retrospective review of 768 patients who received FAC chemotherapy with or without radiation at M.D. Anderson Hospital, reported a significant decrease in local-regional recurrence in all stage II patients and patients with T_3 primary tumors. Patients with 10 or fewer positive nodes had a significant decrease in rates of local-regional recurrence. Patients with 11 or more positive nodes had a decrease in local-regional recurrence rates from 21% to 8% with the addition of radiation; however, the p value for this comparison was .08, presumably because of the small number of patients in this subgroup. Survival results were not presented for either of these two series. Chu and Kiel,[24] in a retrospective review of 101 patients who received postmastectomy cyclophosphamide, methotrexate, 5-fluorouracil, vincristine, and prednisone (CMFVP) with or without radiation, noted no significant improvement in overall or disease-free

Table 11-13 Results of randomized trials comparing postmastectomy chemotherapy (Chemo) with or without adjuvant radiation (R)

	Mayo Clinic[3,75]			University of Arizona[4]		Dana Farber[47]		M.D. Anderson[18,20]		Glasgow[77,94]		
Therapy period	1973-1980			1974-1980		1974-1984		1977-1980		1976-1982		
No. pts.	313			159		206		238		322		
≥4 positive nodes (%)	55			45		60		68		31		
T_3 (%)	NS			0		NS		40		NS		
Chemotherapy	L-PAM, CFP			AC		CMF/MF		FAC ± BCG		CMF		
	L-PAM	**CFP**	**CFP and R**	**Chemo**	**Chemo and R**	**Chemo†**	**Chemo and R†**	**Chemo**	**Chemo and R**	**R**	**R and Chemo**	**Chemo**
Survival (%)												
Overall	56	66	68	—	—	85	77	71	70			
						[.39]		[.71]				
Disease-free	34	48	53	67	63	75	79	52	41	40	51	43
				[.92]		[.71]		[.93]			[.005]	
Follow-up (yr)		5		5		4.4 (median)		5			5	
Distant metastases (%)				18	25	—	—	21	34	41	35	22
								[>.05]				
Local-regional recurrence (%)	26	30	10	11	11	5	2	13	7	16	12	31
						[.61]		[>.05]				

C, cyclophosphamide; M, methotrexate; F, 5-fluorouracil; A, Adriamycin; T, tamoxifen; P, prednisone; [ ], p value for comparison (adjacent columns).
*Premenopausal patients only.
†Results for 1-3 positive nodes only.

survival at 4 years. The incidence of local-regional recurrence was reduced with radiation. Holland and Glidewell[53] reported 100 patients with four or more positive nodes who received vincristine, prednisone, cyclophosphamide, methotrexate, and 5-fluorouracil (VPCMF) postmastectomy with or without radiation. The 5-year survival rate was 37% in the group that received radiation, compared to 80% in the group that received adjuvant chemotherapy. The chest wall was not treated in patients who received radiation; this is the only study that suggests a detrimental effect of adjuvant radiotherapy. Rivkin et al.[88] reported the 10-year results of a randomized trial from the Southwestern Oncology Group (SWOG) in which node-positive patients were randomized to CMFVP vs. L-PAM. Radiotherapy was employed at the discretion of the investigator and local-regional recurrence rate at 10-years was 9% in the group of patients who received chemotherapy and radiation vs. 31% in the group that received chemotherapy only.

PROSPECTIVE RANDOMIZED TRIALS COMPARING POSTMASTECTOMY ADJUVANT CHEMOTHERAPY TO POSTMASTECTOMY ADJUVANT CHEMOTHERAPY AND RADIATION

Nine prospective randomized trials have evaluated the role of postmastectomy radiation and adjuvant chemotherapy in all patients with histologically positive axillary nodes. An additional trial from the Southeastern Cancer Group (SEG) evaluated the role of postmastectomy radiation in patients receiving adjuvant chemotherapy with four or more positive nodes.[74] The results of these trials are presented in Tables 11-13 and 11-14. All of the trials except for one[4] have demonstrated a decrease in the incidence of local-regional recurrence with the addition of radiation to postmastectomy and adjuvant chemotherapy. In the University of Arizona Cancer Center study[4] the randomization to radiotherapy was not strict, and low doses of radiation

British Columbia[86]		**Danish Breast Cancer Cooperative Group[30,84]**		**Piedmont[79]**				**National Cooperative Trial, Israel[13]**		
1979-1986		1982-1989		—				—		
316*		1308*		159				133		
NS		28		48				NS		
NS		15		0				0		
CMF		CMF(T)		L-PAM, CMF				L-PAM, F		
Chemo	**Chemo and R**	**Chemo**	**Chemo and R**	**L-PAM**	**L-PAM and R**	**CMF**	**CMF and R**	**Chemo**	**Chemo and R**	**R**
60	57	68	74	47	60	58	46	48	45	34
[.53]		[.43]								
49	64	51	64							
[.01]		[.004]								
8		4		10				9		
		24	7	35	18	16	8	14	6	3
		[<.0001]			Chemo 25	Chemo and R	13		[.02]	
						[.03]				

Table 11-14 Results of randomized trials comparing postmastectomy chemotherapy (Chemo) with or without adjuvant radiation (R) in patients with ≥4 positive nodes

	SEG[74]			Glasgow[77]			Dana Farber[47]		Arizona[4]	
Treatment period	1976-1981			1976-1982			1974-1984		1974-1980	
No. pts.	295			101			123		72	
Chemotherapy	CMF			CMF			CA		CA	
	CMR × 12 mo	**CMF × 6 mo**	**R and CMF**	**Chemo**	**R and Chemo**	**R**	**Chemo**	**Chemo and R**	**Chemo**	**Chemo and R**
Survival (%)										
Overall	24	37	55				63	59	—	—
							[.27]			
Disease-free	22		36	55	33	25	53	49	59	47
					[.006]		[.22]		[.95]	
Follow-up (yr)		10			5		3.7 (median)		5	
Distant metastases (%)	48	54	42				—	—	24	36
		[.25]								
Local-regional recurrence (%)	16	18	9				20	6	12	18
		[.05]					[.03]			

C, cyclophosphamide; M, methotrexate; F, 5-fluorouracil; A, Adriamycin; [ ], p values for comparison (adjacent columns above).

frequently were employed. In the Dana Farber Cancer Institute study[47] the addition of radiation to adjuvant chemotherapy in patients with one to three positive nodes did not result in a significant reduction in the rates of local-regional recurrence; however, in patients with four or more positive nodes the reduction was significant. None of the studies has demonstrated a significant improvement in the overall survival rates with the addition of adjuvant radiation. However, four of these studies have demonstrated a significant improvement in disease-free survival with the addition of radiation, with follow-up ranging from four to eight years.[4,30,77,84,86,94] In the University of Arizona study[4] a relapse-free survival benefit was noted only in patients with one to three positive nodes who received radiation, despite the fact these patients are typically at low risk for a local-regional recurrence.

The lack of a demonstrable overall survival benefit in these studies is not unexpected. A critical review reveals the same deficiencies as noted in trials evaluating postmastectomy radiation without chemotherapy, i.e., patient selection and inadequate radiotherapy. In five of the trials[4,30,77,79,84] the majority of patients included were at low risk for local-regional recurrence, i.e., they had three or fewer positive nodes. In two of the studies,[13,86] the extent of nodal involvement was not stated. The frequency of T_3 primary tumors often was not stated and in one study[18,20] represented 40% of the patient population. The radiotherapy dose was low in the University of Arizona Cancer Center study,[4] and the chest wall was not treated routinely in the Mayo Clinic trial.[3,75]

The findings from the analysis of the ECOG adjuvant trials[45] offer an explanation for the lack of the survival benefit in all patients with positive axillary nodes receiving adjuvant chemotherapy and radiation. Such a benefit can be expected only in certain subsets of patients, i.e., those with four to seven positive nodes and primary tumors ≥5 cm. Unfortunately, the trials have not performed a separate analysis of these subsets. However, data regarding outcome of patients with four or more positive nodes are available from several trials (see Table 11-14). Two of these trials have demonstrated a significant improvement in the disease-free survival rates with the addition of radiation.[77,94] While the SEG study demonstrated no significant improvement in overall or disease-free survival at 10 years, freedom from recurrence at last follow-up was significantly better in the group of patients who received radiotherapy (52% vs. 40%).[74] In the Glasgow study[77] no overall survival benefit was noted; however, when deaths not related to breast cancer were excluded, the disease-related survival rate was improved significantly in patients with four or more positive nodes who received radiotherapy and chemotherapy (54% vs. 46%, p = .01). In the Piedmont Oncology Group (POG) study[80] 75 patients had four or more positive nodes and were randomized to L-PAM or CMF with or without radiotherapy. The total number of recurrences was least in the group of patients who received radiotherapy in addition to chemotherapy.

Two prospective randomized trials have evaluated the role of postmastectomy radiation specifically in the treatment of operable T_3 primary tumors. These results are presented in Table 11-15. In the Helsinki trial[48,62] patients with operable T_3 tumors were randomized to postmastectomy radiation; vincristine, Adriamycin, and cyclophosphamide (VAC) with or without the addition of levamisole; or a combination of the two. The combined modality arm showed a statistically significant improvement in overall and disease-free survival rates at 5 years. In the ECOG trial[83] patients were randomized to cyclophosphamide, Adriamycin, 5-fluorouracil, tamoxifen, and Halotestin (CAFTH) with or without radiation. With a median follow-up of 3.1 years, a significant reduction in the incidence of local-regional recurrence was observed with radiation without a survival or disease-free survival benefit.

The magnitude of the survival benefit from the addition of postmastectomy radiation to adjuvant chemotherapy in patients with four or more positive nodes or with primary tumors ≥5 cm can be calculated. Without radiation approximately 25% to 30% of these patients will develop a local-regional recurrence (see Table 11-10). With the addition of adequate radiation the local-regional recurrence rate is approximately 10%.[42,44,74] Approximately 30% of the patients with local-regional control develop metastases and do not benefit from the prevention of a local-regional recurrence.[45] Therefore the overall survival benefit with radiation would be 10% to 14% (25% to 30% − 10% = 15% to 20% reduction in local-regional recurrence rates, 0.3 × 15% to 20% = 4.5% to 6% of patients who do not benefit from local-regional control, 15% to 20% − 4.5% to 6% = 10% to 14% total benefit). Assuming a 5-year survival of 50% in these patients (see Table 11-14) and a minimum follow-up of 3 years, a randomized trial comparing adjuvant chemotherapy with or without radiation in this subset of patients would require 328 patients in each arm to demonstrate a significant difference in survival of 10% to 14% with an alpha of .05 and beta of .2. The 14% improvement in the disease-free survival rate with radiation noted at 10 years in the SEG trial of patients with four or more postive nodes may not have achieved statistical significance because of the total sample size (295 patients).[74] The overall survival benefit of 18% to 31% was also not statistically significant. None of the completed randomized trials evaluating postmastectomy radiation in patients receiving adjuvant chemotherapy has had an adequate number of patients in this subset to demonstrate a significant advantage in terms of survival.

In summary, the results of prospective randomized trials evaluating postmastectomy adjuvant chemotherapy and radiation show no overall survival benefit in all patients. In selected subsets of patients there appears to be an improvement in the disease-free survival rates and in a single randomized trial there is evidence for a significant overall survival benefit for patients with operable T_3 primary tumors. Postmastectomy adjuvant radiotherapy should not be abandoned in all patients receiving adjuvant chemotherapy and is indicated in subsets of patients at high risk for local-regional recurrence. These patients can be defined as those with four or more positive nodes or primary tumors

Table 11-15 Results of prospective randomized trials comparing postmastectomy adjuvant chemotherapy (Chemo) with or without radiation (R) for operable T_3 breast cancer

	Helsinki[48,62]			ECOG[83]	
Treatment period	1976-1981			1982-1987	
No. pts.	119			332	
Chemotherapy	VAC ± levamisole			CAFTH	
	R	**Chemo and R**	**Chemo**	**Chemo**	**Chemo and R**
Survival (%)					
Overall	35	95	70	80	78
	[<.001]		[<.01]	[.76]	
Disease-free	25	67	33	61	69
		[<.001]		[.26]	
Follow-up (yr)	5			3.1 (median)	
Distant metastasis (%)	70	28	25	18	18
Local-regional recurrence (%)	18	13	58	16	7

[ ], p values for comparison.

≥5 cm and possibly patients with ER-negative tumors with one to three positive nodes[97] or high-grade node-negative patients.[54,104]

At the University of Pennsylvania, 63 patients with four or more positive nodes or with T_3 primary tumors received postmastectomy radiation and chemotherapy (CMF with or without prednisone or CAF) from 1977 to 1986. The mean and median numbers of positive nodes were 10 and 8 respectively. The median follow-up from the time of surgery was 44 months (range 2 to 116). Radiation was directed to the chest wall and regional nodes. The chest wall received 5000 cGy in 5 weeks. Tissue equivalent bolus was used every other day. The regional nodes received 4400 to 5000 cGy in 4½ to 5 weeks. The internal mammary nodes were not treated routinely, and a direct photon beam field was never employed to treat these nodes. Radiotherapy followed completion of chemotherapy in the majority of patients, and was integrated with chemotherapy in 33%. The overall 5-year survival rate was 52%, with a no evidence of disease (NED) survival rate of 38%. The 5-year actuarial rate of an isolated local-regional recurrence was 4%.

EFFECT OF TAMOXIFEN ON LOCAL-REGIONAL CONTROL IN PATIENTS UNDERGOING MASTECTOMY

Several studies have suggested that the primary effect of tamoxifen is to decrease the incidence of local-regional recurrence. In the Stockholm trial,[91] 1407 postmenopausal women were entered between 1976 and 1984. High-risk patients, classified as those with positive axillary nodes and primary tumor size >3 cm, were randomized to tamoxifen and CMF, tamoxifen and radiation, radiation alone, or CMF alone. Low-risk patients, those with negative axillary nodes or primary tumors ≤3 cm, were randomized to tamoxifen vs. observation. The administration of tamoxifen resulted in a significant decrease in the rates of local-regional recurrence for all patients (13% vs. 8%, $p<.01$) and in both high-risk (20% vs. 13%, $p=.02$), and low-risk (9% vs. 5%, $p=.02$) patients. Tamoxifen therapy did not result in a significant decrease in the incidence of distant metastases in all patients, high-risk patients, or low-risk patients. There was no significant improvement in overall survival rates with tamoxifen; however, there was an improved incidence of relapse-free survival. In the Nolvadex Adjuvant Trial Organization (NATO) trial,[82] 1285 patients (age ≤75 years) were randomized to tamoxifen for 2 years or observation postmastectomy. With a median follow-up of 45 months, tamoxifen resulted in a significant decrease in the death rate and prolongation of the disease-free interval. However, the reduction in recurrence rates was greater for local-regional recurrence or new primary tumors (14% vs. 7%) as opposed to distant metastasis (18% vs. 15%). In the Scottish trial,[15] 1312 postmenopausal node-positive patients and all node-negative patients were randomized to tamoxifen therapy for 5 years vs. observation. The use of tamoxifen resulted in a significant improvement in relapse-free survival and overall survival rates; however, the reduction in rates of local-regional recurrence was greater than that for distant metastasis. For patients with negative axillary nodes, the incidence of local-regional recurrence was decreased from 14% to 7% with tamoxifen, whereas the risk of distant metastases was decreased from 10% to 8%. For node-positive patients, local-regional recurrence rates decreased from 23% to 11% with tamoxifen, and the risk of distant metastases decreased from 35% to 27%. In the Ludwig studies III and IV,[46] postmenopausal patients were randomized to observation vs. prednisone and tamoxifen. With a 4-year median follow-up, rates of local-regional recurrence decreased from 27% to 13%, but the chance of distant metastases decreased from 27% to 24%. Tamoxifen resulted in an improvement of disease-free survival rates but not overall survival rates.

The question arises as to whether either postmastectomy tamoxifen alone or tamoxifen combined with chemotherapy can result in a decrease in the risk of local-regional recurrence, thereby eliminating the need for adjuvant radiation. Two prospective randomized trials have evaluated the addition of tamoxifen to postmastectomy adjuvant radiation.[78,84,92] In the Danish Breast Cancer Group study 77C, 1937 postmenopausal women with positive axillary nodes or T_3 tumors were randomized to radiotherapy alone, radiation therapy and levamisole, or radiation therapy and tamoxifen.[84] The 9-year actuarial rate of local-regional recurrence was 17% in patients receiving radiation and 12% in patients receiving radiation and tamoxifen. In the Stockholm trial[92] 427 postmenopausal women with positive axillary nodes or primary tumor size >3 cm were randomized to postoperative radiotherapy, radiotherapy plus tamoxifen, CMF, or CMF plus tamoxifen. With a mean follow-up of 6.5 years, local-regional recurrence rates were 13% in patients receiving radiation only and 12% in those receiving radiation and tamoxifen. These two trials indicate a minimal benefit from adding tamoxifen to radiation in terms of local-regional recurrence. The Danish Breast Cancer Group in a second trial (82C) randomized 1347 postmenopausal women with positive axillary nodes or T_3 tumors to tamoxifen, radiation and tamoxifen, or CMF and tamoxifen,[84] The 4-year actuarial risk of a local-regional recurrence was 30% for tamoxifen, 23% for CMF and tamoxifen, and 5% for radiation and tamoxifen. This trial suggests that tamoxifen alone is inadequate in preventing local-regional recurrence in this group of patients. In the NSABP B-16[39] trial, node-positive breast cancer patients ≥50 years of age were randomized to tamoxifen for 5 years vs. tamoxifen and chemotherapy. All patients had "tamoxifen responsive" tumors, i.e., age 50 to 59 years and progesterone receptor–positive tumors or age ≥60 years. Chemotherapy consisted of L-PAM and 5-fluorouracil with or without Adriamycin or Adriamycin and cyclophosphamide. The chest wall recurrence rate at 3 years was 3% in the tamoxifen group, compared to 1.6% in the chemotherapy and tamoxifen group. Fifty-four percent of the patients had one to three positive nodes. This study suggests that in postmastectomy patients the addition of chemotherapy to tamoxifen decreases the incidence of chest wall recurrence. The results of prospective randomized trials evaluating the addition of tamoxifen to adjuvant systemic chemotherapy are presented in Table 11-16. While two of the studies[40,92] suggest a benefit in terms of local-regional control for patients receiving tamoxifen in addition to adjuvant systemic chemotherapy, the majority of the studies demonstrate no significant benefit. Rao et al.,[87] in a retrospective review, reported a local-regional recurrence rate of 17% in patients who received L-PAM and 5-fluorouracil and 17% in patients who received L-PAM, 5-fluorouracil, and tamoxifen, with a median follow-up of 5.2 years. A separate analysis for high-risk patients is not available. The present data would therefore suggest that tamoxifen either alone or with adjuvant chemotherapy will not obviate the need for postmastectomy radiation when indicated.

INTEGRATION OF POSTMASTECTOMY ADJUVANT CHEMOTHERAPY AND RADIATION

It has been suggested by some[7,53,68] that postmastectomy radiation may compromise the ability to deliver adjuvant systemic chemotherapy. This may be related to the dose of radiation delivered to the thoracic spine from a direct or angled photon beam field directed to the internal mammary nodes,[68] or may be related to radiation of the mediastinum and circulating blood resulting in a decrease in the peripheral leukocyte count, especially the lymphocytes.[10] Studies that have not employed a direct photon beam field to treat the internal mammary nodes have demonstrated no compromise in the ability to deliver appropriate doses of adjuvant systemic chemotherapy.[44,97] Therefore the radiotherapy technique may influence the ability to deliver optimal doses of chemotherapy, and in patients receiving adjuvant chemotherapy, direct photon beam irradiation of the internal mammary nodes should be avoided.

The optimal sequencing of radiation and chemotherapy remains to be determined. Klefstrom et al.[63] retrospectively reviewed a series of 40 patients who received postmastectomy chemotherapy consisting of six courses of FAC and radiotherapy from 1979 to 1981. The patients had primary T_2 or T_3 tumors and had positive axillary nodes. A significant increase in deaths was noted in the group of patients who received chemotherapy first as opposed to radiotherapy first. The incidence of local-regional recurrence was also increased in the group who received chemotherapy first. Brufman et al.[17] retrospectively reviewed 87 patients who received postmastectomy CMF for stage II breast cancer. The 7-year relapse-free survival rate was 77% for patients who received concurrent chemotherapy

Table 11-16 Incidence of local-regional recurrence in randomized trials of postmastectomy node-positive patients receiving adjuvant chemotherapy with or without tamoxifen

			Local-regional recurrence (%)		
Author	Chemotherapy	Menopausal status	Chemotherapy without tamoxifen	Chemotherapy with tamoxifen	Follow-up (yr)
Fisher et al.[40]	L-PAM, F		27	9	6
	L-PAM, AF		16	8	
Overgaard et al.[84]	CMF		24	33	4
Ingle et al.[57,58]	CFP	Premenopausal	17	16	5.3 (median)
		Postmenopausal	11	13	
Fowble et al.[45]	CMFP	Premenopausal	15	11	3
		Postmenopausal	15	11	3
Rutqvist et al.[92]	CMF	Postmenopausal	32	20	6.5 (mean)

C, cyclophosphamide; F, 5-fluorouracil; A, Adriamycin; P, prednisone; M, methotrexate.

and radiation, compared to 45% in patients who received sequential treatment. The relapse-free survival rate was 77% when chemotherapy was delivered first, compared to 42% when radiotherapy was given first. The Southeastern Cancer Group[68] demonstrated no decrease in survival rates by delaying chemotherapy until after completion of postmastectomy radiation in patients with four or more positive nodes. Stefanik et al.[95] reported only a single local-regional recurrence occurring during chemotherapy given postmastectomy. Chemotherapy consisted of six cycles of CMF. Griem et al.[47] reported only two local-regional recurrences occurring during chemotherapy in a group of 100 patients with four or more positive nodes. However, in both of these series 20% to 28% of the patients who developed a local-regional recurrence did so during adjuvant chemotherapy. A delay of 6 months for adjuvant chemotherapy probably does not increase the risk of local-regional recurrence. There is conflicting data regarding the optimal sequencing, with a single study[17] suggesting that concurrent chemotherapy and radiotherapy resulted in an improved relapse-free survival rate when compared to sequential treatment. The same study suggested that, for patients receiving sequential treatment, it was better to deliver chemotherapy first, whereas a second study[63] suggested that radiotherapy delivered first resulted in improved survival and a decreased local-regional recurrence rate. In patients with a high risk for local-regional recurrence but an even greater risk of distant metastasis, i.e., those with eight or more positive nodes, radiotherapy should be delayed until the completion of chemotherapy. In patients in whom the risk of a local-regional recurrence equals that of a distant metastasis, i.e., those with four to seven positive nodes or with T_3 primary tumors, an initial three to four cycles of chemotherapy followed by radiotherapy with concurrent chemotherapy and then completion of chemotherapy may be an appropriate alternative.

SUMMARY

Patients who are at high risk for local-regional recurrence following radical or modified radical mastectomy are those with T_3 primary tumors or four or more positive nodes. In patients with negative axillary nodes, higher histologic grade also may increase the risk of local-regional recurrence. Young women also appear to have a greater risk of local-regional recurrence following mastectomy. Postmastectomy radiotherapy in high-risk patients results in local-regional recurrence rates of $\leq 10\%$. Despite adjuvant systemic chemotherapy, patients with T_3 primary tumors or four or more positive nodes continue to manifest a high risk of local-regional recurrence. Patients with estrogen receptor–negative tumors and one to three positive axillary nodes also may have an increased risk of local-regional recurrence. Tamoxifen may or may not decrease the risk of local-regional recurrence in patients receiving adjuvant chemotherapy. The potential for a survival benefit from combining adjuvant chemotherapy and radiation exists only in the group of patients where the risk of a local-regional recurrence equals or approaches that of distant metastases. This group has been identified as patients with four to seven positive nodes and those with T_3 primary tumors. Multiple prospective randomized trials evaluating postmastectomy adjuvant chemotherapy with or without radiation have failed to show a survival benefit despite a decrease in local-regional recurrence rates and a significant improvement in disease-free survival in some. These findings are explained readily by the fact that many low-risk patients were included in the trials, and only in a single trial was entry restricted to patients with four or more positive nodes.[74] Two prospective randomized trials have evaluated the role of postmastectomy adjuvant chemotherapy with or without radiation for operable T_3 breast cancer. One of the trials has demonstrated a significant improvement in disease-free and overall survival rates. Postmastectomy radiation should not be employed in all patients receiving adjuvant chemotherapy but should be restricted to those at high risk for local-regional recurrence despite adjuvant chemotherapy.

REFERENCES

1. Aberizk WJ, Silver B, Henderson C, et al: The use of radiotherapy for treatment of isolated locoregional recurrence of breast carcinoma after mastectomy, Cancer 58:1214, 1986.
2. Ahlborn TN, Gump FE, Bodian C, et al: Tumor to fascia margin as a factor in local recurrence after modified radical mastectomy, Surg Gynecol Obstet 166:523, 1988.
3. Ahmann DL, O'Fallon JR, Scanlon PW, et al: A preliminary assessment of factors associated with recurrent disease in a surgical adjuvant clinical trial for patients with breast cancer with special emphasis on the agressiveness of therapy, Am J Clin Oncol 5:371, 1982.
4. Allen H, Brooks R, Jones SE, et al: Adjuvant treatment for Stage II (node positive) breast cancer with adramycin-cyclophosphamide (AC) and radiotherapy (XRT). In Salmon SE and Jones SE, editors: Adjuvant therapy of cancer III, New York, 1981, Grune & Stratton, pp 453-462.
5. Auquier A, Rutqvist LE, Host H, et al: Postmastectomy megavoltage radiation: the Oslo and Stockholm randomized trials. Proceedings of the 17th International Congress of Radiation Oncology, Paris, July 1989, p 47 (abstract).
6. Baker RR, Montague AC, and Childs JN: A comparison of modified radical mastectomy to radical mastectomy in the treatment of operable breast cancer, Ann Surg 189:553, 1979.
7. Banerjee RK, Hoehn JL, Greenlaw RH, and Jacoby C:

Chemotherapy drug dose alteration due to radiation therapy in an adjuvant situation in breast cancer, Am J Clin Oncol 7:437, 1984.
8. Bartelink H, Borger JH, van Dongen JA, and Peterse JL: The impact of tumor size and histology on local control after breast-conserving therapy, Radiother Oncol 11:297, 1988.
9. Beadle GF and Harris JR: The role of post-operative radiotherapy in the treatment of operable breast cancer, Breast Cancer Res Treat 4:159, 1984.
10. Bedwinek J: Adjuvant irradiation for early breast cancer. An ongoing controversy, Cancer 53:729, 1984.
11. Bedwinek JM, Lee J, Fineberg B, and Ocwieza M: Prognostic indicators in patients with isolated local-regional recurrence of breast cancer, Cancer 47:2232, 1981.
12. Berstock DA, Houghton J, Haybittle J, and Baum M: The role of radiotherapy following total mastectomy for patients with early breast cancer, World J Surg 9:667, 1985.
13. Biran S, Brufman G, Robinson E, et al: Ten-year results of a National Cooperative Trial of chemotherapy with and without radiotherapy for stage II breast cancer, Proc Am Soc Clin Oncol 7:40, 1988 (abstract).
14. Bonadonna G, Valagussa P, Tancini G, et al: Current status of Milan adjuvant chemotherapy trials for node-positive and node-negative breast cancer, NCI Monogr 1:45, 1986.
15. Breast Cancer Trials Committee: Adjuvant tamoxifen in the management of operable breast cancer: the Scottish trial, Lancet ii:171, 1987.
16. Brinkley D, Haybittle JL, and Houghton J: The Cancer Research Campaign (King's/Cambridge) trial for early breast cancer: an analysis of the radiotherapy data, Br J Radiol 57:309, 1984.
17. Brufman G, Sulkes A, and Biran S: Effect of timing of onset of chemotherapy on relapse-free survival in stage II breast cancer, Proc Am Soc Clin Oncol 5:62, 1986 (abstract).
18. Buzdar AU, Blumenshein GR, Smith TL, et al: Adjuvant chemotherapy with fluorouracil, doxorubicin and cyclophosphamide, with or without irradiation in operable breast cancer. A prospective randomized trial, Cancer 53:384, 1984.
19. Buzdar AU, McNeese MD, Hortobagyi GN, et al: Is chemotherapy effective in reducing the local failure rate in patients with operable breast cancer? Cancer 65:394, 1990.
20. Buzdar AU, Smith TL, Blumenschein GR, et al: Breast cancer adjuvant therapy trials of MD Anderson Hospital: results of two studies. In Jones SE and Salmon SE, editors: Adjuvant therapy of cancer IV, Orlando, 1984, Grune & Stratton, pp 217-225.
21. Caffier H, Rofte K, and Haeggquist O: Adjuvant chemotherapy versus post-operative irradiation in node negative breast cancer. In Salmon SE and Jones SE, editors: Adjuvant therapy of cancer IV, Orlando, 1984, Grune & Stratton, pp 417-424.
22. Cancer Research Campaign: Management of early breast cancer of the breast. Report of an international multicentre trial, Brit Med J 1:1035, 1976.
23. Cancer Research Campaign Working Party: Cancer Research Campaign (King's/Cambridge) trial for early breast cancer—a detailed update at the tenth year, Lancet ii:55, 1980.
24. Chu AM and Kiel K: Comparison of adjuvant postoperative radiotherapy and multiple-drug chemotherapy (CMF-VP) in operable breast cancer patients with more than four positive axillary lymph nodes, Cancer 50:212, 1982.
25. Crile G: Results of conservative treatment of breast cancer at 10 and 15 years, Ann Surg 181:26, 1975.
26. Crowe JP Jr, Gordon NH, Shenk RR, et al: Local-regional failure after mastectomy: results of a prospective trial, Proc Am Soc Clin Oncol 9:24, 1990 (abstract).
27. Cuzick J, Stewart H, Peto H, et al: Overview of randomized trials of postoperative adjuvant radiotherapy in breast cancer, Cancer Treat Rep 71:15, 1987.
28. Dao TL and Nemoto T: The clinical significance of skin recurrence after radical mastectomy in women with cancer of the breast, Surg Obstet Gynecol 117:447, 1963.
29. Deck KB and Kern WH: Local recurrence of breast cancer, Arch Surg 111:323, 1976.
30. Dombernowsky P, Brincker H, Hansen M, et al: Adjuvant therapy of premenopausal and menopausal high-risk breast cancer patients. Present status of the Danish Breast Cancer Cooperative Group Trials 77B and 82B. Acta Oncol 27:691, 1988.
31. Donegan WL, Perez-Mesa CM, and Watson RF: A biostatistical study of locally recurrent breast carcinoma, Surg Gynecol Obstet 122:529, 1966.
32. Easson EC: Post-operative radiotherapy in breast cancer. In Forrest APM and Kunkler PB, editors: Prognostic factors in breast cancer, Edinburgh, 1968, E&S Livingstone, Ltd, pp 118-135.
33. Elston CW, Gresham GA, Rao GS, et al: The Cancer Research Campaign (King's/Cambridge) Trial for Early Breast Cancer: clinico-pathologic aspects, Br J Cancer 45:655, 1982.
34. Ferguson DJ, Meier P, Karrison T, et al: Staging of breast cancer and survival rates. An assessment based on 50 years of experience with radical mastectomy, JAMA 248:1337, 1982.
35. Fisher B, Fisher ER, and Redmond C: Ten-year results from the National Surgical Adjuvant Breast and Bowel Project (NSABP) clinical trial evaluating the use of L-phenylalanine mustard (L-PAM) in the management of primary breast cancer, J Clin Oncol 4:929, 1986.
36. Fisher B, Montague E, Redmond C, et al: Findings from NSABP protocol no. B-04—comparison of radical mastectomy with alternative treatments for primary breast cancer. I. Radiation compliance and its relation to treatment outcome, Cancer 46:1, 1980.
37. Fisher B, Redmond C, Dimitrov NV, et al: A randomized clinical trial evaluating sequential methotrexate and fluorouracil in the treatment of patients with node-negative breast cancer who have estrogen-receptor-negative tumors, N Engl J Med 320:473, 1989.
38. Fisher B, Redmond C, Fisher ER, et al: Ten year results of a randomized clinical trial comparing radical mastectomy and total mastectomy with or without radiation, N Engl J Med 312:674, 1985.
39. Fisher B, Redmond C, Legault-Poisson S, et al: Post-operative chemotherapy and tamoxifen compared with tamoxifen alone in the treatment of positive-node breast cancer patients aged 50 years and older with tumors responsive to tamoxifen: results from the National Surgical Adjuvant Breast and Bowel Project B-16, J Clin Oncol 8:1005, 1990.
40. Fisher B, Redmond C, Wickerham DL, et al: Doxorubicin-containing regimens for the treatment of stage II breast cancer: the National Surgical Adjuvant Breast and Bowel Project experience, J Clin Oncol 7:572, 1989.
41. Fisher B, Slack NH, Cavanaugh PJ, et al: Post-operative radiotherapy in the treatment of breast cancer: results of the NSABP clinical trial, Ann Surg 172:711, 1970.
42. Fletcher GH, McNeese MD, and Oswald MJ: Long-range results for breast cancer patients treated by radical mastectomy and postoperative radiation without adjuvant chemotherapy: an update, Int J Radiat Oncol Biol Phys 17:11, 1989.
43. Forrest APM, Stewart JH, Roberts MM, and Steele RJC: Simple mastectomy and axillary node sampling (pectoral

node biopsy) in the management of primary breast cancer, Ann Surg 196:371, 1982.
44. Fowble B, Glick J, and Goodman R: Radiotherapy for the prevention of local-regional recurrence in high risk patients post mastectomy receiving adjuvant chemotherapy, Int J Radiat Oncol Biol Phys 15:627, 1988.
45. Fowble B, Gray R, Gilchrist K, et al: Identification of a subgroup of patients with breast cancer and histologically positive axillary nodes receiving adjuvant chemotherapy who may benefit from postoperative radiotherapy. J Clin Oncol 6:1107, 1988.
46. Goldhirsch A and Gelber R: Adjuvant treatment for early breast cancer: the Ludwig breast cancer studies. Proceedings of the NIH Consensus Development Conference on Adjuvant Chemotherapy and Endocrine Therapy for Breast Cancer, Bethesda, MD, 1986, National Cancer Institute, pp 55-70.
47. Griem K, Henderson IC, Gelman R, et al: Post-operative radiotherapy after adjuvant chemotherapy in breast cancer patients: results of a randomized trial, J Clin Oncol 5:1546, 1987.
48. Grohn P, Heinonen E, Klefstrom P, and Tarkkanen J: Adjuvant postoperative radiotherapy, chemotherapy, and immunotherapy in stage III breast cancer, Cancer 54:670, 1984.
49. Haagensen CD: Results with Halsted's radical mastectomy. In Haagensen CD, editor: Diseases of the breast, ed 3, Philadelphia, 1986, WB Saunders Co, pp 903-932.
50. Haagensen CD and Cooley E: Radical mastectomy for mammary carcinoma, Ann Surg 170:884, 1969.
51. Handley RS and Thackray AC: Conservative radical mastectomy (Patey's operation), Ann Surg 170:880, 1969.
52. Haybittle JL, Brinkley D, Houghton J, et al: Postoperative radiotherapy and late mortality: evidence from the Cancer Research Campaign trial for early breast cancer, Br Med J 298:1611, 1989.
53. Holland TF and Glidewell O: Adverse effect of radiotherapy on adjuvant chemotherapy for carcinoma of the breast, Surg Gynecol Obstet 150:817, 1980.
54. Hopton DS, Thorogood J, Clayden AD, and MacKinnon D: Histologic grading of breast cancer: significance of grade on recurrence and mortality, Eur J Surg Oncol 15:25, 1989.
55. Host H, Brennhoud IO, and Loeb M: Post-operative radiotherapy in breast cancer—long term results from the Oslo study, Int J Radiat Oncol Biol Phys 12:727, 1986.
56. Howell A, George WD, Crowther D, et al: Controlled trial of adjuvant chemotherapy with cyclophosphamide, methotrexate, and fluorouracil for breast cancer, Lancet ii:307, 1984.
57. Ingle JN, Everson LK, Wieand S, et al: Randomized trial to evaluate the addition of tamoxifen to cyclosphosphamide, 5 fluorouracil, prednisone adjuvant therapy in premenopausal women with node-positive breast cancer, Cancer 63:1257, 1989.
58. Ingle JN, Everson LK, Wieand HS, et al: Randomized trial of observation versus adjuvant therapy with cyclophosphamide, fluorouracil, prednisone with or without tamoxifen following mastectomy in postmenopausal women with node-positive breast cancer, J Clin Oncol 6:1388, 1988.
59. Janjan JA, McNeese MD, Buzdar AU, et al: Management of locoregional recurrence of breast cancer, Cancer 58:1552, 1986.
60. Jones JM and Ribeiro GG: Mortality patterns over 34 years of breast cancer patients in a clinical trial of post-operative radiotherapy, Clin Radiol 40:204, 1989.
61. Kaae S and Johansen H: Does simple mastectomy followed by irradiation offer survival comparable to radical procedures? Int J Radiat Oncol Biol Phys 2:1163, 1977.
62. Klefstrom P, Grohn P, Heinonen E, et al: Adjuvant postoperative radiotherapy, chemotherapy and immunotherapy in stage III breast cancer, Cancer 60:936, 1987.
63. Klefstrom P, Nuortio L, and Taskinen E: Postoperative radiation therapy and adjuvant chemoimmunotherapy in breast cancer. Aspects of timing and immune competence, Acta Radiol 25:161, 1986.
64. Koyama H, Wada T, Takahashi Y, et al: Surgical adjuvant chemotherapy with mitomycin C and cyclophosphamide in Japanese patients with breast cancer, Cancer 46:2373, 1980.
65. Langlands AO, Prescott RJ, and Hamilton T: A clinical trial in the management of operable cancer of the breast, Br J Surg 67:170, 1980.
66. Lee RO and Lambley DG: Radical mastectomy in the treatment of breast cancer, Br J Surg 58:137, 1971.
67. Lee YN: Breast carcinoma: patterns of recurrence and metastasis after mastectomy, Am J Clin Oncol 7:443, 1984.
68. Levine TF, Coleman CM, Cot RS, et al: The effect of post-operative and primary radiation therapy in delivered dose of adjuvant cyclophosphamide, methotrexate and 5-fluorouracil (CMF) chemotherapy in breast cancer, Cancer 53:237, 1984.
69. Levitt SH, McHugh RB, and Song CW: Radiotherapy in the post-operative treatment of operable cancer of the breast. II. A reexamination of Stjernsward's application of the Mantel-Haenszel statistical method. Evaluation of the effect of radiation on immune response and suggestions for post-operative radiotherapy, Cancer 39:933, 1976.
70. Lythgoe JP, Leck I, and Swindell R: Manchester regional breast study. Preliminary results. Lancet i:744, 1978.
71. Lythgoe JP and Palmer MK: Manchester regional breast study: 5 and 10 year results, Br J Surg 69:693, 1982.
72. Maddox WA, Carpenter JT, Laws HL, et al: A randomized prospective trial of radical (Halsted) mastectomy versus modified radical mastectomy in 311 breast cancer patients, Ann Surg 198:207, 1983.
73. Magno L, Bignardi M, Micheletti E, et al: Analysis of prognostic factors in patients with isolated chest wall recurrence of breast cancer, Cancer 60:240, 1987.
74. Marcial VA, Velez-Garcia E, Bartolucci A, and Carpenter JT: Comparison of adjuvant chemotherapy versus locoregional radiotherapy followed by adjuvant chemotherapy in breast cancer patients with 4 or more positive axillary nodes. A Southeastern Cancer Study Group study, Int J Radiat Oncol Biol Phys 17:180, 1989 (abstract).
75. Martinez A, Ahmann D, O'Fallon J, et al: An interim analysis of the randomized surgical adjuvant trial for patients with unfavorable breast cancer, Int J Radiat Oncol Biol Phys 10(suppl 2):150, 1985 (abstract).
76. Mathews RH, McNeese M, Montague ED, and Oswald NJ: Prognostic implications of age in breast cancer patients treated with tumorectomy and irradiation or with mastectomy, Int J Radiat Oncol Biol Phys 14:659, 1988.
77. McArdle CS, Crawford D, Dykes EH, et al: Adjuvant radiotherapy and chemotherapy in breast cancer, Br J Surg 73:264, 1986.
78. Mouridsen HT, Rose C, Overgaard M, et al: Adjuvant treatment of postmenopausal patients with high risk primary breast cancer. Results from the Danish adjuvant trials DBCG 77C and DBCG 82C, Acta Oncol 27:699, 1988.
79. Muss H, Cooper R, Brockschmidt J, et al: A randomized trial of adjuvant chemotherapy (CT) with and without radiation therapy (RT) for stage II breast cancer: 11 year follow-up of Piedmont Oncology Association Protocol 74176, Breast Cancer Res Treat 14:185, 1989 (abstract).

80. Muss H, Cooper R, Ferree C, et al: Long-term follow-up of L-PAM and CMF with and without radiation therapy as adjuvant treatment for stage II breast carcinoma, Proc Am Soc Clin Oncol 3:117, 1984.
81. Nime FA, Rosen PP, Thaler HT, et al: Prognostic significance of tumor emboli in intramammary lymphatics in patients with mammary carcinoma, Am J Surg Pathol 1:25, 1977.
82. Novaldex Adjuvant Trial Organization: Controlled trial of tamoxifen as single adjuvant agent in management of early breast cancer. Analysis at six years by Nolvadex Adjuvant Trial Organization, Lancet i:836, 1985.
83. Olson JE, Neuberg D, Pandya K, et al: The management of resectable stage III breast cancer. The Eastern Cooperative Oncology Group Trial, Proc Am Soc Clin Oncol 8:23, 1989 (abstract).
84. Overgaard M, Christensen JJ, Johansen H, et al: Postmastectomy irradiation in high risk breast cancer patients. Present status of the Danish Breast Cancer Cooperative Group trials, Acta Oncol 27:707, 1988.
85. Palmer MK and Ribeiro GG: Thirty-four year follow-up of patients with breast cancer in clinical trial of postoperative radiotherapy, Br Med J 291:1088, 1985.
86. Ragaz J, Jackson S, Wilson K, et al: Randomized study of locoregional radiotherapy (XRT) and ovarian ablation in premenopausal patients with breast cancer treated with adjuvant chemotherapy, Proc Am Soc Clin Oncol 7:12, 1988 (abstract).
87. Rao AF, Murthy AK, Hendrickson FR, et al: Analysis of risk factors for loco-regional failure in Stage II breast carcinoma treated with mastectomy and adjunctive chemotherapy, Int J Radiat Oncol Biol Phys 11(suppl 1):151, 1985.
88. Rivkin SE, Green S, Metch B, et al: Adjuvant CMFVP versus melphalan for operable breast cancer with positive axillary nodes: 10 year results of a Southwest Oncology Group study, J Clin Oncol 7:1229, 1989.
89. Rosenman J, Bernard S, Kober C, et al: Local recurrences in patients with breast cancer at the North Carolina Memorial Hospital (1970-82), Cancer 57:1421, 1986.
90. Rubens RD, Knight RK, Fentiman IS, et al: Controlled trial of adjuvant chemotherapy with melphalan for breast cancer, Lancet i:839, 1983.
91. Rutqvist LE, Cedermark B, Fornanader T, et al: The relationship between hormone receptor content and the effect of adjuvant tamoxifen in operable breast cancer, J Clin Oncol 7:1474, 1989.
92. Rutqvist LE, Cedermark B, Glas U, et al: Randomized trial of adjuvant tamoxifen combined with post-operative radiotherapy or adjuvant chemotherapy in postmenopausal breast cancer, Cancer 66:89, 1990.
93. Rutqvist LE, Cedermark B, Glas U, et al: Radiotherapy, chemotherapy and tamoxifen as adjuncts to surgery in early breast cancer: a summary of three randomized trials, Int J Radiat Oncol Biol Phys 15:629, 1989.
94. Smith DC, Crawford D, Dykes EH, et al: Adjuvant radiotherapy and chemotherapy in breast cancer. In Jones SE and Salmon SE, editors: Adjuvant therapy of cancer IV, Orlando, 1984, Grune & Stratton, pp 283-289.
95. Stefanik D, Goldberg R, Bryne P, et al: Local-regional failure in patients treated with adjuvant chemotherapy for breast cancer, J Clin Oncol 3:660, 1985.
96. Stjernsward J: Decreased survival related to irradiation post-operatively in early operable breast cancer, Lancet ii:1285, 1974.
97. Sulkes A, Brufman G, Rizel S, et al: The effect of post-operative radiotherapy on the feasibility of optimal dose adjuvant CMF chemotherapy in stage II breast carcinoma, Int J Radiat Oncol Biol Phys 9:17, 1983.
98. Sykes HF, Sim DA, Wong CJ, et al: Local-regional recurrences in breast cancer after mastectomy and Adriamycin-based adjuvant chemotherapy: evaluation of the role of postoperative radiotherapy, Int J Radiat Oncol Biol Phys 16:641, 1989.
99. Toonkel LM, Fix I, Jacobson LH, et al: Post-operative radiation therapy for carcinoma of the breast: improved results with elective irradiation of the chest wall, Int J Radiat Oncol Biol Phys 8:977, 1982.
100. Tormey DC, Weinberg VE, Holland JF, et al: A randomized trial of five and three drug chemotherapy and chemoimmunotherapy in women with operable node positive breast cancer, J Clin Oncol 1:138, 1983.
101. Turnbull AR, Chant ADB, Buchanan RB, et al: Treatment of early breast cancer, Lancet ii:7, 1978.
102. Valagussa P, Bonadonna G, and Veronesi U: Patterns of relapse and survival following radical mastectomy. Analysis of 716 consecutive patients, Cancer 41:1170, 1978.
103. Wallgren A, Arner O, Bergstrom J, et al: Radiation therapy in operable breast cancer: results from the Stockholm trial on adjuvant radiotherapy, Int J Radiat Oncol Biol Phys 12:533, 1986.
104. Williams MR, Hinton CP, Todd JH, et al: The prediction of local or regional recurrence after simple mastectomy for operable breast cancer, Br J Surg 72:721, 1985.
105. Wood WC, Weiss RB, Tormey DC, et al: A randomized trial of CMF versus CMFVP as adjuvant chemotherapy in women with node-positive stage II breast cancer. A CALGB Study, World J Surg 9:714, 1985.

12 Reconstructive Surgery

Don LaRossa

Almost 100 years ago Halsted espoused his principles for the management of breast carcinoma with the radical mastectomy procedure.[23] The concept of radical mastectomy has been accepted widely and slow to change. It has been only in the last 50 years that the modified radical mastectomy gradually was embraced as an adequate treatment.[33,42] By 1977 only 22% of women underwent radical mastectomies for treatment of their breast cancer.[53] Only in the last 10 to 15 years have less radical procedures such as the total mastectomy been recognized as being acceptable choices for therapy in selected patients. With such a tradition of radical surgical therapy, it is understandable that the concept of breast reconstruction being part of the surgical treatment of breast cancer has evolved only recently. Fueled by a better understanding of the varying biologic behavior of different histologic types of breast cancer, surgical treatment has become less radical. Adjuvant chemotherapy has become more effective. Early detection through enhanced public awareness programs and mammography may result in longer survival for affected women. In this milieu were parallel developments in breast implant technology, skin and skin muscle flap anatomy and physiology, and a greater emphasis on the quality of life. The setting was ripe for the introduction and development of breast reconstruction as part of the complete surgical treatment of the breast cancer patient.

In 1896 Tansini called for attention to the cosmetic outcome from these radical procedures that already had produced good surgical results.[55] His admonitions were not well received at a time when a radical surgical approach was being proposed. In the 1960s there were scattered reports of complicated methods of breast reconstruction using local skin flaps, as well as multistaged procedures using tubed pedicle flaps from the abdomen. These latter methods often were cumbersome, time consuming, or did not produce good results consistently. Hence only the most committed candidates would volunteer for these earlier operations.

Two key events in the evolution of breast reconstruction were the introduction of silicone gel mammary prostheses in 1964 and the description of myocutaneous flaps.[11,38] Although initially used for breast augmentation, silicone implants subsequently were used for breast reconstruction, providing a simpler method with more predictable results. Plastic surgeons already had extensive experience in the use of silicone implants, giving impetus to the field and leading to a broader acceptance by both patients and their treating physicians. The results were not ideal in all cases, nor were all patients candidates for implant-type reconstructions. Reconstructive surgeons sought better solutions through the use of skin muscle flaps and, finally, free tissue transfers in an attempt to create the most natural appearing breasts possible.

The earliest attempts at breast reconstruction were aimed at producing a breast mound that would "look good in clothing."[51] Symmetry, texture, and detail were refinements that had not yet evolved. The next phase of development focused on these refinements in an attempt to create a neobreast that would approximate the natural one more closely. Surgeons focused on nipple and areolar reconstruction and the creation of an inframammary fold and attempts at producing a softer, more ptotic breast. Changes in gel implant technology aimed at reducing capsular contracture and maintaining softness in the reconstructed breast were developed. Sophisticated techniques of flap reconstruction were devised to move tissue composites from the back (latissimus dorsi skin muscle flaps) or abdomen (transverse rectus abdominus skin muscle flaps; TRAM) in an attempt to provide more soft tissue cover or implant-free reconstructions.[7,24,38,48]

Most recently, microsurgical techniques have been used to rebuild a breast solely from autogenous tissue from the buttock (gluteus free flap), abdomen (TRAM flap), and lateral thigh (lateral thigh free flap), capitalizing on the most advanced and sophisticated methods of soft tissue transfer and reconstruction.[15,18,49]

The timing of breast reconstruction also has changed drastically. Initially, only secondary reconstructions were acceptable because of concern about instigating or hiding recurrences. Through a better understanding of the biology of breast cancer and by scrutinizing the potential adverse effects of breast reconstruction, it became evident that neither of these concerns had any scientific basis, and waiting times were shortened.[44] Now, simultaneous reconstruction is gaining widespread acceptance by surgeons, oncologists, and patients. Psychologic studies support early reconstruction as well.[47,54]

Though still in its infancy, the concept of breast reconstruction is taking its place in the total surgical management of the breast cancer patient. Further investigation, creative effort by reconstructive plastic surgeons, and advances in implant technology will enhance future results.

TIMING OF BREAST RECONSTRUCTION

As experience was gained with breast reconstruction the time delay between mastectomy and reconstruction has become shorter. Initially a 2-year waiting period was advised, whereas today many reconstructions are done simultaneous with the mastectomy.[19,26,27,40,57] Timing should be guided by adherence to the highest standards of good oncologic management. Delay is warranted where adjuvant chemotherapy and/or radiation therapy is anticipated, because wound healing complications may delay the start of either of those modalities. There should be a 3- to 6-month delay following completion of chemotherapy to allow the white blood cell count, tissue response, and wound healing metabolism to stabilize. Likewise, healing, stabilization, and softening of the skin should be attained before reconstruction is undertaken following radiation.

Flap reconstructions more commonly are done as secondary procedures because of the length of the operations and the need for patient repositioning to obtain latissimus dorsi flaps and free microvascular gluteus flaps during the operation. However, it is possible for all flap procedures to be performed simultaneously with mastectomy. Operating times can be shortened when a two-team approach is used.

While it was suggested initially by some surgeons that a woman should live with her mastectomy scar so as to better appreciate a less than perfect reconstruction, there is good evidence to support the psychologic benefits of immediate reconstruction.[47,54]

Additional benefits of immediate reconstruction are the potential for a single operation instead of two major procedures, reduced hospitalization and costs, and a shortened period of rehabilitation.[19,26,27,40,57] (See Fig. 12-1.)

PATIENT SELECTION

Like timing, candidacy for breast reconstruction has changed. Whereas only the lowest-risk patients with a good chance for survival were candidates initially, now virtually all patients with breast cancer may be considered. Indeed, selected high-risk patients and some with known metastases may benefit from reconstruction. Implants do not impair the body defenses against cancer.[44] Nor do implants hide local recurrences, as the implant lies deep to the pectoralis and serratus muscles where recurrences virtually never occur. There may be an increased risk of obscuring a recurrence in TRAM (free or pedicled), latissimus dorsi, or free tissue–type reconstruction where a thick soft tissue pad

A

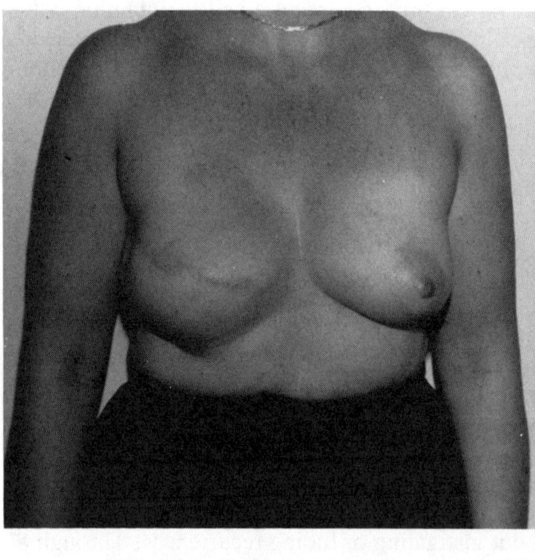

B

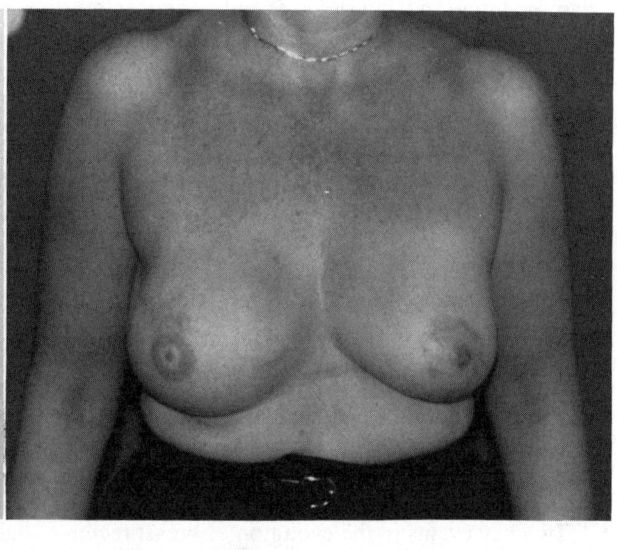

Fig. 12-1 A, Photograph of a patient following immediate reconstruction with a silicone gel prosthesis. **B,** Secondary nipple reconstruction performed 6 months later.

is placed superficial to the pectoralis. Additionally, areas of fat necrosis or fibrosis in pedicled TRAM flaps may masquerade as tumor nodules, occasionally prompting biopsy.

Age is not a factor per se. Instead, general health and the ability to undergo the procedure is the determinant. Older women can receive as much benefit as younger women. Our youngest patient is a 12-year-old girl who had juvenile secretory carcinoma, and our oldest patient was 72 years of age. Both were treated with tissue expansion techniques.

A general psychologic assessment must be included in patient selection. The loss or potential loss of a breast from cancer is a frightening event that women cope with in various ways and with varying degrees of success. Facing additional surgery to reconstruct a breast adds another dimension to the experience. Their preparedness for the reconstruction and its potential risks and their expectations of the final result must be evaluated carefully before the operation. A thorough description of the procedures, rehabilitation, and expected results will usually indicate which individuals are not prepared psychologically.

PRINCIPLES OF BREAST RECONSTRUCTION

Unlike most other mammals, the human has a single pair of breasts that remain fully developed throughout reproductive cycles. They are the symbol of femininity and consequently have received great attention in literature, graphic art, and sculpture. Reduced to its aesthetic essence, the breast is a mound on the chest wall. Ideally it has a nipple and areola affixed to its conical apex. Realistically it is soft, it has some degree of ptosis and an inframammary fold, and it is symmetrical with its mate.

The reconstructive surgeon faces the challenge of recreating this ideal, usually having the remaining normal breast to serve as a model to be emulated.

PHASES OF BREAST RECONSTRUCTION

Breast reconstruction can be divided into two phases. The first is creation of a breast mound and the second is the creation of symmetry. In a rudimentary way, creation of a breast mound is elemental to breast reconstruction. The method used depends on the quality and amount of skin, the size and shape of the opposite breast, and the patient's desires and goals. The patient's general health, age, and body habitus may be factors as well. The method selected may involve the use of an implant, tissue expander, flap transfer or a combination of one or more techniques.

The second phase is to create symmetry, lending realism to the neobreast. It may mean adding a nipple/areolar complex, repositioning or enlarging the breast mound, creating a better defined inframammary fold, or manipulating the remaining breast to match the reconstructed breast by making it smaller, less ptotic, or even larger. The first phase is essential to breast reconstruction, while the second phase is elective.

Phase 1: creation of a breast mound

Implanted prosthetic reconstruction. The simplest methods of creating a breast mound involve placement of a prosthetic implant beneath the skin and muscles of the chest wall. The earliest methods used coverage with only skin and subcutaneous fat, but the results were less than ideal.[51] The breast was subject to capsular contracture, resulting in a firm to hard texture. Without the softening effects of additional soft tissue coverage, these breasts often had a "stuck on, half-grapefruit" appearance. Additionally, they were more subject to exposure of the implant by erosion through the taut skin cover. By placing the implant beneath the pectoralis major and serratus muscles, the contour and texture were softened, resulting in a breast mound with a more natural appearance and feel.[13,14,27] A thicker protective cover had an added benefit, reducing the risk of erosion and implant exposure. Some surgeons have recommended complete muscle coverage of the implant.[13,27] Others favor muscle coverage of the upper portion of the breast, leaving the lower pole in the subcutaneous position.[14] This is the anatomic situation that often exists when secondary reconstructions are done, where the dissection begins in a subpectoral plane but enters the subcutaneous plane at the thinned inferior border of the pectoralis major muscle. We favor this latter technique as it seems to eventuate in the spontaneous development of an inframammary fold more frequently (see Fig. 12-2).

Mammary prostheses used in reconstructive surgery are made of the same materials as those used in augmentation mammoplasty. Five basic types of prostheses are used: saline inflatable silicon shell, gel-inflatable (inner gel and outer reservoir for saline with silicone skin), smooth-surfaced silicone gel, textured-surface silicone gel and polyurethane foam-covered silicone gel. This broad variety of implants has evolved in an attempt to reduce the incidence of capsular contracture, a poorly understood phenomenon of collagen metabolism that results in a breast with a firm to hard texture. Saline-filled implants result in soft breasts more often than smooth-surfaced gel implants, but have an inherent risk of deflation.[21] Smooth-surfaced gel implants have a recognized role in capsular contracture that

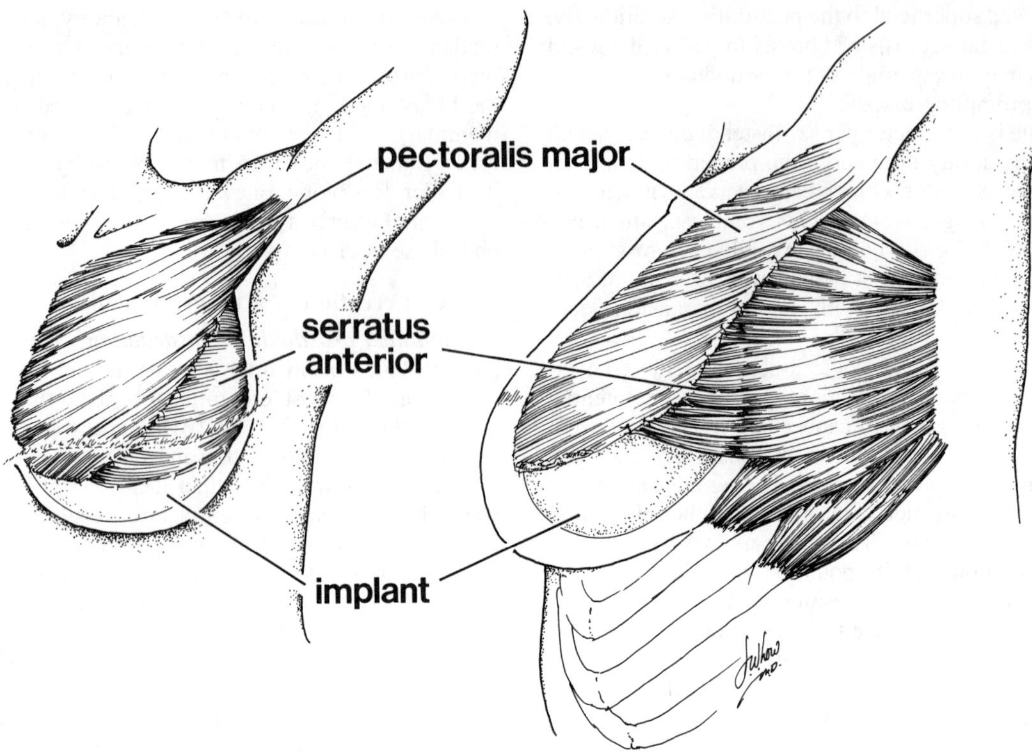

Fig. 12-2 Technique of partial submuscular coverage with pectoralis major-serratus anterior muscle flap. Inferior edge of muscle flap is sutured to the internal surface of the inferior skin flap below the anticipated level of the reconstructed nipple-areola complex. The inferior portion of the prosthesis is subcutaneous.

has been reduced by placement of the implant beneath the pectoralis muscle. Addition of steroids to the external reservoir of gel-inflatable silicone implants has resulted in softer breasts following augmentation mammoplasty, and trials are underway in reconstructive mammoplasty as well by Spear and Little.[52] In the past, others have abandoned the use of steroids because of poor results from thinning of the skin when steroid preparations were used. Manufacturers do not recommend the addition of any medication to the reservoir of gel-inflatable implants.

In an attempt to confuse and control the normal collagen formation and maturation process, silicone surfaces have been textured and polyurethane foam has been used to cover silicone gel implants. Breasts augmented or reconstructed with polyurethane-covered prostheses are softer and remain so for extended periods of time. Therefore some surgeons favor their use in breast reconstruction.[17] However, the composition and fate of the degraded material is unclear. Within 6 months of implant placement a crumbling of the polyurethane covering occurs. After 2 years the foam covering has separated completely from the gel prosthesis, leaving it free floating.[50] In the newer implants, most of the foam remains intact and attached to the gel by an adhesive.[9] Additionally, total removal of the foam material is difficult should an infection occur necessitating implant removal.

Uncertainty regarding these features has led to the development of textured-surface silicone gel prostheses. Long-term results are not available, but these prostheses seem to be a promising alternative.

Because reconstructed breasts do not have the same conical shape as natural breasts, the profile and consistency of gel implants have been modified in prostheses designed specifically for breast reconstruction. Their design is aimed at producing a higher profile or increased projection without sacrificing softness.[6]

The ideal requirements for a reconstructive breast prosthesis is that it be inert and maintain the consistency and texture of a natural breast in all patients. These demands have stimulated considerable research in the field that should be of benefit to future patients undergoing breast reconstruction using implant techniques.

Tissue expanders are an offshoot of implant technology. Originally developed as a means of increasing the amount of skin available for a variety of soft tissue reconstructive problems, they lent themselves quite naturally to breast reconstruction. They are particularly useful when skin is of good quality but of insufficient quantity to match the opposite normal breast, or when patients do not want to undergo more complex soft tissue transfer techniques such as the TRAM or latissimus dorsi flap procedures. Expanders used today in breast reconstruction are of two types: shell and gel-inflatable. The original expanders were of the shell type, composed of a hollow envelope of silicone.[2,40,43] Filling of the implant with injectable saline solution is done through a percutaneous injection into a buried filling port. Older styles such as the Radovan expander have a remote filling port connected by a Silastic tube to the expander. Newer styles contain the filler port within the implants, some with magnetic locating devices that guide the surgeon to the precise location of the valve. The advantage of the latter type of implants is that they are self-contained and more removable than older styles. The disadvantages are the potential risk of accidentally puncturing the expander, and the possibility of repeated needle punctures over the most tightly stretched skin, which may cause erosion of the implant through the skin. These considerations seem more theoretical than real. Other potential complications of expanders are infection, exposure of the implant, tubing, or valve, striae, malpositioning, and chest deformity from pressure[3] (see below).

Expanders are placed beneath the skin or skin and muscle of the chest and are inflated gradually over a period of weeks or months until a breast mound of satisfactory size has been created. The implant must be evacuated totally at the time of insertion because any residual air may cause a sloshing sound and a change in volume with air pressure changes. Saline can be added at surgery to whatever extent the mound and skin will tolerate. This makes expanders particularly useful in immediate or simultaneous reconstructions where poor wound healing of an incision line closed too tightly over an implant can result in exposure and loss of the prosthesis. Following a period of initial healing, inflation is done in the office with the addition of approximately 10% of the final expander volume at each visit. Injections usually are performed on a weekly basis, though more rapid expansion is possible. The process can be started from 1 to 3 weeks postoperatively, depending on the quality of the skin closure and the judgment of the surgeon. In an attempt to create a softer, more ptotic breast, additional soft tissue cover can be developed through overexpansion beyond the desired final breast size. Usually, an additional 30 to 400 ml are added in increments.[21,58] We generally use 150 to 200 ml of overexpansion. Although not recommended by the manufacturer, overexpansion beyond the volume of the Radovan expander can be achieved safely to at least fifteen times the vendor's stated volume.[22] Following overexpansion, the expander is removed and the excess skin is folded beneath the reconstructed breast using an internal or external approach to recreate an inframammary fold.[41,46,56] "Differential" expanders utilizing different shell thicknesses permit varying degrees of differential expansion within the same implant, giving a "breast shape" to the breast mound. Textured silicone vs. smooth-surfaced expanders also are being used in an attempt to reduce capsule formation.

COMPLICATIONS OF TISSUE EXPANSION

1. Infection
2. Exposure
3. Malpositioning
4. Chest deformity

Following the expansion process, shell-type expanders must be removed and replaced with a permanent prosthesis in a second surgical procedure. They are not meant to be permanent devices and eventually will rupture. In an attempt to reduce the number of surgical procedures, the gel-inflatable prosthesis has been developed.[5,20] It has an outer gel envelope with a central reservoir that inflates with saline. If the implant is well positioned, the filling port can be removed through a small incision, often as an office procedure, leaving the implant in place as a permanent prosthesis.[5,20] It is also possible to use implants of this type as primary prostheses by filling them to the desired size and withdrawing the filling tube immediately. This reduces or obviates the need for an inventory of multiple implant sizes. The advantages of permanent expanders are that they potentially reduce the risk from skin ischemic complications during immediate breast reconstruction. Additionally, the patient can participate in the selection of final size, and the surgeon can adjust size conveniently in the postoperative period.[32]

Soft tissue flap breast reconstruction. Soft tissue flaps may be required when there is insufficient skin or it is of poor quality secondary to radiation, poor healing, or thinning, or where soft tissue augmentation of the reconstructive site is needed.[7,12,25,30,36] Historically, local skin flaps have been used. However, more robust skin muscle flaps have largely supplanted their use. Used most commonly are the latissimus dorsi skin muscle unit and, more recently, the TRAM flap.[7,24,37,38,48]

Latissimus dorsi flap. The latissimus dorsi flap usually requires the use of an implant because of its lack of bulk. It is most useful for replacing skin removed during the primary surgery, augmenting thin skin flaps, and in secondary or salvage reconstructions where the soft tissue cover has been impaired seriously[7,37,38,48] (see p. 317).

Categorized as a type V skin muscle unit, the *latissimus dorsi flap* can survive entirely on the blood supply from the thoracodorsal artery and vein[4] or, if the main trunk has been divided in the mastectomy, that from the serratus branch of the thoracodorsal artery.[34] When used with a skin is-

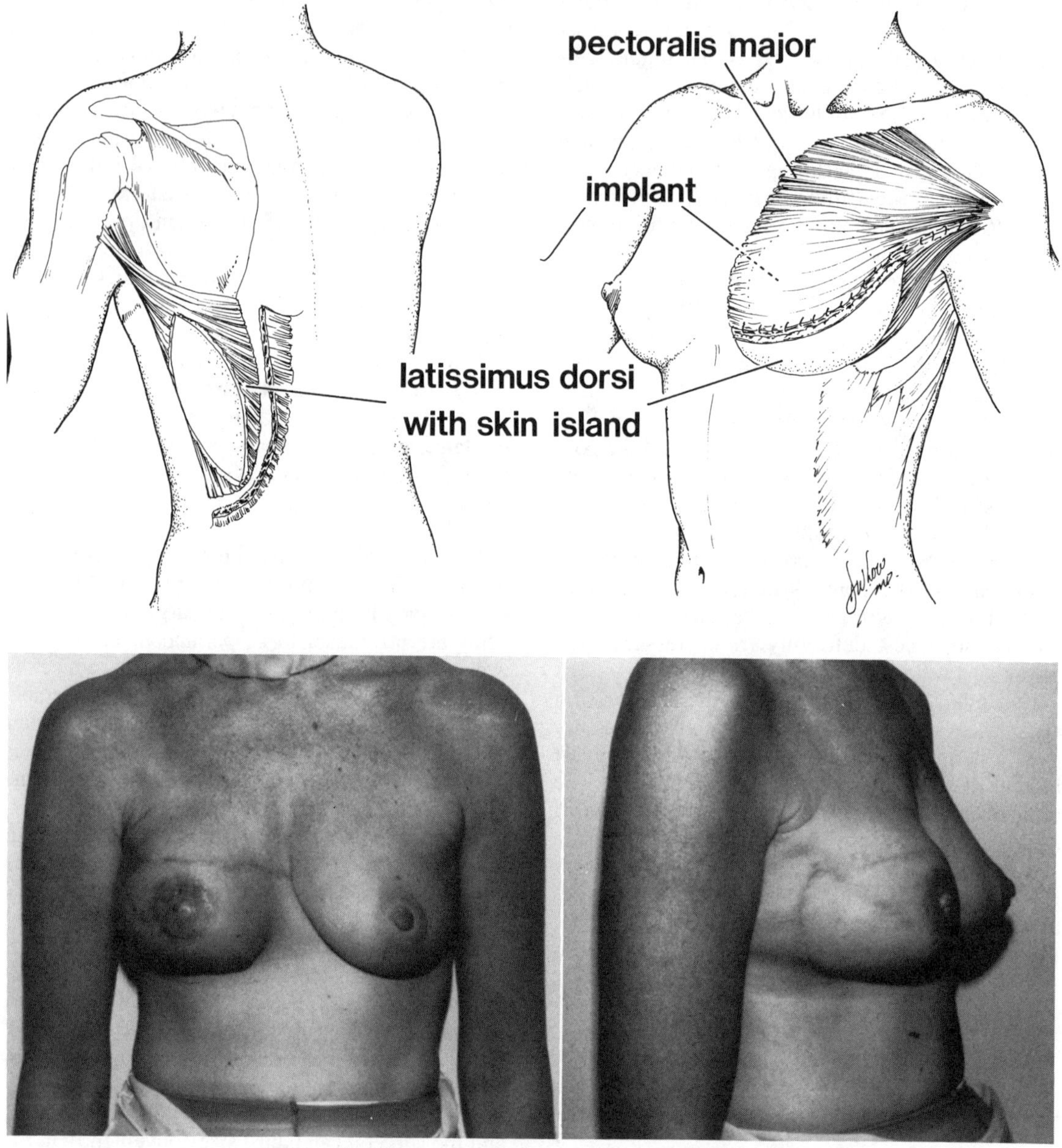

Fig. 12-3 A, Design of a latissimus dorsi skin muscle flap using the inferior margin of the skin paddle to establish the inframammary fold. **B** and **C,** Result following delayed reconstruction using a latissimus dorsi skin muscle flap and gel prosthesis in a patient who had a modified radical mastectomy.

INDICATIONS FOR LATISSIMUS DORSI SKIN MUSCLE FLAPS

1. Poor quality skin cover
   a. Irradiation
   b. Extensive scarring
   c. Thin soft tissue cover
   d. Lack of soft tissue
   e. Failed implant procedures
2. Threatened implant exposure
3. Inability to use TRAM

land, the ellipse is oriented at 90 degrees to the site of insertion. A 7- to 8-cm wide flap permits easy primary closure of the donor site on the back. Careful placement of the donor island will even allow at least partial coverage by low-cut clothing. The skin island can be placed within the mastectomy scar site when the scar is low, near the inframammary fold. However, when the mastectomy scar is located high on the chest wall, the inferior margin of the flap should be used to form the inframammary crease, disregarding the original mastectomy scar (Fig. 12-3). Loss of the latissimus dorsi muscle does not create a functional impairment; most individuals are able to engage in normal levels of activity including athletics. The latissimus dorsi flap can be used in reconstruction of partial mastectomy defects as in melanoma and sarcoma patients, where a generous amount of breast skin may have been removed during the partial mastectomy (Fig. 12-4). Complications involving latissimus dorsi flaps are listed above.

COMPLICATIONS OF LATISSIMUS DORSI FLAPS

1. Partial or complete flap necrosis
2. Hematoma, seroma
3. Brachial plexopathy

Transverse rectus abdominis flap. The TRAM flap, popularized and perfected by Hartrampf et al.,[24] offers a method of breast reconstruction using only autogenous tissue. The transversely oriented skin paddle can be based on either rectus muscle, the contralateral one being the chosen more commonly, particularly in individuals who have had irradiation. The blood supply is the superior epigastric system that forms a racemose system of vessels within the muscle with the stronger, deep inferior epigastric system. The muscle can survive on the blood supplied by the eighth intracostal perforator as well. The blood flow can be augmented by microsurgical anastomosis of the inferior epigastric leash to the thoracodorsal artery and vein (or other suitable vessels) creating the so-called "super-charged" TRAM.

The transverse skin island can be located in the upper, mid, or lower abdomen and is perfused through perforators from the rectus muscle. They are richest in the periumbilical area and should be

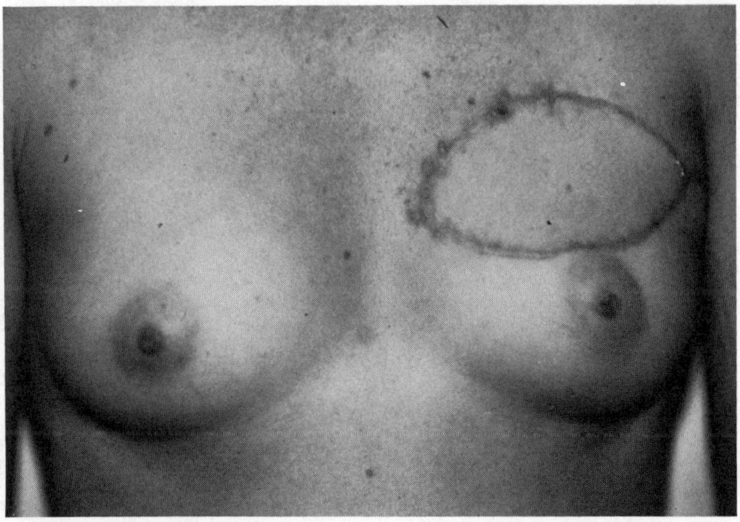

Fig. 12-4 Final result in a patient who had a full thickness wide excision for a high-risk melanoma of the breast skin and immediate reconstruction with a latissimus dorsi skin muscle flap.

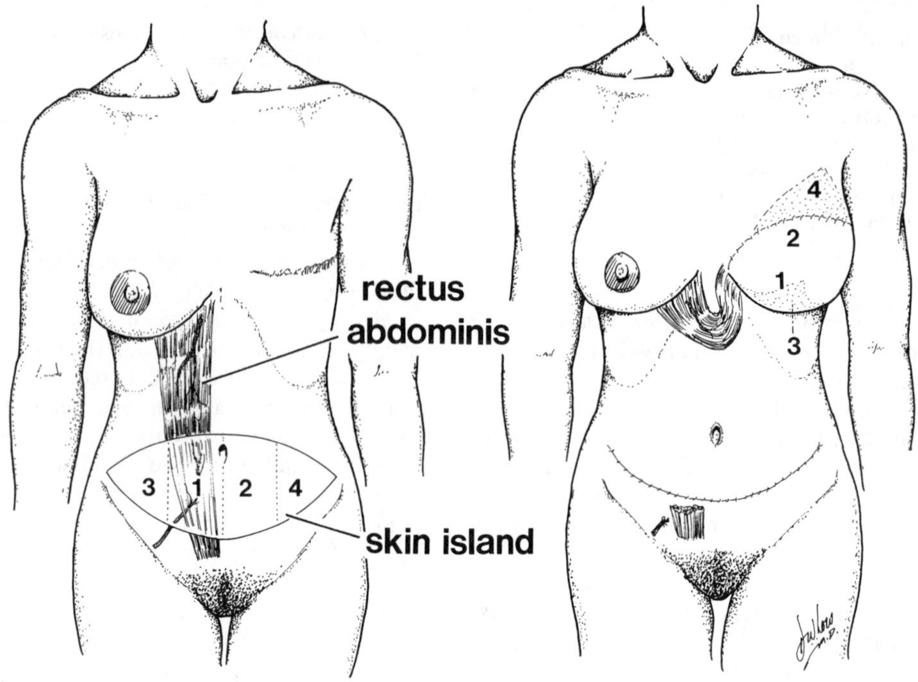

Fig. 12-5 TRAM flap. Contralateral rectus abdominus muscle carries a skin island with zones 1 through 4 in order of decreasing vascularity.

A

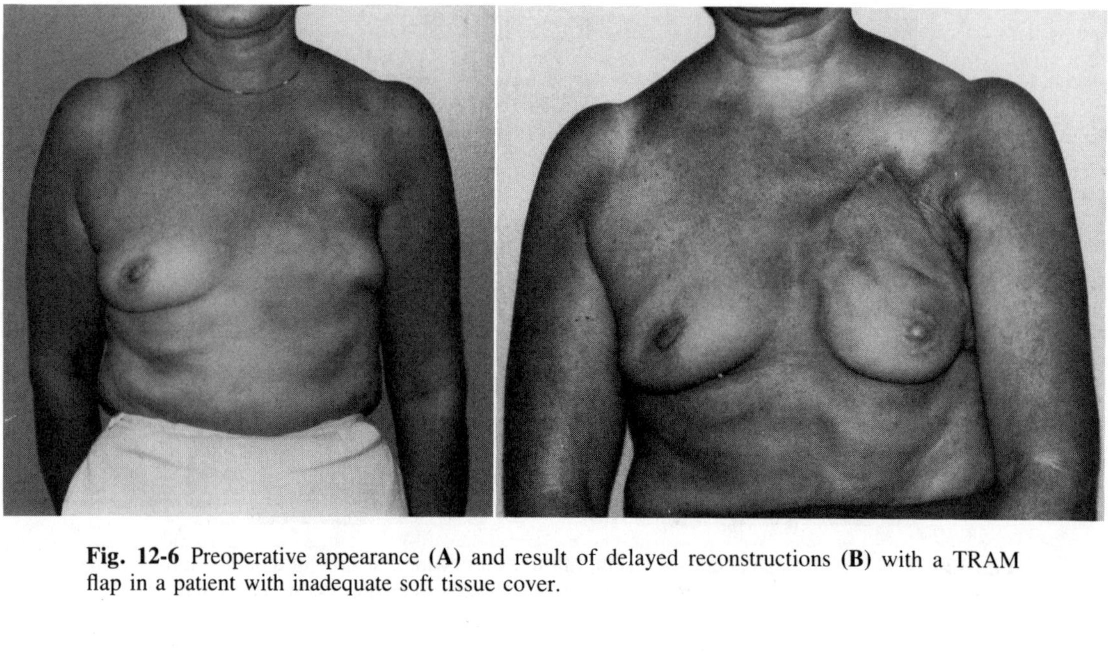

B

Fig. 12-6 Preoperative appearance **(A)** and result of delayed reconstructions **(B)** with a TRAM flap in a patient with inadequate soft tissue cover.

included in the flap. The portion of the skin paddle furthest from the muscle (zone III and zone IV) is the most poorly perfused and is often lost or undergoes spotty fat necrosis (Figs. 12-5 and 12-6). Because of the potential risk to the blood supply, smokers and obese patients have a greater chance of flap loss and may not be candidates for the use of this technique.

Mastectomy incisions can be limited in size and the resultant skin envelope can be filled with a deepithelialized TRAM, leaving a skin island to be exposed at the excised areola and reexcised biopsy sites.

Indications and contraindications for TRAM flaps are listed below at left.

Both rectus muscles also can be used to bolster the blood supply to zone III and zone IV. Likewise, bilateral skin islands can be used for bilateral breast reconstruction. However, this will impair the patient's ability to sit up from a supine position, while loss of a single rectus will permit essentially normal function. The creation of weakness in the abdominal wall and hernia formation are potential risks from harvesting the TRAM. Various surgeons have recommended the use of surgical mesh or creative myofacial closure schemes to reduce this risk. Complications and risks of using TRAM flaps are listed below at right.

Free tissue transfer breast reconstruction. In exploring the possibilities in breast reconstruction, surgeons have employed microvascular techniques to transfer flaps to the breast reconstruction site. Buttock flaps based on the superior or inferior gluteal arteries have been used successfully.[18,49]

The free TRAM flap has been advocated as well. A small segment of the lower rectus is harvested on the inferior epigastric leash. In addition to the enhanced blood supply from the inferior epigastric artery, a smaller defect is left in the abdominal wall, potentially reducing the risk of hernia. The donor sites for both are relatively well hidden and the enhanced blood supply by direct anastomosis to intracostal or thoracodorsal vessels provides a more diffuse vascularity to the flap. Conversely, failure at the anastomosis frequently means complete flap loss.

Most recently, the lateral transverse thigh free flap has been described as an alternative. However, it leaves a more noticeable donor site deformity.[15]

Skin flaps are used infrequently as the modality of choice in breast reconstruction. Rather, they have served as a stepping stone in the evolution of flap reconstructive methods.[25,36]

Phase II: creation of symmetry

The second phase of breast reconstruction is the *creation of symmetry* and it is intended to add realism to the breast mound. Position and size are elementary requirements, although nipple reconstruction, creation of a better-defined inframammary crease, and manipulation of the opposite breast may be needed. Surgical repositioning or change in size of the initial implant may be needed. The relative frequency of repositioning as well as the need to adjust implant size has led many surgeons to use tissue expanders. When TRAM, latissimus dorsi, or free tissue reconstruction are used, initial positioning is critical in preoperative planning. The size of these breasts is fixed unless tissue is removed surgically or an implant is added.

Creation of an inframammary fold. Creation of an inframammary fold often is not an easy matter. Breasts reconstructed using implant techniques are, more often than not, more spherical and firmer than a natural breast. In a clothed individual, this may not be noticeable, but without clothing there are observable differences between the natural breast and the reconstructed one, despite symmetry of size and position.

INDICATIONS AND CONTRAINDICATIONS FOR THE USE OF TRAM FLAPS

Indications

1. Poor quality soft tissue at mastectomy site and adequate abdominal skin and fat
   a. Thin flap
   b. Irradiation
   c. Extensive scarring
   d. Lack of soft tissue
2. Large opposite breast
3. Desire to avoid prosthetic implant
4. Failed prosthetic reconstruction

Contraindications

1. Cigarette smoking (relative)
2. Obesity (relative)
3. Poor physical and psychologic health

COMPLICATIONS AND RISKS OF USING TRAM FLAPS

1. Flap loss, partial or complete
2. Hernia or abdominal wall weakness
3. Functional impairment in bilateral TRAM flaps
4. Hematoma, seroma
5. Infection
6. Fat necrosis and fat fibrosis causing confusing masses on physical examinations

---

When flap-type reconstructions are used. The border of the flap establishes and recreates the fold. However, in implant reconstructions a procedure designed to recreate the fold may be needed. This recreation may be accomplished by internal thinning of the subcutaneous tissue in the region of the fold and suturing of the dermis to the underlying rib, cartilage, and muscle. External approaches utilize a diepithelialization of the skin on either side of the proposed crease, advancing the inferior thoracic skin flap and suturing the infolded dermal flaps to the deep tissues.[41,46]

Overexpansion of a tissue expander and/or the use of differential expanders can be helpful in creating ptosis as well as an inframammary crease.[56]

Implant repositioning, if necessary, and inframammary fold reconstruction should be done before nipple and areolar reconstruction. Likewise, manipulation of the opposite breast should be done in a separate stage to allow time for the opposite breast to "settle down," soften, and assume its final position. The opposite breast may require mastopexy (breast lift), reduction mammoplasty, or even augmentation mammoplasty depending on the patient's desires. One should consider the use of breast reduction and augmentation in higher risk individuals carefully because of the risk of these procedures interfering in subsequent breast examination. Although the surgically reduced breast can be examined by x-ray, calcifications are produced along the internal scar. Therefore a baseline mammogram is recommended 6 months following reduction mammoplasty. Palpable nodules and masses along the internal scars can make breast examinations more confusing. Breast implants are radiopaque, obscuring areas of breast or mammography of an augmented breast. Special techniques and methods of "slipping" the breast off the implant will increase the quantity of breast tissue examined, but it may still be more limited than in the unaugmented breast.

Nipple reconstruction. When final contour symmetry has been achieved, nipple reconstruction puts the finishing, aesthetic touch on the reconstructed breast. A number of techniques have been tried and a few have survived the test of time. Skin grafts from the labia minora and retroauricular area give the darkest and pinkest colored areola skin, respectively.[1,8] More commonly, skin grafts harvested from the opposite areola, when available, or upper inner thigh skin give good color matches with minimal donor site morbidity.[38] Medical tattooing is a relatively easy and painless method, though practice with color blends takes artistry and experience to achieve a natural appearance.[31]

Achieving adequate size and projection with the nipple or papilla is a more difficult problem. Techniques using "quadripod" and "skate flaps" have had most success.[31] Other techniques that have been used and may have selective usefulness are toe tip grafts,[28] earlobe grafts, shared nipple grafts, and ear cartilage implants[8] (Fig. 12-7).

PROPHYLACTIC MASTECTOMY OF THE OPPOSITE BREAST AND RECONSTRUCTION

In selected high-risk individuals prophylactic mastectomy may be warranted (see p. 321).

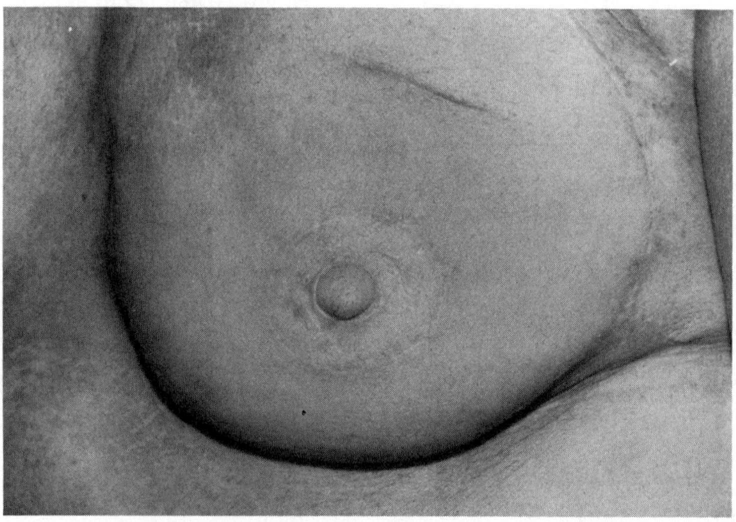

Fig. 12-7 Close-up view of a reconstructed nipple from the patient in Fig. 12-6. A skate flap and skin graft from the upper inner thigh were used.

INDICATIONS FOR PROPHYLACTIC MASTECTOMY

1. Multiple biopsies
2. Difficulty examining breasts
3. Strong family history of breast cancer
4. Breast cancer of the multifocal type—previous cancer in the opposite breast
5. Diffuse calcifications on mammography
6. Cancerophobia

A complete or total mastectomy should be done with sacrifice of the papilla. the areola can be spared in individuals with a small, nonptotic breast. However, in patients with large or ptotic breasts, the nipple and areola may be malpositioned and should be excised totally and reconstructed as a secondary procedure. The prophylactic mastectomy can be done simultaneously with a mastectomy for cancer of the opposite breast or at the time of secondary reconstruction.[17,42]

RECONSTRUCTION IN PREVIOUSLY IRRADIATED PATIENTS

Chest wall irradiation is usually an indication for a flap reconstructive technique rather than one using an implant or expander. However, the choice of techniques seems more related to the quality of the remaining skin cover, the dose of irradiation, and the degree of skin reaction at the time of irradiation.

We attempted delayed or immediate reconstruction in 11 irradiated patients. Eight of the 11 had previous primary lumpectomy and irradiation followed by recurrences necessitating a total mastectomy. The remaining three had postmastectomy irradiation and were seeking secondary reconstructions. Eight of the 11 had successful reconstructions while three failed. One had an infection and implant loss, and two had unsuccessful expansion because of intense fibrosis. All three patients with failed reconstructions had more than 5000 rad (5500 to 6600 rad) and had either a history of moist desquamation during treatment, evidence of radiation-induced hyperpigmentation, or fibrosis of the treated skin. All other patients had minimal evidence of radiation change and their skin responded like unirradiated skin to the expansion process. The surgeon should review the patient's radiotherapy record for documentation of total dose, boost, and history of severe skin reaction including moist desquamation in this patient group. The best candidates had <5000 rad, and had a relatively normal, pliable, soft skin cover with minimal hyperpigmentation. Prosthetic reconstructions are a viable alternative in selected postirradiation patients who decline more complex types of reconstructive procedures[59] (Fig. 12-8).

Conversely, radiation does not seem to affect or change the implant, should radiotherapy be needed after implant reconstruction (see Fig. 12-8).

Surgical treatment of complications following irradiation

In selected patients, radiation therapy is as effective as surgery in treating breast cancer. Patients who have radiation failures often become candidates for mastectomy and breast reconstruction. However, a small group of patients will develop widespread local recurrences; skin, breast, or chest wall necrosis, brachial plexopathy, radiation-induced malignancy, or impaired wound healing following median sternotomy for cardiac procedures. In these individuals, wide resections of involved skin and chest wall and flap reconstructions may be needed.

The management of these complications begins with a careful assessment of the patient and their tumor status. When ulceration is encountered, tumor recurrence or persistence must be ruled out. Likewise, distant disease must be searched for, although its presence is not a contraindication to treatment. In many of these patients, palliation of disease can be successful even though the outcome is not going to be changed. When a patient becomes a candidate for treatment, a wide resection of the involved tissue is essential to insure a healthy bed for wound healing. In cases of tumor recurrence, the resection should attempt to remove all obvious tumor. In patients with radioosteonecrosis, with or without tumor recurrence, the resection should extend to relatively normally vascularized tissue.

The reconstruction should be performed using well-vascularized, arterialized flaps that, in addition to their ability to enhance blood flow into an area of relative ischemia and thus enhance wound healing, can provide for the delivery of chemotherapeutic agents to the area, if there is still a significant tumor risk. Additionally, their use can permit reirradiation of the site if the vascularized tissue that is brought into it has not sustained previous radiation injury. The tissues that are available for reconstruction can be borrowed from the areas peripheral to the anterior chest and include the pectoralis major, latissimus dorsi, and rectus abdominus muscles and the omentum. Of these, the latissimus dorsi is the most valuable, versatile, and reliable either as a skin muscle unit or, more commonly, as a muscle unit covered with a skin graft. In the absence of these commonly available flaps, the omentum can be harvested, based on the right gastroepiploic artery, and transferred to the required area.

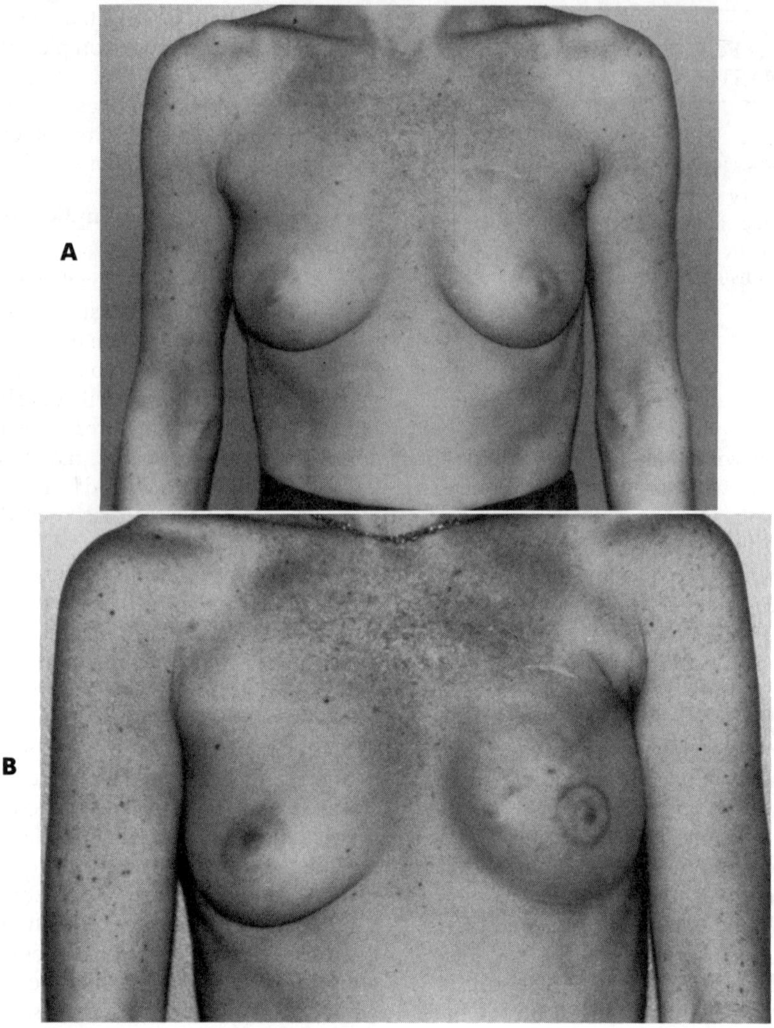

Fig. 12-8 Preoperative view **(A)** and final result **(B)** in a patient with recurrence following lumpectomy and radiation. The reconstruction was done at the same time as mastectomy using a tissue expander. Nipple reconstruction was done secondarily.

For medial defects, the rectus abdominus and pectoralis major muscles are the most valuable. For a central lesion, the pectoralis major muscle is often involved so that the rectus and latissimus muscles are the most useful. For lateral defects, the pectoralis major and the latissimus dorsi muscles are the mainstay of treatment. We treated 12 patients with radiation complications over a 6-year period. In our treatment group there were four patients with radiation necrosis alone, seven patients with tumor recurrence or persistence, and one patient with sternal dehiscence following coronary artery bypass surgery. No instances of malignant degeneration of the skin in the operative area were encountered. In all patients, successfully palliation of disease for up to 72 months after surgery was achieved.

The four patients with radionecrosis alone remained healed and had no evidence of tumor recurrence. Of the seven with tumor present, two died, 4 and 10 months postoperatively; three remained alive with disease; and two were disease free (Tables 12-1 and 12-2).[29]

SUMMARY

Breast reconstruction is still evolving. Its wider acceptance is an impetus for further refinement of technology and techniques. Although results are improving gradually the neobreast often falls short of the mark. Simultaneously, the biology of breast cancer is being better defined. Consequent modifications in surgery, chemotherapy, and radiation therapy are having an impact on end results. The

Table 12-1 Outcome in four patients with radionecrosis without tumor

Patient	Time after surgery (mo)
J.M.	86
L.B.	71
B.N.	33
M.T.	45

Table 12-2 Outcome in seven patients with recurrent or persistent tumor

Patient	Status	Time after surgery (mo)
L.W.	NED	72
S.P.	NED	15
B.D.	AWD	1
B.O.	AWD	20
A.S.	AWD	21
C.M.	DOD	10
G.W.	DOD	4

NED, no evidence of disease; AWD, alive with disease; DOD, dead of disease.

role of breast reconstruction will be better defined by these advances.

REFERENCES

1. Adams WM: Labial transplant for correction of the nipple, Plast Reconstr Surg 4:295, 1949.
2. Argenta LC, Marks MW, and Grubb WC: Selective use of serial expansion in breast reconstruction, Ann Surg 11:188, 1983.
3. Autonyshyn O, Gruss JS, McKinnon SE, and Zuker R: Complications of soft-tissue expansion, Br J Plast Surg 41:239, 1988.
4. Bartlett SP, May JW, and Yarumchuck MJ: The latissimus dorsi muscle: a fresh cadaver study of the primary neurovascular pedicle, Plast Reconstr Surg 67:631, 1981.
5. Becker H: Breast reconstruction using an inflatable breast implant with detachable reservoir, Plast Reconstr Surg 73:678, 1984.
6. Birnbaum L and Olsen JA: Breast reconstruction following radical mastectomy using custom designed implants, Plast Reconstr Surg 61:355, 1978.
7. Bostwick J, Vasconez LO, and Jurklewicz MJ: Breast reconstruction after a radical mastectomy Plast Reconstr Surg 61:682, 1978.
8. Brent B and Bostwick J III: Nipple areolar reconstruction with auricular tissues, Plast Reconst Surg 60:353, 1977.
9. Brody GS: Discussion, Plast Reconstr Surg 73:3, 420, 1984.
10. Crile G Jr: Simplified treatment of cancer of the breast: early results of a clinical study, Am Surg 153:745, 1961.
11. Cronin TD and Gerow FJ: Augmentation mammoplasty: a new natural feeling prosthesis. In Transactions of the Third International Congress of Plastic and Reconstructive Surgeons (International Congress Series no. 60). Amsterdam, 1964, Exerpta Medica, p 41.
12. Cronin TD, Upton J, and McDonough JM: Reconstruction of the breast after mastectomy, Plast Reconstr Surg 59:1, 1977.
13. Dempsey WC and Latham WD: Subpectoral implants in augmentation mammoplasty, Plast Reconstr Surg 42:515, 1968.
14. Dowden RV: Achieving a natural inframammary fold and ptotic affect in the reconstructed breast, Ann Surg 19(6):524, 1987.
15. Elliott LF, Beegle PH, and Hartrampf CR Jr: The lateral transverse thigh free flap: an alternative for autogeneous tissue breast reconstruction, Plast Reconstr Surg 85(2):169, 1990.
16. Eyssen JE, Von Wessowetz AJ, and Middleton GD: Reconstruction of the breast using polyurethane coated prostheses, Plast Reconstr Surg 73(3):415, 1984.
17. Freeman BS and Weiner RD: Total glandular mastectomy, Plast Reconstr Surg 62:167, 1978.
18. Fujino T, Harashmia T, and Enomoto K: Primary breast reconstruction after a standard radical mastectomy by a free flap transfer, Plast Reconstr Surg 58:372, 1976.
19. Georgiade GS, Georgiade NG, McCarty KS, and Seigler H: Rationale for immediate reconstruction of the breast following modified radical mastectomy, Plast Reconstr Surg 8:20, 1982.
20. Gibney J: Use of a permanent tissue expander for breast reconstruction, Plast Reconstr Surg 84(4):607, 1989.
21. Gylbert L, Asplund O, and Jurell G: Capsular contracture after breast reconstruction with silicone-gel and saline-filled implants: a six year follow-up, Plast Reconstr Surg 85(3):373, 1990.
22. Hallock GG: Maximum over-inflation of tissue expanders, Plast Reconstr Surg 80(4):567, 1987.
23. Halstead WS: The results of operations for the cure of cancer of the breast performed at Johns Hopkins Hospital from June 1889 to January 1894, Ann Surg 20:497, 1894.
24. Hartrampf CR, Scheflan M, and Black PH: Breast reconstruction with a transverse abdominal flap, Plast Reconstr Surg 69:216, 1982.
25. Holstrom H and Lossing C: The lateral thoracodorsal flap in breast reconstruction, Plast Reconstr Surg 77(6):933, 1986.
26. Horton CE, Adamson JE, Mladick RA, and Carraway JN: Simple Mastectomy with immediate reconstruction, Plast Reconstr Surg 53:42, 1974.
27. Jarrett JR, Cutter RG, and Teal DT: Subcutaneous mastectomy in small, large or ptotic breasts with immediate submuscular placement of implants, Plast Reconstr Surg 62:702, 1978.
28. Klatsky SA and Manson PN: Toe pulp free grafts in nipple reconstruction, Plast Reconstr Surg 68:245, 1981.
29. LaRossa D and Rosato EF: Personal communications.
30. Lewis JR Jr: Reconstruction of the breast, Surg Clin North Am 51:429, 1971.
31. Little JW: Nipple areolar reconstruction, Clin Plast Surg 11(2):351, 1984.
32. Little JW III: Discussion of the use of a permanent tissue expander for breast reconstruction, Plast Reconstr Surg 84:619, 1989.
33. Madden JL: Modified radical mastectomy, Surg Gynecol Obstet 121:1221, 1965.
34. Maxwell GP, McGibbon BM, and Hoopes JE: Vascular considerations in the use of a latissimus dorsi myocutaneous flap after a mastectomy with axillary dissection, Plast Reconstr Surg 64:771, 1979.
35. Millard DR: Nipple and areolar reconstruction by split graft from the normal side, Plast Reconstr Surg 50:4, 1972.
36. Millard DR Jr: Breast reconstruction after a radical mastectomy, Plast Reconstr Surg 58:283, 1976.
37. Muhlbauer W and Olbrisk R: The latissimus dorsi myocutaneous flap for breast reconstruction, Chir Plast 4:27, 1977.

38. Olivari N: The latissimus flap, Breast J Plast Surg 29:126, 1976.
39. Patey DH and Dyson WH: The prognosis of carcinoma of the breast in relation to the type of operation performed, Breast J Cancer 2:7, 1948.
40. Paul MD: Primary breast reconstruction with a subpectoral silicone tissue expander, Ann Surg 11(5):404, 1985.
41. Pennisi VR: Making a definite inframammary fold under a reconstructed breast, Plast Reconstr Surg 60:523, 1977.
42. Pennisi VR, Capozzi A, and Perez FM: Subcutaneous mastectomy data, Plast Reconstr Surg 59(1):53, 1977.
43. Radovan C: Breast reconstruction after mastectomy using the temporary expander, Plast Reconstr Surg 69:195, 1982.
44. Rosato FE, Horton CE, and Maxwell GP: Post mastectomy breast reconstruction, Curr Prob Surg 17:585, 1980.
45. Rose JH Jr: Carcinoma in a transplanted nipple, Arch Surg 116:1131, 1980.
46. Ryan JJ: A lower thoracic advancement flap in breast reconstruction after mastectomy, Plast Reconstr Surg 70:153, 1982.
47. Schain WS, Willish DK, Pasnau RO, and Landswerk J: The sooner the better: a study of psychological factors in women undergoing immediate versus delayed breast reconstruction, Am J Psychiatry 142:40, 1985.
48. Schneider WJ, Hill HL Jr, and Brown RG: Latissimus dorsi myocutaneous flap for breast reconstruction, Br J Plast Surg 30:277, 1977.
49. Shaw W: Breast reconstruction by superior gluteal microvascular free flaps without silicone implants, Plast Reconstr Surg 72:490, 1983.
50. Smahel J: Tissue reactions to breast implants coated with polyurethane, Plast Reconstr Surg 61:80, 1978.
51. Snyderman RK and Gutherie RH: Reconstruction of the female breast following radical mastectomy, Plast Reconstr Surg 47:565, 1971.
52. Spear S and Little J: Personal communication.
53. Stehlin JS Jr, Evans RA, Gutierez AE, et al: Treatment of carcinoma of the breast, Surg Gynecol Obstet 149:911, 1979.
54. Stevens LA, McGrath MH, Druss RG, et al: The psychological impact of immediate breast reconstruction for women with early breast cancer, Plast Reconst Surg 73:619, 1984.
55. Tansini I: Nuovo processo per l'ampert azione della mammella per cancro, Reforma Med 12:3, 1896.
56. Versaci A: Reconstruction of a pendulous breast utilizing a shaped expander, Ann Surg 23(6):469, 1989.
57. Ward J, Cohen IK, Knaysi GA, and Brown PW: Immediate breast reconstruction with tissue expansion, Plast Reconstr Surg 80(4):559, 1987.
58. Wexler MR and O'Neal RN: Areolar sharing to reconstruct the absent nipple, Plast Reconstr Surg 51:176, 1973.
59. Witham R, Rosen H, and LaRossa D: Personal communications.

13 In Situ Breast Cancer

Barbara Fowble

The term *in situ breast cancer* includes both in situ lobular cancer and in situ ductal (intraductal) cancer. In the past it was thought that in situ lesions eventually would progress to invasive cancers. As a result of this philosophy, mastectomy became the standard treatment. However, recent studies have questioned the malignant potential of in situ cancers and prompted a reevaluation of treatment recommendations. At present, there is no consensus regarding the optimal treatment of in situ breast cancer, be it ductal or lobular carcinoma; however, alternatives to mastectomy clearly exist.[30] Because there are important differences in the behavior of in situ ductal carcinoma and in situ lobular carcinoma that affect treatment recommendations, the two entities will be discussed separately. Patients whose biopsies reveal the simultaneous presence of in situ ductal carcinoma and in situ lobular carcinoma demonstrate a clinical behavior characteristic of in situ ductal carcinoma.[52]

INTRADUCTAL NONINVASIVE BREAST CANCER

Ductal carcinoma in situ (DCIS) by definition represents carcinoma confined to the preexisting duct system of the breast without evidence of penetration of the basement membrane by light microscopy. Intraductal carcinomas that demonstrate microinvasion should be treated as invasive cancer.[31,53,54] With improvements in mammography and an increased emphasis on screening and early detection, the proportion of breast cancers diagnosed as noninvasive is increasing. Approximately 20% to 30% of mammographically detected cancers are ductal carcinoma in situ.[4,23,27,38,54,56] The clinical presentation has changed as well, from primarily that of a palpable mass and/or nipple discharge to that of a mammographically detected lesion characterized most commonly by the presence of microcalcifications[11,56] or of an incidental finding at the time of biopsy of a clinical abnormality that proves to be benign.

The three treatment options for intraductal noninvasive breast cancer are mastectomy, wide excision and radiation, or wide excision alone. The precise role for each treatment has not been defined clearly. Multiple factors have contributed to variations in treatment recommendations and include data based on retrospective series with small patient numbers, variable follow-up time, and divergent clinical presentations, as well as a paucity of data from prospective randomized trials. Differences in the pathologic interpretation also may contribute to the clinical dilemma. The distinction between areas of invasion, atypical ductal hyperplasia, and ductal carcinoma in situ may be difficult. The extension of DCIS into lobules could be mistaken for evidence of invasion or in situ lobular carcinoma. As DCIS is diagnosed with increasing frequency, familiarity with the pathologic entity will help to clarify its definition; the entry of patients into randomized clinical trials will contribute to our knowledge of appropriate treatment choices for the individual patient.

The traditional treatment of intraductal carcinoma has been mastectomy with or without a low axillary dissection. A willingness to depart from this treatment is the result of an increase in the detection of small, clinically inapparent lesions as well as the recognition that conservative surgery and radiation represent a valid alternative to mastectomy for patients with early invasive breast cancer.[3,16,51,66] These two findings have stimulated interest in conservative surgery with or without radiation as an alternative to mastectomy for the treatment of noninvasive intraductal breast cancer.

Mastectomy: rationale and results

The rationale for mastectomy in the treatment of intraductal cancer is related to the observed frequency of multicentric foci of in situ ductal carcinoma, the presence of occult foci of coexistent invasive cancer, the likelihood of residual in situ carcinoma even after wide excision, and a not insignificant breast recurrence rate with either invasive or noninvasive carcinoma after limited surgery. Data regarding the incidence of multicentricity and occult invasion are obtained from mastectomy specimens of patients with intraductal carcinoma. The actual incidence of these findings varies with the thoroughness of the pathologic sampling and examination of the specimen. In most

Table 13-1 Incidence of multicentricity and occult invasive cancer in patients undergoing mastectomy for intraductal carcinoma

Author	No. mastectomy specimens	Multicentricity (separate quadrant; %)	Occult invasive cancer (%)	Method of sectioning
Von Rueden and Wilson[67]	47	38*	11	Multiple random sections
Schuh et al.[53]	51	18	2	Multiple random sections
Carter and Smith[9]	38	66*	18	Multiple random sections
Ashikari et al.[2]	110	32*	0	>1 tissue block
Rosen et al.[49]	53	19	6	Routine random section sampling
Lagios et al.[36]	53	32†	21	Serial subgross and correlated mammographic examination
Fentiman et al[14]	82	23	16	Not stated
Fisher et al[18]	27	0	—	One random section each quadrant
Brown et al[5]	40	33	—	Multiple random sections
Schwartz et al[54]	32	47	—	Multiple random sections
Silverstein et al[57]	97	42	—	Random sections

*Includes multifocal and multicentric foci.
†Multicentricity defined as tumor >5 cm from primary tumor.
Modified from Fowble B: Oncology 3:51, 1989.

series, random sections were obtained from the various breast quadrants. Lagios et al.[36] employed a modification of Egan's technique of serial subgross and correlated mammographic examination. The entire specimen was examined in 2- to 3-mm segments, and tumor extent was documented both with reference to different quadrants and the primary tumor. This is the most thorough but least often employed method. The incidence of multicentricity also varies with the investigators' definition of this term. For the majority of investigators, the presence of cancer in a quadrant separate from that of the primary tumor is regarded as evidence of multicentricity. In contrast, cancer in the vicinity of or at least in the same quadrant as the primary tumor indicates multifocality. Table 13-1 presents the reported incidence of multicentricity in patients with occult invasive cancer from a number of mastectomy series. With the serial subgross and correlated mammographic examination, Lagios et al.[36] reported a 32% incidence of multicentricity and a 21% incidence of occult invasive cancer. The range reported from other series varies from 0 to 47% for multicentricity and 0 to 18% for occult invasion. Fisher et al.[18] commented that their 0 incidence of multicentricity may be an underestimate as only one random section was reviewed from separate quadrants. It appears that approximately one third of patients who undergo mastectomy for intraductal carcinoma have multicentric disease and approximately 20% have areas of occult invasion.

The incidence of residual intraductal carcinoma following a wide excision with negative margins of resection has been reported by the National Surgical Adjuvant Breast Project (NSABP).[18] In the B-06 protocol, 22 patients underwent mastectomy for intraductal noninvasive breast cancer following a wide excision with negative inked margins of resection. Nine (41%) of these patients were found to have residual intraductal carcinoma at the site of the initial excision or within the same quadrant as the excision.

The incidence of breast recurrence following excision alone for intraductal carcinoma is presented in Tables 13-2 through 13-4 and is related to the initial presentation. The results should be interpreted with caution because in certain series it is unlikely that excision was meant to be the sole treatment or that a complete excision was achieved. In the series where intraductal carcinoma was detected as an incidental finding, patients were identified from histologic reviews of biopsy specimens that originally were interpreted as benign. Therefore excision of the entire lesion was not guaranteed, which may account for the relatively high recurrence rate in two of these series.[41,48] For patients presenting with a palpable mass, the completeness of the excision may be assessed by examination of inked margins of the resection specimen. For those whose intraductal carcinoma is detected solely by mammographic microcalcifications with or without an associated mass, the completeness of excision should be assessed both

Table 13-2 Breast recurrence following limited surgery for intraductal carcinoma detected as an incidental finding

Author	Treatment period	No. pts.	Histologic pattern	Breast recurrence (%)	Interval to recurrence (yr)	Dead of disease (%)
Rosen et al.[48]	1940-1950	15	Micropapillary	67	9.7 mean	30
Page et al.[41]	1952-1968	28	Cribriform, micropapillary	25	3-10 6.1 mean	43
Eusebi et al.[12]	1965-1971	28	All	11	3-9	4

Modified from Fowble B: Oncology 3:51, 1989.

Table 13-3 Breast recurrence following limited surgery for intraductal carcinoma detected primarily as a mass

Author	Treatment period	No. pts.	Histologic pattern	Tumor size (cm)	Breast recurrence (%)	Interval to recurrence (yr)	Dead of disease (%)
Lewis and Geschickter[37]	1918-1936	8	Comedo	50% >5 to <9	75	1-4+	0
Kraus and Neubecker[32]	Before 1961	4	Papillary	NS	50	10 + 12	NS
Millis and Thynne[40]	1948-1968	8	All	1-5	25	0.5 + 7	0
Fisher et al.[18]	1976-1984	22	All	2.2 ± 1.3	23	0.3-1.5	0
Price et al.[43]	1972-1982	35	NS	NS	55	NS	NS
Gallagher et al.[22]	1944-1981	13	All	1.6 mean	38	2.4-8	23

NS, not stated.
Modified from Fowble B: Oncology 3:51, 1989.

Table 13-4 Breast recurrence following limited surgery for intraductal carcinoma detected primarily by mammography alone

Author	Treatment period	No. pts.	Histologic pattern	Tumor size (cm)	Breast recurrence (%)	Interval to recurrence (yr)	Dead of disease (%)
Lagios et al.[35]	1972-1987	79	All	0.5 (median)	10	0.75-7.2	0
Arnesson et al.[1]	1978-1984	38	Comedo, cribriform	0.6-1 (median)	13	1-3.8	0
Gallagher et al.[22]	1944-1981	6	All	—	17	—	—

Modified from Fowble B: Oncology 3:51, 1989.

by evaluation of resection margins as well as a postbiopsy mammogram demonstrating no residual calcifications. Only two of the series[18,22] reporting results of intraductal carcinoma presenting as a palpable mass treated solely by local excision assessed margins of resection. All three of the series presenting results of intraductal carcinoma detected primarily by mammography established the completeness of excision by negative margins of resection.[1,22,35] However, only one of these series[35] also established the completeness of excision with a negative postbiopsy mammogram. Given these difficulties, it can be seen that 11% to 67% of patients whose intraductal carcinoma is detected as an incidental finding and who are treated with excision only will develop a breast recurrence. Breast recurrence rates following excision alone for intraductal carcinoma presenting as a palpable mass range from 23% to 75%. Breast recurrence rates following wide excision with negative margins of

Table 13-5 Breast recurrence following wide excision with negative margins of resection for patients with intraductal cancer

Author	No. pts.	Primary method of detection	Tumor size (cm)	Follow-up (yr)	Breast recurrence (%)	Dead of disease (%)
Fisher et al.[18]	22	Mass	2.2 (mean)	3.2 (mean)	23	0
Gallagher et al.[22]	7	Mass	1.6 (mean)	8.3 (median)	57	60
	6	Mammography		8.3 (median)	17	
Arnesson et al[1]	38	Mammography	0.6-1 (median)	5 (median)	13	0
Lagios et al.[35]	79	Mammography	<2.5	3.7 (median)	10	0

resection for intraductal noninvasive breast cancer, detected either as a palpable mass or as a mammographic finding, are summarized in Table 13-5. For lesions detected solely by mammography and with negative margins of resection, the breast recurrence rate ranges from 10% to 17%. Lagios et al.[35] reported the lowest incidence of breast recurrence. This may be related to the fact that completeness of excision also was assessed by a negative postbiopsy mammogram. Arnesson et al.[1] reported a breast recurrence rate of 37% (three of eight patients) for margins ≤5 mm compared to 7% (two of 30 patients) for margins >5 mm. Therefore the breast recurrence rate also may be related to the extent of the negative margin. For patients who present with a palpable mass and undergo wide excision with negative margins of resection, the breast recurrence rate has been reported in one series to be 23% with a mean follow-up of 3.2 years[18] and 57% with a median follow-up of 8.3 years.[22] Therefore in the four series in Table 13-5 where wide excision was meant to be the sole treatment and where completeness of excision was assessed by negative margins of resection, breast recurrence rates range from 10% to 57%. It appears that intraductal carcinoma presenting as a palpable mass has a higher incidence of breast recurrence when treated with wide excision alone than those presenting with mammographic findings only.

The patterns of breast recurrence following wide excision alone for intraductal carcinoma and the results of salvage treatment are presented in Table 13-6. Almost all of the recurrences occur in the vicinity of the original tumor. Approximately 50% recur as an invasive cancer. Virtually all recurrences that are noninvasive are salvaged with subsequent surgery.[1,18,22,35] Salvage of invasive recurrences is less uniformly excellent. In the series of Page et al.[41] only three of seven invasive recurrences were salvaged by subsequent surgery, and in the series of Gallagher et al.,[22] all three of the patients who developed an invasive recurrence subsequently died of metastatic disease. In contrast, Lagios et al.,[35] Arnesson et al.,[1] and Fisher et al.,[18] report 100% salvage of invasive recurrences. The interval to recurrence following limited surgery alone for intraductal carcinoma is somewhat dependent upon the initial clinical presentation. For intraductal carcinomas that are detected as an incidental finding, the mean intervals to recurrence of 6.1 years[41] and 9.7 years[48] have been reported. Where specific information is available regarding the interval to recurrence for patients initially presenting with a palpable mass, six of nine patients

Table 13-6 Results of limited surgery for intraductal carcinoma: patterns of breast recurrence and results of salvage treatment

Author	No. pts.	Location recurrence (% true or marginal recurrence)	Pathology recurrence (% invasive)	No. pts. salvaged: Noninvasive cancer	No. pts. salvaged: Invasive cancer	Dead of disease following recurrence (%)
Gallagher et al.[22]	5	100	60	2/2	0/3	60
Lagios et al.[35]	8	100	50	4/4	4/4	0
Arnesson et al.[1]	5	80	40	3/3	2/2	0
Fisher et al.[18]	5	100	60	2/2	3/3	0
Rosen et al.[48]	10	—	80	5/10		30
Page et al.[41]	7	86	100	—	3/7	43
Farrow[13]	5	100	NS	—	—	—

recurred within 3 years.[18,32,40] Nine of 13 patients whose initial presentation was a mammographic finding only recurred within 3 years.[1,35]

In summary, arguments for mastectomy include the 30% incidence of multicentric disease, the 41% incidence of residual tumor following wide excision with negative margins, the 20% risk of occult invasion, and the 25% incidence of breast recurrence, of which approximately 50% are invasive cancers following limited surgery for intraductal carcinoma.

The success of mastectomy in treating intraductal carcinomas is demonstrated in Table 13-7. Comparison of the various series is difficult because of differences in clinical presentation, tumor size, and follow-up times. For the older series,[2,9,13,40,61] mammograms were not routinely available or performed, and the majority of patients presented with palpable masses. Sunshine et al.[61] state that in their patients the palpable abnormality was frequently benign and the intraductal carcinoma was microscopic. Tumor size was reported in only five series: Lagios et al.,[36] 1 to 160 mm; Millis and Thynne,[40] 1 to 9 cm; Fisher et al.,[18] 2.2 ± 1.3 cm; and Silverstein et al.,[57] 3.8 cm average. Follow-up times vary among the series and in some are not stated. Recurrence rates and survival rates are crude, not actuarial. The percentage of patients dying of disease is given, rather than overall survival rates, because this percentage is one of the most important end points in treatment. Despite these limitations, the incidence of local recurrence ranges from 0 to 4%, and 0 to 8% of patients have died of metastatic breast cancer. These studies indicate that intraductal carcinoma when treated by mastectomy is highly curable.

Wide excision and radiation: rationale and results

With the published results of prospective randomized trials[3,16,51,66] demonstrating that conservative surgery with radiation and mastectomy were equally effective in the treatment of early invasive breast cancer, it appeared logical to extend the conservative approach to intraductal carcinoma. The ability of radiation to decrease the incidence of breast recurrence following wide excision for invasive breast cancer was demonstrated by the NSABP B-06 trial.[16] Tumor multicentricity in patients receiving radiation has not been a significant

Table 13-7 Results of mastectomy for patients with intraductal carcinoma

Author	Treatment period	No. pts.	Presentation: Mass (%)	Presentation: Nipple discharge (%)	Presentation: Positive mammogram (%)	Follow-up (yr)	Local-regional recurrence (%)	Dead of disease (%)
Millis and Thynne[40]	1948-1968	15	94	19	0	<5 to >15	0	0
Farrow[13]	1949-1967	181	80	24	22	—	1	2
Temple et al.[62]	1951-1984	116	—	—	—	7.5 (mean)	0	0
Brown et al.[5]	1952-1975	40	85	2	10	5	0	0
Ashikari et al.[2]	1960-1969	110	54	18	20	1-10	2	1
Sunshine et al.[61]	1960-1972	68	—	15	13	>10	0	4
Carter and Smith[9]	1960-1975	38	—	—	—	—	3	8
Von Rueden and Wilson[67]	1960-1981	47	72	21	8	—	0	0
Schuh et al.[53]	1965-1984	51	33	34	33	5.5 (mean)	0	2
Rosner et al.[50]	1970-1972	182	—	—	—	5	—	2
Kinne et al.[31]	1970-1976	107	—	—	—	11.5 (median)	—	1
Price et al.[43]	1972-1982	19	—	—	20	7 (actuarial)	6	—
Lagios et al.[36]	1975-1980	53	40	—	49	—	4	2
Fentiman et al.[14]	1975-1984	82	54	21	21	4.7 (median)	1	1
Fisher et al.[18]	1976-1984	27	100	—	—	3.2 (mean)	0	4
Arnesson et al.[1]	1978-1984	28	21	4	75	6.4 (median)	0	—
Carpenter et al.[7]	1979-1986	10			100	4.6 (mean)	0	0
Silverstein et al.[57]*	1979-1989	97	—	—	—	4 (median)	1	1

*Includes patients with microinvasion.
Modified from Fowble B: Oncology 3:51, 1989.

clinical problem because the majority of the breast recurrences following conservative surgery and radiation occur in the vicinity of the original tumor.[16,47] It seemed reasonable, therefore, to expect radiation to be equally effective in eradicating multicentric foci of disease and decreasing the risk of a recurrence after wide excision alone for intraductal noninvasive cancer. As breast preservation achieved a more prominent role in the treatment of invasive cancer, mastectomy did not appear to be warranted for treatment for noninvasive cancer.

The first report of results for conservative surgery and radiation for intraductal carcinoma was from the University of Pennsylvania.[15] The initial 14 patients and 6 others were combined with 20 patients treated at the Joint Center for Radiation Therapy in Boston for a second report.[46] Sixty-eight percent of the patients had a palpable mass, and of the 20 patients in whom tumor size was available, 14 had tumors ≤2 cm in size. The 5-year actuarial breast recurrence rate was 10%, and the 5-year survival rate was 100%. Recently we have updated our results at the University of Pennsylvania.[59] From 1978 to 1985, 51 women with intraductal carcinoma of the breast underwent excisional biopsy followed by definitive radiation. Radiation consisted of treatment to the entire breast with 4500 to 5000 cGy followed by a breast boost to a total dose of 6000 to 6600 cGy. The axillary or supraclavicular nodes were not treated. Twenty-two patients underwent a limited axillary dissection; all were found to have negative nodes. Twelve of the 51 patients underwent a reexcision of the primary site and 51% had pathologic assessment of margins with 12 being negative, 10 positive, and 3 close (i.e., ≤2 mm). The primary tumor size was ≤2 cm in 43 patients. Twenty-four patients presented with mammographic findings alone, with the most common finding being microcalcifications. Twenty-one patients presented with a palpable mass, and six patients presented with either bloody nipple discharge or intraductal carcinoma associated with Paget's disease. The median follow-up was 5.7 years. The 5-year actuarial breast recurrence rate was 6%, with a crude rate of 10%. The 5-year rate of survival with no evidence of disease (NED) was 98%. A single patient died from noncancer causes. In five patients, disease recurred in the treated breast at 19, 35, 40, 79, and 119 months. Three of these patients had intraductal carcinoma only, and two patients demonstrated an invasive component. Three of the recurrences were in the vicinity of the original primary tumor and two were in a separate quadrant. All five patients with a breast failure underwent salvage mastectomy, and all are alive NED with follow-up ranging from 6 to 68 months. Analysis was performed to determine if various clinical or pathologic factors could predict for breast recurrence following conservative surgery and radiation for intraductal carcinoma. There was no statistically significant correlation between the risk of breast recurrence and the location of the tumor, the total radiation dose, the final pathology margin, the histologic subtype, the presence of any comedocarcinoma, primary nuclear grade, or worst nuclear grade. The only factor that was significant was the presence of a bloody nipple discharge at presentation. The 5-year actuarial local recurrence rate was 33% in the six patients who presented with bloody nipple discharge, compared to 2% in the 45 patients that did not. Tumor size was not analyzed as a prognostic factor because 91% of the patients had primary tumors ≤2 cm in size. It is difficult to explain the increased incidence of breast cancer in patients who presented with bloody nipple discharge. Both of the two recurrences in this group of six patients had unknown margins of resection, and one had an unknown primary tumor size. We have postulated that intraductal carcinomas presenting with a bloody nipple discharge may be more extensive than what is clinically appreciated. Given the small number of patients in this subgroup, it is difficult to draw definitive conclusions. However, the association of bloody nipple discharge with a breast recurrence also was noted previously in our combined series with the Joint Center for Radiation Therapy.[46] These results suggest that definitive radiation is a valid alternative to mastectomy for selected patients with intraductal carcinoma of the breast. However, we feel that with the long natural history of this disease, further follow-up should provide additional information.

Results from additional published series are presented in Table 13-8. While comparisons with mastectomy series are difficult because of variations in presentation, tumor size, and follow-up, the overall results appear similar. Breast recurrence rates are higher, ranging from 2% to 19%, when compared to chest wall recurrence rates following mastectomy for intraductal carcinoma. However, this higher breast recurrence rate has not affected survival rates adversely, and overall 0 to 5% of patients have died of their disease. Silverstein et al.[57] reported an 11% breast recurrence rate for 54 patients with comedocarcinoma treated with conservative surgery and radiation, compared to a 2% chest wall recurrence rate for 50 patients treated with mastectomy. However, the number of patients dying of breast cancer was similar for the two groups (i.e., one each).

Approximately 50% of the breast recurrences following conservative surgery and radiation for intraductal carcinoma have an invasive compo-

Table 13-8 Results of conservative surgery and radiation for the treatment of noninvasive intraductal carcinoma

Author	Treatment period	No. pts.	Presentation: Mass (%)	Presentation: Nipple discharge (%)	Presentation: Positive mammogram (%)	Follow-up (yr)	Crude local recurrence (%)	Dead of disease (%)
Recht et al.[44]	1976-1985	36	—	—	50	6.6 (median)	19	0
Solin et al.[59]	1978-1985	51	41	12	41	5.7 (median)	10	0
Fisher et al.[18]	1976-1984	29	100	—	—	3.2 (mean)	7	0
Zafrani et al.[71]	1967-1983	54	65	15	24	4.6 (median)	5	2
Kurtz et al.[33]	1975-1985	47	—	—	—	5	4	2
Delouche et al.[10]	1956-1979	18	—	—	—	11 (median)	5	—
Stotter et al.[60]	1958-1987	42	64	26	24	7.7 (median)	7	5
Silverstein et al.[57]*	1979-1989	96	—	—	—	3.5 (median)	7	1
Gallagher et al.[22]	1944-1981	4	—	—	—	8 (median)	0	0

*Includes patients with microinvasion.
Modified from Fowble B: Oncology 3:51, 1989.

nent (Table 13-9). The majority of the recurrences occur in the vicinity of the original primary tumor. The median interval to failure is 5 years in the series in which the interval to failure is reported.[18,33,44,59,60,71] Virtually all of the noninvasive recurrences have been salvaged with subsequent surgery. Ten of 17 invasive recurrences (59%) have been salvaged by subsequent mastectomy. Overall, 79% of all local recurrences following conservative surgery and radiation for intraductal carcinoma have been salvaged.

While these retrospective comparisons provide some evidence for the effectiveness of radiation, the only valid direct comparison between mastectomy and conservative surgery and radiation is the NSABP B-06 prospective randomized trial.[18] This trial was designed for invasive breast cancer; however, histologic review revealed 78 patients with intraductal carcinoma, 29 of whom were randomized to conservative surgery plus radiation and 27 to mastectomy. With a mean follow-up of 39 months, there was no evidence to suggest that one treatment was superior to the other either in terms of survival or local recurrence rates. Breast recurrence was 7% in a group of patients undergoing conservative surgery and radiation, and chest wall recurrence was 0 in a group of patients undergoing mastectomy. None of the patients undergoing wide excision and radiation died of their disease, whereas 4% of the patients undergoing mastectomy died of disease. There are no other prospective randomized trials evaluating the role of mastectomy in the treatment of intraductal noninvasive breast cancer. Therefore long-term follow-up of the lim-

Table 13-9 Conservative surgery and radiation for patients with intraductal carcinoma: patterns of breast recurrence and results of salvage treatment

Author	No. pts.	Location recurrence (% true or marginal recurrence)	Pathology recurrence (% invasive)	No. pts. salvaged: Noninvasive cancer	No. pts. salvaged: Invasive cancer	Dead of disease (%)
Howard et al.[29]	3	100	67	2/2	1/1	0
Stotter et al.[60]	3	NS	100	—	1/3	33
Recht et al.[44]	7	86	57	3/3	3/4	0
Kurtz et al.[33]	3	67	100	—	2/3	33
Zafrani et al.[71]	3	33	33	2/2	0/1	33
Solin et al.[59]	5	60	40	3/3	2/2	0
Fisher et al.[18]	2	100	50	1/1	0/1	0
Silverstein et al.[57]	7	100	28	5/5	1/2	14

NS, not stated.

ited number of patients with intraductal carcinoma entered into the NSABP B-06 randomized trial will provide important information regarding the effectiveness of these two treatments. At the present time there is no evidence to suggest that conservative surgery and radiation for noninvasive breast cancer results in a survival rate inferior to that provided by mastectomy, despite an increased risk of breast recurrence. It appears unlikely that a difference in mortality will appear with longer follow-up.

It has been suggested that intraductal carcinoma may be less radioresponsive than invasive breast cancer. There is no evidence to support this contention (Table 13-10). The breast recurrence rate for intraductal carcinoma as reported by multiple institutions is not significantly different from each institution's overall experience with invasive breast cancer. In the NSABP B-06 protocol,[18] the breast recurrence rate for intraductal carcinoma treated with radiation was not different from that reported for invasive cancers. The Joint Center for Radiation Therapy, however, has identified patients with invasive ductal carcinoma and an extensive intraductal carcinoma component (>25% of the primary tumor and in the surrounding normal breast tissue) as being at high risk for a breast recurrence following conservative surgery and radiation.[47] The 5-year actuarial risk of a breast recurrence in this group of patients was 23%. This figure, however, is greater than the institution's own experience with noninvasive intraductal carcinoma (9%).[44] It is likely that in the case of an invasive cancer with an extensive intraductal component, the high recurrence rate reflects extensive disease in the breast and inadequate surgical excision, rather than a lack of responsiveness to radiation.[45] Holland et al.[27] demonstrated residual tumor in the remainder of the breast in 74% of patients with an invasive ductal carcinoma, and an extensive intraductal component following a limited excision. The 23% breast recurrence rate reported for these patients by the Joint Center for Radiation Therapy is similar to what Van Limbergen et al.[65] and the Joint Center[16] have observed with incisional biopsies and radiation for invasive breast cancer.

Table 13-10 Breast recurrence rates noninvasive intraductal cancer vs. invasive breast cancer in patients undergoing conservative surgery and radiation

	5-year breast recurrence (%)	
Author	Intraductal carcinoma	Invasive carcinoma
NSABP B-06[16,18]	7	7.7
Joint Center for Radiation Therapy[44,47]	9	10
University of Pennsylvania[58,59]	6	6
Marseille Cancer Institute[33]	4	7
Centre de Charlebourg[10]	5	9.7
Curie Institute[6,71]	5	6.5

Modified from Fowble B: Oncology 3:51, 1989.

Guidelines for the evaluation and treatment of patients with intraductal carcinoma with conservative surgery and radiation have been established.[52] Pretreatment mammograms are essential, and postbiopsy mammograms are indicated in patients who present with microcalcifications to evaluate the adequacy of removal of the calcifications. Resection margins and the extent of the intraductal carcinoma within the biopsy specimen should be assessed. Reexcision is recommended for patients with an initial incisional biopsy, a positive or unknown margin of resection, or residual microcalcifications on a postbiopsy mammogram. If extensive residual tumor is identified or reexcision margin(s) are diffusely positive, mastectomy is indicated. Patients with diffuse microcalcifications or multiple areas of malignant calcifications on mammogram, or clinical evidence of gross multicentric disease, are not candidates for conservative surgery and radiation. Mastectomy is the preferred treatment for these patients. To date, the only factor that has been associated with an increased risk of breast recurrence in patients with intraductal carcinoma undergoing conservative surgery and radiation has been the presence of a bloody nipple discharge,[46,59] although this finding may be related to inadequate surgical excision. In these patients the extent of disease should be assessed carefully both clinically and pathologically. In general patients with intraductal carcinoma may be considered candidates for conservative surgery and radiation under the following conditions:

- Tumor size <4 to 5 cm
- No evidence of diffuse microcalcifications on mammogram
- No evidence of gross multicentric disease or multiple areas of calcifications that appear malignant
- Adequate surgical excision demonstrated by negative margins of resection and/or a negative postbiopsy mammogram revealing no residual calcifications

The question arises as to whether an axillary dissection should be part of conservative surgery and radiation for intraductal carcinoma. The incidence of positive nodes at the time of axillary dis-

Table 13-11 Incidence of positive axillary nodes at the time of axillary dissection for patients with intraductal noninvasive breast cancer

Author	No. pts.	Positive nodes (%)
Rosner et al.[50]	210	3.8
Ashikari et al.[2]	113	1
Fentiman et al.[14]	82	0
Silverstein et al.[56]	100	0
Temple et al.[62]	88	0
Lagios et al.[35]	87	2
Rosen et al.[49]	53	0
Sunshine et al.[61]	61	0
Schuh et al.[53]	52	2
Von Rueden and Wilson[67]	32	0
Brown et al.[5]	21	5
Schwartz et al.[54]	18	0
Fowble et al.[20]	15	0
Recht et al.[46]	13	0

From Fowble B: Oncology 3:51, 1989.

section for intraductal carcinoma is presented in Table 13-11. The overall incidence is ≤5%. Therefore routine axillary dissection is not recommended unless there is question of invasion. Gump et al.[25] have correlated the likelihood of positive axillary nodes with the clinical presentation of the intraductal carcinoma. Of patients who presented with a palpable mass, Paget's disease, or bloody nipple discharge (gross DCIS), 2% had positive axillary nodes, compared to 0 of those presenting with mammographic findings only or an incidental pathologic finding (microscopic DCIS). Hardman et al.[26] reported a 4% incidence of positive axillary nodes in patients with the comedo histologic subtype. Lagios et al.[36] reported axillary nodal involvement in none of 29 intraductal tumors ≤2.5 cm in size, and 1 of 25 patients with tumor size >2.5 cm. Although the overall risk of axillary metastases is small, consideration may be given to performing a limited axillary dissection in patients with the histologic subtype of comedocarcinoma, and those who present with palpable masses or evidence of microinvasion. In these patients the risk of axillary metastases appears higher. In patients with microinvasion the incidence has been reported to be 12%.[42] Microinvasion has been noted to be more frequent with comedo histologic subtype tumors,[42,57] high nuclear grade tumors,[42] tumors >2.5 cm in size, and aneuploid tumors. The presence of any of these features also may weigh in the decision to perform an axillary node dissection.

Wide excision alone: rationale and results

Not all patients with intraductal carcinoma have multicentric disease, occult invasion, or recurrence with an invasive or noninvasive cancer following excision alone. Comparisons of outcome for wide excision alone vs. mastectomy are available from two retrospective series[40,50] and a single prospective randomized trial.[18] While breast recurrence rates are higher in the group undergoing wide excision alone, none of these series has demonstrated an increased incidence of patients dying of their disease when surgery less than a mastectomy was employed. As noted in Table 13-5, breast recurrence rates following wide excision alone for intraductal carcinoma, where the wide excision was meant to be the sole treatment and where negative margins of resection were obtained, range from 10% to 57%. Recurrence rates are lowest for those where detection was by mammography alone. A comparison of wide excision alone with wide excision and radiation reveals similar findings. Analysis of patients with intraductal carcinoma entered into the NSABP B-06 trial[18] revealed a breast recurrence rate of 23% for those undergoing wide excision with negative margins, compared to 7% for those undergoing wide excision and radiation. None of the patients who underwent wide excision with or without radiation died of their disease.

As demonstrated in Table 13-6, surgical salvage of breast recurrences following wide excision alone generally has been excellent, although three series[22,41,48] reported 30% to 60% of patients who developed a recurrence (primarily an invasive recurrence) following wide excision alone as having died of their disease. In the series where a significant mortality has been reported, the breast recurrence rate ranges from 25% to 67%,[22,41,48] whereas in the series where salvage results have been excellent,[1,18,35] breast recurrence rates range from 10% to 23%. Therefore there is a valid concern that, as breast recurrence rates increase with wide excision alone, a potential for increased mortality may be seen, as approximately 50% of these recurrences are invasive (see Table 13-6). Recent efforts have been directed towards identifying patients in whom the risk of a breast recurrence is low enough to justify wide excision as the sole treatment.

In identifying patients in whom treatment to less than the entire breast may be appropriate, consideration should be given to the risk of multicentricity and occult invasion. Tables 13-12 and 13-13 present the incidence of multicentricity and occult invasion as noted in mastectomy specimens for intraductal carcinoma related to tumor size, method of detection, and histologic subtype. Multicentricity appears for the most part to be unrelated to

Table 13-12 Multicentricity of intraductal carcinoma related to tumor size/extent, method of detection, and histologic subtype

	Multicentricity (%)					
Tumor characteristics	Lagios et al.[36]	Fentiman et al.[14]	Schwartz et al.[55]	Wobbes et al.[69]	Patchefsky et al.[42]	Gump et al.[25]
Tumor size/extent						
Size						
≤2.5 cm	14					
>2.5 cm	54					
Biopsy specimen (%)						
<75		22				
>75		26				
No. ducts involved						
<10		19				
>10		24				
Method of detection						
Palpable mass		25				
Positive mammogram only		19	38	27		31
Incidental			0			0
Histologic subtype						
Comedo		23			14	
Cribriform		20			27	
Solid		7				
Papillary		24			36	
Micropapillary					86	

tumor size or extent, histologic subtype, or method of detection when comparing palpable lesions to those detected by mammography alone. Lagios et al.,[36] however, noted a 14% incidence of multicentricity with tumors ≤2.5 cm, compared to 54% for tumors >2.5 cm. Fentiman et al.[14] and Patchefsky et al.[42] did not correlate multicentricity with the number of ducts involved. There is no consistent relationship between multicentricity and histologic subtype. Approximately 30% of tumors detected by mammography alone are multicentric,[14,25,55,69] compared to 25% of those that present with a palpable mass.[14] Both Schwartz et al.[55] and Gump et al.[25] reported a 0 incidence of multicentricity in patients in whom the primary lesion was detected as an incidental finding at the time of biopsy for a clinical abnormality that proved to be benign. The apparent inability to correlate multicentricity with tumor extent, method of detection, and histologic pattern may be related to the fact that tumor extent for intraductal carcinoma may be difficult to assess and intraductal carcinomas manifest pathologic diversity. For lesions detected mammographically, the mammogram has underestimated the pathologic extent in 22%[36] and 38%.[28] Lagios et al.[36] reported lesions to be underestimated by an average of 7 mm (range 1 to 20 mm), whereas Holland et al.[28] noted that in 87% of cases the lesions were underestimated by >2 cm. However, this underestimation occurred only with tumors >2 cm size. Lagios et al.[36] noted a greater percentage of overestimation of tumor size[66] by an average of 1.5 cm (median 5 mm). In addition, the size of the lesion is not indicated reliably by the extent of microcalcifications on mammography. Specimen radiography frequently demonstrates more microcalcifications than are seen on the diagnostic mammogram.[11] Holland et al.[28] reported an underestimation of size by >2 cm in 44% of small cell, cribriform, or micropapillary tumors but a relatively accurate assessment of size in comedocarcinomas. Pathologic diversity is not infrequent with more than one histologic pattern being present in 40%,[57] 48%,[71] and 58%[18] of cases. Fisher et al.[18] noted a pure or predominant pattern in 42% of patients with intraductal carcinomas. It must be emphasized, however, that the clinical significance of multicentricity is considerably less frequent than its biologic presence. In patients with intraductal carcinoma treated by excision alone, 80% to 100%

Table 13-13 Occult invasion of intraductal carcinoma related to tumor size/extent, method of detection, and histologic subtype

	Occult invasion (%)				
Tumor characteristics	**Lagios et al.[36]**	**Fentiman et al.[14]**	**Gump et al.[25]**	**Schwartz et al.[55]**	**Hardman et al.[26]**
Tumor size/extent					
Size					
≤2.5 cm	2				
>2.5 cm	29				
Biopsy specimen (%)					
<75		8			
>75		29			
No. ducts involved					
<10		9.5			
>10		18			
Method of detection					
Palpable mass		17	6		
Positive mammogram only		5	0	0	
Incidental			0	0	
Histologic subtype					
Cribriform		13			
Papillary		14			
Solid		28			
Comedo		27			25

of the recurrences occur in the vicinity of the primary tumor (see Table 13-6).

In contrast, the incidence of invasion appears to be related to tumor size and extent, the method of detection, and the histologic subtype (see Table 13-13). It is more common in patients with larger tumors, in those that present with a palpable mass, and in those with a tumor of the solid or comedo histologic subtype. Patchefsky et al.[42] and Silverstein et al.[57] noted the greatest incidence of microinvasion with the comedo histologic subtype. Nuclear grade also has been correlated with histologic subtype, with comedocarcinomas frequently having a high nuclear grade.[42] Because of this relationship, high nuclear grade also is associated more often with microinvasion.[42] Lagios et al.[35] also have correlated high nuclear grade with the comedo and cribriform with necrosis histologic subtypes. Focal invasion also has been associated with ploidy status. Carpenter et al.[7,8] noted that 23 of 26 patients with intraductal carcinoma associated with microinvasion had aneuploid tumors. Four of 12 patients with in situ intraductal carcinoma only had aneuploid tumors.

Additional methods of assessing the biologic aggressiveness of an intraductal carcinoma include thymidine labeling index (TLI) and neu-protein overexpression. Meyer[39] analyzed the TLI in breast cancers where the in situ component was sufficient for a reliable determination. The TLI was significantly lower in the cribriform-papillary intraductal carcinoma than in the comedo subtype. The solid pattern appeared to resemble the cribriform-papillary pattern. Van der Vijver et al.,[63] through immunohistochemical techniques, noted neu-protein overexpression only in the solid or comedo types and not in the small cell papillary or cribriform types. There is no correlation between neu-protein overexpression and tumor size. These findings indicate a higher risk of cell proliferation for the comedo type of intraductal carcinoma. Histologically, tumors with a predominant comedo pattern exhibit the most cellular pleomorphism and mitoses, and have been found more often to have extensive involvement of the biopsy specimen[14,42] and a higher recurrence rate.[57]

Therefore, in selecting patients in whom wide excision alone may be appropriate treatment, patients presenting with palpable masses, large primary tumor size, the comedo or cribriform with necrosis histologic subtype, high nuclear grade, or aneuploidy probably should be excluded based on a higher incidence of occult invasion and their potential biologic aggressiveness. Patients who may be candidates for wide excision alone include those whose lesion is detected as a mammographic finding only, who have primarily diploid tumors, with the papillary or micropapillary subtype or the cribriform subtype without necrosis. Schwartz et al.[55] also have suggested that patients whose diagnosis of intraductal carcinoma is an incidental finding also might be candidates, because the incidence of microinvasion and multicentricity in this group of patients was 0 in their series. However, the older series of Rosen et al.[48] and Page et al.[41] would suggest that breast recurrence rates remain high in this group of patients, although margins of resection were not assessed.

Two recent series have reported results of wide excision alone in the treatment of selected patients with intraductal carcinoma. Lagios et al.[35] established the following criteria for selecting patients to be treated by wide excision alone: patients with occult lesions detected only by mammographic microcalcifications, patients with pathologic size ≤2.5 cm, patients with a negative inked margin of resection, those with no evidence of residual microcalcifications on a postbiopsy mammogram, and patients capable of understanding the risk of treatment as well as being amenable to clinical and mammographic follow-up. Between 1972 and 1987, 79 patients meeting these criteria were treated with wide excision alone. The mean size of the tumor was 6.8 mm, with a median of 5 mm and a range of 1 to 33 mm. With a mean follow-up of 48 months, 10% of the patients had recurrences of disease in the breast and 50% had an invasive recurrence. None of the patients has died of metastatic breast cancer. All of the recurrences were in the same quadrant as the original tumor. Recurrence was related to the histologic subtype. There were no recurrences in 33 patients with a micropapillary pattern, compared to 7 of 36 (19%) with the comedo or cribriform pattern with necrosis. One of 10 patients with a cribriform pattern with anaplasia had a recurrence. In a recent update with a mean follow-up of 68 months, there were recurrences in 10 of these 79 patients (13%).[34] Seven of 31 patients with the comedo pattern have developed a breast recurrence, and 2 of 5 patients with a cribriform or papillary pattern with necrosis have had recurrences, for a total of 9 of 36 patients (25%) in these two histologic subgroups. There have been no further recurrences in patients with the cribriform pattern without necrosis or the micropapillary pattern. This series, although highly selected, would suggest that the breast recurrence rate is significant enough in the comedo and cribriform or papillary types with necrosis following wide excision alone with negative margins to consider treatment to the entire breast either by mastectomy or conservative surgery and radiation. The recurrence rate remains low in the cribriform pattern with anaplasia or the micropapillary pattern, and these patients may be most appropriate for wide excision alone. Arnesson et al.[1] reported 38 patients with a comedo or cribriform histologic subtype detected by mammographic findings alone who underwent wide excision. With a median follow-up of 5 years, the breast recurrence rate was 13%. The interval to recurrence is also shorter for the comedo or cribriform pattern with necrosis; Lagios et al.[35] reported a mean interval to recurrence of 26 months in these patients. The mean interval to recurrence for patients with cribriform or micropapillary patterns has ranges from 73 to 116 months.[35,41,48]

The treatment of a breast recurrence in patients who have undergone wide excision alone as initial treatment for intraductal carcinoma generally has been mastectomy. Mastectomy is the appropriate treatment for patients whose tumors recur with an invasive component.[34] Lagios[34] raised the possibility of reexcision alone as the sole treatment for patients whose recurrence is intraductal carcinoma without invasion. Five patients whose recurrence was in situ carcinoma alone underwent reexcision and remained alive without evidence of disease. Arnesson et al.[1] also recommended repeat wide excision for a recurrence that was in situ and unifocal; however, one of two patients who underwent repeat excision ultimately had a second recurrence necessitating mastectomy. The biologic aggressiveness of the intraductal noninvasive recurrence may impact on further treatment recommendations. In patients whose recurrence is comedo or cribriform with necrosis, aneuploid or high nuclear grade repeat wide excision alone may not be appropriate. The role of reexcision and radiation for a recurrence following initial wide excision alone for an intraductal carcinoma requires further study. It may be considered for patients with small localized recurrences, either invasive or noninvasive, in whom negative margins are achieved. Patients with an invasive recurrence also should undergo an axillary dissection before radiation treatment.

In summary, three treatment options exist for intraductal noninvasive breast cancer. While mastectomy has been standard treatment, there is increasing evidence that conservative surgery with or without radiation represents a valid alternative in selected patients. Candidates for conservative surgery and radiation include those with primary tumors <4 to 5 cm, those who have no evidence of diffuse microcalcifications on a mammogram or evidence of gross multicentric disease demonstrated either clinically or mammographically, and those in whom adequate excision can be achieved as demonstrated by negative margins of resection and postbiopsy mammograms demonstrating no residual microcalcifications. Indications for mastectomy include a tumor size >4 to 5 cm; the presence of diffuse microcalcifications, gross multicentric disease, or multiple areas of calcification that appear malignant; multiple or diffuse positive reexcision margins, and cases in which the patient does not desire conservation therapy. Patients who present with bloody nipple discharge may be at an increased risk for breast recurrence when treated with conservative surgery and radiation, and mastectomy is the preferred treatment in this group of patients. Consideration of wide excision alone as the sole treatment probably should be restricted to patients whose lesions are detected by mammography alone or as an incidental finding and where complete excision is confirmed by negative margins of resection with postbiopsy mammograms demonstrating no residual microcalcifications. Patients with a comedocarcinoma or cribriform pattern with necrosis, and those with aneuploid tumors or high nuclear grade may have a breast recurrence rate following wide excision alone that is high enough to warrant consideration of treatment to the entire breast either by mastectomy or radiation following wide excision. At the present time conservative surgery with or without radiation has resulted in no increase in the incidence of patients dying of their disease when compared to mastectomy, although breast recurrence rates are highest in the group of patients undergoing wide excision without radiation. Currently there are no ongoing randomized trials evaluating the role of mastectomy in the treatment of intraductal breast cancer. There are three ongoing randomized clinical trials comparing wide excision with or without radiation. These include the NSABP B-17,[70] the European Organization for Research and Treatment of Cancer (EORTC) trial,[64] and the Danish Breast Cancer Group trial.[24] The results of these trials will provide further comparisons of wide excision alone with wide excision and radiation.

Treatment recommendations must be based on the clinical and pathologic features of each lesion. The following factors may impact on the selection of a treatment option: the method of detection, the extent of the disease, the histologic subtype, and the adequacy of excision as assessed by margins of resection and postbiopsy mammograms. It must be emphasized that assessment of the extent of disease requires a knowledge of the mammographic, clinical, and pathologic findings. The size of lesion is not indicated reliably by the extent of microcalcifications on the mammogram,[11,36,45] and a specimen radiograph not infrequently demonstrates more microcalcifications.[11]

Management of the contralateral breast in patients with noninvasive intraductal cancer

In patients with in situ ductal carcinoma, the risk of a contralateral breast cancer ranges from 3% to 8%.[2,13,21,68] Frazier et al.[21] have reported a 10-year actuarial risk of 9% in a series of 106 patients. Thus the risk of a contralateral breast cancer in patients with in situ ductal carcinoma is not dissimilar from that of patients with an infiltrating ductal carcinoma. The contralateral breast should therefore be followed with routine physical examinations and yearly mammography.

IN SITU LOBULAR CARCINOMA

Foote and Stewart[84] first employed the term *lobular carcinoma in situ* in 1941 to describe a distinct pathologic entity representing a form of breast cancer that originated in lobules and terminal ducts. In situ lobular carcinoma comprises 1% to 6% of all breast cancers[76,79,91,106-108] and is less common than intraductal noninvasive breast cancer.[107,108] It usually is detected as an incidental finding at the time of biopsy of a clinical or mammographic finding that proves to be benign.[76,84,85,97] The most common clinical presentation is that of a palpable mass.[86,88,95,97,104,115] The mass is characteristically benign in appearance and has been attributed to a breast abscess, fat necrosis, cystic disease, benign cyst, or fibroadenoma.[76,82,87,88,97,104] The most common mammographic finding is the appearance of clustered calcifications,[108] although the calcifications almost always are in benign areas.[90,108] The mammogram demonstrates an abnormality in only 50% of cases.[110] The majority of patients with in situ lobular carcinoma are premenopausal,[74,104,106,107] and their mean age ranges from 44 to 47 years.[72,77,79,80,95,100,102,104,106,117] While it was thought that in situ lobular carcinoma was an estrogen-dependent disease because of age distribution and menopausal status, its presence in postmenopausal women who have not employed exogenous estrogens suggests that the issue is more complex.[106] A positive family history of breast cancer is reported in 15% to 20% of patients.[79,82,104]

Before 1960, treatment was primarily unilateral mastectomy. This approach was based on the documented multifocal and multicentric nature of in situ lobular carcinoma as demonstrated in mastectomy specimens (Table 13-14) and the recognized potential for progression to an invasive lobular carcinoma. Following an excisional biopsy in which in situ lobular carcinoma was identified micro-

Table 13-14 Incidence of residual in situ lobular carcinoma (LCIS) and occult invasion after wide excision in patients undergoing mastectomy

Author	Residual LCIS (%)	Occult invasion (%)
Wanebo et al.[115]	58 [41/70]	4 [3/70]
Carter and Smith[77]	63 [31/49]	6 [3/49]
Rosen et al.[105]	56 [28/50]	4 [2/50]
Benfield et al.[76]	80 [8/10]	0 [0/13]
McDivitt et al.[97]	12 [1/8]	
Schwartz et al.[108]	17 [1/6]	0 [0/6]
Dall'Olmo et al.[79]	56 [14/25]	0 [0/23]
Newman[100]	93 [26/28]	0 [0/28]
Rosen et al.[103]	54 [45/84]	1 [1/84]
Lewison and Finney[95]	62 [21/34]	
Ringberg et al.[102]	69 [11/16]	12 [2/16]
Andersen[73]	47 [9/19]	
Wheeler et al.[117]	—	0 [0/13]
Shah et al.[109]	65 [26/40]	5 [2/40]

[ ], no. pts.

scopically, approximately 60% of patients were found to have residual in situ lobular carcinoma in the mastectomy specimen either in the vicinity of original tumor or separate quadrants. The lower incidence reported by Schwartz et al.[108] and McDivitt et al.[97] may be related to the fact that these authors included only disease noted in a separate quadrant. The simultaneous presence of in situ ductal carcinoma also was noted.[103,105,108] Unlike intraductal carcinoma, the overall incidence of occult invasion is generally <10% (see Table 13-14). Godwin[87] first described the evolution of in situ lobular carcinoma into an invasive carcinoma in a single patient over a period of 12 years. Newman[99] noted the presence of in situ lobular carcinoma in 72 of 73 patients with pure infiltrating lobular carcinoma. Table 13-15 presents the results of treatment of in situ lobular carcinoma with mastectomy. As noted, the incidence of chest wall recurrence following mastectomy is extremely low, and overall ≤3% patients die of their disease.

The bilateral nature of in situ lobular carcinoma was first appreciated in the reports from mastectomy series. Two of the series[103,116] identified a 10% to 20% risk of contralateral breast cancer, although it was more commonly noninvasive breast cancer. Further evidence of the bilateral nature was obtained from the results of contralateral breast biopsies or contralateral prophylactic mastectomies in patients with in situ lobular carcinoma (Table 13-16). Approximately 30% to 40% of patients who underwent a contralateral biopsy were found to have noninvasive breast cancer that was primarily in situ lobular carcinoma and 0 to 9% were found to have an invasive breast cancer. The contralateral biopsy was generally of the upper outer quadrant of the breast and, as advocated by Urban,[112] removed 20% to 25% of the breast parenchyma. Unilateral mastectomy with contralateral breast biopsy was the predominant form of treatment of in situ lobular carcinoma in the 1960s and was advocated by a number of investigators.[76,86,87,91,97,99,104,105] If the contralateral biopsy was positive either for invasive cancer or nonin-

Table 13-15 Results of mastectomy in patients with in situ lobular carcinoma

Author	Treatment period	No. pts.	Local recurrence (%)	Contralateral breast cancer (%)		Dead of disease (%)	Follow-up (yr)
				Invasive cancer	Noninvasive cancer		
Hutter and Foote[91]	1940-1952	6	0	0	0	0	4-27
Benfield et al.[76]	1941-1958	8	0	0	0	0	1-23
Rosen et al.[104]	1940-1950	7	0	0	0	0	24 (mean)
Rosen et al.[103]	1952-1965	84	—	6	14	2	15 (mean)
Dall'Olmo et al.[79]	1952-1971	24	—	—	—	0	2-22
Newman[100]	1953-1961	24	—	—	4	0	—
Giordano and Klopp[86]	1953-1971	105	1	—	—	1	—
Wanebo et al.[115]	1953-1972	49	0	—	—	0	10
Webber et al.[116]	1955-1971	68	—	4	6	—	9 (mean)
Lewison and Finney[95]	1957-1966	37	0	0	0	0	—
Carter and Smith[77]	1960-1975	49	0	0	6	0	8 (mean)
Sunshine et al.[111]	1960-1980	33	—	—	—	3	11.9
Kinne et al.[93]	1970-1976	31	0	0	0	0	11.5 (median)

Table 13-16 Results of contralateral breast biopsy or mastectomy in patients with in situ lobular carcinoma

Author	No. pts.	Negative (%)	Positive (%)	
			Invasive cancer	Noninvasive cancer
Benfield et al.[76]	5	60	0	40
Urban[112]	22	54	5	41
Newman[100]	16	75	0	25
Donegan and Perez-Mesa[80]	7	57	0	43
Rosen et al.[103]	63	52	9	38
Wheeler et al.[117]	7	100	0	0
Carter and Smith[77]	44	61	0	39
Lewison and Finney[95]	15	53	0	47
Sunshine et al.[111]	21	33	0	67
Ringberg et al.[102]	16	6	6	87
Andersen[73]	7	86	0	14

vasive cancer, bilateral mastectomy was performed.

Further evidence for the natural history of in situ lobular carcinoma was provided by the results of series employing wide excision as the sole treatment (Table 13-17). These series again demonstrated the bilateral nature of in situ lobular carcinoma. The risk of development of a subsequent breast cancer in the involved breast, either invasive or noninvasive, was equal to that in the contralateral breast[88,91,103,104] McDivitt et al.[97] reported the risk of an ipsilateral invasive breast cancer following excision only for in situ lobular carcinoma to be 10% at 5 years, 15% at 10 years, 30% at 15 years, and 35% at 20 years. The risk of a contralateral invasive or noninvasive breast cancer was 5% at 5 years, 10% at 10 years, 15% at 15 years, and 25% at 20 years. Haagensen et al.[88] reported a 22% risk of the development of an ipsilateral breast cancer, invasive or noninvasive, after 25

Table 13-17 Results of treatment of in situ lobular carcinoma with excision alone

Author	Treatment period	No. pts.	Subsequent breast cancer (%)				Dead of disease (%)	Follow-up (yr)
			Ipsilateral		Contralateral			
			Invasive cancer	Noninvasive cancer	Invasive cancer	Noninvasive cancer		
Haagensen et al.[88]	1930-1972	192	10	—	10	—	3	1-42
Rosen et al.[104]	1940-1950	84	21	1	15	4	19	24 (mean)
Hutter and Foote[91]	1940-1952	40	25	10	10	5	5	4-27
Benfield et al.[76]	1941-1958	5	0	0	0	0	0	0.5-11
Andersen[72]	1942-1961	44	20	—	9	—	9	15.9 (mean)
Rosen et al.[103]	1952-1965	17	12	47	0	12	12	13 (mean)
Wheeler et al.[117]	1948-1963	25	4	0	3	9	3	17.5 (mean)
Newman[100]	1953-1961	3	33	0	—	—	33	—
Giordano and Klopp[86]	1953-1971	19	10	0	0	0	0	0.5-11
Lewison and Finney[95]	1957-1966	3	0	0	0	0	0	3-10
Carter and Smith[77]	1960-1975	49	2	0	—	—	—	8 (mean)
Eusebi et al.[81]	1965-1971	14	0	0	0	7	0	17 (mean)
Kinne et al.[93]	1970-1976	12	—	—	—	—	0	11.5 (median)
Herrmann[89]	—	5	0	0	0	0	0	1-25

years and a contralateral risk of 25%. Wheeler et al.[117] reported only a 4% risk of an ipsilateral invasive breast cancer at 17.5 years (mean follow-up); a risk of a contralateral invasive breast cancer of 7% at 10 years, 12% at 15 years, and 12% at 20 years. The variations in the estimated risk may be related to the period of follow-up. Rosen et al.[104] reported a mean interval of 16.3 years for the development of an invasive ductal carcinoma and 20.4 years for the development of an invasive lobular carcinoma, either ipsilateral or contralateral. Webber et al.[116] reported contralateral invasive breast cancers occurring over a period of 1 to 16 years with the interval for noninvasive contralateral breast cancer being 0.6 to 5 years. McDivitt et al.[97] reported the interval for the development of an ipsilateral invasive breast cancer to range from 2 to 23 years. Hutter and Foote[91] reported a mean interval for the development of a subsequent breast cancer, either in the ipsilateral or contralateral breast, of 8 years. Therefore the risk appears to increase with time. Variations of the incidence of contralateral breast cancer from the mastectomy series in Table 13-15 also may be related to variation in the follow-up period. These studies also demonstrate that the majority of patients with in situ lobular carcinoma treated with excision only do not develop a subsequent breast cancer.

The role of in situ lobular carcinoma as a precursor or progenitor of invasive breast cancer has been questioned because the risk of development of the subsequent breast cancer is equal for both breasts and the majority of invasive breast cancers that develop are infiltrating ductal carcinomas.[79,84,104,117] Similarly, the clinical significance of the multifocal or multicentric nature of lobular carcinoma appears questionable in light of the bilateral nature of the disease. It has been suggested by others[72,83,88,92,108,114,117] that in situ lobular carcinoma is a marker for a predisposition to the future development of invasive breast cancer in either breast.

The treatment options for in situ lobular carcinoma include unilateral mastectomy with or without contralateral biopsy, bilateral mastectomy, and excision only followed by close observation. Unlike in situ ductal carcinoma, in which the risk for development of a subsequent cancer is primarily unilateral, the bilateral risk associated with in situ lobular carcinoma creates a clinical dilemma. It is clear that unilateral mastectomy ignores the problem of a contralateral breast cancer. A contralateral breast biopsy may be associated with a sampling error and, as noted by Benfield et al.[76] the fact that one biopsy is negative does not provide assurance that a subsequent cancer will not develop in this breast. Rosen et al.[103] reported the risk of development of a subsequent contralateral breast cancer to be the same for patients in whom a contralateral biopsy was not done and in those in whom it was done and was negative or showed atypia. Fourteen of 51 patients who did not have a contralateral breast biopsy subsequently developed a contralateral noninvasive cancer, and four developed a contralateral invasive cancer. Of 29 patients whose contralateral biopsy was negative or showed only atypia, 14 developed a subsequent noninvasive contralateral breast cancer and three developed a contralateral invasive breast cancer. Benfield et al.[76] therefore recommended periodic contralateral breast biopsies. This recommendation can be questioned as the majority of patients will not develop a contralateral breast cancer and periodic biopsies are also subject to sampling error. Bilateral mastectomy with immediate reconstruction, while minimizing the risk of development of a subsequent invasive cancer in either breast, does not appear to be warranted because the majority of patients will not develop subsequent invasive breast cancer. Bilateral mastectomy may be appropriate, however, for the individual patient in whom any risk of the development of a subsequent invasive breast cancer is unacceptable and whose goal is maximal prevention.

The conservative approach, employing unilateral excision only and careful follow-up, gained increasing acceptance in the 1980s.[92,114] The arguments for this approach include the fact that the disease occurs primarily in younger women, a minority of patients ultimately develop an invasive cancer, the interval to the development of an invasive cancer is relatively long (i.e., approximately 15 years) and the percentage of patients dying of their disease when treated with excision alone is relatively low. In a national survey performed by the American College of Surgeons[107] the 5-year NED survival for 33 patients with in situ lobular carcinoma who underwent excision alone was 79%, compared to 93% for 91 patients treated by mastectomy. These differences were not significant. Similarly, recurrence was noted in 3 of the 91 mastectomy patients and none of the 33 patients with excision alone.

The question arises as to whether resection margins must be negative in patients who undergo excision and observation. Rosen et al.[104] state that resection margins are unreliable indicators and do not guarantee that all disease has been removed. Recht et al.[101] also state that negative margins are not mandatory because in situ lobular carcinoma is only a marker of an increased risk for the development of invasive cancer and is not itself malignant. Fisher and Fisher,[83] however, feel that margins of resection should be negative. It appears that excision with careful observation is currently the course given to the majority of patients with in situ lobular carcinoma.[78,92] Conservative surgery and radiation have been employed in a small number of patients with in situ lobular carcinoma.[94] The role of this therapy is limited, as treatment is directed only to the involved breast; radiation is not advised as a preventive measure for the contralateral breast. It may be considered in patients who have undergone a previous mastectomy for breast cancer and in whom the remaining breast demonstrates in situ lobular carcinoma, although results of such treatment are not available. An axillary dissection is not indicated in patients with in situ lobular carcinoma because the likelihood of finding positive axillary nodes ranges from 0 to 4%.[76,77,79,100,105,115]

The question arises as to whether prognostic factors can be identified that will distinguish those women with in situ lobular carcinoma who will develop a subsequent invasive cancer. The majority of in situ lobular carcinomas have a low thymidine labeling index,[98] and most are diploid.[96] The risk of development of subsequent cancer has not been correlated with a positive family history, nulliparity, the number of lobules involved, or the cell type of the in situ lobular carcinoma.[88,104,117] Rosen et al.,[104] however, noted that the combination of large and small cells was associated with an increased risk for the development of a subsequent breast cancer, although the number of patients in this analysis was extremely small. At the present time there are no known factors that can distinguish patients who will develop a subsequent invasive carcinoma from those who will not.

Observation studies have been started in Denmark and Sweden[113] in an effort to improve our knowledge of the natural history and clinical behavior of in situ lobular carcinoma. The NSABP has initiated a registry for patients with in situ lobular carcinoma as part of the B-17 protocol. To date, approximately 100 patients have been registered.[118] The European Organization for Research and Treatment of Cancer has initiated a randomized trial comparing close observation with tamoxifen (20 mg per day) for 5 years.[113] It is hoped that these studies will provide further information that will direct treatment recommendations. Our current philosphy for the treatment of in situ lobular carcinoma is one of unilateral excision only and careful follow-up.

REFERENCES

Intraductal noninvasive breast cancer

1. Arnesson LG, Smeds S, Fagerberg G, and Grontoft O: Follow-up of two treatment modalities for ductal carcinoma in situ of the breast, Br J Surg 76:672, 1989.
2. Ashikari R, Hajdu SI, and Robbins GF: Intraductal carcinoma of the breast, Cancer 28:1182, 1971.
3. Bader J, Lippman M, Swain S, et al: Preliminary report of the NCI early breast cancer study: a prospective randomized comparison of lumpectomy and radiation to mastectomy for Stage I and II breast cancer, Int J Radiat Oncol Biol Phys 13:160, 1987 (abstract).
4. Beahrs DH, Shapiro S, and Smart C: Report of the working group to review the National Cancer Institute—American Cancer Society Breast Cancer Detection Demonstration projects, J Natl Cancer Inst 62:643, 1979.
5. Brown PW, Silverman J, Owens E, et al: Intraductal "noninfiltrating" carcinoma of the breast, Arch Surg 111:1063, 1976.
6. Calle R, Vilcoq JR, Zafrani B, et al: Local control and survival of breast cancer treated by limited surgery followed by irradiation, Int J Radiat Oncol Biol Phys 12:873, 1986.
7. Carpenter R, Boulter PS, Cooke T, and Gibbs NM: Management of screen detected ductal carcinoma in situ of the female breast, Br J Surg 76:564, 1989.
8. Carpenter R, Gibbs N, Mathews J, and Cooke T: Importance of cellular DNA content in pre-malignant breast disease and pre-invasive carcinoma of the female breast, Br J Surg 74:905, 1987.
9. Carter D and Smith RRL: Carcinoma in situ of the breast, Cancer 40:1189, 1977.
10. Delouche G, Bachelot F, Premont M, and Kurtz JM: Conservation treatment of early breast cancer: long term results and complications, Int J Radiat Oncol Biol Phys 13:29, 1987.
11. Dershaw DD, Abramson A, and Kinne DW: Ductal carcinoma in-situ: mammographic findings and clinical implications, Radiology 170:411, 1989.
12. Eusebi V, Foschini MP, Cook MG, et al: Long term follow-up of in situ carcinoma of the breast with special emphasis on clinging carcinoma, Semin Diagn Pathol 6:165, 1989.
13. Farrow JH: Current concepts in the detection and treatment of the earliest of the early breast cancers, Cancer 25:468, 1970.
14. Fentiman IS, Fagg N, Millis RR, and Hayward JL: In situ ductal carcinoma of the breast: implications of disease pattern and treatment, Eur J Surg Oncol 12:261, 1986.
15. Findlay PA and Goodman R: Radiation therapy for treatment of intraductal carcinoma of the breast, Am J Clin Oncol 6:281, 1983.
16. Fisher B, Bauer M, Margolese R, et al: Five-year results of a randomized clinical trial comparing total mastectomy and segmental mastectomy with or without radiation in the treatment of breast cancer, N Engl J Med 312:665, 1985.
17. Fisher ER, Gregorio R, Redmond C, et al: Pathologic findings from the National Surgical Adjuvant Breast Project (protocol 4). I. Observations concerning the multicentricity of mammary cancer, Cancer 35:347, 1975.
18. Fisher ER, Sass R, Fisher B, et al: Pathologic findings from the National Surgical Adjuvant Breast Project (protocol 6). I. Intraductal carcinoma (DCIS), Cancer 57:197, 1986.
19. Fowble B: Intraductal noninvasive breast cancer: a comparison of three local treatments, Oncology 3:51, 1989.
20. Fowble BL, Solin LJ, and Goodman RL: Results of conservative surgery and radiation for intraductal non-invasive breast cancer, Am J Clin Oncol 10:110, 1987 (abstract).
21. Frazier TG, Copeland EM, Gallagher HS, et al: Prognosis and treatment in minimal breast cancer, Am J Surg 133:697, 1977.
22. Gallagher WJ, Koerner FC, and Wood WC: Treatment of

intraductal carcinoma with limited surgery: long term follow-up, J Clin Oncol 7:376, 1989.
23. Gibbs NM: Comparative study of the histopathology of breast cancer in a screened and unscreened population investigated by mammography, Histopathology 9:1307, 1985.
24. Graversen HP, Blechert-Toft M, Dyreberg U, and Andersen J: In situ carcinomas of the female breast. Incidence, clinical findings and DBCG proposals for management, Acta Oncol 27:679, 1988.
25. Gump FE, Jicha DL, and Ozello L: Ductal carcinoma in situ (DCIS): a revised concept, Surgery 102:790, 1987.
26. Hardman PDJ, Worth A, and Lee U: The risk of occult invasive breast cancer after excisional biopsy showing in-situ ductal carcinoma of comedo pattern, Can J Surg 32:56, 1989.
27. Holland R, Connolly J, Gelman R, et al: The presence of an extensive intraductal component following a limited excision correlates with prominent residual disease in the remainder of the breast, J Clin Oncol 8:113, 1990.
28. Holland R, Veling SHJ, Mravunac M, and Hendriks JHCL: Histologic multifocality of Tis, T1-2 breast carcinoma. Implications for clinical trials of breast-conserving surgery, Cancer 56:979, 1985.
29. Howard PW, Locker AP, Dowle CS, et al: In situ carcinoma of the breast, Eur J Surg Oncol 15:328, 1989.
30. Ketcham AS and Moffat FL: Vexed surgeons, perplexed patients and breast cancers which may not be cancer, Cancer 65:387, 1990.
31. Kinne DW, Petrek JA, Osborne MP, et al: Breast carcinoma in situ, Arch Surg 124:33, 1989.
32. Kraus FT and Neubecker RD: The differential diagnosis of papillary tumors of the breast, Cancer 15:444, 1962.
33. Kurtz JM, Jacquemier J, Torhorst J, et al: Conservation therapy for breast cancers other than infiltrating ductal carcinoma, Cancer 63:1630, 1989.
34. Lagios MD: Duct carcinoma in situ: pathology and treatment. Mid-Willamette Valley Cancer Conference, March 1990, Willamette, Ore.
35. Lagios MD, Margolin FR, Westdahl PR, and Rose MR: Mammographically detected duct carcinoma in situ. Frequency of local recurrence following tylectomy and prognostic effect of nuclear grade on local recurrence, Cancer 63:618, 1989.
36. Lagios MD, Westdahl PR, Margolin FR, and Rose MR: Duct carcinoma in situ. Relationship of extent of noninvasive disease to the frequency of occult invasion, multicentricity, lymph node metastases and short-term treatment failures, Cancer 50:1309, 1982.
37. Lewis D and Geschickter CF: Comedo carcinoma of the breast, Arch Surg 36:225, 1938.
38. Margolin FR and Lagios MD: Mammographic detection of early breast cancer, West J Med 144:46, 1986.
39. Meyer JS: Cell Kinetics of histologic variants of in situ breast cancer, Breast Cancer Res Treat 7:171, 1986.
40. Millis RR and Thynne GSJ: In-situ intraduct carcinoma of the breast: a long term follow-up study, Br J Surg 62:957, 1975.
41. Page DL, Dupont WD, Rogers LW, and Landenberger M: Intraductal carcinoma of the breast: follow-up after biopsy only, Cancer 49:751, 1982.
42. Patchefsky AS, Schwartz GF, Finkelstein SD, et al: Heterogeneity of intraductal carcinoma of the breast, Cancer 63:731, 1989.
43. Price P, Sinnett HD, Gusterson B, et al: Duct carcinoma in-situ: can we predict recurrence after surgery? Lancet ii:671, 1989.
44. Recht A, Bornstein B, Connolly JL, et al: Treatment of ductal carcinoma in situ (DCIS) with conservative surgery and radiotherapy. Proceedings of the Fifth European Conference on Clinical Oncology, London, September 1989 (abstract).
45. Recht A, Connolly JL, Schnitt SJ, et al: Conservative surgery and radiation therapy for early breast cancer: results, controversies, and unsolved problems, Semin Oncol 13:434, 1986.
46. Recht A, Danoff BF, Solin LJ, et al: Intraductal carcinoma of the breast: results of treatment with excisional biopsy and irradiation, J Clin Oncol 3:1339, 1985.
47. Recht A, Silen W, Schnitt SJ, et al: Time course of local recurrence following conservative surgery and radiotherapy for breast cancer, Int J Radiat Oncol Biol Phys 15:255, 1988.
48. Rosen PP, Braun DW, and Kinne DE: The clinical significance of pre-invasive breast carcinoma, Cancer 46:919, 1980.
49. Rosen PP, Senie R, Schottenfeld D, and Ashikari R: Noninvasive breast carcinoma: frequency of unsuspected invasion and implications for treatment, Ann Surg 189:377, 1979.
50. Rosner D, Bedwani RN, Vana J, et al: Noninvasive breast carcinoma. Results of a national survey of the American College of Surgeons, Ann Surg 192:139, 1980.
51. Sarrazin D, Le MG, Fontaine MF, and Arriagada R: Conservative treatment versus mastectomy in T_1 or small T_2 breast cancer—a randomized clinical trial. In Harris J, Hellman S, and Silen W, editors: Conservative management of breast cancer, Philadelphia, 1983, JB Lippincott, pp 101-111.
52. Schnitt SJ, Silen W, Sadowsky NL, et al: Ductal carcinoma in situ (intraductal carcinoma) of the breast, N Engl J Med 318:898, 1988.
53. Schuh ME, Nemoto T, Penetrante RB, et al: Intraductal carcinoma. Analysis of presentation, pathologic findings and outcome of disease, Arch Surg 121:1303, 1986.
54. Schwartz GF, Feig SA, Rosenberg AL, et al: Staging and treatment of clinically occult breast cancer, Cancer 53:1379, 1984.
55. Schwartz GF, Patchefsky AS, Finklestein SD, et al: Nonpalpable in situ ductal carcinoma of the breast. Predictors of multicentricity and microinvasion and implications for treatment, Arch Surg 124:29, 1989.
56. Silverstein MJ, Rosser RJ, Gierson ED, et al: Axillary lymph node dissection for intraductal breast carcinoma—is it indicated? Cancer 59:1819, 1987.
57. Silverstein MJ, Waisman JR, Gamagami P, et al: Intraductal carcinoma of the breast (208 cases) clinical factors influencing treatment choice, Cancer 66:102, 1990.
58. Solin LJ, Fowble B, Martz KL, and Goodman RL: Definitive irradiation for early stage breast cancer: the University of Pennsylvania experience, Int J Radiat Oncol Biol Phys 14:235, 1988.
59. Solin LJ, Fowble BL, Schultz DJ, et al: Definitive irradiation for intraductal carcinoma of the breast, Int J Radiat Oncol Biol Phys 19:843, 1990.
60. Stotter AT, McNeese M, Oswald MJ, et al: The role of limited surgery with irradiation in primary treatment of ductal in situ breast cancer, Int J Radiat Oncol Biol Phys 18:283, 1990.
61. Sunshine JA, Moseley HS, Fletcher WS, and Krippaehne WW: Breast carcinoma in situ. A retrospective review of 112 cases with a minimum 10 year follow-up, Am J Surg 150:44, 1985.
62. Temple WJ, Jenkins M, Alexander F, et al: In situ breast cancer in Alberta 1951-1984, Am J Clin Oncol 9:109, 1986 (abstract).
63. Van de Vijver MJ, Peterse JL, Mooi WJ, et al: Neu-protein overexpression in breast cancer. Association with

comedo-type ductal carcinoma in situ and limited prognostic value in stage II breast cancer, N Engl J Med 319:1239, 1988.
64. van Dongen JA, Harris JR, Peterse JL, et al: In-situ breast cancer: the EORTC consensus meeting, Lancet ii:25, 1989.
65. Van Limbergen E, Van der Bogaert W, Van der Schueren E, and Rijnders A: Tumor excision and radiotherapy as primary treatment of breast cancer analysis of patient and treatment parameters and local control, Radiother Oncol 8:1, 1987.
66. Veronesi U, Banfi A, DelVecchio M, et al: Comparison of Halsted mastectomy with quadrantectomy, axillary dissection and radiotherapy in early breast cancer: long-term results, Eur J Cancer Clin Oncol 22:1085, 1986.
67. Von Rueden DG and Wilson WE: Intraductal carcinoma of the breast, Surg Gynecol Obstet 158:105, 1984.
68. Webber BL, Heise H, Neifeld JP, and Costa J: Risk of subsequent contralateral breast carcinoma in a population of patients with in-situ breast carcinoma, Cancer 47:2928, 1981.
69. Wobbes TH, Tinnemans JGM, and van der Sluis RF: Residual tumor after biopsy for non-palpable ductal carcinoma in situ of the breast, Br J Surg 76:185, 1989.
70. Wolmark N: Review noninvasive breast cancer, Oncology 3:42, 1989.
71. Zafrani B, Fourquet A, Vilcoq JR, et al: Conservative management of intraductal breast carcinoma with tumorectomy and radiation therapy, Cancer 57:1299, 1986.

In situ lobular carcinoma

72. Andersen JA: Lobular carcinoma in situ of the breast. An approach to rational treatment, Cancer 39:2597, 1977.
73. Andersen JA: Multicentric and bilateral appearance of lobular carcinoma in situ of the breast, Acta Pathol Microbiol Scand [A] 82:730, 1974.
74. Bedwani R, Vana J, Rosner D, et al: Management and survival of female patients with "minimal" breast cancer: as observed in the long-term and short-term surveys of the American College of Surgeons, Cancer 47:2769, 1981.
75. Beller FK, Nitsch CD, and Nienhaus H: Treatment aspects of minimal breast cancer, Recent Results Cancer Res 106:73, 1988.
76. Benfield JR, Jacobson M, and Warner NE: In situ lobular carcinoma of the breast, Arch Surg 91:130, 1965.
77. Carter D and Smith RL: Carcinoma in situ of the breast, Cancer 40:1189, 1977.
78. Connolly JL, Boyages J, Schnitt SJ, et al: In situ carcinoma of the breast, Ann Rev Med 40:173, 1989.
79. Dall'Olmo CA, Ponka JL, Hern RC, and Riu R: Lobular carcinoma of the breast in situ. Are we too radical in its treatment? Arch Surg 110:537, 1975.
80. Donegan WL and Perez-Mesa CM: Lobular carcinoma—an indication for elective biopsy of the second breast, Ann Surg 176:178, 1972.
81. Eusebi V, Foschini MP, Cook MG, et al: Long term follow-up of in situ carcinoma of the breast with special emphasis on clinging carcinoma, Semin Diagn Pathol 6:165, 1989.
82. Farrow JH: Current concepts in the detection and treatment of the earliest of the early breast cancers, Cancer 25:468, 1970.
83. Fisher ER and Fisher B: Lobular carcinoma of the breast: an overview, Ann Surg 185:377, 1977.
84. Foote FW Jr and Steward FW: Lobular carcinoma in situ. A rare form of mammary cancer, Am J Pathol 17:491, 1941.
85. Frykberg ER, Santiago F, Betsill WL Jr, and O'Brien PH: Lobular carcinoma in situ of the breast, Surg Gynecol Obstet 164:285, 1987.
86. Giordano JM and Klopp CT: Lobular carcinoma in situ. Incidence and treatment, Cancer 31:105, 1973.
87. Godwin JT: Chronology of lobular carcinoma of the breast, Cancer 5:259, 1952.
88. Haagensen CD, Lane N, Lattes R, and Bodian C: Lobular neoplasia (so-called lobular carcinoma in situ) of the breast, Cancer 42:737, 1978.
89. Herrmann JB: Treatment of in situ mammary carcinoma, Int Surg 57:127, 1972.
90. Hutter RVP: The management of patients with lobular carcinoma in situ of the breast, Cancer 53:798, 1984.
91. Hutter RVP and Foote FW Jr: Lobular carcinoma in situ. Long term follow-up, Cancer 24:1081, 1969.
92. Kinne DW: Review of noninvasive breast cancer by Swain SM, Oncology 3:40, 1989.
93. Kinne DW, Petrek JA, Osborne MP, et al: Breast carcinoma in situ, Arch Surg 124:33, 1989.
94. Kurtz JM, Jacquemier J, Torhorst J, et al: Conservation therapy for breast cancers other than infiltrating ductal carcinoma, Cancer 63:1630, 1989.
95. Lewison EF and Finney GG: Lobular carcinoma in situ of the breast, Surg Gynecol Obstet 126:1280, 1968.
96. Ludwig AS, Okagaki T, Richart RM, and Lattes R: Nuclear DNA content of lobular carcinoma in situ of the breast, Cancer 31:1553, 1973.
97. McDivitt RW, Hutter RVP, Foote FW, and Stewart FW: In situ lobular carcinoma. A prospective follow-up study indicating cumulative patient risks, JAMA 201:96, 1967.
98. Meyer JS: Cell kinetics of histologic variants of in situ breast carcinoma, Breast Cancer Res Treat 7:171, 1986.
99. Newman W: Lobular carcinoma of the female breast. Report of 73 cases, Ann Surg 164:305, 1966.
100. Newman W: In situ lobular carcinoma of the breast: report of 26 women with 32 cancers, Ann Surg 157:591, 1963.
101. Recht A, Connolly JL, Schnitt SJ, and Harris JR: Therapy of in situ cancer, Hematol Oncol Clin North Am 3:691, 1989.
102. Ringberg A, Palmer B, and Linell F: The contralateral breast at reconstructive surgery after breast cancer operation: a histopathological study, Breast Cancer Res Treat 2:151, 1982.
103. Rosen PP, Braun DW, Lyngholm B, et al: Lobular carcinoma in situ of the breast: preliminary results of treatment by ipsilateral mastectomy and contralateral breast biopsy, Cancer 47:813, 1981.
104. Rosen PP, Lieberman PH, Braun DW Jr, et al: Lobular carcinoma in situ of the breast. Detailed analysis of 99 patients with average follow-up of 24 years, Am J Surg Pathol 2:225, 1978.
105. Rosen PP, Senie R, Schottenfeld D, and Ashikari R: Noninvasive breast carcinoma. Frequency of unsuspected invasion and implications for treatment, Ann Surg 189:377, 1989.
106. Rosen PP, Senie RT, Farr GH, et al: Epidemiology of breast carcinoma: age, menstrual status, and exogenous hormone usage in patients with lobular carcinoma in situ, Surgery 85:219, 1979.
107. Rosner D, Bedwani RN, Vana J, et al: Noninvasive breast carcinoma. Results of a national survey by the American College of Surgeons, Ann Surg 192:139, 1980.
108. Schwartz GF, Feig SA, and Patchefsky AS: Significance and staging of nonpalpable carcinomas of the breast. Surg Gynecol Obstet 1676:6, 1988.
109. Shah JP, Rosen PP, and Robbins GF: Pitfalls of local excision in the treatment of carcinoma of the breast, Surg Gynecol Obstet 136:721, 1973.
110. Snyder RE: Mammography and lobular carcinoma in situ, Surg Gynecol Obstet 122:255, 1966.

111. Sunshine JA, Moseley HS, Fletcher WS, and Krippachne WW: Breast carcinoma in situ: a review of 112 cases with a minimum 10 year follow-up, Am J Surg 150:44, 1985.
112. Urban JA: Biopsy of the "normal" breast in treatment breast cancer, Surg Clin North Am 49:291, 1969.
113. van Dongan JA, Harris JR, Peterse JL, et al: In-situ breast cancer: the EORTC concensus meeting, Lancet ii:25, 1989.
114. Veronesi U: Clinical management of minimal breast cancer, Semin Surg Oncol 5:145, 1989.
115. Wanebo HJ, Huvos AG, and Urban JA: Treatment of minimal breast cancer, Cancer 33:349, 1974.
116. Webber BL, Heise H, Neifeld JP, and Costa J: Risk of subsequent contralateral breast carcinoma in a population of patients with in-situ breast carcinoma, Cancer 47:2928, 1981.
117. Wheeler JE, Enterline HT, Roseman JM, et al: Lobular carcinoma in situ of the breast. Long-term followup, Cancer 34:554, 1974.
118. Wolmark N: Review of noninvasive breast cancer by Swain SM, Oncology 3:42, 1989.

14 Locally Advanced Breast Cancer

Barbara Fowble** and **Donna Glover

Approximately 20% of breast cancers are locally advanced without evidence of distant metastases at the time of presentation.[136] The term *locally advanced breast cancer,* however, encompasses a heterogeneous group of tumors with a wide range of clinical features and variable biologic behavior. It generally is accepted that tumors with any one of the following characteristics comprise the locally advanced category: primary tumors >5 cm (T_3); tumors of any size with chest wall fixation, edema, skin ulceration, or satellite nodules (T_4); inflammatory carcinoma (T_4); and the presence of fixed ipsilateral axillary nodes (N_2), ipsilateral supraclavicular infraclavicular nodes (N_3), or arm edema (N_3). These criteria are based on the combined International Union Against Cancer–American Joint Committee (UICC-AJC) staging classification of 1983[14] and describe stage III breast cancer. Stage IIIA includes any T_3 tumor with N_0, N_1, or N_2 adenopathy and T_1 or T_2 tumors with fixed axillary nodes. Stage IIIB includes any T_4 tumor and any primary tumor with ipsilateral supraclavicular infraclavicular nodes, or arm edema. The distinction between stage IIIA and stage IIIB generally follows the guidelines for operability as described by Haagensen and Stout.[72] Stage IIIA represents technically operable patients, whereas stage IIIB represents inoperable patients. A revised 1987 staging system[76] now includes T_3N_0 disease in stage II. Supraclavicular nodes are classified as M_1 and therefore represent stage IV disease. N_3 signifies positive internal mammary nodes and remains in stage III. For the most part, the classification in the literature of locally advanced breast cancer still follows the guidelines of the 1983 staging system. Employing this system, approximately two thirds of patients are classified as stage IIIB, and one third are stage IIIA.[136]

In reviewing treatment options for locally advanced breast cancer, it is useful to divide this group into subsets of patients with similar tumor extent and prognosis. The tumors can be divided into three categories: (1) operable, (2) inoperable or borderline resectable (T_4, N_2, or N_3), and (3) inflammatory.

LOCALLY ADVANCED OPERABLE BREAST CANCER

Treatment options and results

Mastectomy. The standard treatment for operable locally advanced breast cancer has been the radical or modified radical mastectomy. The results from surgical series alone, in terms of local-regional recurrence and survival, are presented in Table 14-1. Five year survival rates are approximately 45% to 50%, with a 10-year survival rate of 30%. Approximately 30% of patients experience a local-regional recurrence.

Postmastectomy radiotherapy. Postmastectomy radiotherapy has been employed in the treatment of operable locally advanced breast cancer in an attempt to decrease local-regional recurrence. Table 14-2 presents the results of postmastectomy radiotherapy for operable T_3 lesions. Local-regional recurrence rates have been decreased to approximately 15% in all series except that of Fracchia et al.[64] This decrease in the rates of local-regional recurrence, however, does not appear to result in a significant improvement in 5- or 10-year survival.

Conservative surgery and radiation. Radiotherapy also has been employed as definitive local treatment following an incisional biopsy in this group of patients. Results are presented in Table 14-3. Five- and 10-year survival rates are comparable to those achieved with mastectomy with or without postoperative radiotherapy. However, despite doses of 8000 to 9000 cGy, local-regional recurrence is high, ranging from 22% to 50%. This finding as well as the increasing success of lumpectomy and radiation for stage I and stage II breast cancer prompted the evaluation of excisional biopsy and radiation for operable T_3 breast cancer. Toonkel et al.[155] reported a 12% local-regional recurrence rate in 34 patients undergoing excisional biopsy and definitive radiotherapy. Sheldon et al.[134] reported a 16% local-regional recurrence rate in 54 patients, and Chu et al.[41] reported a 33% local-regional recurrence rate in 15 patients. Clearly the use of an excisional biopsy for selected patients with operable T_3 breast cancer results in a

Table 14-1 Results of mastectomy in the treatment of patients with operable stage III breast cancer

Author	No. pts.	Local-regional recurrence (%)	Survival (%)	
			5 yr	10 yr
Haagensen and Cooley[71]	75	29	37	23
Donegan[53]	130	35	52	30
Baker et al.[9]				
Radical mastectomy	36	8	49	
Modified radical mastectomy	31	39	46	
Butcher[31]	48		48	31
Schottenfeld et al.[129]	62	6	53	34
Arnold and Lesnick[7]	50		40	31
Fracchia et al.[64]	207	25	43	27

Table 14-2 Results of postoperative radiotherapy in the treatment of patients with operable locally advanced breast cancer

Author	No. pts.	Local-regional recurrence (%)	Survival (%)	
			5 yr	10 yr
Atkins and Horrigan[8]	12	17	33	
Bedwinek et al.[15]	93	13		
Arnold and Lesnick[7]	122		33	
Fracchia et al.[64]	179	30	34	13
Toonkel et al.[155]	309	16	55	40
Brown et al.[25]	189	14	45	21

Table 14-3 Results of definitive radiotherapy for patients with operable locally advanced breast cancer

Author	No. pts.	Tumor dose (cGy)	Local-regional recurrence (%)	Survival (%)	
				5 yr	10 yr
Sheldon et al.[134]	83	>6000	—	45 [33]	—
Toonkel et al.[155]	89	6000-7000	47	20	0
Amalric et al.[5]	435	8000	39	[44]	[32]
Calle et al.[35,36]	196	8000	50	59	32
Pierquin[116]	74	8000-8500	16	69	45
Fletcher[62]	229	9000	22	30	—

[ ], disease-free survival.

decreased local-regional recurrence rate when compared to incisional biopsies,[134] although experience with conservative surgery and radiation for operable T_3 breast cancer is extremely limited.

Adjuvant chemotherapy with or without radiation. Approximately 60% of patients with operable T_3 breast cancer will develop distant metastases after treatment with local therapy.[53,129] Systemic chemotherapy has been employed in the treatment of these patients in an attempt to decrease the incidence of distant metastases and to improve survival. A single prospective randomized trial (Helsinki) has evaluated the role of postmastectomy chemotherapy in patients with operable stage III breast cancer.[84] Between 1978 and 1981, 120 patients were randomized to receive either postoperative radiotherapy and/or chemotherapy with or without levamisole. Chemotherapy consisted of six cycles of vincristine, doxorubicin, and cyclophosphamide. The survival rate at 5 years was 35% in the group of patients receiving postoperative radiation only, 70% in the group receiving chemotherapy, and 95% in the group of patients receiving combined modality treatment. The 5-year actuarial disease-free survival rate was 68% for the combined modality group, 33% for the chemotherapy only group, and 25% for the postoperative radiotherapy group. The apparent benefit for the combined modality group, both in terms of disease-free and overall survival, was statistically significant when compared to the chemotherapy only group or the radiotherapy only group. Buzdar et al.,[32] in a retrospective nonrandomized review, compared the 5- and 10-year overall and disease-free survival rates for a group of 145 patients with operable T_3 breast cancer treated with or without FAC (5-fluorouracil, Adriamycin, and cyclophosphamide) chemotherapy. The 5-year survival rate for the FAC group was 56%, with a disease-free survival rate of 48%. The 10-year survival rate was 40%, with a disease-free survival rate of 36%. The 5-year survival rate in the control group was 46% with a disease-free survival rate of 33%. The 10-year survival rate was 26% with a disease-free survival of 28%. The differences in the overall survival rates were significant, with a p value of .05. The differences in disease-free survival rates were significant, with a p value of .03. These series therefore suggest a benefit in terms of disease-free and overall survival for adjuvant systemic chemotherapy in patients with operable stage III breast cancer.

The results of postmastectomy adjuvant chemotherapy for operable stage III breast cancer are limited. In many series, operable T_3 lesions are included in stage II disease, and results are not reported separately. However, Casper et al.[38] reported the results of postmastectomy chemotherapy in 41 patients with operable stage III disease. Following mastectomy, patients were randomized to cyclophosphamide, methotrexate, 5-fluorouracil, vincristine, and prednisone (CMFVP) for 12 cycles, vs. cyclophosphamide, Adriamycin, and 5-fluorouracil (CAF) for six cycles followed by CMFVP for six cycles. Estrogen receptor–positive patients also received tamoxifen. At 48 months, results showed a trend toward an improved disease-free survival rate (30% vs. 3%) with the CAF regimen, although there was no difference in the overall survival rates (35% vs. 34%). Abeloff et al.[1] reported the results of a 16-week, dose-intense adjuvant five-drug chemotherapy regimen in 53 patients with operable breast cancer and 10 or more positive nodes. Thirty percent of these patients had T_3 primary tumors. Chemotherapy consisted of eight cycles (each for 2 weeks) of cyclophosphamide, doxorubicin, vincristine, methotrexate with leukovorin, and 5-fluorouracil on day 1, with a continuous infusion of 5-fluorouracil on days 8 and 9. A 3-year actuarial disease-free survival rate of 61% was reported in this group of patients with a median follow-up of 21 months.

Optimal local-regional therapy in patients receiving adjuvant chemotherapy for operable stage III breast cancer has been evaluated by three prospective randomized trials. Spangenberg et al.[137] reported the results of 131 operable stage III breast cancer patients who were randomized to either postmastectomy irradiation followed by cyclophosphamide for 2 years or chemotherapy consisting of cyclophosphamide, methotrexate, 5-fluorouracil, and vinblastine for 2 years. Among the group of patients receiving radiotherapy, the 5-year relapse-free and overall survival rates were 40% and 62% respectively. The 5-year relapse-free survival rate was 27%, with an overall survival rate of 56% in the group of patients receiving chemotherapy alone. The local-regional recurrence rate was 12% in the group of patients who received radiation, compared to 22% in the group that did not. While there appeared to be a benefit to patients receiving postmastectomy irradiation, the difference was not statistically significant. As previously noted the Helsinki trial[84] randomized 120 patients with operable T_3 breast cancer to postmastectomy irradiation or chemotherapy (consisting of vincristine, Adriamycin, and cyclophosphamide) or a combination of the two with or without levamisole. The combined modality arm had a statistically significant improvement in overall and disease-free survival at 5 years when compared to the chemotherapy only or radiotherapy only arm. The local-regional recurrence rate was 17.5% in the group of patients receiving radiotherapy alone, 13% in the group of patients receiving chemotherapy and radiotherapy, and 58% in the group of patients receiving chemotherapy alone.

The Eastern Cooperative Oncology Group (ECOG) trial[108] randomized 332 women with operable stage III breast cancer to six cycles of cyclophosphamide, Adriamycin, 5-fluorouracil, tamoxifen, and Halotestin with or without radiation therapy. With a median follow-up of 3.1 years, the overall survival rate was 80%, with a disease-free survival rate of 69% in the chemotherapy and radiotherapy group, compared to an overall survival rate of 78% and a disease-free survival rate of 61% in a group of patients receiving chemotherapy alone. These differences were not statistically sig-

Table 14-4 Local-regional recurrence in patients with operable T_3 breast cancer treated by mastectomy and postoperative adjuvant chemotherapy

Author	Chemotherapy	Local-regional recurrence (%)
Fowble et al.[63]	CMFP (T)	19
1-3 positive nodes		12
4-7 positive nodes		31
≥8 positive nodes		15
Stefanik et al.[142]	CMF	27
Rao et al.[118]	CMF, L-PAM ± FT	31
Casper et al.[38]	CAF, CMFVP	18
Sykes et al.[149]	AC	28
Buzdar et al.[32]	FAC	18

C, cyclophosphamide; M, methotrexate; F, 5-fluorouracil; P, prednisone; T, tamoxifen; A, Adriamycin; V, vincristine; L-PAM, melphalan.

nificant. The local-regional recurrence rate was 13% in the group of patients receiving radiotherapy, compared to 20% in the group of patients receiving chemotherapy alone. Therefore two of these trials[108,137] suggest a small benefit in terms of disease-free survival and local recurrence with postmastectomy radiation and chemotherapy for operable stage III breast cancer. The third trial[84] demonstrated a statistically significant benefit in terms of overall and disease-free survival for combined modality treatment.

Retrospective reviews of postmastectomy adjuvant chemotherapy in patients with operable T_3 breast cancer are presented in Table 14-4. With adjuvant chemotherapy there appears to be no significant impact on local-regional recurrence when compared to surgical series alone. Optimal local-regional therapy in patients with operable T_3 breast cancer appears to be a combination of mastectomy and postoperative radiation.

Induction chemotherapy. The role of induction or neoadjuvant chemotherapy before local therapy for the treatment of operable locally advanced breast cancer has been evaluated by several groups. Hortobagyi et al.[79] reported a 29% complete clinical response among 48 patients receiving FAC chemotherapy before modified radical mastectomy. The partial response rate was 60% for a total response rate of 89%. Swain et al.[147] reported a complete response rate of 53% in 30 patients who received cyclophosphamide, Adriamycin, methotrexate, and 5-fluorouracil (CAMF) induction chemotherapy with hormonal synchronization. The partial and total response rates were 37% and 90% respectively. Bonadonna et al.[20] reported a 94% response rate (including complete and partial responses) in 33 patients with T_2 primary tumors ≥3 cm and T_3 tumors with induction chemotherapy consisting of three cycles of cyclophosphamide, methotrexate, and 5-fluorouracil (CMF). However, at the time of quadrantectomy only one of five patients who had a complete clinical response was found to have no evidence of residual tumor. The authors reported that response to induction chemotherapy in this group of patients was unrelated to age, menopausal status, hormone receptors, ploidy, or labeling index. Briffod et al.[24] correlated response to induction chemotherapy in 35 patients with operable T_3 breast cancer. Induction chemotherapy consisted of Adriamycin, vincristine, cyclophosphamide, methotrexate, and 5-fluorouracil (AVCMF) for a total of three cycles followed by

Table 14-5 Results of induction chemotherapy for patients with operable stage III breast cancer

Author	No. pts.	Chemotherapy	Primary local treatment	Local-regional recurrence (%)	Survival (%)	Follow-up
Hortobagyi et al.[79]	48	FAC	S ± R	0	84 [71]	5 yr (actuarial)
					56 [37]	10 yr (actuarial)
Hobar et al.[78]	13	FAC	S ± R	8	85 [85]	34 mo (mean)
Swain et al.[147]	31	CAMF and hormonal synchronization	R, S + R	—	77	3 yr (actuarial)
					0	5 yr (actuarial)

F, fluorouracil; A, Adriamycin; C, cyclophosphamide; M, methotrexate, S, surgery; R, radiation; [ ], disease-free survival.

mastectomy. Total response including complete and partial responses was more common among patients with aneuploid tumors and those demonstrating cytomorphologic changes during chemotherapy as evaluated on cytopuncture material.

The results of induction chemotherapy for operable stage III breast cancer in terms of local-regional recurrence and survival are presented in Table 14-5. The use of hormonal synchronization does not appear to be superior to standard FAC chemotherapy.

Experience with breast preservation employing excisional biopsy and radiotherapy for operable stage III breast cancer is limited. Bonadonna et al.[20] suggested that the use of induction chemotherapy may expand the role of breast preservation in these patients. However, only 20% of their patients who had a complete clinical response to induction chemotherapy had a pathologic complete response demonstrated at the time of quadrantectomy. The Milan group currently is using a regimen of three cycles of FAC chemotherapy followed by quadrantectomy, axillary dissection, and radiation. No further chemotherapy is given unless the axillary nodes are positive. Long-term results from this study will provide further information regarding the role of breast preservation in operable T_3 breast cancer.

Adjuvant chemotherapy plays a major role in the treatment of operable stage III breast cancer. The sequencing of chemotherapy is being evaluated by the NSABP. Patients with operable T_3 breast cancer are randomized to either induction chemotherapy followed by mastectomy or mastectomy followed by chemotherapy. In a nontrial setting, patients with operable T_3 primary tumors and clinically positive axillary nodes may benefit from induction chemotherapy followed by local-regional treatment. An antitumor response to chemotherapy can be expected in the majority of patients. Patients with clinically negative axillary nodes may undergo either mastectomy or chemotherapy first. Before neoadjuvant chemotherapy, a biopsy with sufficient tissue for histologic diagnosis, analysis of hormone receptors, flow cytometry, and other biologic markers should be obtained.

Adjuvant tamoxifen. There are limited data regarding the role of hormonal therapy in the treatment of operable stage III breast cancer. A single prospective randomized trial has evaluated tamoxifen vs. CMF chemotherapy in postmenopausal patients.[3] Following mastectomy and postoperative radiotherapy 71 patients with operable stage III breast cancer were randomized to tamoxifen (40 mg per day) vs. CMF for nine to ten cycles. The 5-year actuarial disease-free survival rate was 27% for the tamoxifen group, compared to 32% for the CMF group. Local-regional recurrences occurred in 18% of the tamoxifen patients, compared to 10% of the chemotherapy patients. These differences were not statistically significant.

Prognostic factors

The most important prognostic factor in patients with operable T_3 breast cancer is the pathologic status of the axillary nodes. Approximately 15% to 20% of patients with operable stage III breast cancer will have histologically negative axillary nodes.[64,65,104] The 5-year survival rate of these patients is 80%, with a 10-year survival rate of approximately 75% (Table 14-6). However, for patients with pathologically positive axillary nodes, the 5-year survival rate decreases to approximately 45%, with a 10-year survival rate of 25% (Table 14-7). Hortobagyi et al.[79] found no correlation with

Table 14-6 Survival rates for operable T_3 pathologic N_0 breast cancer patients

Author	Treatment	Survival (%) 5 yr	Survival (%) 10 yr
Lacour et al.[88]	S	85	—
Sutherland and Mather[144]	S	93	75
Valagussa et al.[159]	S	84	81
Schottenfeld et al.[129]	S	70	43
Garewal et al.[65]	S	87	87
Nemoto et al.[104]	S ± R	[57]	—
Toonkel et al.[155]	S ± R	72	57
Fracchia et al.[64]	S ± R	82	75

S, surgery; R, radiation; [ ], disease-free survival.

Table 14-7 Survival rates for operable T_3 pathologic N_1 breast cancer patients

Author	Treatment	Survival (%) 5 yr	Survival (%) 10 yr
Lacour et al.[88]	S	49	—
Valagussa et al.[159]	S	37	22
Schottenfeld et al.[129]	S	47	31
Garewal et al.[65]	S	33	26
Sutherland and Mather[144]	S		
1-3 positive nodes		60	45
>3 positive nodes		42	25
Nemoto et al.[104]	S ± R	[22]	—
Toonkel et al.[155]	S ± R	45	28
Fracchia et al.[64]	S ± R	44	22

S, surgery; R, radiation; [ ], disease-free survival.

estrogen receptor status, age, primary tumor size, or response to induction chemotherapy in 48 patients with operable stage III breast cancer. The 5-year actuarial survival rate was 93% for patients achieving a complete response to induction chemotherapy, compared to 78% for those achieving a partial response. The corresponding disease-free survival rates were 93% and 55%.

It must be emphasized that a small subset of patients with operable T_3 breast cancer have histologically negative axillary nodes and excellent 5- and 10-year survival rates when treated with local therapy alone. The role of adjuvant systemic therapy in this group of patients has not been clearly established.

Future research

For operable stage III breast cancer the major areas of clinical research appear to be the sequencing of chemotherapy with local-regional treatment (i.e., the role of induction or neoadjuvant chemotherapy), the identification of prognostic factors associated with a poor outcome that will allow for better selection of treatment for various subgroups of patients, and the use of adjuvant hormonal therapy.

LOCALLY ADVANCED INOPERABLE BREAST CANCER

Treatment options and results

Radiotherapy alone. Historically, borderline resectable or technically unresectable breast cancers have been treated by radiotherapy alone. Results in terms of local-regional recurrence and survival are presented in Table 14-8. Five-year survival rates range from 10% to 40%. Local control rates vary from 20% to 70%, depending on the extent of the tumor[153] and the dose of radiotherapy. Generally, increasing doses of radiation are associated with an increase in the local-regional control rate. However, doses in the range of 7000 to 10,000 cGy have been associated with severe breast fibrosis and soft tissue necrosis in approximately 20% of patients.[15,26,138,148] The use of preoperative radiotherapy followed by surgery has the advantage of decreasing the dose of radiation required for local-regional control, with the potential for reducing the incidence of complications and increasing local-regional control. The results of preoperative radiotherapy in the treatment of locally advanced breast cancer are presented in Table 14-9. In the majority of series, local-regional recurrence rates are in the range of 15%, and 5-year survival rates range from 12% to 45%. Following a preoperative dose of radiation ranging from 4500 to 6000 cGy, residual tumor is identified in the breast and/or axilla at the time of mastectomy in 70% of patients.[21,67,91,93,143,158,165] Retrospective comparisons of local therapy in patients with inoperable locally advanced breast cancer not receiving chemotherapy are presented in Table 14-10. The combination of radiotherapy and mastectomy for the most part has resulted in a decrease in local-regional recurrence. Bedwinek et al.[15] reported that there was a statistically significant improvement in local-regional control with the addition of mastectomy to radiation, with a trend toward improved survival rates. Toonkel et al.[155] reported a significant improvement in local-regional control, 5-year overall survival rates, and relapse-free survival rates in patients in whom a definitive surgical procedure removed all gross disease before radiation was given. However, the authors emphasized that some of these differences may be due to patient selection, with patients with

Table 14-8 Results of definitive radiotherapy for patients with locally advanced breast cancer

Author	No. pts.	Tumor dose (cGy)	Local-regional recurrence (%)	5-yr survival (%)
Rubens et al.[123]	184	3600-4000	81	13
Griscom and Wang[69]	97	4000-6000	65	22
Bedwinek et al.[15]	54	4000-7000	61	18
Zaharia et al.[164]	484	6000	75	22
Chu et al.[42]	147	>6000	44	24
Balawajder et al.[10]	38	6500	62	38
Thomas et al.[153]	319	≥6500	44	40
Zucali et al.[165]	321	6000-7000	—	21
Ghossein et al.[66]	22	6000-8000	54	—
Sheldon et al.[134]	121	6000-9000	28	38
Nobler and Venet[105]	36	7000	11	—
Treurniet-Donker et al.[157]	129	≥7000	22	12
Fletcher[62]	144	9000	30	10
Syed et al.[148]	53	9000-10,000	11	—
Alderman[4]	18	10,000	0	—

Table 14-9 Results of preoperative radiotherapy in the treatment of patients with locally advanced breast cancer

Author	No. pts.	Local-regional recurrence (%)	Survival (%) 5 yr	Survival (%) 10 yr
Townsend et al.[156]	53	11		
Stoker and Ellis[143]	23	13		
Terz et al.[151]	35	17		
Zucali et al.[165]	133		45	
Arnold and Lesnick[7]	54		33	17
Pearlman et al.[112]	104	37	12	
Balawajder et al.[10]	17	45	44	
Atkins and Horrigan[8]	23	17	33	

a more favorable prognosis receiving combined-modality treatment.

The use of neutrons has been evaluated as a potential means of improving local-regional control. The lower oxygen-enhancement ratio associated with neutrons makes this form of radiation more effective against hypoxic tumor cells than x-rays. An additional advantage of use of neutrons includes a possible decrease in the capacity of tumor cells to repair injury and less cell cycle–dependent sensitivity.[59] Halpern et al.[74] reported the results of neutron therapy either alone or combined with photons in 28 patients with locally advanced breast cancer. The complete and partial response rates were 32% and 64% respectively. Complications included severe brachial plexopathy in 42%, soft tissue necrosis in 23%, and arm edema in 89%. The high incidence of severe complications that increased with time essentially eliminates neutron therapy as a promising treatment for locally advanced breast cancer.

Chemotherapy. Distant metastases develop in 70% to 80% of patients with inoperable locally advanced breast cancer treated with local therapy alone.[10,15,16,50] Induction chemotherapy or initial chemotherapy before local-regional treatment has been employed not only to decrease the incidence of metastatic disease but also to assess primary

Table 14-10 Retrospective comparisons of local therapy in patients with locally advanced breast cancer not receiving chemotherapy

	No. pts.	Local-regional recurrence (%)	Survival (%) 5 yr	Survival (%) 10 yr
Radiotherapy				
Toonkel et al.[155]	123	47	20	0
Atkins and Horrigan[8]	56	—	11	
Balawajder et al.[10]	38	62	38	
Bedwinek et al.[15]	39	61	—	
Pearlman et al.[112]	28	57	15	
Zucali et al.[165]	321	—	23	
Derman et al.[52]	41	17	—	
Radiotherapy and surgery				
Toonkel et al.[155]	347	16	55	40
Atkins and Horrigan[8]	23	—	33	
Balawajder et al.[10]	17	45	44	
Bedwinek et al.[15]	93	13	—	
Pearlman et al.[112]	16	37	12	
Zucali et al.[165]	133	—	45	
Derman et al.[52]	46	9	—	

[ ], disease-free survival.

tumor response to systemic therapy, and thereby identify an effective regimen. Five prospective randomized trials have evaluated the addition of chemotherapy to local-regional treatment for locally advanced inoperable breast cancer. The results of these trials are presented in Table 14-11.

In the Netherlands trial,[127] 118 patients were randomized to radiotherapy alone, radiotherapy followed by CMF plus tamoxifen, or induction chemotherapy with Adriamycin and vincristine alternating with CMF followed by radiotherapy and further chemotherapy consisting of Adriamycin, vincristine, and CMF. There were no statistically significant differences in 5-year overall or disease-free survival rates. The European Organization for Research and Treatment of Cancer (EORTC) randomized 410 patients to radiotherapy alone, radiotherapy and 12 cycles of CMF, radiotherapy and hormonal therapy, or radiotherapy followed by CMF for a total of 12 cycles and hormonal manipulation.[124] Hormonal therapy consisted of ovarian radiation and prednisolone for premenopausal patients, or radiotherapy and tamoxifen for 5 years for postmenopausal patients. There was a trend toward an improved survival rate in the combined chemotherapy-hormonal treatment arm, but this was not significant. Chemotherapy significantly delayed the time to first progression although the effect was primarily on local-regional progression and not distant metastases. Caceres et al.[34] randomized 87 patients to radiotherapy, radiotherapy and mastectomy, or radiotherapy and CMF. There was no difference in median survival rates among the three treatment groups. The Johannesburg trial[52] randomized 231 patients undergoing local-regional radiotherapy with or without mastectomy to no further treatment or CMF. At 5 years a statistically significant improvement in disease-free survival rates was noted for premenopausal patients receiving CMF, but no difference in overall sur-

Table 14-11 Randomized trials evaluating the addition of chemotherapy to local-regional treatment for patients with locally advanced breast cancer

	Netherlands[127]	EORTC[124]	Caceres et al.[34]	Johannesburg[52]	Serrou et al.[131,132]
Treatment period	1977-1980	1979-1985	—	1978-1985	1975-
No. pts.	118	363	87	231	82
Chemotherapy	CMFT, AV	CMF	CMF	CMF	VCF
Follow-up (yr)	5	6	—	5	4
Local-regional recurrence (%)					
Radiation		81*	—	13	—
Radiation and chemotherapy		58*	—	16	—
Radiation, chemotherapy, and hormonal treatment		50*			
Chemotherapy, radiation, and chemotherapy					
Radiation and surgery					
Survival (%)					
Radiation	37 [14]	27 [7]	20 mo (median)	Premenopausal 30 [18] Postmenopausal 35 [20]	37
Radiation and chemotherapy	37 [23]	24 [15]	25 mo (median)	Premenopausal 58 [40] Postmenopausal 38 [25]	64
Radiation, chemotherapy, and hormonal treatment		31 [20]			
Chemotherapy, radiation, and chemotherapy	37 [23]				
Radiation and surgery			18 mo (median)		
Significant p value	None	Time to first progression		DFS, CMF, premenopausal	None

C, cyclophosphamide; M, methotrexate; F, 5-fluorouracil; T, tamoxifen; A, Adriamycin; V, vincristine; DFS, disease-free survival; [ ], disease free survival.
*Local-regional progression.

vival rates was seen. In the French trial[132] 82 patients were randomized to CMF, bacillus Calmette-Guerin (BCG), or no further treatment following initial radiotherapy with or without mastectomy. Although there was a trend toward improved survival rates with chemotherapy, the differences were not statistically significant.[131,132] Therefore none of these trials has demonstrated benefit in terms of overall survival, although a disease-free survival benefit appears in two of the trials.[52,124]

Retrospective comparisons of radiotherapy with or without chemotherapy for locally advanced breast cancer are presented in Table 14-12. A significant improvement with chemotherapy in the disease-free survival rates has been noted in three series,[16,81,134] with a significant improvement in overall survival rates in two series.[50,81]

Response rates to induction chemotherapy with various regimens are presented in Table 14-13. Approximately 20% of patients will experience a complete clinical response, i.e., complete disappearance of all gross disease. A partial response (i.e., ≥50% regression of gross disease) will occur in 50% to 60% of patients. The best method for assessing tumor response has yet to be determined. Hortobagyi et al.[79] reported a lower incidence of complete response when assessment of response was performed by a combination of physical examination and mammogram as compared to physical examination alone. Segel et al.[130] have defined a complete response mammographically as the absence of evidence of residual tumor. The authors note that calcifications usually do not disappear with induction chemotherapy, and that focal architectural distortion rarely disappears; therefore mammographic assessment in these instances is less reliable. Mammographic response is best when assessing changes in discrete masses. Cocconi et al.[43] compared response to induction chemotherapy (CMF with or without tamoxifen) in 35 patients with locally advanced breast cancer as measured by physical examination and mammography. Physical examination overestimated the response in 22.9% of patients when compared to mammography. Mammography overestimated overall response in 8.6% of patients when compared to physical examination. There were no complete responses as assessed by mammographic criteria, compared to 8% complete responses found with physical examination. Response as measured by physical examination, however, was more likely to correlate with a pathologic complete response. The authors suggest that where there is disagreement between the two methods the most favorable response should be recorded.

Response to induction chemotherapy has not

Table 14-12 Retrospective comparisons of radiotherapy with or without chemotherapy for patients with locally advanced breast cancer

	Hortobagyi et al.[81]	Brufman et al.[27]	Bedwinek et al.[16]	Balawajder et al.[10]	Sheldon et al.[134]	DeLena et al.[50]	Rubens et al.[123]
No. pts.	194	94*	58	61	192	110	24
Chemotherapy	FAC ± BCG	CMF	FAC	CMF	CMF	AV	AV
Follow-up (yr)	5	5	3	5	5	3	3
Local-regional recurrence (%)							
Radiation	23	33	61	62	28	50	
Radiation and chemotherapy	25	26	35	46	24	37	
p value		.002	>.05		>.05		
Disease-free survival (%)							
Radiation	9	30	18	14	26		
Radiation and chemotherapy	43	36	22	41	40		
p value	.007	.0001	<.05		.02		
Survival (%)							
Radiation	27	51	45	38	38	41	39
Radiation and chemotherapy	56	56	43	46	51	53	35
p value	.01	.0003	>.05		>.05	.02	>.05

C, cyclophosphamide; M, methotrexate; F, 5-fluorouracil; A, Adriamycin; V, vincristine.
*Includes patients who received only tamoxifen or estrogens.

Table 14-13 Response rates to induction chemotherapy for patients with locally advanced breast cancer

Author	No. pts.	Chemotherapy	Clinical response (%)	
			Complete	Partial
Thalmo et al.[152]	16	CAF × 2	19	25
Jacquillat et al.[83]	98	VTMFAP infusion	23	68
Hery et al.[77]	25	CAVF × 3	14	64
Morrow et al.[101]	31	CAFT × 2	13	64
Hortobagyi et al.[79]	174	FAC × 3	17	71
Boyages and Langlands[22]	35	CA × 3	14	32
Ragaz et al.[117]	50	ACFM × 3	64	30
Perloff et al.[114]	87	CAFVP × 3	22	55
DeLena et al.[49]	110	AV × 4	15	55
Rubens et al.[125]	12	AV × 4	17	33
Schaake-Konig et al.[127]	39	CMF/AV × 4	26	—
Bedwinek et al.[16]	22	FAC × 2	5	41
Hortobagyi et al.[80]	193	VACP × 3	18	66
Hobar et al.[78]	36	FAC × 3	8	64

C, cyclophosphamide; A, Adriamycin; F, 5-fluorouracil; V, vincristine; T, tamoxifen; P, prednisone; M, methotrexate.

been correlated with estrogen receptor status, histology, nodal status, menopausal status, or age.[147] However, a complete response is more common with stage IIIA disease than stage IIIB disease.[79,147] The majority of patients with inoperable locally advanced breast cancer are rendered operable with induction chemotherapy (Table 14-14). Estrogenic recruitment with or without hormonal synchronization has been employed in an attempt to increase response rates. Swain et al.[147] have reported the results of induction chemotherapy and hormonal synchronization in patients with stage IIIA and stage IIIB breast cancer. Chemotherapy consisted of cyclophosphamide, Adriamycin, methotrexate, and 5-fluorouracil. Tamoxifen, 40 mg per day, was given on days 2 through 6 before the administration of methotrexate and 5-fluorouracil on day 8. Premarin, 0.625 mg, was given orally every 12 hours for three doses on day 7. All drugs were given intravenously and were given to maximal tumor response before local-regional treatment. Patients who experienced a complete response underwent random biopsies of the breast and if no tumor was identified pathologically, they received radiotherapy to the breast and regional nodes. Patients who experienced a partial response underwent mastectomy followed by postoperative radiotherapy. Chemotherapy was continued for an additional 6 months following local therapy. The rationale for the regimen was based on the demonstration that estrogen rescue could reverse the inhibition of breast cancer cell growth by antiestrogens.[54,93,103] Tamoxifen induces a G_1 arrest in MCF-7 human breast cancer cells in culture.[68] Subsequent estrogen treatment could induce DNA synthesis in these cells,[2] resulting in an increased sensitivity of the cells to cytotoxic drugs.[162] The results from this trial are presented in Table 14-15. The overall response rate was 93%, with a complete response rate of 49%. The median number of cycles to maximal response was five. Trucut biopsies before treatment, after tamoxifen administration, and after Premarin administration confirmed that hormonal synchronization occurred, as evidenced by a decrease in the number of cells in the S-phase with tamoxifen and an increase in the number of cells cycling with Premarin. The 4-year survival rate was 50%, with a 5-year survival rate of 17%. Conte et al.[45] reported the results of estrogenic recruitment combined with FAC chemotherapy in the treatment of locally advanced breast cancer. The complete

Table 14-14 Ability of induction chemotherapy to render patients with locally advanced breast cancer operable

Author	Chemotherapy	Operable pts. (%)
Thalmo et al.[152]	CAF	100
Morrow et al.[101]	CAFT	95
Ragaz et al.[117]	ACFM	100
Perloff et al.[114]	CAFVP	81

C, cyclophosphamide; A, Adriamycin; F, 5-fluorouracil; V, vincristine; T, tamoxifen; P, prednisone, M, methotrexate.

Table 14-15 Results of induction chemotherapy with hormonal synchronization/estrogenic recruitment in the treatment of patients with locally advanced breast cancer

	Swain et al.[147]	Conte et al.[45]
No. pts.	76	43
Hormonal synchronization	Tamoxifen	No
Estrogenic recruitment	Premarin	Diethylstilbestrol
Chemotherapy	CAMF	FAC
Complete and partial response (%)	93	64
Complete response (%)	49	—
Survival (%)		
5 yr	17	—
4 yr	50	74 [42]

C, cyclophosphamide; A, Adriamycin; M, methotrexate; F, 5-fluorouracil; [ ], disease-free survival.

and partial response rate was 64%. A 4-year survival rate of 74% with a disease-free survival rate of 42% was reported. A randomized trial of 86 patients[45] comparing FAC chemotherapy to estrogenic recruitment and FAC chemotherapy reported no differences in 4-year overall survival, disease-free survival, or response rates.

Radiotherapy has been combined with induction chemotherapy in an attempt to increase the complete clinical response rate. These results are presented in Table 14-16. The combination of induction chemotherapy and radiation has a higher complete clinical response rate in all series when compared to chemotherapy alone.

Pathologic complete responses (i.e., no evidence of residual disease microscopically) occur in a minority of patients who achieve a complete clinical response with induction chemotherapy. Thalmo et al.[152] reported a pathologic complete response rate of 33% in patients who achieved a complete clinical response with two cycles of CAF chemotherapy. Feldman et al.[58] reported a 54% pathologic complete response rate in 11 patients who achieved a complete clinical response after a minimum of three cycles of FAC chemotherapy. Pathologic complete response in this series, however, was defined as no evidence of macroscopic residual disease. The authors reported no significant difference in disease-free or overall survival rates when they compared patients who had no evidence of microscopic residual disease to those with no evidence of macroscopic residual disease. Morrow et al.[101] reported a 25% pathologic complete response rate in patients receiving CAF chemotherapy with tamoxifen for two cycles before surgery. Piccart et al.[115] obtained a 50% pathologic complete re-

Table 14-16 Response rates to induction chemotherapy and radiation in patients with locally advanced breast cancer

	Complete clinical response (%)		
Author	Chemotherapy	Radiation	Chemotherapy and radiation
Hery et al.[77]			
Breast	14		54
Nodes	27		50
Boyages and Langlands[22]	14		46
Perloff et al.[114]	23		52
DeLena et al.[50]	15		83
Bedwinek et al.[16]	5		78
Rubens et al.[125]	17		42
Schaake-Konig et al.[127]	26	75	64
Shanta et al.[133]		68	77
Zaharia et al.[164]		38	
Thomas et al.[153]		79	
Harris et al.[75]		94	
Meek et al.[99]			50

sponse rate by adding radiation to CMF alternating with Adriamycin and vincristine (AV) chemotherapy. Manji et al.[96] reported a 40% pathologic complete response rate following three cycles of ACMF and radiation before mastectomy. Swain et al.[147] demonstrated a 66% pathologic complete response rate in patients who achieved complete clinical responses with CAMF and hormonal synchronization. However, the pathologic response was determined only by random breast biopsy rather than by examination of mastectomy specimens. Hortobagyi et al.[79] have noted an improved correlation between clinical and pathologic complete response when clinical response was assessed by a combination of physical examination and mammography. None of the nine patients who had a complete response by physical examination and mammogram had residual tumor at the time of mastectomy. Therefore, while 20% of patients will achieve a complete clinical response following induction chemotherapy, approximately two thirds will have residual disease in the breast or axilla at the time of mastectomy.

The sequencing of chemotherapy and local-regional treatment for locally advanced breast cancer has been evaluated in two prospective randomized trials and one retrospective series. In the Netherlands trial there was no difference in the 5-year overall disease-free survival rate of patients who received radiotherapy followed by chemotherapy when compared to patients receiving induction chemotherapy followed by radiation and maintenance chemotherapy.[127] The Eastern Cooperative Oncology Group[140] randomized 113 patients with locally advanced inoperable breast cancer to induction chemotherapy consisting of cyclophosphamide, methotrexate, 5-fluorouracil, and prednisone (CMFP) for two cycles followed by radiation with concurrent chemotherapy followed by an additional 14 cycles of CMFP vs. initial radiotherapy followed by CMFP for 18 cycles. There was no statistically significant difference in median survival time between the two groups or in the percentage of patients experiencing a complete response to initial treatment. Rubens et al.[125] retrospectively reviewed the results of 24 patients who received either four courses of Adriamycin and vincristine followed by radiotherapy and eight courses of CMF, or radiotherapy followed by four courses of Adriamycin and vincristine and eight courses of CMF. There was no difference between the two groups in terms of response rates or survival. Loprinzi et al.[94] reported the results of initial surgery followed by chemotherapy and radiation in 32 patients with stage IIIA and stage IIIB breast cancer. Chemotherapy consisted of cyclophosphamide, methotrexate, 5-fluorouracil, prednisone, and tamoxifen. Ten of the 32 patients had gross residual tumor left behind following initial surgery. The 5-year disease-free survival rate in this group was 9%, compared to 40% of those with no gross residual disease ($p \geq .01$). Bitran et al.[18] reported a 5-year survival rate of 50% with a disease-free survival rate of 28% in 34 patients with locally advanced breast cancer initially treated by radical mastectomy and postoperative radiotherapy followed by 12 cycles of CMF. Shanta et al.[133] reported a significant improvement in 5-year disease-free survival rates in axillary node-positive patients with locally advanced breast cancer who received preoperative chemotherapy (CMF) and radiation when compared to preoperative radiotherapy only (50% vs. 26%, $p = .016$). All patients received postoperative chemotherapy. While some of these studies suggest that there is no statistical advantage to induction chemotherapy before local-regional therapy, induction chemotherapy has several theoretical advantages. Neoadjuvant chemotherapy allows for the early initiation of systemic treatment with the ability to assess primary tumor response and renders the majority of patients with locally advanced inoperable breast cancer operable. Therefore it does not appear appropriate to perform initial definitive surgery beyond an adequate biopsy in patients who are clearly inoperable.

Several series have evaluated regimens employing concurrent chemotherapy and radiotherapy for locally advanced breast cancer (Table 14-17). The toxicity of these regimens has been significant, with marked skin desquamation,[99,115,139] prolongation of the radiation treatment course, delays in initiation of chemotherapy, and decreases in the dose of chemotherapy delivered.[99] There appears to be no advantage to the initial concurrent use of radiotherapy and chemotherapy for the treatment of inoperable locally advanced breast cancer.

The optimal duration of systemic chemotherapy in patients with locally advanced inoperable breast cancer has not been established. Hortobagyi et al.[79] noted no difference in 5-year survival rates when comparing a 2-year program of chemotherapy consisting of FAC followed by maintenance CMF to FAC chemotherapy for 9 months. The majority of programs have employed a 1-year regimen.

Optimal local-regional therapy in patients with locally advanced breast cancer receiving chemotherapy has been evaluated in three prospective randomized trials (Table 14-18). In the Milan trial,[19] 277 patients were randomized following induction chemotherapy with Adriamycin and vincristine to radiotherapy and maintenance chemotherapy, or surgery and maintenance chemotherapy, or radiation without maintenance chemotherapy. There were no statistically significant differences in terms

Table 14-17 Results of concurrent chemotherapy and radiotherapy for patients with locally advanced breast cancer

Author	No. pts.	Regimen	Complete response (%)	Local-regional recurrence (%)	Survival (%)	Follow-up
Piccart et al.[115]	59	AV → CMF and radiotherapy + T × 1 yr and mastectomy	5	12	43	5 yr (actuarial)
Meek et al.[99]	16	CMFP/CMF and radiotherapy with or without surgery CMF/CAF	—	20	—	17 mo (median)
Perez et al.[113]	10	FAC × 2 → FC and radiotherapy → FAC	0	30	[50]	14 mo (median)
Sponzo et al.[139]	6	CFP	83	—	—	—

C, cyclophosphamide; A, Adriamycin; V, vincristine, M, methotrexate; F, 5-fluorouracil; T, tamoxifen; P, prednisone; [ ], disease-free survival.

of overall survival or local-regional recurrence rates among the three treatment arms, although patients undergoing surgery tended to have the lowest incidence of local-regional recurrence. The Cancer and Leukemia Group B (CALGB) study[114] randomized 113 patients to either mastectomy or radiation following induction chemotherapy consisting of Cytoxan, Adriamycin, 5-fluorouracil, vincristine, and prednisone. Three-year results revealed no significant differences in terms of local-regional recurrence, overall, or disease-free survival rates. The Hellenic Breast Cooperative Group (HBCG)[109] randomized 106 patients to surgery vs. surgery and radiation following induction chemotherapy with Cytoxan, Adriamycin, vincristine, methotrexate, and 5-fluorouracil. Postmenopausal patients were randomized to receive tamoxifen or no tamoxifen. Premenopausal patients were randomized to oophorectomy or no oophorectomy. There was no difference in terms of local-regional recurrence at 2 years. However, the results were too preliminary for survival analysis. Therefore two of these trials

Table 14-18 Randomized trials evaluating local therapy in patients with locally advanced breast cancer receiving chemotherapy

	Milan[19]	CALGB[114]	HBCG[109]
No. pts.	277	113	106
Chemotherapy	AV	CAFVP	CAVMF*
Treatment period	1973-1980	1978-1983	1978-1981
Follow-up (yr)	10	3	2
Local-regional recurrence (%)			
Chemotherapy, radiation, and chemotherapy	44	27	
Chemotherapy, surgery, and chemotherapy	28	19	10
Chemotherapy, surgery, radiation, and chemotherapy			8
Chemotherapy and radiation	56		
Survival (%)			
Chemotherapy, radiation, and chemotherapy	26 [14]	54 [37]	
Chemotherapy, surgery, and chemotherapy	28 [22]	55 [37]	
Chemotherapy, surgery, radiation, and chemotherapy			
Chemotherapy and radiation	14		

C, cyclophosphamide; A, Adriamycin; V, vincristine; M, methotrexate; F, 5-fluorouracil; P, prednisone; [ ], disease-free survival.
*With or without tamoxifen or oophorectomy.

have demonstrated no difference when comparing surgery alone to radiotherapy alone for local treatment in patients with locally advanced breast cancer receiving chemotherapy.[19,114] However, local-regional recurrence rates remain high with either modality. This finding has prompted an evaluation of the combination of surgery and radiation in patients receiving chemotherapy. Tables 14-19 to 14-21 present retrospective comparisons of chemotherapy and radiation with chemotherapy, radiation, and mastectomy in the treatment of locally advanced breast cancer. While the combination of surgery and radiation decreases the rate of local-regional recurrence to 15% or less, preliminary

Table 14-19 Results of chemotherapy and radiation for patients with locally advanced breast cancer

Author	Treatment	No. pts.	Local-regional recurrence (%)	Survival (%)	Follow-up (yr)
Balawajder et al.[10]	CMF	53	46	46	5 (actuarial)
Cancer Control Agency[96,117]	ACMF	27	22	57 [22]	4 (actuarial)
Rubens et al.[125]	AV	12	25	50	3 (actuarial)
Boyages and Langlands[22]	CA	35	—	68 [58]	3
Hery et al.[77]	CAVF	25	27	56 [36]	5 (actuarial)
Jacquillat et al.[83]	VTMFAP	98	13	65 [55]	5 (actuarial)
Bedwinek et al.[16]	FAC	22	35	43 [22]	3 (actuarial)
Sheldon et al.[134]	CMF	71	24	51 [40]	5 (actuarial)
Derman et al.[52]	CMF	59	25	—	—

C, cyclophosphamide; M, methotrexate; F, 5-fluorouracil; A, Adriamycin; V, vincristine; T, tamoxifen; P, prednisone; [ ], disease-free survival.

Table 14-20 Results of induction chemotherapy and surgery with or without radiation for patients with locally advanced breast cancer

Author	No. pts.	Chemotherapy	Local treatment	Local-regional recurrence (%)	Survival (%)	Follow-up
Hortobagyi et al.[79]	126	FAC	S ± R	21	44 [33]	5 yr (actuarial)
					26 [30]	10 yr (actuarial)
Hobar et al.[78]	17	FAC	S ± R	19	53 [47]	34 mo (mean)
Swain et al.[147]	41*	CAMF and hormonal synchronization	R, S and R	17	49	3 yr
					25	5 yr
Conte et al.[45]	86	FAC	S, R	—	77 [18]	4 yr
		DES, FAC			74 [42]	

S, surgery; R, radiation; C, cyclophosphamide; A, Adriamycin; F, 5-fluorouracil; M, methotrexate; DES, diethylstilbestrol; [ ], disease-free survival.
*22% of patients stage IIIB.

Table 14-21 Results of chemotherapy, surgery, and radiation for patients with locally advanced breast cancer

Author	Treatment	No. pts.	Local-regional recurrence (%)	Survival (%)	Follow-up (yr)
Morrow et al.[101]	CAFT	31	14	42 mo mean	—
Cancer Control Agency[96,117]	ACMF	41	0	73 [62]	4 (actuarial)
Balawajder et al.[10]	CMF	30	12	38	5 (actuarial)
Piccart et al.[115]	AV, CMFT	59	12	43	5 (actuarial)
Derman et al.[52]	CMF	74	8	—	—

C, cyclophosphamide; A, Adriamycin; F, 5-fluorouracil; T, tamoxifen; M, methotrexate; V, vincristine; [ ], disease-free survival.

comparisons of survival results would suggest no significant improvement.

The role of mastectomy in patients who experience a complete response to induction chemotherapy recently has been questioned. Hortobagyi et al.[79] suggested that breast preservation may be appropriate in these patients. In 126 patients with stage IIIB carcinoma, the local-regional recurrence rate was 10% in those who achieved a complete response to induction chemotherapy, compared to 25% in those who achieved partial response. Fifty-seven percent of the overall group of patients underwent surgery and radiation. The local-regional recurrence rate was not presented for patients who achieved a complete clinical response and were treated with radiotherapy alone. Harris et al.[75] reported a 33% local-regional recurrence rate in patients who had a complete clinical response to radiation. Schaake-Konig et al.[127] reported a 28% local-regional recurrence rate in patients who achieved a complete clinical response to radiotherapy and chemotherapy. Because the majority of patients who achieve a complete clinical response to induction chemotherapy have residual tumor at the time of mastectomy, and because local-regional recurrence rates remain in the range of 30% despite a complete clinical response in those receiving chemotherapy and radiation, it is difficult to recommend the omission of mastectomy in these patients.

Tamoxifen. The role of tamoxifen in the treatment of locally advanced inoperable breast cancer has not been established. Williams et al.[163] reported the results of 87 patients with locally advanced stage III breast cancer who were randomized to receive either radiotherapy or tamoxifen as a first treatment. All patients were postmenopausal. The 3-year survival rate was 72% for the tamoxifen patients, compared to 64% for the radiotherapy patients. Forty-four percent of the tamoxifen patients responded to treatment, compared to 68% of the radiotherapy patients. Fifty-eight percent of the tamoxifen patients required subsequent radiotherapy for progressive local-regional disease. The response to tamoxifen was unrelated to estrogen receptor positivity. It was suggested that tamoxifen alone may be appropriate treatment for women with locally advanced breast cancer who are of advanced age or unable to receive radiotherapy. Veronesi et al.[160] reported a 34% partial response rate with tamoxifen in 41 postmenopausal patients with locally advanced noninflammatory breast cancer. Campbell et al.[37] reported a 40% response rate (complete response 14%) in 51 postmenopausal patients with locally advanced breast cancer treated with tamoxifen alone. Response was unrelated to estrogen receptor status. With a median follow-up of 3 years, 75% of the responders remained in remission. Tamoxifen failures received local-regional radiation of which 64% had an objective response.

In the EORTC randomized trial[124] patients with locally advanced breast cancer randomized to hormonal therapy (tamoxifen for 5 years for postmenopausal women or oophorectomy and prednisolone for premenopausal women) had a significant delay in time to first progression when compared to radiation alone. Hormonal therapy prolonged time to local-regional progression in patients with estrogen receptor–positive tumors. The combination of endocrine therapy and chemotherapy (CMF) appeared to produce the best results in terms of overall survival, but the differences were not statistically significant. Cocconi et al.[44] reported the results of 49 patients with locally advanced breast cancer who were randomized to CMF with or without tamoxifen both before and following mastectomy. The addition of tamoxifen to CMF resulted in a complete response rate of 12%, compared to 4% for CMF alone. Overall response rates (complete and partial) were similar (71% for CMF and 64% for CMF and tamoxifen). There were no significant differences in the time to progression or recurrence; however, the median overall survival was 79.7 months for patients receiving CMF, compared to 41.5 months for patients receiving CMF and tamoxifen ($p = .05$).

Prognostic factors

Prognostic factors for patients with locally advanced breast cancer receiving chemotherapy include response to induction chemotherapy, number of positive nodes at the time of mastectomy, menopausal status, and ploidy. Hortobagyi et al.[79] reported a significant improvement in overall and disease-free survival rates in patients who had a complete response to induction chemotherapy. In a subsequent report,[97] a multivariate analysis for prognostic factors in 136 patients receiving FAC chemotherapy followed by mastectomy revealed the number of positive nodes at the time of mastectomy, tumor stage at initial presentation, clinical response to induction chemotherapy, and menopausal status to be significant. Patients with negative axillary nodes at the time of mastectomy had a 70% 5-year survival rate, compared to 62% for those with one to three positive nodes, 47% for those with four to 10 positive nodes, and 21% for those with >10 positive nodes. Patients whose initial clinical tumor stage was T_1 through T_3 had a 78% 5-year survival rate, compared to 42% for T_4 tumors. Patients who experienced a complete clinical response to chemotherapy had a 5-year survival rate of 94%, compared to a 47% survival rate for those with a partial response and 43% for those with no response. It should be noted that the prognosis for patients who had a partial response was similar to that of those who had no response. Premenopausal patients had a 5-year survival rate of 61%, compared to 45% for postmenopausal patients. The pathologic response of the tumor was a significant prognostic factor in a univariate analysis but not in a multivariate analysis. Patients who had no evidence of residual disease or only microscopic residual disease had a 5-year survival rate of 65%, compared to 49% for those with gross residual tumor. Hobar et al.[78] also correlated survival with response to induction chemotherapy. With a mean follow-up of 34 months, the survival rate was 76% in patients achieving a partial response, compared to 43% in those with less than a partial response. Jacquillat et al.[83] reported the most significant prognostic factor to be a >75% response to induction chemotherapy. Arnerlov et al.[6] correlated survival with ploidy status for 91 patients with stage III breast cancer. The 5-year actuarial survival rate was 64% for patients with diploid tumors, and 36% for patients with aneuploid tumors.

In summary, induction chemotherapy plays a major role in the treatment of inoperable locally advanced breast cancer. Complete response rates are in the range of 20%; however, the great majority of patients are rendered operable. Optimal local-regional treatment appears to be a combination of mastectomy and radiation. The most appropriate sequencing of these two regimens is unknown. Preoperative radiotherapy may promote further tumor regression, allowing for less radical surgery and providing the patient with an additional opportunity to manifest distant metastases, which, if present, would most likely cause the patient to avoid surgery. Postoperative radiotherapy, however, generally is technically easier and may alleviate patient and physician concern related to any delay in initiating definitive surgical treatment. Breast preservation in patients with locally advanced breast cancer who achieve a complete clinical response to chemotherapy requires further study. Preliminary information would suggest that mastectomy is still warranted in these patients. The optimal chemotherapeutic regimen is unknown. A reasonable 5-year survival rate has been reported for the small subset of patients who achieve a complete clinical response with induction chemotherapy; however, patients whose response is partial or less than partial continue to have a relatively poor prognosis.

Future research

Future directions in the treatment of locally advanced breast cancer relate primarily to the development of more effective systemic regimens. Preliminary results of programs employing estrogenic recruitment or hormonal synchronization do not appear to have produced significant improvements.[45,147] The use of high-dose chemotherapy with autologous bone marrow transplantation currently is being investigated by several groups, including the National Cancer Institute, M.D. Anderson Hospital; and Duke University[98] (see Chapter 18). The use of dose-intensive chemotherapy regimens in conjunction with colony-stimulating factors also is being considered. The identification of prognostic factors that determine response to induction chemotherapy will aid in the selection of patients for neoadjuvant regimens. The number of patients available for prospective randomized trials is limited, as a minority of patients present with locally advanced breast cancer. Pilot studies with encouraging results will therefore form the basis of future trials.

INFLAMMATORY BREAST CANCER

Presentation

Approximately 4% of all patients with breast cancer present with inflammatory carcinoma.[11,70,73,86,89,92,95,100,106,121,150] Inflammatory breast cancer represents a distinct clinical entity characterized by the presence of diffuse erythema, increased warmth of the involved skin, edema of the skin (peau d'orange), and induration of the underlying breast tissue with or without a palpable mass.[29,70,90] The extent of erythema that defines inflammatory breast cancer has varied. Haagensen[70] describes inflammatory carcinoma as involving one third or more of the breast. However, the Poussee evolutive system (PEV) introduced by the Institut Gustave-Roussy[51] classifies inflammatory carcinomas into those in which the erythema is localized to the tumor site (PEV2) and those with diffuse erythema (PEV3). Despite the extent of erythema, the breast is usually diffusely enlarged and tender. Typical mammographic changes include an overall increase in the density of the breast, increased thickness of the skin and subcutaneous tissues, and prominent subcutaneous lymphatics manifested by fine streaking perpendicular to the skin surface.[17] In patients with inflammatory breast cancer in whom estrogen and progesterone receptors have been measured, approximately 40% are found to be estrogen receptor positive and one third are found to be progesterone receptor positive.[30,48,106,110,146]

The hallmark of this disease pathologically is the presence of dermal lymphatic invasion.[8] The question arises as to whether the presence of dermal lymphatic invasion is essential for the diagnosis. Ellis and Teitelbaum,[56] in a review of the literature of patients with inflammatory breast cancer, found

Table 14-22 Survival of patients with inflammatory breast cancer related to clinical and pathologic criteria for diagnosis

Author	5-yr survival (%)		
	Clinical criteria only	Clinical and pathologic criteria	Pathologic criteria only
Lucas and Perez-Mesa[95]	3	5	16
Fields et al.[61]	10	23	28
Levine et al.[92]	60*	34*	52*
Hagelberg et al.[73]		25	60

*3-yr results.

eight patients who were disease-free at 5 years. A review of the pathologic material of six of these patients revealed four with negative skin biopsies and no evidence of dermal lymphatic invasion. The authors concluded that the presence of dermal lymphatic invasion was mandatory for the diagnosis of inflammatory breast cancer. Saltzstein[126] suggested that patients with dermal lymphatic invasion without the clinical signs of inflammatory breast cancer also should be included in this category because these patients manifested rapidly progressive disease. In a retrospective review of patients with inflammatory carcinoma at Ellis Fischel State Cancer Hospital, Lucas and Perez-Mesa[95] correlated survival with the clinical and pathologic presentation. Unfortunately, they also included cases of secondary inflammatory carcinoma in which a long-standing tumor resulted in inflammation. The authors concluded that patients with a clinical diagnosis only had a prognosis that was not significantly different from those with a clinical and pathologic diagnosis. Results from this series as well as those of other series are presented in Table 14-22. There is little evidence to suggest that pathologic confirmation of dermal lymphatic invasion is required for a diagnosis of inflammatory breast cancer. Multiple series[30,57,107,128,146] have demonstrated no difference in survival rates between patients with a clinical diagnosis and those with a clinical and pathologic diagnosis. The majority of series reporting results of treatment of inflammatory breast cancer have employed only a clinical diagnosis.[28,30,39,82,85,102,106,122,135,146,154,166]

Treatment options

Local-regional treatment alone. When inflammatory breast cancer is treated with local-regional measures alone, approximately 80% of patients develop distant metastases.[12,13,15,41] Ninety percent of all recurrences occur within 2 years and 80% within 1 year.[12,13] The results of mastectomy with or without postoperative radiotherapy for inflammatory breast cancer are presented in Table 14-23. Five-year survival rates range from 0 to 10%. Radiation became the standard local treatment with the recognition that long-term survival was uncommon with mastectomy alone for inflammatory breast carcinoma. Results of radiotherapy for inflammatory breast carcinoma are presented in Table 14-24. Again 5-year survival rates range from 0 to 14%. Radiotherapy typically involved 6000 to 7000 cGy to the area of gross disease and 5000 to 6000 cGy to the regional nodes. Doses >6000 cGy were required for maximal local control[26,41]; however, the majority of patients continued to manifest local recurrence (Table 14-25). In an attempt to decrease the duration of treatment and prevent the repair of sublethal damage in the tumor, Barker et al.[12] developed a twice daily fractionation schedule. Patients received 5100 cGy to the breast in 4 weeks. Two treatments were given per day separated by 6 to 8 hours. A boost of 2000 cGy in 8 days was then given to the primary with twice-daily fractionation. The authors reported local control in 73% of patients receiving twice-daily treatment, compared to 54% for those patients receiving conventional radiotherapy. Chu et al.[42] also reported improved local control with a twice-daily treatment regimen. Sixty-six percent of patients receiving twice-daily treatment experienced local control, compared to 31% receiving conventional fraction-

Table 14-23 Results of mastectomy with or without radiation as treatment for patients with inflammatory breast cancer

Author	No. pts.	5-yr survival (%)
Haagensen[70]	29	3
Rogers and Fitts[121]	13	8
Barber et al.[11]	50	10
Lucas and Perez-Mesa[95]	36	3
Bozzetti et al.[23]	8	13*
Meyer et al.[100]	63	6
Taylor and Meltzer[150]	6	0

*4-yr actuarial survival.

Table 14-24 Results of radiotherapy in the treatment of patients with inflammatory breast cancer

Author	No. pts.	5-yr survival (%)
Haagensen[70]	30	3
Rogers and Fitts[121]	11	9
Wang and Griscom[161]	23	0
Lucas and Perez-Mesa[95]	18	0
Chu et al.[42]	28	14
Robbins et al.[120]	72	3
Droulias et al.[55]	75	5
Fields et al.[61]	30	7
Zucali et al.[165]	70	28*
Hagelberg et al.[73]	10	10
Rouesse et al.[122]	60	28†
Lee and Tannenbaum[89]	11	0
Barker et al.[13]	69	4
Bruckman et al.[26]	18	[13]

[ ], relapse-free survival.
*3-yr survival.
†4-yr actuarial survival.

Table 14-25 Retrospective comparisons of local-regional control in inflammatory breast cancer patients *not* receiving chemotherapy

	Local-regional control (%)	
Author	Radiation	Mastectomy and radiation
Fields et al.[61]	33	80
Barker et al.[13]	54	35
Bedwinek et al.[15]	48	86
Vaeth et al.[158]	40	66
Chu et al.[42]	31	—
Bruckman et al.[26]	65	—

ation. The addition of mastectomy to radiation also has resulted in improved local-regional control (Table 14-25); however, this has not been translated into an improvement in 5-year survival rates (Table 14-26). Hagelberg et al.[73] reported a 5-year survival rate of 48% in patients undergoing mastectomy, compared to 0 in those treated with radiotherapy alone. However, 87% of the surgery patients also received chemotherapy, compared to 33% of the radiotherapy patients. The difference in 5-year survival rates was statistically significant ($p<.0005$). Fields et al.[60,61] also reported a significantly improved 5-year survival rate for patients who underwent mastectomy vs. those who were treated by radiotherapy (37% vs. 7%, $p=.0004$). In a multivariate analysis[60] chemotherapy was a marginally significant prognostic factor. However, mastectomy was an independent prognostic factor for relapse-free and overall survival.

Combined modality therapy. Combination chemotherapy has become standard treatment for patients with inflammatory breast cancer because the majority of patients develop distant metastases. While patients with inflammatory breast cancer have been included in many of the trials for locally advanced breast cancer, there have been no prospective randomized trials to evaluate the role of chemotherapy in addition to local-regional treatment for the subgroup of patients with inflammatory breast cancer. Results of retrospective com-

Table 14-26 Retrospective comparisons of radiation vs. mastectomy and radiation as treatment for patients with inflammatory breast cancer

	5-yr survival (%)	
Author	Radiation	Mastectomy and radiation
Meyer et al.[100]	0 [10]	6 [63]
Chris[40]	0 [9]	0 [7]
Rogers and Fitts[121]	8 [13]	9 [11]
Spratt and Donegan[141]	0 [17]	0 [11]
Richards and Lewison[119]	0 [6]	0 [6]
Dao and McCarthy[47]	0 [3]	0 [6]
Fields et al.[61]	7 [30]	18 [15]
Bozzetti et al.[23]	0* [12]—cobalt-60 12* [20]—orthovoltage	24* [24]
Barker et al.[13]	4 [69]	0 [17]

[ ], total no. pts.
*4-yr actuarial survival.

parisons are presented in Table 14-27. Fields et al.[61] reported a significant improvement in relapse-free survival and overall survival rates when chemotherapy was given with either radiation or surgery in patients with inflammatory breast cancer. The 5-year relapse-free survival rate for patients receiving chemotherapy was 20%, compared to 5% for those who did not (p=.02). The 5-year actuarial overall survival rates with and without chemotherapy were 23% and 3% respectively (p<.02). Rouesse et al.[122] reported a statistically significant improvement in local-regional control, disease-free survival, and overall survival rates for patients receiving aggressive combination chemotherapy consisting of Adriamycin, vincristine, Cytoxan, methotrexate, and 5-fluorouracil. With the less aggressive regimen of Adriamycin, vincristine, and methotrexate, significant improvement in local-regional control and disease-free survival rates was noted, but not in overall survival rates. Krutchik et al.[87] reported a significant improvement in disease-free and overall survival rates for patients receiving FAC (5-fluorouracil, Adriamycin, and Cytoxan) chemotherapy and BCG compared to a controlled group receiving radiation alone. Subsequent updates of this series[33,57] continue to manifest significant improvements in the disease-free survival rate; however, the benefit has been confined to postmenopausal patients. DeLena et al.[50] reported a 3-year survival rate of 25% in patients with inflammatory breast carcinoma who received Adriamycin and vincristine and compared this figure to a 3-year survival rate of 28% in an historical control group that was treated with radiation alone.[165] Hagelberg et al.[73] reported a trend toward improved survival rates in patients receiving either Cytoxan, methotrexate, and 5-fluorouracil or Cytoxan, Adriamycin, and 5-fluorouracil compared to patients receiving radiotherapy alone, although this difference was not significant. Mourali et al.[102] also reported an improvement in the median metastatic free interval in patients with inflammatory breast carcinoma with the addition of CMF to either surgery or radiation. Therefore sev-

Table 14-27 Retrospective comparisons of local-regional treatment with or without chemotherapy for patients with inflammatory breast cancer

	Fields et al.[61]	Rouesse et al.[122]		Krutchik et al.[87]	Zucali et al.[165] and DeLena et al.[50]	Hagelberg et al.[73]
No. pts.	105	91	79	64	106	28
Chemotherapy	CAF	AVM	AVCMF	FAC and BCG	AV	CMF, CAF
Follow-up (yr)	5	4	4	3	3	5
Local-regional recurrence (%)						
Radiation	66	53	53	22		
Radiation and chemotherapy	52	32	31	22		
Radiation and surgery	20					
Radiation, surgery, and chemotherapy	11					
p value	—	.01	.01			
Disease-free survival (%)						
Radiation	7	16	16	10		
Radiation and chemotherapy	6	28	46	35		
Radiation and surgery	20					
Radiation, surgery, and chemotherapy	37					
p value	.02	<.005	<.0001	<.01		
Overall survival (%)						
Radiation	7	28	28	25	28	10
Radiation and chemotherapy	9	44	66	44	25	37
Radiation and surgery	18					
Radiation, surgery, and chemotherapy	48					
p value	<.02	.17	<.0001	.03		>.05

C, cyclophosphamide; A, Adriamycin; F, 5-fluorouracil; M, methotrexate; V, vincristine.

Table 14-28 Local-regional response to induction chemotherapy in patients with inflammatory breast cancer

Author	No. pts.	Chemotherapy	Response rates (%) Complete	Partial	Total
Israel et al.[82]	25	CF	8	88	96
Crowe et al.[46]	21	CAF or CMFVP	33	53	86
Zylberberg et al.[166]	15	CAVF and melphalan and BCG	20	73	93
Chevallier et al.[39]	64	CMF or AVCF	—	—	47
Burton et al.[30]	22	CAFV	23	73	96
Thoms et al.[154]	61	FAC	16	44	60
Noguchi et al.[106]	28	Mitomycin C, F, or A (intraarterial)	25	64	89
Swain and Lippman[146]	45	CAMF and hormonal synchronization	55	43	98
Mourali et al.[102]	88	CMF	11	51	66
University of Pennsylvania	38	CMF ± PT, CAF ± T	58	21	79

C, cyclophosphamide; F, 5-fluorouracil; M, methotrexate; V, vincristine; P, prednisone; A, Adriamycin; T, tamoxifen.

eral retrospective series have demonstrated a benefit in terms of disease-free and overall survival with the addition of chemotherapy to local-regional treatment.[33,57,61,87,122]

Induction or initial chemotherapy has been employed for the most part in an attempt to decrease the incidence of distant metastases and evaluate local-regional tumor response to systemic therapy. A complete response is defined as complete disappearance of all clinical signs of disease, and a partial response is defined as being 50% or greater regression of the tumor. In most series, induction chemotherapy is followed by maintenance chemotherapy, which is given for a total period of 1 to 2 years. Response rates to induction chemotherapy are presented in Table 14-28. Approximately 20% of patients with inflammatory breast carcinoma will experience a complete response to neoadjuvant chemotherapy. The partial response rate to induction chemotherapy ranges from 21% to 88%, with total response rates (complete and partial) ranging from 47% to 96%. Higher complete response rates have been reported by Swain and Lippman,[146] who employed CAMF with hormonal synchronization (tamoxifen and Premarin). A 55% complete response rate was reported in 45 patients with inflammatory breast carcinoma. The addition of radiation to induction chemotherapy also has resulted in a higher rate of complete response (Table 14-29). Mourali et al.[102] reported an increased complete response rate to induction chemotherapy in patients <50 years of age, compared to older patients. In general induction chemotherapy has been given for a fixed number of regimens;

Table 14-29 Local-regional response to induction chemotherapy with or without radiation for patients with inflammatory breast cancer

			Response rates (%)			
			Chemotherapy		Chemotherapy and radiation	
Author	No. pts.	Chemotherapy	Complete response	Complete and partial response	Complete response	Complete and partial response
Brun et al.[28]	26	AVCF	4	33	12	85
Rouesse et al.[122]	91	AVM and VCF	—	14	—	68
	79	AVCMF and AVM and VCF	—	27	—	80
Sherry et al.[135]	4	CAFT or CMF	—	—	50	
DeLena et al.[50]	34	AV	20	67	73	91

C, cyclophosphamide; A, Adriamycin; V, vincristine; F, 5-fluorouracil; M, methotrexate; T, tamoxifen.

Table 14-30 Pathologic findings at mastectomy in patients achieving a complete clinical response to induction therapy for inflammatory breast cancer

Author	No. pts.	Induction treatment	Pathologic residual tumor (%)
Fastenberg et al.[57]	4	FAC	50 [2/4]
Knight et al.[85]	2	CFP and R	100 [2/2]
Zylberberg et al.[166]	3	CAVF and melphalan and BCG	33 [1/3]
Crowe et al.[46]	7	CAF, CMFVP	100 [7/7]
Thoms et al.[154]	10	FAC	40 [4/20]
University of Pennsylvania	24	CMF ± PT, CAF ± T and R	62 [15/24]

F, 5-fluorouracil; A, Adriamycin; C, cyclophosphamide; P, prednisone; V, vincristine; M, methotrexate; T, tamoxifen; R, radiation.

however, Swain and Lippman[146] have advocated induction chemotherapy given to maximum clinical response followed by local-regional treatment. Zylberberg et al.[166] also employed induction chemotherapy to maximal clinical response as demonstrated by thermographic cooling before local treatment. However, despite a complete clinical response to induction chemotherapy with or without radiation, the majority of patients are found, at the time of mastectomy, to have residual tumor on pathologic examination (Table 14-30).

The results of combined modality therapy for inflammatory breast cancer from multiple series are presented in Table 14-31. Approximately 30% of patients develop a local-regional recurrence. Five-year survival rates range from 30% to 70%, with a disease-free survival rate of 25% to 59%. There appears to be no significant improvement with hor-

Table 14-31 Results of combined modality therapy for patients with inflammatory breast cancer

Author	No. pts.	Chemotherapy	Local-regional treatment	Local-regional recurrence (%)	Survival (%)	Follow-up (yr; actuarial)
Knight et al.[85]	18	CFP	S and R	29	1.75 yr (median)	—
Mourali et al.[102]	112	CMF	S, R	—	2.6 yr (median)	—
Burton et al.[30]	22	CAFV	S and R	—	55 [46]	2
Crowe et al.[46]	21	CAF, CMFVP	S	—	60	2
Chevallier et al.[39]	64	AVCF, CMF	R ± S	—	38	3
DeLena et al.[50]	36	AV	R	—	25	3
Rouesse et al.[122]	91	AVM	R	32	44 [28]	4
	79	AVCMF	R	31	66 [46]	4
Brun et al.[28]	26	AVCF	R ± S	39	[25]	5
Fields et al.[61]	37	CAF	S and R	11	48 [37]	5
Thoms et al.[154]	61	FAC	S ± R	42	35 [27]	5
Sherry et al.[135]	11	CAFT, CMF	R ± S	—	60	5
Zylberberg et al.[166]	15	CAVF and melphalan and BCG	S	—	70	5
Hagelberg et al.[73]	18	CAF, CMF	S ± R, R	28	37	5
Israel et al.[82]	25	CF	S	28	60 [38]	5
Noguchi et al.[106]	28	MMC, F, A, intra-arterial	S	—	63 [59] 47 [53]	5 10
Swain and Lippman[146]	45	CAMF and hormonal synchronization	R ± S	33	30 [28]	5
University of Pennsylvania	38	CMF ± PT, CAF ± T	R and S	8	59 [47]	5

A, Adriamycin; V, vincristine; C, cyclophosphamide; F, 5-fluorouracil; M, methotrexate; P, prednisone; T, tamoxifen; MMC, mitomycin C; S, surgery; R, radiation; [ ], disease-free survival.

monal synchronization as compared to standard induction regimens. Noguchi et al.[106] employed intraarterial chemotherapy, with injections in the internal thoracic and subclavian arteries. They reported a 5-year survival rate of 63%, with a 10-year survival rate of 47%. The intraarterial chemotherapy consisted of mitomycin C, 5-fluorouracil, or Adriamycin, and was followed by an extended radical mastectomy with dissection of the internal mammary and supraclavicular nodes. This regimen has received little attention from other investigators.

Optimal local-regional treatment in patients receiving chemotherapy for inflammatory breast cancer has been evaluated by several retrospective series (Table 14-32). Local-regional recurrence is minimized by a regimen employing both mastectomy and radiotherapy; however, the impact on survival is variable. Fields et al.[61] reported a significant improvement in disease-free and overall survival rates with the combined modality approach employing both mastectomy and radiation. Mourali et al.,[102] in a prospective randomized trial, found no significant difference in 3-year disease-free survival rates when comparing surgery alone to radiation alone following induction chemotherapy of Cytoxan, methotrexate, and 5-fluorouracil. Swain and Lippman[146] also reported no significant improvement in 4-year actuarial survival rates when comparing patients who received radiation to those who received radiation and surgery. Chevallier et al.[39] reported a significant improvement in overall survival rates with the addition of surgery to chemotherapy and radiation in patients with inflammatory breast cancer. Pawlicki et al.[111] reported a significant improvement in survival at 3 years with the addition of mastectomy to induction chemotherapy (CMFV) and radiation (61% vs. 32%, p<.05) in 87 patients with locally advanced breast cancer, 88% of whom had inflammatory breast cancer. The 3-year disease-free survival rate was 38.5% for patients treated with all three modalities, compared to 11.8% for patients treated with chemotherapy and radiation. The combination of mastectomy and radiation therefore minimizes local-regional recurrence but may or may not impact on survival rates. Swain and Lippman[146] suggested that mastectomy was not necessary in patients who experienced a complete clinical response to induction chemotherapy in whom this response

Table 14-32 Retrospective comparisons of local-regional treatment in patients receiving induction chemotherapy for inflammatory breast cancer

Author	No. pts.	Chemotherapy	Local-regional treatment	Local-regional recurrence (%)	Survival (%)		Follow-up (yr)
Brun et al.[28]	13	AVCF	R	54		—	4-9
	10		R and S	20		—	4-9
				p>.05			
Fields et al.[61]	23	CAF	R	52	9	[6]	5 (actuarial)
	37		R and S	11	45	[35]	
					p=.006	p=.0003	
Schafer et al.[128]	21	Chlorambucil and MAF	S	100		—	3.1 (median)
			S and R	12			
Thoms et al.[154]	15	FAC	S	40		—	3 (minimum)
	46		S and R	30			
Mourali et al.[102]*	44	CMF	S	—	[45]		3 (actuarial)
	46		R	—	[59]		
					p>.05		
Swain and Lippman[146]	17	CAMF and hormonal synchronization	R	—	25		4 (actuarial)
	27		R and S	—	32		
					p>.05		
Pawlicki et al.[111]	87	CMFV	R	—	32 [12]		3
			S and R	—	61 [38]		
					p<.05		

A, Adriamycin; V, vincristine; C, cyclophosphamide; F, 5-fluorouracil; M, methotrexate; R, radiation; S, surgery; [ ], disease-free survival.

*Prospective randomized trial.

was confirmed pathologically by negative random Trucut biopsies of the breast. Thoms et al.[154] correlated the incidence of local-regional recurrence with response to induction chemotherapy. The 5-year actuarial risk of a local-regional recurrence was 11% in patients achieving a complete response, 32% in those achieving a partial response, and 67% in those achieving no response. Local-regional treatment consisted of mastectomy with or without radiation. Of the 10 patients who experienced a complete clinical response, a single patient who was treated by surgery alone experienced a local-regional recurrence, compared to none of the nine patients who received surgery and radiation. Therefore in this series, patients who achieved a complete clinical response had a low risk of local-regional recurrence when treated by mastectomy and radiation. Brun et al.[28] reported local-regional recurrence in one of three patients who achieved a complete clinical response following chemotherapy and radiation alone. Chevallier et al.[39] reported local-regional recurrence in 20 of 33 patients who were deemed to have a complete clinical response following induction chemotherapy and radiation. Therefore the use of radiation alone in patients who achieve a complete clinical response with induction chemotherapy has been associated with local-regional recurrence rates of 33% and 61%.[28,39] Additional support for the role of mastectomy in patients with inflammatory breast cancer comes from the finding that clinical response rarely correlates with a pathologic complete response. The majority of patients with a complete clinical response continue to have residual tumor at the time of mastectomy (see Table 14-30).

The University of Pennsylvania initiated a combined modality protocol for the treatment of inflammatory breast cancer in 1982. After metastatic evaluation and surgical biopsy, patients were treated with induction chemotherapy consisting of cyclophosphamide, methotrexate, 5-fluorouracil, prednisone, and tamoxifen. The rationale for tamoxifen was the previously documented response in local-regional disease in 30% to 40% of patients with locally advanced breast cancer.[37,160] Following maximal tumor regression, patients received local-regional radiotherapy to the breast and ipsilateral supraclavicular and axillary lymph nodes. A tumor dose of 5000 cGy was delivered to the breast over a period of 5 weeks and 4600 cGy in 4½ weeks to the regional nodes. Tissue equivalent bolus was employed every third day to the tangential breast fields. During radiotherapy, patients continued to receive cyclophosphamide, 5-fluorouracil, and tamoxifen. Upon the completion of radiotherapy, patients resumed CMFPT chemotherapy for one to three cycles before undergoing modified radical mastectomy. Following mastectomy, chemotherapy was resumed for a total of 10 cycles of CMFPT and 2 cycles of CFT. Tamoxifen was continued indefinitely. Between 1982 and 1988, a total of 38 patients with clinical nonmetastatic inflammatory breast cancer received this combined modality approach. The median age was 48 years. Of the patients, 42% were premenopausal. Dermal lymphatic invasion was documented in 22 breasts, although no skin biopsy was obtained in five of the cases. The median number of chemotherapy cycles before local regional treatment was four, with a range of three to eight. Complete response to induction chemotherapy occurred in 24 patients (58%), a partial response in eight, a less than partial response in three, progression in two, and no response in one. At the time of mastectomy, residual tumor was identified in the breast and/or axilla in 62% of the complete responders and 75% of partial responders. With a median follow-up of 34 months (range 8 to 92), the 5-year actuarial survival rate is 59%, with a relapse-free survival rate of 47%. For complete clinical responders, the 5-year actuarial survival rate was 75%, with a relapse-free survival rate of 65%. The local-regional recurrence rate was 8%. These results compare favorably with other regimens reported in the literature (see Table 14-31).

In summary, the use of induction chemotherapy with maintenance chemotherapy in the treatment of inflammatory breast cancer has resulted in 5-year overall survival rates ranging from 30% to 70%. Optimal local-regional treatment appears to be a combination of mastectomy and radiation. The response to chemotherapy appears to be related to ultimate outcome.

At the present time, initial therapy should consist of induction chemotherapy. For patients who experience a complete clinical response, local-regional treatment should include mastectomy and radiation followed by maintenance chemotherapy. Delays in the initiation of radiation following mastectomy have resulted in an increased local-regional recurrence rate.[154] For patients achieving partial response, local-regional radiotherapy may be employed before mastectomy in an attempt to increase the complete response rate. Chemotherapy should continue during radiation. Following mastectomy, maintenance chemotherapy is employed. For the most part, the currently accepted duration of chemotherapy for inflammatory breast cancer is 1 year.

Prognostic factors

Prognostic factors correlating with outcome in patients receiving chemotherapy for inflammatory breast cancer include response to induction che-

Table 14-33 Survival related to response to induction chemotherapy

Author	Chemotherapy	Disease-free survival (%) Complete response	Partial response	Less than partial response	Follow-up (yr; actuarial)
Rouesse et al.[122]	AVM	60		23	4
	AVCMF	57		43	
Noguchi et al.[106]*	MMC, F, A	66	50	31	5
Thoms et al.[154]	FAC	70	37	0	5
University of Pennsylvania	CMF ± PT, CAF ± T	65	45	—	5

C, cyclophosphamide; A, Adriamycin; M, methotrexate; F, 5-fluorouracil; V, vincristine; MMC, mitomycin C; P, prednisone; T, tamoxifen.
*Pathologic response.

motherapy and the presence of clinically positive supraclavicular nodes. Approximately two thirds of patients who have a complete clinical response to induction chemotherapy are alive with no evidence of disease at 5 years (Table 14-33), compared to approximately 40% for those with a partial response. Chevallier et al.[39] noted that the patient's response to induction chemotherapy significantly correlated with overall and disease-free survival rates in a univariate analysis. However, in a multivariate analysis, initial erythema of the entire breast, persistent erythema after initial chemotherapy, and lymph node involvement were significant prognostic factors for outcome. Brun et al.[28] noted no correlation with outcome and response to induction chemotherapy. Noguchi et al.[106] reported a 5-year disease-free survival rate of 66% in patients who at the time of mastectomy had no residual tumor following intraarterial induction chemotherapy. Mourali et al.[102] noted a significant improvement in the mean disease-free interval for patients with diffuse erythema of the breast who experienced a complete clinical response to induction chemotherapy. Thoms et al.[154] also reported an improved 5-year actuarial disease-free survival rate in patients who achieved a complete clinical response. Rouesse et al.[122] noted no improvement in 4-year disease-free survival rates with induction chemotherapy in patients with fixed axillary nodes or clinically positive supraclavicular nodes. Fields et al.,[61] however, noted no impact on 5-year survival rates in patients who had clinically positive supraclavicular nodes. There has been no correlation with estrogen receptor status and outcome in patients receiving chemotherapy for inflammatory breast cancer.[30,60,110] Paradiso et al.[110] reported an improvement in overall survival rates but not in time to progression for patients with inflammatory breast cancer receiving induction chemotherapy consisting of CMF or CAF who had positive progesterone receptors or a low labeling index. Fastenberg et al.[57] noted an improved relapse-free survival rate in patients ≥50 years of age; however, Israel et al.[82] noted a trend for improved survival in premenopausal patients.

Future research

Future strategies should be directed toward developing more effective systemic regimens as well as increasing the complete response rate to induction therapy. The role of high-dose chemotherapy and autologous bone marrow transplant currently is being investigated by the National Cancer Institute.[146] The role of high-dose chemotherapy in conjunction with colony-stimulating factors requires further evaluation. The identification of prognostic factors for response to chemotherapy will aid in the selection of patients for whom current regimens have produced disappointing results.

REFERENCES

1. Abeloff MD, Beveridge RA, Donehower RC, et al: Sixteen week dose intense adjuvant chemotherapy for operable breast cancer with 10 or more positive nodes, J Natl Cancer Inst 82:570, 1990.
2. Aitken SC and Lippman ME: Hormonal regulation of net DNA synthesis in MCF-7 human breast cancer cells in tissue culture, Cancer Res 42:1727, 1982.
3. Alagaratnam TT and Wong J: Tamoxifen versus chemotherapy as adjuvant treatment in stage III breast cancer, Aust NZ J Surg 56:39, 1986.
4. Alderman S: Combination teletherapy and iridium implantation in the treatment of locally advanced breast cancer, Cancer 38:1936, 1976.
5. Amalric R, Santamaria F, Robert F, et al: Radiation therapy with or without primary limited surgery for operable breast cancer. A 20 year experience at the Marseilles Cancer Institute, Cancer 49:30, 1982.
6. Arnerlov C, Emdin SO, Roos G, et al: Prognostic factors in locally advanced breast cancer (T_3, T_4) with special reference to tumor cell DNA content, Acta Oncol 27:221, 1988.
7. Arnold DJ and Lesnick GJ: Survival following mastectomy for stage III breast cancer, Am J Surg 137:362, 1979.

8. Atkins HL and Horrigan WD: Treatment of locally advanced carcinoma of the breast with roentgen therapy and simple mastectomy, Am J Roentgenol 85:860, 1961.
9. Baker RR, Montague ACW, and Childs JM: A comparison of modified radical mastectomy to radical mastectomy in the treatment of operable breast cancer, Ann Surg 189:553, 1979.
10. Balawajder I, Antich PP, and Boland J: An analysis of the role of radiotherapy alone and in combination with chemotherapy and surgery in the management of advanced breast carcinoma, Cancer 51:574, 1983.
11. Barber KW, Dockerty MO, and Clagett OT: Inflammatory carcinoma of the breast, Surg Gynecol Obstet 112:405, 1961.
12. Barker JL, Montague ED, and Peters LJ: Clinical experience with irradiation of inflammatory carcinoma of the breast with and without elective chemotherapy, Cancer 45:625, 1980.
13. Barker JL, Nelson AJ, and Montague ED: Inflammatory carcinoma of the breast, Radiology 121:173, 1976.
14. Beahrs OH and Myers MH, editors: Manual for staging of cancer, Philadelphia, 1983, JB Lippincott, pp 127-135.
15. Bedwinek J, Rao DV, Perez C, et al: Stage III and localized stage IV breast cancer: irradiation alone vs. irradiation plus surgery, Int J Radiat Oncol Biol Phys 8:31, 1982.
16. Bedwinek JM, Ratkin GA, Philpott GW, et al: Concurrent chemotherapy and radiotherapy for non-metastatic, stage IV breast cancer: a pilot study by the Southeastern Cancer Study Group, Am J Clin Oncol 6:159, 1983.
17. Berger SM: Inflammatory carcinoma of the breast, Am J Roentgenol Radium Ther Nucl Med 88:1109, 1962.
18. Bitran JD, Desser RK, Schifeling D, et al: Multimodality therapy of stage III adenocarcinoma of the breast, J Surg Oncol 22:5, 1983.
19. Bonadonna G, Valagussa P, Zambetti M, and Zucali R: Locally advanced breast cancer: 10 year results after combined treatment, Proc Am Soc Clin Oncol 7:9, 1988 (abstract).
20. Bonadonna G, Veronesi U, Brambilla C, et al: Primary CMF can avoid mastectomy in tumors $\geq$3 cm, Proc Am Soc Clin Oncol 8:20, 1989 (abstract).
21. Bouchard J: Advanced cancer of the breast treated primarily with irradiation, Radiology 84:823, 1965.
22. Boyages J and Langlands AO: The efficacy of combined chemotherapy and radiotherapy in advanced non-metastatic breast cancer, Int J Radiat Oncol Biol Phys 14:71, 1988.
23. Bozzetti F, Saccozzi R, DeLena M, and Salvadori B: Inflammatory cancer of the breast: analysis of 114 cases, J Surg Oncol 18:355, 1981.
24. Briffod M, Spyratos F, Tubiana-Hulin M, et al: Sequential cytopunctures during preoperative chemotherapy for primary breast. Cytomorphologic changes, initial tumor ploidy and tumor regression, Cancer 63:631, 1989.
25. Brown OR, Horiot JC, Fletcher GH, et al: Simple mastectomy and radiation therapy for locally advanced breast cancers technically suitable for radical mastectomy, Am J Roentgenol 120:67, 1974.
26. Bruckman JE, Harris JR, Levene MB, et al: Results of treating stage III carcinoma of the breast by primary radiation therapy, Cancer 43:985, 1979.
27. Brufman G, Melad Y, and Biran S: Adjuvant hormonal versus chemotherapy in stage III breast cancer, Proc Am Soc Clin Oncol 3:115, 1984 (abstract).
28. Brun B, Otmezguine Y, Feuilhade F, et al: Treatment of inflammatory breast cancer with combination chemotherapy and mastectomy versus breast conservation, Cancer 61:1096, 1988.
29. Bryant T: Diseases of the breast, Wood's Med Surg Monogr 4:35, 1889.
30. Burton GV, Cox EB, Leight GS, et al: Inflammatory breast carcinoma. Effective multimodal approach, Arch Surg 122:1329, 1987.
31. Butcher HR: Radical mastectomy for mammary carcinoma, Ann Surg 170:883, 1969.
32. Buzdar AU, Kau SW, Smith TL, and Hortobagyi GN: Ten-year results of FAC adjuvant chemotherapy trial in breast cancer, Am J Clin Oncol 12:123, 1989.
33. Buzdar AU, Montague ED, Barker JL, et al: Management of inflammatory carcinoma of breast with combined modality approach—an update, Cancer 47:2537, 1981.
34. Caceres B, Zaharia M, and Lingan M: Combined therapy of stage III adenocarcinoma of the breast, Proc Am Acad Cancer Res 798:199, 1980.
35. Calle R, Pilleron JP, Schlienger P, and Vilcoq JR: Conservative management of operable breast cancer. Ten years experience at the Foundation Curie, Cancer 42:2045, 1978.
36. Calle R, Vilcoq JR, Pilleron JP, et al: Conservative treatment of operable breast carcinoma by irradiation with or without limited surgery—ten-year results. In Harris J, Hellman S, and Silen W, editors: Conservative management of breast cancer, Philadelphia, 1983, JB Lippincott, pp 3-9.
37. Campbell FC, Morton AL, Bishop HM, et al: The management of locally advanced carcinoma of the breast by Nolvadex (tamoxifen): a pilot study, Br Assoc Surg Oncol 10:111, 1984.
38. Casper ES, Guidera CA, Bosi GJ, et al: Combined modality treatment of locally advanced breast cancer: adjuvant combination chemotherapy with and without doxorubicin, Breast Cancer Res Treat 9:39, 1987.
39. Chevallier B, Asselain B, Kunlin A, et al: Inflammatory breast cancer. Determination of prognostic factors by univariate and multivariate analysis, Cancer 60:897, 1987.
40. Chris SM: Inflammatory carcinoma of the breast: report of 20 cases and review of the literature, Br J Surg 38:163, 1950.
41. Chu AM, Cope O, Doucette J, and Curran B: Non-metastatic locally advanced cancer of the breast treated with radiation, Int J Radiat Oncol Biol Phys 10:2299, 1984.
42. Chu AM, Wood WC, and Doucette JA: Inflammatory breast carcinoma treated by radical radiotherapy, Cancer 45:2730, 1980.
43. Cocconi G, DiBlasio B, Alberti G, et al: Problems in evaluating response of primary breast cancer to systemic therapy, Breast Cancer Res Treat 4:309, 1984.
44. Cocconi G, di Blasio B, Bisagni G, et al: Neoadjuvant chemotherapy or chemotherapy and endocrine therapy in locally advanced breast cancer. A prospective, randomized study, Am J Clin Oncol 13:226, 1990.
45. Conte PF, Gardin G, Miglietta L, et al: Chemotherapy with estrogenic recruitment in locally advanced and metastatic breast cancer: results of two randomized trials, Proc Am Soc Clin Oncol 9:43, 1990 (abstract).
46. Crowe J, Hakes T, Rosen P, et al: Changing trends in the management of inflammatory breast cancer: a clinicopathologic review of 69 patients, Am J Clin Oncol 8:21, 1985 (abstract).
47. Dao TL and McCarthy JD: Treatment of inflammatory carcinoma of the breast, Surg Gynecol Obstet 113:729, 1961.
48. Delarue JC, May-Levin F, Mouriesse H, et al: Estrogen and progesterone cytosolic receptors in clinically inflammatory tumors of the human breast, Br J Cancer 44:911, 1981.

49. DeLena M, Varini M, Zucali R, et al: Multimodal treatment for locally advanced breast cancer, Cancer Clin Trials 4:229, 1981.
50. DeLena M, Zucali R, Viganotti G, et al: Combined chemotherapy-radiotherapy approach in locally advanced (T3b-T4) breast cancer, Cancer Chemother Pharmacol 1:53, 1978.
51. Denoix P: Treatment of malignant breast tumors. In Recent results in cancer research, New York, 1970, Springer-Verlag, pp 245-257.
52. Derman DP, Browde S, Kessell IL, et al: Adjuvant chemotherapy (CMF) for stage III breast cancer: a randomized trial, Int J Radiat Oncol Biol Phys 17:275, 1989.
53. Donegan WL: Staging and primary treatment. In Donegan WL and Spratt JS, editors: Cancer of the breast, ed 3, Philadelphia, 1988, WB Saunders, pp 336-402.
54. Donehower R, Allegra JC, Lippman ME, and Chabner B: Combined effects of methotrexate and 5-fluoropyrimidine on human breast cancer cells in serum-free culture, Eur J Cancer 16:665, 1980.
55. Droulias CA, Swell CW, McSweeney MB, and Powell RW: Inflammatory carcinoma of the breast. A correlation of clinical radiologic and pathologic findings, Ann Surg 184:217, 1976.
56. Ellis DL and Teitelbaum SL: Inflammatory carcinoma of the breast—a pathologic definition, Cancer 33:1045, 1974.
57. Fastenberg NA, Buzdar AU, Montague ED, et al: Management of inflammatory carcinoma of the breast. A combined modality approach, Am J Clin Oncol 8:134, 1985.
58. Feldman LD, Hortobagyi GM, Buzdar AV, et al: Pathologic assessment of response to induction chemotherapy in breast cancer, Cancer Res 46:2578, 1986.
59. Field SB and Fowler JF: The biologic basis for neutron therapy, J Eur Radiother 3:170, 1984.
60. Fields JN, Kuske RR, Perez CA, et al: Prognostic factors in inflammatory breast cancer. Univariate and multivariate analysis, Cancer 63:1225, 1989.
61. Fields JN, Perez CA, Kuske RR, et al: Inflammatory carcinoma of the breast: treatment results on 107 patients, Int J Radiat Oncol Biol Phys 17:249, 1989.
62. Fletcher GH: Clinical dose-response curves of human malignant epithelial tumors, Br J Radiol 46:1, 1973.
63. Fowble B, Gray R, Gilchrist K, et al: Identification of a subgroup of patients with breast cancer and histologically positive axillary nodes receiving adjuvant chemotherapy who may benefit from postoperative radiotherapy, J Clin Oncol 6:1107, 1988.
64. Fracchia AA, Evans JF, and Eisenberg BC: Stage III carcinoma of the breast—a detailed analysis, Ann Surg 192:705, 1980.
65. Garewal HS, Takasugi B, Jones SE, et al: Is $T_3N_0M_0$ breast cancer with pathologically negative nodes truly stage III? J Clin Oncol 2:242, 1984.
66. Ghossein NA, Stacey P, Alpert S, et al: Local control of breast cancer with tumorectomy plus radiotherapy or radiotherapy alone, Radiology 121:455, 1976.
67. Golding P: The treatment of inoperable carcinoma of the breast in Portsmouth, 1960-69, Proc Soc Med 69:701, 1976.
68. Green MD, Whybourne AM, Taylor IW, and Sutherland RL: Effects of antiestrogens on the growth and cell cycle kinetics of cultured human mammary carcinoma cells. In Sutherland RL and Jorna VC, editors: Non-steroidal antiestrogens, New York, 1981, Academic Press, pp 397-413.
69. Griscom NT and Wang CC: Radiation therapy of inoperable breast carcinoma, Radiology 79:18, 1962.
70. Haagensen CD: Inflammatory carcinoma. In Haagensen CD, editor: Diseases of the breast, ed 2, Philadelphia, 1971, WB Saunders, pp 566-584.
71. Haagensen CD and Cooley E: Radical mastectomy for mammary carcinoma, Ann Surg 170:884, 1969.
72. Haagensen CD and Stout AP: Carcinoma of the breast. II. Criteria of operability, Ann Surg 118:859, 1943.
73. Hagelberg RS, Jolly PC, and Anderson RP: Role of surgery in the treatment of inflammatory breast carcinoma, Am J Surg 148:125, 1984.
74. Halpern J, Maor MH, Hussey DH, et al: Locally advanced breast cancer treated with neutron beams: long term follow-up in 28 patients, Int J Radiat Oncol Biol Phys 18:825, 1990.
75. Harris JR, Sawicka J, Gelman R, and Hellman S: Management of locally advanced carcinoma of the breast by primary radiation therapy, Int J Radiat Oncol Biol Phys 9:345, 1983.
76. Hermanek P and Sobin LH, editors: UICC international union against cancer: TNM classification of malignant tumors, 4th ed, Berlin, 1987, Springer-Verlag, pp 93-99.
77. Hery M, Namer M, Moro M, et al: Conservative treatment (chemotherapy/radiotherapy) of locally advanced breast cancer, Cancer 57:1744, 1986.
78. Hobar PC, Jones RC, Schouten J, et al: Multimodality treatment of locally advanced breast carcinoma, Arch Surg 123:951, 1988.
79. Hortobagyi GN, Ames FC, Buzdar AU, et al: Management of Stage III primary breast cancer with primary chemotherapy, surgery and radiation therapy, Cancer 62:2507, 1988.
80. Hortobagyi G, Holmes F, Frye D, et al: Comparison of two adjuvant chemotherapy programs for locally advanced breast cancer, Proc Am Soc Clin Oncol 9:21, 1990 (abstract).
81. Hortobagyi GM, Spanos W, Montague ED, et al: Treatment of locoregionally advanced breast cancer with surgery, radiotherapy and combined chemoimmunotherapy, Int J Radiat Oncol Biol Phys 9:643, 1983.
82. Israel L, Breau J-L, and Morere J-F: Two years of high-dose cyclophosphamide and 5-fluorouracil followed by surgery after 3 months for acute inflammatory breast carcinomas. A phase II study of 25 cases with a median follow-up of 35 months, Cancer 57:24, 1986.
83. Jacquillat C, Baillet F, Weil M, et al: Results of a conservative treatment combining induction (neoadjuvant) and consolidation chemotherapy, hormonotherapy, and external and interstitial irradiation in 98 patients with locally advanced breast cancer (IIIA-IIIB), Cancer 61:1977, 1988.
84. Klefstrom P, Grohn P, Heinonen E, et al: Adjuvant postoperative radiotherapy, chemotherapy and immunotherapy in stage III breast cancer. II. 5-year results and influence of levamisole, Cancer 60:936, 1987.
85. Knight CD Jr, Martin JK, Welch JS, et al: Surgical considerations after chemotherapy and radiation for inflammatory breast cancer, Surgery 99:385, 1986.
86. Koyama H, Nishizawa Y, Wada T, et al: Intra-arterial infusion chemotherapy as an induction therapy in multidisciplinary treatment for locally advanced breast cancer. A long term follow-up study, Cancer 56:725, 1985.
87. Krutchik AN, Buzdar AU, Blumenschein GR, et al: Combined chemoimmunotherapy and radiation therapy of inflammatory breast carcinoma, J Surg Oncol 11:325, 1979.
88. Lacour J, Bucalossi P, Cacers E, et al: Radical mastectomy vs. radical mastectomy plus internal mammary dissection. Five year results of an international cooperative study, Cancer 37:206, 1976.
89. Lee BJ and Tannenbaum NE: Inflammatory carcinoma of the breast, Surg Gynecol Obstet 39:580, 1924.

90. Lee BJ and Tannenbaum NE: Inflammatory carcinoma of the breast: a review of twenty-eight cases from the breast clinic of the Memorial Hospital, Surg Gynecol Obstet 39:580, 1924.
91. Lenz M: Tumor dosage and results in roentgen therapy of cancer of the breast, Am J Roentgenol Radium Ther 56:67, 1946.
92. Levine PH, Steinhorn SC, Ries LG, and Aron JL: Inflammatory breast cancer: the experience of the Surveillance, Epidemiology and End Results (SEER) program, J Natl Cancer Inst 74:291, 1985.
93. Lippman ME, Bolan G, and Huff K: The effects of estrogens and antiestrogens on hormone-responsive human breast cancer in long-term tissue culture, Cancer Res 36:4595, 1976.
94. Loprinzi CL, Rasmussen PW, Tormey DC, and Carbone PP: Combined modality treatment of local regionally advanced breast cancer patients. 5 to 10 year follow-up, Am J Clin Oncol 12:208, 1989.
95. Lucas FV and Perez-Mesa C: Inflammatory carcinoma of the breast, Cancer 41:1595, 1978.
96. Manji M, Ragaz J, Worth A, et al: Is mastectomy indicated in patients with Stage III breast cancer treated with preoperative (neoadjuvant) therapy? Proc Am Soc Clin Oncol 7:36, 1988 (abstract).
97. McCready DR, Hortobagyi GN, Kau SW, et al: The prognostic significance of lymph node metastases after preoperative chemotherapy for locally advanced breast cancer, Arch Surg 124:21, 1989.
98. McGuire WL, Abeloff MD, Hortobagyi GN, and Swain SM: Treatment of stage III breast cancer, Breast Cancer Res Treat 13:225, 1989.
99. Meek AG, Order SE, Abeloff MD, et al: Concurrent radiochemotherapy in advanced breast cancer, Cancer 51:1001, 1983.
100. Meyer AC, Dockerty MB, and Harrington SW: Inflammatory carcinoma of the breast, Surg Gynecol Obstet 87:417, 1948.
101. Morrow M, Braverman A, Thelmo W, et al: Multimodal therapy for locally advanced breast cancer, Arch Surg 121:1291, 1986.
102. Mourali N, Tabbane F, Muenz LR, et al: Preliminary results of primary systemic chemotherapy in association with surgery or radiotherapy in rapidly progressing breast cancer, Br J Cancer 45:367, 1982.
103. Nawata H, Chong M, Bronzert D, and Lippman ME: Estradiol independent growth of a subline of MCF-7 human breast cancer cell line in culture, J Biol Chem 256:6895, 1981.
104. Nemoto T, Vana J, Bedwani RN, et al: Management and survival of female breast cancer: results of a national survey by the American College of Surgeons, Cancer 45:2917, 1980.
105. Nobler MP and Venet L: Twelve years experience with irradiation as the primary treatment for breast cancer, Int J Radiat Oncol Biol Phys 7:33, 1981.
106. Noguchi S, Miyauchi K, Mishizaua Y, et al: Management of inflammatory carcinoma of the breast with combined modality therapy including intraarterial infusion chemotherapy as an induction therapy, Cancer 61:1483, 1988.
107. Nussbaum H, Kagan AR, Gilbert H, et al: Management of inflammatory breast carcinoma, Breast, Diseases of the Breast 1:25, 1977.
108. Olson JE, Neuberg D, Pandya K, et al: The management of resectable stage III breast cancer. The Eastern Cooperative Oncology Group Trial. Proc Am Soc Clin Oncol 8:23, 1989 (abstract).
109. Papaioannou A, Lissaios B, Vasilaros S, et al: Pre- and postoperative chemoendocrine treatment with or without postoperative radiotherapy for locally advanced breast cancer, Cancer 51:1284, 1983.
110. Paradiso A, Tommasi S, Brandi M, et al: Cell kinetics and hormonal receptor status in inflammatory breast carcinoma. Comparison with locally advanced disease, Cancer 64:1922, 1989.
111. Pawlicki M, Skolyszewski J, and Brandys A: Results of combined treatment of patients with locally advanced breast cancer, Tumor 69:249, 1983.
112. Pearlman NW, Guerra O, and Fracchia AA: Primary inoperable cancer of the breast, Surg Gynecol Obstet 143:909, 1976.
113. Perez CA, Presant C, Philpott G, and Ratkin G: Phase I-II study of concurrent irradiation and multi-drug chemotherapy in advanced carcinoma of the breast: a pilot study by the Southeastern Cancer Study Group, Int J Radiat Oncol Biol Phys 5:1329, 1979.
114. Perloff M, Lesnick GJ, Korzun A, et al: Combination chemotherapy with mastectomy or radiotherapy for stage III breast carcinoma: a cancer and Leukemia Group B study, J Clin Oncol 6:261, 1988.
115. Piccart MJ, DeValeriola P, Paridaens R, et al: Six-year results of a multimodality treatment strategy for locally advanced breast cancer, Cancer 62:2501, 1988.
116. Pierquin B: Conservative treatment for carcinoma of the breast: experience of Creteil—ten year results. In Harris J, Hellman S, and Silen W, editors: Conservative management of breast cancer, Philadelphia, 1983, JB Lippincott, pp 11-14.
117. Ragaz J, Manji M, Olivotto I, et al: Role of mastectomy in preoperative (neoadjuvant) combined modality therapy of locally advanced breast cancer, Proc Am Soc Clin Oncol 6:55, 1987 (abstract).
118. Rao AF, Murthy AK, Hendrickson FR, et al: Analysis of risk factors for loco-regional failure in Stage II breast carcinoma treated with mastectomy and adjunctive chemotherapy, Int J Radiat Oncol Biol Phys 11(suppl 1):151, 1985 (abstract).
119. Richards GJ and Lewison EF: Inflammatory carcinoma of the breast, Surg Gynecol Obstet 113:729, 1961.
120. Robbins GF, Shah J, Rosen P, et al: Inflammatory carcinoma of the breast, Surg Clin North Am 54:801, 1974.
121. Rogers CS and Fitts WT: Inflammatory carcinoma of the breast: a critique of therapy, Surgery 39:367, 1956.
122. Rouesse J, Friedman S, Sarrazin D, et al: Primary chemotherapy in the treatment of inflammatory breast carcinoma: a study of 230 cases from the Institut Gustave-Roussy, J Clin Oncol 4:1765, 1986.
123. Rubens RD, Armitage P, Winter PJ, et al: Prognosis in operable stage III carcinoma of the breast. Eur J Cancer 13:805, 1977.
124. Rubens RD, Bartelink H, Engelsman E, et al: Locally advanced breast cancer: the contribution of cytotoxic and endocrine treatment to radiotherapy, Eur J Cancer Clin Oncol 25:667, 1989.
125. Rubens RD, Sexton S, Tong D, et al: Combined chemotherapy and radiotherapy for locally advanced breast cancer, Eur J Cancer 16:351, 1980.
126. Saltzstein SL: Clinically occult inflammatory carcinoma of the breast, Cancer 34:382, 1974.
127. Schaake-Konig C, van der Linden EH, Hart G, and Engelsman E: Adjuvant chemo- and hormonal therapy in locally advanced breast cancer: a randomized clinical study, Int J Radiat Oncol Biol Phys 11:1759, 1985.
128. Schafer P, Alberto P, Forni M, et al: Surgery as part of a combined modality approach for inflammatory breast cancer, Cancer 59:1063, 1987.
129. Schottenfeld D, Nash AG, Robbins GF, and Beattlie EJ: Ten-year results of the treatment of primary operable

breast carcinoma. A summary of 304 patients evaluated by the TNM system. Cancer 28:1001, 1976.
130. Segel MC, Paulus DD, and Hortobagyi GM: Advanced primary breast cancer: assessment at mammography of response to induction chemotherapy, Radiology 169:49, 1988.
131. Serrou B, Sancho-Garnier H, Cappelaere P, et al: Follow-up results from a randomized trial for T_3 and T_4 breast cancer patients: previous BCG improves response to chemotherapy in the relapse patient, Rec Results Cancer Res 80:157, 1982.
132. Serrou B, Sancho-Garnier H, Cappelaere P, et al: Results of a randomized trial of prophylactic chemotherapy in $T_{3\text{-}4}$ breast cancer patients previously treated by radiotherapy. In Bonadonna G, Mathe G, and Salmon SE, editors: Adjuvant therapies and markers of post-surgical minimal residual disease II. Adjuvant therapies of the various primary tumors, New York, 1979, Springer-Verlag, pp 105-108.
133. Shanta V, Krishnamurthi S, Sastry DVLN, and Menon R: Multimodal approach in the therapy of stage III female breast cancers, J Surg Oncol 28:134, 1985.
134. Sheldon T, Hayes DF, Cady B, et al: Primary radiation therapy for locally advanced breast cancer, Cancer 60:1219, 1987.
135. Sherry MM, Johnson DH, Page DL, et al: Inflammatory carcinoma of the breast. Clinical review and summary of the Vanderbilt experience with multimodality therapy, Am J Med 79:355, 1985.
136. Sorace RA and Lippman ME: Locally advanced breast cancer. In Lippman ME, Lichter A, and Danforth DN, editors: Diagnosis and management of breast cancer, Philadelphia, 1988, WB Saunders, pp 272-295.
137. Spangenberg JP, Nel CJC, Anderson ID, and Doman MJ: A prospective study of the treatment of stage III breast cancer, S Afr J Surg 24:57, 1986.
138. Spanos WJ, Montague ED, and Fletcher GH: Late complications of radiation only for advanced breast cancer, Int J Radiat Oncol Biol Phys 6:1473, 1980.
139. Sponzo RW, Cunningham TJ, Caradonna RR, and Antemann R: Management of non-resectable (stage III) breast cancer, Int J Radiat Oncol Biol Phys 5:1475, 1979.
140. Sponzo RW, Gray R, Damsker I, et al: The management of non-resectable (Stage III) breast cancer, Proc Am Soc Clin Oncol 2:110, 1983.
141. Spratt JS and Donegan WL: Cancer of the breast, Philadelphia, 1967, WB Saunders, p 167.
142. Stefanik D, Goldberg R, Bryne P, et al: Local-regional failure in patients treated with adjuvant chemotherapy for breast cancer, J Clin Oncol 3:660, 1985.
143. Stoker TAM and Ellis H: Post-irradiation toilet mastectomy in the management of locally advanced carcinoma of the breast, J Radiol 45:851, 1972.
144. Sutherland CM and Mather FJ: Long-term survival and prognostic factors in patients with regional breast cancer (skin, muscle and/or chest wall attachment), Cancer 55:1389, 1985.
145. Swain S, Bagley C, Boder J, et al: Treatment of locally advanced breast cancer using primary induction chemotherapy with hormonal synchronization followed by radiation therapy with or without debulking surgery, Proc Am Soc Clin Oncol 6:50, 1987 (abstract).
146. Swain SM and Lippman ME: Treatment of patients with inflammatory breast cancer, Important Adv Oncol 129, 1989.
147. Swain SM, Sorace RA, Bagley CS, et al: Neoadjuvant chemotherapy in the combined modality approach of locally advanced non-metastatic breast cancer, Cancer Res 47:3889, 1987.
148. Syed AMN, Puthawala A, Fleming P, et al: Combination of external and interstitial irradiation in the primary management of breast carcinoma, Cancer 46:1360, 1980.
149. Sykes HF, Sim DA, Wong CJ, et al: Local-regional recurrences in breast cancer after mastectomy and Adriamycin-based adjuvant chemotherapy: evaluation of the role of postoperative radiotherapy. Int J Radiat Oncol Biol Phys 16:641, 1989.
150. Taylor GW and Meltzer A: Inflammatory carcinoma of the breast, Am J Cancer 33:33, 1938.
151. Terz JJ, Romero CA, Kay S, et al: Preoperative radiotherapy for stage III carcinoma of the breast, Surg Gynecol Obstet 147:497, 1978.
152. Thalmo W, Sand J, Marti J, et al: Clinical and pathological findings in locally advanced breast cancer treated with cyclophosphamide-Adriamycin-5-FU, Proc Am Soc Clin Oncol 3:127, 1984 (abstract).
153. Thomas F, Arriagada R, Mouriesse H, et al: Radical radiotherapy alone in non-operable breast cancer: the major impact of tumor size and histologic grade on prognosis, Radiother Oncol 13:267, 1988.
154. Thoms WW Jr, McNeese MD, Fletcher GH, et al: Multimodal treatment for inflammatory breast cancer, Int J Radiat Oncol Biol Phys 17:739, 1989.
155. Toonkel LM, Fix I, Jacobson LH, et al: Locally advanced breast carcinoma: results with combined regional therapy, Int J Radiat Oncol Biol Phys 12:1583, 1986.
156. Townsend CM, Abston S, and Fish JC: Surgical adjuvant treatment of locally advanced breast cancer, Ann Surg 201:604, 1985.
157. Treurniet-Donker AD, Hop WCJ, and Den Hoed-Sijtsema S: Radiation treatment of stage III mammary carcinoma: a review of 129 patients, Int J Radiat Oncol Biol Phys 6:1477, 1980.
158. Vaeth JM, Clark JC, Green JP, et al: Radiotherapeutic management of locally advanced carcinoma of the breast, Cancer 30:107, 1972.
159. Valagussa P, Bonadonna G, and Veronesi U: Patterns of relapse and survival following radical mastectomy. Analysis of 716 consecutive patients, Cancer 41:1170, 1978.
160. Veronesi A, Frustaci S, Tirelli U, et al: Tamoxifen therapy in postmenopausal advanced breast cancer: efficacy at the primary tumor site in 46 evaluable patients, Tumor 67:235, 1981.
161. Wang CC and Griscom NT: Inflammatory carcinoma of the breast: results following orthovoltage and supervoltage radiation therapy, Clin Radiol 15:168, 1964.
162. Weichselbaum RR, Hellman S, Piro AJ, et al: Proliferation kinetics of a human breast cancer cell line in vitro following treatment with 17b-estradiol and 1-b-D-arabinofuranosylcytosine, Cancer Res 38:2339, 1978.
163. Williams MR, Gilson D, Marsh L, et al: The early results from a randomized study of radiotherapy versus Nolvadex (tamoxifen) as initial treatment for stage III breast cancer, Eur J Surg Oncol 14:235, 1988.
164. Zaharia M, Caceres E, Valdivia S, et al: Radiotherapy in the management of locally advanced breast cancer, Int J Radiat Oncol Biol Phys 13:1179, 1987.
165. Zucali R, Uslenghi C, Kenda R, and Bonadonna G: Natural history and survival of inoperable breast cancer treated with radiotherapy and radiotherapy followed by radical mastectomy, Cancer 37:1422, 1976.
166. Zylberberg B, Salat-Baroux J, Ravine JH, et al: Initial chemoimmunotherapy in inflammatory carcinoma of the breast, Cancer 49:1537, 1982.

15 Local-Regional Recurrence Following Definitive Treatment for Operable Breast Cancer

Barbara Fowble and Fred Schwaibold

LOCAL-REGIONAL RECURRENCE FOLLOWING CONSERVATIVE SURGERY AND RADIATION

A local recurrence following conservative surgery and radiation is one that occurs in the treated breast. Local recurrences can be further subdivided into true or marginal recurrence, which occur in the vicinity of the original primary tumor, or recurrences that occur elsewhere, i.e., in a quadrant separate from the original primary. Regional recurrences include those in the ipsilateral axilla, supraclavicular, or internal mammary nodes.

Local recurrence

Recurrence in the ipsilateral breast following conservative surgery and radiation occurs in 5% to 10% of patients at 5 years and 10% to 15% at 10 years (Table 15-1). Risk factors for recurrence following conservative therapy and radiation can be divided into three categories: (1) clinical factors; (2) histopathologic factors; and (3) treatment-related factors. A detailed discussion of risk factors for breast recurrence is presented in Chapter 5. Briefly, clinical factors include patient age, tumor size, tumor location, gross multicentricity, mammographic evidence of diffuse microcalcifications, and estrogen and progesterone receptor status. There is no evidence to suggest that tumor size is related to breast recurrence in patients with stage I or stage II disease provided that an excisional biopsy has been performed.[7,8,14,21,53,71] Similarly, there is no increased risk of a breast recurrence when comparing tumors in the central or inner quadrant locations with those in an outer quadrant.[2,7,8,78] The presence of gross multicentric or multifocal disease has been associated with an increased risk of breast recurrence in patients undergoing conservative surgery and radiation.[12,36,42] The impact of estrogen and progesterone receptor status on breast recurrence in patients undergoing conservative surgery and radiation is uncertain. An increased risk of breast recurrence has been identified in young women with estrogen receptor–negative tumors,[41] and Ryoo et al.[65] also reported an increased risk of breast recurrence in all women with negative estrogen receptors. Others, however, have found no correlation between estrogen receptor status and breast recurrence.[23,34,49] Similarly, the existence of negative progesterone receptors has been correlated with breast recurrence in one study[34] and not in three others.[23,41,49]

The association between young age and an increased risk of breast recurrence is controversial. Several series[24,41,48,60] have reported an increased risk of breast recurrence in women under the age of 35 to 40 years who undergo conservative surgery and radiation, while others have found no increased risk in these young women.[14,52,72] The increased risk of a breast recurrence in young women has been attributed to inadequate surgery for the primary tumor[24] and a greater prevalence of tumors demonstrating an extensive intraductal component.[24,37,60] However, the relative importance of young age as a prognostic factor for breast recurrence can be modified by treatment. Rose et al.[64] reported a breast recurrence rate of 9% in women <35 years of age who were treated with conservative surgery, radiotherapy, and multiagent adjuvant chemotherapy, compared to 26% for those who did not receive chemotherapy. Adequate surgery for the primary also has decreased the breast recurrence rate in young women.[24,72] Kurtz et al.,[37] however, failed to note a significant decrease in the rate of breast recurrence in young women receiving adjuvant chemotherapy, although most of the patients received only perioperative single-agent treatment. Similarly, the authors failed to note a decrease in breast recurrence rates in young women with negative margins of resection who had either an extensive intraductal component or a major cellular reaction.[37] At the University of Pennsylvania there has been no increased risk of breast recur-

Table 15-1 Breast recurrence following conservative surgery and radiation at 5, 10, and 15 years

Author	No. pts.	Breast recurrence (%)		
		5 yr	10 yr	15 yr
Clarke et al.[14]	436	5	7	
Recht et al.[63]	607	10	16	
Haffty et al.[29]	278	9	20	
Leung et al.[43]	493		10	
Clark et al.[12]	1130	10	14	
Pierquin[56]				
T_1	99	3	8	
T_2	235	6	7	
Kurtz et al.[35]	1593	7	14	18
Fourquet et al.[24]	518	7	11	18
Stotter et al.[77]	490	9	19	
Greco et al.[28]	1232	—	7	
University of Pennsylvania	697	8	18	

rence associated with young age; perhaps this is a reflection of the emphasis on complete gross excision of the primary tumor with reexcision where indicated, assessment of resection margins, and the use of adjuvant systemic chemotherapy in all premenopausal node-positive patients.[72]

Histopathologic factors that have been analyzed for their ability to predict for a breast recurrence following conservative surgery and radiation include histologic or nuclear grade, tumor necrosis, vascular lymphatic invasion, inflammatory infiltrate, the presence of intraductal noninvasive cancer in association with an invasive ductal cancer, status of the margins of resection, histology other than infiltrating ductal carcinoma, and the pathologic nodal status. Knowledge of the histopathologic factors that significantly correlate with a breast recurrence is evolving. Factors associated with an increased risk of breast recurrence in patients treated in a contemporary manner (i.e., preoperative mammograms, complete excision, assessment of resection margins and reexcision where indicated, axillary dissection, and adjuvant systemic therapy) remain to be determined. It appears that, in patients whose tumors have an extensive intraductal component and in whom adequate excision is not achieved, there is an increased risk of breast recurrence with conservative surgery and radiation.[36,63,81] In series where margins of resection have been assessed and are negative,[3,23,81] an extensive intraductal component has not been a prognostic factor for breast recurrence. Kurtz et al.,[37] however, reported that negative margins of resection did not decrease the risk of a breast recurrence significantly in women <40 years of age with either a major cellular reaction and/or more than 50% intraductal carcinoma within the tumor. However, margin assessment was not performed by routine inking of the specimen but was retrospectively assessed by reviewing routine sections taken from the tumor and at the periphery. In this series, an extensive intraductal component predicted for a breast recurrence only in premenopausal women. A higher risk of breast recurrence also has been reported for histologic grade III tumors.[36,45] However, this has not been found to be a prognostic factor in other series,[7,24,34,47,68] and in the NSABP B-06 trial[23] histologic grade was not an important prognostic factor for breast recurrence in patients who underwent excision with negative margins. The presence of a moderate or marked inflammatory infiltrate has been reported by some to be associated with an increased risk of breast recurrence,[36,45] but not by others.[7,23,47,68] The presence of lymphatic or vascular invasion has been correlated with an increased risk of breast recurrence in two series,[24,34] but not in five others.[7,23,36,45,47,68] Mate et al.[47] reported an increased risk of breast recurrence in patients whose tumors demonstrated necrosis within the invasive component. Lindley et al.[45] reported an increased risk of breast recurrence for tumors demonstrating necrosis in the noninvasive component of the tumor. Three additional series have noted no influence of the presence of necrosis on breast recurrence following conservative surgery and radiation.[7,23,36,68] Patients with infiltrating lobular carcinomas do not appear to have an increased risk of breast recurrence when compared to those with infiltrating ductal carcinoma.[38,69] The risk of a breast recurrence appears small for patients with medullary or colloid carcinomas.[38] There appears to be no increased risk of a breast recurrence in patients with histologically positive axillary nodes when compared to those with histologically negative axillary nodes.[4,14,18,21,63,71,78] This finding is in contrast to the risk of a chest wall recurrence following mastectomy, where the histologic status of the axillary node significantly correlates with a chest wall recurrence.

Treatment-related factors that may impact on the risk of a breast recurrence include the extent of the surgical resection of the primary tumor, the radiation technique, and the use of adjuvant systemic chemotherapy or hormonal therapy. Incisional biopsies arc associated with a threefold to fourfold increase in the risk of a breast recurrence.[4,10,61,78] Patients who have grossly positive margins of surgical resection have an increased risk of breast recurrence[81] compared to those with grossly negative margins. In contrast, patients with microscopically positive margins of resection do not appear to have an increased risk of breast recurrence provided that a boost dose of radiation is employed.[3,14,33,65,67] At the University of Pennsylvania, the 5-year actuarial risk of a breast recurrence for patients with microscopically positive margins of resection was 2%, compared to 7% for those with negative margins and 9% for those with unknown margins. However, patients with an extensive intraductal component may require negative margins of resection to minimize the risk of a breast recurrence. Radiotherapy factors that have been correlated with an increased risk of breast recurrence include a delay in initiation of radiation,[30,76] the use of weekly doses of <800 cGy,[39,54] and the omission of a boost in patients with microscopically positive margins of resection.[65] The addition of adjuvant systemic chemotherapy to radiation has been associated with a decreased risk of breast recurrence at 5 years.[6,21,64,71] The omission of radiation in node-positive patients receiving chemotherapy who have undergone wide excision alone results in an increased risk of breast recurrence.[21,44] Delays in the initiation of radiation for the administration of chemotherapy have also been associated with an increased risk of breast recurrence.[31] Tamoxifen therapy has resulted in a significant decrease in the rates of breast recurrence in node-negative, estrogen receptor (ER)–positive patients undergoing conservative surgery and radiation when compared to those who did not receive tamoxifen (2% vs. 0).[20]

The method of detection of a breast recurrence following conservative surgery and radiation is presented in Table 15-2. The majority of recurrences are detected by physical examination, with approximately one third being detected by a positive mammogram only. The mammographic finding of microcalcifications associated with a mass is virtually always indicative of a recurrence.[73,76] Approximately two thirds of patients whose sole mammographic finding is the appearance of new microcalcifications have biopsy-proven recurrence.[59,74,76] The finding of a mass only on mammogram was reported by Stomper et al.[76] to be associated with a biopsy-proven recurrence in 33% of patients; however, Solin et al.[73] reported a 62% incidence of biopsy-proven recurrence in a similar group of patients.

The majority of recurrences following conservative surgery and radiation are true or marginal (i.e., in the vicinity of the original primary tumor) (Table 15-3). Twenty percent to 30% of recurrences occur in a separate quadrant from the original primary (see Table 15-3). The incidence of recurrences elsewhere may be related to the extent of the initial primary surgery as well as the time interval to recurrence. In the NSABP B-06 trial, all breast recurrences following segmental mastectomy with negative resection margins were in the area of the original primary tumor.[23] Veronesi et al.[79] reported that 50% of the recurrences following quadrantectomy and radiation were in the original quadrant and 50% were in a separate quadrant. The incidence of recurrences in a quadrant separate from the primary tumor appears to increase with the time interval to recurrence. Kurtz et al.[40] noted that 32% of recurrences after 5 years were elsewhere compared to 14% before 5 years. The majority of the recurrences after 10 years were elsewhere.[35] Recht et al.[63] reported a 1% actuarial risk

Table 15-2 Detection of breast recurrence after conservative surgery and radiation

<table>
<tr><th>Author</th><th>Mammography positive, physical examination negative</th><th>Physical examination positive, mammography negative or not done</th><th>Positive physical examination and mammography</th></tr>
<tr><td>Stomper et al.[76]</td><td>35</td><td>39</td><td>26</td></tr>
<tr><td>Bartelink et al.[3]</td><td>27</td><td colspan="2">73</td></tr>
<tr><td>Haffty et al.[29]</td><td>25</td><td>25</td><td>50</td></tr>
<tr><td>Fowble et al.[26]</td><td>29</td><td>50</td><td>21</td></tr>
</table>

Table 15-3 Location of breast recurrence following conservative surgery and radiation

Author	Recurrence (%)	
	True/marginal	Elsewhere
Veronesi et al.[79]	50	50
Fourquet et al.[24]	46	54
Ray et al.[58]	66	33
Leung et al.[43]	66	25
Haffty et al.[29]	67	33
Kurtz et al.[35]	79	21
Nobler and Venet[53]	80	20
Recht et al.[63]	80	20
Peterse et al.[55]	80	20
Clarke et al.[14]	82	18
Clark et al.[12]	94	6
NSABP B-06[23]	100	0
Fowble et al.[26]	65	35
Stotter et al.[77]	78	22

for an elsewhere recurrence at 5 years with a 4% risk at 10 years. In the University of Pennsylvania series, 23% of the breast recurrences occurring before 5 years were elsewhere compared to 46% after 5 years.[26] The location of the recurrence also has been related to the histology of the primary tumor. Schnitt et al.[69] reported all invasive lobular recurrences to be true or marginal compared to 80% for invasive ductal cancers. However, Kurtz et al.[38] found only 3 of 12 invasive lobular recurrences to be in the vicinity of the original primary, while the remainder were elsewhere or involved more than one quadrant. In the University of Pennsylvania series[26] 6 of 8 invasive lobular recurrences were true or marginal, 1 was elsewhere, and 1 was diffuse. Of the 36 invasive ductal cancers, 24 were true or marginal, 11 were elsewhere, and 1 was diffuse.

The median interval to a breast recurrence is presented in Table 15-4. Overall, the median interval is approximately 3 years. The interval to recurrence is related to the location of the recurrence with true or marginal recurrences tending to

Table 15-4 Interval to breast recurrence (months) following conservative surgery and radiation

Author	All pts.	True/marginal	Elsewhere
Pierquin et al. (Groupe European)[57]	24		
Sarrazin et al.[66]	37		
Bluming et al.[5]	37		
Haffty et al.[29]	44		
Fourquet et al.[24]	53		
Fowble et al.[26]	34	38	46
Boyages et al.[7]	37	48/35	58
Veronesi et al.[79]		48	66
Bartelink et al.[3]		29	83
Recht et al.[63]		38	68

Table 15-5 Interval to breast recurrence for stage I and stage II breast cancer following conservative surgery and radiation

Author	Recurrence (%)		
	<5 yr	5-10 yr	>10 yr
Delouche et al.[15]	70	25	5
Leung et al.[43]	67	28	5
Spitalier et al.[75]	76	20	4
Veronesi et al.[79]	50	50	0
Kurtz et al.[40]	60	32	8
Clarke et al.[14]	73	18	9
Montague[51]	71	23	6

occur earlier than those located elsewhere (see Table 15-4). Approximately 70% of breast recurrences occur within 5 years (Table 15-5), although late local recurrences have been reported.[30,39] The risk of a breast recurrence within 5 years has been estimated to be 1.5% to 2.5% per year, diminishing to 1% per year after 8 to 10 years.[35,63] Recurrences within the first year following treatment are uncommon.[51,63] The appearance of a palpable mass and/or induration beneath the biopsy site with or without associated inflammation within the first year is more characteristic of fat necrosis.[13]

Approximately 10% of patients with a breast recurrence following conservative surgery and radiation will have simultaneous or antecedent distant metastases.[14,26,35,43,47,62] Eighty-five percent to 90% of those presenting without distant metastases are surgically operable (Table 15-6). Approximately one third of patients with an invasive breast recurrence at the time of salvage mastectomy and axillary dissection will have positive axillary nodes.[29,35,43,62]

At the time of salvage mastectomy, 85% to 90% of the patients with breast recurrences have an invasive histology.[26,62] Recht et al.[62] reported 10 of 79 patients with operable breast recurrences to have noninvasive intraductal cancer and an additional 10 patients to have predominantly intraductal cancer with focal areas of invasion. Peterse et al.[55] reported 3 of 15 breast recurrences to be predominantly or exclusively intraductal carcinoma. Noninvasive recurrences more commonly are detected by mammography alone.[26,70] Paget's disease is an uncommon presentation of breast recurrence following conservative surgery and radiation.[26,46,50,70]

The standard treatment of a breast recurrence following conservative surgery and radiation is mastectomy. Salvage mastectomy has resulted in subsequent local-regional control in 90% of patients.[26,35,40,43,62] Reconstruction following salvage mastectomy, either immediate or delayed, has not been associated with a significant incidence of complications.[26,62] Five-year actuarial rates following salvage mastectomy are presented in Table 15-7 and appear to be excellent. Two series have demonstrated no difference in 10-year survival rates between patients who developed an isolated breast recurrence and underwent salvage mastectomy and those who did not develop such a recurrence.[8,11] Clarke et al.[14] noted a 5-year disease-free survival rate of 81% for patients who developed an isolated breast recurrence, compared to 84% for those who did not. Kurtz et al.[40] reported that recurrences occurring after 5 years had no adverse effect on prognosis up to 15 years after initial treatment. Recurrences within 5 years, however, were associated with a decreased survival rate at 5, 10, and 15 years after initial treatment when compared to patients who did not develop a recurrence. Stotter et al.[77] reported a 5-year survival rate of 78% following initial treatment for patients with a local failure, compared to 88% for those who did not develop a recurrence.

The role of surgical procedures less than mastectomy in the treatment of an isolated breast recurrence following conservative surgery and radiation has been evaluated by Kurtz et al.[35,40] The authors reported the results of wide excision alone for the breast recurrence in a select group of patients. Local-regional control was 64% in those whose recurrence was within 5 years and 78% for those whose recurrence was after 5 years. While local-regional control appeared less with breast-sparing procedures when compared to mastectomy, there was no adverse impact on overall survival rates. However, patient selection for the two procedures may have influenced the results. In an attempt to identify a subset of patients for whom wide excision alone would be appropriate treatment for breast recurrence, pathologic findings from pa-

Table 15-6 Operability of isolated breast recurrence following conservative surgery and radiation

Author	Operable (%)
Delouche et al.[15]	75
Mate et al.[47]	83
Calle et al.[8]	96
Fowble et al.[26]	93
Kurtz et al.[35]	89
Leung et al.[43]	90
Sarrazin et al.[66]	73
Spitalier et al.[75]	91
Recht et al.[63]	88

Table 15-7 Survival rates following salvage surgery for an isolated breast recurrence

Author	No. pts.	5-yr survival (%)
Calle et al.[8]	20	75
Kurtz et al.[35]	159	69
Clark et al.[12]	87	55
Stotter et al.[77]	49	63
Clarke et al.[14]	11	81
Osborne et al.[54]	12	50
Recht et al.[63]	65	63
Haffty et al.[29]	25	48
Dubois et al.[17]	30	70
Fowble et al.[26]	52	84

tients undergoing salvage mastectomy at the University of Pennsylvania were reviewed.[26] At the time of salvage mastectomy, 13 of 31 patients whose initial biopsy for recurrence was excisional had no residual tumor as determined by random sections from quadrants separate from the recurrence and multiple sections from the area of recurrence. Detailed sectioning of the breast was not performed. No significant factors could be identified that would predict for patients who would have no residual tumor. However, the finding of no residual tumor was observed more commonly in patients whose initial age was >35 years, those who had no axillary involvement at the time of recurrence, those whose recurrence was true or marginal, and those whose recurrence had no associated intraductal component. Schnitt et al.[69] reported that 4 of 6 patients with invasive lobular cancer had involvement of all four quadrants of the breast at the time of salvage mastectomy, compared to 3 of 16 patients with ductal cancers who had involvement beyond the initial quadrant. In the University of Pennsylvania experience,[26] 4 of 8 patients with invasive lobular cancer had tumor extending beyond the initial quadrant. Peterse et al.[55] noted that 4 of 6 patients wtih initial lymphatic invasion had multicentric disease at the time of salvage mastectomy. Lymphatic invasion at the time of recurrence has been correlated with extensive disease in the breast in the University of Pennsylvania series. Based on these limited data, it would appear that patients who are not candidates for surgical procedures less than mastectomy at the time of recurrence are those with invasive lobular cancer, a recurrence elsewhere in the breast, an associated intraductal component, lymphatic invasion, positive axillary nodes, and an initial age ≤35. Further attempts at breast preservation result in higher local-regional recurrence rates when compared to mastectomy. This finding, in conjunction with the inability to identify factors that will predict for no residual tumor following an excisional biopsy at the time of recurrence, would suggest that mastectomy should remain the preferred local treatment.

The role of chemotherapy in the treatment of a breast recurrence following conservative surgery and radiation is unknown. For the most part it has been reserved for patients with positive axillary nodes, extensive involvement of the breast, or dermal lymphatic, vascular lymphatic, or lymphatic invasion.[26,62] Chemotherapy is not indicated for patients whose recurrence is purely noninvasive intraductal carcinoma. It may not be indicated for patients whose prognosis following salvage mastectomy for an isolated breast recurrence is good (i.e., those whose interval to recurrence is >5 years, initial tumor size is T_1, or whose recurrence is located elsewhere). Adjuvant chemotherapy may be beneficial in patients whose recurrences are associated with an unfavorable prognosis (i.e., positive axillary nodes, interval to recurrence <5 years, initial T_2 tumor size, or a diffuse recurrence).

A number of factors have been analyzed for their ability to predict survival following an operable breast recurrence: the time interval to recurrence; initial age; initial tumor size; initial pathologic nodal status; the location of the recurrence; the method of detection; the histology of the recurrence; the presence of residual tumor at the time of salvage mastectomy; the presence of skin, dermal lymphatic, or vascular lymphatic invasion; and the pathologic nodal status of the recurrence. The time interval to recurrence appears to be a significant factor in determining prognosis. Fourquet et al.[24] reported a 5-year actuarial survival rate for recurrences within 3 years of initial treatment of 45%, compared to 87% for those after 3 years. Earlier recurrences tended to be more aggressive and were associated more often with simultaneous nodal or distant metastases.[24,78] Kurtz et al.[35] also identified the most important prognostic factor for operable recurrences as being the disease-free interval of time from initial treatment. Recurrences within 2 years had a 5-year survival rate of 48%, compared to 84% for those after 5 years. For recurrences within 5 years, additional prognostic factors included histologic grade and anatomic extent. For recurrences after 5 years, the most important factor was the extent of the recurrence.[40] Those with axillary node involvement had a 5-year survival rate of 34% compared to 87% for those without. Prognosis also has been correlated with the extent of the recurrence.[14,29] Localized recurrences (i.e., those <2 to 3 cm) have been associated with an improved prognosis.[14,29,35,77] The presence of diffuse involvement or skin involvement is associated with a worse prognosis.[29,35,77] There is a trend towards a decreased survival rate in patients with histologically positive axillary nodes at the time of recurrence.[30,35,40,43,62] The histology of the recurrence also affects prognosis; patients with a predominantly or exclusively noninvasive recurrence have the best prognosis.[62] In the University of Pennsylvania series of operable breast recurrences,[26] the only significant factor associated with prognosis was the initial clinical tumor size. Initial T_2 tumors more often recurred within 3 years, had three or four quadrants of the breast involved, and were associated with skin, dermal lymphatic, or vascular invasion. Haffty et al.[29] noted that patients whose initial tumor size was T_2 more often had diffuse recurrences associated with a worse prognosis. Stotter et al.[77] correlated initial stage II disease with advanced local recurrences. The

5-year survival rate was 40% for an advanced recurrence, compared to 74% for a less advanced local recurrence. In the University of Pennsylvania series, an observed trend toward improved survival rates was noted with a longer interval to recurrence, initial age >35 years, initial pathologic nodal status negative or unknown, a noninvasive recurrence, no residual tumor at the time of mastectomy, and the absence of skin dermal lymphatic, vascular lymphatic, or muscle invasion, although these findings were not statistically significant.[26] Overall the prognosis of an isolated breast recurrence is superior to that of a chest wall recurrence following mastectomy (see following section).

The University of Pennsylvania experience consists of 65 patients who developed a recurrence in the treated breast from the overall population of 948 women who underwent conservative surgery and radiation between the years 1978 and 1986.[26] Nine of the recurrences were associated with simultaneous or antecedent distant metastases. Twenty-nine percent of the recurrences were detected by mammography alone, 50% by physical examination alone, and 21% by both physical examination and mammography. The median interval to recurrence was 34 months. Sixty-five percent of the recurrences were in the vicinity of the original tumor, although for recurrences occurring after 5 years 54% were in a separate quadrant. Ninety-five percent of the recurrences unassociated with distant metastases were operable and subsequent pathology revealed noninvasive cancer in only 10%. Fifty-two patients underwent salvage mastectomy. The 5-year actuarial overall and disease-free survival rates for patients undergoing salvage mastectomy were 84% and 59% respectively. The 5-year actuarial overall and disease-free survival rates for all patients were 73% and 44% respectively. The only significant prognostic factor for survival was the initial clinical tumor size, which was related to the extent of the recurrence.

Regional node recurrence following conservative surgery and radiation

Regional node failure following conservative surgery and radiation is defined as a failure in the ipsilateral axillary, infraclavicular, supraclavicular, or internal mammary nodes. The incidence of regional node failure following conservative surgery and radiation is presented in Table 15-8. Overall, <5% of patients develop a recurrence in the regional nodes. The incidence of regional node recurrence following conservative surgery and radiation for stage I and stage II is not dissimilar from that observed following mastectomy as demonstrated by three prospective randomized trials comparing these two treatments.[1,19,80]

The most common site for regional node recurrence following conservative surgery and radiation is the axilla with or without a simultaneous breast failure.[14,15,25,30,43,57] The incidence of simultaneous breast and axillary recurrence ranges from 0.7% to 4.6%.[8,15,25,30,43,57] The second most common site for a regional failure is the supraclavicular nodes. Internal mammary node recurrences are infrequent following conservative surgery and radiation, with the overall incidence ranging from 0 to 0.1%.[43,57,66,80]

The interval to development of a regional node recurrence following conservative surgery and radiation is related to the site of recurrence. The median interval for an isolated axillary failure is approximately 15 months,[25,57] although others have reported longer intervals of 24 and 31 months.[16,75] The median interval for a simultaneous breast and axillary failure is approximately 2 years.[25,57] The median interval for a supraclavicular failure is approximately 3 years.[25,57]

Table 15-8 Incidence of regional node relapse following conservative surgery and radiation for stage I and stage II breast cancer

Author	Total no. pts.	Follow-up	Regional node relapse (%)
Veronesi et al.[80]	352	8 yr (median)	2.3
Pierquin et al.[57]	3353	>5 yr (median)	3
Sarrazin et al.[66]	592	78 mo (median)	2
Leung et al.[43]	493	10 yr (mean)	1.2
Mate et al.[47]	180	5 yr (actuarial)	5
Van Limbergen et al.[78]	235	80 mo (median)	3
Fisher et al.[19]	625	38.9 mo (mean)	2.2
Delouche et al.[15]	410	11 yr (median)	1.2
Calle et al.[8]	324	5 yr (minimum)	2.1
Fowble et al.[25]	990	5 yr (actuarial)	3

From Fowble B et al: Int J Radiat Oncol Biol Phys 17:707, 1989.

The risk of a regional node failure is related to the extent of the initial axillary surgery and the extent of the region(s) treated with radiation. For patients with histologically negative axillary nodes, the risk of an axillary recurrence is ≤3% for patients who undergo either a limited axillary dissection or a complete axillary dissection.[9,16,25,27,32,80] In patients with histologically positive axillary nodes, Dewar et al.[16] reported a 5-year actuarial recurrence rate of 33% in patients who underwent a limited axillary dissection without radiation. The addition of axillary radiation to a limited axillary dissection in patients with histologically positive nodes decreases the risk of an axillary recurrence to 0 to 1.6%.[16,25,32] Patients with histologically positive axillary nodes who undergo a complete axillary dissection with or without radiation have an extremely low risk of axillary recurrence.[16,27,80] Fisher et al.[22] reported a correlation between the number of axillary nodes removed and axillary recurrence in patients undergoing mastectomy. The axillary recurrence rate was 21% for patients having no nodes identified, 11% for those with 5 or fewer nodes, 5% for 6 to 9 nodes, and <1% for 10 or more nodes. At the University of Pennsylvania,[25] patients who had 3 or fewer histologically negative axillary nodes removed at the time of the limited axillary dissection and who did not receive axillary radiation had a 33% (1 of 3) axillary node failure rate. Pierquin et al.[57] correlated supraclavicular recurrence with omission of supraclavicular irradiation. The overall incidence of regional node failure following conservative surgery and radiation has not been correlated with primary tumor size, pathologic nodal status, or treatment with chemotherapy.[80] In the University of Pennsylvania experience,[25] nodal relapse correlated only with the number of axillary nodes removed and patient age. Supraclavicular recurrences were found to be more common in younger women.

The treatment of a regional node relapse following conservative surgery and radiation is related to the site of failure. Isolated axillary failures are best treated with repeat axillary dissection. At the University of Pennsylvania, 1 of 11 patients undergoing a repeat axillary dissection for a recurrence developed a subsequent axillary recurrence. However, 1 of 2 patients undergoing excisional biopsy developed an axillary recurrence. Dewar et al.[16] reported regional control in only 1 of 4 patients with an axillary recurrence treated with radiation and chemotherapy. Therefore maximum regional control for an axillary recurrence appears to be achieved with axillary dissection whenever feasible. There is no role for mastectomy in patients with an isolated axillary recurrence who have no clinical or mammographic evidence of a breast recurrence.[25] The role of adjuvant chemotherapy following an axillary recurrence is unknown, although it generally is recommended. Patients who develop a simultaneous breast and axillary failure are best managed by mastectomy including axillary dissection. Supraclavicular recurrences should be treated by excisional biopsy where possible followed by regional radiation provided that this area has not received prior irradiation. Pierquin et al.[57] reported regional control in 77% of patients with a supraclavicular recurrence. Adjuvant systemic therapy may be indicated in patients with a supraclavicular recurrence because this pattern of failure is associated with a poor prognosis.

Survival rates following a regional node recurrence after conservative surgery and radiation are presented in Table 15-9. The overall survival rate ranges from 15% to 57% and is related to the site of recurrence. Isolated axillary recurrences have

Table 15-9 Survival following a regional node recurrence after conservative surgery and radiation

		NED survival (%) related to regional node recurrence			
Author	All pts.	Breast and axilla	Axilla	Supraclavicular	Follow-up (yr)
Fowble et al.[25]	57	83	50	0	3
Calle et al.[8]		60	80	0	5
Kurtz et al.[40]		[34]			5
Veronesi et al.[80]				33	—
Clarke et al.[14]	15				3
Mate et al.[47]	20				5
Leung et al.[43]	35				
Clark et al.[12]			57		5

NED, no evidence of disease; [ ], metastasis-free survival.

been associated with a relatively good prognosis,[8,12,25] while supraclavicular recurrences have a very poor prognosis.[8,25,80] A relatively good prognosis also has been associated with a simultaneous breast and axillary failure.

In summary, breast recurrence following conservative surgery and radiation occurs in 5% to 10% of patients at 5 years and 10% to 15% at 10 years. The majority of recurrences occur within 5 years of initial treatment. Ten percent to 15% present with simultaneous distant metastases, and 90% of isolated breast recurrences are operable. Salvage mastectomy has resulted in 5-year survival rates of 50% to 84% and prognosis appears to be related to the interval to recurrence, the extent of the recurrence, and the pathology of the recurrence. Regional node failures following conservative surgery and radiation are infrequent. The majority occur within 5 years. The most common site is the axilla with or without a simultaneous breast failure, followed by the supraclavicular nodes. Salvage treatment is effective for an isolated axillary recurrence and should include a repeat axillary dissection. Mastectomy with an axillary dissection is the appropriate treatment for patients with a simultaneous breast and axillary failure. Supraclavicular failures are best managed by excisional biopsy followed by radiation, provided that no prior radiation therapy has given. The role of chemotherapy in the treatment of a local-regional recurrence following conservative surgery and radiation remains to be determined; however, possible indications include positive axillary nodes, the presence of vascular lymphatic invasion, dermal lymphatic or skin invasion, ER-negative recurrence, or recurrence that is aneuploid or associated with a high S-phase tumor.

LOCAL-REGIONAL FAILURE FOLLOWING MASTECTOMY

The overall incidence of local-regional recurrence following mastectomy with or without adjuvant chemotherapy for operable breast cancer is approximately 10%, with 30% of all first recurrences presenting as local-regional.[94,118,125,127,185,187] Local-regional recurrences may cause significant morbidity, bleeding, ulceration, and pain. Bedwinek et al.[90] reported that 62% of patients with uncontrolled local-regional recurrence experienced one or more distressing symptoms for the duration of their life. While the optimal treatment of a local-regional recurrence following mastectomy is unknown, multimodality therapy commonly is employed.

Definition of local-regional recurrence

In general a local-regional recurrence refers to a recurrence in the chest wall within the skin, subcutaneous tissue, or muscle. The surgical definition of a local recurrence also may include the axilla, as this region is included in the operative field. Regional failure refers to a recurrence within the axillary, parasternal, or supraclavicular lymph nodes. It is not always possible to distinguish between a local and a regional failure. A mass in the interpectoral region or parasternal area may appear to be a local recurrence, but may actually represent enlarged internal mammary or retropectoral nodes. A mass in the infraclavicular region may represent either enlarged apical axillary nodes or a chest wall recurrence. An isolated local-regional failure is a recurrence without evidence of distant metastases confirmed by routine metastatic work-up.

Risk factors for local-regional recurrence

Several factors have been associated with an increased risk of local-regional recurrence following mastectomy. These can be divided into clinical factors, pathologic factors, and treatment-related factors. Clinical factors include primary tumor size, patient age, and hormonal receptor status. Pathologic factors include the pathologic axillary nodal status, tumor grade, histologic type, and status of the resection margin. Treatment-related factors include the extent of surgery and the use of adjuvant systemic chemotherapy and/or tamoxifen.

Clinical factors. The risk of a local-regional recurrence following mastectomy increases with increasing tumor size, as presented in Table 15-10. It is greatest for T_3 primary tumors (i.e., those >5 cm in diameter). Conway and Neumann[102] reported a 50% incidence of local recurrence for tumors ≥7 cm vs. a 4% incidence for tumors <3 cm. Age at the time of surgery has been reported to influence local-regional recurrence postmastectomy. Lewis and Rienhoff[152] reported a higher incidence of local-regional recurrence in women ≤40 years of age when compared to those >40 years of age. Forty-four percent of the young women who died had a local recurrence, compared to 24% of the older women. Donegan et al.[112] reported a 46% incidence of local-regional recurrence at 5 years in women <40 years of age, compared to 12% in women >40 years of age. Mathews et al.[160] and Bartelink et al.[3] also have noted a higher incidence of local-regional recurrence following mastectomy in young women.

Receptor status has been correlated with the risk of local-regional recurrence following mastectomy. Campbell et al.[98] noted an increased risk of regional recurrence in ER-negative patients when compared to ER-positive patients (15% vs. 7.5%, respectively). However, no difference in the frequency of chest wall recurrences was reported. Sykes et al.[186] also identified patients who had histologically

Table 15-10 Incidence of local-regional recurrence following mastectomy related to primary tumor size

		Local-regional recurrence (%)			
Author	Surgery	T_1	T_2	T_3	Follow-up (yr)
Donegan et al.[112]	RM	7 [73]	16 [398]	30 [135]	5
Rosenman et al.[174]	RM/MRM	8 [51]	18 [87]	32 [44]	2-14
Dao and Nemoto[106]	RM	6 [36]	6 [70]	24 [29]	1.3-3+
Baker et al.[87]	MRM			39 [31]	5
	RM			9 [36]	5
Maddox et al.[155]	MRM			20 [20]	3-5
	RM			6 [16]	

RM, radical mastectomy; MRM, modified radical mastectomy; [ ], total no. pts.

positive axillary nodes and estrogen receptor–negative tumors to be at high risk for a local-regional recurrence despite adjuvant Adriamycin and cyclophosphamide chemotherapy. The risk of a local-regional recurrence was 23% at 20 months in patients with ER-negative tumors and one to three positive nodes and it was 31% for patients with ER-negative tumors and four or more positive nodes. Rosenman et al.[174] reported that initial progesterone receptor status predicted for local-regional recurrence in node-positive patients. The incidence of local-regional recurrence was 28% in progesterone negative patients vs. 0 in progesterone receptor–positive patients ($p = .017$).

Pathologic factors. The most important pathologic predictor for local-regional recurrence following mastectomy for operable breast cancer is the histologic status of the axillary nodes (Table 15-11). The risk for a local-regional recurrence is greater for node-positive patients and increases as the number of positive nodes increases. Haagensen[132] reported a 40% risk of local-regional recurrence when eight or more nodes were involved at the time of radical mastectomy. Tumor type and differentiation also may influence the risk of a local-regional recurrence. Lewis and Rienhoff[152] reported that patients with scirrhous carcinomas have a higher risk of recurrence than those with medullary or adenocarcinomas (i.e., 34% vs. 23.5% and 28.5%, respectively). Donegan et al.[111] reported a direct correlation with increasing tumor grade and the risk of a local recurrence. The risk was 0 and 11.1% for grade I and grade II tumors vs. 18.2% and 34% for grade III and grade IV tumors. Patients with negative axillary nodes and grade III tumors have a risk of local-regional recurrence that approaches 20% and appears higher than those with grade I tumors for whom the risk is <10%.[139,195]

The correlation between the status of the margin of resection and local-regional recurrence is controversial. Ahlborn et al.[83] reported a slightly higher incidence of local-regional recurrence (5.7%) in patients with a close margin (i.e., ≤4

Table 15-11 Incidence of local-regional recurrence following radical mastectomy (RM) or modified radical mastectomy (MRM) related to the axillary nodal status

		Local-regional recurrence (%)				
			Positive nodes			
Author	Surgery	Negative nodes	All	1-3	≥4	Follow-up (yr)
Haagensen[132]	RM	3	—	4	22	10-37
Donegan et al.[112]	RM	6	27	12	38	5
Fisher et al.[120]	RM	8	24	24	31	5
Valagussa et al.[191]	RM/MRM	8	27	—	—	10
Rosenman et al.[174]	RM/MRM	4	—	17	22	2-14
Lee[151]	RM/MRM	6	—	11	37	4.4 median
Dao and Nemoto[106]	RM	0	16	—	—	1.3-3+
Deck and Kern[107]	RM/MRM	4	11	—	—	3+

mm who underwent modified radical mastectomy for T_1 or T_2 tumors with histologically negative axillary nodes and received no adjuvant therapy). The incidence of local-regional recurrence was 3.4% for those whose margins were >4 mm. Twenty-seven percent of the 322 patients had a close deep margin. Mentzer et al.[162] were unable to correlate the incidence of local-regional recurrence with margin status in 100 patients with stage II breast cancer who underwent mastectomy. Fifty-nine percent had positive axillary nodes. The deep margin, however, was measured grossly in 67% of patients and only 39 patients had microscopic assessment. In patients who received no postoperative radiotherapy, none of 4 with a positive margin had a local-regional recurrence, and 3 of 25 patients with a margin of ≤2 mm had a local-regional recurrence. Five of 45 patients with a margin ≤5 mm had a local-regional recurrence, compared to 1 of 33 with a margin >5 mm. Overall, 35% of patients had ≤2 mm margins of resection. Therefore patients with close margins but with an intact pectoral fascia have a somewhat higher, but not significantly increased, risk of local-regional recurrence. Pectoral fascia involvement has been associated with a 28% to 29% risk of local-regional recurrence.[112,125]

Treatment-related factors. The extent of the surgical procedure may impact on the incidence of local-regional recurrence. There is some evidence that radical mastectomy is associated with a decreased risk of local-regional recurrence when compared to modified radical mastectomy (Table 15-12). Baker et al.[87] and Maddox et al.[155] reported a decreased risk of local-regional recurrence for patients with T_3 tumors with radical mastectomy (see Table 15-10). Of the two prospective randomized trials comparing modified radical mastectomy with radical mastectomy, Maddox et al.[156] reported a statistically significant decrease in rates of local-regional recurrence in the radical mastectomy group (11% vs 6%, p = .04) at 10 years. However, in the second trial[190] no significant difference in the risk of a local-regional recurrence was associated with radical mastectomy. In a retrospective intrainstitutional comparison of the two surgical procedures, Rosenman et al.[174] reported that the 7-year actuarial risk of local-regional recurrence for patients undergoing radical mastectomy was 23%, compared to 28% for those undergoing modified radical mastectomy. Donegan[111] and Williams et al.[194] also reported no significant increase in the incidence of local-regional recurrence with the modified radical mastectomy. The technical aspects of surgery such as the size and thickness of the skin flap and the margin around the primary tumor do not appear to be important factors influencing local-regional recurrence.[106-108,112,162,168,197] The type of wound closure also does not appear to influence local-regional recurrence rates when comparing skin grafts versus primary closure.[112]

The risk of an axillary recurrence is related to the extent of the axillary surgery. In the clinically negative undissected axilla, the incidence of axillary recurrence ranges from 17% to 37% with the majority of the recurrences occurring within two years.[88,103,106,119,124,148] Clinically positive nodes in an undissected axilla will progress in 48% of patients within 2 years.[88] The risk of an axillary recurrence also has been correlated with the number of axillary nodes removed. Fisher et al.[121] reported axillary failure in 21% of patients with no nodes

Table 15-12 Local-regional recurrence following mastectomy related to surgical procedure

Author	Local-regional recurrence (%)			Follow-up
	RM		MRM	(yr)
Prospective randomized trials				
Turner et al.[190]	25	[.4]	21	5
Maddox et al.[156]	6	[.04]	11	10
Retrospective comparisons				
Williams et al.[194]	33		20	10
Baker et al.[87]				
Stage I	9	[>.05]	13	5
Stage II	10	[>.05]	9	
Stage III	8	[.009]	39	
Donegan[111]	14	[.64]	20	12
Rosenman et al.[174]	23	[>.05]	28	7

RM, radical mastectomy; MRM, modified radical mastectomy.
[ ], p values for comparison (adjacent columns).

removed, 11% with five or fewer nodes, 5% with six to 10 nodes, and <1% for more than 10 nodes. Graverson et al.[129] reported a 5-year probability of axillary recurrence of 10% in patients with 1 to 2 negative nodes vs. 5% with 3 to 4 negative nodes, and 3% for the removal of 5 to 10 negative nodes. Fowble et al.[125] correlated the number of axillary nodes removed and examined with the risk of an isolated local-regional recurrence in patients receiving adjuvant systemic chemotherapy. At 3 years, 15% of patients with 10 or fewer nodes examined had a local-regional recurrence, compared to 10% for those with more than 10 nodes.

The impact of adjuvant systemic chemotherapy on the risk of a local-regional recurrence following mastectomy is variable and is discussed in detail in Chapter 11. Four prospective randomized trials have failed to demonstrate a significant decrease in the rate of local-regional recurrence with the addition of chemotherapy to surgery alone.[95,125,147,176] In four additional prospective randomized trials, the addition of postmastectomy chemotherapy resulted in a decreased risk of local-regional recurrence.[118,127,140,141] Table 15-13 presents the incidence of local-regional recurrence in node-positive patients receiving postmastectomy adjuvant chemotherapy. Overall the risk for patients with four or more positive nodes or T_3 tumors does not appear dissimilar from that reported for surgery alone.

The impact of tamoxifen administration on local-regional recurrence following mastectomy requires further investigation. Several studies have suggested that the primary effect of tamoxifen is to decrease the incidence of local-regional recurrence, with less of an effect on distant metastases. In the Stockholm trial,[177] 1470 postmenopausal women were randomized to tamoxifen and CMF cyclophosphamide, methotrexate, 5-fluorouracil (CMF), tamoxifen and radiation, radiation alone, or CMF alone if they were classified as high risk (primary tumor size >3 cm or positive axillary nodes) or tamoxifen vs. observation if they were classified as low risk (negative axillary nodes, primary tumor size ≤3 cm). Tamoxifen resulted in a significant decrease in local-regional recurrence for all patients (13% vs. 8%, $p<.01$), but no significant decrease in the incidence of distant metastasis in all patients. There was no significant improvement in overall survival rates with tamoxifen; however, there was an improved relapse-free survival rate. In the Nolvadex adjuvant trial,[167] 1285 patients were randomized to tamoxifen for 2 years or observation following mastectomy. With a median follow-up of 45 months, tamoxifen resulted in a significant decrease in the death rate and prolongation of the disease-free interval. However, the reduction in recurrences was greater for local-regional recurrence or new primary tumors as opposed to distant metastases. A similar finding was noted in the Scottish trial[96] in which 1312 postmenopausal node-positive patients and all node-negative patients were randomized to tamoxifen for 5 years vs. observation. Tamoxifen resulted in a significant improvement in relapse-free survival and overall

Table 15-13 Incidence of local-regional recurrence in node-positive patients receiving adjuvant chemotherapy following mastectomy

		Local-regional recurrence (%)				
Author	**Chemotherapy**	**All pts.**	**1-3 positive nodes**	**≥4 positive nodes**	**T_3**	**Follow-up (yr)**
Bonadonna et al.[95]	CMF	9	5	14† [21]	—	8
Stefanik et al.[185]	CMF	19	9	36	27	5
Tormey et al.[188]	CMF	—	—	18	—	2.8 median
	CMFVP	—	—	10	—	
Fowble et al.[125]	CMF (PT)	11	7	15	19	3
Rao et al.[173]	CMF	18	6	24	31	5.2 median
	PFT					
Lee[151]	CMF, L-PAM	20	9	27	—	4.4 median
Goldhirsch and Gelber[127]*	CMFP	11	8	15	—	4 median
Griem et al.[130]	CMF/MF	14	5	—	—	4.4 median
	CA			20	—	
Sykes et al.[186]	AC	—	10	10	28	2.9
Buzdar et al.[97]	FAC	12	7	14† [21]	18	5

[ ], >10 positive nodes.
*Premenopausal pts. only.
†4-10 positive nodes.

survival rates; however, again the reduction in local-regional recurrence was greater than that for distant metastases. In the Ludwig studies III and IV,[127] postmenopausal women were randomized to observation vs. prednisone and tamoxifen. With a 4-year median follow-up, the incidence of local-regional recurrence decreased from 27% to 13%, but that of distant metastases decreased from 27% to 24%. Tamoxifen resulted in an improvement in disease-free survival but not overall survival rates. Therefore tamoxifen may decrease the risk of a local-regional recurrence following mastectomy, although its impact in high-risk patients (i.e., those with T_3 primary tumors or four or more positive nodes) is unknown. A detailed discussion of the role of tamoxifen in the prevention of local-regional recurrence following mastectomy is presented in Chapter 11.

Clinical presentation and site(s) of involvement

Sites of involvement for local-regional recurrence following mastectomy are presented in Table 15-14. The chest wall is the most common site of failure either as a single site or as a component of multiple-site failure. The second most common site is the supraclavicular node region, followed by the axilla. Internal mammary node recurrences are infrequent. The majority of recurrences involve a single site. Multiple sites are involved in 8% to 29% of patients.

For the most part, chest wall recurrences present as a single asymptomatic nodule in or around the mastectomy scar.[126] Pawlias et al.[171] noted the greatest number of recurrences to be medial to the scar. Damaree[108] reported similar results. Haagensen[131] noted that the majority of recurrences were in the grafted sites. Donegan[111] reported that 42% of recurrences involved the scar. An erythematous rash may be the only sign of recurrence. Carcinoma en cuirasse is an unusual presentation of advanced local recurrence. The entity was initially described by Velpeau in 1838.[136] The clinical presentation includes swelling, redness, pruritus, and brawny induration of the chest wall.[136] The changes may extend across the midline or inferiorly to involve the abdominal skin.

At the time of a local-regional recurrence, approximately 30% of patients will have antecedent distant metastasis[90,92,117,159] and 25% will develop distant metastasis within several months of the diagnosis of a local-regional recurrence.[126,159] Therefore only half of the patients who develop a local-regional recurrence will have no evidence of distant metastases.

Interval to recurrence

The majority of local-regional recurrences present within 2 years of surgery, and by 5 years 80% to 90% have become manifest.[108,110,111,168,171,182,183,197] The peak incidence is seen in the second year.[111] However, late recurrences have been reported, with the longest interval occurring at 50 years.[104] Montague[164] reported that 34% of local-regional recurrences following mastectomy occurred after 5 years, with 10% occurring after 10 years.

The interval to the development of a local-regional recurrence is influenced by the initial tumor stage, the type of surgery, the histologic axillary nodal status, and the histologic grade. Shorter intervals are reported for increasing clinical stage.[85,126,131,187,189] For clinical stage I, the mean interval to local-regional recurrence following mastectomy has been reported to be 6 to 7 years, compared to 2 years for clinical stage III disease.[89,126] A shorter interval to recurrence also has been reported for histologically node-positive patients[191] and for patients undergoing modified

Table 15-14 Site of involvement of local-regional recurrence

		Single sites (%)				Multiple sites (%)		
Author	No. pts	Chest wall	Axilla	Supraclavicular node	Internal mammary node	Chest wall + nodes	Regional nodes	Other
Chu et al.[101]	215	49	5.5	13	2	24	4	<1
Chen et al.[100]	194	55	7	12	10			16
Halverson et al.[135]	224	60	7.5	13	6	10	4	<1
Bedwinek et al.[90]	129	46	8	19	8	12	4	
Toonkel et al.[187]	124	63	12	0	5	10	4	2
University of Pennsylvania	28	67	4	8	3	17		3
Aberizk et al.[82]	90	50						
Andry et al.[85]	128	65	6	25	4	8		
Deutsch et al.[109]	107	44	7	17	10	11	<2	3
Danoff et al.[105]	72	69	3	0	3	22		1

radical mastectomy when compared to those undergoing radical mastectomy.[155,170] However, Turner et al.[190] found no difference in time to recurrence in a randomized trial comparing radical mastectomy patients to modified radical mastectomy patients. Increasing histologic grade also has been associated with a shorter interval to recurrence.[85]

Treatment of local-regional recurrence following mastectomy

Surgery. A biopsy is indicated to confirm the diagnosis of a local-regional recurrence and allows for the determination of the receptor status of the recurrence. The receptor status for the recurrence is concordant with that of the original primary tumor in only 80% of patients.[84,99] For patients with extensive lesions, an incisional biopsy is adequate to establish the diagnosis. For patients with nodal or chest wall recurrences that can be excised, excisional biopsy is preferred. Excisional biopsy before irradiation reduces the tumor burden and in some series has resulted in an improvement in local control. Aberizk et al.[82] reported a 57% local control rate at 5 years in patients who had undergone total gross excision, compared to 24% without prior excision. Stadler and Kogelnik[184] also reported improved local control with the use of excisional biopsy as well as an improvement in overall survival rates. Beck et al.[89] reported a 5-year survival rate of 63% for recurrences that were excised vs. 24% for those that were not. It is difficult to determine whether excision alone is responsible for the improved survival in these series, because the extent of the disease is related to its resectability as well as the overall prognosis. However, the use of an excisional biopsy before irradiation has resulted in improved local control and permits the use of lower doses of radiation.[82]

Excision alone as the sole treatment for local-regional recurrence has resulted in subsequent local failure in 57% to 76% of patients (Table 15-15). Although it has been suggested that excision alone may be appropriate in patients with a long disease-free interval,[137] there are no data to suggest that these patients have long-term control with this treatment. Excision alone does not appear to represent optimal treatment for a local-regional recurrence.

Radical resections of the chest wall have been employed for selected patients. The resection may include the full thickness of the chest wall, skin, subcutaneous tissue, and muscle as well as the bony chest wall, including ribs and sternum. The deep margin of resection may extend to the parietal pleura. The resultant defect may be closed with vicryl or similar materials or a myocutaneous flap. Candidates for radical surgical resections include patients with persistent disease or recurrence after aggressive radiation, and those with a long disease-free interval and no evidence of distant metastases. Symptomatic chest wall recurrences have been resected in patients with limited distant metastases (i.e., those whose life expectancy is >1 year and those who do not have evidence of brain, bone marrow, or extensive bulky visceral disease). Results of radical surgical resection are presented in Table 15-16. Local control ranges from 60% to 88% with major complications ranging from 0 to 33%. Five-year survival rates range from 31%[181] to 50%[197] depending on patient selection.

Radiotherapy. Radiotherapy has been the primary treatment for local-regional recurrence following mastectomy. The results achieved have been variable and often reflect a heterogeneous group of patients as well as significant variations in the region(s) treated, use of prior surgical resection, and total radiation dose.

The optimal radiotherapy technique for a post-mastectomy local-regional recurrence has not been defined. For chest wall recurrences confined to the chest wall, the use of small fields results in significant failure rates of 18% to 43%.[91,100,142,157,184] Treatment of the entire chest wall with elective treatment of the draining nodal areas has resulted in improved local control,[90,101,135,157,170,184,187] with the majority of studies demonstrating an improved 5-year survival rate.[135,170,187] Omission of the chest wall for regional node failures results in a subsequent recurrence rate in the chest wall of 30% to 43%.[124,133] The available data would therefore suggest that for a chest wall or nodal failure the entire

Table 15-15 Local failure rates after excision alone

Author	Treatment period	No. pts.	Local failure after excision alone (%)
Tough[189]	1944-1977	15	57
Donegan et al.[112]	1948-1958	15	73
Bedwinek et al.[90]	1964-1977	25	76
Andry et al.[85]	1969-1979	35	57
Beck et al.[89]	1970-1974	11	73

Table 15-16 Chest wall resections

Author	Treatment period	No. pts.	Mean disease-free interval* (yr)	Local control (%)	Major complications (%)	Operative mortality (%)	Survival (%)	Follow-up (yr)
Shah and Urban[181]	1950-1972	47	5.2	†			31	5
Nieminin et al.[166]	1972-1975	26	3.4	62	0	0	77	2
Zoetmulder and van Dongen[197]	1974-1986	30	9.5‡	93	33	0	50	5
McKenna et al.[161]	1977-1982	32	6.7	88	12.5	5	9	3.3
Larson et al.[150]	1979-1981	10				10	—	—

*From initial treatment to chest wall resection.
†No evidence of disease in 30% at 5 years.
‡Median.

chest wall should be treated as well as the appropriate lymphatics. Elective treatment of the axilla is probably not indicated as recurrence rates in this region without axillary radiation have been ≤6%.[90,135] Elective irradiation of the axilla also results in an increased incidence of arm edema.[135] Similarly, elective irradiation of the internal mammary nodes probably is not indicated because subsequent failure rates in this site are ≤4%.[90,135] Omission of elective treatment of the supraclavicular region has resulted in supraclavicular failure rates of 16%[90] and 28%.[135] Therefore, for patients with a chest wall failure, elective irradiation of the supraclavicular region is indicated, and for patients with a regional node failure elective irradiation of the chest wall is indicated.

The recommended dose of radiation is dependent on the volume of the disease and the extent of prior surgery. For electively treated sites, a dose of 4500 cGy results in 90% control.[122] Table 15-17 presents local control related to the presence or absence of gross residual disease and radiation dose. For patients who have undergone complete excision of their recurrent disease, doses in the range of 4500 to 5000 cGy result in 90% control. A boost dose of an additional 1000 to 1500 cGy may be considered in patients who have positive margins of resection or unknown margins. The presence of gross residual disease requires higher doses.

Local control is related to the size of the gross residual tumor. For tumors in the range of 1 to 3 cm, Halverson et al.[135] reported that 15 of 15 patients were controlled with doses >6000 cGy and 16 of 21 patients were controlled with doses <6000 cGy. The recommended dose for lesions measuring 1 to 3 cm, therefore, is a minimum of 6000

Table 15-17 Local-regional control related to extent of surgery and radiation dose

Dose	Author	Local-regional control (%)	
		Complete excision	Gross residual tumor
≤4000 cGy	Patanaphan et al.[170]	—	48
	Magno et al.[157]	50	—
	Bedwinek et al.[90]	50	27
	Chu et al.[101]	—	48
≥4000 cGy	Patanaphan et al.[170]	—	70
	Aberizk et al.[82]	57	24
4000 to 5000 cGy	Bedwinek et al.[90]	96	61
	Halverson et al.[135]	88	47
5000 to 6000 cGy	Bedwinek et al.[90]	100	80
	Halverson et al.[135]	96	70
	Chu et al.[101]	—	77
	Chen et al.[100]	—	73
	University of Pennsylvania	78	—
>6000 cGy	Halverson et al.[135]	83	71
	Bedwinek et al.[90]	—	67
	University of Pennsylvania	—	62

Table 15-18 Local control related to radiation technique

Author	Treatment period	No. pts.	Local control (%)	
			Adequate radiation*	Inadequate radiation†
Chu et al.[101]	1950s-1960s	215	77	48
Chen et al.[100]	1956-1981	194	66	
Patanaphan et al.[170]	1963-1977	133	70	48
Bedwinek et al.[90]	1964-1977	157	72	28
Toonkel et al.[187]	1966-1978	121	71	50
Stadler and Kogelnik[184]	1970-1978	149	50	33
Magno et al.[157]	1973-1979	162	50	32

*Adequate radiation: large fields, at least 5500 cGy to site(s) of gross disease.
†Inadequate radiation: small volumes or ≤5000 cGy for gross disease.

cGy.[90,135] For patients with larger recurrences, doses in the range of 6000 to 7000 cGy result in 50% control.[135] Local control does not appear to increase with doses in excess of 7000 cGy. Local control rates are lower for recurrences that involve both the chest wall and regional nodes. Halverson et al.[135] reported local control in 41% of patients with a chest wall and nodal recurrence and Aberizk et al.[82] reported local control in 10% of patients with chest wall and nodal involvement. For patients presenting with regional node recurrences, excision should be considered before radiation. Regional control is improved with the use of excision before radiotherapy. Halverson et al.[135] reported regional node control in 82% of patients who underwent excision before radiation, compared to 66% for those who had gross residual tumor. Fletcher and Montague[123] reported that doses of 5000 cGy followed by a boost of 1000 to 2000 cGy controlled 87% of patients with palpable axillary disease and 98% of those with supraclavicular adenopathy. However, complications related to treatment were reported in 26% of patients. These included arm edema and brachial plexopathy. Therefore, while doses of 6000 to 8000 cGy result in control in approximately two-thirds of nodal recurrences, the complications from treatment are considerable. Excision before radiation results in an improved regional control and allows for the use of lower doses of radiation that are associated with a lower risk of complications. Local control related to radiation technique is presented in Table 15-18. Adequate radiation is defined as treatment to the entire chest wall and elective irradiation of the regional node sites with a minimum dose of 5500 cGy to site(s) of gross disease. Inadequate irradiation is defined as the use of small volumes or doses ≤5000 cGy for gross disease. Local control is clearly improved with the use of adequate radiotherapy techniques. Adequate radiation also has resulted in an improved survival rate in the majority of series (Table 15-19).

Complete response rates to radiation therapy as well as the rates of ultimate local-regional failure are presented in Tables 15-20 and 15-21. Complete response rates range from 63% to 97%. Despite these relatively high complete response rates, recurrences after radiation are common, ranging from 40% to 47%.[82,105,109,157] As previously noted, the local-regional control achieved with radiation is influenced by the extent of the disease, prior surgical resection, and the dose employed. Local-regional control rates range from 40% to 69%[82,90,184] in patients who have had an excisional biopsy followed by radiation; these rates are similar to those achieved in patients with gross residual disease who achieve a complete response with radiation.

Several authors have emphasized the importance of computerized tomography (CT) scans before the initiation of radiation for local-regional recurrence to determine the extent of the disease.[153,163,165,175,196] A thoracic CT scan may identify previously unsuspected disease in patients with large-volume disease or a parasternal recurrence. Table 15-22 presents the incidence of unsuspected disease in

Table 15-19 Survival related to radiation technique

Author	5-yr survival (%)	
	Chest wall and regional node irradiation	Chest wall irradiation
Patanaphan et al.[170]	42	35
Toonkel et al.[187]	54	27
Halverson et al.[135]	53	35
Deutsch et al.[109]	36	54

Table 15-20 Initial complete response rates after radiotherapy

Author	Treatment period	No. pts.	Initial complete response (%)
Donegan et al.[112]	1940-1958	24	79
Jackson[142]	1949-1955	81	60
Chu et al.[101]	1950s	215	67
Chen et al.[100]	1956-1981	194	64
Patanaphan et al.[170]	1963-1977	133	44
Bedwinek et al.[90]	1964-1977	157	70
Toonkel et al.[187]	1966-1978	121	66
University of Pennsylvania	1967-1988	128	74
Aberizk et al.[82]*	1968-1978	90	97
Beck et al.[89]	1970-1979	121	63
Deutsch et al.[109]	1970-1979	107	78
Stadler and Kogelnik[184]	1970-1978	149	69
Danoff et al.[105]	1972-1980	72	71
Janjan et al.[144]	1972-1983	57	40
Magno et al.[157]*	1973-1979	162	73

*Includes excised patients.

Table 15-21 Local failure rates after radiotherapy

			Subsequent local-regional failure (%)	
Author	Treatment period	No. pts.	All pts.	Pts. with complete tumor response or no gross residual
Jackson[142]	1949-1955	81	40	
Chu et al.[101]	1950s	215	33	
Chen et al.[100]	1956-1981	194	36	
Halverson et al.[135]	1964-1986	224	43	
Bedwinek et al.[90]	1964-1977	157	61	
Toonkel et al.[187]	1966-1978	121	54	
Janjan et al.[144]	1972-1983	57	35	
University of Pennsylvania	1967-1988	128	59	57
Aberizk et al.[82]	1968-1978	90	58	45
Deutsch et al.[109]	1970-1979	107	59	47
Danoff et al.[105]	1972-1980	72	46	40
Magno et al.[157]	1973-1979	162	50	43

Table 15-22 Impact of CT scans in patients with local-regional recurrence

Author	No. pts.	Unsuspected local-regional recurrence (%)	Unsuspected distant metastases (%)	Change in treatment (%)
Rosenman et al.[174]	33	37 [9]*	39 [13]	30 [10]
Lindfors et al.[153]	42	50 [21]†	24 [10]	70
Zeinreich et al.[196]	25			64
Meyer and Munzenrider[163]	18	72 [13]‡		39
Vilari et al.[193]	19	42	26	

[ ], no. pts.
*5 ipsilateral axilla, 4 internal mammary.
†12 internal mammary.
‡All had CT evidence of IM involvement; 5 were evident on routine chest x-ray.

patients with local-regional recurrences undergoing CT scans. This includes both unsuspected local-regional disease as well as unsuspected distant metastases. A change in the radiotherapy treatment plan occurred in 30% to 70% of patients based on these findings. Therefore CT scans may improve radiotherapy treatment planning, and the identification of unsuspected sites of distant metastases may alter treatment recommendations significantly.

Chemotherapy. The role of chemotherapy in the treatment of local-regional recurrence following mastectomy remains to be determined. Its potential use is related to the fact that the majority of patients with an isolated local-regional recurrence ultimately develop distant metastases.[82,91,135,182,184] Table 15-23 presents the results of chemotherapy and/or radiation in the treatment of local-regional recurrences following mastectomy. Local control rates with chemotherapy alone range from 29% to 46%. Janjan et al.[143] reported the results of 50 patients receiving chemotherapy alone for local-regional recurrences. Treatment consisted of 8 to 10 cycles of 5-fluorouracil, Adriamycin, and cyclophosphamide. The local-regional recurrence rate was 54% for patients treated with chemotherapy alone vs. 35% with radiation therapy alone. The differences were statistically significant. The Southwest Oncology Group (SWOG) reported a 34% complete response rate employing Adriamycin-based chemotherapy without radiation for local disease.[138] Beck et al.[89] reported improvement in local control at 3 years in a group of patients who received radiation alone when compared to a group of patients who received either chemotherapy alone or hormonal treatment alone. Therefore chemotherapy alone results in a lower incidence of local-regional control when compared to radiation with or without chemotherapy. The combination of chemotherapy and radiotherapy, however, appears to improve local-regional control rates. Olson et al.[169] reported the results of a randomized trial of radiation and actinomycin D vs. radiation alone. The rate of local control was 80% in the chemotherapy/radiation group (15 patients), compared to 59% in the radiation alone group (17 patients). The differences were statistically significant. A larger retrospective series by the same authors noted similar results.[169] Janjan et al.[143,144] reported a local control rate of 65% for radiation alone vs. 67% for patients treated with chemotherapy and radiation. Bedwinek et al.[90] found no difference in local-regional control rates for patients treated with combined radiation and chemotherapy vs. radiation alone.

The impact of systemic therapy on survival in patients with an isolated local-regional recurrence following mastectomy requires further investigation. There are no prospective randomized trials that have evaluated the effects of the combination of chemotherapy and radiation. The results from retrospective reviews have been variable. Janjan et al.[144] reported the results of treatment for 164 patients with isolated local-regional recurrence at M.D. Anderson Hospital. Patients were treated with radiation alone, chemotherapy alone consisting of 5-fluorouracil, Adriamycin, and Cytoxan, or a combination or chemotherapy and radiation. The overall 5-year survival rate was 45% for the combined modality group, compared to 47% for the radiation alone group, with disease-free survival rates of 33% and 22%, respectively. The differences were not statistically significant.

Table 15-23 Local-regional control and survival rates with chemotherapy and/or radiation

		Local-regional control (%)			5-year survival (%)		
Author	No. pts.	Chemotherapy	Radiation	Chemotherapy and radiation	Chemotherapy	Radiation	Chemotherapy and radiation
Olson et al.[169]	124	—	60	79	(16 mo; median)	(18 mo; median)	
Janjan et al.[143,144]	107	46	65	67	60	47	45
			[.049]				
Beck et al.[89]*	110	14	37	—	—	18	38
		[≤.05]				[≤.05]	
Bedwinek et al.[90]	31	29	79	70	—	—	—
Toonkel et al.[187]*	121	—	—	—	—	35	38
Deutsch et al.[109]	107	—	—	—	—	32	38
University of Pennsylvania	128	—	35	57	—	47	54
			[.23]			[.57]	

[ ], p value for comparison (adjacent columns).
*Includes hormonal therapy.

Local-regional control, however, was statistically improved in the combined modality group. Beck et al.[89] compared the results of treatment of a local-regional recurrence following mastectomy with biopsy and radiation vs. biopsy and hormonal therapy or vs. biopsy and chemotherapy. The 5-year disease-free survival rate was 25% for the systemically treated group compared to 6% for the group that received radiation only. The overall 5-year survival rate was 38% for the chemotherapy group vs. 18% for the radiation alone group. Toonkel et al.[187] reported a 5-year survival rate of 35% for patients who received radiation for an isolated local-regional recurrence, compared to 38% for those who received radiation and adjuvant systemic therapy. Deutsch et al.[109] also reported a nonsignificant improvement in 5-year survival rates with the addition of systemic therapy (39% vs. 32%). Olson et al.[169] reported no significant differences in median survival for patients treated with radiation with or without actinomycin D. These series suggest some benefit to systemic therapy in terms of survival, although for the most part they are retrospective and variations in patient characteristics and tumor extent could account for the observed treatment differences.

Hormonal therapy. Data regarding the role of hormonal therapy alone in the treatment of local-regional recurrence following mastectomy is limited. Andry et al.[85] reported 15 patients receiving hormonal therapy for local-regional recurrences. Six local-regional recurrences appeared in nine patients who had prior complete excision. None of the five patients treated with hormonal therapy following an incisional biopsy experienced a complete response. As previously noted, Beck et al.[89] reported significantly improved local control in patients treated with radiation alone when compared to patients treated with systemic therapy (i.e., hormonal management in 30 patients, chemotherapy in 12). Bedwinek et al.[90] noted no difference in local-regional control rates in patients treated with hormonal therapy and radiation (62%) vs. radiation alone (79%). Seven of 11 patients treated with hormonal therapy alone had uncontrolled local-regional disease. Tamoxifen may play a role in the treatment of patients with local-regional recurrence who are estrogen receptor positive, although this should be combined with radiation.

Survival and prognostic factors

Survival results for the treatment of local-regional recurrence following mastectomy are presented in Table 15-24. The majority of series have employed radiation as the primary treatment. Five-year survival rates range from 10% to 50%, with 10- year survival rates of 5% to 26%. The 5-year ease-free survival rate is approximately 25%, with 10-year disease-free survival rates of 10% to 15%.

The prognosis of a patient with local-regional recurrence following mastectomy is related to several factors, including the disease-free interval, the initial nodal status, the initial tumor size, hormone

Table 15-24 Survival following treatment for a local-regional recurrence following mastectomy

			Survival (%)	
Author	Treatment period	No. pts.	5 yr	10 yr
Shimkin et al.[182]	1918-1947	98	10	
Gilliand et al.[126]	1944-1977	60	18	5
Fentiman et al.[117]	1948-1975	73	30	13
Jackson[142]	1949-1955	81	10	
Chu et al.[101]	1950-1960s	215	21	5
Di Pietro et al.[110]	1955-1965	120	28	
Halverson et al.[135]	1964-1986	224	43 [25]	26 [15]
Bedwinek et al.[91]	1964-1977	157	36	
Toonkel et al.[187]	1966-1978	121	38 [26]	26 [15]
University of Pennsylvania	1967-1988	128	49	23
Aberizk et al.[82]	1968-1978	90	50	26 [7]
Karabali-Dalomaga et al.[146]	1968-1976	150	26	
Beck et al.[89]	1970-1979	121	37 [21]	23 [12]
Deutsch et al.[109]	1970-1979	107	35	
Stadler and Kogelnik[184]	1970-1978	149	22	
Danoff et al.[105]	1972-1980	72	50	
Magno et al.[157]	1973-1979	162	34	

[ ], disease-free survival.

Table 15-25 Five-year survival rates related to disease-free interval

Author	Treatment period	No. pts.	5-yr survival (%) Disease-free interval <24 mo	Disease-free interval >24 mo	p value
Di Pietro et al.[110]	1955-1965	120	10	70	<.001
Patanaphan et al.[170]	1963-1977	133	25	57	NS
Bedwinek et al.[91]	1964-1977	157	17	56	.0001
University of Pennsylvania	1967-1988	128	30	67	.0027
Aberizk et al.[82]	1968-1978	90	33	58	.04
Andry et al.[85]*	1969-1979	86	13	37	<.001
Deutsch et al.[109]†	1970-1979	107	29	57	NS
Danoff et al.[105]	1972-1980	72	39	63	.02
Magno et al.[157]	1973-1979	162	20	50	

NS, not stated.
*<12 mo vs. >12 mo.
†<5 mo vs. >5 yr.

receptor status, the size of recurrence, the number of sites involved, and the use of surgery and adequate radiation. The most important factors appear to be the disease-free interval between primary treatment and the recurrence, the initial disease extent as reflected in the initial tumor size and histologic nodal status, and the extent of the recurrence. Survival related to the disease-free interval is presented in Table 15-25. Patients whose recurrence is manifest within 2 years of initial treatment have a decreased 5-year survival rate that in the majority of series is statistically significant. Survival also has been correlated with the initial tumor stage. Shimkin et al.[182] reported the median survival rate after local recurrence to be 38% for stage I disease, 22% for stage II, and 9% for stage III. Disease-free interval and stage appear to be interrelated in that patients with stage I or stage II disease have a longer disease-free interval than those with stage III disease.[89,126,129] Survival rates related to the initial pathologic nodal status are presented in Table 15-26. The 5-year survival rate for node-negative patients ranges from 45% to 64% vs. 30% to 42% for node-positive patients. The extent of nodal involvement also correlates with prognosis.[90,157]

Survival is also influenced by the extent of recurrent disease. A single nodule on the chest wall is associated with a 5-year survival rate of 40% to 60% compared to a 5-year survival rate ranging from 10% to 26% for multiple nodules.[91,117,144,157,184] The size of the largest recurrence is also a predictor for survival. Bedwinek et al.[91] noted a 5-year survival rate of 51% for a recurrence ≤1 cm vs. 18% for those of 1 to 3 cm. Magno et al.[157] noted a significantly improved survival rate when comparing patients with lesions ≤1 vs. those with lesions >1 cm. The involvement of multiple sites is associated with decreased survival rates. Halverson et al.[135] noted a superior 5-year survival rate for patients with a chest wall recurrence as compared to those with a chest wall and nodal recurrence. Deutsch et al.[109] reported a 5-year survival rate of 25% for patients with involvement of the chest wall and regional nodes, compared to 37% when a single site was involved. Patients with nodal failures have been reported to have a diminished rate of 5-year survival when

Table 15-26 Five-year survival rates after recurrence related to initial nodal status

Author	Treatment period	No. pts.	5-yr survival (%) Node-negative pts.	Node-positive pts.	Pts. with 1-3 nodes	Pts. with ≥4 nodes
Di Pietro et al.[110]	1955-1965	120	64	42		
Chen et al.[100]	1956-1981	194	[48]	—	[29]	[11]
Andry et al.[85]	1969-1979	86	53	—	28	
Beck et al.[89]	1970-1979	121	59	34		
Magno et al.[157]	1973-1979	162	45	30	42	18

[ ], 5-year disease-free survival.

Table 15-27 Survival rates related to controlled vs. uncontrolled local-regional disease

Author	Treatment period	No. pts.	5-yr survival (%)	
			Controlled	Uncontrolled
Chu et al.[101]	1950-1960	215	26	7
Chen et al.[100]	1956-1981	194	63	34
Halverson et al.[134]	1964-1986	224	63	22
University of Pennsylvania	1967-1988	128	64	35
Stadler and Kogelnik[184]	1970-1978	149	45	20
Danoff et al.[105]	1972-1980	80	62*	0*
Janjan et al.[144]	1972-1983	164	60	37
Magno et al.[157]	1973-1979	162	42	5

*3-yr survival.

compared to those with recurrences in the chest wall.[109,135,187] However, others have reported no such difference.[89,91,101,116] The initial histologic grade of the primary tumor may predict for survival after a local-regional recurrence. Fentiman et al.[116] reported patients with grade I lesions as having an improved survival rate when compared to those with grade III lesions (i.e., 44% vs. 0). Andry et al.[85] noted similar findings, patients with grade I lesions having a 2-year survival rate of 88% and those with grade III lesions having a 2-year survival rate of 54%. The use of adequate radiotherapy has resulted in an improvement in local-regional control, as demonstrated in Table 15-17, and in some series has resulted in an improvement in survival.[135,187] While the use of excisional biopsy before radiation has been associated with improved survival,[89,184] this finding may be related to the extent of the recurrence. Several series have suggested that patients who are locally controlled have a superior survival rate when compared to uncontrolled patients. Table 15-27 presents 5-year survival rates related to the status of local-regional disease. Controlled patients appear to have an improved rate of survival.

TREATMENT AFTER RADIATION THERAPY FAILURE

Treatment options for patients developing a local-regional recurrence after irradiation are limited. However, effective therapy may still be possible with surgery, reirradiation, or radiation combined with hyperthermia. For those patients with a small localized recurrence, wide excision alone may be considered with or without systemic therapy. Radical chest wall resections have been employed and were discussed previously.

The role of radiotherapy alone in treating previously irradiated patients for chest wall recurrence is not well established. Elkort et al.[115] described an aggressive approach of surgical debridement, skin grafting, and irradiation. The second course of radiation consisted of treatment to the area of the recurrence plus a margin. Total doses ranged from 4000 to 5000 cGy plus a boost of 1000 to 1500 cGy. Four to 6 meV electrons were employed. At death or at last follow-up, five of seven patients had a complete response to treatment and six of seven patients had stable or controlled disease. No complications were reported. Laramore et al.[149] reported on reirradiation with doses of 4000 to 5000 cGy with 7 meV electrons in patients previously treated with adjuvant radiation therapy. Local control was obtained in 8 of 13 patients. Systemic therapy also was employed. No soft tissue necroses were reported.

The role of low-dose reirradiation in combination with hyperthermia is currently under investigation. The complete response rates with hyperthermia and radiation for recurrent chest wall disease range from 35% to 74%.[93,128,154,172,178-180] The response rate is influenced by the size of the recurrent tumor.[128,172,178,179] Perez et al.[172] reported that patients with lesions ≤3 cm had a higher complete response rate than those with larger tumors. The adequacy of heat treatment and total dose of radiation also correlate with response rates.[114,128,178,179,192] Dragnovic et al.[113] reported 30 previously irradiated patients with recurrences who were treated with 6 to 9 meV electrons to a dose of 3200 cGy, utilizing 400-cGy fractions. Radiation was given twice weekly followed by hyperthermia treatment. The overall complete response rate was 57%, 81% for patients with lesions <5 cm and 29% for those >5 cm. Six of the 16 evaluated patients later developed either a true in-field or marginal recurrence, and two patients developed a nonhealing ulcer. The overall rate of ulceration was 11%. Seegenschmiedt et al.[180] reported on 13 patients treated for recurrence after previous radiotherapy. Complete response at 1 month was 48%. The complication rate was 41% and consisted of skin blisters and ulceration. Perez et al.[172] reported 48 patients treated with 9 to 16 meV electrons to total doses of 2000 to 4000 cGy, delivered in 400-cGy fractions twice weekly followed by hyperthermia treatment. Complete response was obtained in 12 of 15 patients whose tumors measured 1 to 3 cm. For patients with larger lesions the complete response rate was 65%. Ulceration developed in 25% of patients. Scott et al.[178] reported the results of a phase I-II Radiation Therapy/Oncology Group (RTOG) trial investigating definitive radiotherapy and hyperthermia in 133 patients with recurrent cancer. Thirty-three patients had recurrent breast cancer. Treatment consisted of conventional radiation therapy with total doses ranging from 6000 to 7000 cGy. Hyperthermia was delivered twice a week for a total of 12 sessions. Complete response was observed in 85% of the breast patients. Acute toxicity consisted of thermal blisters in 70% and late toxicity (i.e., after 6 months) occurred in 16% and consisted of ulceration or necrosis. These results have led to a randomized phase III trial with definitive radiation and hyperthermia in previously untreated patients. Hyperthermia plus radiation should be considered for the treatment of local-regional recurrence in symptomatic patients previously irradiated who are not candidates for surgical resection. For previously untreated patients, the superiority of hyperthermia plus radiation over radiation alone is unproven and is the subject of a prospective randomized trial.

Table 15-28 Characteristics of patients treated at the University of Pennsylvania for isolated local-regional recurrence of breast cancer

Total no. pts.	128
Age	
Median	57
Range	31-83
Menopausal status	
Premenopausal	30
Postmenopausal	83
Perimenopausal	9
Unknown	6
Initial T stage	
T_1	19
T_2	41
T_3	19
T_4	8
T_{is}	2
Unknown	39
No. of involved nodes	
0	54
1-3	24
4-7	19
>7	23
Unknown	8
Adjuvant systemic therapy	
Chemotherapy	51
Hormonal therapy	19
Disease-free interval	
Median	33 mo
Range	1-234 mo
Follow-up	
Median	33 mo
Range	1-164 mo

UNIVERSITY OF PENNSYLVANIA EXPERIENCE

Between 1967 and 1986, 128 patients with an isolated local-regional recurrence following mastectomy were treated with definitive radiation therapy. Table 15-28 illustrates the clinicopathologic characteristics of these patients and Table 15-29 presents the site(s) of involvement. Statistical comparisons between survival curves were performed using the Mantel-Cox test.[158] Survival and local-regional control rates were determined by the Kaplan-Meier method.[145]

Interval to recurrence

Factors that influenced the time to recurrence were the initial T stage, nodal status, and type of surgery. The median time interval to recurrence for patients with T_1 and T_2 tumors was 29 and 25 months,

Table 15-29 Distribution of local-regional failures

Site	No. pts.
Total	128
Single sites	
Chest wall only	86
Axilla only	5
Supraclavicular nodes only	11
Internal mammary nodes only	4
Infraclavicular nodes	2
Multiple sites	
Chest wall and axilla	9
Chest wall and supraclavicular nodes	9
Chest wall and infraclavicular nodes	1
Chest wall and infraclavicular and supraclavicular nodes	1

respectively, vs. 17 and 14 months for those patients with T_3 and T_4 lesions (p = .0054). When comparing node-negative patients to node-positive patients, no difference was evident. However, patients with ≤3 (including 0) nodes involved vs. those with ≥4 had a median time to recurrence of 24 and 16 months respectively (p = .016). Patients having radical mastectomy had a median time to recurrence of 33 months vs. 22 months for those undergoing modified radical mastectomy (p = .016).

Sites of recurrence

The recurrence was confined to a single site in 109 patients (85%). The chest wall was the most common location, in 84 patients. The second most common site was the supraclavicular fossa. As Table 15-29 demonstrates, there were multiple sites in 20 patients, all involving the chest wall. Fifty one percent of the patients with chest wall failures alone presented with a single nodule, and 62% of the recurrences involved the scar.

Treatment

Surgical treatment consisted of excision of all gross disease in 78 patients and incisional biopsy in 49 patients. One patient was treated without biopsy. Radiation therapy was directed to the entire chest wall in 19% of patients with isolated chest wall recurrences and to the chest wall and regional nodes in 81%. In 23 patients with isolated nodal recurrences, treatment was directed to the nodal site and chest wall in 87% and regional nodes in 13%. Patients with multiple sites of involvement received treatment to the chest wall and regional nodes in all cases.

Treatment to the chest wall or regional nodes consisted of 4600 to 5000 cGy in 4½ to 5 weeks with or without a boost to sites of gross disease. Eighty five percent of those with an excised chest wall failure received a boost dose of 500 to 2000 cGy for a median total dose of 6000 cGy. The median dose to gross disease in chest wall failures alone was 6100 cGy, the range being 2000 to 8000 cGy. Sixty-two percent of patients with excised nodal failures received a boost of 500 to 2000 cGy (median total dose 5000 cGy). Patients with gross disease in nodal sites only received a median dose of 5600 cGy (range 4000 to 6800). At the time of recurrence, 23 patients received chemotherapy (CMF or CAF), 35 received tamoxifen, and 8 patients received both chemotherapy and tamoxifen.

Local control

The 5-year actuarial rate of local-regional control was 43% for the entire group. In a univariate analysis, local control was significantly related to the extent of surgery for recurrence, menopausal status, initial nodal status, disease-free interval, and estrogen receptor status of the recurrence. Patients undergoing excision of gross disease had a local-regional control rate of 48% vs. 34% for those not excised (p < .003). The size of the recurrence was not a factor in local-regional control in patients who underwent total gross excision before radiation. The addition of chemotherapy in excised patients resulted in a 78% local-regional control rate, compared to 38% in patients not receiving chemotherapy. However, this observation did not reach statistical significance (p = .15).

For patients with gross disease, the initial complete response rate to radiation was 74%. The size of the recurrence and total dose influenced local control in this group of patients. When gross disease measured ≤4 cm and doses of ≥6000 cGy were delivered, the control rate was 57% vs. 15% for lower doses. For larger recurrences, no dose response was evident. The use of systemic therapy at the time of recurrence resulted in a local control rate of 57%, compared to 35% for those treated with radiation alone (p = .23).

In a multivariate analysis only the estrogen receptor status of the recurrence was significant as a predictor for local-regional control. This factor, however, proved to be a global indicator for patients who underwent excision of the recurrence, had an initial negative axillary nodal status, and a disease-free interval of >2 years.

Survival and prognostic factors

The 5-year actuarial survival rate following treatment for recurrence for all patients was 49%, with a relapse-free survival rate of 23%. In a univariate analysis the following factors correlated significantly with an improved overall rate of survival: initial nodal status of ≤3 positive nodes vs. ≥4, initial estrogen receptor positive, disease-free interval ≥24 months, recurrent tumor size ≤2 cm, estrogen receptor– and progesterone receptor–positive recurrence, excision of all gross disease, ultimate local-regional control, and the use of hormonal therapy in patients with gross disease. Patients with 0, 1 to 3, or ≥4 positive axillary nodes had a 5-year survival of 52%, 69%, and 29%, respectively (p = .03). Patients undergoing excision before radiation therapy had an overall survival rate at 5 years of 54% vs. 40% in patients not excised (p = .003). Patients achieving local control had a superior survival rate than uncontrolled patients, 64% vs. 34%, respectively. For all patients the administration of systemic therapy at the time of recurrence resulted in a 5-year survival rate of 54%, compared to 47% in those not systemically treated (p = .57). In patients undergoing gross excision, the addition of chemotherapy resulted in a 5-year survival rate of 72% vs. 48% in those who did not receive chemotherapy. The addition of hormonal therapy had no impact on survival rates in all patients or in those who underwent gross excision. However, in patients with gross disease the addition of hormonal therapy resulted in a 5-year survival rate of 73% vs. 25% for those who did not receive hormones ($p = .05$). Patients with initial estrogen receptor–positive primary tumors had a 5-year survival rate of 78% vs. 48% in patients with estrogen receptor–negative tumors ($p = .02$). The initial estrogen and progesterone receptors and the recurrent receptors were concordant in 69% and 74% of patients, respectively. A prognostic factor not reported previously was the recurrent tumor's estrogen and progesterone receptors. Patients whose recurrent tumors were estrogen receptor positive had a 5-year survival rate of 66% vs. 41% for estrogen receptor–negative patients ($p = .01$). Patients having positive progesterone receptors in the recurrent tumor had a better 5-year survival rate (88%) than progesterone receptor–negative patients (46%) ($p = .006$).

The disease-free interval was a strong predictor of a patient's survival after recurrence. Patients with a disease-free interval ≥24 months had a 5-year survival rate of 67% vs. 30% for those with a shorter interval ($p = .003$). Regional node and chest wall presentations had similar prognoses. The number, size, and location of recurrences on the chest were examined for their prognostic value. Patients with a single nodule on the chest wall had an overall 5-year survival rate of 77% vs. 44% for those with multiple nodules ($p = .021$). The size of the largest recurrence also predicted for survival; when the recurrent tumor measured ≤2 cm, the 5-year survival rate was 70% vs. 39% for those with larger recurrences ($p = .021$).

In a univariate analysis the following factors significantly correlated with relapse-free survival: initial nodal status, disease-free interval, hormone receptor status of the recurrence, excisional biopsy, ultimate local-regional control, and the use of hormones at the time of recurrence in patients with gross disease. The 5-year relapse-free survival rate was 53% for patients who underwent gross excision and received chemotherapy, compared to 19% for those who did not ($p = .30$). For all patients the 5-year relapse-free survival rate was 34% with chemotherapy, compared to 17% without ($p = .62$). Hormonal therapy significantly improved the 5-year relapse-free survival rate in patients with gross disease (28% vs. 4%, $p = .004$).

In an attempt to identify independent prognostic factors, the data were subjected to a multivariate analysis. For overall survival, the disease-free interval, use of excisional biopsy, and ultimate local-regional control remained significant. For relapse-free survival, the initial pathologic status of the axillary nodes, the disease-free interval, and the use of an excisional biopsy were significant. The subgroup of patients with a disease-free interval ≥24 months, excision of gross disease before radiation, and local-regional control, had a 5-year actuarial survival rate of 61% and a relapse-free survival rate of 59%. This group represented 18% of the entire population. Thus, although the prognosis for patients with a local-regional recurrence is generally poor, a subset with a reasonable prognosis exists. A nihilistic approach to all patients is not justified.

Summary

Approximately 30% of all first recurrences after mastectomy with or without adjuvant chemotherapy are local-regional only, with the chest wall being the most common site and the supraclavicular region the next most common. Axillary and internal mammary nodal recurrences are less common. If uncontrolled, such a recurrence can be the source of substantial morbidity. Recurrence is seen most commonly in the first 2 years after mastectomy, but late recurrences are seen up to 50 years after initial surgery.

The clinical and pathologic risk factors that predict for local-regional recurrence include the primary tumor size, the histologic status of the axillary lymph nodes, tumor grade, and receptor status. Treatment-related factors include the extent of surgery and the use of adjuvant chemotherapy or hormonal treatment.

The primary treatment of a local-regional recurrence is radiation therapy. The use of adequate radiation results in complete response rates of 40% to 79% and an overall local control rate of 50% to 77%. Local control is influenced by the volume of disease and the extent and total dose of radiation. Patients who have local control have improved survival. Systemic therapy commonly is employed because of the substantial risk of metastatic disease. Several retrospective studies have suggested that an improvement in disease-free and overall survival rates can be achieved when systemic therapy is combined with local treatment, but there are no randomized trials available to confirm this observation. The addition of chemotherapy to radiation has resulted in some improvement in local control rates. Radiation appears to be the most single effective treatment modality for postmastectomy local-regional recurrences.

Survival rates following a local-regional recurrence range from 10% to 50% at 5 years and are influenced by several factors. The most important are the disease-free interval, initial nodal status, the extent of the recurrence, and the hormone receptor status. Treatment-related factors influencing survival rates are related to local control. Patients having excisional biopsy and controlled local regional disease (maximized by adequate radiation therapy) have a superior survival rate when compared to patients with uncontrolled disease. When local-regional disease is controlled, the 5-year survival rate ranges from 26% to 68% vs. 0 to 43% with uncontrolled disease.

Treatment recommendations for a postmastectomy local-regional recurrence include the use of an excisional biopsy, where feasible, followed by adequate radiotherapy. Adequate radiation is defined as treatment to the entire chest wall and supraclavicular nodal region. Elective treatment of the axillary or internal mammary nodes does not appear necessary in terms of local-regional control or survival. The dose for prophylactic irradiation is 4500 to 5000 cGy. A boost dose of 1000 cGy may be given to the site of recurrence. For patients with gross residual disease, doses in the range of 6000 to 6500 cGy have resulted in local control in 70% of patients. The use of higher doses has not resulted in improved control and must be weighed against the potential for complications. Patients who may benefit from adjuvant systemic therapy include those who have been identified as having a relatively poor prognosis (i.e., disease-free interval <2 years, unresectable disease, multiple sites of involvement, recurrence in the supraclavicular region, initial positive axillary nodes, or estrogen receptor–negative disease). In the University of Pennsylvania experience, patients who had undergone excision of all gross disease and received chemotherapy had a trend toward an improved overall survival, relapse-free survival, and local regional control. Hormonal therapy was most beneficial in those with gross residual disease and resulted in a significant improvement in overall, relapse-free survival.

Treatment for patients who present with a local-regional recurrence and simultaneous or antecedent distant metastases is primarily systemic therapy. Radiation may be considered in symptomatic patients with a reasonable life expectancy.

Treatment options for patients who develop a local-regional recurrence following radiation include excisional biopsy alone, chest wall resection, low-dose reirradiation plus hyperthermia, or systemic chemotherapy or hormonal therapy.

REFERENCES

Local-regional recurrence following conservative surgery and radiation

1. Bader J, Lippman M, Swain S, et al: Preliminary report of the NCI early breast cancer study: a prospective randomized comparison of lumpectomy and radiation to mastectomy for Stage I and II breast cancer, Int J Radiat Oncol Biol Phys 13:160, 1987 (abstract).
2. Balawajder I, Antich PP, and Boland J: The management of breast carcinoma by primary radiotherapy at Mount Sinai Hospital from 1962-1979, Cancer 49:1587, 1982.
3. Bartelink H, Border JH, van Dongen JA, and Peterse JL: The impact of tumor size and histology on local control after breast-conserving therapy, Radiother Oncol 11:297, 1988.
4. Bedwinek JM, Perez CA, Kramer S, et al: Irradiation as the primary management of stage I and II adenocarcinoma of the breast, Cancer Clin Trials 3:11, 1980.
5. Bluming AZ, Dosik G, Lowiz B, et al: Treatment of primary breast cancer without mastectomy. The Los Angeles community experience and review of the literature, Ann Surg 204:136, 1986.
6. Borger JH and Keijser AH: Conservative breast cancer treatment: analysis of cosmetic results and the role of concomitant adjuvant chemotherapy, Int J Radiat Oncol Biol Phys 13:1173, 1987.
7. Boyages J, Recht A, Connolly J, et al: Factors associated with local recurrence as a first site of failure following conservative treatment of early breast cancer, Recent Results Cancer Res 115:92, 1989.
8. Calle R, Vilcoq JR, Zafrani B, et al: Local control and survival of breast cancer treated by limited surgery followed by irradiation, Int J Radiat Oncol Biol Phys 12:873, 1986.
9. Cedermark B, Askergren J, Alveryd A, et al: Breast-conserving treatment for breast cancer in Stockholm, Sweden 1977 to 1981, Cancer 53:1253, 1984.
10. Chu AM, Cope O, Russo R, and Lew R: Patterns of local-regional recurrence and results in stages I and II breast cancer treated by irradiation following limited surgery, Am J Clin Oncol 7:221, 1984.
11. Clark RM, Wilkinson RH, Mahoney LJ, et al: Breast cancer: a 21 year experience with conservative surgery and radiation, Int J Radiat Oncol Biol Phys 8:967, 1982.
12. Clark RM, Wilkinson RH, Miceli PN, and MacDonald WD: Breast cancer: experiences with conservation therapy, Am J Clin Oncol 10:461, 1987.
13. Clarke D, Curtis JL, Martinez A, et al: Fat necrosis of the breast simulating recurrent carcinoma after primary radiotherapy in the management of early stage breast carcinoma, Cancer 52:442, 1983.
14. Clarke DH, Le MG, Sarrazin D, et al: Analysis of local-regional relapse in patients with early breast cancers treated by excision and radiotherapy. Experience of the Institut Gustave-Roussy, Int J Radiat Oncol Phys 11:137, 1985.
15. Delouche G, Bachelot F, Premont M, and Kurtz JM: Conservation treatment of early breast cancer: long term results and complications, Int J Radiat Oncol Biol Phys 13:29, 1987.
16. Dewar JA, Sarrazin D, Benhamou E, et al: Management of the axilla in conservatively treated breast cancer: 592 patients treated at Institut Gustave-Roussy, Int J Radiat Oncol Biol Phys 13:475, 1987.
17. Dubois JB, Gary-Bobo J, Pourquier H, and Pujol H: Tumorectomy and radiotherapy in early breast cancer: a report on 392 patients, Int J Radiat Oncol Biol Phys 15:1275, 1988.
18. Durand JC, Poljicak M, LeFranc JP, and Pilleron JP: Wide excision of the tumor, axillary dissection and post-operative radiotherapy as treatment of small breast cancers, Cancer 53:2439, 1984.
19. Fisher B, Bauer M, Margolese R, et al: Five-year results of a randomized clinical trial comparing total mastectomy and segmental mastectomy with or without radiation in the treatment of breast cancer, N Engl J Med 312:665, 1985.
20. Fisher B, Costantino J, Redmond C, et al: A randomized clinical trial evaluating tamoxifen in the treatment of pa-

tients with node-negative breast cancer who have estrogen-receptor-positive tumors, N Engl J Med 320:479, 1989.

21. Fisher B, Redmond C, Poisson R, et al: Eight-year results of a randomized clinical trial comparing total mastectomy and lumpectomy with or without irradiation in the treatment of breast cancer, N Engl J Med 320:822, 1989.
22. Fisher B, Wolmark N, Bauer M, et al: The accuracy of clinical nodal staging and of limited axillary dissection as a determinant of histologic nodal status in carcinoma of the breast, Surg Gynecol Obstet 152:765, 1981.
23. Fisher ER, Sass R, Fisher B, et al: Pathologic findings from the National Surgical Adjuvant Breast Project (Protocol 6). II. Relation of local breast recurrence to multicentricity, Cancer 57:1717, 1986.
24. Fourquet A, Campana F, Zafrani B, et al: Prognostic factors in the conservative management of early breast cancer. A 25 year follow-up at the Institut Curie, Int J Radiat Oncol Biol Phys 17:719, 1989.
25. Fowble B, Solin LJ, Schultz DJ, and Goodman RL: Frequency, sites of relapse and outcome of regional node failures following conservative surgery and radiation for early breast cancer, Int J Radiat Oncol Biol Phys 17:703, 1989.
26. Fowble B, Solin LJ, Schultz DJ, et al: Breast recurrence following conservative surgery and radiation: patterns of failure, prognosis and pathologic findings from mastectomy specimens with implications for treatment, Int J Radiat Oncol Biol Phys 19:833, 1990.
27. Gerard JP, Montbarbon JF, Chassard JL, et al: Conservative treatment of early carcinoma of the breast: significance of axillary dissection and iridium implant, Radiother Oncol 3:17, 1985.
28. Greco M, Sacchini V, Merson M, and Galimberti V: Risk of local failure in conservative treatment of breast cancer, Breast Cancer Res Treat 12:116, 1988.
29. Haffty BG, Goldberg NB, Fischer D, et al: Conservative surgery and radiation therapy in breast carcinoma: local recurrence and prognostic implications, Int J Radiat Oncol Biol Phys 17:727, 1989.
30. Harris JR, Recht A, Amalric R, et al: Time course and prognosis of local recurrence following primary radiation therapy for early breast cancer, J Clin Oncol 2:37, 1984.
31. Harter K, Goldberg R, Bryne P, et al: Local recurrence of breast cancer following lumpectomy in patients receiving adjuvant chemotherapy prior to definitive breast irradiation, Proc Am Soc Clin Oncol 3:125, 1984 (abstract).
32. Hery M, Namer M, Verschoore J, et al: Conservative treatment of breast cancer. A report of 108 patients, Int J Radiat Oncol Biol Phys 10:2185, 1984.
33. Hunig R, Walther E, Harder F, et al: The Basel lumpectomy protocol: 5 year experience with a prospective study for conservative treatment of breast cancer. In Harris JR, Hellman S, and Silen W, editors: Conservative management of breast cancer, Philadelphia, 1983, JB Lippincott, pp 23-35.
34. Koper PCM, van Putten WLJ, Wijnmaalen AJ, et al: Breast conserving surgery and radiotherapy in early stage breast cancer, Int J Radiat Oncol Biol Phys (in press).
35. Kurtz JM, Amalric R, Brandone H, et al: Local recurrence after breast-conserving surgery and radiotherapy. Frequency, time course and prognosis, Cancer 63:1912, 1989.
36. Kurtz JM, Jacquemier J, Amalric R, et al: Risk factors of breast recurrence in pre- and postmenopausal patients with ductal cancers, Cancer 65:1867, 1990.
37. Kurtz JM, Jacquemier J, Amalric R, et al: Why are local recurrences after breast conserving therapy more frequent in young patients? J Clin Oncol 8:591, 1990.
38. Kurtz JM, Jacquemier J, Torhorst J, et al: Conservation therapy for breast cancers other than infiltrating ductal carcinoma, Cancer 63:1630, 1989.
39. Kurtz JM, Spitalier J, and Amalric R: Late breast recurrence after lumpectomy and irradiation, Int J Radiat Oncol Biol Phys 9:1191, 1983.
40. Kurtz JM, Spitalier J, Amalric R, et al: The prognostic significance of late local recurrence after breast conserving therapy, Int J Radiat Oncol Biol Phys 18:87, 1990.
41. Kurtz JM, Spitalier JM, Brandone H, et al: Mammary recurrences in women younger than forty, Int J Radiat Oncol Biol Phys 15:271, 1988.
42. Leopold KA, Recht A, Schnitt SJ, et al: Results of conservative surgery and radiation for multiple synchronous cancers of one breast, Int J Radiat Oncol Biol Phys 16:11, 1989.
43. Leung S, Otmezguine Y, Calitchi E, et al: Local regional recurrences following radical external beam irradiation and interstitial implantation for operable breast cancer—a twenty three year experience, Radiother Oncol 5:1, 1986.
44. Levine M, Goodyear M, Gent M, et al: Systemic adjuvant chemotherapy reduces ipsilateral breast recurrence following lumpectomy: results from a randomized trial, Proc Am Soc Clin Oncol 9:33, 1990 (abstract).
45. Lindley R, Bulman A, Parsons P, et al: Histologic features predictive of an increased risk of early local recurrence after treatment of breast cancer by local tumor excision and radical radiotherapy, Surgery 105:13, 1989.
46. Markopoulos C and Gazet TC: Paget's disease of the nipple occurring after conservative management of early breast cancer, Eur J Surg Oncol 14:77, 1988.
47. Mate TP, Carter D, Fischer DB, et al: A clinical and histopathologic analysis of the results of conservation surgery and radiation therapy in Stage I and II breast carcinoma, Cancer 58:1995, 1986.
48. Mathews RH, McNeese M, Montague ED, and Oswald NJ: Prognostic implications of age in breast cancer patients treated with tumorectomy and irradiation or with mastectomy, Int J Radiat Oncol Biol Phys 14:659, 1988.
49. Maylin C, Socie G, Clot PH, et al: Five years local control after conservative treatment in breast cancer with intraoperative brachytherapy. Uni- and multivariate analysis of 410 cases stage I-II. UICC, St. Louis Hospital experience—Paris. Proceedings of the Seventeenth International Congress of Radiation Oncology, Paris, 1989, p. 49 (abstract).
50. Menzies D, Barr L, and Ellis H: Paget's disease of the nipple occurring after wide local excision and radiotherapy for carcinoma of the breast, Eur J Surg Oncol 15:271, 1989.
51. Montague ED: Conservative surgery and radiation therapy in the treatment of operable breast cancer, Cancer 53:700, 1984.
52. Muscolino G, Luini A, Bedini AV, et al: Impact of young age on local recurrence risk in patients with early breast cancer who have undergone Q.U.A.R.T. Breast Conference, San Antonio, Texas, 1988 (abstract).
53. Nobler MP and Venet L: Prognostic factors in patients undergoing curative irradiation for breast cancer, Int J Radiol Oncol Biol Phys 11:123, 1985.
54. Osborne MP, Ormiston N, Harmer CL, et al: Breast conservation in the treatment of early breast cancer, Cancer 53:349, 1984.
55. Peterse JL, Van Dongen JA, and Bartelink H: Recurrence of breast carcinoma after breast conserving treatment, Eur J Surg Oncol 14:123, 1988.
56. Pierquin B: Conservative treatment for carcinoma of the breast. Experience of Creteil—ten year results. In Harris J, Hellman S, and Silen W, editors: Conservative man-

agement of breast cancer, Philadelphia, 1983, JB Lippincott, pp 11-14.
57. Pierquin B, Mazeron J, and Glaubiger D: Conservative treatment of breast cancer in Europe: report of the groupe Europeen du Curietherapie, Radiother Oncol 6:187, 1986.
58. Ray GR, Fish VJ, Lee RH, et al: Biopsy and definitive radiation therapy in stages I and II carcinoma of the female breast, Int J Radiat Oncol Biol Phys 9:23, 1983.
59. Rebner M, Pennes DR, Adler DD, et al: Breast microcalcifications after lumpectomy and radiation, Radiology 170:691, 1989.
60. Recht A, Connolly JL, Schnitt SJ, et al: The effect of young age on tumor recurrence in the treated breast after conservative surgery and radiotherapy, Int J Radiat Oncol Biol Phys 14:3, 1988.
61. Recht A, Connolly JL, Schnitt SJ, et al: Conservative surgery and radiation therapy for early breast cancer: results, controversies, and unsolved problems, Semin Oncol 13:434, 1986.
62. Recht A, Schnitt SJ, Connolly JL, et al: Prognosis following local or regional recurrence after conservative surgery and radiotherapy for early stage breast carcinoma, Int J Radiat Oncol Biol Phys 16:3, 1989.
63. Recht A, Silen W, Schnitt SJ, et al: Time course of local recurrence following conservative surgery and radiotherapy for early stage breast cancer, Int J Radiat Oncol Biol Phys 15:255, 1988.
64. Rose MA, Henderson IC, Gelman R, et al: Premenopausal breast cancer patients treated with conservative surgery, radiotherapy and adjuvant chemotherapy have a low risk of local failure, Int J Radiat Oncol Biol Phys 17:711, 1989.
65. Ryoo ME, Kagan AR, Wollin M, et al: Prognostic factors for recurrence and cosmesis in 393 patients after radiation therapy for early mammary carcinoma, Radiology 172:555, 1989.
66. Sarrazin D, Dewar JA, Arriagada R, et al: Conservative management of breast cancer, Br J Surg 73:604, 1986.
67. Schmidt-Ullrich R, Wazer DE, Tercilla O, et al: Tumor margin assessment as a guide to optimal conservation surgery and irradiation in early stage breast cancer, Int J Radiat Oncol Biol Phys 17:733, 1989.
68. Schnitt SJ, Connolly JL, Harris JR, et al: Pathologic predictors of early local recurrence in Stage I and II breast cancer treated by primary radiation therapy, Cancer 53:1049, 1984.
69. Schnitt SJ, Connolly JL, Recht A, et al: Influence of infiltrating lobular histology on local tumor control in breast cancer patients treated with conservative surgery and radiotherapy, Cancer 64:448, 1989.
70. Schnitt SJ, Connolly JL, Recht A, et al: Breast relapse following primary radiation therapy for early breast cancer. II. Detection, pathologic features and prognostic significance, Int J Radiat Oncol Biol Phys 11:1277, 1985.
71. Solin LJ, Fowble B, Martz KL, and Goodman RL: Definitive irradiation for early stage breast cancer: the University of Pennsylvania experience, Int J Radiat Oncol Biol Phys 14:235, 1988.
72. Solin LJ, Fowble B, Schultz DJ, and Goodman RL: Age as a prognostic factor for patients treated with definitive irradiation for early stage breast cancer, Int J Radiat Oncol Biol Phys 16:373, 1989.
73. Solin LJ, Fowble BF, Schultz DJ, et al: The detection of local recurrence after definitive irradiation for early stage carcinoma of the breast: an analysis of the results of breast biopsies in the post-irradiated breast, Cancer 65:2497, 1990.
74. Solin LJ, Fowble BL, Troupin RH, and Goodman RL: Biopsy results of new calcifications in the postirradiated breast, Cancer 63:1956, 1989.
75. Spitalier JM, Gambarelli J, Brandone H, et al: Breast conserving surgery with radiation therapy for operable mammary carcinoma: a 25 year experience, World J Surg 10:1014, 1986.
76. Stomper PC, Recht A, Berenberg AL, et al: Mammographic detection of the recurrent cancer in the irradiated breast, AJR 148:39, 1987.
77. Stotter AT, McNeese MD, Ames FC, et al: Predicting the rate and extent of locoregional failure after breast conservation therapy for early breast cancer, Cancer 64:2217, 1989.
78. Van Limbergen E, Van der Bogaert W, Van der Schueren E, and Rijnders A: Tumor excision and radiotherapy as primary treatment of breast cancer analysis of patient and treatment parameters and local control, Radiother Oncol 8:1, 1987.
79. Veronesi U, Banfi A, DelVecchio M, et al: Comparison of Halsted mastectomy with quadrantectomy, axillary dissection and radiotherapy in early breast cancer: long-term results, Eur J Cancer Clin Oncol 22:1085, 1986.
80. Veronesi U, Zucali R, and DelVecchio M: Conservative treatment of breast cancer with the Q.U.A.R.T. technique, World J Surg 9:767, 1985.
81. Zafrani B, Vielh P, Fourquet A, et al: Conservative treatment of early breast cancer: prognostic value of ductal in situ component and other pathologic variables on local control and survival, Eur J Cancer Clin Oncol 25:1645, 1989.

Local-regional failure following mastectomy

82. Aberizk WJ, Silver B, Henderson IC, et al: The use of radiotherapy in patients with isolated locoregional recurrence of breast carcinoma after mastectomy, Cancer 58:1214, 1986.
83. Ahlborn TN, Gump FE, Bodian C, et al: Tumor to fascia margin as a factor in local recurrence after modified radical mastectomy, Surg Gynecol Obstet 166:523, 1988.
84. Allegra JC, Barlock A, Huff KK, and Lippman ME: Changes in multiple or sequential estrogen receptor determinations in breast cancer, Cancer 45:792, 1980.
85. Andry G, Suciu S, Vico P, et al: Locoregional recurrences after 649 modified radical mastectomies: incidence and significance, Eur J Surg Oncol 15:476, 1989.
86. Arriagada A, Le MG, Mouriesse H, et al: Long-term effect of internal mammary chain treatment. Results of multivariate analysis of 1195 patients with operable breast cancer and positive axillary nodes, Radiother Oncol 11:213, 1988.
87. Baker RR, Montague ACW, and Childs JN: A comparison of modified radical mastectomy to radical mastectomy in the treatment of operable breast cancer, Ann Surg 189:553, 1979.
88. Baum M and Coyle PJ: Simple mastectomy for early breast cancer and the behavior of the untreated axillary nodes, Bull Cancer Paris 64:603, 1977.
89. Beck TM, Hart NE, Woodard DA, and Smith CE: Local or regionally recurrent carcinoma of the breast: results of therapy in 121 patients, J Clin Oncol 1:400, 1983.
90. Bedwinek JM, Fineberg B, Lee J, and Ocwieza M: Analysis of failures following local treatment of isolated local regional recurrence of breast cancer, Int J Radiat Oncol Biol Phys 7:581, 1981.
91. Bedwinek JM, Lee J, Fineberg B, and Ocwieza M: Prognostic indicators in patients with isolated local regional recurrence of breast cancer, Cancer 47:2232, 1981.
92. Bedwinek JM, Munro D, and Fineberg B: Local regional treatment of patients with simultaneous local regional recurrence and distant metastases following mastectomy, Am J Clin Oncol 6:295, 1983.
93. Bicher HI, Wolfstein RS, Lewinsky BS, et al: Microwave

hyperthermia as an adjuvant to radiation therapy: summary experience of 256 multifraction treatment cases, Int J Radiat Oncol Biol Phys 12(9):1667, 1986.
94. Bonadonna G, Valagussa P, Rossi A, et al: Ten year experience with CMF-based adjuvant chemotherapy in resectable breast cancer, Breast Cancer Res Treat 5:95, 1985.
95. Bonadonna G, Valagussa P, Tancini G, et al: Current status of Milan adjuvant chemotherapy trials for node-positive and node-negative breast cancer, NCI Monogr 1:45, 1986.
96. Breast Cancer Trials Committee: Adjuvant tamoxifen in the management of operable breast cancer: the Scottish trial. Lancet ii:171, 1987.
97. Buzdar AU, McNeese MD, Hortobagyi GN, et al: Is chemotherapy effective in reducing the local failure rate in patients with operable breast cancer? Cancer 65:394, 1990.
98. Campbell FC, Blamey RW, Elston CW, et al: Oestrogen-receptor status and sites of metastasis in breast cancer, Br J Cancer 44:456, 1981.
99. Campbell FC, Elston CW, Blamey RW, et al: Quantitative oestradiol receptor values in primary breast cancer and response of metastases to endocrine therapy, Lancet ii:1317, 1981.
100. Chen KKY, Montague ED, and Oswald MJ: Results of irradiation in treatment of locoregional breast cancer recurrence, Cancer 56:1269, 1985.
101. Chu FCH, Lin FJ, Kim JH, et al: Locally recurrent carcinoma of the breast: results of radiation therapy, Cancer 37:2677, 1976.
102. Conway H and Neumann CG: Evaluation of skin grafting in the technique of radical mastectomy in relation to local recurrence of carcinoma, Surg Gynecol Obstet 88:45, 1949.
103. Crile G Jr: Results of simplified treatment of breast cancer, Surg Gynecol Obstet 118:517, 1964.
104. Danckers UF, Hamann A, and Savage JL: Postoperative recurrence of breast cancer after 32 years: a case report and review of the literature, Surgery 47:656, 1960.
105. Danoff BF, Coia LR, Cantor RI, et al: Locally recurrent breast carcinoma: the effect of adjuvant chemotherapy on prognosis, Radiology 147:849, 1983.
106. Dao TL and Nemoto T: The clinical significance of skin recurrence after radical mastectomy in women with cancer of the breast, Surg Gynecol Obstet 117:447, 1963.
107. Deck KB and Kern WH: Local recurrence of breast cancer, Arch Surg 111:323, 1976.
108. Demaree EW: Local recurrence following surgery for cancer of the breast, Ann Surg 134:863, 1951.
109. Deutsch M, Parsons JA, and Mittal BB: Radiation therapy for local regional recurrent breast carcinoma, Int J Radiat Oncol Biol Phys 12:2061, 1986.
110. Di Pietro S, Bertario L, and Piva L: Prognosis and treatment of loco-regional breast cancer recurrences: critical considerations on 120 cases, Tumori 66:331, 1980.
111. Donegan WL: Local and regional recurrence. In Donegan WL and Spratt JS, editors: Cancer of the breast, Philadelphia, 1988, WB Saunders Co, pp 648-663.
112. Donegan WL, Perez-Mesa CM, and Watson FR: A biostatistical study of locally recurrent breast carcinoma, Surg Gynecol Obstet 122:529, 1966.
113. Dragnovic J, Seydel HC, Sandhu T, et al: Local superficial hyperthermia in combination with low dose radiation therapy for palliation of locally recurrent breast carcinoma, J Clin Oncol 7:30, 1989.
114. Dunlop PR, Hand JW, Dickinson RJ, and Field SB: An assessment of local hyperthermia in clinical practice, Int J Hyperthermia 2(1):39, 1986.
115. Elkort RJ, Kelly W, Mozden PJ, and Feldman MI: A combined treatment program for the management of locally recurrent breast cancer following chest wall irradiation, Cancer 46:647, 1980.
116. Fentiman IS, Lavelle MA, Caplan D, et al: The significance of supraclavicular fossa node recurrence after radical mastectomy, Cancer 57:908, 1986.
117. Fentiman IS, Matthews PN, Davison OW, et al: Survival following local skin recurrence after mastectomy, Br J Surg 72:14, 1985.
118. Fisher B, Fisher ER, and Redmond C: Ten year results from the National Surgical Adjuvant Breast and Bowel Project (NSABP). Clinical trials evaluating the use of L-phenylalanine mustard (L-Pam) in the management of primary breast cancer, J Clin Oncol 4:929, 1986.
119. Fisher B, Redmond C, Fisher ER, et al: Ten year results of a randomized clinical trial comparing radical mastectomy and total mastectomy with or without radiation, N Engl J Med 312:674, 1985.
120. Fisher B, Slack NH, Cavanaugh PJ, et al: Post-operative radiotherapy in the treatment of breast cancer: results of the NSABP clinical trial, Ann Surg 172:711, 1970.
121. Fisher B, Wolmark N, Bauer M, et al: The accuracy of clinical nodal staging and of limited axillary dissection as a determinant of histological nodal status in carcinoma of the breast, Surg Gynecol Obstet 152:765, 1981.
122. Fletcher GH: Local results of irradiation in the primary management of localized breast cancer, Cancer 29:545, 1972.
123. Fletcher GH and Montague ED: Radical irradiation of advanced breast cancer, Am J Roentgenol 93:573, 1965.
124. Forrest ADM, Stewart HJ, and Roberts MM: Simple mastectomy and axillary node sampling in the management of breast cancer, Ann Surg 196:371, 1982.
125. Fowble B, Gray R, Gilchrist K, et al: Identification of a subgroup of patients with breast cancer and histologically positive nodes receiving adjuvant chemotherapy who may benefit from postoperative radiotherapy, J Clin Oncol 6:1107, 1988.
126. Gilliand MD, Barton RM, and Copeland EM: The implications of local recurrence of breast cancer as the first site of therapeutic failure, Ann Surg 197:284, 1983.
127. Goldhirsch A and Gelber R: Adjuvant treatment for early breast cancer: the Ludwig breast cancer studies. In NCI Monogr: 55:55, 1986.
128. Gonzalez D, vanDijk JD, and Blank LE: Chest wall recurrences of breast cancer: results of combined treatment with radiation and hyperthermia, Radiother Oncol 12(2):95, 1988.
129. Graverson HP, Toft MB, Anderson JA, and Zelder K: Breast cancer: risk of axillary recurrence in node negative patients following partial dissection of the axilla, Eur J Surg Oncol 14:407, 1988.
130. Griem KL, Henderson IC, Gellman R, et al: Postoperative radiotheray after adjuvant chemotherapy in breast cancer patients: results of a randomized trial, J Clin Oncol 5:1546, 1987.
131. Haagensen CD: Diseases of the breast, ed 2, Philadelphia, 1971, WB Saunders Co, pp 913-914.
132. Haagensen CD: Results with Halsted's radical mastectomy. In Haagensen CD, editor: Diseases of the breast, ed 3, Philadelphia, 1986, WB Saunders Co, pp 903-932.
133. Halsted WS: The results of operations for the cure of cancer of the breast performed at the Johns Hopkins Hospital from June 1889 to January 1894, Medical Classics 3:441, 1938.
134. Halverson KJ, Perez CA, Kuske RR, et al: Management of isolated locoregional recurrent breast cancer after mastectomy, Int J Radiat Oncol Biol Phys 17:180, 1989 (abstract).

135. Halverson KJ, Perez CA, Kuske RR, et al: Isolated local-regional recurrence of breast cancer following mastectomy: radiotherapeutic management, Int J Radiat Oncol Biol Phys 19:851, 1990.
136. Handley WS: The pathology of cancerous pachydermia (so called "Cancer en Cuirasse"). In Handley WS, editor: Cancer of the breast and its treatment, ed 2, New York, 1922, Paul B Hoeber, p 165.
137. Henderson IC: Cancer of the breast. In DeVita VT, Hellman S, and Rosenberg SA, editors: Cancer principles and practice of oncology, Philadelphia, 1989, JB Lippincott, p 1259.
138. Hoogstraten B, Gad-El-Mawla N, Maloney TR, et al: Combined radiation therapy for first recurrence of breast cancer. A Southwest Oncology Group study, Cancer 54:2248, 1984.
139. Hopton DS, Thorogood J, Clayden AD, and MacKinnon D: Histologic grading of breast cancer: significance of grade on recurrence and mortality, Eur J Surg Oncol 15:25, 1989.
140. Howell A, George WD, Crowther D, et al: Controlled trial of adjuvant chemotherapy with cyclophosphamide, methotrexate, and fluorouracil for breast cancer, Lancet ii:307, 1984.
141. Ingle JN, Everson LK, Wieand HS, et al: Randomized trial of observation versus adjuvant therapy with cyclophosphamide, fluorouracil, prednisone with or without tamoxifen following mastectomy in postmenopausal women with node-positive breast cancer, J Clin Oncol 6:1388, 1988.
142. Jackson SM: Carcinoma of the breast—the significance of supraclavicular lymph node metastases, Clin Radiol 17:107, 1966.
143. Janjan NA, McNeese MD, Buzdar AU, et al: Locoregional recurrent breast cancer treated with radiation or a combination of radiation and chemotherapy, Int J Radiat Oncol Biol Phys 2(suppl) 1):152, 1985 (abstract).
144. Janjan NA, McNeese MD, Buzdar AU, et al: Management of locoregional recurrent breast cancer, Cancer 58:1552, 1986.
145. Kaplan EL and Meier P: Non-parametric estimation from incomplete observation, J Am Stat Assoc 53:457, 1958.
146. Karabali-Dalomaga S, Souhami RL, O'Higgins NJ, et al: Natural history and prognosis of recurrent breast cancer, Br Med J 2:730, 1978.
147. Koyama H, Wada T, Takahashi Y, et al: Surgical adjuvant chemotherapy with mitomycin C and cyclophosphamide in Japanese patients with breast cancer, Cancer 46:2373, 1980.
148. Kyle J, Norman JN, Carr J, et al: Management of early cancer of the breast: report of an international multicenter trial supported by the Cancer Research Campaign, Br Med J 1:1035, 1976.
149. Laramore GE, Griffin TW, Parker RG, and Gerdes AJ: The use of electron beams in treating local recurrence of breast cancer in previously irradiated fields, Cancer, 41:991, 1978.
150. Larson DL, McMurtrey MJ, Howe J, and Irish EC: Major chest wall reconstruction after chest wall irradiation, Cancer 49:1286, 1982.
151. Lee NY: Breast carcinoma: pattern of recurrence and metastasis after mastectomy, Am J Clin Oncol 7:443, 1984.
152. Lewis D and Rienhoff WF Jr: A study of the results of operations for the cure of cancer of the breast, performed at Johns Hopkins Hospital from 1889 to 1931, Ann Surg 95:336, 1932.
153. Lindfors KK, Meyer JE, Busse PM, et al: CT evaluation of local and regional breast cancer recurrence, Am J Roentgenol 145:833, 1985.
154. Lindholm CE, Kiellen E, Nilsson P, and Hertzman S: Microwave-induced hyperthermia and radiotherapy in human superficial tumors: clinical results with a comparative study of combined treatment versus radiotherapy alone, Int J Hyperthermia 3(5):393, 1987.
155. Maddox WA, Carpenter JT, Laws HL, et al: A randomized perspective trial of radical mastectomy versus modified radical mastectomy in 311 breast cancer patients, Ann Surg 198:207, 1983.
156. Maddox WA, Carpenter JT, Laws HT, et al: Does radical mastectomy still have a place in the treatment of primary operable breast cancer? Arch Surg 122:1317, 1987.
157. Magno L, Bignardi M, Micheletti E, et al: Analysis of prognostic factors in patients with isolated chest wall recurrence of breast cancer, Cancer 60:240, 1987.
158. Mantel M: Evaluation of survival data and two new rank order statistics arising in its consideration, Cancer Chemother Rep 50:163, 1966.
159. Marshall KA, Redfern A, and Cady B: Local recurrences of carcinoma of the breast, Surg Gynecol Obstet 139:406, 1974.
160. Mathews RH, McNeese M, Montague ED, and Oswald NJ: Prognostic implications of age in breast cancer patients treated with tumorectomy and irradiation or with mastectomy, Int J Radiat Oncol Biol Phys 14:659, 1988.
161. McKenna RJ, Mountain CF, McMurtrey MJ, et al: Current techniques for chest wall reconstruction: expanded possibilities for treatment, Ann Thorac Surg 46(5):508, 1988.
162. Mentzer SJ, Osteen RT, and Wilson RE: Local recurrence and the deep resection margin in carcinoma of the breast, Surg Gynecol Obstet 163:513, 1986.
163. Meyer JE and Munzenrider JE: Computed tomographic demonstration of internal mammary lymph node metastasis in patients with locally recurrent breast carcinoma, Radiology 139:661, 1981.
164. Montague ED: Conservative surgery and radiation in the treatment of operable breast cancer, Cancer 53:700, 1984.
165. Munzenrider JE, Tchakarova I, Castro M, and Carter B: Computerized body tomography in breast cancer, Cancer 43:137, 1979.
166. Nieminen S, Hietanen T, and Nordman E: Surgical treatment of local recurrences of breast carcinoma in the skin and subcutaneous tissues, Acta Chir Scand 145:463, 1979.
167. Novaldex Adjuvant Trial Organization: Controlled trial of tamoxifen as single adjuvant agent in management of early breast cancer. Analysis at six years by Nolvadex Adjuvant Trial Organization, Lancet i:836, 1985.
168. Oliver DR and Sugarbaker ED: The significance of skin recurrences following radical mastectomy, Surg Gynecol Obstet 85:360, 1947.
169. Olson CE, Ansfield FJ, Richards MJ, et al: Review of soft tissue recurrence of breast cancer irradiated with and without actinomycin D, Cancer 39:1981, 1977.
170. Patanaphan V, Salazar OM, and Poussin-Rosillo H: Prognosticators in recurrent breast cancer: a 15 year experience with irradiation, Cancer 54:228, 1984.
171. Pawlias KT, Dockerty MB, and Ellis FH: Late local recurrent carcinoma of the breast, Ann Surg 148:192, 1958.
172. Perez CA, Kuske RR, Emani B, and Fineberg B: Irradiation alone or combined with hyperthermia in the treatment of recurrent carcinoma of the breast in the chest wall: a randomized comparison, Int J Hyperthermia 2:179, 1986.
173. Rao AF, Murthy AK, Hendrickson FR, et al: Analysis of risk factors for loco-regional failure in stage II breast carcinoma treated with mastectomy and adjunctive chemotherapy, Int J Radiat Oncol Biol Phys 11(suppl 1):151, 1985.

174. Rosenman J, Bernard S, Kober C, et al: Local recurrences in patients with breast cancer treated at the North Carolina Memorial Hospital, Cancer 57:1421, 1986.
175. Rosenman J, Churchill CA, Macro MA, et al: The role of computed tomography in the evaluation of postmastectomy locally recurrent breast cancer, Int J Radiat Oncol Biol Phys 14:57, 1988.
176. Rubens RD, Knight RK, Fentiman IS, et al: Controlled trial of adjuvant chemotherapy with melphalan for breast cancer, Lancet i:839, 1983.
177. Rutqvist LD, Cedermark B, Fornanader T, et al: The relationship between hormone receptor content and the effect of adjuvant tamoxifen in operable breast cancer, J Clin Oncol 7:1474, 1989.
178. Scott R, Gillespie B, Perez CA, et al: Hyperthermia in combination with definitive radiation therapy: Results of a phase I/II RTOG study, Int J Radiat Oncol Biol Phys, 15(3):711, 1988.
179. Scott RS, Johnson RJR, Story KV, and Clay L: Local hyperthermia in combination with definitive radiotherapy: increased tumor clearance and reduced recurrence rate in extended follow-up, Int J Radiat Oncol Biol Phys 10:2119, 1984.
180. Seegenschmiedt MH, Brady LW, and Rossmeissl G: External microwave hyperthermia combined with radiation therapy for extensive superficial chest wall recurrences, Recent Results Cancer Res 107:147, 1988.
181. Shah JP and Urban JA: Full thickness chest wall resection for recurrent breast cancer involving the bony chest wall, Cancer 35:567, 1975.
182. Shimkin MB, Lucia EL, Low-Beer VA, and Bell HG: Recurrent cancer of the breast: analysis of frequency, distribution and mortality at the University of California Hospital, 1918 to 1947, inclusive, Cancer 7:29, 1954.
183. Spratt JS: Locally recurrent cancer after radical mastectomy, Cancer 20:1051, 1967.
184. Stadler B and Kogelnik D: Local control and outcome of patients irradiated for isolated chest wall recurrences of breast cancer, Radiother Oncol 8:105, 1987.
185. Stefanik D, Goldberg R, Byrne P, et al: Local regional failure in patients treated with adjuvant chemotherapy for breast cancer, J Clin Oncol 3:660, 1985.
186. Sykes HF, Simm DA, Wong CJ, et al: Local-regional recurrences in breast cancer after mastectomy and adriamycin-based adjuvant chemotherapy: evaluation of the role of postoperative radiotherapy, Int J Radiat Oncol Biol Phys 16:641, 1989.
187. Toonkel LN, Fix I, Jacobson LH, and Wallach CB: The significance of local recurrence of carcinoma of the breast, Int J Radiat Oncol Biol Phys 9:33, 1983.
188. Tormey DC, Weinberg VE, Holland JF, et al: A randomized trial of five and three drug chemotherapy and chemoimmunotherapy in women with operable node positive breast cancer, J Clin Oncol 1:138, 1983.
189. Tough ICK: The significance of recurrence in breast cancer, Br J Surg 53:897, 1966.
190. Turner L, Bell WGT, Hartley RC, et al: Radical versus modified radical mastectomy for breast cancer, Ann R Coll Surg Engl 63:239, 1981.
191. Valagussa P, Bonadonna G, and Veronesi U: Patterns of relapse and survival following radical mastectomy: analysis of 716 consecutive patients, Cancer 41:1170, 1978.
192. Van Der Zee J, Treurniet-Donker AD, The SK, et al: Low dose reirradiation in combination with hyperthermia: a palliative treatment for patients with breast cancer recurring in previously irradiated areas, J Radiat Oncol Biol Phys 15:1407, 1988.
193. Vilari R, Fargroli R, and Munga R: CT evaluation of chest wall recurrences of breast cancer, Eur J Radiol 5:206, 1985.
194. Williams JG, Murley RS, and Curwen MP: Carcinoma of the female breast: conservative and radical surgery, Br Med J 2:788, 1953.
195. Williams MR, Hinton CP, Toddy JH, et al: The prediction of local or regional recurrence after simple mastectomy for operable breast cancer, Br J Surg 72:721, 1985.
196. Zeinrich ES, Fishman EK, Jacobs CG, et al: CT evaluation of recurrent breast carcinoma: impact on treatment planning, Radiology 53:270, 1984.
197. Zoetmulder FAN and van Dongen JA: Chest wall resection in the treatment of local recurrence of breast cancer, Eur J Surg Oncol 14:127, 1988.

16 Metastatic Breast Cancer

Daniel G. Haller, Kevin R. Fox, and Lynn M. Schuchter

Treatment of Metastatic Breast Cancer*

Although the vast majority of women who develop breast cancer present with localized, potentially curable disease, a substantial proportion of patients will ultimately develop metastases. Adjuvant therapy has significantly decreased this risk, although the absolute number of patients who will require treatment for metastases remains quite high. The goal of treatment for patients with metastatic breast cancer is almost always palliative, and the heterogeneity of this population requires a level of individualization of therapy unmatched by almost any other malignant disease. The wide variety of treatment modalities available, therefore, makes the selection of therapy a critical and often complicated step in the management of patients with metastatic breast cancer. This section addresses systemic chemotherapy and hormone therapy for patients with metastatic breast cancer.

EVALUATION OF METASTATIC DISEASE

In order to determine prognosis and to choose the best therapy for patients with metastatic breast cancer, the treating physician must undertake an adequate evaluation to assess the patient's symptoms and the potential sites of metastases. Although metastatic breast cancer may involve virtually every organ system, there are sites where metastases are relatively more common, which require the most complete evaluation. In large series of patients, the most frequent sites of metastases from metastatic breast cancer are bone, lung, pleura, soft tissue, and liver.[80] Both symptomatic and asymptomatic patients should have these common sites assessed by appropriate physical examination or radiographic studies, and symptomatic patients should have additional diagnostic evaluations appropriate to the suspected origin of their symptoms.

A complete physical examination should not be overlooked in patients suspected of having recurrent or metastatic breast cancer. Since the chest wall and regional lymph nodes are a relatively common site of recurrence, physical examination may not only confirm the presence of metastases but may suggest easily accessible sites of tumor for obtaining tissue for histologic confirmation and for special studies such as the determination of estrogen and progesterone receptor status. Because the lung, pleura, and liver are also common sites of metastases, appropriate physical examination of the chest and abdominal cavities is warranted.

Radiographic studies are utilized extensively in the diagnosis and evaluation of patients with a suspected recurrence of breast cancer. Radiographs of the chest, done either for routine follow-up or for evaluation of symptoms, merit inclusion in the list of appropriate studies of these patients, based on their availability and relatively low cost. Radionuclide scans are highly appropriate in the evaluation of patients with symptoms suggestive of skeletal metastases, but their relative high sensitivity and low specificity make bone scans less useful in patients who are asymptomatic. For example, in an evaluation of more than 1600 patients with node-positive operable breast cancer who had bone scans performed 12 months after surgery, 50 scans were required to identify each of the 136 patients with a first relapse to bone.[107] The low predictive value of this study in the asymptomatic patient would, therefore, limit its use in this population outside of clinical trials.

For the evaluation of liver metastases, CT scans and MRI scans are both more sensitive and specific than are physical examination, liver function tests, or radionuclide scans of the liver. As liver metastases frequently may be asymptomatic, the presence or absence of such metastases should be documented sufficiently during the initial evaluation of patients with metastatic disease, both for additional prognostic information and for the impact that the presence of visceral metastases will have on the choice of therapy.

In contrast to the radiographic evaluation of patients for liver metastases, studies such as CT or MRI scans are unlikely to find central nervous sys-

*The section on treatment of metastatic breast cancer is authored by Daniel G. Haller.

temic involvement in an asymptomatic patient, and they therefore should be reserved for patients with specific neurologic symptoms.[100] In addition to space-occupying metastases of the central nervous system, patients with breast cancer may also develop carcinomatous meningitis. The diagnosis of carcinomatous meningitis requires a high index of suspicion, as the symptoms are frequently subtle. Although MRI scans may suggest the diagnosis of carcinomatous meningitis, lumbar punctures for cytologic evaluation are required for accurate diagnosis. The diagnosis and management of this specific site of metastasis will be described in further detail later in this chapter.

In addition to radiographs, routine evaluations of laboratory studies in patients with metastatic breast cancer frequently are obtained. Although baseline measurements of renal and hepatic function are easy to obtain and are relatively inexpensive, their sensitivity and specificity are of low predictive value for the presence of metastases. In order to improve on the sensitivity and specificity of the laboratory evaluation of patients with metastatic breast cancer, various tumor-associated serum markers have been evaluated. Unfortunately, the routine clinical application of such markers remains controversial, either when used as screening or diagnostic tools or as methods for monitoring patients who are receiving treatment. Of the commonly used tumor markers, carcinoembryonic antigen (CEA) has been most extensively evaluated. In general, CEA levels reflect changes in disease status, but widespread use of CEA is limited by its suboptimal sensitivity and specificity.[89,137] Newer tumor markers also are under evaluation. CA 15-3 is a circulating tumor antigen that can be identified in the blood in patients with breast cancer by immunoradiometric assay. Initial studies of CA 15-3 suggest reasonable specificity, with <10% of normal controls having elevated antigen levels.[57] In the same study, 73% of 158 patients with known metastatic breast cancer had elevated (>22 U/ml) levels of CA 15-3. CA 15-3 appears to be somewhat more sensitive than CEA for breast cancer, but the suboptimal specificity for both of these tumor markers limits their usefulness in the routine staging and follow-up of patients with metastatic breast cancer.

PROGNOSTIC FACTORS

In patients with breast cancer, there are a number of categories for prognostic factors that may be considered in predicting outcome as well as in choosing therapy. One such set of factors, more pertinent to the adjuvant therapy of primary breast cancer, includes characteristics of the primary tumor and the determination of the growth potential of tumor cells reflected by lymph node status, estrogen and progesterone receptor status, and flow cytometry data. In patients with metastatic breast cancer, there are two important sets of prognostic factors that must be considered. The first is the expected natural history of the metastatic disease as determined by the biologic and clinical features of the tumor at the time of presentation with metastases. The second group of prognostic factors in patients with metastatic breast cancer includes those features that influence selection of therapy, as well as those that help to predict outcome once a particular treatment program has been instituted. For example, the presence or absence of hormone receptors may influence the decision to institute chemotherapy or hormonal therapy as initial management, and the relative positivity of the receptor status also may influence the survival of a patient once treatment has been instituted. Factors influencing the outcome of treatment will be further discussed in the sections addressing specific treatment programs.

Once metastases have occurred, there are certain characteristics of the mode of recurrence that reflect the biologic growth potential of the tumor and that can predict survival after recurrence. The extreme heterogeneity of patients with breast cancer requires that some form of multivariate analysis of potential prognostic factors be performed to create an optimal predictive index for the survival of patients with recurrent, metastatic breast cancer. A series of 1015 patients with recurrent breast cancer were analyzed and reported by Clark et al. in 1987.[25] Factors that were significantly correlated with poorer survival in a univariate analysis were increasing number of axillary nodes and size of primary tumor at presentation, negative estrogen receptor status, absence of any prior adjuvant therapy, shorter disease-free interval, and visceral metastases. In a multivariate analysis, the site of recurrence, the estrogen receptor status, the axillary lymph node status at diagnosis, and the disease-free interval all correlated with patient survival, but the primary tumor size, the administration of adjuvant therapy, and the number of metastatic sites lost prognostic significance. Most of these predictors are in general agreement with other studies of prognostic variables in patients with metastatic breast cancer. In particular, the disease-free interval has been observed to be an excellent surrogate for predicting the biologic aggressiveness of metastases.[35]

Although there is some disagreement among studies concerning the influence of sites of metastases, patients with brain, liver, or lung metastases generally fare considerably worse than patients who present with soft tissue, pleural, or osseous metastasis. Wide variations in median survival may be observed in patients according to the metastatic sites at initial presentation, with some series showing a range in median survival of 4 months for patients with widespread metastases to visceral organs, 29 months for those with bone involvement, and 44 months for those with pleural metastases alone.[126] In particular the group of patients with dominant osseous metastases at relapse is a particularly favorable subgroup, with median survivals in most studies in excess of 2 years, compared to median survivals of a year or less in patients with visceral metastases.[38,108]

Independent of the site of recurrence and the choice of treatment for recurrence, estrogen receptor status significantly affects survival. Not only are patients with visceral metastases more likely to have estrogen receptor–negative tumors, those patients with visceral metastases and absent estrogen receptors have a significantly worse survival than those patients with visceral metastases and positive estrogen receptors.[25] Newer markers for the biologic growth potential of metastatic breast cancer, such as aneuploidy and growth fraction by flow cytometry, may add to this list of prognostic variables that influence survival after relapse.

The choice of therapy for patients with metastatic breast cancer, however, does not rest solely on an arbitrary list of factors that relate to response to therapy or to overall prognosis. Appropriate palliative management of these patients also requires that the treating physician be acutely aware of the symptoms at presentation and of the potentially life-threatening complications of the disease, which may be documented in an asymptomatic patient during the staging process. Fig. 16-1 illustrates a decision tree for the management of patients with metastatic breast cancer. Implicit in this decision-making process is the balance between the available, effective treatment modalities and the actual or potential symptomatic manifestations of the disease. For example, patients with local symptoms, best treated by specific measures such as radiation therapy or orthopedic procedures for lytic bone metastases, require acute management. These may be instituted concurrently with systemic therapy, or may be of such urgency that immediate local measures are taken first, with delay of hormonal therapy or chemotherapy. In contrast, some patients may present with few if any symptoms, with prognostic factors indicating an indolent growth pattern and with no life-threatening local complications. These patients may best be treated with simple hormone therapies, without additional local treatment. It is the balance among all of these factors that is most important in the selection of treatment for the individual patient.

HORMONAL THERAPY FOR METASTATIC BREAST CANCER

As surgery historically represents the first treatment for primary breast cancer, hormonal manipulation represents the first systemic therapy for many patients with metastatic breast cancer. In the century since oophorectomy was first observed to lead to responses in premenopausal women with inoperable breast cancer, there has been an explosion of information concerning the mechanisms of action of hormonal treatments, as well as an ever-growing list of therapeutic alternatives.[11] Beyond the simple observation that estrogen deprivation leads to a response in breast tumor cells, there is not universal agreement about the mechanisms of action of various hormone manipulations. Preclinical data from tissue cultures and animal models support the concept that estrogen-responsive cells secrete growth factors that are stimulated by estrogen via estrogen receptors.[87] These growth factors appear to work through both autocrine and paracrine stimulation of breast cancer cells. Tumors that are hormone-independent may secrete these growth factors in the absence of estrogen stimulation. In addition to the support of breast cancer cells by estrogen, the effects of other hormones such as androgens and progestational agents suggests alternative mechanisms of action for these hormones.

Selection of patients for hormone therapy

Before the advent of routine measurement of hormone receptors in patients with breast cancer, the selection of patients for hormonal therapy was primarily based on clinical factors that reflect the intrinsic biology of the tumor in an individual patient. The two most commonly used clinical criteria for selecting patients for hormone therapy are the disease-free interval from the diagnosis of the primary tumor to the appearance of metastases and the sites of metastatic spread. Those patients with a relatively long disease-free interval (i.e., >2 years) and with tumor confined to prognostically favorable sites, such as bone and soft tissue, are recognized to have hormone-responsive tumors and an indolent course of disease. Therefore, patients are most often selected for initial hormone therapy alone if they have a tumor with prognostic criteria consistent with an indolent growth pattern and if they have disease that is confined primary to nonvisceral sites, such as soft tissue, lymph nodes, or pleura. Typically, hormonal therapy may require 2 to 3 months to result in an objective or subjective response, so that patients with significant symptoms from their metastases should be considered for treatment with chemotherapy in addition to hormones to achieve more rapid palliation (see Fig. 16-1).

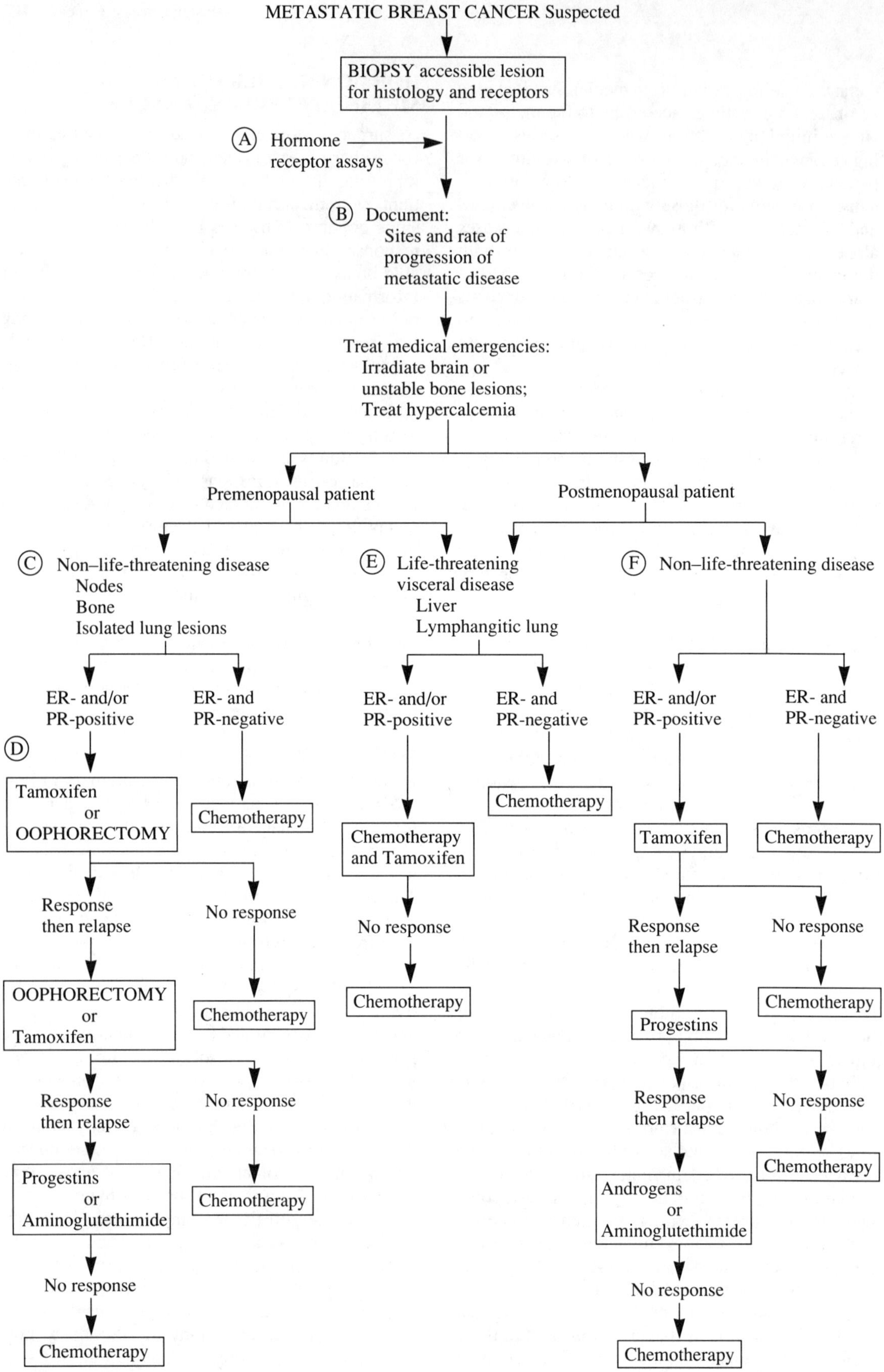

Fig. 16-1 Decision tree for management of patients with metastatic breast cancer. (Reprinted with permission from Glick JH: Metastatic breast cancer. In Schein PS, editor: Decision making in oncology, Philadelphia, 1989, BC Decker, p 113.)

During the 1970s the identification of estrogen and progesterone receptors in breast cancer cells, and the relationship of these receptors to the results of hormone manipulation, greatly advanced the rational use of hormonal therapy.[65,72,147] Initial summaries of objective responses to various hormone manipulations by estrogen receptor status suggested that more than 50% of patients with ER-positive (≥10 fmol/mg protein) tumors would respond to such treatment, compared to <10% of patients with negative estrogen receptors[147] (Table 16-1). Progesterone receptors also have been shown to be useful in predicting response to hormone therapy, with a response rate of 71% in patients who have tumors that are both ER and PR positive, compared to 32% in patients whose tumors are ER positive and PR negative.[24] It has been further shown that the quantification of estrogen receptors has predictive ability for response to hormonal therapy, with higher receptor levels associated with an increased chance of response.[103] Although measurements of estrogen and progesterone receptors have improved the selection of patients for hormone therapy greatly, the well-recognized clinical features of patients with hormone-dependent tumors, including the disease-free interval and sites of metastases, remain extremely useful in practice.[17]

In spite of the ability to recognize and quantify hormone receptors in the tumors of patients with metastatic breast cancer, there are a number of reasons why the ability to predict response remains imperfect. First, patients with breast cancer typically have a disease that is not monoclonal, which means that from site to site and within sites there are cells with varying degrees of biologic potential, including receptor expression. Therefore, characterizing a patient's chance of response based on the receptor status of a single site may be misleading. In addition, the choice of hormone therapy frequently is based on the receptor status of the patient at the time of primary diagnosis, rather than on the receptor status of the metastases at time of relapse. In general, receptor positivity—and therefore hormone dependency—decreases from measurements in the primary tumor to those in metastatic sites.[4,101] Although this decline in receptor positivity may be seen in the setting of prior hormone therapy or chemotherapy, such changes also may be noted in the absence of intervening treatment, implying the evolution of cell lines with higher biologic aggressiveness.

Table 16-1 Relationship between receptor status and response to hormonal therapy

	ER-positive	ER-negative
PR-positive	78% (135/174)	45% (5/11)
PR-negative	34% (55/164)	10% (16/165)
Total	58% (190/329)	12% (21/176)

Modified from Witliff JL: Cancer 53:630, 1984.

When faced with imperfect, metachronous receptor data, clinicians frequently must rely on traditional clinical predictors of response to hormone treatment. In patients already receiving hormone therapy, response to a previous endocrine manipulation frequently is considered as a surrogate for a favorable receptor status. Independent of the hormone therapy initially used, a response to primary hormonal treatment is an excellent predictor of response to second- or third-line hormonal therapy.[61] As would be expected, the duration and completeness of the response to previous hormonal therapy directly relates to the chance of response to second- or third-line treatment, no doubt reflecting the quantity of estrogen receptor present in the metastatic tumor sites.

Specific endocrine therapies

In the discussion of the specific endocrine therapies available, it is useful to recall that there may be a number of criteria of response upon which comparisons of these therapies may depend. Typically, the objective response rate, combining both complete and partial responses by standard definitions, is the most accurate and reproducible of these criteria. However, older trials are likely to have applied the definitions of response less stringently, so that historical comparisons are frequently misleading. In addition, it is the very group of hormonally responsive patients who also have sites of disease that are the most difficult to measure and document objectively. Although osseous, pleural, and soft tissue metastases are the sites most commonly associated with hormone response, they are frequently only considered as evaluable, rather than measurable, sites. Ironically, although treatment or prevention of symptoms is the ultimate goal of palliative therapy for metastatic breast cancer, subjective improvement and measurements of quality of life are even more difficult to obtain, and rarely are accepted as measures of efficacy in clinical trials. Duration of response to therapy and overall patient survival are useful in defining an objective response, as it is expected that treatments associated with higher degrees of tumor cytotoxicity should also have prolonged durations of response and improvement in survival. Clinical trials of hormonal therapy and chemotherapy may not report all of these possible criteria of response, making comparisons among treatments more difficult.

Oophorectomy. As previously noted, oophorectomy has been utilized as a hormone manipulation for premenopausal women with breast cancer for nearly 100 years. Ablation of ovarian function may be achieved by either surgical castration or by radiation therapy.[40] Although these two methods have not been directly compared, series of patients suggest that effective ablation of ovarian function may be achieved with either technique. Surgical castration is most often performed, because it is only the rarest patient—otherwise eligible for hormone manipulation—who could not undergo a simple oophorectomy. Collected series of unselected patients who have undergone surgical castration suggest an overall response rate in excess of 30%.[131] In two recent trials, responses to oophorectomy were seen in 21% and 37% of premenopausal patients[15,70] (Table 16-2). The higher response rate was reported from the series in which estrogen receptor–negative patients were excluded, whereas the lower overall response rate was reported from the series in which patients were treated regardless of receptor status. As one would expect, patients who have been selected for castration based on a positive estrogen receptor have a significantly higher rate of response.[36] In addition to considering traditional and biochemical parameters for prediction of response, the menopausal status of the patient also must be taken into account when considering oophorectomy. Based on their intrinsically estrogen-deprived status, postmenopausal women have less than one chance in ten of responding to oophorectomy.[42,142] Oophorectomy should, therefore, be reserved for premenopausal women with a relatively high likelihood of response based on clinical data and on receptor status.

Adrenalectomy. As neither menopause nor oophorectomy completely eliminate the secretion of estrogens, alternative methods of hormone ablation have been investigated. After cessation of ovarian hormone function by whatever cause, the chief source of estrogen in the postmenopausal female is the adrenal gland, secreting estrone and androstenedione, which is peripherally metabolized to estrone.[50] Surgical adrenalectomy has been associated with response rates equivalent to those seen with other endocrine manipulations for comparable groups of patients.[121] However, the risks of surgery and of permanent steroid replacement, as well as the advent of simpler hormonal manipulations, including inhibition of steroidogenesis with aminoglutethimide, has rendered surgical adrenalectomy an obsolete procedure for the treatment of patients with metastatic breast cancer.

Hypophysectomy. Hypophysectomy was introduced as an alternative means by which ablation of adrenal function could be achieved. When directly compared in a randomized trial, hypophysectomy and adrenalectomy were equally effective in terms of response, although hypophysectomy was associated with longer survival.[58] As with adrenalectomy, surgical morbidity and the availability of equivalently effective and less toxic therapies have eliminated the need for hypophysectomy.

Estrogens. Until the mid-1970s, the use of the synthetic estrogen diethylstilbestrol (DES), was the most common additive therapy for patients with metastatic breast cancer. Because the first hormonal treatments for patients with breast cancer were all aimed at decreasing estrogen levels, the response of these patients to pharmacologic doses of estrogen seems paradoxical. It is not known by what mechanism high doses of estrogen become antiestrogenic in action. In other respects, however, additive estrogen therapy is similar to other hormone manipulations. The patient who traditionally has responded to estrogen therapy is clinically similar to other patients with hormone-dependent tumors, and the overall response rate to estrogens in large series of patients ranges up to 38%.[59] Although higher doses of estrogen (>10 to 15 mg/day) have been associated with improved response rates, toxicity also prohibitively increases at higher dose levels.[22] These toxicities include nausea and vomiting, anorexia, fluid retention, and dysfunctional uterine bleeding. Additive estrogen therapy is rarely used today, so that the previously described

Table 16-2 Tamoxifen versus oophorectomy in premenopausal women

	Ingle et al.[70]		Buchanan et al.[15]	
	Tamoxifen (20 mg/day)	Oophorectomy	Tamoxifen (40 mg/day)	Oophorectomy
No. pts.	26	27	55	52
Response rate	27%	37%	24%	21%
Median duration of response (mo)	15	16	20	7
Median survival (mo)	30	18	15	25

phenomenon of withdrawal response after successful estrogen therapy is now a historical footnote to the hormonal treatment of breast cancer.[10]

Androgens. The mechanisms by which androgens manifest antiestrogenic effects are also uncertain. Since the initial observations more than 50 years ago that male hormones could inhibit the growth of tumors in the laboratory, much effort has been directed toward the elucidation of potential mechanisms of action. It has been proposed that androgens may have two mechanisms of action relevant to their antitumor effect in female breast cancer.[113] The first of these potential mechanisms is the blocking of pituitary gonadotropin release, resulting in decreased ovarian function. Second, there may be a direct antiestrogenic effect, which may be modulated via hormone receptors. The largest series of patients treated with androgens was a group of 564 postmenopausal women given testosterone proprionate.[31] An overall response rate of 21% was observed, with the highest responses seen in the subgroups of patients traditionally associated with hormone responsiveness. When androgen and estrogen therapies have been directly compared, the response rate to androgen therapy has typically been significantly inferior.[31] This lesser activity, coupled with the propensity of these drugs to cause virilization, has relegated androgen therapy to a small subgroup of patients as third-line hormonal therapy. When used, it is typically instituted after successful therapy with tamoxifen and progestational agents, and is administered as Halotestin (fluoxymesterone), 10 mg orally, twice daily.

Glucocorticoids. The mechanism of action of glucocorticoids in metastatic breast cancer is also unknown. Early clinical trials of glucocorticoids suggested that true objective regressions of tumor may occur.[77] In particular, high doses of glucocorticoids have been associated with response rates of up to 15%, although responses generally were observed to be of short duration.[46] At the present time, it is difficult to be certain whether such responses are nonspecific effects of steroids, or specific cytolytic effects on breast cancer cells. In this regard, a preliminary report of a higher objective response rate when prednisolone was added to either tamoxifen or oophorectomy is encouraging, although further studies are warranted.[114] For the moment, glucocorticoids probably should be reserved for the nonspecific supportive care of patients with metastatic breast cancer.

Aminoglutethimide. Although aminoglutethimide is significantly too toxic as an anticonvulsant, its ability to block adrenal function has caused it to be used as an effective anticancer therapy. Aminoglutethimide is an indirect antiestrogen that has at least two major biochemical functions.[118] It can inhibit steroidogenesis in the adrenal gland by blocking the conversion of cholesterol. More importantly, it also can inhibit the peripheral conversion of androstenedione to estrone. When given at a standard dose of 250 mg qid, glucocorticoid replacement therapy in doses of 25 to 40 mg of hydrocortisone daily is also given to both decrease levels of ACTH released from the pituitary gland and to prevent adrenal crisis. A total daily dose of 500 mg is adequate to suppress estrogen,[117] and a dose of 250 mg bid appeared to be as effective clinically as 250 mg qid in a randomized trial.[133] When used at standard doses of 500 to 1000 mg daily, lethargy, drug rash, and dizziness are among the common initial side effects of aminoglutethimide. These can be ameliorated by initiating therapy at a lower dose range, although typically these symptoms also decrease with continued therapy even at higher dose levels.[60] In spite of these toxicities, aminoglutethimide remains useful and effective for endocrine manipulation, with an average objective response rate of 31%, equivalent to that of other hormone treatments.[134] As a second-line hormonal therapy for patients previously treated with tamoxifen, an overall response rate of 34% has been reported; a 25% response rate was seen in patients who failed to respond to prior tamoxifen administration.[14] At least one trial has reported the superiority of aminoglutethimide to tamoxifen when response in osseous metastases alone was considered.[128] Because this drug has no effect on ovarian estrogen function, its use is limited to postmenopausal patients, in whom the majority of circulating estrogen is derived from products of the adrenal gland. However, aminoglutethimide could be considered a second-line therapy for premenopausal women who have responded to oophorectomy and/or tamoxifen administration.

Progestational agents. There are two progestational agents that are commonly used in the treatment of advanced breast cancer: megestrol acetate (MA) and medroxyprogesterone acetate (MPA).[54] Since the late 1960s, these synthetic derivatives of progesterone have been reported to have activity in metastatic breast cancer,[130] but the mechanism of action of these agents remains uncertain. In preclinical studies, progestins have been shown to have both direct cytotoxicity and the capability of abolishing stimulating effects of estrogen on tumor cell lines.[5] In spite of a lack of specific knowledge of the mechanism of action of these agents, they are useful as both first- and second-line therapies for hormone-responsive patients. In randomized trials of megestrol acetate compared to tamoxifen as first-line therapy, MA appears equivalent to tamoxifen in overall response rates.[95,98] In the largest comparative trial of MA 40 mg qid vs. tamoxifen 10 mg bid in receptor-positive or receptor-unknown patients, the overall objective response rates for the two agents were 29% and 31% respectively.[98] Although responses were seen with equal frequency in most sites, 7 of 19 (37%) patients with visceral disease responded to tamoxifen, compared to none of 18 patients treated with MA. Time to progression was similar between the two regimens, but the median survival time after adjustment for pretreatment characteristics favored tamoxifen ($p = .0037$).

Medroxyprogesterone acetate also has been tested at wide dose ranges, with a combined objective response rate of 41% (range, 28% to 66%) in a collected series of 696 unselected patients.[92] Higher dose ranges of MPA have been associated with higher response rates, although time-to-disease progression and survival have generally not been prolonged. In a randomized comparison of megestrol acetate and medroxyprogesterone acetate, responses were more frequent in the MPA-treated group (43% vs. 25%), but median progression-free survival and overall survival rates were not different.[146] The most common side effect of progestational therapy, weight gain, was more frequently seen in patients treated with medroxyprogesterone acetate (1000 mg PO daily) compared to megestrol acetate (160 mg PO daily).

Although wide ranges of dose for both of these agents have been tested, the standard doses for megestrol acetate (40 mg PO qid), and medroxyprogesterone acetate (400-600 mg PO daily), seem reasonable when balancing toxicity and efficacy. Because increasing numbers of women are receiving tamoxifen as adjuvant therapy for primary breast cancer, it is likely that many women will experience their first relapse while receiving that drug. Progestational agents, therefore, assume a greater role as first-line therapy for metastatic breast cancer.

Tamoxifen. When choosing an appropriate hormone therapy, the efficacy of the treatment must be balanced against its toxicity profile. Of the previously described hormone manipulations, most in current use have limited side effects when balanced against their excellent palliative capabilities, particularly when compared with other forms of cancer therapy. Based on this algorithm, however, the antiestrogen tamoxifen is the first-line treatment of choice for patients with hormone-responsive metastatic breast cancer because of its near-absence of side effects and its efficacy, which is equivalent to that of other agents used for hormone manipulations.

Tamoxifen is a nonsteroidal antiestrogen, which is known to bind to estrogen receptors, where it competes with circulating estradiol. However, this antiestrogenic activity does not account for all of the physiologic effects of tamoxifen, and some estrogenic manifestations of the drug may be seen in women undergoing therapy.[44] By preventing tumor cells from entering the cell cycle, tamoxifen is considered to be a cytostatic rather than a cytotoxic drug.[73] The reversibility of the estrogen blockade, and, therefore, of cytostasis has led to the development of dose schedules that are both continuous and long term. By virtue of its antiestrogenic effects, tamoxifen can increase pituitary gonadotropin levels and plasma estradiol levels through the negative feedback mechanism.[84] Clinically this results in the persistence of menstrual cycles in many premenopausal women while taking tamoxifen.

Since the introduction of tamoxifen in the early 1970s, the efficacy of this treatment in hormone-responsive patients has been substantiated extensively. Its activity is similar to that of other agents used for hormone manipulations, with an overall response rate of 34% (ranging as high as 78% in estrogen and progesterone receptor–positive patients, and as low as 14% in unselected patients

Table 16-3 Representative trials of tamoxifen vs. other hormone therapies in postmenopausal women

	No. pts.	Response rate (%)	Response duration (mo)	Reference
Tamoxifen	143	41	7.9	69
DES		33	13.1	
Tamoxifen	79	30	NS	145
Fluoxymesterone		19	—	
Tamoxifen	110	29	NS	98
Megestrol acetate		31	NS	
Tamoxifen	117	30	20	128
Aminoglutethimide		30	16	

without hormone receptor data)[106] (Table 16-3). The broad range of response to tamoxifen, as with other hormone treatments, is no doubt attributable to the previously described prognostic variables that impact on response in patients treated with hormone manipulation. When reported, the complete response rate to tamoxifen therapy, even in highly selected series of estrogen receptor–positive patients, is approximately 10%.[71,98] Duration of response to tamoxifen treatment also varies widely. Recent trials in both premenopausal and postmenopausal women with estrogen receptor–positive tumors or tumors of unknown status have demonstrated median durations of response in excess of 1 year, with significantly longer durations in postmenopausal patients with higher estrogen receptor values.[71]

The majority of patients treated with tamoxifen in clinical trials have been postmenopausal patients, in whom the highest response rate would be expected. However, tamoxifen also has been demonstrated to be effective in potentially hormone-responsive premenopausal women as well.[111] Tamoxifen has been compared to surgical oophorectomy in two randomized trials of premenopausal women with metastatic breast cancer (Table 16-2).[15,70] A total of 176 patients were entered into these two trials, and taken together they failed to show a significant difference in response rate or median survival rate between tamoxifen and surgical oophorectomy. In the larger trial of 122 patients, the response rate to tamoxifen was 24% and to oophorectomy was 21%.[15] Although median survival was longer in those patients who underwent oophorectomy (25 months vs. 15 months), the duration of response was longer for tamoxifen (20 months vs. 7 months); neither of these differences were statistically significant. In the smaller trial from the Mayo Clinic, the response rate to oophorectomy and to tamoxifen were also similar (37% and 27%, respectively).[70] In this trial, however, patients were crossed over on failure of the initial treatment. Crossover responses were seen in 5 of 15 patients treated with oophorectomy, including three responses in 10 prior tamoxifen nonresponders. Only 2 of 18 patients treated with tamoxifen after oophorectomy responded. In this trial, patients with visceral sites appeared to respond more often with oophorectomy, although the small number of patients precludes definitive judgment. These limited data would seem to indicate that tamoxifen is an acceptable alternative to oophorectomy as initial hormone therapy in appropriately selected premenopausal women with metastatic breast cancer. Second-line responses with either modality may be observed sequentially, although oophorectomy performed after tamoxifen appears to be more efficacious than tamoxifen given after oophorectomy.

The standard dose of tamoxifen in the United States is 10 mg orally twice daily. Studies of dose response in postmenopausal women have failed to demonstrate a significant advantage for higher doses.[67] Because premenopausal women treated with tamoxifen frequently have marked elevations in estradiol levels, resulting in persistent menses, higher doses of tamoxifen have been evaluated in these patients.[90] Although these studies have demonstrated the ability of higher doses of tamoxifen to suppress menses, doses of >40 mg daily were not associated with higher response rates. In all patients, doses of 20 to 40 mg of tamoxifen daily appear to be optimal. Although tamoxifen is most frequently given on a twice-daily schedule, the serum half-life of the drug is extremely long, and daily dosing is, therefore, permissible.[37] As the long half-life of tamoxifen may cause it to be detectable 6 weeks or more after discontinuing therapy, this aspect of its pharmacology must be kept in mind when obtaining tissue for biochemical estrogen receptor assays, which may give false negative results in the presence of circulating tamoxifen.

The toxicity of tamoxifen is minimal. Initial randomized trials in which tamoxifen therapy was compared with other hormonal agents typically demonstrated that tamoxifen was equally active and significantly less toxic.[69] In trials that have carefully evaluated patients for toxicity from tamoxifen, transient nausea and hot flashes are the most common symptoms. Transient leukopenia and thrombocytopenia are observed very rarely, but these virtually never are associated with clinically important complications, and do not require careful monitoring. An increased risk of venous thrombosis and thrombophlebitis also has been described with tamoxifen therapy, although the risk of this complication is considered to be <3%.[88] This complication also has been observed when tamoxifen has been administered with adjuvant chemotherapy of breast cancer, suggesting that systemic anticancer therapy, rather than breast cancer itself, is responsible for this increased risk of thrombogenesis.[83] Recently, reports have appeared suggesting that tamoxifen may be associated with an increased risk of endometrial carcinoma, particularly when it is given over long periods of time in the adjuvant setting.[52] This potential complication may be a reflection of the estrogenic manifestations of tamoxifen activity. Although the exact risk of this complication is not known, it seems prudent for patients on long-term tamoxifen therapy to continue routine gynecologic care, including Pap smears.

Included among the toxicities of tamoxifen is the

occasional flare reaction, which is in reality a phenomenon associated with tumor response. This reaction typically occurs during the initiation of tamoxifen therapy and is associated with increased bone or tumoral pain and hypercalcemia.[110] It is unclear whether the flare reaction represents a peculiar inflammatory manifestation of tumor response, or whether it represents early unbalanced estrogenic stimulation by tamoxifen.[13] Because the tumor flare is considered to be a reflection of tumor response, it is important that tamoxifen therapy not be discontinued. The duration of the flare reaction is usually <1 to 2 weeks and patients with increased bone pain or hypercalcemia may be given appropriate supportive care.

Newer hormone therapies. Given the overall efficacy and lack of toxicity for the antiestrogen tamoxifen, it is not surprising that there has been research directed toward the development of other antiestrogens. One such agent is toremifene, a triphenylethylene derivative related chemically and pharmacologically to tamoxifen.[73] At low doses, which are as comparably antiestrogenic as tamoxifen, toremifene has less intrinsic estrogenic activity than tamoxifen. At higher doses, estrogenic effects increase, but cytolytic activity—independent of its primary hormonal effect—is also documented. Early clinical trials of toremifene suggests that it is as active as tamoxifen, but randomized clinical trials are underway to establish its ultimate role relative to the more established drug.[51,62]

Based on the observation that interruption of pituitary function (hypophysectomy) has a beneficial effect on patients with metastatic breast cancer, medical inhibitors of pituitary function also are under evaluation. Danazol, a synthetic steroid that inhibits pituitary function, has been shown in limited trials to have efficacy in postmenopausal women with metastatic breast cancer.[28] More recent efforts have been directed toward the investigation of luteinizing hormone–releasing hormone (LHRH) analogues. These agonist drugs, including leuprolide, goserelin, and buserelin, cause decreased FSH and LH excretion, decreased prolactin excretion, and decrease in circulating sex hormones.[78] Both premenopausal and postmenopausal women with advanced breast cancer have been treated with LHRH agonists, with activity documented for all of these analogues. Preliminary data for leuprolide indicate that premenopausal women achieve medical castration with continued therapy; in one trial, this treatment was associated with objective response in 11 of 25 (44%) evaluable patients.[56] Combined therapy with tamoxifen and LHRH analogues is now being tested in both advanced disease and in the adjuvant setting. In premenopausal patients, the goal of such combined therapy is to suppress elevated estradiol levels caused by gonadotropin stimulation secondary to tamoxifen therapy.

Combined endocrine therapy. There are multiple reasons why combining endocrine therapies may be theoretically attractive. First, as most endocrine manipulations do not involve major toxicities, it would not be expected that combined hormonal therapies would produce untoward or unexpected side effects. Second, when hormone therapies are associated with toxicity, these side effects frequently are not overlapping. Third, based on our current state of knowledge of the mechanisms of hormone therapy, there may be both additive and synergistic effects of two or more combined hormones.[74,132] Considering the large number of drugs and other hormone manipulations currently used for treatment, it is not surprising that there are many combinations of hormone treatments that have not yet been investigated. Based on measures of efficacy and toxicity, there are some combinations that are more attractive than others, and for which some clinical data are available.

In particular, tamoxifen has been compared to combinations of tamoxifen with other hormonal drugs. Tamoxifen plus fluoxymesterone (Halotestin) has been shown to have a significantly better response rate (38% vs. 15%) than tamoxifen alone, but there was no prolongation of duration, response, or median survival for the overall population of patients.[139] In a more recent trial of tamoxifen alone compared to tamoxifen plus fluoxymesterone in postmenopausal patients with metastatic breast cancer, the overall response rates to the two treatments were 42% and 54%, respectively.[71] Time to disease progression was better for the combined treatment (11.6 vs. 6.5 months), although the durations of response and the median survival times were similar. In the subgroup of patients 65 years of age and older, and with positive estrogen receptors, the combination of tamoxifen and fluoxymesterone was better than tamoxifen alone in median survival (42.9 months vs. 27.8 months; $p = .06$). Because fluoxymesterone as a single agent was allowed as crossover treatment for patients who failed on tamoxifen, the survival benefit cannot be entirely attributed to sequential hormone response. Of the 53 patients who received second-line fluoxymesterone after tamoxifen, 21 (40%) responded, with a higher proportion of responses observed in prior tamoxifen responders. Although these data are intriguing, a prospective comparison of tamoxifen alone to tamoxifen plus fluoxymesterone in the subgroup of patients 65 years and older with positive estrogen receptors is warranted.

The glucocorticoid prednisolone has been observed to have a dampening effect on the rise in sex hormone–binding globulin associated with tamoxifen therapy.[144] In a large trial of the effects of prednisolone, premenopausal patients initially were treated with ovarian irradiation and postmenopausal patients with tamoxifen; subsequently, these patients were randomized to receive either no additional treatment or prednisolone 5 mg bid.[115] The response rate in the group treated with prednisolone was significantly higher (49% vs. 30%), and both the median duration of response and median time to disease progression were prolonged. Median survival also was prolonged significantly by 4 months in the group receiving prednisolone. Further confirmation of these benefits is required.

As noted earlier, there is theoretical support for the combination of LHRH agonists and tamoxifen in premenopausal women with metastatic breast cancer.[78,112] Initial trials of such combinations have demonstrated transient stimulation of FSH over the first 2 weeks of therapy, followed by subsequent low gonadotropin levels. Ultimately, castrate levels of serum estradiol and progesterone levels are reached. Whether such combination therapy will prove to be significantly better than tamoxifen or oophorectomy alone in premenopausal patients will need to be determined by randomized clinical trials.

Combinations of tamoxifen and progestational agents have not been extensively studied. In one trial in which tamoxifen alone was compared to tamoxifen plus medroxyprogesterone acetate (MPA), a higher response rate was seen with single agent tamoxifen, although the median duration of response was similar in both arms.[141] Sequential tamoxifen and medroxyprogesterone acetate also has been investigated, based on the ability of tamoxifen to induce the synthesis of progesterone receptors in hormone-responsive breast cancers. Although a preliminary phase II trial of sequential tamoxifen-MPA therapy demonstrated a response rate of 56% in 30 patients, a subsequent randomized trial comparing sequential tamoxifen-MPA therapy to tamoxifen alone failed to demonstrate a difference in initial response between the sequential combination and tamoxifen (24% vs. 26%).[9,93] To date, combinations of tamoxifen plus aminoglutethimide have failed to demonstrate significant superiority compared to tamoxifen alone.[32]

Summary

For appropriately selected patients, hormone therapies remain the treatment of choice for metastatic breast cancer. For most hormone manipulations in current use, efficacy is equivalent for most populations of patients, with toxicity profiles that compare very favorably with most cancer treatments. Table 16-4 briefly describes the most commonly used hormone treatments, with positive and negative aspects of each treatment. By virtue of its lack of toxicity and its comparable efficacy, tamoxifen is the single hormonal treatment of choice. In both premenopausal and postmenopausal patients, progestational agents are assuming a greater role, because many patients may have received tamoxifen as adjuvant therapy and may have experienced relapse while receiving that drug. Although there are some minor toxicities associated with the use of progestins, they do not usually require dose modification or cessation of the drug.

For premenopausal women surgical oophorec-

Table 16-4 Commonly used hormonal therapies for metastatic breast cancer

Options	Favorable	Unfavorable
Tamoxifen	Effective in premenopausal and postmenopausal women	Minimal toxic effects, including hot flashes, amenorrhea, mild nausea
Progestins	Effective in premenopausal and postmenopausal women As effective as tamoxifen Effective in tamoxifen failures	Toxicity includes weight gain and fluid retention
Androgens	Effective in premenopausal and postmenopausal women	Masculinizing effects
Aminoglutethimide	Effective in postmenopausal women, or in women after oophorectomy	Initial toxicities include lethargy, skin rash Usually requires additional glucorticoid therapy
LHRH analogues	Effective in premenopausal women	Menopausal symptoms including hot flashes, amenorrhea
Glucocorticoids	May have additive effects with tamoxifen or oophorectomy	Toxicities include cushingoid effects
Oophorectomy	Equally effective as tamoxifen Effective in premenopausal patients	Requires surgery or radiation therapy Hot flashes, amenorrhea

tomy or medical oophorectomy with the LHRH analogues may represent an appropriate alternative to tamoxifen therapy, although there are no convincing data from randomized trials to suggest that either of these treatment approaches are superior to tamoxifen alone. For postmenopausal women, in whom ablation of ovarian function is inappropriate, suppression of estrogen formation by aminoglutethimide remains a reasonable option. Androgen therapy and glucocorticoid therapy generally have been relegated to third-line treatment as single agents because of their overall low activity and higher risks of toxicity.

Combined hormonal therapy remains investigational. Although there are data suggesting that the addition of Halotestin, prednisolone, or progestational agents to tamoxifen may result in improved response rates compared to tamoxifen alone, both the lack of improved durations of response or survival and the increased toxicity make these combinations inappropriate for general use. Sequential, rather than combined, hormonal therapy is therefore preferred in the hormone-responsive patient.

CHEMOTHERAPY

In the palliative management of women with metastatic breast cancer, the role of chemotherapy has been intensively investigated and its clinical use is widespread. Like endocrine therapy, the principle goal of chemotherapy is palliation, and the endpoints by which successful treatment are measured—efficacy and toxicity—are the same. However, the overall toxicity for either single agent or combination chemotherapy is greater than that for most hormone therapies, and therefore the decision to treat or not treat a patient with metastatic breast cancer with chemotherapy frequently requires different selection criteria. Therefore, careful selection of patients is a critical initial step in choosing and initiating treatment.

Selection of patients for chemotherapy

In the management of patients with endocrine therapies for breast cancer, both excellent clinical criteria and biochemical criteria exist for proper patient selection. Both the presence of estrogen receptors and the clinical parameters that describe a slow-growing tumor help to predict for response to hormone manipulation. However, if one excludes those factors that are well known to be associated with a good response to chemotherapy treatments in all solid tumors, there are no specific clinical or biochemical parameters that are associated with a higher chance of response in breast cancer. Like most other solid tumors, better outcomes are achieved in patients who have had limited prior chemotherapy or radiation therapy, good or excellent performance status, minimal tumor burden, and lack of involvement of visceral sites.

Because patients who previously have responded well to endocrine manipulation are likely also to have more indolent disease, it is not surprising that patients with prior successful hormone therapy also have better survival rates after treatment with chemotherapy, compared to those patients who initially failed to respond to primary hormonal therapy.[129] This observation clearly reflects patient selection, because the response rate of patients treated with chemotherapy after hormone therapy is equal between hormone nonresponders and responders.[81] Neither age nor menstrual status appear to affect response to chemotherapy in metastatic breast cancer.[33] Estrogen receptor status also has been used in the selection of patients for chemotherapy, based on the potential surrogate value of estrogen receptor for tumor growth rate. Although it is true that a lack of estrogen receptor may be associated with a higher growth rate, the ability of estrogen receptor to predict for a response to chemotherapy would require that faster growing tumors would always and uniformly respond more completely and quickly to chemotherapy. In collected series of patients in whom estrogen receptor status and response to chemotherapy have been analyzed, this does not appear to be the case.[33] Further evaluations of more specific determinants of cell kinetics, such as S-phase fraction by flow cytometry, are needed.

More specifically related to the success or failure of chemotherapy may be the presence of membrane glycoproteins such as P-170, which are expressed as a result of the multidrug-resistant (MDR) phenotype. Quantitative measurement of such intrinsic or acquired resistance to chemotherapy drugs might be extremely useful in the selection of patients for chemotherapy.[104] Initial studies of P-170 in patients with breast cancer have suggested that strong positive staining for this glycoprotein was correlated significantly with poor initial response to chemotherapy and with a shorter progression-free survival.[143]

As with the selection of patients for hormone therapy, it is important for clinicians to recognize that it is a global evaluation of the patient with metastatic breast cancer, rather than any single determinant, which will support the use of chemotherapy as primary treatment (see Fig. 16-1). Patients with life-threatening or visceral metastases should virtually always be considered for chemotherapy as initial treatment, because meaningful clinical responses to hormonal therapy in these patients are usually quite rare. Chemotherapy also may be considered as part of the initial management of patients with potentially hormone-responsive tumors, when there are symptoms that require rapid and complete relief. In patients with more indolent disease, and without life-threatening disease manifestations, chemotherapy should be reserved for the time when hormonal treatments are no longer successful.

Single-agent chemotherapy

Given the frequency of metastatic breast cancer and the responsiveness of breast tumor cells to chemotherapeutic agents, it is not surprising that virtually every new cytotoxic drug has been tested in this disease. Historically, alkylating agents such as cyclophosphamide and antimetabolites such as 5-fluorouracil and methotrexate have had the most extensive testing and clinical use. Each of these agents was evaluated in a randomized trial more than 25 years ago, and the response rates observed were quite comparable to those currently accepted.[135] On initial treatment, 22% of patients randomized to cyclophosphamide and 37% of patients randomized to 5-fluorouracil responded. Non–cross resistance between these drugs was also documented. Methotrexate, one of the first antimetabolites in general clinical use, was first described as having activity in metastatic breast cancer as early as 1959.[148] Methotrexate has been tested at many dose levels, particularly in combination chemotherapy regimens, but no specific dose or schedule appears to be superior.

The anthracyclines are among the most extensively tested classes of drugs active in metastatic breast cancer. Early clinical trials of doxorubicin demonstrated that this drug was not only active in metastatic breast cancer but was also non–cross resistant with other drugs, such as cyclophosphamide, methotrexate, and 5-fluorouracil. Other anthracycline drugs also have been tested in patients with metastatic breast cancer. 4′-Epidoxorubicin was synthesized as a less cardiotoxic drug than doxorubicin, and preliminary reports suggest a favorable comparison to doxorubicin when it is used in combination therapy.[7] Other anthracyclines such as esorubicin and idarubicin are also active in metastatic breast cancer, and their comparability to doxorubicin as single agents and in combination chemotherapy is being determined.[91,99]

In addition to traditional bolus schedules of doxorubicin, both infusional and weekly doxorubicin regimens have been designed to decrease both myelosuppression and cardiotoxicity. Four-day continuous infusions of doxorubicin, now made more practical by ambulatory infusion devices, have been shown to be at least as effective as bolus doxorubicin therapy, with less cardiac toxicity.[82] Similarly, weekly doses of doxorubicin appear to have efficacy similar to that of bolus therapy, but with less risk of cardiac toxicity.[23]

Although ifosfamide was demonstrated to have single-agent activity in metastatic breast cancer more than 25 years ago, its clinical usefulness was limited by severe urothelial toxicity.[1] The ability of mesna to protect against this toxicity has stimulated further clinical trials of this drug. Recent trials of ifosfamide, as a single agent and in combination chemotherapy programs, have confirmed the activity of this drug, but its overall role remains to be determined.[94,116]

Mitoxantrone, an anthracene derivative, also has been extensively tested and compared with doxorubicin. This synthetic DNA intercalating agent was designed to be equally effective but less cardiotoxic than doxorubicin, and it demonstrated sufficient single-agent activity in phase II trials to be compared to doxorubicin in phase III randomized trials. On the whole, these trials have suggested that mitoxantrone is associated with somewhat less hematologic and cardiotoxicity than doxorubicin, as well as slightly lower response rates, but with similar durations of response and median survival.[53] For patients in whom either overall toxicity or cardiac toxicity are not a major factor in selecting first- or second-line chemotherapy, doxorubicin remains the drug of choice, and mitoxantrone does not represent an acceptable alternative. However, for patients in whom such toxicities are overriding concerns, mitoxantrone is a useful single agent.

The vinca alkaloids vinblastine and vincristine are also used in patients with metastatic breast cancer. Vincristine historically was incorporated in a number of combination chemotherapy programs because of its lack of significant myelosuppression at standard doses. When prospectively evaluated, however, vincristine appears to have little efficacy in treating advanced breast cancer.[119] Vinblastine probably has more significant activity as a single agent, although rigorous phase II trials of this drug in single agent bolus therapy have not been reported. In an attempt to minimize myelosuppression, this drug has been administered by 5-day continuous infusions, with a response rate of 37% in a single large trial of >100 patients, most of whom had received prior therapy.[43] Subsequent published trials of continuous infusion vinblastine generally have failed to substantiate this observation, with no responses recorded in a total of 32 patients treated in two other trials.[68,136] Further evaluation of this myelosuppressive and cumbersome regimen are required before it can be recommended for routine clinical practice.

Cisplatin, introduced into clinical practice at the time when combination chemotherapy of breast cancer became standard, has had remarkably little phase II evaluation as a single agent. Initial studies in heavily pretreated patients showed modest activity in 4 of 37 patients, with responses limited to those treated at 120 mg/m^2.[41] These data have been confirmed in later studies, with responses generally seen only at higher dose levels of cisplatin.[125] A single trial of cisplatin in patients previously untreated with chemotherapy reported a response in nine of 19 evaluable patients, treated with 30 mg/m^2 daily for 4 days.[124] The requirement for high dose levels of cisplatin, with associated organ toxicities, limits the usefulness of this drug in standard practice, either as a single agent or in combination therapy.

Etoposide (VP-16) has demonstrated little single-agent activity in metastatic breast cancer, although it almost always has been evaluated in patients who have had extensive prior chemotherapy. In this population of patients, the overall response rate in a collected series has been reported to be only 6.6%.[123] In vitro synergy of cisplatin and etoposide would suggest that this combination may have greater activity than either drug used alone, although this combination has not been tested prospectively in large clinical trials.

Mitomycin is extensively utilized in second- and third-line chemotherapy in clinical practice, with its overall use limited by cumulative myelosuppression. As a single agent, mitomycin has modest activity; in a trial of this drug given at a dose of 20 mg/m^2 every 6 weeks to 43 previously treated patients, there were five (12%) partial responses observed.[105] In an attempt to ameliorate the cumulative myelosuppression caused by this drug, mitomycin also has been tested at lesser dose intensity. In a trial of 90 patients treated with 10 mg/m^2 every 28 days, a response rate of 18% was observed.[34] Lesser degrees of myelosuppression were seen with this dose schedule, although frequent dose escalations were required.

Combination chemotherapy

Early observations of improved response rates seen in certain solid tumors and lymphomas with combination therapy led to the study of similar combinations of active agents in breast cancer. Initial response rates for combinations of thiotepa plus methotrexate and of cyclophosphamide, methotrexate, 5-fluorouracil, vincristine, and prednisone (CMFVP) were remarkably high, perhaps reflecting the less stringent criteria for complete and partial responses of that era.[29,49] Further investigations of the CMFVP regimen have failed to confirm the very high complete response rate initially reported, although the efficacy of the CMF moiety subsequently has been well documented. As noted previously, when vincristine has been evaluated specifically as a variable in randomized trials, it appears to add little but toxicity to combination chemotherapy.[119] Although prednisolone appears to improve the response to primary endocrine treatments such as oophorectomy or tamoxifen,[115] the overall role of the glucocorticoids in chemotherapy programs is uncertain. When combined with CMF, prednisone has been associated with slightly longer durations of response and survival than CMF alone.[138] These benefits may have been related to the higher doses of CMF given with prednisone, and these modest improvements must be balanced against the additional toxicity of steroid therapy. These data suggest that the CMF moiety of the CMFVP regimen is responsible for most of the demonstrated clinical activity. When CMF is administered to patients with metastatic breast cancer, the overall response rate is usually in excess of 50%, with 10% to 15% of patients achieving a clinical complete response.[176] The median duration of response may range from 6 to 9 months, with the median survival typically ranging from 12 to 15 months.[138]

Early clinical trials sought to establish the superiority of combination chemotherapy to monotherapy and to sequential single-agent therapy. Comparisons of CMF to L-phenylalanine mustard (L-PAM), CMFVP to cyclophosphamide, and CMFVP to 5-fluorouracil all demonstrated significantly improved response rates and median duration of response for the combination chemotherapy programs, although median survival was not always significantly prolonged.[18,21,96] Trials also have been performed in which combination chemotherapy programs have been compared to combination therapy with the constituent drugs of the programs administered as single agents in sequential fashion. In general, these evaluations have confirmed the superiority of combination chemotherapy to single-agent therapy in treating metastatic breast cancer.[127]

When doxorubicin was introduced into clinical practice, it was both compared to and combined with standard CMF combinations. When compared to combination therapy with either CMF or CMFVP, doxorubicin alone proved similar to overall response rate.[19,63] When substituted for methotrexate in combination chemotherapy programs such as FAC or CAF (Table 16-5), doxorubicin invariably has been associated with improved overall response rates, duration of response, and median survival time, although these differences are not always statistically significant.[2,140] One of the earliest comparisons of CMF to CAF showed a superior response rate for CAF (82% vs. 62%), but no difference in the median duration of response.[16] In later cooperative group data, the efficacy of CAF

Table 16-5 Commonly used combination chemotherapy regimens in metastatic breast cancer

Regimen	Dosage	Frequency
CMF		
Cyclophosphamide	100 mg/m² PO day 1-14	Repeated every 28 days
Methotrexate	40 mg/m² IV day 1 and 8	
5-Fluorouracil	600 mg/m² IV day 1 and 8	
CAF		
Cyclophosphamide	100 mg/m² PO day 1-14	Repeated every 28 days
Doxorubicin	30 mg/m² day 1 and 8	
5-Fluorouracil	500 mg/m² day 1 and 8	
FAC		
5-Fluorouracil	500 mg/m² IV day 1 and 8	Repeated every 21 days
Doxorubicin	50 mg/m² IV day 1	
Cyclophosphamide	500 mg/m² day 1	

was further substantiated, with an overall response rate of 62% (23% complete remission) and with median durations of response and survival of 11.4 and 20.2 months respectively.[39] In a randomized trial comparing CAFVP to CMFVP, the doxorubicin-containing regimen was superior in response rate (71% vs. 50%), median remission duration (14 vs. 7 months) and median survival (19 vs. 13 months).[140] Based on these cumulative data for CMF and CAF combination chemotherapy, it can be concluded that either regimen represents acceptable combination chemotherapy treatment for patients with advanced breast cancer. Only toxicity varies slightly between the two regimens, with more myelosuppression and alopecia reported with doxorubicin-containing combinations.

Second-line chemotherapy

With an expanding list of active single agents, better supportive care, and a continued need for palliation of patients with metastatic breast cancer, multiple second- and third-line chemotherapy regimens have been devised and evaluated. Presuming that standard guidelines for treatment have been met, such as adequate performance status, there is reasonable rationale for such palliative treatment. In patients who have been treated previously with CMF, drugs such as doxorubicin, vinblastine, mitomycin, and cisplatin all have been shown to have sufficient activity for second-line therapy, as single agents or as part of combination chemotherapy programs.

The combination of vinblastine, doxorubicin, thiotepa and fluoxymesterone (VATH) initially was reported to induce objective responses in half of all patients previously treated with chemotherapy for up to 1 year.[55] The VATH combination subsequently was compared to the same regimen, but with the investigational alkylating agent dibromodulcitol substituted for thiotepa (DAVH).[122] Of 184 patients randomized to these two regimens, 32% of patients treated with DAVH and 38% of patients treated with VATH achieved an objective response. Durations of response were similar, as were median survivals. For patients who have not received doxorubicin during recent adjuvant therapy or for metastatic disease, such doxorubicin-containing regimens are acceptable options. However, with increasing numbers of women who have received adjuvant doxorubicin or who have been treated with doxorubicin for a first relapse, there is a need for second-line regimens that do not contain this drug. In such patients, other combinations, including mitomycin plus vinblastine, have been reported in single trials to have response rates as high as 40%, although median durations of response generally have been short (4 to 6 months).[45,79] It is expected that innovative combinations employing cisplatin, ifosfamide, and newer anthracycline drugs also will be reported, but large-scale testing of such combinations will be required before they can be considered in standard clinical practice. The need for better second-line regimens is real, as most patients with metastatic breast cancer will require continued palliative management after CMF or CAF. Unfortunately, there is no standard regimen for these patients, and the choice must be based on a multitude of factors, including the type of drugs previously used, the goals of palliation, and the adequacy of cardiac, renal, and bone marrow functions. The wide variability of these factors means that the development of a single approach to second- or third-line therapy is unlikely.

Variations in chemotherapy programs

Although there are relative standard doses and schedules for both CMF and CAF combination chemotherapy, many potentially important variations in treatment have not been explored systematically. These variations include the frequency of treatment, the optimal dose of chemotherapy, the overall duration of treatment, and the sequence of drugs in combination chemotherapy. When combination chemotherapy programs have been designed, practical issues unrelated to drug pharmacology or tumor kinetics frequently have dictated the choice of dose and schedule.

When frequency of chemotherapy has been investigated systematically, there appears to be no consistent benefit to the use of intermittent treatments compared with more continuous (weekly) treatments. Dose intensity has been evaluated both retrospectively and prospectively in combination chemotherapy programs for metastatic breast cancer. In a metaanalysis of CMF and CAF regimens, overall response rates and—to a lesser degree—survival times were correlated with increasing dose intensity.[66]

There are few prospective, randomized controlled trials that address the issue of dose intensity. In one study in which patients were randomized to doses of doxorubicin ranging from 25 to 75 mg/m^2, no significant differences in response rate were observed.[102] A second trial randomized patients to receive either standard-dose FAC chemotherapy (see Table 16-5) or high-dose FAC (100% to 260% higher than standard) for the first three cycles of therapy. There were no significant differences in response rates, median duration of response, or median survival times between these two treatment groups.[64] The results of these studies do not negate the possibility that dose intensity and dose escalation are important in treating metastatic breast cancer, as the high-dose regimens were only modestly more intense than standard-dose regimens. The issue of autologous bone marrow transplantation as an alternative, potentially more effective, means of dose intensification is discussed in Chapter 18.

Little attention has been paid to the optimal duration of chemotherapy for patients with metastatic breast cancer. This remains an important issue, because the goal of treatment is prolonged palliation and maintenance of quality of life. Continuation of toxic chemotherapy programs past the time when tumor cells are already becoming resistant may simply add side effects without necessarily conferring benefits in terms of prolongation of response or median survival. Clearly, in clinical models where duration of therapy can be more successfully addressed—such as testicular cancer, Hodgkin's disease, and certain lymphomas—maintenance chemotherapy after optimal cytoreduction appears to convey little added benefit. One early study addressing the issue of duration of chemotherapy in metastatic breast cancer suggested no detrimental effects if CMFVP was discontinued in responding patients after 6 months of therapy.[127] However, the number of patients evaluated in this trial was relatively small. A more recent randomized trial compared continuously administered CMFP or AC (doxorubicin plus cyclophosphamide) to the same regimens given for three induction cycles, and then repeated only upon evidence of disease progression.[26] By comparisons of objective response, response duration, and survival, patients who received intermittent therapy fared considerably worse than those who were treated with continuous chemotherapy. In addition, quality of life improved during the first three cycles when all patients received treatment. However, patients who received intermittent therapy subsequently developed a decreased sense of well-being and a poorer quality of life index compared to those patients who were maintained on continuous therapy. Although this study did not specifically address the optimal duration of chemotherapy, the results suggest that very short, intermittent treatment cycles are not appropriate. Maintaining an objective response appears to be a worthwhile objective, because significant palliative benefits are achieved.

There are both practical and theoretical limits on the number of drugs that can be administered at the same time in a given combination chemotherapy program, with myelosuppression as the chief limitation. A retrospective evaluation of response rate and duration of response compared to the number of drugs in combination chemotherapy program suggested that a plateau is reached when three drugs are combined, with no added benefits for combinations of four or more drugs.[20] In an attempt to maintain optimal doses of each drug, and to reduce the risk of drug resistance, alternating, non–cross resistant chemotherapy programs have been proposed.[48] Unfortunately, the theoretical advantage of this approach has not translated into demonstrable clinical benefits, in spite of a rather large series of randomized trials.[60]

COMBINED CHEMOHORMONAL THERAPY

Tumor heterogeneity and the availability of both effective chemotherapy and hormonal therapy have provided a compelling rationale for investigating the role of combined chemohormonal therapy in patients with advanced breast cancer. Early evaluations of such chemohormonal trials are difficult to evaluate because of relatively small sample

Table 16-6 Chemotherapy alone versus chemotherapy plus tamoxifen

Regimen	No. pts.	Response (%) All pts.	Response (%) ER-positive pts.	Median duration of response (mo)	Median duration of survival (mo)
CMF[27]	133	51	46	11.7	27.8
CMF + tamoxifen		74	80	12.8	19.5
CMF[47]	220	49	—	12	19
CMF + tamoxifen		75	—	18	24
CAF[75]	419	55	50	14.6	—
CAF + tamoxifen		62	47	17.3	—
AC[8]	226	45	—	—	18
AC + tamoxifen		51	—	—	20

sizes, variable chemotherapy-hormone therapy combinations and incomplete data concerning estrogen receptor status.[120] A review of these early studies of chemohormonal therapy suggest a higher response rate for combined treatment compared to chemotherapy alone, but without significant differences in median duration of response or in overall survival (Table 16-6).[85] In a recent prospective trial of patients in whom estrogen receptor values were known, CAF was compared to CAF plus tamoxifen in advanced breast cancer. The addition of tamoxifen conferred no significant advantages, independent of estrogen receptor or menopausal status.[109] The response rates of estrogen receptor–positive and estrogen receptor–negative patients to chemotherapy were identical, suggesting that both chemotherapy and hormonal therapy compete for the same pool of sensitive cells, thereby potentially explaining the failure of combined treatment to result in additive or synergistic effects.

Sequential endocrine therapy and chemotherapy also has been evaluated, based on preclinical data that estrogens may increase the growth rate of breast cancer cells, rendering them potentially more sensitive to chemotherapy.[3] A pilot study of 25 patients treated with Premarin followed by chemotherapy (methotrexate and 5-fluorouracil) demonstrated an overall response rate of 72% with a high proportion of complete responses.[6] A subsequent randomized trial of tamoxifen and Premarin recruitment plus CAMF chemotherapy compared to CAMF chemotherapy alone failed to demonstrate a significant difference in response rates between the two treatment programs.[86] The group receiving hormone pretreatment had nonsignificant prolongation of median duration of response and survival. Further confirmation of the potential benefits of sequential hormonal-chemotherapy will be documented in randomized controlled trials.

Chemohormonal therapy, while not of value for most patients, may be useful in a select group of patients with receptor-positive tumors and with life-threatening visceral disease presenting with rapid progression. In such patients, the increased response rates observed with combined chemotherapy and endocrine approaches may translate into a more rapid and complete response, leading to more effective symptom palliation. In patients with less rapidly growing tumors and with less serious consequences of tumor growth, sequential therapy with hormones followed by chemotherapy represents a more appropriate treatment option.

CONCLUSION

While the presentation of patients with metastatic breast cancer may vary widely, and the number of available therapies seem endless, the goal in every patient remains the same: palliation of symptoms, prolongation of the symptom-free interval and—when possible—improvement in overall survival. Fig. 16-1 displays a flow chart that describes various steps in choosing appropriate therapy for an individual with metastatic breast cancer.[47] Initially, a biopsy should be obtained of accessible lesions, where possible, to confirm recurrence and to obtain tissue for hormone receptor assays (Fig. 16-1, *A*). Once recurrence has been confirmed, an overall evaluation of the patient must be obtained, to document sites of metastases and to evaluate signs and symptoms attributable to these metastases (Fig. 16-1, *B*), as well as the tempo of the patient's metastatic disease.

Frequently, patients with metastatic breast cancer present with either a single site of recurrence that can be treated with local measures (such as radiotherapy, described later in this chapter), or with dominant, life-threatening manifestations (e.g., brain metastases, pending fractures from bone metastases, or hypercalcemia) requiring immediate or specific local therapy. When it has been determined that systemic therapy alone is necessary, it is convenient to categorize patients according to the presence or absence of life-threatening or visceral-predominant sites of metastases (Fig. 16-1, *E*). Independent of menopausal status, these patients most often have disease that is hormone insensitive; initial chemotherapy is most often considered. Isolated reports exist of patients successfully treated with hormone therapy for liver or lymphangitic lung metastases, but such therapy is not reasonable unless patients are at high risk from complications of chemotherapy. When life-threatening disease is not present, it is convenient to categorize patients by menopausal status when considering systemic therapy. Premenopausal patients who are proven to be hormone receptor positive or who have clinical characteristics that would suggest receptor positivity should be considered for initial therapy with tamoxifen or surgical oophorectomy. If a response of significant duration occurs after such hormonal therapy, the alternate hormonal approach should be considered upon relapse (Fig. 16-1, *D*). Third-line hormonal therapy in these patients is not often used, but progestational agents, aminoglutethimide, and LHRH agonists could all be considered in selected patients. In premenopausal patients who fail to respond to hormone therapy, or who achieve short durations of response, systemic chemotherapy should be instituted.

The decision tree for postmenopausal patients with non–life threatening metastatic disease is similar to that for premenopausal patients, except that oophorectomy is not an appropriate option (Fig. 16-1, *F*). Patients known to be hormone receptor positive or who have clinical characteristics consistent with receptor positivity initially should be treated with tamoxifen therapy. If a significant response occurs on tamoxifen, or if patients relapse while receiving adjuvant tamoxifen, one of the progestational agents represents the best option for second-line therapy. Postmenopausal patients frequently have indolent tumors with high levels of estrogen receptor positivity, and therefore may respond to more than two hormones given sequentially. In these instances, aminoglutethimide or fluoxymesterone represent legitimate options. In patients without significant ovarian function, LHRH agonists are not likely to be beneficial. To patients who fail to respond to hormone therapy, or who have only transient objective responses, combination chemotherapy should be administered. There appears to be no standard role for combined chemohormonal therapy in most patients, particularly when indolent, non–life threatening disease is present.

Metastatic breast cancer is one of the most common diseases treated by oncologists. Although some patients manifest recurrent disease with predominantly solitary or local sites of metastases, the vast majority will develop widespread metastases requiring systemic management. Recognizing that palliation of symptoms is the most important consideration, the oncologist must balance the likelihood of achieving this goal against the risks of treatment. This process is greatly aided not only by the knowledge of the natural history of metastatic breast cancer, but also by the proper selection of patients for the wide variety of available therapies.

Special Complications of Metastatic Disease*

GENERAL PRINCIPLES AND MANAGEMENT OF SPECIFIC COMPLICATIONS

This section examines specific structural and metabolic complications of metastatic breast cancer. Breast cancer is capable of metastasizing to virtually any organ or site; certain sites are at relatively higher risk than others, and only the more frequently encountered complications are considered in this section. Many, but not all, of these complications present urgently or emergently, and the speed and precision of the requisite clinical assessment vary greatly among patients. The general approach to the oncologic urgency or emergency has been discussed eloquently by Glover and Glick[210]; their outline of management considerations holds true for breast cancer patients as well (see p. 421). As in any malignant disease, the diagnostic and therapeutic interventions must be applied only after careful regard for all facets of the patient's clinical, psychologic, and social situation.

Each of the special complications in this section presents with its own array of symptoms and signs, many of which overlap, rendering the complications indistinguishable from one another. Nonetheless, a detailed knowledge of each clinical syndrome provides the oncologist or internist with a factual base from which to guide his work-up. The speed or tempo with which each symptom presents is as important an indicator of need for emergent evaluation as the symptom itself. Clearly, the metastatic breast cancer patient with chronic low back pain who is neurologically intact does not require the urgent evaluation appropriate to the patient with

*The section on special complications is authored by Kevin R. Fox and Lynn M. Schuchter.

MANAGEMENT CONSIDERATIONS IN THE TREATMENT OF METASTATIC BREAST CANCER AND SPECIFIC COMPLICATIONS

1. Symptoms
2. Tempo of symptoms and disease progression
3. Natural history of specific breast cancer
   a. Interval between treatment of the primary lesion and development of metastases and/or the oncologic emergency
   b. Status of the primary and other metastatic sites
   c. End-stage disease
4. Responsiveness to available antineoplastic therapy
5. General medical condition
   a. Age
   b. Nutrition
   c. Performance status
   d. Concurrent medical problems
   e. Psychologic status
6. Goals of therapy
   a. Palliative versus curative
   b. Quality of life
   c. Objectives of the patient and family
   d. Toxicity of treatment

the subacute onset of dyspnea, or the acute onset of dysarthria. The speed with which the metastatic complication occurs relative to the original diagnosis of breast cancer is also extraordinarily important in clinical decision making. The patient who develops multiple pulmonary metastases and a solitary cerebral metastasis while receiving adjuvant chemotherapy for stage II breast cancer with 12 positive axillary nodes and negative estrogen receptors might not be a good candidate for craniotomy and resection, whereas a patient with a solitary cerebral nodule occurring 4 years after diagnosis *in the absence* of other metastatic disease who is receiving tamoxifen for a stage II, node-negative, estrogen receptor–positive breast cancer might be an appropriate candidate for surgical resection.

The concurrent or preexisting development of metastatic disease in other sites and the patient's overall disease status must be considered in the diagnostic and therapeutic maneuvers to be undertaken. The development of multiple cranial nerve abnormalities in the absence of metastatic disease in a patient with a known history of breast carcinoma should prompt an aggressive and exhaustive search for leptomeningeal carcinomatosis, while the same search would be of dubious value in a bedridden patient with multiple treated brain metastases and paraplegia from epidural metastases. The patient who is deemed to be terminally ill as a result of widespread metastatic disease may only achieve transient symptom relief from emergency intervention, with an accompanying prolongation in survival that may be meaningless.

As breast cancer stands as one of the more responsive solid tumors to systemic therapy, a patient's therapeutic history is of extraordinary importance in the decision analysis. A variety of hormonal and chemotherapeutic agents may be applied in succession and control metastatic disease for substantial periods of time. A precise knowledge of the patient's previous therapies, her response or failure to respond to these therapies, and the degree of toxicity to the patient is always required. The patient with small moderately symptomatic pleural effusions might be a candidate only for tamoxifen therapy if there is no prior history of metastatic disease and the patient's primary tumor is known to be hormone receptor positive. The patient with progressive pleural effusions (even in the absence of other metastatic disease) that have responded and then progressed in the face of multiple hormonal and chemotherapeutic treatments is probably best treated with insertion of a chest tube and pleurodesis, rather than an attempt at a third or fourth-line chemotherapeutic regimen that has little chance of working.

Naturally, the patient's general condition and factors not directly related to the cancer itself must be evaluated before any aggressive diagnostic and therapeutic plan is initiated. Age alone is a very difficult criterion on which to base these decisions. There is no convincing evidence that age-dependent differences exist in the natural history of breast cancer,[325] or that younger patients, often assumed to have inherently "more aggressive" breast cancers might in turn benefit more from aggressive therapies. Although the hematologic toxicity of chemotherapy is more pronounced in older patients and the risk of anthracycline-induced cardiotoxicity may be greater in older patients,[168] the subjective toxicities of therapy should not be assumed to be greater with increasing age.[345] The coexistence of other significant medical illnesses may be more common in older patients, and may prohibit aggressive diagnostic maneuvers, surgery, or chemotherapy. If the presence of end-stage obstructive lung disease or ischemic cardiomyopathy predict for limited survival, the treatment of site-specific metastatic cancer may be either contraindicated on toxicity grounds, or be totally irrelevant. Severe impairment of performance status or nutritional status, whether from metastatic cancer or unrelated conditions, influences prognosis and response to therapy and limits quality of life.

The final element, and perhaps the most important element, in managing urgent or emergent complications is a precise examination of the goals of therapy and the psychologic state of the patient and family with whom these goals are discussed. Metastatic breast cancer is a disease that is virtually never cured. Emergent complications demand intervention for relief of symptoms and perhaps prolongation of life, but such intervention are ultimately only palliative. Fortunately, palliative therapeutic maneuvers will occasionally beget long periods of symptom-free or disease-free survival. A thorough understanding of goals of therapy by the patient and her family will provide the greatest foundation for all subsequent clinical decisions. The patient may wish to remain optimistic, and request all possible diagnostic and therapeutic measures to maintain this optimism despite a limited likelihood of success or even short-term benefit. The physician may be required to relent and submit to the patient's demands, even if they are contrary to the best medical judgment. Conversely, a patient may deny therapeutic intervention if she deems such intervention unworthy of the short- or long-term benefit it will provide. The withholding of therapy under such circumstances may be appropriate despite a reasonable chance of palliation and improvement in quality of life.

CEREBRAL METASTASES

Metastatic disease to the brain is relatively common in patients with breast cancer. Breast cancer is probably the second most common cause of metastatic disease in the brain in all patients, after lung cancer[311,343] (Table 16-7). The actual prevalence of metastatic disease to the brain varies from series to series, with autopsy studies showing a prevalence of up to 25%,[320] while antemortem studies show an expected lower prevalence of approximately 10%.[187] Factors that may predict for a greater likelihood of developing parenchymal brain metastasis include age, the presence of concurrent metastatic disease, and the estrogen-receptor status of the primary tumor. The risk appears to be greatest in premenopausal patients or patients within 5 years of menopause,[321] and in patients with estrogen receptor–negative tumors.[326]

Table 16-7 Sites of origin of metastatic disease to brain

Tumor	No. cases: Veith and Odom[343]	Shehata et al.[311]
Lung	86 [28]	40 [49]
Breast	51 [16]	15 [18.5]
Melanoma	49 [16]	—
Unknown	44 [14]	4 [5]
Genitourinary	22 [7]	3 [4]
Other	61 [19]	19 [23.5]

[ ], % pts.

The natural history of brain metastases from breast cancer differs little, if at all, from that of other tumor types. Brain metastases are rarely the presenting manifestation of breast cancer; synchronous presentations at the time of diagnosis of the primary breast cancer are slightly more common; metachronous presentations, occurring sometime after the original diagnosis, will be found in the vast majority of patients.[204] The median time from diagnosis of the primary tumor to the development of brain metastases was approximately 1½ years in one series of patients with a variety of malignancies. Breast cancer patients typically develop metachronous cerebral metastases after a longer interval.[204] When metastases do develop, approximately half of breast cancer patients will have solitary metastases as detected by computed tomographic scanning.[313] This figure is consistent with the findings of published series in which all tumor types are considered.[289]

Presenting manifestations

Brain metastases generally present in the supratentorial cerebrum, with cerebellar metastases accounting for only 8% to 15% of all parenchymal lesions.[289,343] Brainstem metastases are uncommon. The presenting signs and symptoms in breast cancer patients do not differ from those of patients with other diseases. Symptoms are produced by actual destruction of brain tissue by carcinoma, by obstruction to CSF flow and resulting hydrocephalus, by peritumoral edema, or, rarely, by hemorrhage into the brain parenchyma. Peritumoral edema or hemorrhage may cause frontal or temporal herniation. Clinical symptoms and signs will evolve over a period of a few days to several weeks. Acute (stroke-like) symptoms other than seizures occur relatively infrequently, in <10% of patients.[287] Headache is the most common presenting symptom, occurring in 45% or more of patients.[207] These headaches are usually generalized and eventually become unremitting. Global behavioral and mental status changes occur in approximately one third of patients, although in-depth testing of cognitive and intellectual function will increase this finding to over half of patients.[288] Focal weakness is a presenting complaint in 20% to 40% of patients, and can be elicited on physical examination in two thirds.[172,207] Seizures occur in up to 20% of patients, and are more typically generalized than localized.[204,207] Physical findings other than the frequently elicited impairments of cognitive function and focal weakness are relatively uncommon. Aphasia and gait ataxia occur in less than one fifth of patients, while papilledema, which is associated with a sustained increase in intracranial pressure, is found in only 15% to 25% of patients at presentation.[204,286] Other manifestations of elevated intracranial pressure may include somnolence, nausea, vomiting, and disturbances in pulse or blood pressure.

Diagnostic work-up

When symptoms or signs of cerebral metastasis are present, the computed tomographic scan of the head or magnetic-resonance imaging scan remain the diagnostic procedures of choice. Until detailed comparative studies of CT and MRI are done to establish the superiority of one modality over the other, the contrast-enhanced CT scan of the head remains the preferred procedure. Either or both of these modalities will aid in excluding nonmetastatic causes of neurologic dysfunction, including cerebrovascular accidents, dural hemorrhages, abscesses, or primary brain tumors. Smith et al.[319] have described an unusual association between breast cancer and meningioma, the latter a relatively common cerebral neoplasm most often found in middle-aged females. If meningioma is suspected on the basis of location, high CT scan density, and relative paucity of peritumoral edema, arteriography may be an invaluable diagnostic step in distinguishing this tumor from metastatic breast cancer.[207] Such a distinction is of particular importance as approximately half of breast cancer brain metastases are solitary, and because cerebral metastasis may be the sole manifestation of metastatic disease in as many as 16% of patients.[313]

Cerebral metastases from breast cancer will have a low-density appearance on precontrast scans in approximately three fourths of patients, with high-density lesions or calcifications appearing much less frequently.[313] After contrast administration, virtually all lesions will demonstrate contrast enhancement, including those that were originally hyperdense.

The relative superiority of CT scanning vs. MRI remains to be worked out. The merits of MRI scanning include the potential for greater sensitivity using gadolinium enhancement and superior visualization of the brainstem and cerebellum. When the diagnosis remains in doubt, neurosurgical exploration may be required to confirm the diagnosis. Fine-needle aspiration of deep-seated lesions may be used under circumstances where the morbidity of neurosurgical exploration would be prohibitive.[315]

Treatment

The primary goals of treatment of cerebral metastases are relief of symptoms and improvement or preservation of neurologic function translating into improved quality of life. The use of corticosteroids, radiation therapy with or without surgery, chemotherapy, and anticonvulsants plays a significant role in management, and each is discussed separately.

Steroids, in the form of dexamethasone, methylprednisolone, or prednisone act by reducing peritumoral edema via mechanisms that are poorly understood. The primary role of steroids is symptom relief, and between 60% and 80% of patients will obtain prompt and occasionally complete symptomatic relief with steroid administration.[285,350,358] Focal neurologic signs will respond less well to steroid therapy. The accepted dose of corticosteroid is equivalent to at least 16 mg/day of dexamethasone in four divided doses,[350] with some experts recommending a loading dose of 10 mg.[207] As a substantial minority of patients fail to respond to steroids at these doses; the use of higher doses of up to 100 mg/day of dexamethasone is justified.[189] Should neurologic status deteriorate rapidly despite steroid therapy or before steroid therapy has time to be effective (usually 6 hours to 2 days), intravenous infusions of mannitol or glycerol, hyperventilation, or emergency craniotomy may be required (these are discussed elsewhere).[210,356]

As steroids are of little value as cytolytics in breast cancer, an antitumor effect of steroids alone should not be anticipated, and significant prolongation of survival will not result without institution of appropriate therapy.[174] Radiation therapy remains the mainstay of treatment of all patients except those in whom uncontrolled systemic metastases preclude meaningful quality of life. The optimum dosing scheme and schedule of treatment has been the subject of much scrutiny. A series of clinical trials conducted by the Radiation Therapy Oncology Group (RTOG) stand as the best reference studies from which an optimum dose and schedule can be gleaned. The initial study compared four treatment programs: 30 Gy in 2 weeks or 3 weeks, and 40 Gy in 3 weeks or 4 weeks.[166] No significant differences in response or survival were noted, and a randomized trial to evaluate shorter treatment schedules was undertaken. In this second trial, intensified dosing schemes of 20 Gy in a week or 12 Gy in 2 days were compared to the more conventional schemes of 30 Gy in 2 weeks or 40 Gy in 3 weeks. The lower dosing schemes were generally inferior with respect to the rapidity and duration of response.[166] Despite other reports that demonstrate the effectiveness of single, high-dose fractions,[229] the administration of 30 Gy over a 2-week period remains the standard therapy for breast cancer patients.[210,356] The issue of retreatment at the time of relapse of neurologic symptoms is a difficult one, as no standards of care exist. A single study by Kurup et al.[249] provides some fairly compelling data. In this study, 15 breast cancer patients were represented in a group of 56 patients all of whom were retreated with doses of 5 to 46 Gy over periods of 1 day to 4 weeks. Clinical responses were seen in 75% of the group, with responses of >6 months duration in four patients. Most patients, however, responded for periods of <3 months, and median survival for the responding group was 3.5 months. Complications such as brain necrosis and leukoencephalopathy were not reported. Older studies confirm the utility of single retreatment doses of 10 Gy in eliciting clinical responses in the majority of patients.[311] It seems reasonable to retreat patients, on the basis of this data, if other systemic metastases are well controlled, and if a transient but legitimate improvement in quality of life is desirable.

The role of surgery in the treatment of brain metastases remains controversial, although a wealth of nonrandomized data exists. Most analyses make retrospective comparison of survival data in surgically treated patients to that of patients treated with radiotherapy alone. Some of these studies do show some survival advantage in the surgically treated group, while others do not, including a recent review of the neurosurgical experience at the Memorial Sloan-Kettering Cancer Center.[204] Any comparison of this type is obviously and automatically flawed in that the selection criteria are probably quite different for the surgical group. Most of these patients had solitary metastases, and one must assume that their overall physical and neurologic condition was superior to the group receiving radiotherapy alone.

In 1990 Patchell et al. at the University of Kentucky published results of the first randomized trial of surgery plus radiotherapy vs. radiotherapy alone for patients with solitary brain metastases.[278] In this trial 48 patients (37 of whom had primary lung cancer) were randomized to undergo resection followed by 36 Gy of whole-brain radiotherapy vs. stereotaxic needle biopsy followed by the same dose of radiation. Patients were required to be capable of independent self-care, have surgically accessible lesions, and not be in need of emergency therapy to prevent neurologic deterioration. Patients with radiosensitive tumors (small-cell lung cancer, myeloma, lymphoma, leukemia, and germ-cell tumors) were excluded. All patients underwent both computed tomographic and magnetic resonance imaging of the brain to exclude multiple metastases preoperatively. Overall survival was superior for the surgically treated group (40 weeks median vs. 15 weeks median).

The local recurrence rate of tumor in the primary tumor bed also was reduced significantly (20% vs. 52%), while the median length of time from treatment to the recurrence of the original tumor was increased (>59 weeks vs. 21 weeks). No difference in the rate of occurrence of metastases elsewhere in the brain was noted. The incidence of deaths from systemic disease rather than brain metastases was considered: 71% of the surgically treated group and 50% of the radiation-treated group died of systemic illness. This difference was not significant. Maintenance of an independent level of self-care was also greater for the surgically treated group (38 weeks vs. 8 weeks). The patient results of this study are summarized in Table 16-8.

This study redefines the criteria for surgical intervention in patients with brain metastases (see p. 425). There is little argument that surgery should be undertaken if there is any level of diagnostic uncertainty. When Posner reviewed autopsy findings in a series of patients treated preoperatively

Table 16-8 Results of the University of Kentucky study comparing surgery plus radiotherapy to radiotherapy alone in solitary metastasis to the brain

	Surgery and radiotherapy (n = 25)	Radiotherapy alone (n = 23)
Overall survival duration	40 weeks	15 weeks (p<.01)
Rate of local recurrence	20%	52% (p<.02)
Time to local recurrence	>59 weeks (n = 5)	21 weeks (n = 12)
Rate of death from systemic illness	71%	50% (p = .26)
Duration maintaining independent quality of life	38 weeks	8 weeks (p<.005)

From Patchell et al: N Engl J Med 322:494, 1990.

CRITERIA FOR CONSIDERATION OF SURGICAL RESECTION OF CEREBRAL METASTASIS IN BREAST CANCER PATIENTS

1. Diagnostic uncertainty
   a. Meningioma
   b. Possibility of benign disease
2. Treatment of acute complications
   a. Hemorrhage
   b. CSF obstruction
   c. Rapid deterioration of neurologic status
3. Radioresistant tumor producing symptoms
4. Solitary metastasis, providing the following conditions are met
   a. Ambulatory performance status
   b. Surgically accessible lesion in noncritical location
   c. Control of systemic metastatic disease

with radiation therapy for cerebral metastatic disease, over one third of the patients had an erroneous premorbid diagnosis.[285] In the University of Kentucky series, six of the original 54 randomized patients (11%) proved to have nonmetastatic disease.[278] Patients who have acute complications with rapid neurologic deterioration may be considered for surgical resection. Patients who fail to respond to radiotherapy or who progress with surgically resectable disease may achieve additional survival with resection.[278] The data in Table 16-8 suggest that a population of patients clearly exists in whom surgical resection of solitary metastases is appropriate. Optimum medical care requires that the fairly rigid selection criteria of Patchell et al.[278] be applied. This rigorous selection probably excludes a substantial number of patients with solitary metastasis, although the precise frequency of exclusion is unclear.

Systemic chemotherapy is clearly capable of producing clinical responses in patients with cerebral metastases. The relative impenetrability of the blood brain barrier to chemotherapeutic agents seems to be altered by the presence of malignant lesions in the brain parenchyma. Rosner et al.[303] treated 66 breast cancer patients who had brain metastases but had not received primary radiotherapy. Patients received a variety of chemotherapeutic regimens, all of which contained some combination of Cytoxan, methotrexate, 5-fluorouracil, vincristine, and prednisone. Thirty-four of 66 patients demonstrated a radiographic response, with a median survival time of 13 months for responders and 3 months for nonresponders. Although these results are intriguing, the role of chemotherapy in the treatment of cerebral metastases is unclear and cannot be considered part of standard management at this time.

The use of anticonvulsant therapy is relatively straightforward. The prophylactic use of anticonvulsant medication is not recommended for seizure-free patients,[180,207] as the duration of action of dexamethasone may be decreased by the concurrent use of diphenylhydantoin,[175,222,286] and as one retrospective analysis showed no reduction in the incidence of seizure activity.[180] When seizures do occur, diphenylhydantoin remains the drug of choice in doses necessary to maintain a steady blood level of 10 to 20 μg/ml (usually 300 to 400 mg/day).

Impact on functional survival

The essential role of treatment of cerebral metastases is the improvement or preservation of neurologic function and maintenance of an acceptable quality of life.

Radiation therapy will partially relieve symptoms in most patients (69% to 86% in the RTOG studies), and will produce complete resolution of symptoms in one third to two thirds.[166] Despite these improvements, the prognosis is dismal, with up to half of treated patients ultimately dying within a few months of recurrent cerebral metastases, and the remainder from complications of systemic malignant disease.[166,278]

The potential for survival of breast cancer patients deserves particular mention. Two recent reviews of surgical series demonstrate that breast cancer patients have a longer survival relative to patients with other tumor types, with a median survival of 13 months in one series[205] and 14 months in another,[354] with the latter showing a 2-year survival of 48%. The time between the diagnosis of the primary lesion and the subsequent development of brain metastasis is significant. Several studies demonstrate a longer survival for patients with longer intervals between primary diagnosis and brain metastasis,[202,278,334] and that patients with breast cancer tend to have relatively long intervals until the diagnosis of brain metastasis is rendered.[278,334] When compared to other tumor types this information does not imply that breast cancer patients with brain metastases have a uniquely superior prognosis, but it simply reinforces the notion that long-term survival is a possibility in selected patients, and a thoughtful approach to treatment in light of potential gains should remain the standard of care.

CARCINOMATOUS MENINGITIS

Carcinomatous meningitis, or leptomeningeal carcinomatosis, occurs when malignant cells seed the

Table 16-9 Solid tumors associated with leptomeningeal carcinomatosis

	% pts.		
	Wasserstrom et al.[349] **(n = 90)**	**Spiers et al.**[322] **(n = 45)**	**Theodore and Gendelman**[336] **(n = 33)**
Breast	51	58	64
Lung	25	29	15
Melanoma	12		15
Genitourinary	6	4	
Other	6	9	6

leptomeningeal membranes anywhere along the craniospinal neuraxis and produce a broad spectrum of neurologic symptoms and signs. This remains a relatively uncommon condition, occurring in approximately 10% of breast cancer patients at autopsy[359]; the incidence of the diagnosis antemortem may be somewhat lower.[233] Most experts agree that the incidence of carcinomatous meningitis is increasing, owing presumably to superior systemic therapies that are incapable of treating the CSF space adequately.[210,270,349,359] A sound working knowledge of the natural history of this complication is essential in breast cancer patients for two reasons. First, most published series suggest that breast cancer is the most common cause of carcinomatous meningitis in adults (see Table 16-9). Second, the series of Yap et al.[359] emphasizes the occurrence of carcinomatous meningitis as the sole manifestation of metastatic disease in 16% of patients in whom the diagnosis was ultimately rendered. Furthermore, 30% of the entire group had control of systemic metastatic disease at the time of diagnosis of meningitis. The variety of successful systemic cytotoxic and hormonal therapies at our disposal for treating breast cancer increases the likelihood that this condition will become more prevalent in the future.

Carcinomatous meningitis may develop by a number of mechanisms, some or all of which might conceivably occur in any given patient. Direct hematogenous spread via arachnoid vessels has been demonstrated in leukemia,[294] and provides the most logical mechanism in most patients. Other mechanisms include hematogenous spread to the choroid plexus and dissemination into the CSF,[215] direct invasion of the CSF space by expanding cerebral parenchymal metastases,[349] or perineural invasion retrograde into the spinal CSF space by paravertebral tumor masses.[218] All of those mechanisms emphasize the inadequacy of systemic chemotherapy in sterilizing malignant cells in the CSF space. Whatever the mechanism the malignant cells will progress in a thin and widespread layer or will grow in a nodular pattern that may be multifocal and interrupted by regions of normal leptomeningeal membrane.[349] The complexity of symptoms and signs that arise from such an unpredictable pathologic process is not surprising.

The extensive clinical study by Wasserstrom et al. in 1982[349] remains the central reference work in any discussion of carcinomatous meningitis. Glover and Glick[210] have combined the presenting symptoms and signs in three of the larger clinical studies,[272,349,359] including those of Wasserstrom et al. and the series of Yap et al.,[359] the latter study confined to patients with breast cancer.

These findings are summarized in Tables 16-10 to 16-12 according to the presumed site of meningeal pathology: cerebrum, cranial nerve, or spine. Several conclusions may be drawn from these figures. First, the variety of possible presenting symptoms and signs is substantial, and reinforces the well-known clinical axiom that "the clinical diagnosis of meningeal carcinomatosis rests upon the finding of neurologic signs and symptoms at more than one level of the neuraxis."[349] Second, a relative comparison of symptoms vs. signs suggests that clinical findings equal or exceed symptoms at presentation, particularly in those patients with spinal cord manifestations. No particular region appears to predominate in any series, and according to Wasserstrom et al.[349] only 17 of 90 patients presented with symptoms or signs in a single area of the neuraxis. Headaches, lower extremity weakness and paresthesias, and complaints referable to cranial nerve dysfunction (diplopia, hearing loss, visual loss, and facial numbness) appear to be the most common initial complaints. Classic signs of meningeal irritation (nuchal rigidity and back pain on straight-leg raising) appear to be uncommon, presenting in 8% and 12% of cases in one series of 90 patients.[349] Seizures and papilledema were also relatively uncommon in this series (fewer than 6% of patients at presentation, although papilledema was reported in over 20% of patients in one smaller series).[336]

Table 16-10 Frequency of cerebral symptoms and signs in patients with carcinomatous meningitis

	Frequency (%)
Symptoms	
Headache	38-52
Change in mental status	17-48
Persistent nausea or vomiting	8-14
Dizziness or lightheadedness	12-16
Transient loss of consciousness	3-6
Aphasia	2
Diabetes insipidus	2
Signs	
Abnormal mental status examination	31-56
Positive Babinski sign	32-50
Papilledema	6-20
Ataxic gait	13
Hemiparesis	2

Derived from Glover and Glick,[210] compiled from Wasserstrom et al.,[349] Yap et al.,[359] and Olsen et al.[272]

Table 16-11 Frequency of cranial nerve dysfunction in patients with carcinomatous meningitis at presentation

	Frequency (%)
Symptoms	
Diplopia	8-24
Hearing loss	6-24
Facial numbness	6
Decreased visual acuity	6-36
Blindness	3
Dysarthria	0-8
Loss of taste	3
Tinnitus	2-8
Hoarseness	2
Dysphagia	2
Vertigo	1-2
Signs	
Ocular muscle paresis	20-46
Facial weakness	17-42
Hearing loss	10-30
Visual loss—optic neuritis	2-6
Trigeminal neuropathy	6-12
Hypoglossal neuropathy	6-8
Blindness	0-4
Decreased gag reflex	4-16

Derived from Glover and Glick,[210] compiled from Wasserstrom et al.,[349] Yap et al.,[359] and Olsen et al.[272]

The diagnosis of carcinomatous meningitis rests on the evaluation of the CSF in any patient whose complaints and/or physical findings arouse suspicion. In one series, 97% of patients had some abnormality in the CSF on first examination,[349] another series detected abnormalities in 85%.[336] Expected abnormalities include an increased opening pressure, elevated protein levels, decreased glucose levels, pleocytosis consisting primarily of lymphocytes, and positive cytologic examination for malignant cells. Table 16-13 summarizes the findings of Wasserstrom et al.[349] and emphasizes one crucial point in the diagnostic work-up. In this series, despite the almost uniform finding of some chemical, cellular, or hydrostatic abnormality on initial CSF examination, a firm diagnosis of malignancy could only be made on cytologic grounds in 54% of patients. A second lumbar puncture increased the cytologic yield to 84%; two additional patients eventually yielded a positive CSF after three and seven lumbar punctures. The value of repeated lumbar punctures in optimizing the diagnostic yield has been observed by others and is clearly the standard of diagnosis.[248,272,336,349]

Although a positive CSF cytology is the quintessential requirement in making the diagnosis of carcinomatous meningitis, the fact remains that a minority of patients never demonstrate evidence of malignant cells despite repeated lumbar punctures. These patients represent <10% of the total in most series, but pose a significant diagnostic and therapeutic dilemma. Several explanations may ac-

Table 16-12 Frequency of spinal cord symptoms and signs in patients with carcinomatous meningitis

	Frequency (%)
Symptoms	
Weakness	33
Paresthesias	31
Back pain	25
Radicular pain	19
Bowel/Bladder dysfunction	13
Signs	
Reflex asymmetry	67
Weakness	64
Cauda equina syndrome	33
Sensory loss	31
Straight-leg raising	13
Decreased rectal tone	12
Nuchal rigidity	11

Derived from Glover and Glick,[210] compiled from Wasserstrom et al.,[349] Yap et al.,[359] and Olsen et al.[274]

Table 16-13 CSF findings in patients with leptomeningeal metastases from solid tumors (n = 90)

Finding	No. pts. Initial finding	Subsequent finding
Pressure >160 mm CSF	45	64
Cells >5 mm^3	51	65
Protein >50 mg/dl	73	80
Glucose <40 mg/dl	28	37
Positive cytology	49	82
Normal	3	1

From Wasserstrom WR et al: Cancer 49:759, 1982.

count for the failure of lumbar puncture to reveal malignant cells. First, it is presumed that tumor deposits in some patients will be strongly adherent to the meninges, and will never shed cells into the CSF proper. Second, malignant cells may fail to reach the lumbar region because of disturbances of flow in a craniocaudal fashion. Grossman et al.,[219] using ^{111}Indium-DTPA flow scans, established a significant incidence of impairment of flow from the ventricles to the spinal canal, either by ventricular outlet obstruction (4 of 27 patients) or spinal canal obstruction (7 of 27 patients). All patients who demonstrated spinal canal obstruction had concurrent evidence of epidural cord compression by myelography. These findings explain the ability to diagnose carcinomatous meningitis by ventricular or cisternal tap in some patients with a negative lumbar puncture, as demonstrated in four patients by Wasserstrom et al.[349] Murray et al.[269] confirmed the potential and sometimes marked disparity between CSF findings in the ventricles and lumbar spaces, even in the absence of spinal epidural block. Clearly, cisternal puncture should be considered when the lumbar puncture yields no diagnosis and clinical suspicion is high.

Alternative methods may increase the index of suspicion when cytologic examination is negative. Wasserstrom et al.[349] evaluated a variety of biochemical markers in a limited number of patients in their series. Seventeen breast cancer patients had levels of carcinoembryogenic antigen (CEA) or β-glucuronidase in the CSF. Thirteen patients had β-glucuronidase levels elevated above 80 mu/L, while 10 of 17 had elevation of the CEA above 1 μg/ml with a concurrent serum level of <100 ng/ml. Abnormal LDH-isoenzyme patterns (LDH 5/LDH 1 >15%) were noted in 9 of 12 breast cancer patients. The true diagnostic value of these tumor markers has not been firmly established and should, if abnormal, provoke a more diligent search for evidence of meningeal carcinoma rather than be taken as an indication for treatment.

The value of radiologic evaluation with computed tomography of the head, myelography, or MRI scanning as an adjunct to CSF analysis or as a diagnostic test in a cytologically negative patient is controversial. Patients with suspected or established carcinomatous meningitis should undergo CT scanning of the brain, as cerebral metastases will coexist with meningitis in as many as one fourth of patients.[349] In addition, several characteristic CT scan findings have been described in patients with documented carcinomatous meningitis, and may therefore strengthen the diagnosis when the CSF is negative. These findings include hydrocephalus, enhancement of the basal cisterns, enhancement of the cortical sulci, and enhancement of the tentorium, and they may be present in more than a third of patients.[242,250,349] The high incidence of hydrocephalus in these analyses raises the question of whether the CT scan should be performed before or after lumbar puncture in patients with suspected carcinomatous meningitis. Given the relative ease and negligible morbidity of brain CT scanning and the uncertain risk of the lumbar puncture in hydroencephalus, recent recommendations suggest that the CT scan should be performed first.[208]

Myelography is also of considerable importance in the initial evaluation of these patients. Like CT scanning of the brain, myelograms are abnormal in substantial numbers of patients. In one series[349] myelograms were abnormal in 27 of 49 patients, with 13 patients showing unique features of irregular subarachnoid filling resulting from thickening and nodularity of nerve roots. It is plausible to consider this unique myelographic change sufficient evidence of meningeal involvement by carcinoma if cytologic examination of the CSF remains normal. The value of spinal MRI scanning purely as a diagnostic aid is uncertain. A more compelling indication for myelography is the detection of epidural metastases. Fourteen of 49 patients in one series had myelographic evidence of epidural metastasis on initial evaluation.[349] It seems prudent to perform myelography (or spinal MRI scanning) as part of the initial evaluation in any patient who manifests signs or symptoms of spinal involvement,[212,349] even without frank evidence of spinal cord compression. Here, the relative value of MRI scanning vs. myelography is emerging, and will be discussed in the next section.

The treatment of carcinomatous meningitis is relatively straightforward. Some combination of radiation therapy and/or chemotherapy, with or without the use of steroids, is recommended. Radiation therapy, while not appropriate for every patient, is typically given to the whole brain if cerebral symptoms occur, to the base of the skull if cranial nerve symptoms occur, and to selected areas of the spinal cord that correlate with clinical symptoms and signs.[208,210,349] Irradiation to the entire spine is probably unwise because of excessive exposure to a significant amount of bone marrow; this accentuates the need for myelographic or MRI imaging in patients with spinal symptoms or signs so that appropriate radiation portals can be devised. Some authors[208] do not treat the base of skull selectively, but will treat the entire brain and skull base even if cranial nerve signs are the sole manifestation of disease. The doses to the whole brain (and skull base) are consistent with those used to treat brain metastases (≤30 Gy over 2 weeks), while the doses to the spine are sometimes higher (≤40 Gy).

Although radiotherapy may be the most effective means of palliation of symptoms if localized symptoms are present, the diffuse nature of carcinomatous meningitis usually requires some form of "systemic" therapy. Unfortunately, conventional chemotherapeutic agents at standard doses will not attain cytocidal concentrations in the CSF. This requires direct installation of chemotherapy into the CSF, either by lumbar puncture or, preferably, via an intraventricular (Ommaya) reservoir.[273] This subcutaneous device typically is inserted through a burr hole into the frontal horn of one of the lateral ventricles, this is done with an almost negligible complication rate.[201,271]

Intraventricular chemotherapy administration has several practical and theoretical advantages over lumbar chemotherapy. It is technically simpler, virtually painless for patients, and ensures (in the absence of abnormal CSF flow) distribution of the drug evenly in a craniocaudal direction in concentrations that are cytotoxic.[162,310] Methotrexate is the drug used most frequently in the intraventricular treatment of carcinomatous meningitis. Cytosine arabinoside and thiotepa have been used as well, but to a lesser extent in published series. Combinations of methotrexate and thiotepa have been used with considerable success in small series of patients,[341] but a prospective, randomized trial of methotrexate vs. methotrexate and cytosine arabinoside showed no advantage to the combination.[236] A combination of all three drugs appeared to produce unacceptable hematologic toxicity in a group of 22 patients treated at Vanderbilt University.[205] The treatment paradigm of Wasserstrom et al.[349] using methotrexate alone represents the most widely accepted approach to treatment with intraventricular chemotherapy.[208,210] Methotrexate in doses of 7 mg/m^2 (standard total dose 12 to 15 mg) is given twice weekly for five doses, or longer, until clinical improvement or stabilization is evident and evidence of a clearing of malignant cells is seen. Chemotherapy was instilled weekly thereafter, and if continued improvement or stabilization was seen, the interval between injections was lengthened up to 4 weeks. Therapy was continued until the time of relapse, and several patients were treated for over a year. Patients who fail to respond within the first several weeks should be considered for treatment with alternate drugs; chances for success are uncertain but should probably be small under these circumstances. Each dose of methotrexate should be accompanied by oral leukovorin calcium (approximately 10 mg) at 6-hour intervals for two to six doses after each treatment. Standard doses of alternate agents are 10 to 15 mg for thiotepa and 30 to 100 mg for cytosine arabinoside.

Results of treatment, toxicity, and survival expectations

Carcinomatous meningitis is an incurable condition, and treatment should be directed at the relief of symptoms, stabilization or improvement of neurologic deficits, and prolongation of life. Survival without therapy is limited, generally only 1 to 3 months. Although transient clinical responses may be observed with steroids alone, significant neurologic remission should not be expected.[336] The use of intrathecal methotrexate clearly induces clinical responses and stabilizes or improves neurologic symptoms in the majority of breast cancer patients (Table 16-14). A consistent survival advantage has been demonstrated in responders vs. nonresponders, with occasional long-term survival.[336,349,358] In the series of Wasserstrom et al.[349] breast cancer patients had the longest survival and highest response rate of patients with all major tumor types. Fifteen percent of the breast cancer patients survived for more than a year. In the series of Yap et al.,[358] which examined only breast cancer patients, five patients survived beyond 48 weeks, with one patient alive at 70 weeks of follow-up. Nonresponding patients had a median survival of 4 weeks in this series.

Relapse of leptomeningeal disease, although inevitable, does not necessarily account for the death of patients if other systemic disease is uncontrolled. In one series, only 43% of patients who died had death ascribed solely to neurologic causes; systemic disease accounted for death in 22%, and some combination of neurologic and systemic disease in 20%.[349] In the series of Yap et al., recurrent neurologic disease was accountable for death in 70% of patients with breast cancer, while 30% were in neurologic remission at the time of death.[358]

The toxicity of intrathecal chemotherapy (with or without radiotherapy) is usually modest but must

Table 16-14 Response rates and survival in breast cancer patients with carcinomatous meningitis treated with intrathecal methotrexate with or without radiotherapy

	Wasserstrom et al.[349]	Yap et al.[359]	Theodore and Gendelman[336]
Response or stabilization	28/46 (61%)	27/39 (67%)	8/11 (73%)
Median survival in months for responders	7.2 (range: 1-29)	6 (range: 1-70+ weeks)	7 (range: NS)

be understood thoroughly by the practitioner. The acute effects of intraventricular or intrathecal administration appear in a minority of patients. An acute meningoencephalopathy characterized by fever, confusion, disorientation, and nuchal rigidity occurred in 9 of 90 patients treated with methotrexate one series.[349] This phenomenon was not necessarily accompanied by changes in the cell count or protein content of the CSF, it resolved within 72 hours, and it never recurred, despite subsequent treatment with the same drug. In the series of Hitchins et al.,[236] 8 of 22 patients developed nausea and vomiting, and four cases of bacterial meningitis occurred. Systemic toxicities of methotrexate (pancytopenia, mucositis) occur infrequently, probably owing to the concurrent administration of leukovorin calcium, but deaths from infection and marrow suppression have been reported in the absence of other possible causes.[336,349]

The chronic effects of intrathecal or intraventricular methotrexate administration are usually irrelevant in these patients because of their short-term survival in most cases. However, as long-term survival does occur in occasional breast cancer patients, these toxicities must likewise be appreciated. Wasserstrom et al.[349] reported four cases of leukoencephalopathy, characterized in three patients by diminished cognitive function. Each of these patients had survived for >6 months, had received more than 140 mg of intrathecal methotrexate, and had received whole-brain radiotherapy. This condition is presumed to be very uncommon in patients receiving intrathecal chemotherapy alone, but may be more likely in patients receiving concurrent systemic methotrexate for metastatic disease.[161] This complication is felt to be reversible with cessation of methotrexate therapy.

We should expect no diminution in the incidence of carcinomatous meningitis over the next decades as our systemic therapies for breast cancer continue to improve. Our present treatments for this dire metastatic complication are inadequate, but do have an impact on the well-being of most patients, if only for short periods of time. There is no role for prophylactic CNS therapy in breast cancer patients, nor are there prognostic factors that allow us to identify patients at highest risk for leptomeningeal disease. Until superior therapies are identified, patients will derive the greatest benefit from thorough pretreatment evaluation, both medical and psychologic, and the judicious application of available therapies.

SPINAL CORD COMPRESSION

Spinal cord compression occurs when tumor invades the epidural or intradural space, causing pressure on and/or ischemic injury to the spinal cord or nerve roots. It is a relatively uncommon but well-recognized clinical phenomenon in cancer patients. Epidural (and very rarely intradural) metastases are recognized in approximately 5% of cancer patients[152]; the true incidence of spinal cord compression in breast cancer is not known. Whereas brain metastases and carcinomatous meningitis are dire complications of metastatic disease and may occasionally present with rapid neurologic deterioration, the finding of cord compression in any patient with breast cancer constitutes a true medical emergency. Preservation of neurologic function is always greatest when the patient is ambulatory with minimal to absent neurologic dysfunction; this fact alone provides a compelling reason for swift and accurate diagnostic and therapeutic action in any patient with epidural metastatic disease.

The contribution of breast cancer to this clinical problem in oncology has been reviewed exhaustively by Stillman and Foley.[327] In their analysis of nine studies ranging from 1959 to 1983 and covering more than 2000 patients, between 9% and 28% of cases were caused by breast cancer; only carcinoma of the lung accounted for as many or more cases on a consistent basis. The relative frequency of this problem in breast cancer is not surprising, given the frequency of bony involvement in patients with metastatic breast cancer, a figure that may be as high as 61% in one study of the vertebral column alone.[193] This correlation presumes that spinal cord compression in breast cancer patients will occur by what is presumed to be the most common pathophysiologic mechanism: tumor originating in the vertebral body or neural arch will extend into the spinal canal and press against the dural sac, resulting in cord compression. Other mechanisms are probably less important in breast cancer: tumor may reach the epidural space by direct hematogenous spread, may seed directly from meningeal deposits, or may invade the neural foramina directly from adjacent (paravertebral) masses. The most common site of epidural cord compression in all oncology patients is the thoracic spine (70%),[160,170,210] and this is probably no different in breast cancer, with the lumbar spine accounting for most of the remaining sites of disease (20%).[160,210,323,327]

The clinical presentation of spinal cord compression will involve a variety of signs and symptoms that may be present for months before the diagnosis is rendered. Gilbert et al.[206] describe the extraordinary variability in duration of presenting symptoms. In their series of 130 patients, the median duration of symptoms was 2 months, with a range of 5 days to 2 years before diagnosis. In one series of patients with breast cancer the duration of symptoms before diagnosis was approximately 2 months.[178] Spinal cord compression theoretically may be the first presentation of metastatic disease; however, in the series of Gilbert et al.,[206] of the 8% of patients who presented in this fashion, none had breast cancer. The remarkable latency period that may occur between primary diagnosis and cord compression in breast cancer is illustrated in the same series; of 28 patients with breast cancer, 3 developed epidural metastatic disease at 12, 14, and 19 years after diagnosis and treatment of the primary lesion.

The presenting signs and symptoms in the 130 patients reported by Gilbert et al. are summarized in Table 16-15. Pain is the most reliable presenting symptom of cord compression, and has been consistently present in over 85% of patients in clinical series for the last 30 years.[160,170,206,210,340] The pain may be localized or radicular, the latter predominantly in the lumbar or cervical regions. Many authors describe the pain as slowly progressive and likely to increase with maneuvers such as coughing, sneezing, straining, or movement. Recumbency tends to aggravate the pain, a feature that is most helpful in distinguishing the back pain of benign (disc) origin. In one series the localization of the pain correlated strongly with the eventual myelographic site of epidural disease. Most patients, however, will develop additional symptoms and signs by the time the diagnosis is rendered; only 12 of 130 patients (9%) in this series continued to have pain exclusively during the prodromal period.[206]

Weakness either as a subjective complaint or an objective finding was rarely the only presenting complaint, but was present in over 75% of patients at the time of diagnosis. Neurologic examination elicited weakness in a larger majority (87%).[206] Of the small but significant number of patients who presented with frank paraplegia (14% of 126); all had pain as a presenting symptom (i.e., none experienced paraplegia in the absence of pain).

Sensory disturbances, defined as either subjective sensory change (numbness, paresthesia) or objective findings on neurologic examination were present in 51% and 78% of patients at diagnosis, respectively, in this series, but these were never isolated presenting complaints. Anatomic dysfunction, defined as subjective dysfunction of bowel or bladder, were likewise never an isolated presenting complaint, but were reported in over half of patients. In its most dramatic form the patients developed the rapid onset of urinary retention and obstipation. Subtler complaints of nocturia, hesitancy, and urgency incontinence should not be ignored, however.

The range of differential diagnostic possibilities is broad in the cancer patient with back, neck, or interscapular pain or weakness, with or without neurologic signs. Benign disc disease with or without spinal stenosis, paraneoplastic syndromes (Eaton-Lambert syndrome), vertebral collapse from

Table 16-15 Signs and symptoms at diagnosis in 130 patients with spinal cord compression as reported by Gilbert et al.[206]

Symptoms or sign	No. pts. with symptom or sign at diagnosis	No. pts. with only this symptom as initial complaint
Pain	125 [96]	125 [96]
Subjective weakness	99 [76]	2 [2]
Objective weakness	113 [87]	
Subjective sensory change	66 [51]	0
Objective sensory change	101 [78]	
Bowel/Bladder dysfunction	74 [57]	0

[ ], % pts.

osteoporosis, paraspinous abscess, radiation myelopathy (including the Lhermitte syndrome), herpes zoster, brachial plexopathy, spinal cord ischemia, or epidural hematoma may all present in a fashion indistinguishable from epidural metastasis and spinal cord compression. Thorough diagnostic evaluation rarely should fail to detect these conditions.

Diagnostic evaluation

When epidural metastasis is expected, the work-up should proceed in a precise and efficient manner. A thorough physical and neurologic examination occasionally discloses findings that heighten suspicion but should never, if normal, completely deter some radiologic work-up. Obviously, frank extremity weakness or the detection of a sensory "level" of dysfunction reinforces the need for further evaluation. When the patient complains of pain, various maneuvers such as neck flexion, back percussion, or straight-leg raising may augment the pain and aid in localization of the potential epidural lesion. Spasticity in the absence of frank weakness and disturbances in the deep tendon reflexes may be the only signs of impending cord compression. The examiner must remember that deep tendon reflexes may be diminished or absent in a lesion involving the cauda equina, while these reflexes may be abnormally brisk in a true cord lesion. However, an acute compression of the lumbar spine may produce decreased reflexes, and predominant nerve root involvement of the lumbar cord may do the same.

If suspicion remains high at this point, it is entirely appropriate to begin dexamethasone therapy as the work-up continues. If the work-up ultimately proves to be negative for spinal cord compression and has been carried out expeditiously, then the patient's exposure to unnecessary corticosteroid will be negligible, with nominal risk of toxicity. The conventional steroid dose is similar to that used in the treatment of brain metastases, using 4 mg every 6 hours,[350] with some authorities using a 10-mg intravenous loading dose.[302] Higher doses of steroids in the range of 100 mg/day of dexamethasone have been used in prospective fashion, but have not resulted in a dramatic change in outcome.[217] The impact of steroids on neurologic outcome is unknown, but their prompt use is of unquestioned value in reversing neurologic progression and relieving pain.[217,290,350]

The value of plain radiographs of the spine in patients with suspected spinal cord compression is considerable, and abnormalities on plain radiographs have been demonstrated in over two thirds of patients who ultimately were diagnosed with spinal cord compression. This incidence actually may be higher in patients with breast cancer.[228] In an important prospective study of plain radiographs in aiding the diagnosis of cord compression, Rodichok et al.[301] demonstrated a high correlation between plain film abnormalities and the eventual diagnosis of epidural lesion by myelogram (Table 16-16). Plain x-ray abnormalities suggestive of metastatic disease predicted epidural cord compression in over 80% of patients. The predictive value was as high as 68% in patients with pain, but without neurologic findings. In 18 patients with normal x-rays but with neurologic findings, myelograms were positive in four patients. The negative plain x-ray–positive myelogram sequence did not occur in 10 patients without neurologic findings in this study. These data suggest that further work-up (see below) *is* indicated in any patient with a known malignancy and back pain or neurologic complaints *if* the plain films are abnormal, or if the neurologic examination is abnormal and plain films are normal. A more difficult situation arises when both plain films and neurologic examination are intact; prudence suggests continuation of work-up if clinical suspicion is high. Two studies performed in U.S. Army hospitals encourage the use of spinal CT scanning in the evaluation of such patients.[275,295] This study was performed in 60 patients with known malignancies who had new spinal abnormalities on bone scanning, with or without back pain, and normal results from neurologic examinations. Eighteen of these patient had normal plain films of the spine. Subsequent spinal CT scanning was directed at each abnormal area on bone scan. Twelve of 18 patients were found to have metastatic disease of vertebral bodies by this method, and all 12 underwent myelography. Evidence of epidural cord compression was noted in three patients (17% of the entire group), none of whom had breast

Table 16-16 Diagnostic correlation between plain radiographs of the spine and myelogram findings in patients with suspected cord compression

	Normal myelogram	Abnormal myelogram
Pts. with neurologic findings (n = 48)		
Normal x-ray	14	4
Abnormal x-ray	3	27
Pts. with no neurologic findings (n = 29)		
Normal x-ray	10	0
Abnormal x-ray	7	15

Modified from Rodichok LD et al: Am J Med 70:1181, 1981.

cancer. Of the nine patients with breast cancer in this group, spinal CT scanning demonstrated abnormalities in seven, but none of these had spinal cord compression on subsequent myelography.

These studies are important in that they fail to identify a subgroup of patients with breast cancer who are at risk for epidural cord compression who have back pain, normal plain films but positive bone scans, and a normal neurologic examination results. Although older studies have reported occasional patients with epidural lesions but normal plain x-rays, this number is hypothetically quite small.[228,323] A sensible approach to a patient who is neurologically and radiographically normal, but in pain, would be expectant management while further diagnostic work-up (bone scanning and/or spinal CT scanning) is undertaken.

Although myelography has been the standard of care in the definitive diagnosis of spinal cord compression, the introduction of CT scanning and MRI have augmented and perhaps confounded present care standards. Myelography carries the distinct advantage of relatively prompt visualization of entire spinal canal, thereby detecting the presence of multiple sites of epidural compression, a phenomenon that may occur in more than 15% of patients.[186,351] If complete epidural block exists, as it did in nearly three fourths of 130 patients in one series,[206] then the rostral extent of the lesion can only be discerned by alternative measures such as cervical myelography or CT scanning. An additional risk of myelography is the possibility of acute neurologic deterioration following lumbar puncture in patients with complete epidural block. This has been reported in up to 14% of patients in one series,[237] and may be minimized by not removing cerebrospinal fluid if a complete block is demonstrated.[210]

CT scanning after the installation of metrizamide, a water-soluble contrast agent, can provide excellent axial views that supplement, but do not replace, myelographic imaging. Weissman et al.[350] demonstrated a strong but imperfect correlation between myelogram and CT scan in establishing the presence of epidural metastases. Evaluation of the full caudal-rostral extent of any epidural lesion may not be possible by CT scanning alone in 20% to 30% of patients,[224,346,351] and therefore would not permit appropriate treatment planning.

MRI scanning of the spine is an attractive alternative to myelography as it is noninvasive, obviating the risk and discomfort of lumbar puncture. Theoretically, sagittal MRI images of the entire spine would always estimate the true rostral-caudal extent of an epidural lesion. Studies of MRI scanning in patients with suspected epidural cord compression have been conducted in both prospective and retrospective fashion, making a true assessment of the relative value of MRI scanning vs. myelography difficult. Sarpel et al.[308] evaluated 16 patients prospectively, none of whom had breast cancer, but all of whom had malignant disease and the new onset of back pain. MRI scanning demonstrated evidence of metastatic bony involvement despite negative plain films in six patients, negative bone scans in six others (three of whom also had negative plain x-rays), and normal neurologic examinations in four. Involvement of the thecal sac with compression was detected in three patients, all of whom had had negative myelograms. A retrospective analysis of patients at the University of Iowa[212] included 22 patients who underwent both MRI scanning and myelography as part of evaluation for spinal metastatic disease. In 19 cases, myelography and MRI scanning disclosed the same abnormality. In one of the three discordant cases MRI failed to diagnose an intradural metastasis. MRI scanning contributed additional information to myelography in nine cases, including demonstration of the rostral extent of metastasis in four cases in lieu of a cervical puncture, paraspinous involvement in three cases where the cord was normal, and additional areas of cord involvement in two cases.

In an important study conducted at Vanderbilt University by Hagenau et al.,[221] 31 patients underwent both MRI and myelography in cases of back pain or myelopathy and suspected spinal cord compression. The results of this study are summarized in Table 16-17. In eight cases of complete cord compression, the MRI scan and myelogram identified epidural lesions "adequately" in six patients. In all eight patients, myelography correctly identified the presence of cord compression, but failed to define the full extent of the lesion in two cases. In patients with noncompressive epidural defects or nerve root impingement, myelography detected abnormalities missed by MRI scanning in 9 of 19 (47%) cases.

One must not assume that MRI scanning is a perfect substitute for myelography. Prospective studies comparing the two modalities will be difficult to perform. Despite the efforts of the investigators at Vanderbilt to perform both studies in all patients with suspected cord compression, this was successfully carried out in only 33% of patients presenting at that hospital over a 16-month period.[221] These studies suggest that using MRI scanning as the first diagnostic step for diagnosing cord compression is not wrong, but that a negative scan may not obviate the need for subsequent myelography. Proper scanning of the entire spine may take up to 3 hours, an unacceptable length of time for some patients in pain. Limiting the length of spinal

Table 16-17 A comparison of myelography and MRI scanning in patients suspected of having spinal cord compression

Symptom	No. pts. with lesions adequately defined	
	MRI	Myelogram
Cord compression	6/8 [75]	6/8 [75]
Noncompressive epidural defects	10/19 [53]	18/19 [94]

[ ], % pts.
Modified from Hagenau C et al: J Clin Oncol 5:1663, 1987.

cord evaluation may save time, but may compromise the ability to detect clinically relevant epidural metastases at distant sites.[165,221] Contrast enhancement with gadolinium DTPA will not always heighten the sensitivity of MRI scanning.[333] At this time, these studies should be considered complimentary to one another, and it would be unwise to suggest that MRI scanning effectively has replaced myelography in the evaluation, as some have suggested.[253]

Treatment

The ultimate goal of therapy in the treatment of epidural spinal cord compression is relief of pain, preservation of ambulatory neurologic function, attainment of superior neurologic function in patients who are nonambulatory, and improving or preserving sphincter function. As is the case with other neurologic complications of breast cancer, a significant prolongation in survival is not possible. A wealth of clinical data reinforces the observation that therapeutic outcome rests heavily on the pretreatment ambulatory status of the patient. This irrefutable clinical fact mandates that any patient with demonstrable epidural cord compression should receive emergency radiotherapeutic or neurosurgical consultation without delay. The data of Gilbert et al.[206] emphasizes the relationship between pretreatment ambulatory status and posttreatment outcome (Table 16-18). Although not shown here, the outcome for patients with relatively radioresistant tumors, including breast carcinoma, did not differ dramatically from the group as a whole. The general trend for improved therapeutic outcome with superior pretreatment ambulatory status has been demonstrated in older, surgical series,[252,357] and several general conclusions may be drawn: from two thirds to three quarters of patients who are ambulatory will remain ambulatory, from one fourth to one half of paraparetic patients will attain ambulatory status, while fewer than one tenth of paraplegic patients will become ambulatory.[257]

Following the institution of dexamethasone therapy, the appropriate therapy consists of external beam radiotherapy, decompressive neurosurgery, or both. The debate over the relative superiority of one mode vs. another has continued for decades, and is no less heated now than before. Clearly, neurosurgical intervention is appropriate under certain circumstances, and these are listed on p. 435. Patients with an uncertain diagnosis or no prior tissue diagnosis of cancer should undergo neurosurgical exploration or decompression, as should patients who progress neurologically despite radiation therapy or who have recurrence of epidural cord compression in the field of previous radiation treatment. Spinal instability from extensive tumor destruction of anterior or posterior vertebral elements must be stabilized neurosurgically to main-

Table 16-18 Treatment outcome of patients with epidural spinal cord compression based on pretreatment ambulatory status[206]

Pretreatment condition	Surgery and radiation therapy		Radiation therapy alone	
	No. treated	Ambulatory (%)	No. treated	Ambulatory (%)
Ambulatory	22	64	58	79
Paraparetic	33	45	83	45
Paraplegic	10	10	29	3

From Gilbert RW et al: Ann Neurol 3:40, 1978.

INDICATIONS FOR NEUROSURGICAL INTERVENTION IN PATIENTS WITH SPINAL CORD COMPRESSION

1. Need for tissue diagnosis or an uncertain diagnosis
2. Neurologic progression despite radiation therapy
3. Recurrence of disease in a previously radiated area
4. Spinal instability
5. Bony invasion of the spinal cord

Table 16-19 Results of treatment of spinal cord compression as reviewed by Black[160]

	No. pts.	% pts. improved
Surgery alone	327	30 (range: 14-42)
Radiation therapy alone	405	46 (range: 34-50)
Surgery plus radiation	216	51 (range: 43-61)

tain freedom from pain and neurologic deterioration. Finally, patients with invasion of the epidural space by bony fragments that have retropulsed from collapsed vertebral bodies will not be expected to respond significantly to radiation therapy.

The relative merits of surgery vs. radiation therapy have been reviewed extensively by Black in 18 clinical series involving over 900 patients before 1978.[160] These results are summarized in Table 16-19, showing percentages of patients who were considered "improved" after therapy of a particular type. This table and other retrospective analyses of large patient groups[178,206,217,261] emphasize that the combination of surgery with radiation therapy holds no particular advantage over radiation therapy alone. The only prospective series randomizing patients to surgery (laminectomy) plus radiotherapy or radiotherapy alone involved a relatively small number of patients, and showed no difference in outcome.[361]

The plight of neurosurgery, its relative inadequacy, and its evolving role in the treatment of spinal cord compression has been given an eloquent historical perspective by Delaney and Oldfield.[186] These authors posit, as do others[160,210,327] that the historical failure of surgery to provide better clinical results stems from the inherent inadequacy of older surgical technique. The posterior laminectomy, the standard neurosurgical decompressive procedure, is unlikely to produce adequate results in patients whose tumors are anterior to the cord (i.e., within the vertebral body). The inferior results of posterior laminectomy in patients with anteriorly located tumors is well documented.[223,357] As over 80% of episodes of spinal cord compression will be from tumors arising in the anterior vertebral body, limitation of posterior laminectomy to patients with tumors situated in the posterior elements or the neural arch seems appropriate, as does the development of superior techniques for treatment of anteriorly situated lesions. To this end, complete resection of the involved vertebral body through an anterior approach for cervical and lumbar lesions or a conventional transthoracic approach for thoracic lesions, followed by spinal stabilization with pins or intervening rods and methylmethacrylate injection, has been utilized. Several studies to date, in patients with vertebral collapse, neurologic progression following radiotherapy, relatively radioresistant tumors, no tissue diagnosis, or spinal instability, demonstrated encouraging results with vertebral body resection.[167,226,262,314,332] These studies have reported improvement in neurologic function from nonambulatory to amulatory status in 70% of 46 patients,[332] 80% of 44 patients,[314] and 62% of 26 patients.[262] Pain relief was obtained (regardless of ambulatory status) in 85%,[332] 56%,[314] and 71%,[262] respectively.

Despite these encouraging advances in neurosurgical techniques, radiation therapy remains the mainstay of treatment for epidural spinal cord compression, with maintenance or improvement in neurologic function anticipated in approximately 50% of patients depending on pretreatment ambulatory status. Standard doses of 30 Gy to 40 Gy delivered over 2 to 4 weeks are delivered to the tumor site plus two vertebral bodies above and below the affected site; no standard dosing schedule has shown superiority over another. Although Gilbert et al.[206] showed a distinctly better outcome for patients with radiosensitive tumors (seminoma, myeloma, lymphoma, neuroblastoma, Ewing's sarcoma), one must not assume that breast cancer is inherently radioresistant. In one study confined to breast cancer patients,[178] pain relief was obtained in 72% of 26 patients; it is not possible to say that treatment outcome is necessarily better for breast cancer patients compared to other patients with carcinoma or other radioresistant tumors. Despite the relative chemosensitivity and hormone sensitivity of metastatic breast cancer, the use of cytotoxic combination chemotherapy or hormonal therapy cannot be recommended in the initial management of epidural spinal cord compression in breast cancer patients.

Management guidelines for patients with suspected spinal cord compression are complex. Useful algorithms for the diagnostic and therapeutic approach in breast cancer patients have been published elsewhere.[327] Several general principles should be applied to each patient:

1. Patients who present with symptoms or signs that arouse any suspicion of epidural cord compression should be treated emergently.
2. Dexamethasone therapy is best administered promptly as the work-up proceeds.
3. Patients with back pain and neurologic findings of myelopathy and/or radiculopathy should undergo immediate conventional x-ray study. A definitive study (myelography or MRI scanning) should be performed, even if plain radiographs are normal.

   The optimum diagnostic study for patients with symptoms of brachial or lumbar plexopathy, and not myelopathy, is unclear when plain x-rays of the cervical or lumbosacral spine are normal. CT scanning of the pelvis or cervical spine may be considered if it can be performed promptly.
4. Patients with neurologic findings but without pain are uncommon, but should be subjected to the same diagnostic scrutiny as patients with pain and neurologic findings.
5. Patients with pain but without neurologic findings should undergo immediate plain x-ray evaluation. Positive x-rays predict for epidural metastasis in a substantial number of patients, and further diagnostic workup should proceed.
6. Normal plain x-rays in a patient with pain and no neurologic findings permit expectant management. Compulsive neurologic follow-up is indicated. Bone scanning may identify areas of metastasis, and CT scanning through the affected site will reveal epidural metastasis in a small number of patients.
7. The decision to utilize MRI scanning versus myelography is difficult. Evolving MRI technology predicts that this diagnostic method will supersede myelography. At this time, the decision must rest on the speed with which the diagnostic study can be obtained, the patient's ability to remain comfortably still for MRI scanning, and the clinician's confidence in the interpretation of MRI scan results by his radiologists. A normal MRI scan does not eliminate the need for myelography if neurologic signs persist or worsen
8. Evaluation of the entire spinal column is mandatory if the MRI scan is used. The clinician must be mindful of the occurrence of multiple epidural lesions.
9. Definitive therapy must be instituted without delay. Indications for neurosurgery are listed on p. 435. If none of these conditions exist, the choice between radiotherapy or definitive neurosurgery depend on the location of the lesion, the availability of radiotherapy, and the availability and experience of the surgeon.
   a. Patients who are in poor medical condition should probably not undergo surgery unless it is mandated by the conditions listed on p. 435.
   b. Posterior laminectomy cannot be considered optimal primary therapy for lesions that are situated anteriorly.
   c. Radiation therapy remains the treatment of choice. Despite the encouraging results from vertebral body resection and spinal stabilization, this procedure should be limited to institutions with extensive surgical experience.

HYPERCALCEMIA

Hypercalcemia was identified in the early 1920s as a metabolic complication of malignancies.[363] Much has been learned over the past decade about the pathophysiology of the hypercalcemia of malignancy and newer, more effective treatments are now available. Breast cancer is one of the most common neoplasms associated with hypercalcemia and this is the most frequent metabolic complication of breast cancer, occurring in 30% of patients.[152,199,234] When hypercalcemia does occur, it tends to be a late complication and is often associated with widespread bony metastases.[199] In one study, hypercalcemia was the cause of death in 3% of patients.[220] The mean survival after diagnosis of hypercalcemia in these patients is 3 months.

Pathophysiology

Normal calcium homeostasis depends upon the integration of three systemic hormones acting on the gut, kidney, bone, and the extracellular fluid. This includes parathyroid hormone (PTH), 1,25-dihydroxyvitamin D [1,25-$(OH)_2$–vitamin D], and calcitonin, each of which controls the level of ionized serum calcium. PTH raises serum calcium concentration levels by stimulating bone resorption and renal calcium resorption by indirectly stimulating production of 1,25-$(OH)_2$–vitamin D by the kidney. Intestinal calcium absorption is increased by 1,25-$(OH)_2$–vitamin D. Calcitonin inhibits bone resorption and therefore acts as a counter-regulator to PTH. Ordinarily, net absorption of calcium from the gut is equal to the amount of calcium excreted in the urine.[265]

Generally, hypercalcemia in breast cancer and other malignancies has been separated into two etiologic categories: metastatic disease to bone, resulting in osteolytic bone destruction[195,265,324] and

MEDIATORS OF HYPERCALCEMIA OF MALIGNANCY

Parathyroid hormone–related protein (PTHrP)
Transforming growth factors alpha and beta
Prostaglandin E_2
Interleukin-1
Tumor necrosis factors alpha and beta
1,25-dihydroxyvitamin D

humoral hypercalcemia.[183,240,264] The latter was suggested by reports of hypercalcemia occurring in cancer patients in the absence of bone metastases, and the observation that some patients with extensive bony metastases do not develop hypercalcemia. Therefore osteoclast activity and proliferation may be stimulated directly by osseous metastases or indirectly by tumor derived products. These factors are summarized above.

In breast cancer patients, skeletal destruction by bony metastases is the predominant mechanism responsible for hypercalcemia.[264] The mechanism of bone destruction includes direct effects of tumor cells on bone and activation of osteoclasts by factors released by tumor cells including prostaglandins and transforming growth factor alpha and beta.[198]

It has been postulated for many years that PTH or PTH-like factors could be involved in the hypercalcemia of malignancy. Data suggests that parathyroid hormone–related protein (PTHrP) mediated bone resorption may be a dominant mechanism. PTHrP has recently been isolated and the DNA sequenced, identified, and cloned from tumors associated with humoral hypercalcemia, including breast cancer.[169,172] The amino acid sequence has striking homology to parathyroid hormone and interacts with parathyroid hormone receptors.[173] PTHrP is produced commonly by many solid tumors. Plasma levels of PTHrP can now be measured with immunoassays and may be useful in the differential diagnosis of hypercalcemia. Early data suggests that 50% of patients with hypercalcemia of malignancy have increases in PTHrP. Whether PTHrP has a role in normal calcium homeostasis remains to be clarified.

The role of PTHrP in hypercalcemia of breast cancer is not clear. Isales et al.[240] have evaluated prospectively 17 patients with hypercalcemia and breast cancer and found that 6 of the 17 patients (32%) had increased levels of nephrogenous cAMP, which is a marker for humoral hypercalcemia. Four of these six patients had no evidence of bony metastases. In addition, PTHrP was detected in breast cancer tissue, suggesting a purely humoral component in these patients. These observations suggest that humoral, tumor-derived products may play a role in the hypercalcemia of breast cancer.[240] In addition, breast cancers also could stimulate the production of factors such as lymphotoxin, tumor necrosis factor, or interleukin-1 as part of the cell-mediated immune response to the presence of metastatic tumor. These factors are all powerful bone resorbing factors.[195,198,214]

Ultimately, the final common pathophysiologic pathway of hypercalcemia of malignancy is increased osteoclastic stimulation resulting in bone resorption. Infrequently, increased gastrointestinal absorption of calcium or impaired renal excretion of calcium may play a role.[264] In some patients with breast cancer, co-existing primary hyperparathyroidism has been reported.[328]

Hormonal treatment of metastatic breast cancer may actively precipitate hypercalcemia as part of the flare response that may also include worsening bone pain. This complication occurs in 15% of ER-positive breast cancer patients with extensive bone metastases.[246] The use of estrogens, androgens, progestin, and tamoxifen have all been reported.[246,252,277] If symptoms occur, appropriate treatment of hormone-induced hypercalcemia consists of discontinuing the hormonal therapy and instituting glucocorticoids.

Clinical presentation

Hypercalcemia occurs when the corrected serum calcium level is elevated above a normal value, usually >10.5 mg/dl. The clinical presentation is determined by the level of hypercalcemia, the rate at which it develops, and factors such as performance status, age, and other organ dysfunction. Patients with serum calciums >14 mg/dl are generally symptomatic. Patients with hypercalcemia associated with malignancy tend to be more symptomatic than patients with nonneoplastic causes of hypercalcemia. The symptoms of hypercalcemia are often subtle and nonspecific and reflect alterations in cellular function affecting neurologic, gastrointestinal, renal, cardiovascular, and musculoskeletal systems.[267,316] The earliest symptoms include nonspecific complaints of fatigue, anorexia, nausea, and constipation. Hypercalcemia results in a renal tubular defect that causes loss of urinary concentrating ability, mimicking nephrogenic diabetes insipidus.[362] As a result, patients develop polyuria, polydipsia, and nocturia, which promote dehydration, thereby worsening hypercalcemia and perpetuating a vicious cycle. Neurologic manifestations include confusion, lethargy, weakness, depression, decreased deep tendon reflexes, which may progress to seizures, stupor, coma, and ultimately death.[179] Gastrointestinal symptoms include anorexia, nausea, intractable vomiting, and constipation. Cardiovascular consequences include electrocardiographic changes characterized by slowed conduction (prolongation of PR and QRS intervals, and shortening of QT intervals).[267] As serum calcium levels increase, bradyarrthymias develop, which can progress to complete heart block with cardiac arrest.[300]

Treatment

The most effective measure of correcting hypercalcemia of malignancy is reduction of the tumor burden by effective therapy. In asymptomatic patients early in the course of breast cancer with mild hypercalcemia, such therapy may be successful. However, hypercalcemia tends to be a late complication of breast cancer, occurring when systemic chemotherapy and hormonal therapy are less effective.[199] Therefore, preventive measures and specific antihypercalcemic therapy is necessary. Preventive measures, which have some limited value, include maintaining adequate fluid and salt intake, avoidance of immobilization and thiazide diuretics, and control of nausea and vomiting.[267,316]

When mild hypercalcemia is precipitated by hormonal therapy for breast cancer, the hormone can be continued as long as patients are monitored closely. Concurrent therapy with hydration, steroids, and antihypercalcemic agents should be initiated. If severe hypercalcemia develops after hormonal therapy, the hormone should be discontinued until the serum calcium level normalizes. Hormonal therapy can then be reinstituted cautiously.[252]

Therapeutic maneuvers are directed at decreasing calcium resorption from bone and increasing urinary excretion of calcium. The mainstay of initial treatment of hypercalcemia is vigorous hydration with normal saline. This results in corrrection of dehydration and volume depletion, and increases glomerular filtration, which enhances urinary calcium excretion.[239] The rate of intravenous fluid administration depends on the severity of dehydration, the serum calcium level, and the cardiovascular status of the patient. Three to 4 L/day is generally sufficient, and urine output is maintained to avoid volume overload. Loop diuretics such as furosemide further decrease renal tubular resorption of calcium. Careful attention to electrolyte balance is required.[331] Clinical improvement in mental status and modest decreases in calcium usually are seen following adequate hydration. For complete response and long-term control, additional measures directed at inhibiting osteoclastic resorption must be initiated. These agents are summarized below at left.

AGENTS TO TREAT HYPERCALCEMIA

Biphosphonates	Glucocorticoids
Plicamycin	Inorganic phosphates
Calcitonin	Prostagladin inhibitors
Gallium nitrate	WR-2721

Biphosphonates. The biphosphonates represent a new therapeutic approach to the treatment of malignancy-associated hypercalcemia. Development of these agents stems from the identification that pyrophosphate, an endogenous substance, binds to hydroxyapatite and prevents the dissolution of hydroxyapatite crystals.[192] Biphosphonates are stable, structural analogues of pyrophosphate and exert their antihypercalcemic effects by inhibiting normal osteoclast function and activity and effects on osteoclast precursors.[192] Three compounds have been studied extensively; clodronate, etridronate, and pamidronate; but only etriodonate is currently approved and available for clinical use.[164,241,245,256] However, additional biphosphonates will be available in the next year. Success rates have varied depending on dose, duration of treatment, and route of administration. Because these agents are poorly absorbed from the gastrointestinal tract, clinical trials have focused principally on intravenous administration. These agents are extremely effective in reducing serum calcium with >65% of patients achieving eucalcemia in a number of clinical trials.[164,256] Normocalcemia occurs in 2 to 3 days. Randomized studies comparing the various biphosphonates demonstrate that the second-generation agent pamidronate is more effective than clodronate and etridonate in reducing serum calcium levels.[298] These agents are well tolerated. Side effects include fever, mild renal insufficiency, both hypophosphatemia and hyperphosphatemia, transient asymptomatic hypocalcemia, and osteomalacia.[298] Etridronate disodium is available for oral and intraveneous administration. The recommended intravenous dose is 7.5 mg/kg/day administered over 2 hours for 3 to 7 days. Oral etridronate is poorly absorbed and its role in the management of hypercalcemia has yet to be defined.[297] The biphosphonates should be considered as a first-line treatment of hypercalcemia; they are at least as effective as other agents and are less toxic. In the future, oral biphosphonates will be available that will be a useful adjunct for the chronic, outpatient management of hypercalcemia.

Because skeletal metastases are present in about 70% of patients with breast cancer, several studies have attempted to assess the benefit of biphosphonates in these patients. These studies have demonstrated a significant reduction in tumor-related morbidity, hypercalcemia, bone pain, analgesic requirements, pathologic fractures, and need for additional therapeutic interventions.[263]

Gallium nitrate. Gallium nitrate is a newly approved agent for the treatment of cancer-related symptomatic hypercalcemia. Gallium nitrate exerts a hypocalcemic effect by inhibiting calcium resorption from bone, although the precise mechanism has not been determined.[348] Results of a randomized double-blind trial comparing gallium nitrate to calcitonin demonstrated that more patients treated with gallium nitrate achieved normocalcemia (75% vs. 27%), and the duration of response was 7.5 times longer with gallium nitrate than with calcitonin (7.5 days vs. 1 day, respectively).[347] Ninety-two percent of patients treated with gallium nitrate had a decrease in serum calcium >2.0 mg/dl compared to 54% of patients treated with calcitonin. The recommended dose is 200 mg/m^2 for 5 days, given as a continuous infusion. Controlled studies have not been performed to evaluate the safety or effectiveness of retreatment with gallium nitrate. The only contraindication of gallium nitrate is renal impairment (serum creatinine >2.5 mg/dl). Concurrent use of gallium nitrate with potentially nephrotoxic drugs (aminoglycosides) may increase the risk of developing severe renal toxicity and is not recommended. Reported side effects incude mild hypocalcemia in 38% of patients, rises in BUN and creatinine levels in 12.5% of patients, and mild asymptomatic decreases in blood pressure. Gallium nitrate should be discontinued if the serum creatinine exceeds 2.5 mg/dl.

Plicamycin. Plicamycin (mithramycin) initially was used as an antineoplastic agent in the 1960s. Hypocalcemia was a frequent side effect of therapy, which led to its clinical investigation as an antihypercalcemic agent. Numerous trials have confirmed its effectiveness at reducing serum calcium levels, presumably as a result of toxic effects on osteoclasts, thereby inhibiting bone resorption.[190] It appears to be equally effective in the presence or absence of bone metastases.[281] Plicamycin is administered as an intravenous bolus at a dose of 25 μg/kg. Reduction in serum calcium is obtained within 36 to 48 hours, and most patients ecome eucalcemic after a single dose.[190] The dose may be repeated if no detectable hypocalcemic effect is seen within 48 hours. The duration of response is unpredictable and may last days to weeks or longer.[264] Repeated treatments are effective, but should be withheld until hypercalcemia recurs.

The major disadvantages of plicamycin are the adverse effects associated with its use related to dose and frequency of administration. Plicamycin causes nausea and vomiting, hepatocellular dysfunction, bleeding diathesis, nephrotoxicity, and proteinuria in dehydrated patients. Plicamycin is a vesicant drug with the potential to cause necrosis of soft tissue if extravasation occurs. It should be used only in those patients with normal or near-normal renal function.

Calcitonin. Calcitonin is a hormone secreted by the parafollicular cells of the thyroid gland.[265] It derives its hypocalcemic activity primarily from inhibition of osteoclastic bone resorption and enhanced renal excretion of calcium by inhibiting absorption in the distal tubule.[267] Calcitonin is extremely effective in reducing serum calcium levels. Approximately 80% of treated patients show improvement, which is usually evident within a few hours. However, the antihypercalcemic effect is short lived, lasting only several days.[265] The tachyphylaxis significantly limits its clinical usefulness. The advantage of calcitonin is its rapid onset of action and safety in patients with dehydration and renal insufficiency.[268] Calcitonin can be utilized in combination with glucocorticoids, which may prolong the hypocalcemic effect.[329]

Salmon calcitonin is the most potent and most frequently utilized preparation. The recommended dose is 4 MRC units/kg every 12 hours by either subcutaneous or intramuscular injection.[268] Side effects are minimal and include nausea, vomiting, and flushing. Allergic reactions have been reported, albeit rarely; skin testing is recommended before beginning treatment.

Glucocorticoids. While glucocorticoids are effective in treating hypercalcemia associated with hematologic malignancies, they are rarely useful in solid tumors.[268] Breast cancer is an exception. Steroids are effective, especially when hypercalcemia is a consequence of hormonal therapy.[252,280] The hypocalcemic effects of steroids include blocking bone resorption by inhibition of cytokine release (IL-1), reduced intestinal absorption of calcium, and increasing urinary calcium excretion.[280] Relatively high doses of prednisone are required (40 to 100 mg/day) to reduce serum calcium levels. The long-term use of steroids for the management of hypercalcemia is limited by toxicities associated with their chronic use.

Prostaglandin synthesis inhibitors. Prostaglandins, especially PGE_2, have been implicated in the pathogenesis of hypercalcemia of malignancy.[195,264] However, attempts to utilize nonsteroidal antiinflammatory agents to treat hypercalcemia have been disappointing. Indomethacin (75 to 100 mg/day in divided doses) can be administered to patients with refractory hypercalcemia who have failed on all other measures.[268]

Phosphates. Intravenous phosphate is indicated to control life-threatening hypercalcemia that is refractory to more conventional measures. The decline in serum calcium levels reflects precipitation of calcium in the extracellular fluid with phosphate.[268] Doses should not exceed 1.5 g of phosphorous infused over 6 to 8 hours. Calcification of vital organs, hypotension, and renal failure limit its usefulness.[188]

Oral phosphates may be useful in the outpatient management of chronic hypercalcemia following successful reduction of serum calcium levels with other measures as described above. It interferes with absorption of calcium from the gastrointestinal tract. The usual starting dose is 1 g/day in divided doses.[188,268] It should not be administered to patients when serum phosphate levels are >4 mg/dl. Oral phosphates are used rarely today because of associated nausea and vomiting.

WR-2721. WR-2721, an organic thiophosphate, is an experimental agent used clinically to protect against the myelosuppressive and neurotoxic effects of chemotherapy. Calcium-lowering effects were seen in early clinical study.[209] The hypocalcemic effects are mediated by inhibition of PTH secretion and renal tubular calcium reabsorption. WR-2721 has been effective in lowering the serum calcium in patients with parathyroid carcinoma.[211] WR-2721 may have potential as an antihypercalcemic drug.

Summary

Hypercalcemia is a common and often life-threatening complication of metastatic breast cancer. Excessive resorption of bone is the primary mechanism underlying hypercalcemia of malignancy. If untreated or inadequately treated, it leads to progressive dehydration, anorexia, polyuria, lethargy, coma, and death. Rehydration, mobilization, and initiation of effective treatment of the breast cancer are recommended, but these measures often fail to normalize serum calcium levels. The agents currently available to control hypercalcemia—biphosphonates, gallium nitrate, plicamycin, calcitonin, and glucocorticoids—exert their hypocalcemic effects by inhibiting bone resorption, with varying degrees of success.

PLEURAL EFFUSIONS

Malignant pleural involvement is most commonly associated with metastatic breast cancer. Indeed, 50% of patients with breast cancer will develop a pleural effusion during the course of their disease.[251] Effusions are a significant cause of morbidity; however, the quality of patients' lives can be greatly improved by successful management.

Pathophysiology

Under normal physiologic conditions, the pleural space contains approximately 5 to 20 ml of fluid with a protein content of <2 g/dL. This is the result of a dynamic equilibrium between hydrostatic and colloidal osmotic pressures, lymphatic drainage, and capillary permeability. Any imbalance in these factors can lead to accumulation of fluid in the pleural space.[159,194,247]

Most malignant pleural effusions are caused by metastatic pleural involvement to the visceral or parietal pleural surfaces. In breast cancer, this can be the consequence of hematogenous spread or local-regional invasion through the chest wall via lymphatic pathways.[191] As a result, capillary permeability increases due to inflammation and disruption of capillary endothelium, as well as impaired lymphatic drainage secondary to obstruction by tumor.

A number of other tumor-related factors can contribute to the development of pleural effusions, including extensive mediastinal node invasion, parapneumonic effusion from obstructive pneumonia, prior mediastinal radiation therapy, pericardial effusion (malignant or postradiation), malignant ascites, malnutrition (hypoalbuminemia) and pulmonary embolism.[230]

Clinical presentation

Patients with pleural effusions typically present with dyspnea that is exacerbated in the supine position. Nonproductive cough and a sense of heaviness in the chest also are reported. Pleuritic chest pain is associated with smaller effusions and generally is less of a factor as an effusion enlarges, unless there is parietal pleural or chest wall involvement with tumor.[177,230] Physical examination reveals dullness to percussion and decreased or absent breath sounds, egophony above the effusion and findings secondary to the underlying cancer. A pleural friction rub may be heard over areas of neoplastic pleural involvement. Contralateral tracheal deviation also is observed with significant pleural effusions.[150]

While these physical findings are helpful in diagnosis, the chest radiograph remains the most useful screening tool for the assessment of pleural fluid. The chest radiograph (PA and lateral) will detect as little as 175 to 500 ml of pleural fluid. The lateral decubitus films can detect as little as 100 ml of fluid and should be performed on all patients to determine if fluid layers out or is loculated.[355] Other imaging procedures (ultrasound, CT scan) are seldom needed.[306]

Pleural effusions are frequently the first manifestation of metastatic breast cancer and there is often a long interval between the initial diagnosis and the development of the effusion. The survival of patients with breast cancer and pleural effusions is longer compared to all other tumor types.[230] In one series, median survival was 48 months in breast cancer patients with no other evidence of metastatic disease.[289] In other series, the median survival of malignant pleural effusions in patients with breast cancer ranges from 7.3 months to 20 months.[177] Pleural effusion tend to develop ipsilaterally supporting local-regional spread as an important factor in the pathogenesis.

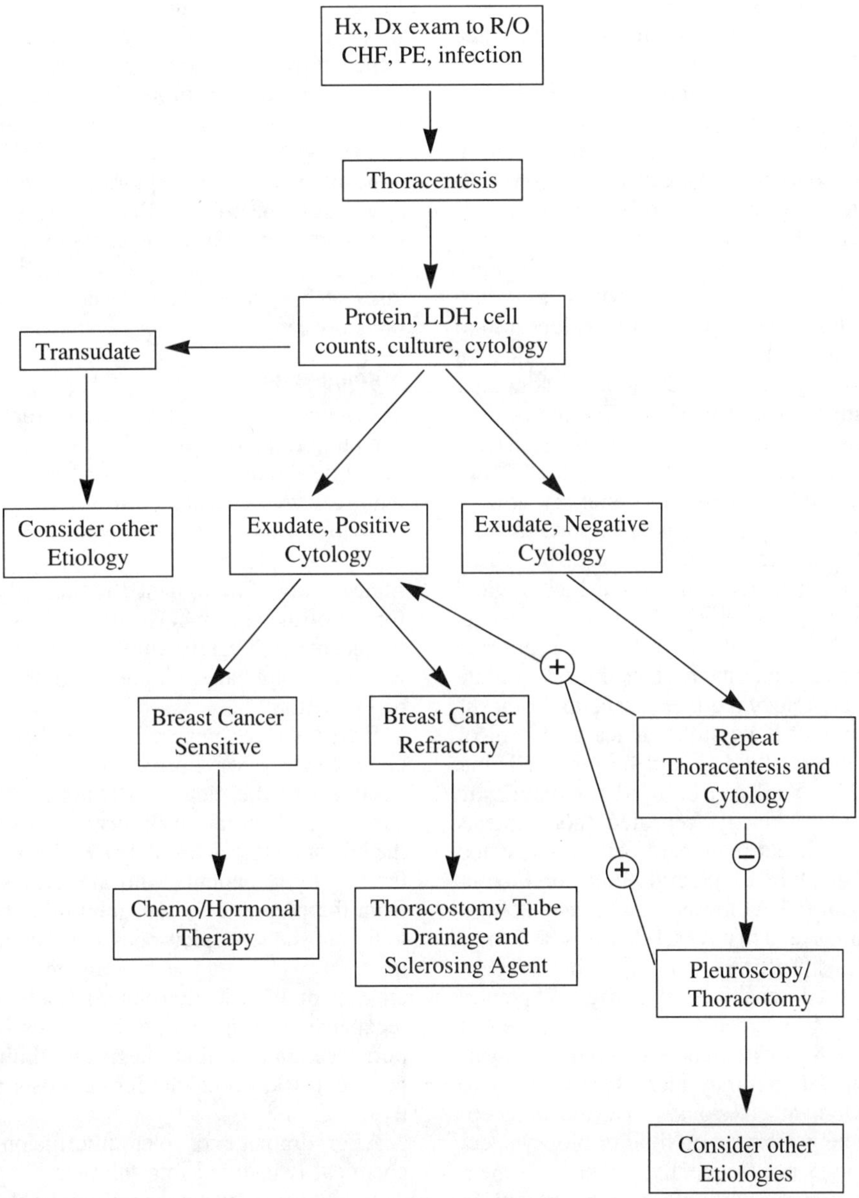

Fig. 16-2 Approach to diagnosis and treatment of pleural effusions in breast cancer patients.

Diagnostic evaluation

The first step after radiographic confirmation of a pleural effusion is to perform a thoracentesis for the relief of symptoms and for diagnostic purposes. Pleural effusions that develop in patients with breast cancer are not always malignant. Effusions can develop as a consequence of therapy including radiation therapy, congestive heart failure secondary to anthracyclines, or infections as a result of immunosuppression or chemotherapy-induced neutropenia. Therefore diagnostic evaluations should include a careful history and physical examination and restaging for breast cancer. A diagnostic and treatment approach is outlined in Fig. 16-2. The fluid obtained should be heparinized and analyzed for cytology, cell count, protein, glucose, lactic dehydrogenase (LDH), and appropriate cultures.[230,232] Concurrent determinations of serum protein and LDH levels are needed as well. Pleural effusions secondary to breast cancer are almost always exudates, except if caused by lymphatic obstruction. Exudative pleural effusions generally have the following characteristics: protein content >3.0 g/dl or ratio of pleural fluid to serum protein of >0.5; LDH >200 U/ml or pleural fluid LDH to serum LDH ratio >0.6; and a specific gravity >1.015 g/ml.[232,254] Cell counts generally reveal primarily mononuclear cells, but are of little diagnostic value. Malignant pleural effusions are occasionally hemorrhagic with >100,000 RBC/mm^3. Pleural fluid glucose is generally low.[151] Pleural fluid cytology is the most important diagnostic test and is positive in 70% to 80% of malignant effusions; it generally has a higher yield than pleural biopsies.[154,293] False-positive results are very rare. False-negative cytology does not rule out the diagnosis of malignant effusion. An exudate with negative cytology requires a second thoracentesis for cytology. If possible, at least 250 ml of heparinized pleural fluid should be removed, but as little as 3 to 5 ml can be used for diagnostic purposes.[293] Occasionally, repeated thoracentesis are required to detect malignant cells. In selected cases, determination of pleural fluid carcinoembryonic antigen (CEA) levels may be useful. Malignant effusions tend to have CEA levels >10 mg/ml but false-positive titers do occur in benign conditions. Reported sensitives in malignant pleural effusion range from 25% to 57%.[299] The use of cytogenetics or flow cytometry (searching for aneuploid cell populations) may increase the ability to diagnose malignant effusions.[292] Hormone receptors also can be performed on fluid or biopsy specimens. Although not frequently performed, measurement of pleural fluid pH can be useful in managing patients. Sahn and Good reported that those patients with malignant effusions from breast cancer whose pleural fluid pH was low (<7.3) had a shorter mean survival and a poor response to pleurodesis.[307]

If diagnosis cannot be obtained by thoracentesis, then percutaneous needle biopsy of the parietal pleural can be performed. When multiple specimens are taken, a positive diagnosis can be expected in 50% to 75% of cases.[304] The presence of pleural fluid facilitates needle biopsy but is not absolutely necessary. Pleural biopsy carries a greater risk of complication than thoracentesis and so should be reserved for difficult diagnostic cases. In cases where a pleural needle biopsy, fluid cytology, and special studies are negative, then it may be necessary to perform an open pleural biopsy, which provides a larger piece of tissue. Pleuroscopy with biopsy is probably the best procedure as it is less risky than a thoracotomy and has a diagnostic yield of 93% to 96%.[292,304] The final diagnostic approach is exploratory thoracotomy, but it is rarely necessary. Pleural effusions with repeated negative cytologies and biopsies are usually caused by mechanisms other than pleural metastases such as lymphatic obstruction or elevated venous pressure.

Management

Thoracentesis is utilized initially for palliation of symptoms and diagnosis. The volume aspirated the first time should not exceed 1 L. However, patients with recurrent effusions can often tolerate removal of 3 to 4 L. In the majority of patients, without therapy, the pleural fluid will rapidly reaccumulate. In one study of malignant effusions, the mean time for the effusion to recur was 4.2 days.[274] Repeated thoracentesis is rarely an effective approach and it is often complicated by pneumothorax, empyema, or loculation.[230]

Breast cancer generally is highly sensitive to chemotherapy or hormonal therapy. Therefore treatment of the pleural effusion should be thoracentesis and initiation of systemic therapy. When the breast cancer is unlikely to respond to systemic therapy or in patients who are very symptomatic from the pleural effusion, then tube thoracostomy with subsequent pleurodesis is the appropriate treatment. This approach is aimed at reducing the amount of fluid in the pleural space and requires reexpansion of the lung to be successful. Most reports recommend that chest tube drainage should be under 100 ml/24 hr for sclerosis to be effective.[304]

After drainage of pleural effusion an irritant chemical is instilled into the pleural space to produce pleural irritation, thereby stimulating fibrous adhesion of parietal and visceral pleural surfaces. A number of agents have been used for sclerosis

TREATMENT AGENTS FOR MALIGNANT PLEURAL EFFUSION

Tetracycline
Bleomycin
Thiotepa, nitrogen mustard, 5-FU
Quinacrine
Talc
Radioactive phosphorus or gold

and are summarized above.[216,235,276,279,330,335] These agents differ in sclerosing properties and side effects. The two agents most commonly employed are bleomycin and tetracycline.[216,276] Both agents control malignant pleural effusions in approximately 70% of patients and are not myelosuppressive nor as toxic as many other agents reported. However, each one has certain advantages and limitations. The advantage of tetracycline is that it is safe, effective, and inexpensive. Disadvantages are the reported side effects, which included pleuritic chest pain and elevated temperatures in many patients.[344] Reports on the use of bleomycin confirm that it is well tolerated by patients and possibly more effective than tetracycline with few patients experiencing pain or other side effects. However, this agent is far more costly. The instillation of talc into the pleural space creates an intense pleuritis and likely is the most effective sclerosing agent. It should be reserved for refractory effusions because the morbidity and mortality are greater with this method.

Should this approach fail, pleurectomy may be considered in patients who can tolerate surgery and have a significant life expectancy. However, this is associated with a high incidence of complications and a 10% mortality rate.[258]

Summary

Malignant pleural effusions are a common complication of metastatic breast cancer. A stepwise approach to diagnosis and treatment, which should lead to control of the effusion and relief of symptoms, is outlined in Fig. 16-2.

PERICARDIAL DISEASE

Pericardial disease is the most prominent type of cardiac involvement in patients with cancer.[157] Breast cancer, lung cancer, and hematologic malignancies are the most common cancers that involve the heart or pericardium. Autopsy studies have shown that the pericardium is involved in up to 35% of patients with metastatic breast cancer.[220,291] While the pericardial disease may remain subclinical, in many, severe or life-threatening symptoms of cardiac tamponade will develop. Malignant pericardial effusions are the most common cause of pericardial tamponade. However, of importance is the fact that 50% of cancer patients with symptomatic pericardial disease have nonmalignant pericardial disease.[337]

Pathophysiology

Generally, metastases to the heart and pericardium result from retrograde dissemination of tumor cells from involved mediastinal lymph nodes into the lymphatic channels of the heart and pericardium. In addition, tumor cells can invade the pericardium by hematogenous spread.[296,337] Neoplastic pericardial effusions result from pericardial invasion, which leads to exudation of fluid. Spread to the rich epicardial vascular and lymphatic networks tend to block lymphatic flow from the heart, further contributing to the development of a pericardial effusion. Obstruction of lymphatic flow by mediastinal or hilar adenopathy can also lead to accumulation of fluid in the pericardial sac. Radiation therapy to the left breast can result in three types of cardiac injury, asymptomatic pericardial effusion, acute pericarditis, and constructive pericarditis.[181] These syndromes generally are seen with doses in excess of 3500 rad and can develop weeks or months after therapy or as a chronic form up to 20 years later.

Cardiac tamponade results from either accumulation of fluid within the pericardial sac or pericardial constriction by tumor or radiation pericarditis. The severity of tamponade depends on the rapidity of development and volume of fluid. As pericardial fluid accumulates, intrapericardial pressure rises until one or both ventricular diastolic pressures are equilibrated with it. Further increments in intrapericardial pressure cause a sharp fall in stroke volume and blood pressure and an increase in heart rate.

Clinical presentation

Malignant pericardial effusions generally develop gradually over days or several weeks, but can cause tamponade and represent an oncologic emergency requiring pericardiocentesis. Many of the signs and symptoms result from increases in ventricular diastolic pressure. Patients with malignant pericardial effusion without tamponade can be asymptomatic or complain of dyspnea, pleuritic chest pain, orthopnea, or dysphagia.[318,337] Physical examination can reveal distant heart sounds, cardiac enlargement, and pleural effusion. Patients with cardiac tamponade or constrictive pericarditis present with dyspnea, cough, and chest pain, which is often relieved by leaning forward. Vague gastrointestinal symptoms from visceral congestion can occur. Decreased cerebral perfusion can result in confusion or coma. Examination may demonstrate jugular venous distention, pericardial friction rub, distant heart sounds, pulsus paradoxus, sustained tachycardia, arrhythmias, and hypotension. As venous pressure increases, peripheral edema, ascites, hepatomegaly, and hepatojugular reflux may develop.[296,337]

Diagnostic evaluation begins with a standard chest radiograph. Accumulation of more than 200 ml of pericardial fluid results in enlargement of the cardiac silhouette. Displacement of the pericardial fat pad, mediastinal widening, or hilar adenopathy also can be seen.[255] Cardiac size may be normal in patients with pericardial effusion and in patients with constrictive pericarditis. Echocardiography is currently the most sensitive technique for detecting the presence of pericardial fluid. As little as 15 ml may be detected. An echo-free space develops between the epicardial echo of the posterior left ventricular wall and the denser pericardial fluid echo. Echocardiography also may detect the presence of tumor deposits in and around the heart. Although echocardiography allows detection of pericardial fluid, it does not establish the diagnosis of pericardial tamponade, which is established by clinical and hemodynamic criteria.[337] Thoracic CT scans also have become important radiographic tools in diagnosing pericardial effusions.[213] Electrocardiogram findings include low voltage, tachycardia, nonspecific ST-T wave changes. Elevation of the S-T segment that is characteristic of acute pericarditis is not usually present with neoplastic pericardial effusions. Electrical alternans—alternating high- and low-voltage P waves or ventricular complexes—is associated with large effusions. Sinus bradycardia and heart block have been noted in some patients, associated with tumor invasion of the conducting system. Finally, right heart cardiac catheterization can be performed when the differentiation between pericardial disease and myocardial disease is important. The hemodynamic hallmark is equilibration of the diastolic pressures in the four cardiac chambers.[337]

Diagnostic evaluation

The use of percutaneous pericardiocentesis guided by two-dimensional echocardiography permits diagnostic assessment of the fluid and usually rapid relief of symptoms; it is indicated when a significant pericardial effusion is present in a patient with cancer. This procedure is associated with a high diagnostic yield and a low frequency of complications.[158,282] Pericardiocentesis may not be necessary, however, when an asymptomatic moderate effusion is detected. The characteristics of the pericardial fluid can often give immediate clues to its cause. Hemorrhagic fluid is commonly associated with a positive pericardial fluid cytology. The pericardial fluid obtained should be analyzed for culture, cell count, and cytologic examination. The cytologic analysis of malignant pericardial effusions from breast cancer is positive with malignant cells in 30% to 58% of cases.[338,360] Thus, a negative cytologic report does not rule out the diagnosis of malignant pericardial effusion. Importantly, 50% of patients with symptomatic pericardial disease and underlying cancer may have nonmalignant pericardial disease, including radiation-induced pericarditis, idiopathic pericarditis, drug-induced pericarditis, infection, hypothyroidism, or autoimmune disorders.[337] If cytologic examination of the pericardial fluid is negative and histologic diagnosis is important to plan overall management, a pericardial biopsy may be obtained under local anesthesia. When pericardiocentesis is required, a flexible, indwelling catheter may be left in place. This catheter facilitates the collection of additional fluid if initial culture and cytology are nondiagnostic and also provides access for instillation therapy if cytology is positive.

Management

The management of malignant pericardial effusions remains controversial. As stated above, it is important initially to confirm that the effusion is in fact malignant. In patients who have had prior radiation therapy it can often be difficult to distinguish radiation-induced pericarditis from malignant pericardial disease. When planning for treatment of malignant pericardial effusions one must consider the performance status of the patient, the extent of metastatic disease, the availability of effective systemic therapy, and other underlying medical conditions. Two basic therapeutic approaches are (1) the use of systemic chemotherapy directed at controlling the metastatic breast cancer and (2) local therapy for the palliation of the local pericardial process.

If systemic hormonal or cytotoxic therapy is expected to be effective and there is no evidence of tamponade, a trial of systemic therapy should be undertaken before local therapy begins.[296] Local treatment of malignant pericardial effusion is necessary only when cardiac tamponade appears to be imminent, a suspected infectious etiology of breast cancer is refractory to systemic therapy, or in those patients in whom the diagnosis of recurrent cancer cannot be made any other way. Local therapy may be accomplished by radiotherapy, instillation therapy, or surgery.[158,255,318] There is no consensus as to the optimal application of these treatment modalities. Unless definitive local therapy to prevent recurrent tamponade is initiated, tamponade generally recurs within 24 to 48 hours following pericardiocentesis.[255,337] Generally, instillation therapy is the initial treatment of choice; it can be accomplished with an indwelling catheter into the pericardial space. This will induce an inflammatory response, fibrosis, and prevent reaccumulation of pericardial fluid.[255] A variety of sclerosing agents and radioisotopes have been used. Tetracycline is one of the most frequently used agents. Between 500 to 1000 mg is inserted through the catheter into the pericardial sac, with local anesthetic administered before tetracycline injection. This procedure is repeated every 2 to 3 days until sclerosis is complete, as measured by <25 ml of drainage during the previous 24 hours. Complications include low grade fever and local chest pain.[185,312] Pericardial sclerosis with instillation of bleomycin also has been shown to be effective in controlling malignant pericardial effusions. This approach may have advantages over tetracycline, with fewer adverse effects reported and pain-free instillation.[342] Other agents such as quinacrine, talc, 5-FU, nitrogen mustard, MTX, and gold-198 have all been used, but complications are more frequent.[337]

If drainage and instillation therapy fails, then surgical management should be considered. Surgical management includes placement of a pericardial window or pericardiectomy, designed to provide permanent drainage.[260] A window can be either pericardiocutaneous or pleural-pericardial with a higher frequency of closure and recurrent effusion with the latter. Overall success is 70% to 80% likely.[255,260,337] Pericardiectomy is rarely indicated for malignant pericardial effusions because of the high mortality and morbidity rates associated with the procedure and the short life expectancy of patients with extensive metastases to the pericardium.[337]

Radiation therapy can be extremely effective in the treatment of malignant pericardial effusions.[176] Generally, 150 to 200 rad/day are delivered to a total dose of 2500 to 3000 cGy over a 3- to 4-week period. Approximately 70% of malignant pericardial effusions related to breast cancer will respond to this approach.[171,255] Radiation therapy is indicated when pericardiocentesis with instillation therapy has failed and for patients in whom a surgical window is contraindicated. Previous or planned doxorubicin use is considered a relative contraindication to radiation therapy because of the potential risk for congestive heart failure.

Corticosteroids have been reported to be of benefit in patients with radiation-induced pericardial effusions; whether their use prevents or delays the development of constriction is unknown.[156] Pericardiectomy is the treatment of choice for radiation-induced pericardial disease that does not respond to conservative medical treatment.[260,291]

Summary

Patients with breast cancer and pericardial effusions have a better overall prognosis than patients with other solid tumors.[171] Median survival time is approximately 1 year if tamponade does not occur. In patients with tamponade, the survival time is substantially less, generally on the order of weeks to months, although some long-term survivors have been reported.

The development of pericardial effusion in a patient with breast cancer is not an infrequent occurrence. Patients with minimal pericardial involvement may be asymptomatic but even more extensive involvement may not be suspected clinically, as the symptoms are nonspecific, including fatigue and weakness. They are often attributed to the systemic effects of the underlying malignancy. The clinician must maintain a high index of suspicion, because pericardial effusion can be a fatal complication. Following pericardiocentesis, definite treatment depends on the sensitivity of the breast cancer. As outlined above, effective therapy is available that can provide excellent palliation and prolong survival.

SKELETAL METASTASES/PATHOLOGIC FRACTURES

Skeletal metastases occur in almost 70% of patients with breast cancer and breast cancer is the most common tumor associated with bone metastases.[149,353] Median survival in this subgroup of patients is almost 6 months, with 20% of patients surviving for more than 1 year. This is generally a longer time than is seen in patients with other solid tumors.[259]

The most common sites of bony metastases from breast cancer are spine, pelvis, femur, and humerus, in that order. Pathologic fractures are a devastating complication of metastatic breast cancer to bone, associated with severe pain, loss of function and mobility, and shortening of life expectancy. However, mean life expectancy following a pathologic fracture of a long bone is 23 months.[259] Management focuses on two aspects, prophylactic management of skeletal lesions and surgical intervention of documented fractures. New advances in joint repalcement and development of newer bone cements such as polymethylmethacrylate have permitted reliable methods of treating patients with pathologic fractures.[184,227]

Pathophysiology

Skeletal metastases develop primarily in the axial skeleton and the lower extremities as a result of hematogenous dissemination, or, rarely, contiguous extension.[149,197] There are no lymphatic channels in bone. The breast drains principally by the azygous venous sytem, communicating with Batson's paravertebral plexus, initially in the thoracic region.[155] The thoracic spine is the most common site for skeletal metastases and the vertebral body is typically affected first. Metastatic bone disease predominantly involves the red bone marrow, which is related to the special hemodynamic and microanatomic aspects of its vasculature.[155] The pattern of metastases to bone is not fully understood but is usually selective and dependent on anatomic aspects of vasculature, special characteristics of bone, and specific properties of the tumor cells themselves.[155] Tumor cells may destroy bone directly, or produce mediators such as prostaglandins (PGE_1 and PGE_2), and transforming growth factors, or stimulate IL-1, which can stimulate resorption of bone by osteoclasts.[196,200,266]

Clinical presentation

The development of bone metastases is common and often a catastrophic manifestation of metastatic breast cancer, compromising patients' quality of life by causing severe pain, neurologic deficits, pathologic fractures, immobility, and occasionally hematologic compromise.[259] Pain, which is the hallmark of bone metastases, characteristically is initially intermittent and gradually over weeks to months becomes more severe and unrelenting. Percussion tenderness at the site of involvement is common. Careful neurologic examination of patients with back pain is crucial because metastatic disease to vertebral bodies is associated with extradural spinal disease, which contributes to spinal cord compression. Sudden worsening of pain or functional impairment suggest fracture. Nonspecific laboratory abnormalities include elevation of serum alkaline phosphatase and mild anemia.

Diagnostic evaluation

Generally, multiple bone lesions are seen in metastatic breast cancer patients. A solitary lesion occasionally occurs, which can present as a diagnostic dilemma, at times requiring a biopsy. Painful bony areas in a patient with breast cancer must undergo radiographic evaluation. The radionuclide bone scan with ^{99m}Tc-diphosphonate is currently the best method for detecting skeletal metastases. The accuracy of bone scan ranges from 80% to 95%.[231,238] In general bone scans detect metastases before they are seen on plain x-rays. However, a positive bone scan (increased area of activity) is not specific for bone metastases.[266] Radiographs help to distinguish benign from malignant processes and aid in evaluating the structural integrity of bone. Metastatic breast cancer to bone is typically osteolytic but an osteoblastic or a mixed pattern can be seen.[196] Typically, x-rays reveal multiple small-to-medium sized lesions with a moth-eaten appearance. Osteoblastic lesions are sclerotic, tend to be smaller, and have increased radiographic density. Pathologic fractures occur less frequently in association with osteoblastic metastases as compared to osteolytic lesions.[196] Computed tomography is a useful tool for evaluating lesions of the pelvis and spine when bone scan and radiographs are equivocal.

The sensitivity of MRI may exceed that of other imaging modalities, and sometimes reveals tumor infiltration of bone before physiologic changes have occurred.[284] MRI may be useful in patients with a normal bone scan and persistent, unexplained pain or positive bone scans with negative plain films and CT scans.[197,284]

Management

Bone metastases require treatment to palliate pain and improve mobility. A multimodality approach that employs the expertise of medical, surgical, and radiation oncologists is the optimal approach. Symptomatic skeletal metastases not associated with fracture generally respond to treatment with radiation therapy, chemotherapy, or hormonal therapy. Radiation therapy is recommended for sites of disease unresponsive to treatment or bony metastases in weight bearing areas such as the femoral neck or vertebral bodies where complication of tumor progression can be devastating. Radiation therapy is extremely effective in reducing pain in patients with metastatic breast cancer.[259] It is generally given on an outpatient basis, as high-dose, fractionated treatment. Therapy is well tolerated with little morbidity. For patients with extensive skeletal metastases, hemibody irradiation has been utilized to relieve pain. Complications include moderate gastrointestinal toxicity and myelosuppression.[339]

Prophylactic surgical fixation of impending pathologic fractures is controversial, with no randomized prospective trials available to date. Surgical series have identified subgroups of patients at high risk for fracture who might benefit from prophylactic surgery. In weight-bearing bones recommendations are (1) a lytic lesion >50% of the cross-sectional diameter of the bone; (2) painful lytic lesions involving >2.5 cm of cortex in axial length, (3) persistent pain despite irradiation, and (4) pathologic avulsion fracture of the lesser trochanter.[224,309] In non–weight bearing bones (humerus, ulna, radius) lytic lesions involving >50% of the cross-sectional area of cortical bone or longer than 5 cm should be considered for prophylactic fixation.[317]

The morbidity associated with prophylactic fixation is substantially lower than that experienced with patients with pathologic fractures. Once prophylactic fixation of the affected bone has been achieved, radiotherapy should be initiated.[225,305,339]

Pathologic fractures that require surgical intervention occur in approximately 9% of patients with metastatic bony disease.[184] Once a fracture has occurred, healing and pain relief are poor unless aggressive local therapy with orthopedic stabilization and local radiation therapy are performed.[225,227] Postoperative radiation therapy is necessary because continued growth and bone destruction by the tumor will eventually weaken the bone despite fixation.[225] Generally, treatment of pathologic fractures of the lower extremity requires extensive surgery; therefore patients should be medically stable, with a life expectancy of more than one month.[225] Hip fractures occur in 10% of patients with metastatic breast cancer, which is one of the most common sites of pathologic fractures and one of the most difficult regions to repair.[225,244] Depending upon the location, hip replacement, hip screw, or rods, supplemented with cement, have been used successfully. Because prophylactic procedures are the same as those used after pathologic fracture, the advantages of reduced morbidity with prophylactic fixation do not apply.[184,309] Generally, postoperative complications are quite serious, including a 40% morbidity rate, although surgical fixation of pathologic fracture results in relief of pain and secure ambulation. Fracture of the femoral shaft can be treated with intramedulary rods with cement followed by radiation therapy.

For pathologic fractures of the upper extremity, surgical management depends primarily on the location of the lesion in the bone, the extent of destruction, and the general condition of the patient. Often pathologic fractures of the upper extremity can be treated conservatively with a nonoperative approach.[317] This includes immobilization with a functional brace followed by extensive physical therapy. Indications for operative management of a pathologic humeral fracture includes those patients who are expected to live more than 3 months, those who require the upper extremity for weight bearing, and those in whom conservative, nonoperative therapy has failed.[317]

The biphosphonates are potent inhibitors of osteoclastic bone resorption that may have a role in managing skeletal metastases. Experimental evidence suggest that the biphophonates decrease tumor-induced osteolysis as measured by calcium kinetics and calcium balance.[243,244] Pamidronate disodium, one of the new biphosphonates, has been evaluated in patients with symptomatic bone metastases from breast cancer. Preliminary data demonstrates significant reduction in tumor-related morbidity, including hypercalcemia, bone pain, pathologic fractures, and the need for surgical or radiotherapeutic intervention.[182] Sclerosis of lytic lesions occurs in approximately 20% of treated patients.[263] Clodronate has been evaluated in a randomized, placebo-controlled trial in which reduction in the formation of new bone metastases and a statistically significant improvement in overall survival was demonstrated in the clodronate-treated group. Preliminary data suggests that these agents' clinical effects are primarily in patients with lytic bone metastases.

Summary

The management of skeletal metastases and pathologic fractures must be individualized. Although treatment in metastatic bone disease is palliative, aggressive medical and surgical treatment yields very satisfactory results, which significantly improve the quality of life of patients by providing relief of pain and improvement in function. Future studies evaluating the new biphosphonates could have a major impact on managing this common complication of breast cancer.

REFERENCES

Treatment of metastatic breast cancer

1. Ahmann DL, Bisel HF, and Hahn RG: Phase II clinical trial of isophosphamide (NSC-109724) in patients with advanced breast cancer. Cancer Chemother Rep 58:861, 1974.
2. Aisner J, Weinberg V, Perloff M, et al: Chemotherapy versus chemoimmunotherapy (CAF v CAFVP v CMF each plus/minus MER) for metastatic carcinoma of the breast: a CALBG study, J Clin Oncol 5:1523, 1987.
3. Aitken SC and Lippman ME: Hormonal regulation of net DNA synthesis in MCF-7 human breast cancer cells in tissue culture, Cancer Res 42:1727, 1982.
4. Allegra JC, Barlock A, Huff KK, et al: Changes in multiple or sequential estrogen receptor determinations in breast cancer, Cancer 45:792, 1980.
5. Allegra JC and Kiefer SM: Mechanisms of actions of progestational agents, Semin Oncol 12:3, 1985.
6. Allegra JC, Woodcock TM, Richman SP, et al: A phase II trial of tamoxifen, premarin, methotrexate and 5-fluorouracil in metastatic breast cancer, Breast Cancer Res Treat 2:93, 1982.
7. Armand JP, Hurteloup P, Hayat M, et al: Phase III chemotherapy comparing FAC vs FEC in advanced breast cancer, Proc Am Soc Clin Oncol 3:118, 1984.
8. Australian and New Zealand Breast Cancer Trials Group (ANZBCTG): A randomized trial in postmenopausal patients with advanced breast cancer comparing endocrine and cytotoxic therapy given sequentially or in combination, J Clin Oncol 4:186, 1986.
9. Ayme Y, Brandone H, and Brandone JM: Antiestrogenotherapie cyclique dans les cancers du sein en phase avancee: association sequentielle tamoxifen-medroxyprogesterine, Cancerologie 44:1984.
10. Baker LH and Vaitkevicius VK: Reevaluation of rebound regression in disseminated carcinoma of the breast, Cancer 29:1268, 1972.
11. Beatson GT: On the treatment of inoperable cases of carcinoma of the mamma: suggestion for a new method of treatment, Lancet ii:162, 1896.

12. Brambilla C, DeLena M, Rossi A, et al: Response and survival in advanced breast cancer after two non-cross-resistant combinations, Br Med J 1:801, 1976.
13. Brooks BJ and Lippmann ME: Tamoxifen flare in advanced endometrial carcinoma, J Clin Oncol 3:222, 1985.
14. Brufman G and Biran S: Second-line hormonal therapy with aminoglutethimide in metastatic breast cancer, Acta Oncol 29:717, 1990.
15. Buchanan RB, Blamey RW, Durrant KR, et al: A randomized comparison of tamoxifen with surgical oophorectomy in premenopausal patients with advanced breast cancer, J Clin Oncol 4:1326, 1986.
16. Bull JM, Tormey DG, and Li SH: A randomized comparative trial of Adriamycin versus methotrexate in combination drug therapy, Cancer 41:1649, 1978.
17. Byar D, Sears M, and McGuire W: Relationship between estrogen receptor values and clinical data in predicting the response to endocrine therapy for patients with advanced breast cancer, Eur J Cancer 15:299, 1979.
18. Canellos GP, Pocock SJ, Taylor SG, et al: Combination chemotherapy for metastatic breast carcinoma: prospective comparison of multiple drug therapy with L-phenylalanine mustard, Cancer 35:1882, 1976.
19. Carbone PP, Bauer M, Band P, et al: Chemotherapy of disseminated breast cancer, Cancer 39:2916, 1977.
20. Carbone PP and Tormey DL: Combination chemotherapy for advanced disease. In McGuire WL, editor: Breast cancer. Advances in research and treatment, vol 1, New York, 1977, Plenum Press, p 165.
21. Carmo-Pereira J, Costa FO, and Henriques E: Single-drug versus combination cytotoxic chemotherapy in advanced breast cancer, Eur J Cancer 16:1621, 1980.
22. Carter AC, Sedransk N, Kelley RM, et al: Diethylstilbestrol: recommended dosages for different categories of breast cancer patients, JAMA 237:2079, 1977.
23. Chlebowski RT, Paroly WS, and Pugh RP: Adriamycin given as a weekly schedule without a loading course, Cancer Treat Rep 64:47, 1980.
24. Clark GM and McGuire WL: Progesterone receptors and human breast cancer, Breast Cancer Res 3:157, 1983.
25. Clark GM, Sledge GW, and Osborne CK: Survival from first recurrence: relative importance of prognostic factors in 1,015 breast cancer patients, J Clin Oncol 5:55, 1987.
26. Coates A, Gebski V, Bishop JF, et al: Improving the quality of life during chemotherapy for advanced breast cancer: a comparison of intermittent and continuous treatment strategies, N Engl J Med 317:1490, 1987.
27. Cocconi G, DeLisi V, Boni C, et al: Chemotherapy versus combination of chemotherapy and endocrine therapy in advanced breast cancer, Cancer 51:581, 1983.
28. Coombes RC, Dearnaley D, Humphreys J, et al: Danazol treatment of advanced breast cancer, Cancer Treat Rep 64:1073, 1980.
29. Cooper RG: Combination chemotherapy in hormone resistant breast cancer, Proc Am Assoc Cancer Res 10:15, 1969.
30. Cooperative Breast Cancer Group: Results of studies of the Cooperative Breast Cancer Group 1961-1963, Cancer Chemother Rep 41:1, 1964.
31. Cooperative Breast Cancer Group: Testosterone proprionate therapy in breast cancer, JAMA 188:1069, 1964.
32. Corkery J, Leonard RCF, Henderson IC, et al: Tamoxifen and aminoglutethimide in advanced breast cancer, Cancer Res 42:3409, 1982.
33. Corle DK, Sears ME, and Olson KB: The relationship of quantitative estrogen receptor level and clinical response to cytotoxic chemotherapy in advanced breast cancer: an extramural analysis, Cancer 54:1554, 1984.
34. Creech RH, Catalano RB, Shah MK, et al: An effective low-dose mitomycin regimen for hormonal- and chemotherapy-refractory patients with metastatic breast cancer, Cancer 51:1034, 1983.
35. Cutler SJ: Classification of extent of disease in breast cancer, Semin Oncol 1:91, 1974.
36. Dao TL and Nemoto T: Steroid receptors and response to endocrine ablations in women with metastatic cancer of the breast, Cancer 46:2779, 1980.
37. Fabian C, Sternson L, El-Serafi M, et al: Clinical pharmacology of tamoxifen in patients with breast cancer: correlation with clinical data, Cancer 48:876, 1981.
38. Falkson G, Gelman RS, Leone L, et al: Survival of premenopausal women with metastatic breast cancer. Long-term follow-up of Eastern Cooperative Oncology Group and Cancer and Leukemia Group B studies, Cancer 66:1621, 1990.
39. Falkson G, Gelman RS, Tormey DC, et al: The Eastern Cooperative Oncology Group experience with cyclophosphamide, Adriamycin and 5-fluorouracil (CAF) in patients with metastatic breast cancer, Cancer 56:219, 1985.
40. Fitzpatrick PJ and Garrett PG: Metastatic breast cancer. Ovarian ablation with lower half body radiation, Int J Radiat Oncol Biol Phys 7:1523, 1981.
41. Forastiere AA, Hakes TB, Wittes JT, et al: Cisplatin in the treatment of metastatic breast carcinoma: a prospective randomized trial of two dosage schedules, Am J Clin Oncol 5:243, 1982.
42. Fracchia AA, Farrow JH, DePalo AJ, et al: Castration for primary inoperable or recurrent breast carcinoma, Surg Gynecol Obstet 128:1226, 1969.
43. Fraschini G, Yap HY, and Hortobabyi GN: Five-day continuous infusion vinblastine in the treatment of breast cancer, Cancer 56:225, 1985.
44. Furr BJA and Jordan VC: The pharmacology and clinical uses of tamoxifen, Pharmacol Ther 25:127, 1984.
45. Garewal HS, Brooks RJ, and Jones SE: Treatment of advanced breast cancer with mitomycin-C combined with vinlastine or vindesine, J Clin Oncol 1:772, 1983.
46. Geimer NF and Donegan WL: Role and mechanisms of corticosteroid therapy in breast cancer, Rev Endocrine-Related Cancer 6:5, 1980.
47. Glick JH: Metastatic breast cancer. In: Schein PS, editor: Decision making in oncology, Philadelphia, 1989, BC Decker, p 112.
48. Goldie JH, Coldman AJ, and Gudauskas GA: Rationale for the use of alternating non-cross resistant chemotherapy, Cancer Treat Rep 66:439, 1982.
49. Greenspan EM, Fieber M, Lesnick G, et al: Response of advanced breast carcinoma to the combination of the antimetabolite methotrexate and the alkylating agent thio-TEPA, J Mt Sinai Hosp 30:246, 1963.
50. Grodin JM, Siiteri PK, and MacDonald PC: Source of estrogen production in postmenopausal women, J Clin Endocrinol 36:207, 1973.
51. Gundersen S: Toremifene, a new antiestrogenic compound in the treatment of metastatic mammary cancer. A phase II study, J Steroid Biochem 36:233, 1990.
52. Gusberg SB: Tamoxifen for breast cancer: associated endometrial cancer, Cancer 65:1463, 1990.
53. Haller D, Andersen J, and Muggia F: Chemohormone therapy with Adriamycin or mitoxantrone combinations in advanced breast cancer: an ECOG trial, Proc Am Soc Clin Oncol 7:19, 1988.
54. Haller DG and Glick JH: Progestational agents in advanced breast cancer: an overview, Semin Oncol 13:2, 1986.
55. Hart R, Perloff M, and Holland J: One day VATH therapy for advanced breast cancer refractory to chemotherapy cancer, Cancer 48:1522. 1981.

56. Harvey HA, Lipton A, Max DT, et al: Medical castration produced by the GNRH analogue leuprolide to treat metastatic breast cancer, J Clin Oncol 3:1068, 1985.
57. Hayes DF, Zurawski VR, and Kufe DW: Comparison of circulating CA15-3 and carcinoembryonic antigen levels in patients with breast cancer, J Clin Oncol 4:1542, 1986.
58. Hayward JL, Atkins JHB, Falconer MA, et al: Clinical trials comparing transfrontal hypophysectomy with adrenalectomy. In Joslin CAF and Gleave AN, editors: The clinical management of advanced breast cancer, Cardiff, 1970, Alpha Omega Alpha Publishing, p 50.
59. Henderson IC and Canellos GP: Cancer of the breast: the past decades, N Engl J Med 302:17, 1980.
60. Henderson IC, Hayes DF, Comes S, et al: New agents and new medical treatments for advanced breast cancer, Semin Oncol 14:34, 1987.
61. Henderson IC: Selection of therapy for metastatic breast cancer. In Santen RJ and Henderson IC, editors: A comprehensive guide to the therapeutic use of immunoglutethimide, Basel 1982, Karger, p 47.
62. Hindi I, Juho SE, Szanto J, et al: Effect of toremifene in breast cancer patients. Preliminary communication, J Steroid Biochem 36:255, 1990.
63. Hoogstraten B, George SL, and Samal B: Combination chemotherapy and Adriamycin in patients with advanced breast cancer, Cancer 38:13, 1976.
64. Hortobabyi GN, Bodey GP, and Buzdar AU: Evaluation of high-dose versus standard FAC chemotherapy for advanced breast cancer in protected environment units: a prospective randomized study, J Clin Oncol 5:354, 1987.
65. Horwitz KB, McGuire WL, Pearson OH, et al: Predicting response to endocrine therapy in human breast cancer: a hypothesis, Science 989:726, 1975.
66. Hryniuk W and Bush H: The importance of dose intensity in chemotherapy of metastatic breast cancer, J Clin Oncol 2:1281, 1984.
67. Ingle JN: Additive hormonal therapy in women with advanced breast cancer, Cancer 53:766, 1984.
68. Ingle JN, Ahmann DL, Gestner JG, et al: Evaluation of vinblastine administered by 5-day continuous infusion in women with advanced breast cancer, Cancer Treat Rep 68:803, 1984.
69. Ingle JN, Ahmann DL, Green ST, et al: Randomized clinical trial of diethylstilbestrol versus tamoxifen in postmenopausal women with advanced breast cancer, N Engl J Med 304:16, 1981.
70. Ingle JN, Krook JE, Green SJ, et al: Randomized trial of bilateral oophorectomy versus tamoxifen in premenopausal women with metastatic breast cancer, J Clin Oncol 4:178, 1986.
71. Ingle JN, Twito DI, Schaid DJ, et al: Combination hormonal therapy with tamoxifen plus fluoxymesterone versus tamoxifen alone in postmenopausal women with metastatic breast cancer, Cancer 67:886, 1991.
72. Jensen EV, Block GE, Smith S, et al: Estrogen receptors and breast cancer. Response to adrenalectomy. Prediction of response in cancer therapy, Natl Cancer Inst Monogr 34:55, 1971.
73. Jordan VC: Laboratory studies to develop general principles for the adjuvant treatment of breast cancer with antiestrogen: problems and potential for future clinical applications, Breast Cancer Res Treat 3:73, 1983.
74. Jordan VC and Tormey DC: Antiestrogen therapy for breast cancer: current strategies and future prospects, Cancer Treat Res 39:97, 1988.
75. Kardinal CG, Perry MC, Korzun AH, et al: Response to chemotherapy or chemoendocrine therapy in patients with advanced breast cancer previously treated with adjuvant chemotherapy, Breast Cancer Res Treat 6:185, 1985.
76. Kardinal CG, Perry MC, Weinberg V, et al: Chemoendocrine therapy vs. chemotherapy alone for advanced breast cancer in postmenopausal women: preliminary report of a randomized study, Breast Cancer Res Treat 3:365, 1983.
77. Kelley RM: Hormones and chemotherapy in breast cancer, Cancer 28:686, 1971.
78. Klijn JGM, DeJung FH, Blankenstein MA, et al: Antitumor and endocrine effects of chronic LHRH agonist treatment (buserelin) with or without tamoxifen in premenopausal metastatic breast cancer, Breast Cancer Res Treat 4:209, 1984.
79. Konits P, Aisner J, Van Echo D, et al: Mitomycin-C and vinblastine chemotherapy for advanced breast cancer, Cancer 48:1295, 1981.
80. Lee YN: Breast carcinoma: patterns of recurrence and metastases after mastectomy, Am J Clin Oncol 7:443, 1984.
81. Legha S, Buzdar A, Smith T, et al: Response to hormonal therapy as a prognostic factor for metastatic breast cancer treated with combination chemotherapy, Cancer 46:438, 1980.
82. Legha SS, Benjamin RS, Mackay B, et al: Adriamycin therapy by continuous infusion in patients with metastatic breast cancer, Cancer 49:1762, 1982.
83. Levine MN, Gent M, Hirsh J, et al: The thrombogenic effect of anticancer drug therapy in women with stage II breast cancer, N Engl J Med 318:401, 1988.
84. Lippman ME: Antiestrogen therapy of breast cancer, Semin Oncol 10:11, 1983.
85. Lippman ME: Efforts to combine endocrine chemotherapy in the management of breast cancer: do two and two equal three? Breast Cancer Res Treat 3:117, 1983.
86. Lippman ME, Cassidy J, Wesley M, et al: A randomized attempt to increase the efficacy of cytotoxic chemotherapy in metastatic breast cancer by hormonal synchronization, J Clin Oncol 2:28, 1984.
87. Lippman ME, Dickson RB, Kasid A, et al: Autocrine and paracrine growth regulation of human breast cancer, J Steroid Biochem 24:187, 1986.
88. Lipton A, Harvey HA, and Hamilton RW: Venous thrombosis as a side effect of tamoxifen treatment, Cancer Treat Rep 68:887, 1984.
89. Loprinzi C, Tormey D, and Rasmussen P: Prospective evaluation of carcinoembryonic antigen levels and alternating chemotherapeutic regimens in metastatic breast cancer, J Clin Oncol 4:46, 1986.
90. Manni A and Pearson OH: Antiestrogen-induced remissions in premenopausal women with stage IV breast cancer: effects on ovarian function, Cancer Treat Rep 64:779, 1980.
91. Martoni A, Piana E, and Guaraldi M: Comparative phase II study of idarubicin versus doxorubicin in advanced breast cancer, Oncology 47:427, 1990.
92. Mattson W: Current status of high dose progestin treatment in advanced breast cancer, Breast Cancer Res Treat 3:231, 1983.
93. Mauriac L, Durand M, and Bonichon F: Sequential hormone therapy (tamoxifen-MPA) vs tamoxifen in metastatic breast cancers: preliminary results, Bull Cancer (Paris) 72:11, 1985.
94. Millward MJ, Haris AL, and Cantwell BM: Phase II study of doxorubicin plus ifosfamide/mesna in patients with advanced breast cancer, Cancer 65:2421, 1990.
95. Morgan LR: Megestrol acertate v. tamoxifen in advanced breast cancer in postmenopausal patients, Semin Oncol 12:43, 1985.
96. Mouridsen HT, Palshof T, Brahm M, et al: Evaluation of single drug versus multiple drug chemotherapy in the

treatment of advanced breast cancer, Cancer Treat Rep 61:47, 1977.
97. Mouridsen HT, Rose C, Engelsman E, et al: Combined cytotoxic and endocrine therapy in postmenopausal patients with advanced breast cancer. A randomized study of CMF vs CMF plus tamoxifen, Eur J Clin Oncol 21:219, 1985.
98. Muss HB, Paschold EH, and Black WR: Megestrol acetate v. tamoxifen in advanced breast cancer: a phase III trial of the Piedmont Oncology Association (POA), Semin Oncol 12:55, 1985.
99. Muss HB, Van Echo D, and Korzun AH: Esorubicin in advanced breast cancer. A phase II study of the CALGB, Am J Clin Oncol 13:233, 1990.
100. Muss HB, White DR, and Cowan RJ: Brain scanning patients with recurrent breast cancer, Cancer 38:1574, 1976.
101. Nomura Y, Tashiro H, and Shinozuka K: Changes of steroid hormone receptor content by chemotherapy and/or endocrine therapy in advanced breast cancer, Cancer 55:546, 1985.
102. O'Bryan RM, Baker LH, Gottlieb JE, et al: Dose response evaluation of adriamycin in human neoplasia, Cancer 39:1940, 1977.
103. Paradaens R, Sylvester RJ, Ferrazzi E, et al: Clinical significance of the quantitative assessment of estrogen receptors in advanced breast cancer, Cancer 46:2889, 1980.
104. Pastan I and Gottesman M: Multiple drug resistance in human cancer, N Engl J Med 316:1388, 1987.
105. Pasterz RB, Buzdar AU, Hortobagyi GN, et al: Mitomycin in metastatic breast cancer refractory to hormonal and combination chemotherapy, Cancer 56:2381, 1985.
106. Patterson JS, Battersby LA, and Edwards DG: Review of the clinical pharmacology and international experience with tamoxifen in advanced breast cancer, Rev Endocrine-Related Cancer 9:563, 1982.
107. Pedrazzini A, Gelber R, Isley M, et al: First repeated bone scan in the observation of patients with operable breast cancer, J Clin Oncol 4:389, 1986.
108. Perez JE, Machiavelli M, Leone MA, et al: Bone-only versus visceral-only metastatic patterns in breast cancer: analysis of 150 patients. A GOCS study, Am J Clin Oncol 13:294, 1990.
109. Perry MC, Kardinal CG, Korzun A, et al: Chemohormonal therapy in advanced carcinoma of the breast. CALGB protocol 8081, J Clin Oncol 5:1534, 1987.
110. Plotkin D, Lechner J, Jung WE, et al: Tamoxifen flare in advanced breast cancer, JAMA 240:2644, 1978.
111. Pritchard K, Thomson DS, Myers RE, et al: Tamoxifen therapy in premenopausal patients with metastatic breast cancer, Cancer Treat Rep 64:787, 1980.
112. Robertson JF, Walker KJ, Nicholson RI, et al: Combined endocrine effects of LHRH agonist (Zoladex) and tamoxifen (Nolvadex) therapy in premenopausal women with breast cancer, Br J Sur 76:1262, 1989.
113. Rochefort H: Biochemical basis of breast cancer treatment by androgens and progestins. In Gurpide E, Calandra R, and Levy C, editors: Hormones and cancer, New York, 1984, Alan R. Liss, p 79.
114. Rubens RD and Knight RK: The contribution of prednisolone to primary endocrine therapy in advanced breast cancer, Proc Am Soc Clin Oncol 4:53, 1985.
115. Rubens RD, Tinson CL, Coleman RE, et al: Prednisolone improves the response to primary endocrine treatment for advanced breast cancer, Br J Cancer 58:626, 1988.
116. Sanchiz F and Milla A: High dose ifosfamide and mesna in advanced breast cancer. A phase II study, Cancer Chemother Pharmacol 26:591, 1990.
117. Santen RJ, Boucher AE, Santner SJ, et al: Inhibition of aromatase as treatment of breast carcinoma in postmenopausal women, J Lab Clin Med 109:278, 1987.
118. Santen RJ, Samojlik E, and Worgul TJ: Aminoglutethimide. In Santen RJ and Henderson IC, editors: A comprehensive guide to the therapeutic use of aminoglutethimide, Basel, 1982, Karger, p 101.
119. Segaloff A, Carter AC, Escher GC, et al: An evaluation of the effect of vincristine added to cyclophosphamide, 5-fluorouracil, methotrexate and prednisone in advanced breast cancer, Breast Cancer Res Treat 5:311, 1985.
120. Sheth SP and Allegra JC: What role for concurrent chemohormonal therapy in breast cancer? Oncology 1:19, 1987.
121. Silverstein MJ, Byron RL, Yonemoto RH, et al: Bilateral adrenalectomy for advanced breast cancer: a 21 year experience, Surgery 77:825, 1975.
122. Skeel RT, Andersen JW, Tormey DC, et al: Combination chemotherapy of advanced breast cancer. Comparison of dibromodulcitol, doxorubicin, vincristine and fluoxymesterone to thiotepa, doxorubicin, vinblastine, and fluoxymesterone: an Eastern Cooperative Oncology Group study, Cancer 64:1393, 1989.
123. Sledge GW: Etoposide in the management of metastatic breast cancer, Cancer 67:266, 1991.
124. Sledge GW, Loehrer PJ, Roth BJ, et al: Cisplatin as first-line therapy for metastatic breast cancer, J Clin Oncol 6:1811, 1988.
125. Sledge GW and Roth BT: Cisplatin in the management of breast cancer, Semin Oncol 16:110, 1989.
126. Smalley RV, Lefante J, Bartolluci A, et al: A comparison of cyclophosphamide, Adriamycin and 5-fluorouracil (CAF) and cyclophosphamide, methotrexate, vincristine, and prednisone (CMFVP) in patients with advanced breast cancer, Breast Cancer Res Treat 3:209, 1983.
127. Smalley RN, Murphy S, Huguley CM, et al: Combination versus sequential five-drug chemotherapy in metastatic carcinoma of the breast, Cancer Res 36:3911, 1976.
128. Smith ILE, Harris EL, Morgan M, et al: Tamoxifen vesus aminoglutethimide versus combined tamoxifen and aminoglutethimide in the treatment of advanced breast cancer, Cancer Res 42:3430, 1982.
129. Steiner R, Stewart JF, and Rubens RD: Results of endocrine therapy do not predict response to chemotherapy in advanced breast cancer, Eur J Cancer Clin Oncol 19:1559, 1983.
130. Stoll BA: Progestin therapy of breast cancer: comparison of agents, Br Med J 3:338, 1967.
131. Stoll BA: Castration and oestrogen therapy. In Stoll BA, editor: Endocrine therapy in malignant disease, London, 1972, Saunders, p 139.
132. Stoll BA: Combination endocrine therapy in breast cancer, Eur J Cancer Clin Oncol 21:413, 1985.
133. Stuart-Harris R, Bozek T, Gazet JC, et al: Low-dose aminoglutethimide in treatment of advanced breast cancer, Lancet ii:604, 1984.
134. Stuart-Harris RC and Smith IE: Aminoglutethimide in the treatment of advanced breast cancer, Cancer Treat Rev 11:189, 1984.
135. Talley RW, Vaitkevicius VK, and Leighton GA: Comparison of cyclophosphamide and 5-fluorouracil in the treatment of patients with metastatic breast cancer, Clin Pharmacol Ther 6:740, 1965.
136. Tannock I, Ehrlichman C, Perrault D, et al: Failure of 5-day vinblastine infusion in the treatment of patients with advanced refractory breast cancer, Cancer Treat Rep 66:1783, 1982.
137. Tormey D and Waalkes T: Clinical correlation between CEA and breast cancer, Cancer 42:1507, 1978.

138. Tormey DC, Gelman R, Band PR, et al: Comparison of induction chemotherapies for metastatic breast cancer, Cancer 50:1235, 1982.
139. Tormey DC, Lippman ME, Edwards BK, et al: Evaluation of tamoxifen doses with and without fluoxymesterone in advanced breast cancer, Ann Intern Med 98:139, 1983.
140. Tormey DC, Weinberg VE, Leone LA, et al: A comparison of intermittent vs continuous and of Adriamycin vs methotrexate 5-drug chemotherapy for advanced breast cancer, Am J Clin Oncol 7:231, 1984.
141. Van Veelen H, Willemse PH, and Sliejfer DT: Adrenal suppression by oral high-dose medroxyprogesterone acetate in breast cancer patients, Cancer Chemother Pharmacol 12:83, 1984.
142. Veronesi U, Pizzocaro G, and Rossi A: Oophorectomy for advanced carcinoma of the breast, Surg Gynecol Obstet 141:569, 1975.
143. Verrelle P, Meissonniere F, Fonck Y, et al: Clinical relevance of immunohistochemical detection of multidrug resistance P-glycoprotein in breast carcinoma, J Natl Cancer Inst 83:111, 1991.
144. Wang DY, Rubens RD, Clark GM, et al: Effects of prednisolone on sex hormone binding globulin during primary endocrine treatment of advanced breast cancer, Breast Cancer Res Treat 11:67, 1988.
145. Westerberg H: Tamoxifen and fluoxymesterone in advanced breast cancer: a controlled clinical trial, Cancer Treat Rep 64:117, 1980.
146. Willense PH, Van der Ploeg E, Sleijfer DT, et al: A randomized comparison of megestrol acetate and medroxyprogesterone acetate in patients with advanced breast cancer, Eur J Cancer 26:337, 1990.
147. Wittliff JL: Steroid-hormone receptors in breast cancer, Cancer 53:630, 1984.
148. Wright JC, Cobb JP, Golomb FM, et al: Chemotherapy of disseminated carcinoma of the breast, Ann Surg 150:221, 1959.

Complications of metastatic disease

149. Abrams HL, Spiro R, and Goldstein N: Metastases in carcinoma: analysis of 1000 autopsied cases, Cancer 23:74, 1950.
150. Austin EH and Flye MW: The treatment of recurrent malignant pleural effusion, Ann Thoracic Surg 28:190, 1979.
151. Barbor LM: Glucose level in pleural fluid as a diagnostic aid, Dis Chest 31:680, 1957.
152. Barrons KD, Mirano A, Araki S, et al: Experiences with metastatic neoplasms involving the spinal cord, Neurology 9:91, 1959.
153. Batson OV: Role of vertebral veins in metastatic processes, Ann Intern Med 16:38, 1942.
154. Benedict WF and Porter JH: The cytogenetic diagnosis of malignancy in effusions, Acta Cytol 16:304, 1972.
155. Berrettoni BA and Carter JR: Mechanisms of cancer metastasis to bone, J Bone Joint Surg 68:308, 1986.
156. Biran S: Corticosteroids in radiation-induced pericarditis, Chest 74:96, 1978.
157. Biran S, Brufman G, Klein E, and Hochman A: The management of pericardial effusion in cancer patients, Chest 71:182, 1977.
158. Bitran JD, Evans R, and Brown C: The management of cardiac tamponade in patients with breast cancer, J Surg Oncol 27:42, 1984.
159. Black LF. The pleural space and pleural fluid, Mayo Clin Proc 47:493, 1978.
160. Black P: Spinal metastases: current status and recommended guidelines for management, Neurosurgery 5:726, 1979.
161. Bleyer WA: The clinical pharmacology of methotrexate, Cancer 41:36, 1978.
162. Bleyer WA and Poplack DG: Intraventricular versus intralumbar methotrexate for central nervous system leukemia: prolonged remission with the Ommaya reservoir, Med Pediatr Oncol 6:207, 1979.
163. Blomquist GP: Malignant hypercalcemia—a hospital survey, Acta Med Scand 220:455, 1986.
164. Body JJ, Borkowski A, Cleeren A, et al: Treatment of malignancy-associated hypercalcemia with intravenous aminohydroxypropylidine diphosphonate, J Clin Oncol 4:1177, 1986.
165. Bonner JA, Lichter AS: A caution about the use of MRI to diagnose spinal cord compression, N Engl J Med 322:446, 1988 (letter).
166. Borgelt B, Gelber R, Kramer S, et al: The palliation of brain metastases: final results of the first of two studies by the radiation therapy oncology group, Int J Radiat Oncol Biol Phys 6:1, 1980.
167. Bosley TM, Cohen DA, Schotz NV, et al: Comparison of metrizamide computed tomography and magnetic resonance imaging in the evaluation of lesions at the cervicomedullary junction, Neurology 35:485, 1985.
168. Bristow MR, Mason JW, Billingham ME, et al. Doxorubicin cardiomyopathy: evaluation by phonocardiography, cardiomyocardial biopsy, and cardiac catheterization, Ann Intern Med 88:168, 1978.
169. Broadus AE, Mangia M, Ikeda K, et al: Humoral hypercalcemia of cancer. Identification of a novel parathyroid hormone-like peptide, N Engl J Med 319:556, 1988.
170. Bruckman JE and Bloomer WD: Management of spinal cord compression, Semin Oncol 5:135, 1978.
171. Buck M, Ingle JN, Giuliani ER, et al: Pericardial effusion in women with breast cancer, Cancer 60:263, 1987.
172. Burtis WJ, Brady TG, Orloff JJ, et al: Immunochemical characterization of circulating parathyroid hormone-related protein in patients with humoral hypercalcemia of cancer, N Engl J Med 322:1106, 1990.
173. Burtis WJ, Wu T, Bunch C, et al: Identification of a novel 17,000-dalton parathyroid hormone-like adenylate cyclase-stimulating protein from a tumor associated with humoral hypercalcemia of malignancy, J Biol Chem 262:7151, 1987.
174. Cairncross JG, Kim JH, and Posner JB: Radiation therapy for brain metastases, Ann Neruol 7:529, 1980.
175. Chalk JB, Ridgeway K, Brophy T, et al: Phenytoin impairs the bioavailability of dexamethasone in neurological and neurosurgical patients, J Neurol Neurosurg Psychiatry 47:1087, 1984.
176. Cham WC, Freiman AH, Carsters PH, et al: Radiation therapy of cardiac and pericardial metastases, Radiation 114:701, 1975.
177. Chernow B and Sahn SA: Carcinomatous involvement of the pleura, Am J Med 63:695, 1977.
178. Cobb C, Leavens ME, and Eckles N: Indications for nonoperative treatment of spinal cord compression due to breast cancer, J Neurosurg 47:653, 1977.
179. Cogan MG, Covey CM, Arieff AI, et al: Central nervous system manifestations of hyperparathyroidism, Am J Med 65:693, 1978.
180. Cohen N, Strauss G, Lew R, et al: Should prophylactic anticonvulsants be administered to patients with newly-diagnosed cerebral metastases? A retrospective analysis, J Clin Oncol 6:1621, 1988.
181. Cohn KE, Stewart JR, Fajands LF, et al: Heart disease following radiation, Medicine 46:281, 1967.
182. Coleman RE, Woll PJ, Miles M, et al: Treatment of bone metastases from breast cancer with APD, Br J Cancer 58:621, 1988.

183. Coleman RL, Fogelman I, and Rubens RD: Hypercalcemia and breast cancer: an increased humoral component in patients with liver metastases, Eur J Surg Oncol 14:428, 1988.
184. Coran AG, Banks HH, Aliapoulios MA, et al: The management of pathologic fractures in patients with metastatic carcinoma of the breast, Surg Gynecol Obstet 127:1225, 1968.
185. Davis S, Rambotti P, and Grignani F: Intrapericardial tetracycline sclerosis in the treatment of malignant pericardial effusion: an analysis of thirty-three cases, J Clin Oncol 2:631, 1984.
186. Delaney TF and Oldfield EH: Spinal cord compression. In DeVita VT, Hellman S, and Rosenberg SA, editors: Cancer: principles and practice of oncology, Philadelphia, 1989, JB Lippincott, pp 1978-1986.
187. DiStefano A, Yap HY, Hortobagyi GN, et al: The natural history of breast cancer patients with brain metastases, Cancer 44:1913, 1979.
188. Dudley FJ and Blackburn CRB: Extraskeletal calcification complicating oral neutral phosphate therapy, Lancet ii:628, 1970.
189. Ehrenkranz JR and Posner JB: Adrenocorticosteroid hormones. In Weiss L, Gilber HA, and Posner JB, editors: Brain metastases, Boston 1980, Hall, pp 340-363.
190. Elias EG, Reynoso G, and Mittelman A: Control of hypercalcemia with mithramycin, Ann Surg 175:431, 1972.
191. Fentiman IS, Rubens RD, and Hayward JL: Control of pleural effusions in patients with breast cancer, Cancer 52:737, 1983.
192. Fleisch H, Russell RGG, and Francis MD: Diphosphonates inhibit hydroxyapatite dissolution in vitro and bone resorption in tissue culture and in vivo, Science 165:1262, 1969.
193. Fornasier VL and Horne JG: Metastases to the veretebral column, Cancer 36:590, 1975.
194. Friedman MA and Slater E: Malignant pleural effusions, Cancer Treat Rev 5:49, 1978.
195. Galasko CSB: Mechanism of bone destruction in the development of skeletal metastases, Nature 263:507, 1976.
196. Galasko CSB: Mechanisms of lytic and blastic metastatic disease of bone, Clin Orthop 169:20, 1982.
197. Glasako CSB: Skeletal metastases, Clin Orthop 210:18, 1986.
198. Galasko CSB and Bennett A: Relationship of bone destruction in skeletal metastases to osteoclast activation and prostaglandins, Nature 263:508, 1976.
199. Galasko CSB and Burn JL: Hypercalcemia in patients with advanced mammary cancer, Br Med J 3:573, 1971.
200. Galasko CSB, Samuel AW, Rushton S, et al: The effect of prostaglandin synthesis inhibitors and diphosphonates on tumor induced osteolysis, Br J Surg 67:493, 1980.
201. Galicich JH and Guido LJ: Ommaya device in carcinomatous and leukemic meningitis: surgical experience in 45 cases. Surg Clin North Am 54:915, 1974.
202. Galicich JH, Sundaresan N, Arbit E, et al: Surgical treatment of single brain metastases: factors associated with survival, Cancer 45:381, 1980.
203. Galicich VH, French LA, and Melby JC: Use of dexamethasone in the treatment of cerebral edema associated with brain tumors, J Lancet 81:46, 1961.
204. Gamache FW, Posner JB, and Galicich JH: Treatment of brain metastases by surgical extirpation. In Weiss L, Gilber HA, and Posner JB, editors: Brain metastases, Boston, 1980, Mall, pp 390-414.
205. Giannone L, Greco FA, and Hainsworth JD: Combination intraventricular chemotherapy for meningeal neoplasia, J Clin Oncol 4:68, 1986.
206. Gilbert RW, Kim JH, and Posner JB: Epidural spinal cord compression from metastatic tumor: diagnosis and treatment, Ann Neurol 3:40, 1978.
207. Glass JP and Foley KM: Brain metastases in patients with breast cancer. In Harris JR, Hellman S, Henderson IC, et al, editors: Breast diseases, Philadelphia, 1987, JB Lippincott, pp 480-488.
208. Glass JP and Foley KM: Carcinomatous meningitis. In Harris JR, Hellman S, Henderson IC, et al, editors: Breast diseases, Philadelphia, 1987, JB Lippincott, pp 497-505.
209. Glover D, Riley L, Carmichael K, et al: Hypercalcemia and inhibition of parathyroid hormone secretion after administration of WR-2721 (a radioprotective and chemoprotective agent), N Engl J Med 309:1137, 1983.
210. Glover DJ and Glick JH: Oncologic emergencies and special complication. In Schein P, Rosenberg S, and Calabrese P, editors: Medical Oncology, New York, 1985, Macmillan, pp 1261-1326.
211. Glover DJ, Shaw L, Glick JH, et al: Treatment of hypercalcemia in parathyroid cancer with WR-2721, S-2-(3-aminopropyl) ethyl-phosphorothioic acid, Ann Intern Med 103:55, 1985.
212. Godersky JC, Smoker WRK, and Knutzon R: Use of magnetic resonance imaging in the evaluation of metastatic spinal disease, Neurosurgery 21:676, 1987.
213. Golding RD and Zanten TEG: Computed tomography in malignant conditions affecting the pericardium, J Belge Radiol 67:371, 1984.
214. Gowen M, Wood OD, Ihrie EJ, et al: An interleukin-1 like factor stimulates bone resorption in vitro, Nature 306:378, 1983.
215. Grain GO and Karr JP: Diffuse leptomeningeal carcinomatosis. Clinical and pathologic characteristics, Neurology 5:706, 1955.
216. Gravelyn TR, Michelson MK, Gross BH, and Sitrin RG: Tetracycline pleurodesis for malignant pleural effusions, Cancer 59:1973, 1987.
217. Greenberg HS, Kim J-H, and Posner JB: Epidural spinal cord compression from metastatic tumor: results with a new treatment protocol, Ann Neurol 8:361, 1980.
218. Griffin JW, Thompson RW, Mitchinson MJ, et al: Lymphomatous leptomeningitis, Am J Med 51:200, 1971.
219. Grossman SA, Trump DL, Chen DCP, et al: Cerebrospinal fluid flow abnormalities in patients with neoplastic meningitis. An evaluation using III-Indium DTPA ventriculography, Am J Med 73:641, 1982.
220. Hagemeister FB, Buzdar AU, Luna MA, et al: Causes of death in breast cancer. A clinicopathologic study, Cancer 46:162, 1980.
221. Hagenau C, Grosh W, Currie M, et al: Comparison of spinal magnetic resonance imaging and myelography in cancer patients, J Clin Oncol 5:1663, 1987.
222. Hague N, Thrasher K, Werk E, et al: Studies on dexamethasone metabolism in man: effect of diphenylhydantoin, J Clin Endocrinol Metabol 34:44, 1972.
223. Hall AJ and MacKay NN: The results of laminectomy for compression of the cord and cauda equina by extradural malignant tumor, J Bone Joint Surg 55:497, 1973.
224. Harper G, Cooper G, Rodichok L, et al: Value of myelography for planning radiation treatment of spinal epidural metastases, Proc Am Soc Clin Oncol 3:5, 1984 (abstract).
225. Harrington KD: New trends in the management of lower extremity metastases. Clin Orthop 169:53-61, 1982.
226. Harrington KD: Anterior cord compression and spinal stabilization for patients with metastatic disease of the spine, J Neurosurg 61:107, 1984.
227. Harrington KD, Sim FH, Enis JE, et al: Methylmethacrylate as an adjunct in internal fixation of pathological fractures, J Bone Joint Surg 58A:1047, 1976.

228. Harrison KM, Muss HB, Ball MR, et al: Spinal cord compression in breast cancer, Cancer 55:2839, 1985.
229. Harwood AR and Simpson WF: Radiation therapy of cerebral metastases. A randomized prospective clinical trial, Int J Radiat Oncol Biol Phys 2:1091, 1977.
230. Hausheer FH and Yarbo JW: Diagnosis and treatment of malignant pleural effusions, J Clin Oncol 12:54, 1985.
231. Hayward RB and Frazier TG: A re-evaluation of bone scans in breast cancer, J Surg Oncol 28:111, 1985.
232. Health and Public Policy Committee, ACP: Diagnostic thoracentesis and pleural biopsy in pleural effusions, Ann Intern Med 103:799, 1985.
233. Henderson IC, Harris JR, Kinne DW, et al: Cancer of the breast. In DeVita VT, Hellman S, and Rosenberg SA, editors: Cancer: principles and practice of oncology, Philadelphia, 1989, JB Lippincott, pp 1197-1268.
234. Hickey RC, Samaan NA, and Jackson GL: Hypercalcemia in patients with breast cancer, Arch Surg 116:545, 1981.
235. Hickman JA and Jones MC: Treatment of neoplastic pleural effusions with local instillation of quinacrine hydrochloride, Thorax 25:226, 1970.
236. Hitchins RN, Bell DR, Woods RL, et al: A prospective randomized trial of single-agent versus combination chemotherapy in meningeal carcinomatosis, J Clin Oncol 5:1655, 1987.
237. Hollis PH, Malis LI, and Zappullo RA: Neurological deterioration after lumbar puncture below complete spinal subarachnoid block, J Neurosurg 64:253, 1986.
238. Hortobagyi GN, Lipshitz HI, and Seabold JE: Osseous metastases of breast cancer. Clinical, biochemical, radiographic, and scintigraphic evaluation of response to therapy, Cancer 53:577, 1984.
239. Hosking DJ, Cowley A, and Bucknall CA: Rehydration in the treatment of severe hypercalcemia, Q J Med 200:473, 1981.
240. Isales C, Carcangiu ML, and Stewart AF: Hypercalcemia in breast cancer: reassessment of the mechanism, Am J Med 82:1143, 1987.
241. Jacobs TP, Siris ES, Bilezikian JP, et al: Hypercalcemia of malignancy: treatment with intravenous dichloromethylene diphosphonate, Ann Intern Med 94:312, 1981.
242. Jaeckle KA, Krol G, and Posner JB: Evolution of computed tomographic abnormalities in leptomeningeal metastases, Ann Neurol 17:85, 1985.
243. Jung A, Bartholdi P, Mermillod B, et al: Critical analysis of methods for analyzing human calcium kinetics, J Theor Biol 73:131, 1978.
244. Jung A, Chantraine A, Donath A, et al: Use of dichloromethylene diphosphonate in metastatic bone disease, N Engl J Med 308:1499, 1983.
245. Kanis JA, Urwin GH, Gray RES, et al: Effects of intravenous etidronate disodium on skeletal and calcium metabolism, Am J Med 82:55, 1987.
246. Kennedy DJ, Tibbits DM, Nathanson IT, et al: Hypercalcemia: a complication of hormone therapy in advanced breast cancer, Cancer Res 13:445, 1953.
247. Kinasewitz GT and Fishman AP: Influence of alterations in Starling forces on visceral pleural fluid movement, J Appl Physiol 51:671, 1981.
248. Kirkwood JM and Bankole DO: Carcinomatous meningitis at Yale 1970-1980, Proc Am Assoc Cancer Res and Am Soc Clin Oncol 22:633, 1981.
249. Kurup P, Reddy S, and Hendrickson FR. Results of re-irradiation for cerebral metastases, Cancer 46:2587, 1980.
250. Lee YY, Glass JP, Geoffray A, et al: Cranial computed tomographic abnormalities in leptomeningeal metastasis, Am J Neurol Radiol 5:559, 1984.
251. Leff A, Hopewell PC, and Costello J: Pleural effusions from malignancy, Ann Intern Med 88:532, 1978.
252. Legha SS, Powell K, Buzdar AU, et al: Tamoxifen-induced hypercalcemia in breast cancer, Cancer 47:2803, 1981.
253. Lien HH, Blomlie V, and Heimdal K: Magnetic resonance imaging of malignant extradural tumors with acute spinal cord compression, Acta Radiol 31:187, 1990.
254. Light RW: Pleural effusions, Med Clin North Am 64:1339, 1977.
255. Lokich JJ: The management of malignant pericardial effusions, JAMA 224:1401, 1973.
256. Mannix KA, Carmichael J, Harris AL, et al: Single high-dose (45 mg) infusions of aminohydroxypropylidine diphosphonate for severe malignant hypercalcemia, Cancer 64:1358, 1989.
257. Martenson JA, Evans RG, Lie MR, et al: Treatment outcome and complications in patients treated for malignant epidural spinal cord compression (SCC), J Neurooncol 3:77, 1985.
258. Martin N, Bains MS, and Beattie EJ: Indications for pleurectomy in malignant effusion, Cancer 35:734, 1975.
259. Miller F and Whitehill R: Carcinoma of the breast metastatic to the skeleton, Clin Orthop 184:121, 1984.
260. Miller JI, Mansour KA, and Hatcher CR: Pericardiectomy: current indications, concepts, and results in a university center, Ann Thorac Surg 34:40, 1982.
261. Mones RJ, Dozier D, and Berrett A: Analysis of medical treatment of malignant extradural spinal cord tumors, Cancer 19:1842, 1966.
262. Moore A and Utley D: Anterior decompression and stabilization of the spine in malignant disease, Neurosurgery 24:713, 1989.
263. Morton AR, Cantrill JA, Pillai GU, et al: Sclerosis of lytic bone metastases after disodium aminohydroxypropylidene biphosphonate (APD) in patients with breast cancer, Br Med J 297:772, 1988.
264. Mundy GR: Hypercalcemia of malignancy revisited, J Clin Invest 82:1, 1988.
265. Mundy GR: Pathophysiology of cancer-associated hypercalcemia, Semin Oncol 17:10, 1990.
266. Mundy GR, Ibbotson KJ, and D'Souza SM: Tumor products and hypercalcemia of malignancy, J Clin Invest 76:391, 1985.
267. Mundy GR, Ibbotson KJ, D'Souza SM, et al: The hypercalcemia of cancer: clinical implications and pathogenic mechanisms, N Engl J Med 310:1718, 1984.
268. Mundy GR and Martin JT: The hypercalcemia of malignancy: pathogenesis and management, Metabolism 31:1247, 1982.
269. Murray JJ, Greco FA, Wolff SN, et al: Neoplastic meningitis. Marked variation of cerebrospinal fluid composition in the absence of extradural block, Am J Med 75:289, 1983.
270. Nugent JL, Bunn PA, Matthews MJ, et al: CNS metastases in small cell bronchogenic carcinoma-increasing frequency and changing patterns with lengthening survival, Cancer 44:1885, 1979.
271. Obbens EAMT, Leavens ME, Beal JW, et al: Ommaya reservoirs in 387 cancer patients: a 15-year experience, Neurology 35:1274, 1985.
272. Olsen ME, Chernik NL, and Posner JB: Infiltration of the leptomeninges by systemic cancer, Arch Neurol 30:122, 1974.
273. Ommaya AK: Subcutaneous reservoir and pump for sterile access to ventricular cerebrospinal fluid, Lancet ii:983, 1963.
274. O'Neill W, Spurr C, Muss H, et al: A prospective study of chest tube drainage and sclerosis versus chest tube drainage alone in the treatment of malignant pleural effusion, Proc Am Soc Clin Oncol 23:C-120, 1980.

275. O'Rourke T, George CB, Redmond J III, et al: Spinal computed tomography and computed tomographic metrizamide myelography in the early diagnosis of metastatic disease, J Clin Oncol 4:576, 1986.
276. Ostrowski MJ, and Halsall GM: Intracavitary bleomycin in the management of malignant effusions: a multicenter study, Cancer Treat Rep 66:1903, 1982.
277. Otteman LA and Long HJ: Hypercalcemic flare with megestrol acetate, Cancer Treat Rep 68:1420, 1984.
278. Patchell RA, Tibbs PA, Walsh JW, et al: A randomized trial of surgery in the treatment of solitary metastases to the brain, N Engl J Med 322:494, 1990.
279. Pearson FG and MacGregor DC: Talc poudrage for malignant pleural effusion, J Thorac Cardiovasc Surg 51:732, 1966.
280. Percival RC, Yates AJP, Gray RES, et al: Role of glucocorticoids in management of hypercalcemia, Br Med J 289:287, 1984.
281. Perlia CP, Gubisch NJ, Wolter J, et al: Mithramycin treatment of hypercalcemia, Cancer 25:389, 1970.
282. Piehler JM, Pluth JR, Schaff HV, et al: Surgical management of pericardial disease, J Thorac Cardiovasc Surg 90:506, 1985.
283. Poe RH, Qaz R, Israel RH, et al.: Survival of patients with pleural involvement by breast cancer, Am J Clin Oncol 6:523, 1983.
284. Porter BA, Shields AF, and Olson DO: Magnetic resonance imaging of bone marrow disorders, Radiol Clin North Am 24:269, 1986.
285. Posner JB: Diagnosis and treatment of metastases to the brain, Clin Bull 4:47, 1974.
286. Posner JB: Management of central nervous sytem metastases, Semin Oncol 4:81, 1977.
287. Posner JB: Neurological complications of systemic cancer, Med Clin North Am 63(4):783, 1979.
288. Posner JB: Clinical manifestations of brain metastases. In Weiss L, Gilbert HA, and Posner JB, editors: Brain metastases, Boston, 1980, Hall, pp 189-207.
289. Posner JB and Chevnik NL: Intracranial metastases from systemic cancer, Adv Neurol 19:575, 1978.
290. Posner JB, Howieson J, and Cvitkovic E: "Disappearing" spinal cord compression: oncolytic effect of glucocorticoids (and other chemotherapeutic agents) on epidural metastases, Ann Neurol 2:409, 1977.
291. Posner MR, Cohen GI, and Skarin AT: Pericardial disease in patients with cancer, Am J Med 71:407, 1981.
292. Prakash UBS and Dines DE: Thoracentesis, pleural biopsy and pleuroscopy, Semin Respir Med 3:42, 1981.
293. Prakash UBS and Reiman HM: Comparison of needle biopsy with cytologic analysis for the evaluation of pleural effusion: analysis of 414 cases, Mayo Clin Proc 60:158, 1985.
294. Price RA and Johnson WW: The central nervous system in childhood leukemia. I. The arachnoid, Cancer 31:520, 1973.
295. Redmond J, Friedl KE, Cornett P, et al: Clinical usefulness of an algorithm for the early diagnosis of spinal metastatic disease, J Clin Oncol 6:154, 1988.
296. Reynolds PM and Byrne MJ: The treatment of malignant pericardial effusion in carcinoma of the breast, Aust NZ J Med 7:169, 1977.
297. Ringenberg QS and Ritch PS: Efficacy of oral administration of etidronate disodium in maintaining normal serum calcium levels in previously hypercalcemic cancer patients, Clin Ther 9:1, 1987.
298. Ritch P, Gucalp R, Wiernik P, et al: Pamidronate (APD) and etidronate disodium (EHDP) in hypercalcemia of malignancy—preliminary report of a comparative multicentre trial. In Rubens RD, editor: The management of bone metastases and hypercalcemia by osteoclast inhibition, Bern, Switzerland, 1990, Hans Hueber Publishers, pp 46-49.
299. Rittgers RA, Loewenstein MS, Feinerman AE, et al: Carcinoembryonic antigen levels in benign and malignant pleural effusions, Ann Intern Med 88:631, 1978.
300. Roberts WC and Waller BF: Effect of chronic hypercalcemia on the heart: an analysis of 18 necropsy patients, Am J Med 71:371, 1981.
301. Rodichok LD, Harper GR, Ruckdeschel JC, et al: Early diagnosis of spinal epidural metastases, Am J Med 70:1181, 1981.
302. Rodriguez M and Dinapoli RP: Spinal cord compression with special reference to metastatic epidural tumors, Mayo Clin Proc 55:442, 1980.
303. Rosner D, Nemoto T, Pickren J, et al: Management of brain metastases from breast cancer by combination chemotherapy, J Neurooncol 1:31, 1983.
304. Ruckdeschel J: Management of malignant pleural effusion. An overview, Semin Oncol 15:24, 1988.
305. Ryan JR, Rowe DE, and Salcicuolio GG: Prophylactic internal fixation of the femur for neoplastic lesions, J Bone Joint Surg 58A:1071, 1976.
306. Sahn SA: Malignant pleural effusions, Semin Respir Med 9:43, 1987.
307. Sahn SA and Good JT: Pleural fluid pH in malignant effusions, Ann Intern Med 108:345, 1988.
308. Sarpel S, Sarpel G, Yu E, et al: Early diagnosis of spinal-epidural metastasis by magnetic resonance imaging, Cancer 59:1112, 1987.
309. Schurman DS and Amstutz HC: Orthopaedic management of patients with metastatic carcinoma of the breast, Surg Gynecol Obstet 137:831, 1973.
310. Shapiro WR, Young DF, and Mehta BM: Methotrexate: distribution in cerebrospinal fluid after intravenous, ventricular and lumbar injection, N Engl J Med 293:161, 1975.
311. Shehata WM, Hendrickson FR, and Hindo WA: Rapid fractionation technique and re-treatment of cerebral metastases by irradiation, Cancer 34:257, 1974.
312. Shepard FA, Ginsberg JS, and Evans WK: Tetracycline sclerosis in management of malignant pericardial effusion, J Clin Oncol 3:1678, 1985.
313. Shi M-L, Wallace S, Libshitz HI, et al: Cranial computed tomography of breast carcinoma, J Comput Assist Tomogr 6:77, 1982.
314. Siegal T and Siegal T: Surgical decompression of anterior and posterior malignant epidural tumors compressing the spinal cord: a prospective study, Neurosurgery 17:424, 1985.
315. Silverman JF: Cytopathology of fine-needle aspiration biopsy of the brain and spinal cord, Diagn Cytopatho 2:312, 1986.
316. Silverman P and Distelhorst CW: Metabolic emergencies in clinical oncology, Semin Oncol 16:504, 1989.
317. Sim FH and Pritchard DJ: Metastataic disease in the upper extremity, Clin Orthoped 169:83, 1982.
318. Smith FE, Lane M, and Hudgins PT: Conservative management of malignant pericardial effusion, Cancer 33:47, 1974.
319. Smith FP, Slavik M, and MacDonald JS: Association of breast cancer with meningioma: report of two cases and review of the literature, Cancer 42:1992, 1978.
320. Smith IE: Recurrent disease. In Harris JR, Hellman S, Henderson IC, et al, editors: Breast diseases, Philadelphia, 1987, JB Lippincott, pp 369-384.
321. Sparrow GEA and Rubens RD: Brain metastases from breast cancer: clinical course, prognosis, and influence on treatment, Clin Oncol 7:291, 1981.

322. Spiers ASD, Cameron RA, and Morton J: Meningeal carcinomatosis as the initial presentation of cancer, Proc Am Assoc Can Res 23:160, 1982.
323. Stark RJ, Henson RA, and Evans SJW: Spinal metastases, a retrospective survey from a general hospital, Brain 105:189, 1982.
324. Stewart AF, Horst R, Deftos LJ, et al: Biochemical evaluation of patients with cancer associated with hypercalcemia: evidence for humoral and non-humoral groups, N Engl J Med 303:1377, 1980.
325. Stewart JA and Foster RS: Breast cancer and aging, Semin Oncol 16:41, 1989.
326. Stewart JF, King RJB, Sexton S, et al: Oestrogen receptors sites of metastatic disease and survival in recurrent breast cancer, Eur J Cancer Clin Oncol 17:449, 1981.
327. Stillman M and Foley KM: Breast cancer and epidural spinal cord compression: diagnostic and therapeutic strategies. In Harris JR, Hellman S, Henderson IC, et al, editors: Breast diseases, Philadephia, 1987, JB Lippincott, pp 488-497.
328. Strodel WE, Thompson NW, Eckhauser FE, et al: Malignancy and concomitant primary hyperparathyroidism, J Surg Oncol 37:10, 1988.
329. Strumpf M, Kowalski MA, and Mundy GR: Effects of glucocorticoids on osteoclast-activating factor, J Lab Clin Med 92:772, 1978.
330. Suhrland LG and Weisberger NS: Intracavitary 5-fluorouracil in malignant effusions, Arch Intern Med 116:431, 1965.
331. Suki WN, Yium JJ, Von Minden M, et al: Acute treatment of hypercalcemia with furosemide, N Engl J Med 283:836, 1970.
332. Sundaresan N, Galicich JH, Lane JM, et al: Treatment of neoplastic epidural cord compression by vertebral body resection and stabilization, J Neurosurg 63:676, 1985.
333. Sze G, Krol G, Zimmerman RD, et al: Malignant epidural spinal tumors: MR imaging with Gd-DTPA, Radiology 167:217, 1988.
334. Takakura K, Sano K, Hojo S, et al: Metastatic tumors of the central nervous sytem, Tokyo, 1982, Igaku-Shoin, p 113.
335. Tattersall MHN: Intracavitary Adriamycin, nitrogen mustard and tetracycline in the control of malignant effusions: a randomized study, Med J Aust 2:447, 1980.
336. Theodore WH and Gendelman S: Meningeal carcinomatosis, Arch Neurol 38:696, 1981.
337. Theologides A: Neoplastic cardiac tamponade, Semin Oncol 5:181, 1978.
338. Thurber DC, Edioards JE, and Achor RWP: Secondary malignant tumors to pericardium, Circulation 26:228, 1962.
339. Tong D, Gillick L, and Hendrickson FR: The palliation of symptomatic osseous metastases—final results of the study by the Radiation Therapy Oncology Group, Cancer 50:893, 1982.
340. Torma T: Malignant tumors of the spine and the spinal epidural space: a study based on 250 histologically verified cases, Acta Chir Scand 225:1, 1957.
341. Trump DL, Grossman SA, Thompson G, et al: Treatment of neoplastic meningitis with intraventricular thiotepa and methotrexate, Cancer Treat Rep 66:1549, 1982.
342. VanBelle SJP, Bolckaert A, Taeymans Y, et al: Treatment of malignant pericardial tamponade with sclerosis induced by instillation of bleomycin, Int J Cardiol 16:155, 1987.
343. Veith RG and Odom GL: Intracranial metastases and their neurosurgical treatment, J Neurosurg 23:375, 1965.
344. Wallach HW: Intrapleural tetracycline for malignant pleural effusions, Chest 68:510, 1975.
345. Walsh SJ, Begg CB, and Carbone PP: Cancer chemotherapy in the elderly, Semin Oncol 16:66, 1989.
346. Wang AM, Lewis ML, Rumbaugh CL, et al: Spinal cord or nerve root compression in patients with malignant disease: CT evaluation, J Comput Assist Tomogr 8:420, 1984.
347. Warrell RP, Israel R, Frisone M, et al: Gallium nitrate for acute treatment of cancer-related hypercalcemia: a randomized, double-bind comparison to calcitonin, Ann Intern Med 108:669, 1988.
348. Warrell RP, Issacs M, Alcock NW, et al: Gallium nitrate for treatment of refractory hypercalcemia from parathyroid carcinoma, Ann Intern Med 107:683, 1987.
349. Wasserstrom WR, Glass JP, and Posner JB: Diagnosis and treatment of leptomeningeal metastases from solid tumors: experience with 90 patients, Cancer 49:759, 1982.
350. Weissman DE: Glucocorticoid treatment for brain metastases and epidural spinal cord compression: a review, J Clin Oncol 6:543, 1988.
351. Weissman DE, Gilbert M, Wang H, et al: The use of computed tomography of the spine to identify patients at high risk for epidural metastases, J Clin Oncol 3:1541, 1985.
352. White WA, Patterson RH, and Bergland RM: Role of surgery in the treatment of spinal cord compression by metastatic neoplasm, Cancer 27:558, 1971.
353. Wilner D: Cancer metastases to bone. In Wilner D, editor: Radiology of bone tumors and allied disorders, Philadelphia, 1982, WB Saunders, p 3646.
354. Winston KR, Walsh JW, and Fischer EG: Results of operative treatment of intracranial metastatic tumors, Cancer 45:2639, 1980.
355. Woodring JH: Recognition of pleural effusion on supine radiographs, Am J Roentgenol 142:59, 1984.
356. Wright DC and Delaney TF: Treatment of metastatic cancer to the brain. In DeVita VT, Hellman S, and Rosenberg SA, editors: Cancer: principles and practice of oncology, Philadelphia, 1989, JB Lippincott, pp 2245-2261.
357. Wright RL: Malignant tumors in the spinal extradural space: results of surgical treatment, Ann Surg 157:227, 1963.
358. Yap HY, Yap BS, Rasmussen S, et al: Treatment for meningeal carcinomatosis in breast cancer, Cancer 50:219, 1982.
359. Yap HY, Yap BS, Tashima CK, et al: Meningeal carcinomatosis in breast cancer, Cancer 42:283, 1978.
360. Yazdi HM, Hajdu SI, and Melamed MR: Cytopathology of pericardial effusions, Acta Cytol 24:401, 1980.
361. Young RF, Post EM, and King GA: Treatment of spinal epidural metastases: randomized prospective comparison of laminectomy and radiotherapy, J Neurosurg 53:741, 1980.
362. Zefren JL and Heinemann HO: Reversible defect in renal concentrating mechanism in patients with hypercalcemia, Am J Med 33:54, 1962.
363. Zondek H, Petow H, and Sieben W: Die Bedeutung der Calcium best-immung im Blute fur die Diagnose der Nierreninsuffizienz, Z Klin Med 99:129, 1924.

17 Management of the Effects of Breast Cancer Therapy and Progressive Disease

Rosemary C. Polomano, Gloria A. Hagopian, *and* ***Mary Dee McEvoy***

While improved detection and treatment methods have led to cure and high survival rates, women with breast cancer must live with cancer or the thought of it recurring and must adapt their lives accordingly. For some, it will mean long-term follow-up care, while for others it means living with a chronic illness involving periodic exacerbations and remissions. Efforts to manage the effects of therapy and/or progressive disease are an integral part of any treatment plan; they are aimed toward minimizing distress and maximizing the patient's quality of life, educating patients, and offering opportunities for patients and their families to participate in decision making.

The effectiveness of any symptom management plan for cancer patients depends on several factors. First, health professionals must be knowledgeable about the potential and actual outcomes of cancer and its therapy. Myths and misconceptions regarding cancer care must be relinquished when sound research proves them wrong. For example, an overwhelming concern regarding the consequence of addiction in cancer patients requiring medicinal narcotics for pain still prevails in light of evidence to support that the potential for addiction in these patients is exceedingly small.

Second, a strong collaborative working relationship between physicians and nurses lays the foundation for effective communication and joint responsibility for patient care. Mutual respect between physician and nurse is important, as is respect for the discipline to which each belongs. Physicians need to recognize that, just as medical practice in the area of cancer care has become specialized, so too has nursing practice. Cancer nursing has evolved as a major subspecialty of nursing, offering tremendous role diversity and opportunity for professional growth. Specialization in oncology has afforded nurses the opportunity to develop in-depth knowledge in certain aspects of cancer care. Moreover, it is apparent that the role of nurses in patient care is expanding not only in inpatient facilities, but outpatient and community settings as well.

Third, it is imperative that physicians and nurses agree upon common goals for the patient and family. Furthermore, patient and family participation in formulating such goals is crucial. Even though physicians and nurses share a bond of commitment to cancer patients, their specific goals and priorities of care may at times be dissimilar.

The last important aspect relating to the effectiveness of symptom management efforts is the issue of sensitivity to quality of life parameters, information sharing with patients and families, and encouraging active patient participation in decision making. All too often such issues are overlooked in the management of cancer patients. Nurses possess the ability to assess these aspects of care and to offer suggestions and interventions for promoting self-care behaviors that restore optimal functioning and, to the extent that is possible, minimize disruptions in daily living. The advanced education of nurses at the graduate level and, more specifically, the doctoral level has sparked considerable research in these areas of care. Therefore physicians should use findings from nursing research for the purposes of guiding clinical practice in symptom management and gaining new perspectives in cancer care. Because quality of life, patient education, and patient decision making are believed to form the common grounds on which physicians and nurses should ideally base their practices, a discussion of these issues follows.

QUALITY OF LIFE

Quality of life issues for women with breast cancer remain important considerations for health professionals. Although there is general agreement that the domains of quality of life need to be assessed, especially for patients involved in clinical trials, there is little evidence to demonstrate that health professionals caring for cancer patients reliably and consistently evaluate quality of life indices. In fact, studies have shown a particularly low compliance rate with standard quality of life measures used in clinical trials.[66] Belcher[5] stresses that patients' perceptions of quality of life should now more than ever be a growing concern as patients are living longer, being subjected to a variety of treatments, and struggling in a changing society and economic climate. Unfortunately, the capabilities of health professionals to assess or evaluate dimensions of quality of life are limited by the variety of interpretations for quality of life, the diversity of instruments used to measure quality of life, and lack of the time necessary for an accurate appraisal of the dimensions of quality of life. Judgments regarding quality of life indicators should be made by those in whom quality of life is being measured. Given the assumption that the meaning of "quality of life" is highly subjective and individualized, some acceptable standards and concensus for measuring this phenomenon are necessary. After reviewing several quality of life instruments, Cella and Tulsky[11] outline 10 distinct categories of importance for assessment, including among others physical concerns, functional ability, spirituality, treatment satisfaction, sexuality-intimacy, and occupation-related issues.

Quality of life has been defined in many ways: those things that make life worth living[51]; the degree of satisfaction with perceived life circumstances[74]; and the degree to which one has self-esteem, a purpose in life, and a minimum of anxiety.[41] Welch-McCaffery[72] has identified social, physiologic, and psychologic factors that may affect a patient's quality of life. The social factors include social dependence, life-style changes, time spent within the medical system, and ability to return to work. Physiologic factors that may affect quality of life include symptom distress, performance level, freedom from pain, and sexual activity. Behavior, morale, freedom from stress, degree of happiness, degree of satisfaction, purpose of life, anxiety, and self-esteem are psychologic factors that can affect an individual's perceived quality of life.

While there are several tools to measure quality of life, the Karnofsky Index, a 100-point scale, is used in most clinical trials. The Functional Living Index—Cancer (FLIC) represents a more comprehensive evaluation of functional mobility and commonly is employed in quality of life studies. However, it is important to keep in mind that both of these scales only measure physical performance and do not take into account the patient's perceptions of the quality of life. Another tool, the Quality of Life Index, provides a multidimensional operational definition of quality of life.[51] Cella and Tulsky[11] have provided a comprehensive review of quality of life measures appropriate for cancer patients. As the discussion of symptom control proceeds, the impact of side effects and management plans needs to be considered carefully in the context of quality of life domains.

PATIENT EDUCATION

Often patients and families are expected to make decisions about their care and to participate to a certain degree in this care without adequate knowledge of their disease, treatment options, and outcomes. The process of educating patients and families is of the utmost importance. Informing patients of their options for treatment and the associated effects of therapy requires planning and sensitivity to issues surrounding information sharing such as timeliness, appropriateness, and the degree of information given. Although there may not be an ideal time to discuss treatments with patients, high anxiety levels may interfere with learning. Furthermore, the amount of information conveyed to patients varies according to the patient's cognitive ability, state of health, and receptiveness to teaching.

The physician and nurse should discuss the goals of therapy and the available treatment options with the patient and family, giving the risks and benefits of each one, and the treatment schedules. Decisions for selecting a particular treatment may be based on convenience and the potential that the treatment offers for the least disruption in daily routines. Unless patients are informed and understand the information presented to them, decisions should not be made. There are certain safeguards to ensure that information is delivered in the best possible manner. Oncology nurses able to work with patients over period of time can be a powerful force in assessing and intervening in matters pertaining to patients' learning needs. Assessment also allows time for the nurse to establish good rapport with the patient and create the trusting, open climate that is an essential condition for learning. Patients need information so they can cope with their disease and treatment, manage side effects and symptoms, and use available resources.

Readiness to learn

The timing of teaching is important and is often determined by readiness for learning. If any of the following factors are lacking, the patient's readiness to learn may be impaired:

1. Comfort—both physical and psychologic factors can interfere with learning.
2. Energy—patients who lack energy may have a decreased ability to learn.
3. Motivation—learning will be enhanced if patients are motivated to learn.
4. Capacity—a patient's capacity for learning depends on both physical and cognitive capabilities.[30]

Principles of teaching and learning

There are several principles of teaching and learning that should be applied, including the following:

1. Heredity and environment as well as goals, aspirations, and desires influence learning. The more that is known about the patient's background and goals, the more likely it is that teaching can be planned to help the patient.
2. A comfortable, quiet environment enhances learning.
3. People are more likely to learn those things that interest them or things they believe are important.
4. Teaching requires good communication skills.
5. A specific time should be set aside for teaching.
6. Teaching sessions should be kept short and meaningful.
7. The learner should be actively involved.
8. Build on what the patient already knows.
9. Provide reinforcement and positive feedback.

By using these principles of teaching and learning, health professionals can provide teaching at the most opportune time and in a way that will promote learning. Patients are then able to participate in their care, feel in control, and make informed decisions and choices.[30]

Educational resources

There are two major sources of educational resources for patients and families: The National Cancer Institute (NCI) and the American Cancer Society (ACS). The NCI publishes numerous pamphlets and brochures about cancer. In addition, it sponsors the Cancer Information Service (CIS), a nationwide toll-free telephone program. Trained specialists are available through the CIS to answer questions about cancer from the public, patients with cancer, the families of patients, and health professionals. By calling the toll-free number 1-800-4-CANCER, the caller automatically will be connected to the CIS in the local area. The staff can provide information and can mail free NCI publications on all aspects of cancer. They also may know about cancer-related services in local areas. Some of the NCI publications related to breast cancer are listed above at right.

The American Cancer Society offers a variety of services to patients with cancer and their families, as well as pamphlets and brochures. Information can be obtained from the national headquarters or a local chapter.

BREAST CANCER PAMPHLETS AVAILABLE FROM NATIONAL CANCER INSTITUTE*

Breast biopsy: what you should know	87-657
Breast cancer: understanding treatment options	87-2675
Mastectomy: a treatment for breast cancer	87-658
Radiation therapy: a treatment for early stage breast cancer	87-659
Adjuvant therapy: facts for women with breast cancer	87-2877
After breast cancer: a guide for follow up care	87-2400
Breast reconstruction: a matter of choice	88-2151
Breast exams: what you should know	89-2000
Breast lumps: questions and answers	88-2401
When cancer recurs: meeting the challenge again	
Breast cancer: we're making progress every day	88-2409
What you need to know about breast cancer	88-556
When someone in your family has cancer	88-2685
Taking time: support for people with cancer and the people who care for them	87-2059
Advanced cancer: living each day	87-856
Chemotherapy and you	88-1136

*For a complete list of available NCI publications, write to the National Cancer Institute, Building 31, Room 10A24, Bethesda, Md. 20892.

DECISION MAKING

Increased consumer awareness of health care choices has highlighted the importance of patient choice and their decision-making capabilities. Often patients and families are expected to make decisions regarding treatment options. The choice between breast conservation surgery or mastectomy has received attention since the early 1980s. Currently there is evidence that both treatments are equally efficacious.[19] However, women who choose conservative breast surgery may do so out of fear of body image changes and sexuality concerns associated with the loss of a breast. Increasingly, choices are given to patients regarding chemotherapy regimens. However, the ability to choose chemotherapy options becomes more and more limited as standard therapies are exhausted.

Several authors have studied how patients make choices.[14,49] Consideration of the outcome and weighing the risks and benefits of each choice are involved. However, the benefits of adjuvant therapy are theoretical and future-oriented (i.e., reducing the risk of relapse with no immediate benefit evidence to the patient). Patients never know if they would have relapsed anyway, regardless of a particular treatment choice. The difficulty of comprehending the risks of treatment compounds the problems associated with making choices. Health professionals can only describe symptoms associated with treatment, and the meaning that any given symptom will hold for an individual patient cannot be conveyed by the health professional nor appreciated by the patient until it is experienced. For example, the trauma associated with some symptoms, such as hair loss, can never be explained fully.

Each patient will address the discussion of treatment option differently. In a study of participation in treatment decisions, Cassileth et al.[10] found that the majority of the 256 patients studied desired to participate in treatment decisions. Degner and Russell,[14] however, found that patients essentially fell into three major categories of preference: those who wished to give away control of the treatment decision, those who wished to maintain control of the treatment decision, and those who wished to share control. Careful attention to verbal cues of patients aids the clinician in discussing treatment choices.

MANAGING THE EFFECTS OF SURGICAL INTERVENTION

The role of surgical intervention and the routine surgical care of breast cancer patients undergoing mastectomy or lumpectomy with axillary node dissections are discussed elsewhere in this text. Surgical complications such as wound infections and postoperative morbidity are addressed in the section on surgical management. Recommended exercises for women following lymph node dissections are outlined in Chapter 22. However, there are effects of surgery, particularly mastectomy, that are often overlooked and rarely addressed.

Phantom breast syndrome

Phantom-like phenomena related to the loss of a limb are well described in the literature. Comparatively, the phantom experience following the loss of a breast rarely is mentioned despite its common occurrence after mastectomy. Phantom breast syndrome (PBS) is characterized by the acute awareness of perceptual phenomena in the absent breast. Classically the descriptions of breast phantoms are somewhat vague and not described as vividly as those associated with limb loss. Poor perceptual definitions of breast phantoms make them difficult to describe and hamper efforts to study them.[65] These sensations, some of which are painful, range from the vague feeling that the entire breast is present to distinct sensations arising from specific parts of the amputated breast. It is estimated that anywhere from 25% to 66% of women have phantom sensations at one time or another after a mastectomy,[38,45,67] yet women seldom freely voice complaints about breast phantoms unless asked whether or not they have been experienced and reassured that they are normal. Most women are relieved and comforted by the opportunity to discuss phantom experiences, as many women feel that their mind is playing tricks on them.

As early as the 1950s several descriptive studies on breast phantoms appeared in the literature.[6,13] Physicians acknowledged that breast phantoms existed; however, traditionally little or nothing had been done to prepare women for this experience, and today, women undergoing mastectomy rarely are informed of PBS. Possibly it was because some believed that knowledge of a particular outcome will predict its occurrence. In addition, the paucity of research on this topic hampered the dissemination of information to the surgical community.

Unfortunately the perceived threats associated with PBS are underestimated, as it often is viewed as a benign syndrome and the value of discussing it with patients is questioned by many. It is certainly not justified to ignore the opportunities to discuss this experience with patients, as some patients are frightened when they experience breast phantoms and often do not understand what is happening to them. To avoid and minimize such distress, routine surgical management of women undergoing mastectomy should include preparatory information on incidence and characteristics of breast phantoms.

Certain trends have been observed with the incidence and frequency of breast phantoms. Some studies have shown that younger women tend to experience more phantoms than older women.[67] However, in a more recent study, investigators found no relationship to age.[38] Younger women who experienced phantoms are more likely to continue to experience them as time goes on,[67,71] and no significant decline in the number of phantom experiences over the first year after mastectomy has been shown.[38] According to Kroner et al.[38] patients with premastectomy pain are more likely to have painful phantoms that are believed to represent the former premastectomy pains. Age, menstruation, weather conditions, and breast prostheses have also been shown to elicit phantoms. Laterality and histiologic type of tumor do not correlate with the incidence of breast phantoms.

Characteristically, phantoms have been described as a general awareness of the whole breast, or as itching, burning, tingling, or pain in any part of the breast. In a study of 218 women, 35% experienced painful phantoms.[45] Rarely do phantom breast pains cause the same distress that accompanies phantom limb pain, and seldom do breast phantoms require treatment. Characteristically, the pains are described as sharp, shooting pains or twinges that last only a few seconds. Because many women experience chest wall pain and pain in the axilla area, it is important to differentiate phantom breast pains from pain associated with postmastectomy syndrome to the greatest extent possible.

Postmastectomy syndrome

Entrapment of the intercostobrachial nerve following mastectomy may lead to persistent pain, referred to as postmastectomy pain syndrome (PMPS). The overall incidence of PMPS varies from 4% to 14%, depending on the source.[24,69] Before a diagnosis of PMPS is made, certain features of the pain, such as duration, location, and character or quality must be explored in order to distinguish this pain syndrome from normal postoperative pain, painful phantom breast sensations, and local tumor infiltration of the brachial plexus.

Persistent pain in the area or areas of the chest wall, axilla, and medial upper arm is expected immediately after a mastectomy as a result of swelling, skin tightness, and muscle stiffness. However, if the pain continues for >3 months after allowances for healing and optimal mobility are made, a diagnosis of PMPS can be considered. PMPS usually is described as a burning, hyperesthetic, dysesthetic, and painful numbing of the upper arm, axilla, and/or chest wall. Sometimes disturbances in skin sensations are more noticeable when the patient begins to wear a prosthesis. Chest tightness or a banding type of pain originating in the anterior chest wall also may be experienced.

The decision to spare or dissect the intercostobrachial nerve remains an issue of great controversy among surgeons. Although dissection of the nerve is believed to reduce the possibility of PMPS, sparing the intercostobrachial nerve without subjecting it to unnecessary damage may prove equally beneficial. PMPS is believed to result from traumatic insult to the nerve, either from inadvertent damage with an electrocautery device, ligation of the nerve, or partial dissection of the nerve. Neuroma formation of the intercostobrachial nerve is a consequence of such trauma, and it is likely to elicit the painful stimuli.[35]

Treatment of PMPS usually consists of therapy with nonsteroidal antiinflammatory drugs, antidepressant therapy (amitriptyline [Elavil] usually 25 to 75 mg per day), neuroleptics, anticonvulsants, and transcutaneous nerve stimulation (TENS). Because the nature of this type of pain is neuropathic, narcotic analgesics are seldom of any benefit.[3] Rarely are surgical approaches undertaken. More recently, encouraging results in the treatment of PMPS have been obtained with the topical application of capsaicin (Zostrix), a substance P inhibitor.[70] In time, PMPS may resolve or become less apparent and distressing to the patient.

Lymphedema

Some women may develop lymphedema after treatment by surgery and radiation therapy. It is seen most often in women who have had radical mastectomies, extensive lymph node dissection, or a combination of axillary dissection and radiation to the axilla. It is caused by loss or damage to lymph nodes and their connecting vessels. The circulation of lymph fluid in the affected arm is slowed, and the ability to fight infection is impaired. Weight loss, exercise, and use of a light elastic sleeve may be helpful. If swelling does not respond to these interventions, the patient may need to be referred to the physical therapy department for special exercises or pneumomassage treatment with an inflatable sleeve. If the lymphedema is severe, patients should be advised to wear a MediAlert bracelet inscribed "Caution—Lymphedema Arm." Bracelets cost about $10.00 and order blanks for bracelets can be found in pharmacies. Accumulation of fluid can be aggravated by strenuous exercise, injury, or infection. Steps to help prevent infection that should be taught to the patient are found above. A detailed discussion of the management of lymphedema is presented in Chapter 22.

STEPS TO PREVENT INFECTION

- Avoid burns while cooking and smoking. Wear a mitt when reaching into the oven.
- Avoid sunburn.
- Have all injections, vaccinations, blood samples, and blood pressure readings done on the unaffected arm.
- Use only an electric razor for underarm shaving.
- Carry heavy packages or handbags with the unaffected arm.
- Wash cuts promptly, treat them with antibacterial agents, and cover them with sterile gauze. Check for redness, soreness, or elevated temperature.
- Wear gloves when gardening or using strong detergents.
- Use a thimble when sewing.
- Avoid harsh chemicals.
- Use insect repellant to avoid bites and stings.
- Avoid elastic cuffs.
- Never cut cuticles. Use hand cream or lotion.
- Wear watches or jewelry loosely, if at all, on the affected arm.
- Call your doctor if your arm swells, becomes red, or feels hot.

CARING FOR THE PATIENT RECEIVING RADIATION THERAPY

Radiation therapy

With new equipment and technologic innovations, patients who undergo a course of radiation therapy usually tolerate the treatment, experiencing minimal side effects and few disruptions in their lives.

Patients need to learn about the radiation therapy department, its routines, and what to expect during treatment. More importantly, they need to be instructed as to how to manage the side effects they will encounter. Patients in the early stage of disease may experience fatigue and some skin changes during treatment. During later stages of disease, patients need specific information on the site being treated. Health professionals should identify appropriate interventions to prevent or minimize symptom distress, so that patients can tolerate treatment with little interference in their daily lives.

Introduction to the radiation therapy department

Patients who will be undergoing a course of radiation therapy need to know both the purpose of the therapy and the procedural aspects of the treatment. They need to know that a simulation or treatment planning session will be done at the beginning and again toward the end of treatment; this is done to mark the treatment field clearly. Initially, the affected breast and possibly the adjacent lymph node area are treated. Later in treatment, a boost dose of radiation is delivered to the tumor bed. During the simulation procedure, tattoos or small permanent marks are made on the patient around the area to be treated. A special immobilization device called a cast is made to keep patients in position during the treatment. This allows them to be supported in a comfortable position, and the radiation can be delivered more accurately as patients are in the same position each day.

Patients will be in the department about 30 minutes each day. Although the treatment itself only lasts 1 to 2 minutes, the preparation and positioning on the table can take 10 to 15 minutes. Patients are alone in the room during the treatment, but are under constant observation through a window or television screen. Although the machine generally makes a whirring noise, patients will not feel anything during the treatment.

It is important to recognize that during the first few visits to the department the patient may be anxious and may not remember some of the information. Reteaching may be necessary. Misconceptions should be clarified. Patients sometimes have misconceptions, but may not ask questions for a number of reasons. Patients should be told that they will not become radioactive, that they can have sexual relations, that they can go to the hairdresser, and that they will not lose scalp hair from radiation to the breast.

While under treatment, weekly assessments will be performed by the physician and nurse. These assessments should include response to treatment and tumor status, presence and management of side effects, anticipatory guidance, and coping abilities. A blood count to monitor hemoglobin, hematocrit, white blood cells, and platelet count should be performed weekly. Patients are weighed each week to monitor nutritional status.

There are two NCI publications pertaining to radiation therapy that may be helpful to patients. One is an NCI fact sheet, *Radiation Therapy for Cancer,* designed to provide patients with a brief introduction. The second, *Radiation Therapy and You,* provides more detailed information about treatment and side effects.

Skin

With the use of megavoltage equipment it is rare to see patients with either severe acute or chronic skin reactions.[26] The maximum dose that can be delivered has increased because of the skin-sparing effect of high energy rays. However, the electron beam does not have this skin-sparing effect. Radiation therapy may cause skin changes such as dryness, redness, tanning, and peeling in the areas in the treatment field. Patients need to be taught what skin changes to expect as the treatment progresses and how to care for their skin. They need to know that skin changes may persist for several weeks after treatment has started. Patients may notice that their skin is red and feels sunburned. Skin care instructions for patients are listed at top of p. 463.

Erythema and dry desquamation. There are a number of skin care products that can be used for erythema and dry desquamation. It is important to keep in mind that any substance should be used sparingly to avoid a build-up that could act as a bolus and increase the dose to the skin. Also, patients should be informed that these products should be washed off before treatment. Baby powder often relieves pruritus. Cornstarch relieves pruritus and reduces moisture build-up in skin folds. Several products provide moisture: hydrophilic creams (Eucerin) and ointments (Aquafor), A & D Ointment, Lanolin, and Lubriderm.

Moist desquamation. A number of treatments can be instituted for moist desquamation. Steroid ointments can be used to decrease itching but also may increase thinning and consequently the possibility of injury. Gentian violet is an antiseptic and antifungal agent that has a drying effect, but it is messy. Washing with hydrogen peroxide and water and applying A & D Ointment can also be done. Hydrogen peroxide always should be diluted, because full-strength hydrogen peroxide interferes with granulation. If a dressing is applied, it should be removed before treatment to reduce the bolus effect. Moisture vapor–permeable (MVP) dressings have been used successfully on a variety of

SKIN CARE INSTRUCTIONS FOR PATIENTS UNDERGOING RADIATION THERAPY

1. Wash skin in treatment field with lukewarm water only and blot dry with a soft towel.
2. Do not wash the treated area with soap or apply any ointment, salve, deodorant, perfume, cologne, lotion, cosmetic, or self-remedy during the treatment period.
3. Do not rub, scrub, or scratch skin in the treatment field. If the skin becomes dry and/or itches, tell your nurse. If necessary your doctor may order a medication for this problem.
4. Do not shave in the treated area throughout the treatment period and until any skin reaction that may have occurred has disappeared.
5. Do not use hot water bottles, heating lights, electric heating pads, or hot packs to the treated area.
6. Keep the treated areas out of the sun. Prevent sunburn throughout the treatment period. Continue to take precautions after the treatment has ended by using a sunscreen with a 15 or greater sun protective factor.
7. Radiation therapy frequently causes skin changes such as dryness, redness, tanning, and peeling. Do not be alarmed by these reactions. They are temporary and will disappear within a few weeks after the treatment has ended.
8. Keep your skin clean, dry, and open to the air as much as possible.
9. Wear only loose-fitting cotton clothing over the skin in the treatment field to avoid further reaction.
10. Report any skin reactions to your nurse or doctor.

surgical incisions, skin grafts, and pressure sores, which suggests that they may be used for radiation therapy skin reactions. In a pilot study comparing patients treated with a MVP dressing (n = 8) and those treated conventionally with hydrous lanolin gauze (n = 8), those treated with an MVP dressing healed in an average of 19 days, compared to 24 days for those given conventional treatment. Although these results were not statistically significant, they do suggest that further study is warranted.[64] Patient instructions for moist desquamation are listed at right.

Other changes

Once treatment has been completed, the redness will subside gradually. It may be replaced with darker skin. The pores may enlarge. The breast may feel thickened and firmer.

Nutrition

Patients should be taught the importance of a balanced diet to help maintain strength, prevent tissues from breaking down, and help rebuild normal tissues that have been damaged by treatment. Generally, protein and calorie needs are greater than normal during illness and treatment.

Fatigue

Many patients undergoing radiation therapy will experience a mild fatigue. However, this usually does not interfere with activities, and most women are able to carry out their normal routines. Fatigue is a subjective feeling of increased tiredness and decreased efficiency, resulting from a variety of physiologic, psychologic, and situational factors. It can vary in intensity and duration. Fatigue often is associated with activities that increase the expenditure of energy. Activity and rest patterns can play a significant role in its cause and alleviation.[56]

PATIENT INSTRUCTIONS FOR MOIST DESQUAMATION RESULTING FROM RADIATION THERAPY

1. Gently wash area under breast and arm with peroxide and water. Use a gauze pad for this and do not scrub.
2. Pat these areas dry. Use a gauze pad for this.
3. Put A & D Ointment on the shiny side of Telfa or nonstick dressing. Spread ointment on the dressing with a knife or tongue blade. Apply Telfa underneath your breast.
4. Repeat this three to four times a day, particularly at bed time.
5. Do not apply ointment before treatments.
6. Do not use deodorant, soaps, powders, or lotions on the treated area. Please see your doctor or nurse before using products you are not sure about.

Equipment

½ cup peroxide
½ cup water
Gauze pads
Knife or tongue blade
Telfa
A & D Ointment

Other symptoms, such as pain, dyspnea, nausea, or vomiting may occur with fatigue. It has been suggested that fatigue may be the common denominator in these and other protective phenomena. Control of symptoms may reduce or prevent fatigue.[48] Psychologic stressors such as depression and anxiety may at times influence fatigue. Fatigue can prevent the individual from engaging in valued activities that give meaning to one's life and can lead to a loss of hope. For a person with cancer, any new or persistent weakness may be viewed as a sign of impending decline and death and therefore may be terrifying.

It is important to assess and elicit information about the pattern of fatigue, including its onset, duration, intensity, aggravating and alleviating factors, impact on lifestyle, and the presence of other signs and symptoms. If the fatigue is severe, it may affect mobility and nutrition.[36] An instrument to measure and record fatigue is the Rhoten Fatigue Scale. The Rhoten Scale consists of 10 increments of fatigue ranging from zero (not tired, full of energy) to 10 (total exhaustion) measured over a 24-hour period. Activities also are recorded to pinpoint sources of excessive energy use.[1,8]

Careful management is required to prevent patients from being overwhelmed by fatigue. Patients should be taught energy conservation measures that include rest, activity, priority setting in activities that are important, and the delegation of nonessential tasks. They need to be taught to manage emotional stress by using support systems. Reliance on support systems also can help to conserve energy. Exercise can conserve energy by increasing tolerance for physical activity. There is evidence that many patients with cancer may benefit from exercise behaviors similar to those of the general population.

End of treatment

Patients should be prepared for the end of treatment and the beginning of follow-up care. Although most patients look forward to the end of their daily visits to the department, some experience anxiety, because they will miss the daily contact with health professionals. Preparing patients ahead of time may help, along with reminding the patient that health professionals are available by telephone if necessary.

Follow-up care

Once treatment is completed, patients will continue to be monitored by their radiation oncologist. An initial appointment is made for 2 to 4 weeks after the completion of treatment, to monitor the skin response. If there has been a problem during treatment, an appointment may be made within a week or two to inspect the skin. Follow-up appointments are then scheduled at 3-month intervals for 1 year, at 3 to 4-month intervals for the second and third years, and then at 6-month intervals. A mammogram, bone scan, chest x-ray, and laboratory work that includes a complete blood count and liver function tests are done yearly. Patients should continue to perform a self-breast examination monthly.

It is important to keep in mind that fearful, anxious, or uninformed patients can sometimes misinterpret symptoms and think the cancer has metastasized. It is important that patients realize that they may suffer from symptoms caused by colds, muscle strains, and ordinary physical problems, and that these symptoms should be kept in perspective.

Late reactions to radiation therapy to the breast can include rib fractures and chest wall discomfort. Radiation pneumonitis occurs in $\leq 1\%$ of patients and is accompanied by fever, malaise, and cough; it may occur generally within 2 to 3 months. A mild reaction should clear within a few weeks. Fibrotic changes may be seen on x-ray.

Other symptoms

Between follow-up examinations, patients should be taught to report symptoms that may be indicative of recurrent disease. These symptoms to report are listed below.

UNDERSTANDING AND MANAGING THE EFFECTS OF CHEMOTHERAPY

Most chemotherapeutic regimens produce at least one, and often times several, side effects. Moreover, the severity of these side effects tends to differ and is subject to a variety of factors. Certainly the most important predictors of the incidence and severity of any given side effect are related to the drug used and the dosage and frequency of its administration. However, there are both physiologic and psychosocial determinants that contribute to

SYMPTOMS TO REPORT

- Changes in the breast or scar during self-examination, especially lumps, thickening, or inflammation
- Persistent pain in breast, shoulder, hip, lower back, or pelvis
- Persistent cough or hoarseness
- Nausea, vomiting, diarrhea, or heartburn persisting for several days
- Loss of weight or unexplained weight change
- Changes in menstrual flow or cycle
- Persistent dizziness, blurred vision, severe and frequent headaches, and difficulty in walking

the actual severity of side effects and the perceived distress associated with untoward symptoms. Age, disease status, prior administration of chemotherapy, past or concurrent treatment with radiation, psychologic status, and social supports are among the many but not all of the factors shown to influence side effects and reactions to chemotherapeutic agents. For example, older patients have been shown to experience less distress, difficulty with treatment, and worry than younger patients.[47] Specific to patients with breast cancer, Ehlke[17] measured symptom distress among women receiving adjuvant chemotherapy and found that women with an external focus of control reported greater symptom distress than those with an internal focus of control. Additionally, women with negative perceptions of illness had more symptom distress than those with positive ones. Data correlating the multitude of variables associated with incidence and severity of side effects support the need for pharmacologic as well as behavioral approaches to managing these effects.

While patients have been exposed to the initial treatment modalities of surgery and radiotherapy, the role of chemotherapy may be less clear, especially that of adjuvant chemotherapy. Criteria used to determine the need for adjuvant chemotherapy coupled with the benefits derived from this type of therapy are often difficult concepts for patients to understand. Reassurance can be offered to women anticipating adjuvant chemotherapy for breast cancer, as there is some evidence to show that the side effects associated with this form of therapy are easily tolerated by most women. Glass et al.[23] report only 3% to 5% of patients receiving a 2-year course of treatment discontinued their therapy secondary to side effects. Even with the knowledge that this form of chemotherapy is well tolerated by the majority of patients, myths and misconceptions regarding chemotherapy do prevail and may evoke unnecessary fears and concerns.

Table 17-1 outlines many of the chemotherapeutic agents used in the treatment of breast cancer. Effective management of the accompanying side effects is dependent on an understanding of the physiologic and psychologic basis for the occurrence of such effects, astute assessment skills, knowledge of appropriate interventions, and the optimal participation of informed patients. Selected cutaneous, gastrointestinal, and bone marrow toxicities are discussed in detail below, along with certain drugs and regimens that produce side effects.

Cutaneous toxicities

Alopecia. The most obvious and one of the most distressing effects of chemotherapy is alopecia. Although the degree of epilation caused by specific chemotherapeutic agents differs, the effects of cytotoxic agents on hair loss, if any, almost universally begin to occur 2 to 4 weeks after therapy is initiated. The amount of epilation is compounded by the use of multiple agents that cause hair loss. Even with continued treatment, regrowth of hair may be evident approximately 3 to 6 months from the onset of therapy. Several studies conducted in attempts to prevent or retard the loss of hair are summarized by Joss et al.[33] The ability to interpret the results of these studies is hampered by several methodologic limitations. Nonrandomized samples are used for many of these studies. When randomization is employed, the sample sizes are extremely small. Moreover, methods of measuring hair loss pose several validity threats, because standardized reliable grading systems are not used, and observers often are not consistent.

Scalp hypothermia, with or without tourniquet application to the scalp, is among the most commonly employed techniques to prevent hair loss associated with chemotherapy treatments. However, this technique should not be used in diseases where soft tissue metastasis is possible and, in circumstances where such metastasis is likely, should only be used with palliative treatments. Because patients are unable to withstand the application of cold to the scalp or to wear the apparatus continuously, this technique is not effective for epilation resulting from oral and continuous-infusion cytotoxic therapy. Hypothermia caps are commercially available (Kold Cap, Spenco Hypothermia Cap).

Unfortunately, the most dramatic results from scalp hypothermia have been observed with doxorubicin as a single agent; the success of combination regimens with doxorubicin has not been documented. Giaccone et al.[22] randomly assigned patients receiving Adriamycin-containing regimens to scalp hypothermia or a control group. Significantly less hair loss ($p < .025$) was found as a result of scalp hypothermia in 37% of patients. According to another study,[33] as many as 50% to 70% of patients receiving single-agent doxorubicin can expect good to excellent results with this technique. The use of oral tocopherol has been studied with much less success and popularity.[43] Some have suggested that topical minoxidil, successful in preventing male pattern baldness, ought to be evaluated for its efficacy with chemotherapy-induced alopecia.[33]

Patients receiving cytotoxic agents with high potentials for epilation (daunorubicin, doxorubicin, cyclophosphamide, and etoposide) and moderate epilation (methotrexate, 5-fluorouracil, vincristine, vinblastine, and mitomycin) should be forewarned. Although reassurance that hair regrowth will occur

Table 17-1 Common chemotherapeutic agents

Classification	Dosage/route	Adverse reactions	Special precautions
Alkylating agents			
Cyclophosphamide (Cytoxan)	500-1000 mg/m^2 IV every 3 weeks 60-100 mg/m^2 PO every day	Nausea and vomiting begins 4-8 hours after IV administration, chronic nausea with daily oral administration	Administer antiemetics Encourage small frequent meals
		Nadir 7-14 days	Monitor for signs of infection; instruct patient regarding infection precautions
		Alopecia after 3-4 weeks; thinning or complete loss	Purchase a wig or head covering
		Hemorrhagic cystitis	Instruct patient to drink 3-4 L of fluids daily; void frequently Discontinue use if hematuria develops
		Nasal stuffiness during IV administration	
Ifosfamide (Ifex)	50 mg/kg/day × 5 days IV	Hematuria	IV hydration before administration; instruct patient to drink 3-4 L of fluids daily
		Nausea; increased at higher doses, begins several hours after infusion, extends 3 days	Administer antiemetics
		Alopecia; begins 2-4 weeks	Purchase wig or head covering
		Phlebitis at injection site with potential extravasation	Monitor signs of pain during injection, redness and swelling
Antibiotics			
Doxorubicin (Adriamycin)	60-75 mg/m^2 IV every 3 weeks	Nausea and vomiting; 1-3 hr after infusion, extending 24 hours	Administer antiemetics
		Nadir 10-14 days	Monitor for signs of infection; instruct patient regarding infection precautions
		Irritant to veins	Administer through free-flowing IV
		Vesicant, tissue necrosis and damage if extravasation occurs	For suspected or actual extravasation, immediately apply ice to area and appropriate measures (refer to p. 471)
		Alopecia; 2-5 weeks	Purchase wig or head covering
		Stomatitis	Instruct patient regarding oral hygiene measures and early signs and symptoms of stomatitis
		Cardiomyopathy	Monitor ECG abnormalities Observe for signs of congestive heart failure Monitor cardiac ejection fraction

Table 17-1 Common chemotherapeutic agents—cont'd

Classification	Dosage/route	Adverse reactions	Special precautions
Mitomycin (Mutamycin)	2 mg/m² × 5 days 15 mg/m² IV every 6-8 weeks	Vesicant/tissue damage or necrosis if extravasation occurs	Administer free flowing IV For suspected or actual extravasation, immediately apply ice to area and institute appropriate measures (refer to p. 471)
		Nausea and vomiting; 1-2 hours postinfusion extending 3-4 days	Administer antiemetics Monitor for signs of infection
		Nadir delayed 4-5 weeks	Instruct patient regarding infection precautions
Mitotic inhibitors			
Vincristine (Oncovin)	0.4-1.4 mg/m² IV weekly	Irritant	Administer free flowing IV
		Alopecia	Purchase wig early
		Paresthesias of hands and feet	
		Constipation	Begin bowel regimen (see p. 480)
		Jaw pain, hoarseness	Pain medications; may require narcotics
		Vesicant severe tissue damage and necrosis if extravasation occurs	For suspected or actual extravasation, immediately apply heat and inject Wydase (hyaluronidase) locally into area (refer to p. 471)
Vinblastine (Velban)	3-4 mg/m² IV every 7-14 days 6 mg/m² IV weekly 1-1.3 mg/m²/day IV × 5-7 days every 3 weeks by continuous intravenous infusion	Irritant	Administer free-flowing IV
		Nadir 4-10 days	Monitor for signs of infection Instruct patient regarding infection precautions
		Peripheral paresthesia; jaw pain	Pain medication
		Constipation	Begin bowel regimen (see p. 480)
		Alopecia	Instruct patient to purchase wig or head covering
Antimetabolites			
5-fluorouracil	12-15 mg/m² IV	Mild nausea and vomiting	Administer antiemetics
		Stomatitis	Instruct patient regarding oral hygiene measures and early signs and symptoms of stomatitis
		Diarrhea	Drink 2 liters of fluid daily, administer antidiarrheal medication
		Nadir 7-14 days	Instruct patient regarding infection precautions
		Alopecia	Purchase wig or head covering (common with 5-day infusions)
		Photosensitivity; increase skin pigmentation	Avoid exposure to the sun; use sunblock (protection factor >15) Warn patient regarding possible skin and nail changes

Continued.

Table 17-1 Common chemotherapeutic agents—cont'd

Classification	Dosage/route	Adverse reactions	Special precautions
Methotrexate	30-40 mg/m² IV 100-7500 mg/m² IV (high dose with leucovorin rescue)	Nausea and vomiting mild	Administer antiemetics
		Stomatitis	Instruct patient regarding oral hygiene measures and early signs and symptoms of stomatitis
		Nadir 6-9 days	Instruct patient regarding infection precautions
		Alopecia; may be only thinning	Purchase wig or head covering (common with 5-day infusions)
Miscellaneous agents			
Megestrol acetate (Megace)	40 mg QID PO	Mild nausea and vomiting Weight gain Alopecia	
Mitoxantrone	4-12 mg/m² IV × 5 days	Irritant; drug is blue, blue staining along vein	Administer slowly through a free-flowing IV
		Nausea and vomiting; mild Nadir 7-14 days Alopecia Green urine	
Tamoxifen	10-20 mg PO BID	Mild nausea and vomiting	Reassure patient that nausea usually subsides after 2 weeks of therapy
		Vaginal discharge/dryness	Instruct patient to use lubricant during intercourse
		Hot flashes Flare bone and tumor pain	

does not necessarily ameliorate or minimize the psychologic distress accompanying hair loss, it reaffirms for the patient the temporary nature of the situation and may make coping with it somewhat easier. The texture and color of new hair regrowth following chemotherapy may differ from the original hair characteristics. Patients at risk for hair loss should be advised to do the following:

1. Shop for a wig (if so desired) before hair loss is significant, in order to select a wig that closely resembles the color, texture, and style of the patient's real hair. Otherwise, the patient should be instructed to bring a picture of themselves when shopping for a wig.
2. Avoid hair dyes or coloring, permanents, hot air blow-drying, electric curlers, perfumed shampoos, alcohol-containing hair products, scalp exposure to the sun, and brushes with hard bristles.
3. Keep scalp clean by shampooing with a mild shampoo. Moisturizing shampoos are particularly useful to prevent scalp dryness.
4. Avoid extreme temperature on scalp when washing.
5. Insure that wigs fit properly and are removed at intervals during the day and at night.
6. Purchase scarves, turbans, or hats in addition to or in place of a wig.
7. Check insurance coverage for the purchase of a wig. Wigs for patients undergoing chemotherapy are reimbursable items by some third-party insurance carriers and Medicare. If coverage is not available, the local American Cancer Society may be helpful in procuring a wig.

Dermatologic effects. In addition to alopecia, there are other dermatologic effects associated with administration of chemotherapy. Chemotherapy-induced photosensitivity to ultraviolet rays and tissue damage accompanying the extravasation of vesicant agents are among the most serious of these effects. Photosensitivity to sunlight has been reported in patients receiving 5-fluorouracil, methotrexate, and vincristine.[2,7] It is necessary to alert patients who receive these drugs to the potential consequences of exposure to the sun's rays. These patients should be instructed to stay out of the sun and avoid indirect exposure through windows and

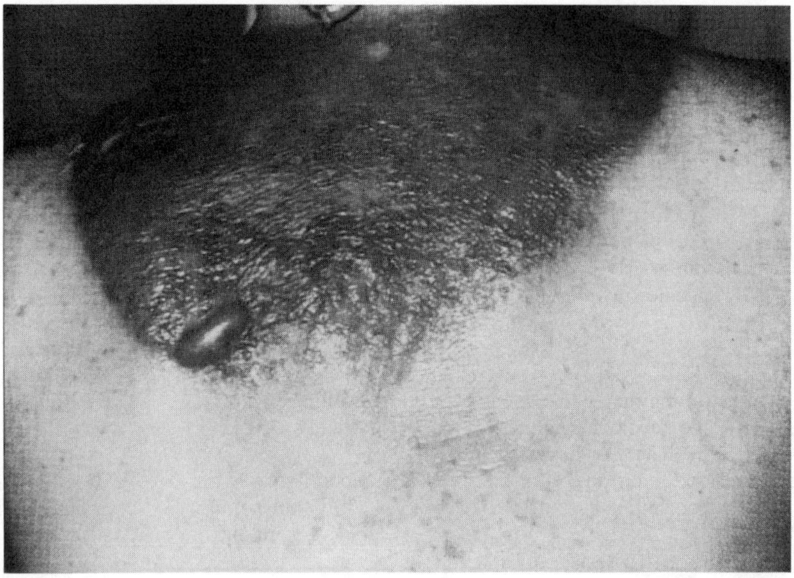

Fig. 17-1 Acute reaction after exposure to the sun in a client who had received high-dose methotrexate a few days previously. (From Yasko JM: Cutaneous reactions related to treatment with chemotherapy. In Yasko JM, editor: Nursing management of symptoms associated with chemotherapy, Columbus, Ohio, 1984, Adria Laboratories Inc, p 23.)

skylights. If patients must be or insist on being outdoors, protective head coverings, sun visors, and clothing should be worn. Patients should not be misled by cloudy days, as ultraviolet rays may still penetrate the skin even if the sun is not shining. Fig. 17-1 shows the consequences of sunlight exposure in a woman who received methotrexate a short time before going outdoors. The use of sunscreen with a high sun-protection factor often is recommended; however, its application may provide a false sense of security as sunscreens have not been shown to limit chemotherapy-induced photosensitivity reactions.

If vesicants or sclerosing agents extravasate into the tissues during administration, tissue damage and necrosis may result. Unlike chemical irritants that potentially can lead to phlebitis and inflammation of tissues—effects that tend to be reversible—vesicants that leak into the tissues can cause progressive irreversible damage and functional impairments. To help distinguish the difference between irritants and vesicants the Oncology Nursing Society[50] provides the definition that a vesicant is an "agent capable of causing or forming a blister and/or causing tissue destruction" whereas an irritant is "capable of producing venous pain at the side and along the vein with or without an inflammatory reaction." Certainly the degree of tissue impairment and loss of mobility from the leakage of vesicants into tissue depend on the location of the extravasation and the amount of drug that has been introduced into the tissues.

Administration of vesicants through a free-flowing, recently inserted peripheral intravenous catheter is imperative. Selection of peripheral veins should include the forearm and upper hand veins. Antecubital veins and those in the wrist area should be avoided, as joint mobility potentially can be affected should extravasations with vesicants occur. Table 17-2 provides a useful guide to distinguishing the local effects of chemical irritants vs. vesicant agents on peripheral veins and soft tissues. When the extravasation of a vesicant is suspected, specific local measures that differ depending upon the drug must be instituted promptly. In fact, it is advisable that an institutional policy or written protocol be available to health professionals who might encounter such problems. See pp. 470-471 for an example of institutional guidelines for the treatment of extravasations, taken from the Hospital of the University of Pennsylvania, which was developed from selected references.[15,39,50] Any patient with an actual or suspected extravasation from a chemotherapy vesicant should be evaluated by a plastic surgeon within 1 week after the occurrence for possible excision and skin grafting. Fig. 17-2 shows an ulceration on the forearm caused by an extravasation of Adriamycin.

Table 17-2 Nursing assessment of extravasation vs. other reactions

Assessment parameter	Extravasation	Irritation of the vein	Flare reaction
Pain	Pain, burning, or stinging are common and can occur while the drug is being given and around the needle site	Aching and tightness along the vein	Itching
Redness	Redness may occur around the needle site	The full length of the vein may be reddened or darkened	Either red blotches or red streaks can occur as the drug is given. The blotches/streaks appear along the vein
Swelling	Swelling may occur around the needle site, either immediately or hours later	Swelling is not likely	Swelling is not likely
Blood return	Blood return may still be present	Blood return is usually, but not always, present	Blood return is usually, but not always, present

From Cancer chemotherapy guidelines: module V recommendations for the management of extravasation anaphylaxis, Oncology Nursing Society, Pittsburgh, Penn, p 6. Reprinted with permission from the Oncology Nursing Society, Pittsburgh, Penn.

Other cutaneous side effects such as hyperpigmentation, nail changes, and interactions with radiotherapy are summarized by Hood.[27]

Stomatitis. Stomatitis, an inflammation of the mouth, results from the direct cytotoxic effects of certain chemotherapeutic agents.

The antimetabolite classification to which methotrexate and 5-fluorouracil belong tends to be among the most likely group of drugs to cause stomatitis. Also, stomatitis is observed with doxorubicin therapy. Patients receiving any chemotherapeutic agent or agents with the propensity to damage the oral mucosa must be informed of this potential side effect and be adequately prepared to institute measures to prevent occurrences and minimize severity. Good oral hygiene practices should begin before the start of chemotherapy. Patients at risk for stomatitis are instructed to (1) use a soft toothbrush and nonabrasive toothpaste; (2) avoid the use of commercially available mouth wash preparations, as many of these contain phenol and alcohol; (3) rinse with physiologic saline solution frequently; (4) make sure dentures fit properly, as the slightest amount of weight loss may affect denture grip; (5) avoid the ingestion of mechanically rough, hot, and spicy foods; and (6) be alert for early signs and symptoms of stomatitis. Gingivitis and heavy plaque formation around teeth predispose patients to stomatitis; therefore routine professional cleaning of the oral cavity before chemo-

HOSPITAL OF THE UNIVERSITY OF PENNSYLVANIA PROTOCOL FOR THE TREATMENT OF EXTRAVASATION OF ANTINEOPLASTIC AGENTS[15, 39, 50]

The following is a list of antineoplastic agents classified as vesicants, along with recommendations regarding treatment in the event of extravasation. All personnel involved in dispensing or administration of chemotherapy are advised to follow these recommendations. Extravasation kits containing instructions and antidote medications are located in the main pharmacy, pharmacy satellites, oncology pharmacy, and nursing units in which chemotherapy is administered. If a vesicant antineoplastic drug extravasates during administration, the physician shall give an order to administer the appropriate antidotes. The physician or nurse will administer the antidote(s). Treatment and follow-up of the extravasation will be documented by the nurse and/or physician using the extravasation documentation treatment record in the kit.

Prepared by Jeffrey E. Ball, Pharm.D., Oncology Pharmacist, Hospital of the University of Pennsylvania, Philadelphia, Penn. Reprinted with permission from the Hospital of the University of Pennsylvania, Philadelphia, Penn.

HOSPITAL OF THE UNIVERSITY OF PENNSYLVANIA PROTOCOL FOR THE TREATMENT OF EXTRAVASATION OF ANTINEOPLASTIC AGENTS—cont'd

Vesicants

Caution: if pain or swelling persists after 72 to 96 hours of the following treatment, plastic surgery should be consulted regarding the extravasation injury. The patient must be seen by the plastic surgeon within 1 to 2 weeks.

Antibiotics

Dactinomycin (Cosmegen)—elevate extremity for 24 to 48 hours, then encourage normal use of extremity. Apply cold packs for 20 minutes, four times daily, for 72 hours.
Mitomycin (Mutamycin)—elevate extremity for 24 to 48 hours, then encourage normal use of extemity. Apply cold packs for 20 minutes, four times daily, for 72 hours.
Plicamycin (mithramycin, Mithracin)—elevate extremity for 24 to 48 hours, then encourage normal use of extremity. Apply cold packs for 20 minutes, four times daily, for 72 hours.

Anthracycline antibiotics

Daunorubicin (Cerubidine)—elevate extremity for 24 to 48 hours, then encourage normal use of extremity. Apply cold packs for 20 minutes, four times daily, for 72 hours.
Doxorubicin (Adriamycin)—elevate extremity for 24 to 48 hours, then encourage normal use of extremity. Apply cold packs for 20 minutes, four times daily, for 72 hours.

Vinca alkaloids

Vinblastine (Velban)—subcutaneously (SC) inject hyaluronidase (Wydase) into the affected site as follows:

- *Antidote preparation*—to one vial containing 150 U, add 1 ml preservative-free normal saline (NS) to provide a solution containing 150 U/ml

One vial = 150 U = 1 ml

- *Method of administration*—inject five 1-ml doses of hyaluronidase (150 U/ml) SC into the extravasated site with multiple injections.

Warm compresses should be applied to the affected site for 20 minutes, four times daily for 72 hours.

Vincristine (Oncovin)—subcutaneously inject hyaluronidase (Wydase) into the affected site as follows:

- *Antidote preparation*—to one vial containing 150 U, add 1 ml preservative-free NS to provide a solution containing 150 U/ml.

One vial = 150 U = 1 ml

- *Method of administration*—inject five 1-ml doses of hyaluronidase (150 U/ml) SC into the extravasation site with multiple injections.

Warm compresses should be applied to the affected site for 20 minutes, four times daily for 72 hours.

Etoposide, VP-16 (VePesid)—subcutaneously inject hyaluronidase (Wydase) into the affected site as follows:

- *Antidote preparation*—to one vial containing 150 U, add 1 ml preservative-free NS to provide a solution containing 150 U/ml.

One vial = 150 U = 1 ml

- *Method of administration*—inject five 1-ml doses of hyaluronidase (150 U/ml) SC into the extravasation site with multiple injections.

Warm compresses should be applied to the affected site for 20 minutes, four times daily for 72 hours.

Alkylating agents

Mechlorethamine, nitrogen mustard (Mustargen)—use sodium thiosulfate as follows:

- *Antidote preparation*—draw up 1.6 ml of 25% of sodium thiosulfate solution; mix with 8.4 ml sterile water for injection to yield 10 ml solution.
- *Method of administration*—inject 5 ml IV through the existing line.

Apply *cold* compresses to the affected site for 20 minutes, four times daily, for 72 hours.

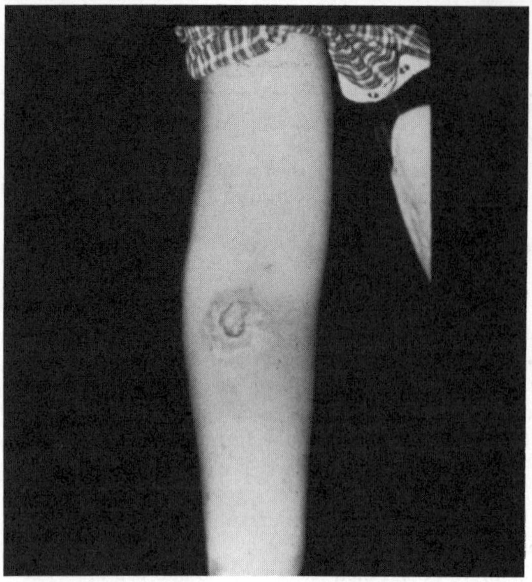

Fig. 17-2 Adriamycin extravasation on forearm.

therapy and during therapy is recommended. It is imperative that patients inform their dentists or dental hygienists that they are undergoing cancer chemotherapy and avoid any dental procedure before or during the anticipated nadir. Leukocyte counts must be within acceptable ranges, with an absolute neutrophil count of >1500 mm^3 before dental procedures can be safely undertaken.

Early manifestations of stomatitis include a sensitivity to hot and cold foods, a slight burning sensation in the mouth, a dry mouth, erythema of the oral mucosa, pain when eating or drinking, and a feeling of thick or swollen mucous membranes. Once isolated or diffuse ulcerations appear, stomatitis has progressed beyond the early stages and more meticulous oral care usually is required. It is essential to keep the oral membranes clean and moist, as the accompanying decrease in saliva alters the normal environment for oral tissues. Frequent rinsing with physiologic saline, half-strength hydrogen peroxide, or quarter-strength Dakin's solution (one part liquid household bleach to 40 parts water) helps to remove oral debris and denuded cells. Chlorhexidine gluconate 0.12% (Peri-dex) is an excellent oral rinse. If oral rinsing is not possible secondary to the pain often encountered with very severe cases of stomatitis, oral lavage with an irrigation set should be considered.

Topical anesthetic agents such as Dyclone 0.5% and diphenhydramine 0.5%, viscous xylocaine, and lidocaine solution can be used to promote comfort. Aluminum and/or magnesium hydroxide (Maalox, Mylanta, Milk of Magnesia) solutions or kaolin pectin (Kaopectate) solutions can be applied to oral tissues to soothe them, and they serve as a nice vehicle for administration of some topical anesthetic preparations. Severe stomatitis is extremely painful and often warrants systemic narcotic therapy. Mouth moisturizers, either in the form of a water-soluble gel or a solution similar to the consistency of human saliva, relieve the accompanying dry mouth. If eating is problematic, mechanically soft diets or liquid diets are recommended. Gravies and liquids added to solid foods assist with mastication and swallowing should decreased saliva and mouth dryness be experienced.

Nausea and vomiting

The exact causes of chemotherapy-induced nausea and vomiting remain unclear. There is, however, some consensus that a multitude of effects ranging from direct central and peripheral mechanisms caused by drug metabolites to behavioral responses, as seen with anticipatory nausea and vomiting, are likely initiators. Whatever the case, an estimated 10% to 30% of patients refuse chemotherapy treatments because of the distress caused by nausea and vomiting.[40,54] Successful control of chemotherapy-induced nausea and vomiting is dependent on a thorough understanding of the possible causes as well as the utilization of pharmacologic and behavioral approaches.

Patients who experience nausea and vomiting with their initial treatment tend to continue the pattern.[53] Patterns related to nausea and vomiting can be assessed with respect to timing, frequency, and duration as well as the degree of distress associated with the symptoms. Timing of nausea and vomiting refers to time of onset. Patients experiencing anticipatory nausea and vomiting may experience these well in advance or immediately before the administration of therapy. Some predictability regarding the onset of nausea and vomiting is appreciated by knowledge of the particular agent or agents and the emetogenic properties. Once a pattern has been established, antiemetic therapy can be instituted at appropriate times to maximize its benefit. Duration of nausea and vomiting can be categorized as either acute, occurring during the first 24 hours following treatment, or delayed, persisting up to 7 days after the therapy.[42] Precipitation of acute chemotherapy-induced nausea and vomiting is affected by the emetogenic potential to the drugs, prior experience, and the antiemetic regimen used. Rhodes et al.[62] offer a comprehensive model for assessing patterns of nausea, vomiting, and distress accompanying treatment with antineoplastic therapy.

Prolonged nausea and infrequent vomiting may be associated with oral cyclophosphamide therapy used for adjuvant purposes. Strategies to control the nausea include a three times daily dosing schedule so that smaller doses are taken more frequently, bedtime administration to minimize nausea during the waking hours, frequent ingestion of carbohydrates, and regular dosing of an antiemetic such as prochlorperazine (Compazine). If patients do consume the total dose at bedtime, advise them to drink plenty of fluid before going to sleep in order to prevent hemorrhagic cystitis. As the chemotherapy cycle progresses, patients may find it increasingly difficult to swallow the oral tablets because of their size. Taking medications with soft foods such as pudding or ice cream may make them easier to ingest.

Anticipatory nausea and vomiting occur from behavioral conditioning, whereby perceptual phenomena, such as visual and olfactory stimuli, spark the awareness of nausea that can ultimately lead to spontaneous vomiting. Experience with events associated with the chemotherapy treatment like venipuncture for the insertion of an intravenous line, certain smells, the sight of caregivers administering the therapy, or even just sitting in the chemotherapy room have been known to elicit anticipatory nausea and vomiting. Age is an important consideration in predicting anticipatory nausea and vomiting, with patients under the age of 50 years more likely to develop this problem.[31,44] Anxiety also increases the risk of anticipatory sequelae.[31,44,46] Interestingly, Nerenz etal.[46] also have identified drug taste, which is particularly strong for patients receiving cyclophosphamide and doxorubicin, as a predictor for anticipatory nausea and vomiting.

Interventions for anticipatory nausea and vomiting are aimed at reducing the offensive stimuli or distracting the patient from it and alleviating or reducing anxiety. More importantly, effective control of these symptoms at the onset of the chemotherapeutic regimen limits the degree of behavioral conditioning associated with nausea and vomiting. The administration of lorazepam (Ativan) helps reduce anxiety and interferes with the process of recalling events and experiences related to the treatment.

In general the most powerful defense against chemotherapy-induced nausea and vomiting is antiemetic therapy. Table 17-3 outlines a survey of antiemetics currently used for chemotherapy-related nausea and vomiting. For highly or moderately emetogenic drugs, a combination of antiemetics for premedication purposes is useful. Occasionally, the use of prochlorperazine or metoclopramide may precipitate extrapyramidal symptoms; more commonly they produce dystonic reactions of the face and mouth, and sometimes generalized severe muscle twitching and rigidity. Although these reactions are not harmful to patients, they are quite uncomfortable and distressing. These symptoms can be reversed quickly with the administration of parenteral diphenhydramine (Benadryl).

A number of behavioral strategies such as hypnosis and relaxation therapy have been investigated for control of chemotherapy-related nausea and vomiting. Cotanch and Strum[12] used progressive relaxation therapy for 20 patients receiving multiple-course, highly emetogenic chemotherapy regimens, and compared ranked self-reports of nausea and vomiting to patients in a placebo control group and a no-treatment group. Progressive relaxation made a significant difference ($p = .03$) in the management of vomiting but no difference in the sensation of nausea among patients.

The efficacy of hypnosis has been well established for chemotherapy-induced emesis, especially anticipatory emesis.[60] Aerobic exercise has been shown to be a useful adjunctive measure for controlling nausea in women with breast cancer who are receiving chemotherapy.[73] Such an approach encourages self-management of nausea and can improve physical stamina.

Weight gain

Weight gain rarely is encountered with most chemotherapeutic regimens, except for those involving the administration of corticosteroids and hormones. However, weight gain often is observed in women receiving adjuvant chemotherapy for breast cancer even in the absence of corticosteroids and hormonal therapy. The exact cause or causes for such observations remain unclear.

In a review of 87 outpatient clinic records of women receiving adjuvant chemotherapy, Knobf et al.[37] calculated a >10-lb gain in weight over an average of 15.4 months in 45% of their sample. Similarly, Hunnington[29] reported that 50% of 29 patients experienced weight gain associated with adjuvant chemotherapy for breast cancer. In fact, women receiving cyclosphosphamide, methotrexate, and 5-fluorouracil (CMF) alone gained more weight while undergoing treatment than those with vincristine and prednisone added to the regimen.

Few investigators have been able to find significant correlations between sample characteristics and weight gain. Foltz[20] identified five factors thought to be related to weight gain and proceeded to study them in 34 women receiving adjuvant chemotherapy. Neither activity, depression, intake, metabolic rate, nor estradiol levels showed any significant relationship to weight gain among her study population. Admittedly her sample size was small and limitations on estradiol measurements and dietary histories were encountered. Some

Text continued on p. 478.

Table 17-3 Survey of antiemetics in current use for chemotherapy-related nausea (N) and vomiting (V)

	Proposed mechanism of action	Duration of action	Availability	Recommended dose/schedule	Side effects/comments
Phenothiazines					
Prochlorperazine (Compazine)	Dopamine antagonist CTZ, ?VC	3-4 hr 3-4 hr 10-12 hr 3-4 hr 3-4 hr	Soln: 5 mg/ml Tabs: 5, 10, 25 mg Sustained release (Compazine spansules): 10, 15, 30 mg Suppositories: 2.5, 5, 25 mg Parenteral 5 mg/ml	Low dose: 10 mg PO/IM, 25 mg PR q 4 hr or ½° AC and HS High dose: 20-40 mg slow IV 30 min before, 3 hr and 6 hr after chemo For delayed N&V: 30 mg TID day 1* 30 mg BID day 2* 15 mg BID days 3 thru 6* *plus dexamethasone	Most common s.e.: EPS (akathisia and dystonic rxn) and sedation ▪ Children more prone to EPS ▪ Dehydration may increase risk of akathisia ▪ Treat akathisia with benzodiazepine (diazepam or lorazepam) ▪ Treat dystonic rxn with diphenhydramine or benztropine Hypotension may occur, particularly with 1st parenteral dose ▪ Do not exceed 5 mg/min with IV dose ▪ Administer IV doses of >10 mg over 20-30 min to recumbent patient Hypotension and other CV effects (i.e., tachycardia) usually resolve within ½-2 hr ▪ monitor VS Other common side effects: CNS (drowsiness, anxiety, HA, etc); anticholinergic (dry mouth, constipation, etc.) ▪ Use SR capsules on regular basis for delayed/persistent N&V
Thiethylperazine (Torecan)	Dopamine antagonist CTZ, ?VC	up to 4 hr	Tabs: 10 mg Suppositories: 10 mg Parenteral: 5 mg/ml	10 mg q 4 hr	See prochlorperazine for side effects
Butyrophenones					
Haloperidol (Haldol)	Dopamine antagonist (CTZ)	2-6 hr	Soln: 2 mg/ml Tabs: 0.5, 1, 2, 5 mg Parenteral: 5 mg/ml	Doses variable: 1 mg BID-TID PRN 2 mg IM 3 mg IV q 2° × 5 Starting 30 min prior to chemotherapy	Use lowest effective dose. Similar in structure to phenothiazines; may be as effective May have additive effects with other CNS depressants, i.e., opioid analgesics, sedatives, barbiturates

					Side effects: EPS (treat as with phenothiazines), sedation, tachycardia, hypotension, anticholinergic
Droperidol (Inapsine)	Dopamine antagonist (CTZ)	2-4 hr	Parenteral: 2.5 mg/ml (IM, IV)	Doses variable: 1 mg IVP q hr × 6 15 mg IV, then 7.5 mg IV q 2° × 7	See haloperidol Sedation may persist for up to 12 hr Hypotension: consider hypovolemia ▪ Monitor I & O ▪ Monitor VS ▪ Administer IV Fluids PRN
Substituted benzamide					
Metoclopramide (Reglan)	Dopamine antagonist (CTZ) ▪ ?5HT_3 antagonist in GI tract ▪ Accelerates gastric emptying and small bowel transit	?2-3 hr (peak—30 min-2 hr.)	Soln: 5 mg/ml Tabs: 5 mg, 10 mg Parenteral: 5 or 10 mg/ml	2-3 mg/kg IV or PO q 2-3 hr × 3-5 3 mg IV 30 min before and 90 min after chemo 2 mg/kg PO or IV q 2° × 3, then 1 mg/kg q 2° × 3	Administer IV doses slowly (over 15 min) to prevent transient, intense anxiety Compatible with dexamethasone in IV soln May have additive effects with other CNS depressants Side effects: EPS ▪ Treat as with phenothiazines ▪ More common in children, adolescents and young adults ▪ More common with PO administration over several days Sedation, HA, fatigue, restlessness, diarrhea, decreased renal plasma flow ▪ Monitor I & O ▪ Monitor VS

CTZ, chemoreceptor trigger zone; VC, vomiting center; EPS, extrapyramidal symptoms; HA, headache; CNS, central nervous system; PG, prostaglandin; AP, anterior pituitary; VS, vital signs; LOC, level of consciousness; ANS, anatomic nervous system.
From Wickham R: Oncol Nurs Forum 16(4):566, 1989.

Continued.

Table 17-3 Survey of antiemetics in current use for chemotherapy-related nausea (N) and vomiting (V)—cont'd

	Proposed mechanism of action	Duration of action	Availability	Recommended dose/schedule	Side effects/comments
Steroids					
Dexamethasone (Decadron) Methylprednisolone (Solu-Medrol)	?inhibition of PG synthesis in AP ?alter permeability of blood brain barrier	Unknown		Doses variable: ▪ Methylprednisolone 500 mg IV q 6° × 4 ▪ Dexamethasone 10-20 mg IV prior to chemo ▪ Dexamethasone 80-150 mg IV × 1 ▪ Dexamethasone 20 mg IV × 6 2 hr before chemo and 3, 6, 9, and 12 hr post chemotherapy ▪ Dexamethasone 8 mg PO TID day 1, 8 mg BID day 2, and 4 mg BID days 3-6 for delayed N&V	Rapid IV administration may be accompanied by transient perineal, rectal, or vaginal burning Side effects: insomnia, anxiety, euphoria
Cannabinoid					
Dronabinol (Marinol)	Unknown ▪ Alter PG synthesis ▪ Binds to opiate receptors and inhibits VC	4-6 hr	Tabs: 2.5, 5, 10 mg	5 mg/kg q 4-6 hr	Schedule II drug, generally used as second line antiemetic Side effects: ▪ CNS—sedation, dizziness, disorientation, impaired concentration, anxiety, dysphoria ▪ ANS—orthostatic hypotension, dry mouth ▪ CV—tachycardia

Benzodiazepine					
Lorazepam (Ativan)	Anxiolytic Anterograde amnesia CNS depressant	4-8 hr (duration of sedation)	Tabs: 0.5, 1, 2 mg (PO or sublingual) Parenteral: 2 or 4 mg/ml	Doses variable: ▪ 0.5-2 mg PO or IV × 1 or repeat PRN 1.5 mg/m^2 IV before chemo (3 mg max) ▪ 0.05 mg/kg *before chemo (4 mg max) and q 4° PRN × 4 ▪ 0.05 mg/kg *sublingual before chemo *protocol amended to 0.025 mg/kg	Sublingual provides rapid plasma levels and greater bioavailability than PO administration Side effects: sedation, amnesia May have additive effect with other CNS depressants, i.e., opioids, sedatives, etc. Use cautiously in patients with hepatic or renal dysfunction (organs of metabolism and excretion) Use cautiously in debilitated patients or those with compromised pulmonary function (may lead to underventilation and hypoxia) ▪ Monitor labs ▪ Monitor VS ▪ Monitor LOC ▪ Administer small dose and repeat to desired effect

have speculated that a decrease in activity secondary to fatigue is likely to be responsible for increased weight, rather than an increase in appetite. However, accurate diet histories and evaluation of activity patterns in well-designed studies are necessary before such conclusions can be inferred.

Grindel et al.[25] studied the food intake patterns of healthy women and women with breast cancer receiving adjuvant chemotherapy. With a convenience sample of 19 women receiving adjuvant chemotherapy (six receiving CMF alone, while the majority received CMF plus tamoxifen, vincristine, and/or prednisone) matched with healthy controls, a statistically significant difference ($p<.01$) using repeated measures analysis of variance (ANOVA) was found with respect to dietary intake. Women with breast cancer consumed more calories over a 3-day period than healthy control subjects. Interestingly, no significant difference in weight between the two groups over a 6-month period was noted.

The consequences of weight gain further complicates psychologic distress and negative body image that already may be apparent from the diagnosis of cancer and primary treatment. Patients should be informed and prepared for a change in weight associated with therapy. Dietary counseling should be offered and encouraged.

Hemorrhagic cystitis

Hemorrhagic cystitis characterized by acute or insidious diffuse vesical bleeding[16] is an untoward effect of systemic drug therapy with oxazaphosphorine alkylating compounds, to which cyclophosphamide and structurally related isophosphamide belong. A metabolite of these drugs, rather than the active drugs themselves, appear to be the likely cause of bladder damage and subsequent bleeding.[55] Repeated exposure to the metabolite from long-term oral therapy or intermittent contact with the metabolite from high-dose therapy of cyclophosphamide increase the risk for hemorrhagic cystitis.

Forni et al.[21] describe the cytologic and histologic changes observed with cyclophosphamide treatment in detail. Fibrosis of the bladder wall causing low compliance lead to symptoms of urinary frequency and urgency. As mucosa damage and sloughing progress, microscopic or macroscopic hematuria is evident. In the past, efforts to prevent or retard the resultant effects of cyclophosphamide metabolite on bladder tissue were aimed toward hydration. By diluting the metabolite and enhancing elimination through frequent voiding or Foley catheterization, contact with the bladder wall is minimized. Unfortunately, the incidence of hemorrhagic cystitis increases with more aggressive and prolonged chemotherapy regimens, making these measures alone unsuccessful.

Today the administration of drugs such as n-acetylcysteine, mesna, and more recently prostaglandins, appears to be a more promising alternative for preventing the occurrence of hemorrhagic cystitis associated with cyclophosphamide therapy.[16] Hydration still remains an acceptable measure to mitigate the effects of the metabolite-induced bladder mucosal changes. Patients receiving oral cyclophosphamide therapy should be instructed to drink at least 2 quarts of fluids each day. Those who take their therapy before bed need to be especially cautious that they are well hydrated before sleeping. Accompanying symptoms of frequency, urgency, pain, or bleeding with cyclophosphamide or ifosfamide therapy must be reported to the physician or nurse promptly.

Neutropenia

The neutrophil component of the white blood cells serves as the first line of defense against infection. In the healthy individual, absolute neutrophil counts range from 2500 to 6000 cells/mm^3, comprising 54% to 62% of the total leukocyte count. Neutrophil counts of <1000 cells/mm^3 constitute neutropenia. The neutrophil count is determined by the following formula:

$$\text{ANC (absolute neutrophil count)} = \frac{\%\text{ neutrophils} \times \text{total WBC}}{100}$$

$$\text{ANC} = \text{total WBC} \times (\%\text{ segmented} + \%\text{ band})\text{ cells}$$

Neutropenia increases the patient's risk for infection. The majority of infections acquired from neutropenia stem from endogenous bacterial sources, such as *Escherichia coli, Klebsiella pneumoniae* and *Pseudomonas aerogenes*.[63] Potential sites of infection include the lung, gastrointestinal tract, urinary tract, blood, and skin. Prevention, early detection, and aggressive management are the standards of care for neutropenic patients.

Neutropenia may be the result of the disease itself or the result of treatment, as in the nadir period of chemotherapy. Careful monitoring of the neutrophil count is essential to ascertain the risk potential for infection. Although neutrophil counts of <1000/mm^3 increase the likelihood of acquiring life-threatening complications, this risk is increased dramatically with counts of <500/mm^3. The neutropenic patient who is also febrile has a $>60\%$ chance of harboring a bacterial infection of some sort. Fungal infections are common secondary sources. Usually neutropenia resulting from cancer treatments resolves spontaneously. However, during the nadir and recovery period, patients must be instructed in taking precautionary measures and watching for signs and symptoms. Routine instructions for patients at risk for neutropenia include the following: (1) avoid crowds, people with colds or infectious illnesses, and children who may have recently been exposed to the varicella or chicken pox virus; (2) monitor temperature at least once a day; (3) report immediately any fever greater than 100.5° F, chills, redness or swelling in any body part, burning or frequent urination, persistent cough, and soreness or tenderness in the rectal area. Sexual intercourse is permissible; however, should the neutrophil count fall below 500/mm^3, it is recommended that patients seek the advice of their health care providers.

Patients must be forewarned of the potential hazardous complications of neutropenic fevers. All fevers of 100.5° should be reported immediately to the physician. The telephone numbers of emergency on-call personnel should be given to patients in writing as well as the names and dosages of the medications they are receiving. Fevers during the nadir period will necessitate a visit to the clinic or emergency room, including a complete blood count with differential.

Detection of infectious sources involves a complete history and physical examination, with particular attention being paid to common sources of infection. Female patients should be advised to wipe from front to back after having a bowel movement. The pharynx, lung, skin, perineum, fingernails, and toenails must be examined carefully, and cultures should be taken. Blood, urine, and sputum cultures should be obtained, and a chest x-ray performed. Vascular access devices should be examined carefully, obtaining blood cultures from the catheter lumen as well as a peripheral site. The incidence of catheter infections range from 0 to 0.8 infections per 100 catheter days.[59,61]

If neutropenic patients develop a fever, prompt, aggressive treatment empirically with broad-spectrum antibiotic coverage should be initiated before the results of the cultures are known, as the progression from local infection to disseminated sepsis may be rapid. Hughes et al.[28] conducted an extensive review of the various types of antiinfective agents recommended for treatment by the Infectious Disease Society of America. They conclude that combination drug treatment with an aminoglycoside (gentamicin, tobramycin, or amikacin), an antipseudomonal penicillin (mezlocillin) or a cephalosporin (ceftazidime) was sufficient. Vancomycin may be added to the regimen if organisms like coagulase-negative staphylococci, *S. aureus, Corynebacterium* spp., and α-hemolytic streptococci are suspected as in patients with central venous catheters.[59]

Antibiotic therapy for the management of neutropenia is continued for a minimum of 7 days, until the patient is free of the signs and symptoms of infection, and the granulocyte count is >500/mm^3. Persistent fevers of 3 days or more warrant reassessment of therapy and sometimes reculturing for infectious sources. In these circumstances, the following approaches are recommended.[28] If the patient's condition has not changed and the neutropenia is expected to resolve in approximately 5 days, the initial antibiotics may be continued. For patients whose conditions worsen and whose initial treatment included the three-drug approach, consideration may be given to changing to a third-generation cephalosporin such as ceftazidime. Finally, the addition of amphotericin B may be considered assuming the existence of a systemic fungal infection.

During the hospital course, strict attention is given to the granulocyte count, anticipating an upward trend. Strict handwashing before and after contact with the patient is essential. Protective isolation has not been shown to reduce the risk of infection. Additionally, this type of isolation is costly, consumes health professionals' time in gowning and wearing a mask, and may physically isolate patients from staff. In circumstances where prolonged neutropenia is evident, the benefits of protective isolation are controversial. The use of agents such as granulocyte colony–stimulating factor (G-CSF) are currently under investigation.[32]

MANAGING RECURRENT AND ADVANCED DISEASE

When cancer recurs, patients will sometimes experience fear, anxiety, anger, and guilt. It is important to encourage communication and the expression of feelings. Although they already may have been exposed to one or more treatments in the initial stage of their illness, patients probably will need to be retaught about the side effects of treatment. Along with the psychologic adjustment to illness, patients are faced with coping with a set of new physiologic insults.

Nutrition

With recurrent disease, good nutrition is essential. Anorexia may be a problem at this time, for cancer and its treatment can interfere with usual dietary patterns. The high rate of tumor metabolism and treatment can cause an increased demand for nutrients. *Eating Hints,* an NCI publication, discusses the need for good nutrition during treatment for cancer. Common digestive problems and what to do about them, advice on meal planning, and recipes are included in this publication. The nurse should monitor the patient's weight and energy levels and suggest ways to increase the intake of calories and protein.

Brain metastases

Patients who receive cranial irradiation for brain metastases will lose their hair during treatment and may need assistance in obtaining a wig. Alopecia has been discussed earlier in this chapter. The family may need help in learning how to communicate with the patient who has brain metastases. In addition, the family may need to take extra safety precautions, as the patient with brain metastases may have an unsteady gait, become forgetful, and show inappropriate judgment, thus exposing himself or herself to dangerous situations.

Bone metastases

Bone metastases occur in about 80% of women who develop metastatic disease. The first sign is bone tenderness and pain. Most often, the vertebrae, pelvic bones, ribs, or skull will be affected. Bone scans often will show the presence of metastases before they become painful, and up to 1 year before disease can be detected by conventional x-rays. Radiation therapy can effectively relieve pain. Patients should be cautioned to avoid lifting heavy objects, climbing, falling, making twisting motions, or placing any undue stress on bones. Those patients who have difficulty walking may need assistive devices such as walkers or wheelchairs.

Pain syndromes

Like other patients with progressive cancer, women with metastatic breast cancer are plagued with diffuse pain. Bony pain from skeletal tumor involvement is the most common somatic source of pain. Visceral pain is often evident from metastases to the liver. Various forms of neuropathic pain syndromes such as brachial plexus involvement from tumors occur from tumor spread. In addition to the direct effects of tumors, pain syndromes also result from cancer treatment. Portenoy[57] summarizes the various causes of pain in patients with cancer.

The pharmacologic management of mild cancer pain should proceed with the use of weak narcotic analgesics, acetaminophen, aspirin, or nonsteroidal antiinflammatory drugs (NSAIDs). For the management of bony pain secondary to tumor infiltration, NSAIDs are particularly effective. As tumor invades the bone, prostaglandins, hyperanalgesic substances, are released. Inhibition of these pain-promoting substances by NSAIDs appear to make the receptors in the bone less vulnerable to painful stimuli. Sometimes, for control of mild pain, a combination of a weak narcotic and nonnarcotic is useful. As cancer pain worsens, more potent narcotic analgesics may be necessary such as hydromorphone, levorphanol, morphine, or methadone.

Inturrisi[34] provides a comprehensive overview of the pharmacologic management of cancer patients. Reluctance to give the patient stronger narcotic analgesics should not be based on concerns about analgesic tolerance. Rarely is tolerance to narcotic analgesics a clinical problem. If tolerance develops, it is most likely a function of the pain worsening, rather than the result of repeated exposure to narcotics.[52] Furthermore, safe escalation of narcotic analgesics is recommended to accommodate increased narcotic requirements. Likewise, the fear of addiction should not color the prescribing patterns of physicians, because the incidence of addiction among cancer patients, and for the most part all hospitalized patients, is exceedingly low.[58] Constipation is an expected outcome of narcotic analgesic therapy. Therefore measures to both prevent and manage constipation are necessary (see at left).

More recently, long-acting oral morphine has been introduced for the management of chronic cancer pain. Its use requires longer dosing intervals and fewer doses than shorter-acting opioids. Quality of life measurements of patients using controlled-released oral morphine (MS Contin) were significantly better than those of patients receiving shorter-acting narcotics.[18] Even though several advantages do exist with these preparations, a combination of a short-acting opioid with a longer-acting one may be required for the control of

---

BOWEL REGIMEN FOR PREVENTION AND MANAGEMENT OF CONSTIPATION

Prevention plan

1. Increase fiber in diet (fruits, vegetables, bran).
2. Drink eight glasses of liquid each day.
3. Drink hot liquids.
4. Use a bulk product (Metamucil).
5. Consider a stool softener (dioctyl sodium sulfosuccinate [Colace])

If constipated

1. Add oral laxative to above plan:
   - Milk of Magnesia (magnesium hydrochloride) 30 to 60 ml daily
   - Dioctyl sodium sulfosuccinate with casanthranol (Pericolace) 1 tablespoon daily up to TID
   - Senna (Senokot) 2 to 4 tablespoons daily up to BID
   - Chronulac (lactulose) 15-60 ml daily or BID
2. Consider suppositories and enemas:
   - Glycerin suppository 1 PR daily to BID
   - Bisacodyl suppository 1 PR daily
   - Tap water 500 to 1000 ml
   - Fleets enema 1 to 2 as needed

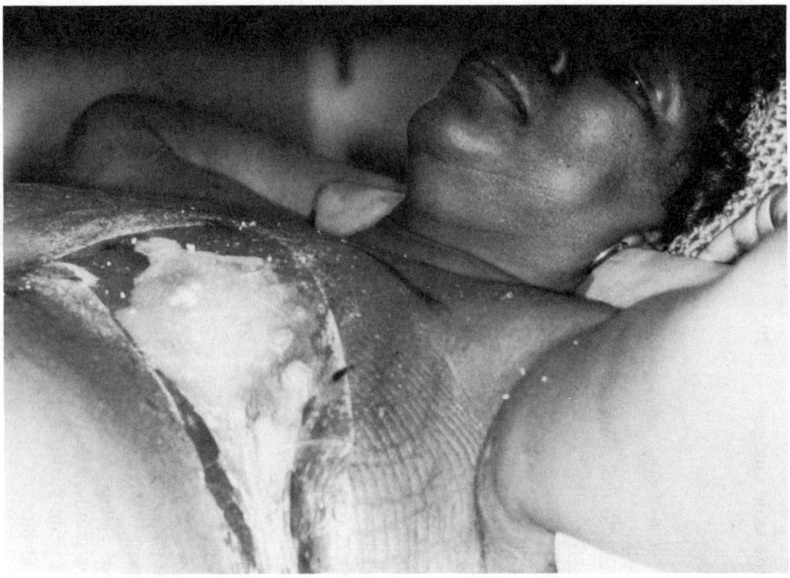

Fig. 17-3 Patient undergoing radiation for ulcerating chest wall lesion from local recurrence of breast carcinoma following mastectomy. Local care regimen included daily irrigations with Dakin's solution, with the application of Bard absorption dressing and moisture vapor–permeable dressing.

acute exacerbations or bouts of pain, as with the pain of bony metastases. Brooks et al.[9] outline the principles of pain management with long-acting oral morphine.

Narcotic infusional therapy can be used when patients are no longer able to tolerate oral pain medication or if dosages cannot be ingested easily. Innovative approaches such as continuous infusion therapy with patient-controlled analgesia have been used for the management of cancer pain.[4]

Neuropathic pain syndromes, like the pain accompanying brachial plexopathies, are notoriously unresponsive to systemic narcotic analgesics.[3] In order to ameliorate such pain, a combination of antidepressants, anticonvulsants, neuroleptics, steroids, NSAIDs, and transcutaneous nerve stimulations (TENS) may be effective.

Hypercalcemia

Metastatic invasion of the bone by tumor may cause elevated serum calcium levels. The normal serum calcium level ranges between 8.5 and 10.1 mg/dl in women. In addition to an elevated calcium level, the patient may exhibit changes in mental status such as lethargy and confusion, muscle weakness, fatigue, coma, and, if not corrected, cardiac arrest. Adequate hydration is usually necessary, as patients are often dehydrated because of a combination of nausea, vomiting, poor fluid intake, and polyuria. Once the patient has been hydrated, diuretics may be given to enhance calcium excretion. Thiazide diuretics are contraindicated because they inhibit urinary excretion of calcium.[68] Immobilization should be avoided because it tends to increase bone resorption of calcium, and it enhances hypercalcemia. Care of hypercalcemic patients involves monitoring levels of calcium, fatigue, and assessing mental and neurologic status.

Ulcerating chest wall skin lesions

Ulcerating chest wall lesions can result from recurrent locally invasive tumors when systemic chemotherapy and local radiation are no longer effective in controlling local tumor spread. The frequency of occurrence for ulcerating chest wall lesions is unknown. Moreover, not all local tumors progress to fungating lesions. When local skin and underlying tissues in the chest wall are affected by tumor and are unresponsive to therapy, numerous problems with infection, bleeding, odor, and drainage can arise.

A comprehensive approach to the care of these lesions includes provisions for keeping the wound clean, preventing infection, removing necrotic tissue by debridement, controlling odor, minimizing potential for and controlling bleeding and providing a comfortable covering to contain drainage and conceal the lesion. If patients are receiving local radiotherapy to the chest wall concurrently, skin care products must be evaluated so that they do not interfere with skin penetration or enhance skin toxicity. Fig. 17-3 shows an ulcerating chest wall le-

Text continued on p. 486.

Table 17-4 Skin care products for ulcerating chest wall lesions

	Properties/action	Application	Advantages	Disadvantages
Antiinfective agents				
Acetic acid solution 0.25%-5%	Solution with bactericidal properties against topical pseudomonas at concentrations of ≥1%	Irrigate or soak lesion with solution 2-3 times per day (10-15 min soaks are preferrable if pseudomomas organisms are present)	Easy to make from white table vinegar	Vinegar odor Burns in concentrations >1%
Chlorhexidine (Hibiclens)	Antiseptic, antimicrobial skin cleanser Exerts an antimicrobial effect with broad-spectrum activity on organisms including *Pseudomonas aerogenes* Antiseptic rinse (Hibistat) contains 70% isopropyl alcohol and should not be used on open lesions of this type	Apply a small amount on lesion and gently scrub; rinse thoroughly	Helps deodorize wound Effective in removing drainage and/or exudate	Produces suds that may be difficult to remove Residue or film may accumulate Requires gentle friction on application
Hexachlorophene (pHisoHex 3%, Septi-Soft 0.25%, Septisol [solution] 0.25%)	Skin cleanser Bacteriostatic agent against gram-positive bacteria like staphylococci	Dilute liquid soap to solution <1% and irrigate wound gently Rinse thoroughly with water or saline Discontinue use if redness, swelling or irritation occurs	With repeated use, bacteriostatic action lingers for several days	Must rinse thoroughly Systemic absorption of hexachlorophene is problematic Must be diluted Can cause skin and tissue irritation
Antibiotic ointment/solution				
(Polysporin, Neosporin, Triple antibiotic, Garamycin)	Topical ointment or solution Broad spectrum Bactericidal action	Apply ointment to lesion and/or dressing	Broad-spectrum action for many preparations against common gram-negative and gram-positive organisms	Resistant organisms may develop with continued use Caution must be exercised with neomycin solution as systemic absorption is possible when used on open wounds Bacitracin may cause contact dermatitis Tetracycline-containing compounds may stain clothing
Nystatin (Mycostatin, Nilstat)	Ointment or cream-based preparation Exerts fungicidal and fungistatic actions on variety of yeasts and yeast-like organisms	Apply ointment/cream to area 2 to 3 times per day after cleansing and/or irrigation with debriding agents	Well tolerated even with prolonged administration	

Hydrogen peroxide (3% solution)	Oxidizing agent with bactericidal	Irrigate wound with solution and rinse with water	Removes drainage and exudate	Must dilute to ≤1.5% May cause burning Expensive for large-volume use Must rinse solution after use Continued use may cause fungal overgrowth
Silver sulfadiazine (Silvadene)	Cream with bactericidal properties against gram-negative and gram-positive organisms	Apply a small amount on lesion directly over infected or necrotic areas 1-2 times per day	Effective against microbial growth in necrotic tissue or eschar Acts on bacteria resistant to antibiotic therapy	Difficult to remove Inhibits lymphocyte migration to tissue
Topical hemostatic agents				
Absorbable gelatin sponge (Gelfoam)	Foam-like sponge material capable of absorbing and containing blood Also available in powder form	Break off appropriate size of sponge exceeding the desired area of hemostasis Leave in place; apply dry or moistened with saline	Easy to apply Effectively maintains hemostasis Stops small vessel bleeds	If left in place for an extended time may be a source of infection Not indicated for large vessel bleeds
Microfibrillar collagen hemostat (MCH) (Ativene)	Absorbable topical hemostatic agent prepared as a dry, sterile, water-insoluble salt Attracts platelets and increases adherence to fibrils	Apply directly to area, use dry	More effective for bleeds that are difficult to localize	May interfere with healing May heal over a site and conceal underlying bleeding Hemostatic capability impaired if moistened with saline or thrombin
Oxidized cellulose (Oxycel, Surgicel)	Absorbable hemostatic agent; exact mechansim of action unclear Contact with blood produces a dark tenacious adhesive cellulose Swells upon contact to enhance hemostatic control by pressure	Use sparingly over sites Caution: do not precede its use with silver nitrate or escharotic chemicals Remove with sterile water or saline once bleeding has stopped If in place for 24-48 hr forms gelatinous substance that is easy to remove	Possesses bactericidal properties Can leave in place for extended period of time	Expensive
Silver nitrate	Allows for cauterization of tissue Caustic	Apply tip of silver nitrate stick to bleeding area	Useful for small vessel bleed Provides immediate hemostasis Accurate application possible	Difficult to use over extensive area

Continued.

Table 17-4 Skin care products for ulcerating chest wall lesions—cont'd

	Properties/action	Application	Advantages	Disadvantages
Topical thrombin (Thrombinar)	Thrombin directly converts fibrinogen to fibrin with no physiologic agent for its action Speed of hemostasis depends on concentration	Wipe lesion gently until free from blood Sprinkle dry thrombin over lesion Avoid manipulation once hemostasis is maintained	Effective for large areas Can be used with absorbable gelatin sponge	Requires preparation of lesion Useful only for minor bleeding and when vessels are accessible Expensive
Wound exudate/drainage absorption dressings				
Bard absorption dressing	Hydroxylated starch that absorbs 30 times its weight in drainage	Granules must be mixed with water at ratio of 5 to 25 parts; available premixed	Absorbs drainage Controls odor Prevents necrotic tissue formation More infrequent dressing changes required Easy to remove; dissolves with water irrigation	Expensive but cost effective May not adhere to superficial lesions Weight of dressing may be painful to extremely sensitive tissues
Vigilon (maufacturer C.R. Bard)	Protective moisture hydrogel dressing	Peel off coverings on each side and apply directly to lesion	Absorbs bacteria and can be used with topical ointments Easily conforms to superficial lesions Secondary dressing not necessary Soothes and comforts exudated tissue	Absorption capacity limited May not conform to concave or convex lesions May be difficult to secure Expensive Pseudomonas infections may develop under dressing
Aluminum acetate solution (Burow's or modified Burow's solution)	Astringent wet dressing for relief of inflammatory conditions of the skin	Add 1-2 Domeboro tablets to 1 pint of water Soak lesion for 10-15 min and air dry	Relieves itching Soothing to surrounding skin Dries weepy lesions	Enzyme action of topical collagenase may inhibit aluminum acetate solution Irrigate
Calcium alginate (Kaltostate, Sorbean)	Rapidly and effectively removes exudate while maintaining a moist physiologic environment	Forms a soft alginate hydrogel on contact with wound absorbing 20 times its weight in drainage	Nonadherent, easy to remove, rinses with saline Prevents drying Provides barrier to infection Reduces frequency of dressing changes May remain in place for extended periods >24 hr	Expensive yet cost effective Secondary dressing necessary

Agents for debridement				
Collagenase (Biozyme-C, Santyl)	Enzyme is contained in white petroleum that digests collagen in the appropriate pH range	Apply directly to necrotic areas	Collagen in healthy tissue is unaffected making continued use possible if granulation of new tissue is present Compatible with most topical antibiotic preparations Can be used very effectively with Dakin's solution Infrequent application (once a day is possible)	Enzymatic activity is altered by topical use of tincture of iodine, hexachlorophene nitrofurazone, and heavy metal ions such as silver nitrate Cannot be used with Burow's solution Difficult to remove excess ointment
Dakin's solution				
Sodium hypochlorite; 0.25% (½ strength, 1 part to 20 parts H_2O); 0.125% (¼ strength, 1 part to 40 parts H_2O)	Extends a weak germicidal action on bacteria and on some fungi, while removing necrotic tissue and exudate	Use generously either by soaking lesion for 10-15 min or irrigating lesion Apply 2-3 times a day	Inexpensive Easily prepared from household bleach Effective debriding agent Requires no rinsing after use Controls odor	Dissolves clots and therefore may precipitate bleeding Without the addition of a sodium bicarbonate buffer, stability of solution is lost after 24 hr May cause burning and irritation of tissues
Fibrinolysin and desoxyribonuclease (Elase)	Available as dry powder for reconstitution or ointment that digests fibrinous material such as exudate	Can be used as an irrigant applied as a wet-to-dry dressing Ointment should be applied 3-4 times per day	Removes purulent exudate	Expensive
Sutilains	Ointment-based biochemical debriding agent exerting proteolytic action on necrotic soft tissue	Use sparingly over necrotic wound areas 3-4 times per day	Effectively removes necrotic tissue with continued use	Thorough cleansing/rinsing of wound is necessary before application to remove any topical agents that may denature the enzyme activity such as hexachlorophene, iodine, and nitrofurazone Mild pain and dermatitis may be experienced Expensive Ointment must be refrigerated at 2°-8° C

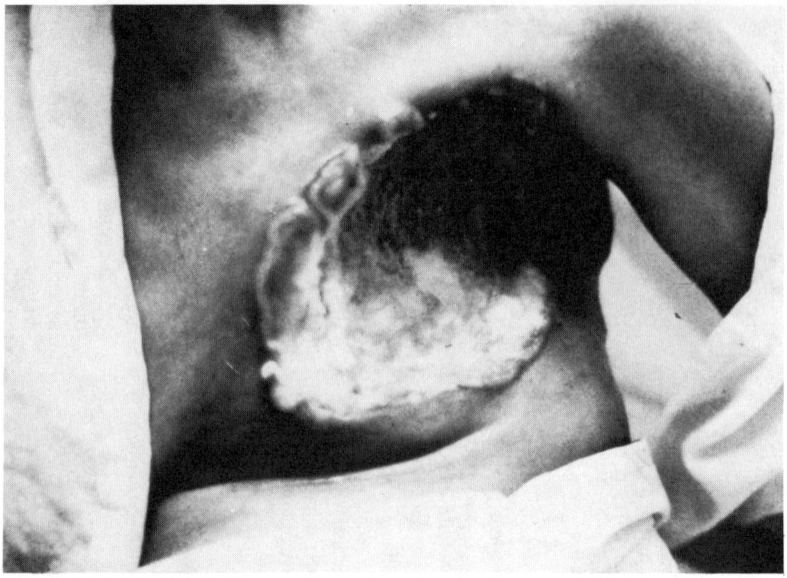

Fig. 17-4 A 68-year-old female with locally aggressive breast carcinoma resulting in an extensive chest wall lesion.

sion in a woman receiving radiation therapy, managed with daily Dakin's irrigation, the application of a Bard absorption dressing to absorb drainage, and the application of a moisture vapor–permeable dressing. In addition, measures to maintain skin integrity around the perimeter of the lesion must be implemented as wound exudate and topical agents may irritate intact skin areas. Table 17-4 provides a summary of topical agents useful for local care, along with their advantages and disadvantages.

Because of tissue destruction and necrosis, increased drainage and exudate, and impaired circulation as a result of the tumor, local measures to keep the lesion clean, debrided, and free of topical infection are important. Topical infections are almost inevitable with these lesions, as prolonged exposure of tissues—especially if tissue necrosis is evident—poses several risks for the growth of microorganisms. Aggressive local care is imperative for immunologically impaired patients, as life-threatening systemic infections may originate in these lesions.

Ulcerating breast cancer lesions are highly vascular and susceptible to bleeding even with the most careful manipulation. Therefore care must be taken to prevent unnecessary trauma and irritation. The following actions are important considerations in devising a local care regimen:

1. Avoid rubbing or actually manipulating tissues.
2. Do not allow the lesion to become dry and crusty.
3. Use a nonadherent dressing directly over the lesion. If the dressing is dry, moisten it before removal.
4. Instruct the patient to protect the chest wall by avoiding unnecessary pressure from seat belts, tight protective coverings or undergarments, and lying on the chest area.

Whatever the local care regimen, provisions for debridement are necessary to prevent infection and bleeding, control odor, and reduce drainage. Both mechanical and chemical debridement techniques can be successful. Gentle mechanical debridement with vigorous syringe irrigations or showering is preferred to surgical or wet-to-dry procedures, because the latter technique can cause uncontrollable bleeding. Chemical debridement with Dakin's solution or proteolytic enzymes is safer and, on a continued basis, provides a more reliable means of removing necrotic tissue. Fig. 17-4 illustrates extensive tissue erosion from highly locally invasive breast carcinoma that was effectively debrided with Dakin's solution.

Skin breakdown around the perimeter of the lesion is problematic, necessitating measures to protect intact skin from the caustic effects of some topical agents, wound exudate, and the tape used to secure dressings. Skin barriers used by ostomy patients to prevent irritation from excrement are helpful. The application of skin protectors such as salves and creams provides a barrier to resist further insult to normal skin. Sprays are available that provide a moisture-resistant barrier. However, caution must be exercised to avoid application of these products directly to the lesion.

REFERENCES

1. Alistars J: Fatigue in the cancer patient: a conceptual approach to a clinical problem, Oncol Nurs Forum 14(16):25, 1987.
2. Anderson KE and Lindskov R: The recall of UVB-induced erythema in breast cancer patient receiving multiple drug therapy, Photodermatol 1(3):129, 1984.
3. Arner S and Meyerson BA: Lack of analgesic effect of opioids on neuropathic and idiopathic forms of pain, Pain 33:11, 1988.
4. Barkas G and Duafala ME: Advances in cancer pain management: a review of patient-controlled analgesics, J Pain Symptom Management 3(3):150, 1988.
5. Belcher AE: Nursing aspects of quality of life enhancement in cancer patients, Oncology 4(5):197, 1990.
6. Bressler B, Cohen SI, and Magnussen F: The problem of phantom breast and phantom pain, J Nerv Ment Dis 123(2):181,1956.
7. Breza TS, Halprin KM, and Taylor JR: Photosensitivity reaction to vinblastine, Arch Dermatol 111(9):1168, 1975.
8. Britton D: Fatigue. In Yasko JM, editor: Guidelines for cancer care, Reston, Va, 1983, Reston Publishing Co, pp 33-37.
9. Brooks I, DeJager R, Blumenreich M, et al: Principles of cancer pain management: use of long acting oral morphine, Journal Fam Pract 28(3):275, 1989.
10. Cassileth B, Zupksin R, Sutton-Smith K, and March V: Information and participation preferences among cancer patients, Ann Intern Med 92:832, 1980.
11. Cella DF and Tulsky DS: Measuring quality of life today: methodologic aspects, Oncology 4(5):29, 1990.
12. Cotanch PH and Strum S: Progressive muscle relaxation as antiemetic therapy for cancer patients, Oncol Nurs Forum 14(1):33, 1987.
13. Crone-Munzerbrock A: Phantomgefuhl and Phantomschmerz nach Mammaamputation, Langenbecks Arch U Dtsch Z Chir 266:569, 1950.
14. Degner L and Russell C: Preferences for treatment control among adults with cancer, Res Nurs Health 11:367, 1988.
15. Desai MH and Teres D: Prevention of doxorubicin-induced skin ulcers in the rat and pig with dimethyl sulfoxide (DMSO), Cancer Treat Rep 66:1371, 1982.
16. DeVries CR and Freiha FS: Hemorrhagic cystitis: a review, J Urol 143(1):1, 1990.
17. Ehlke G: Symptoms distress in breast cancer patients receiving chemotherapy in the outpatient setting, Oncol Nurs Forum 15:343, 1988.
18. Ferrell B, Wisdom C, and Wenzl C: Quality of life as an outcome variable in the management of cancer pain, Cancer 63(11):2321, 1989.
19. Fisher B, Redmond C, Poisson R, et al: Eight year results of a randomized trial comparing total mastectomy and lumpectomy with or without radiation in the treatment of breast cancer, N Engl J Med 320:822, 1989.
20. Foltz AT: Weight gain among stage II breast cancer patients: a study of five factors, Oncol Nurs Forum 12(3):21, 1985.
21. Forni AM, Koss LG, and Geller W: Cytological study of the effects of cyclophosphamide of the epithelium of the urinary bladder in man, Cancer 17:1348, 1964.
22. Giaccone G, DiGiulio FD, Morandini MP, and Calciata A: Scalp hypothermia in the prevention of doxorubicin-induced hair loss, Oncol Nurs Forum 11(3):170, 1988.
23. Glass A, Wieand S, Fisher B, et al: Acute toxicity during adjuvant chemotherapy for breast cancer: the National Surgical Adjuvant Breast and Bowel Project experience from 1717 patients receiving single and multiple agents, Cancer Treat Rep 65:363, 1981.
24. Granek I, Ashikari R, and Foley KM: The post-mastectomy pain syndrome, Proc Am Soc Clin Oncol 3:122, 1983.
25. Grindel CG, Cahill CA, and Walker M: Food intake of women with breast cancer during their first six months of chemotherapy, Oncol Nurs Forum 16(3):401, 1989.
26. Hassey KM and Rose CM: Altered skin integrity in patients receiving radiation therapy, Oncol Nurs Forum 9(4):44, 1982.
27. Hood AF: Cutaneous side effects of cancer therapy, Med Clin North Am 70(1):187, 1986.
28. Hughes W, Bodey G, Feld R, et al: Guidelines for use of antimicrobial agents in neutropenic patients with unexplained fever, J Infect Dis 161:381, 1990.
29. Hunnington MO: Weight gain in patients receiving adjuvant chemotherapy for carcinoma of the breast, Cancer 56(3):472, 1985.
30. Hymovich DP and Hagopian GA: The teaching role of the office nurse, Office Nurse 2(5):30, 1989.
31. Ingle RJ, Burish TG, and Wallston KA: Conditionability of cancer chemotherapy patients, Oncol Nurs Forum 11(4):97, 1984.
32. Jakubowski A, Souza L, Kelly F, et al: Effects of Leman granulocyte colony stimulating factor in a patient with idiopathic neutropenia, N Engl J Med 320:38, 1989.
33. Joss RA, Kiser J, Weston S, and Brunner KW: Fighting alopecia in cancer chemotherapy. Supportive care in cancer patients, Recent Results Cancer Res 108:117, 1988.
34. Inturrisi CE: Management of cancer pain: pharmacology and principles of management, Cancer 63(11):2308, 1989.
35. Kanner R: Postsurgical pain syndrome, management of cancer pain. Syllabus of the Post Graduate Course, Memorial Sloan-Kettering Cancer Center, New York, 1985, p 65.
36. Kellum MD: Fatigue. In Jacobs MM, editor: Signs and symptoms in nursing: interpretation and management, Philadelphia, 1980, JB Lippincott, pp 103-118.
37. Knobf MK, Mullen JC, Xistris D, et al: Weight gain in women with breast cancer receiving adjuvant chemotherapy, Oncol Nurs Forum 10(2):28, 1983.
38. Kroner K, Krebs B, Kov J, and Jorgensen HS: Immediate and long term phantom breast syndrome after mastectomy: incidence, clinical characteristics and relationship to premastectomy pain, Pain 36(3):327, 1989.
39. Larson DL: What is appropriate management of tissue extravasation by antitumor agents? Plast Reconstr Surg 75:397, 1985.
40. Laszlo J: Emesis as limiting toxicity in cancer chemotherapy. In Laszlo J, editor: Antiemetics and cancer chemotherapy, Baltimore, 1983, Williams & Wilkins, pp 1-5.
41. Lewis FM: Experienced personal control and quality of life in late stage cancer patients, Nurs Res 31(2):113, 1982.
42. Lindley CM, Bernard S, and Fields SM: Incidence and duration of chemotherapy-induced nausea and vomiting in the outpatient oncology population, J Clin Oncol 7(8):1142, 1989.
43. Martin-Jimenez M, Diaz-Rubio E, and Gonzalez Larriba JE: Failure of high dose tocopherol to prevent alopecia induced by doxorubicin, N Engl J Med 315:894, 1986
44. Morrow GR: Clinical characteristics associated with the development of anticipatory nausea and vomiting in cancer patients undergoing chemotherapy treatments, J Clin Oncol 2(10):1170, 1984.
45. Nail L, Jones LS, Giuffre M, and Johnson JE: Sensations after mastectomy, Am J Nurs 84(9):1121, 1984.

46. Nerenz DR, Leventhal H, Easterling DV, et al: Anxiety and drug taste as predictors of anticipatory nausea and vomiting in cancer chemotherapy, J Clin Oncol 4(2):224, 1986.
47. Nerenz DR, Love RR, Leventhal H, et al: Psychosocial consequences of cancer chemotherapy for elderly patients, Health Serv Res 20:961, 1986.
48. Norris MC: Tiredness and fatigue. In Norris CM, editor: Concept clarification in nursing, Rockville, Md, 1982, Aspen Systems Corp, pp 263-275.
49. O'Conner A, Boyd N, Tritchler D, et al: Eliciting preferences for alternative cancer drug treatment: the influence of framing, medium and rater variables, Med Decis Making 5(4):453, 1985.
50. Oncology Nursing Society Clinical Practice Committee: Cancer chemotherapy guidelines: module V recommendations for the management of extravasation and anaphylaxis, Pittsburgh, 1988, Oncology Nursing Society, p 7.
51. Padilla GV and Grant M: Quality of life as a cancer nursing outcome variable, Adv Nurs Sci 8(1):45, 1985.
52. Paice JA: The phenomenon of analgesic tolerance in cancer pain management, Oncol Nurs Forum 15(4):455, 1988.
53. Pater J and William A: Methodologic issues in trials of antiemetics, J Clin Oncol 2:484, 1984.
54. Penta J, Poster D, and Bruno S: The pharmacologic treatment of nausea and vomiting caused by cancer chemotherapy: a review. In Laszlo J, editor: Antiemetics and cancer chemotherapy, Baltimore, 1983, Williams & Wilkins, pp 53-92.
55. Philips FS, Sternberg SC, Cronin AP, and Vidal PM: Cyclophosphamide and urinary bladder toxicity, Cancer Res 21:1577, 1961.
56. Piper B, Lindsey A, and Dodd M: Fatigue mechanisms in cancer patients: developing nursing theory, Oncol Nurs Forum, 14(16):17, 1987.
57. Portenoy RK: Cancer pain: epidemiology and syndromes, Cancer 63(11):2298, 1989.
58. Porter J and Jick H: Addiction rare in patients treated with narcotics, N Engl J Med 302:123, 1980.
59. Press OW, Ramsey PG, Larson EB, et al: Hickman catheter infections in patients with malignancies, Medicine 63:189, 1984.
60. Redd W, Anderson G, and Minagawa R: Hypnotic control of anticipatory emesis in patients receiving chemotherapy, J Consult Clin Psychol 50(3):14, 1982.
61. Reed WP, Newman KA, DeJong C, et al: Prolonged venous access for chemotherapy by means of the Hickman catheter, Cancer 52:185, 1983.
62. Rhodes VA, Watson PM, Johnson MH, et al: Patterns of nausea, vomiting and distress in patients receiving antineoplastic drug protocols, Oncol Nurs Forum 14(4):35, 1987.
63. Rolston K: Management of febrile episodes during neutropenia caused by chemotherapy, Am J Clin Oncol 13(2):171, 1990.
64. Shell JA, Stanutz F, and Grimm J: Comparison of moisture vapor permeable (MVP) dressings to conventional dressings for management of radiation skin reactions, Oncol Nurs Forum 13(1):11, 1986.
65. Simmel ML: A study of phantoms after computation of the breast, Neuropsychologia 4:331, 1966.
66. Skeel RT: Quality of life assessment in cancer clinical trials—it's time to catch up, J Nat Cancer Inst 81(14):472, 1989.
67. Staps T, Hoogenhaut J, and Wobbs T: Phantom breast sensations following mastectomy, Cancer 56:2898, 1985.
68. Therault RL: Hypercalcemia of malignancy, Am J Clin Oncol 12(4):361, 1989.
69. Watson CPN and Evans RJ: Intractable pain with breast cancer, Can Med Assoc J 126:263, 1982.
70. Watson CPN, Evans RJ, and Watt VR: The post-mastectomy pain syndrome and the effect of topical capsaicin, Pain 38:177, 1989.
71. Weinstein S, Vetter RJ, and Sersen EA: Phantoms following breast amputation, Neuropsychologia 8:185, 1956.
72. Welch-McCaffrey D: Cancer, anxiety, and quality of life, Cancer Nurs 9(3):151, 1985.
73. Winningham ML and MacVicar MG: The effects of aerobic exercise on patient reports of nausea, Oncol Nurs Forum 15(4):447, 1988.
74. Young K and Longman A: Quality of life and persons with melanoma: A pilot study, Cancer Nurs 6(3):219, 1983.

18 Bone Marrow Transplantation for Breast Cancer

Edward A. Stadtmauer

Approximately 50% of women with resectable breast cancer will be cured when treated with surgery, hormonal therapy, radiation, or chemotherapy, used alone or in combination.[4,43] Additionally, the majority of patients with metastatic or recurrent disease achieve objective responses with systemic treatments.[43] Despite these encouraging results, many poor-prognosis patients with primary disease are destined to relapse. The median survival after first documentation of advanced disease remains approximately 2 years.[13] Less than 3% of patients who developed systemic breast cancer remain in long-term remission, including those with objective complete responses.[47]

Breast cancer in experimental and clinical systems, like most therapy-response malignancies, shows a steep relationship between therapy dose and tumor response.[32] Prolonged myelosuppression limits dose escalation for most alkylating agents and radiation. Infusion of hematopoietic stem cells successfully overcomes this toxicity and allows for significant increases in the maximally tolerated doses of therapeutic agents. This combination of high-dose therapy with donor bone marrow rescue is termed "allogeneic bone marrow transplantation" (AlloBMT). AlloBMT is now the treatment of choice for a variety of hematologic diseases, including chronic myelogenous leukemia,[42,116] acute myelogenous leukemia,[14] aplastic anemia,[106] and congenital immunodeficiency.[82]

Autologous bone marrow transplantation (ABMT) is the combination of high-dose therapy with the patient's own bone marrow. ABMT first was performed successfully in the late 1970s. Since then, significant response rates have been reported in such hematologic malignancies as non-Hodgkin's lymphoma, Hodgkin's disease, and acute leukemia.[12] More recently, solid tumors, including neuroblastoma, testicular cancer, small-cell lung cancer, and breast cancer have been treated with increased frequency. Approximately 5000 autotransplants were performed in 1990.

This chapter reviews the general principles of bone marrow transplantation and the experience and the future role of this high-dose therapy in the treatment of breast cancer.

PRINCIPLES OF BONE MARROW TRANSPLANTATION

The general principles of high-dose therapy are listed below.

Steep dose-response relationship

The alkylating agents and radiation commonly are employed in high-dose treatment regimens. They have a broad spectrum of antitumor activity and myelosuppression is the initial dose-limiting toxicity. The alkylating agents and radiation demonstrate clear dose-response relationships in both in vivo and in vitro systems.[33,36,57] The relationship between tumor cell kill and dose is log-linear over a certain dose range followed by a flattening of the curve. A small change in dose can thereby produce a significantly increased response.

Early work by Kaplan in Hodgkin's disease showed the log-linear relationship of radiation dose to freedom from local relapse.[57] Similar in vitro work with alkylating agents in murine and human tumor systems (including the MCF-7 breast

GENERAL PRINCIPLES OF HIGH DOSE THERAPY

Combination of active single agents

Steep dose-response relationship for each agent
Activity in conventional doses for each agent
Myelosuppression is primary initial toxicity
Nonmyelosuppressive secondary toxicities of each agent do not overlap

Proper patient selection

Early disease
Minimal disease
Responding disease
Poor prognosis disease with conventional-dose therapy

cancer cell line) generally shows log-linear dose-response curves. For nonalkylating agents, the plot is curvilinear with substantial loss of activity after the first log of cell kill.[32,34,35,36]

Hryniuk and Bush[48] and Hryniuk and Levine[49] have conducted retrospective analyses of dose intensity (dose of drug/m^2 body surface area/unit time) for chemotherapy in both metastatic and resectable breast cancer. These studies suggest a relationship of dose to response in patients with breast cancer. The inferential nature of this literature has been criticized by Gelman and Henderson[37] and Henderson et al.[44] Two randomized controlled trials have evaluated prospectively the dose-response relationship. These trials included patients with chemotherapy-untreated metastatic disease. Tannock et al. compared standard-dose cyclophosphamide, methotrexate, and 5-fluorouracil (CMF) to half-dose CMF and showed a higher response rate and a survival advantage for the more dose-intensive arm ($p = .03$).[112] In another study, patients were assigned randomly to treatment with 5-fluorouracil, doxorubicin, and cyclophosphamide (FAC) at standard doses or high doses following a dose escalation schedule. The two groups showed no difference in overall response, duration of response, or survival rates.[46] A Cancer and Leukemia Group B (CALGB) adjuvant trial designed to further explore the effect of dose intensity is currently underway.

The most commonly used agents in high-dose regimens are listed in Table 18-1. Virtually all of these agents provide activity against breast cancer at conventional doses. The initial dose-limiting toxicity of these agents is myelosuppression, with the exception of cis-platinum. As can be seen in Table 18-1, significant dose escalation becomes possible when these agents are combined with bone marrow support. The agents have different nonmyelosuppressive toxicities that allow for their combination in many regimens.

Combination therapy

Nonsurgical curative therapy has depended primarily on the use of combinations of antineoplastic agents.[31,76] Combinations are chosen to include agents with different mechanisms of action and different mechanisms of resistance. Malignancies in which combination chemotherapy is a curative therapeutic modality include Hodgkin's disease, diffuse large-cell lymphoma, testicular cancer, and acute myeloid leukemia. The first positive study of bone marrow transplantation was reported by Thomas et al.[115] Investigators used a high-dose combination of cyclophosphamide and total body irradiation to treat patients with acute leukemia that was refractory to available therapy. Ten percent of these patients remain in long-term disease-free remission.

The favorable dose-response relationship for alkylating agents has led to the combination of two or more of these drugs in high-dose regimens. Experimental work has now shown little cross resistance among alkylating agents in high-dose regimens. In fact, a synergistic relationship frequently can be demonstrated.[93,94,113] Various combinations of high-dose alkylating agents and total body irradiation have now cured patients with acute and chronic leukemia and Hodgkin's and non-Hodgkin's lymphoma.[105]

Patient selection

Bone marrow transplantation remains a very toxic treatment modality, with significant potential morbidity, mortality, and financial cost. Small phase I and phase II studies to establish dose, toxicity, and initial response data have been essential in the development of bone marrow transplantation as a treatment option. The stage is now set for well-designed randomized phase III trials to compare this modality to more conventional treatment. All bone marrow transplantation should be considered investigational until these studies have been com-

Table 18-1 Characteristics of agents used in high-dose therapy

Agent	Conventional dose (mg/m^2)	Maximum dose without ABMT (mg/m^2)	Maximum dose with ABMT (mg/m^2)	Dose escalation	Limiting toxicity
Cyclophosphamide	1000	8000	8000	8	Cardiac
Melphalan	40	140	225	6	Mucositis
Thiotepa	40	180	1135	28	Mucositis
Cis-platinum	100	200	200	2	Renal
Carmustine	200	600	1200	6	Hepatic
Busulfan	1.5 mg/kg	6 mg/kg	16 mg/kg	10	Hepatic
Ifosfamide	8000	18000	18000	2.25	Renal
Carboplatinum	400	1600	2000	5	Hepatic
Etoposide	300	2700	3000	10	Mucositis
Radiation	150 cGy	300 cGy	1500 cGy	10	Lung

Table 18-2 Three-year disease-free survival in intermediate non-Hodgkin's lymphoma and acute myeloid leukemia treatment with autologous bone marrow transplantation

Disease status	Disease-free survival (%)
Non-Hodgkin's lymphoma	
Refractory relapse	<5
Sensitive relapse	20-25
Second/Later remission	35-45
First remission	>65
Acute myeloid leukemia	
Refractory relapse	<1
Second/Later remission	20-30
First remission	45-50

pleted. Patients selected for bone marrow transplantation should have disease that carries with it a poor prognosis when treated with conventional therapy. High-dose treatment should result in long-term disease-free survival or cure in a significant fraction of patients chosen for treatment. Given the potential morbidity and expense of this procedure, short-term palliation is an inappropriate therapeutic goal.

Extensive experience with hematologic malignancies has generated other general principles of patient selection. Approximate results of autologous bone marrow transplantation for acute myeloid leukemia and non-Hodgkin's lymphoma are shown in Table 18-2. These data suggest that once a patient is deemed to have a poor prognosis with conventional therapy, high-dose therapy is most effective early in the natural history of the disease, at the time of minimal disease, and while disease still responds to conventional-dose therapy. This has led to the common conventional dose cytoreduction treatment to identify responding disease before high-dose therapy.

PROCEDURE FOR BONE MARROW TRANSPLANTATION

Fig. 18-1 diagrams the procedure for bone marrow transplantation. Patients and physicians must see bone marrow transplantation as a process, rather than as a single procedure, as it can take up to a year or more from initiation to completion.

Cytoreduction

As previously discussed, cytoreduction is the use of conventional-dose therapy in patients with a poor prognosis. The goal is to demonstrate sensitivity to conventional-dose therapy and to render the patient in remission (minimal disease) before high-dose cytoablative therapy. Examples include induction therapy for acute leukemia, salvage chemotherapy for relapsed Hodgkin's disease, and combination chemotherapy for patients with metastatic breast cancer. Patients unresponsive to cytoreduction have a dismal prognosis with bone marrow transplantation treatment and should be excluded.

Stem cell harvest and storage

At some point during or after cytoreduction and before high-dose therapy, stem cells must be harvested. These may be derived from an allogeneic or syngeneic donor, or the patient's own autologous stem cells.

Allogeneic transplantation uses stem cells derived most commonly from a human leukocyte antigen (HLA) identical sibling, although more recently HLA-mismatched transplants and HLA-identical unrelated donors have been used. AlloBMT has provided long-term disease-free survival in a select group of young patients with acute myeloid leukemia, acute lymphoid leukemia, chronic myelogenous leukemia, and aplastic anemia, and other nonmalignant bone marrow disorders. Donor marrow contains lymphocytes potentially immunologically active against the recipient tissues. AlloBMT is therefore complicated by acute and chronic graft vs. host disease (GVHD). Acute GVHD occurs within 3 months of bone marrow infusion, is modulated by donor cytotoxic T cells, and primarily affects the skin, mucous membranes, gastrointestinal tract, and liver. It also acts as a risk factor for infection and other unique bone marrow transplantation toxicities such as interstitial pneumonitis. This disease is a major contributor to death in up to 50% of patients in whom it develops.[27] The incidence and severity of GVHD are age related, limiting AlloBMT bone marrow transplantation mainly to patients <45 years old.

Twenty to thirty percent of patients who survive beyond 3 months develop chronic GVHD.[27] This syndrone is similar to an autoimmune disease and can involve virtually any organ. Chronic GVHD disease carries substantial morbidity, but it is responsive to steroids and is less commonly a direct cause of death.

Other problems with AlloBMT include graft rejection and limited donor availability. Graft rejection occurs in up to 14% of patients and is related to the number of stem cells infused.[31] Attempts to modulate GVHD with T cell depletion have been limited by increased graft rejection.

Each sibling has only a 1 in 4 chance of HLA identity to recipient. Statistical analysis has shown that only 10% of patients with acute leukemia have suitable donors and ultimately go on to receive

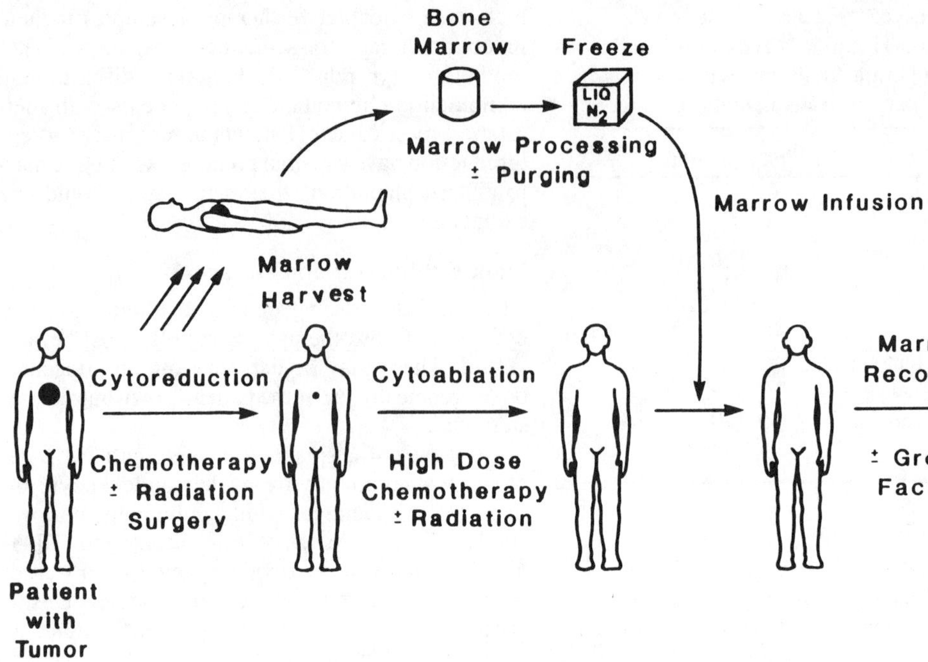

Fig. 18-1 Schema for autologous bone marrow transplantation.

AlloBMT.[28] The National Bone Marrow Transplant Registry in time will allow for more HLA-matched unrelated donors. Initial studies, however, show significantly increased toxicity with this procedure when compared to the use of related sibling donors. One potential benefit of allogeneic bone marrow transplantation is an immunologic graft vs. tumor effect. This has been demonstrated for leukemia and possibly lymphoma. No data exists for a graft vs. breast cancer effect. Attempts to induce GVHD in autologous bone marrow transplantation patients are under early investigation.

Autologous stem cells have been the preferred source for patients treated with high-dose chemotherapy. Comparison of allogeneic and autologous transplantation is shown at left. Autologous transplantation is uncomplicated by GVHD or the need to obtain a donor. Additionally, autologous cells have been transplanted successfully in patients age 60 years or older. Autologous transplantation is complicated, however, by possible contamination with viable clonogenic tumor cells. There is also no possible beneficial graft vs. tumor effect.

Autologous stem cells may be obtained by either bone marrow harvest or peripheral stem cell harvest. Marrow harvest usually is performed under general anesthesia with patients in the prone position. Between 400 and 2000 ml of bone marrow is obtained by multiple aspirations from bilateral illiac crests. Usually, 10^8 to 10^9 nucleated cells per kg body weight are harvested. Marrow is placed into a heparinized tissue culture medium and filtered through wire mesh to mix and remove bone and tissue fragments. Stem cells are separated in a Ficoll-Hypaque gradient and then properly diluted with autologous plasma.

Preservation of marrow is required while patients undergo further therapy. This involves controlled-rate freezing with liquid nitrogen to − 196° C in the presence of the cryoprotectant dimethylsulfoxide (DMSO). DMSO prevents ice crystal formation inside cells during freezing. Bone marrow is stored in 50 to 100 ml aliquots in the liquid or vapor phase of liquid nitrogen.

AUTOLOGOUS BONE MARROW TRANSPLANTATION COMPARED TO ALLOGENEIC BONE MARROW TRANSPLANTATION

Advantages of ABMT

Applicable to older patients
No limitation due to donor availability
No graft rejection
No graft vs. host disease

Disadvantages of ABMT

Possible contamination with clonogenic tumor cells
Potential loss of graft vs. tumor effect
Delayed engraftment from purging technique

Experimental animal and human studies reveal the presence of autologous stem cells in peripheral blood that were capable of restoring normal hematopoiesis.[7,71,75] Recently, peripheral stem cells have been a successful source of autologous hematopoietic rescue in patients treated with cytoablative chemotherapy.[6,37,60] Additionally, combinations of peripheral and marrow stem cells have been used.[39] Peripheral stem cells are obtained in multiple 4-hour leukophereses and may be enriched by chemotherapy or growth factor augmentation. This material is then processed in a fashion similar to bone marrow.

Stem cell purging

Many diseases treated with high-dose therapy and autologous stem cell rescue have the potential for bone marrow contamination with tumor cells. Leukemia, lymphoma, and breast cancer, even when in clinical remission by microscopic examination of bone marrow, are likely to have residual clonogenic tumor cell involvement. Various immunologic, physical, and chemical attempts to purge bone marrow of these tumor cells have been made and are listed below. The use of 4-hydroperoxycyclophosphamide (4-HC) as a purging agent has been widespread. This derivative of cyclophosphamide is a stable crystal that readily metabolizes to the active phosphoramide mustard once exposed to bone marrow, without need for hepatic metabolism. Doses of 60 to 100 μg/ml have been shown to remove detectable clonogenic tumor cells and still allow for consistent stem cell engraftment in experimental and human studies.[91,98]

The role of bone marrow purging remains speculative. To date, no study has demonstrated a significant benefit to purging. Statistical analysis has shown that a clinical study to prove benefit is prohibitively large and may never be conducted. On the other hand, unpurged, grossly involved bone marrow has been used successfully to treat patients with refractory leukemia and lymphoma, producing a number of long-term disease-free survivors. Purging techniques have been shown to prolong time to engraftment and length of hospitalization significantly when compared to treatment without purging.

Positive stem cell selection is far more conceptually appealing. Surface antigen markers of hematopoietic stem cells recently have been identified. Techniques such as long-term cell culture may enrich for stem cells or monoclonal antibody–laden columns may allow for specific separation of stem cells from the rest of the harvested material. These techniques are under active investigation.

BONE MARROW PURGING TECHNIQUES

Chemical

Cyclophosphamide derivatives (4-HC)
Etoposide
Glucosteroids
Cytosine arabinoside derivatives
Platinols

Immunologic

Polyclonal or monoclonal antibodies
- Complement-mediated lysis
- Toxin or drug-linked lysis
- Magnetic bead linked lysis

Adoptive immunotherapy (i.e., LAK cells)
Interferon

Physical

Agglutination
Centrifugation
Counterflow elutriation
Photoradiation
Radioisotopes

Cytoablation

The general principles of the high-dose cytoablative regimen have been discussed earlier. The regimen consists of a combination of alkylating agents with each individual agent possessing a steep dose-response relationship in the particular tumor at both conventional and high doses. Myelosuppression should be the primary initial toxicity of each agent and the nonmyelosuppressive secondary toxicities of each agent should not overlap. Such successful regimens include busulfan and cyclophosphamide for myeloid leukemias and total body irradiation and cyclophosphamide for lymphoid malignancies.

Stem cell reinfusion

Stem cells are reinfused once cytoablative therapy is completed and the requisite time for active metabolites to be excreted has passed. Individual bags are removed from the freezer and placed in a 40° C waterbath, usually at the patient's bedside. DMSO is toxic to stem cells at room temperature, so thawed marrow is infused rapidly via central venous catheters into the recipient. Patients usually are pretreated with diphenylhydramine, steroids, mannitol, bicarbonate, and intravenous hydration to lessen the potential histamine release from DMSO or renal toxicity from infusion of lysed erythrocytes. Infusion frequently is complicated by transient chest tightness, flushing, and bradycardia. Autopsy studies have shown that stem cells initially lodge in the lungs and then circulate to the bone marrow where engraftment and replication proceeds.

Supportive care

The entire process of stem cell harvest, cytoablative therapy, and bone marrow infusion is usually completed in <10 days. The ensuing long hospitalization is necessitated by profound marrow aplasia with resultant infections, bleeding, and complicating toxicity from the agents in the high-dose regimen. The preeminent risk factor for infection in the bone marrow transplantation patient is profound neutropenia. Other risk factors include humoral and cell-mediated immune defects, injured barriers to infections (skin, mucous membranes, and gut) and indwelling central venous catheters. Supportive care during the neutropenic period is therefore similar to that required for other aggressively treated cancer patients. Bacterial infections remain the initial life-threatening concern of neutropenic fever. Techniques of ultraisolation including laminer airflow rooms, skin sterilization, sterile diet, or gut sterilization by oral and intravenous antibiotics have demonstrated no clear survival advantage for these patients. Most patients are treated with routine hospital single-room isolation, with masks and handwashing. Broad-spectrum antibacterial coverage for the febrile neutropenic patient is essentially the same as that used for leukemic patients.

Prolonged neutropenia and broad spectrum antibiotic administration become major risk factors for the development of fungal infections. The most common isolates are *Candida* species and *Aspergillus*, but more recently the incidence of other organisms has increased. The development of fevers despite days of broad-spectrum antibacterial therapy strongly suggests occult fungal infection and necessitates the institution of systemic antifungal therapy (i.e., amphotericin). Unlike antibacterial prophylaxis, antifungal prophylaxis with high-efficiency air filters for mold spores and the use of topical or oral azole antifungal agents has decreased the incidence of systemic fungal infections.

Human herpes viruses commonly are reactivated in the course of bone marrow transplantation and can result in significant morbidity and mortality (Table 18-3). Prophylactic acyclovir has been shown to decrease the incidence of reactivation of herpes simplex virus and cytomegalovirus (CMV).[74,92,120] CMV seronegative blood products and leukocyte filtration also decrease the incidence of CMV infection. The use of prophylactic intravenous immunoglobin is less well established.

Prophylactic blood transfusions are used to prevent bleeding complications of cytopenias. A platelet count of approximately 20,000/mm^3 usually is maintained by platelet transfusion from random donors. Patients refractory to random donor platelets require single-donor, HLA-identical, or family member platelets. Packed red blood cell transfusions are used to maintain a hemoglobin of approximately 8.0 g/dl. There is no role for prophylactic granulocyte transfusion, but therapeutic granulocyte transfusion may be appropriate for the selected neutropenic patient with clear bacterial or fungal infection unresponsive to conventional therapy. All granulocyte, platelet, or packed red blood cell transfusions for transplant patients must be irradiated with 2000 to 3000 cGy to inactivate lymphocytes that may engraft and produce GVHD. The incidence of viral hepatitis and HIV infection has dropped dramatically in the transplant patient with the advent of serologic viral testing.

Table 18-3 Herpes virus latency and reactivation

Virus	Population latently infected (%)	BMT patients with reactivation (%)
HSV-1	40-90	>50
HSV-2	30-50	>50
VZV	80-90	7-35
CMV	50-70	50-90
EBV	80-90	50-80

HSV, herpes simplex virus; VZV, varicella zoster virus; CMV, cytomegalovirus; EBV, Epstein-Barr virus.
Adapted from Croen KD: The immunocompromised host 6:3, 1989.

Organ toxicity

There are many potential toxic complications from high-dose therapy (see p. 495). Two such disorders will be reviewed in further detail.

Venoocclusive disease (VOD) of the liver can occur after high-dose therapy even without bone marrow transplantation. Patients usually develop right upper quadrant pain, weight gain, jaundice, hepatomegaly, ascites, and hyperbilirubinemia 2 to 4 weeks after completion of therapy. Pathologically, patients have obstruction of small intrahepatic venules. Supportive care with close monitoring of fluid status is the standard of care. The majority of patients show complete resolution of VOD by the end of their hospital course. Twenty to thirty percent die, however, at least in part as a result of VOD. Patients with pretreatment elevated serum transaminases or recent antineoplastic treatment are more likely to develop VOD.

Interstitial pneumonitis (IP) is a major problem in AlloBMT, but it also complicates autologous

TOXICITY OF HIGH DOSE THERAPY WITH AUTOLOGOUS STEM CELL RESCUE

Skin
Desquamation
Maculopapular rash
Erythematous exanthem
Hyperpigmentation
Alopecia

Musculoskeletal
Arthralgia

Hematologic
Myelosuppression and aplasia
Autoimmune thrombocytopenia
Autoimmune hemolytic anemia

Central nervous system
Seizure
Polyneuropathy
Paralysis of cranial nerves
Encephalopathy
Encephalomyelitis
Meningitis
Cerebral hemorrhage
Mental and behavioral changes

Gastrointestinal system
Nausea and vomiting
Diarrhea
Anorexia
Loss of weight
Mucositis
Stomatitis
Ascites
GI hemorrhage
Esophagitis
Mallory-Weiss syndrome
Gastric and duodenal ulcer
Ileus
Cholecystitis
Hepatitis
Hepatic failure

Respiratory system
Pulmonary edema/capillary leak syndrome
Pulmonary hemorrhage
Pulmonary fibrosis
Interstitial pneumonitis (idiopathic)

Genitourinary system
Renal insufficiency
Hemorrhagic cystitis
Vaginal bleeding
Urinary tract infection
Renal failure

Cardiovascular system
Cardiac arrhythmia
Hypotension
Cardiomyopathy
Carditis
Congestive heart failure
Venous thrombosis
Cardiac arrest

Adapted from Cheson BD et al: Ann Intern Med 110:51, 1989.

bone marrow transplantation. Infection (usually CMV but also Pneumocystis or fungal organisms) is implicated in about 50% of patients. The syndrome is felt to be related to the high-dose therapy in the other patients. Total body irradiation, busulfan, or carmustine (BCNU) has been implicated most frequently. Most recently, diffuse alveolar hemorrhage has been noted in autologous bone marrow recipients. Clinically, IP occurs within 6 months of therapy and is characterized by a nonproductive cough, fever, interstitial infiltrates, hypoxia, and a markedly decreased diffusing capacity. Open lung biopsy shows only a nonspecific infiltrate or fibrosis. IP frequently progresses; it is fatal in the vast majority of patients despite mechanical ventilatory support. Recently, the use of ganciclovir and intravenous gamma globulin have significantly decreased mortality from CMV pneumonitis.[25,87] Alveolar hemorrhage may respond to high-dose corticosteroid therapy. Patients with low diffusing capacity at the time of transplantation or with significant previous pulmonary irradiation or potentially pulmonary toxic drug exposure are at greatest risk.

HIGH-DOSE THERAPY IN RELAPSED AND REFRACTORY ADVANCED BREAST CANCER PATIENTS

Single-agent pilot studies

The development of high-dose therapy for breast cancer has paralleled the development of autologous bone marrow transplantation for other diseases. Initial studies involved women with refractory, end-stage, and metastatic disease. These phase I studies determined toxicity and maximum dose for a number of individual agents. Results of 17 studies with alkylating and nonalkylating agents are summarized in Table 18-4.

The number of patients treated with any particular agent was limited. Highest response rates were seen with the alkylating agents melphalan, thiotepa, cyclophosphamide, and carboplatinum.

Table 18-4 Single-agent high-dose studies in relapsed and refractory breast cancer patients

	No. pts.	Complete response	Partial response	Overall response (%)	Dose (mg/m²)	Reference
Nonalkylators						
Etoposide	21	0	2	10	900-2700	30, 78, 123
Amsacrine	16	0	2	13	600-750	111
Hydroxyurea	8	0	3	3	40,000	5
Alkylators						
Melphalan	20	5	11	80	120-225	16, 45, 61, 62, 65, 69, 70
Mitomycin-C	17	0	1	5	30-60	95, 96, 110
Thiotepa	20	1	9	50	180-1575	11, 26, 64, 66
Cyclophosphamide	8	0	4	50	5-7.8*	15, 99
Dibromodulcitol	7	0	1	14	1500-4800	1
Carboplatin	2	0	1	50	500-2400	97
Total	119	6	34	33		

*Unit of measure is g/m².

Overall response rates of 33% (5% complete remission) were reported. Very few long-term disease-free survivors were documented.

Combination-agent pilot studies

The next generation of studies combined active agents. Early studies combined high-dose chemotherapy with total body irradiation in light of success with this regimen in hematologic malignancies. Studies with total body irradiation have included only 19 patients. Responses were frequent (63%) with median duration of response <10 months with no long-term disease-free survivors.[17,79,104]

Regimens containing two or more alkylating agents are used more commonly to treat metastatic breast cancer. The conceptual basis for this lies in studies in both murine and human in vitro breast cancer systems that have demonstrated therapeutic synergy with lack of cross resistance for selected alkylating agents when used in combination. Programs at the Dana-Farber Cancer Institute, Duke University, University of Chicago, and other centers have set out to design effective combination regimens for high-dose therapy. The first and most extensively used combination alkylating agent regimen, cyclophosphamide, carmustine, and cis-platinum (CBP or STAMP I) was designed at the Dana-Farber Cancer Institute and then used extensively at Duke.[21] This combination was instigated by laboratory models suggesting synergy and additive cytotoxicity with these agents. Attempts to add melphalan to this regimen were unsuccessful because of resultant renal toxicity. The maximum tolerated dose in this combination was 5.625 g/m² of cyclophosphamide, 600 mg/m² carmustine, and 165 mg/m² cis-platinum and further dose escalation was limited by fatal hepatic venoocclusive disease. In 14 patients with metastatic breast cancer, the overall response rate was 71% with rapid tumor regression and three complete remissions. Median duration of response was 5 months.[1]

The favorable response to CBP in metastatic breast cancer prompted investigation into regimens that contained more active and less toxic agents. The combination of cyclophosphamide and thiotepa was tested vigorously in vivo and in vitro.[114] In human and murine breast tumor systems, significant synergy and additive cytotoxicity was demonstrated for these agents. The combination of cyclophosphamide and thiotepa was studied as either a continuous infusion or bolus dosing in a phase I manner at two centers.[20,81] The maximally tolerated continuous infusion dose was 6 g/m² of cyclophosphamide and 720 mg/m² thiotepa. The maximally tolerated bolus dose was 7.5 g/m² cyclophosphamide and 700 mg/m² thiotepa. No significant dose of melphalan could be added. The dose-limiting toxicity was mucositis.

Other more complex regimens were devised including the addition of agents with less capacity for dose escalation such as anthracyclines (mitoxantrone and doxorubicin) and etoposide, without significantly greater response rates. Most recently, carboplatinum has been added to high-dose regimens. Carboplatinum has demonstrated similar efficacy and cytotoxic activity to cis-platinum. The dose-limiting toxicity of carboplatinum is

Table 18-5 Combination agent high-dose therapy for relapsed and refractory breast cancer patients

Regimen	No. pts.	Complete response	Partial response	Overall response (%)	Reference
CB ± P	24	5	13	75	21, 100
CT ± H ± L	28	2	19	74	2, 20, 77, 78
CTP	15	2	7	60	54, 82
CTCb	4	0	4	100	22, 23
CTL ± B	19	2	12	75	8, 9, 55, 56
LE	4	2	2	100	1
CL ± P ± M	19	9	8	79	1, 63, 69
TM ± E	52	10	28	73	1, 18
CPE ± B	10	0	6	60	1, 51
BC	4	1	0	25	1
CD	3	0	1	33	117
FMV	1	0	1	100	88
BP	3	0	0	0	1
DCH/EP	16	1	6	43	1
MC or L	2	2	0	100	73
Total	202	36 (17%)	107	70	

C, cyclophosphamide; B, BCNU; P, cis-platinum; T, thiotepa; H, hydroxyurea; L, L-PAM; Cb, carboplatin; E, etoposide; M, mitoxantrone; D, doxorubicin.

myelosuppression; this contrasts markedly with cis-platinum in allowing for a significant dose escalation when used with stem cell hematopoietic rescue. The Dana-Farber investigators have incorporated carboplatinum successfully into a continuous-infusion regimen with cyclophosphamide and thiotepa. The current regimen (CTCb or STAMP V) contains cyclophosphamide 6 g/m^2, thiotepa 500 mg/m^2, and carboplatinum 800 mg/m.[2,21]

The results of all nonradiation combination-agent pilot studies are summarized in Table 18-5. High response rates (70%) and complete response (CR) rates (17%) were obtained after treatment of 202 patients with advanced breast cancer who had progressed after conventional chemotherapy. Responses, however, were not durable, and relapses occurred within a median of 5 months with <1% remaining in unmaintained remission beyond 2 years.[1] These studies laid the foundation for the current evaluation of these regimens in more potentially favorable groups of patients with early, minimal, and responding breast cancer.

Untreated advanced breast cancer

Fifty-three patients have been treated in four studies with high-dose therapy for newly diagnosed inflammatory or metastatic breast cancer previously untreated for advanced disease. The results are summarized in Table 18-6. An overall response rate of 75% was noted, with a number of patients in continuous, unmaintained clinical remission. In one study, Duke investigators treated 22 premenopausal patients with estrogen receptor–negative resectable metastatic breast cancer.[84] Twelve of these patients (54%) achieved a complete response. Median duration of response in patients obtaining a CR was 9 months.[52] Median survival time from transplant was 14 months. Relapses occurred pri-

Table 18-6 High-dose therapy for untreated advanced breast cancer patients

Institution	Regimen	No. pts.	Complete response	Partial response	Overall response %	Continuous complete response	Reference
Duke University	CBP	21	11	3	66	2	84
Dana-Farber Cancer Institute	CBP	4	3	1	100	1	21
Tokai University	CAU	23	7	10	74	4	107, 108
Rush Medical Center	CTP	5	4	1	100	2	54
Total		53	25	15	75	9 (16%)	

C, cyclophosphamide; B, BCNU; P, cis-platinum; T, thiotepa; A, doxorubicin; U, 5-fluorouracil.

Table 18-7 High-dose therapy for responding advanced breast cancer patients

Regimen	No. pts.	After induction: Complete response	After induction: Partial response	After induction: Overall response (%)	After ABMT: Complete response	After ABMT: Partial response	After ABMT: Overall response (%)	Continuous complete response	Toxic death	Reference
C/TBI	19	6	11	89	13	3	84	3	3	1, 40, 41, 68
L	16	8	7	93	13	0	81	1	3	1, 119
CL ± M	23	7	9	69	16	1	73	12	2	1
CPE	58	20	29	84	31	17	82	13	2	11, 18, 19, 102
CBP	44	17	23	91	25	13	86	10	8	52, 53, 121
CT ± H	54	17	34	94	24	27	94	11	4	1, 9, 58, 59, 87
CTCb	29	10	19	100	13	16	100	11	1	3
CMC	9	4	3	77	6	2	88	0	0	8, 90
CETam	10	10	0	100	10	0	100	3	1	72, 122
CB	11	5	6	100	7	4	100	6	2	101
Total	273	104	141	89	158	83	88	75 (30%)	26 (9%)	

C, cyclophosphamide; TBI, total body irradiation; P, cis-platinum; L, L-PAM; M, mitoxantrone; E, etoposide; Tam, tamoxifen; H, hydroxyurea; B, BCNU; MC, mitomycin C.

marily in sites of bulk disease or in areas of prior radiation therapy. Toxicity was substantial, and five patients (23%) died of therapy-related conditions including hemorrhagic myocarditis, acute renal failure, and toxic hepatitis. Three patients (14%) are in an unmaintained remission at 3.3, 4.7, and 6.4 years.[52]

High-dose therapy in responding advanced breast cancer

Conventional chemotherapy and radiation has been used as a cytoreduction before high-dose chemotherapy in patients with advanced breast cancer. In these studies, patients who obtain remission went on to high-dose therapy. Unresponsive patients generally were excluded from further therapy. Induction regimens have included such combinations of conventional dose therapy as CMF or CAF with 10% to 20% complete remission rates and 40% to 70% response rates. More dose-intensive induction regimens such as AFM (doxorubicin 25 mg/m^2 daily for 3 days, 5-fluorouracil 750 mg/m^2 as a continuous infusion over 5 days, and methotrexate 250 mg/m^2 as a single dose), FAC (cyclophosphamide 600 mg/m^2, doxorubicin 60 mg/m^2, 5-fluorouracil 600 mg/m^2), or a 16-week multidrug regimen, have resulted in higher response rates in a number of small series with short follow-up.

Results of a number of high-dose regimens when used in 273 patients responding to induction therapy is shown in Table 18-7. A total of 58% of these patients achieved complete response and 30% are in continuous unmaintained remission at a median duration of 2 years.

The largest clinical experience exists at Duke and the Dana-Farber Cancer Institute. At Duke, 44 patients with measurable metastatic breast cancer that was estrogen receptor–negative or progressive with hormonal therapy were treated.[83] AFM was given for 3 weeks until maximal tumor shrinkage, toxicity, or maximal doxorubicin dose. Overall response rate was 91% (38% CR). Of these responding patients, 39 went on to treatment with CBP and ABMT. The response rate was 97%, with a CR of 64%. Ten patients (22%) remained free from progression at a median of 20 months after bone marrow infusion.

At the Dana-Farber Cancer Institute, 29 patients with responding metastatic or unresectable breast cancer were treated. Standard-dose therapy was given before CTCb high-dose therapy with ABMT. The response rate was 100%, with a CR of 44%. Eight patients (27%) remained progression-free at short follow-up (<18 months).

The major limitation to this high-dose therapy approach is the significant toxicity and associated morbidity and mortality. Treatment-related death with CBP occurred in 21% of treated patients. Mortality was related directly to infection, bleeding, or specific regimen toxicity. Mortality with the CTCb regimen was 3% and was caused by hemorrhagic cystitis in the single patient who died.

High-dose therapy in poor-prognosis primary breast cancer

Experience with high-dose therapy and advanced breast cancer allowed for the development of high-dose regimens with predictable toxicity and response rates. The greatest potential curative role for high-dose therapy, however, exists in the treatment of poor-prognosis primary breast cancer patients. Retrospective analyses of prospective surgical trials have demonstrated a number of poor prognostic factors. Patients with 10 or more histologically involved axillary lymph nodes have relapse rates greater than 85%.[29,118] Additionally, patients with unresectable inflammatory breast cancer or stage III primary tumors, especially if hormone receptor–negative, have a poor prognosis.[43]

High-dose chemotherapy and autologous bone marrow transplantation recently has been incorporated into experimental investigation of the adjuvant therapy of these high-risk breast cancer patients. Patients first receive a number of cycles of conventional-dose adjuvant therapy. This is followed by high-dose consolidation of initial remission. Table 18-8 lists the results of such studies. Fifty-six patients with unresectable disease (inflammatory and stage III disease) have been reported in five studies. A total of 79% of these patients were in complete remission after standard-dose treatment, and 89% were in complete remission after the high-dose consolidation. Only 54% are in continued clinical remission at the time of most recent analysis with short follow-up.

Eighty-nine breast cancer patients with 10 or more axillary lymph nodes involved have been treated with high-dose adjuvant therapy. Eighty-eight percent of these patients were in clinical complete remission at time of last report, with a very short follow-up. High-dose therapy for primary breast cancer will remain an active area of investigation for the next decade.

INVESTIGATIONAL ISSUES

Bone marrow involvement

The use of autologous stem cells for high-dose therapy may be complicated by the frequent bone involvement in breast cancer patients. Standard pathologic examination of bone marrow biopsy and aspiration specimens reveal involvement in >40% of patients with nonosseous metastatic breast cancer.[50] Fifty-five percent of patients with positive bone scans or bone x-rays have bone marrow in-

Table 18-8 High-dose therapy for poor prognosis primary breast cancer patients

Primary investigator	Regimen	No. pts.	Complete response after induction	Complete response after ABMT	Continuous complete response	Deaths	Reference
Inflammatory/stage III							
Gisselbrecht	C/TBI	9	9	9	3	0	40, 41
Mulder	CET	18	18	17	12	1	78, 122
Maraninchi	CL ± M	11	4	0	4	0	70
Gisselbrecht	CLM	13	12	11	6	1	1
Gianni	L/TBI	5	1	5	5	0	10
Total		56	44 (78%)	50 (89%)	30 (54%)	2 (3%)	
>10 lymph nodes							
Gianni	L	14			14	0	10
Fay	CT	5			5	0	26
Peters	CBP	52			47	4	81
Tajima	CAU	18			12	0	107-109
Total		89			78 (87%)	4 (4%)	

C, cyclophosphamide; TBI, total body irradiation; P, cis-platinum; L, L-PAM; M, mitoxantrone; E, etoposide; Tam, tamoxifen; H, hydroxyurea; B, BCNU; A, doxorubicin; U, 5-fluorouracil.

volvement.[50] New techniques involving either monoclonal antibodies or cell cultures have shown up to 30% of otherwise negative bone marrow samples may have involvement with malignant cells.[24,86] The impact of bone marrow contamination with clonogenic tumor cells on high-dose therapy is unknown. Initial in vivo and in vitro studies of bone marrow purging in breast cancer have been conducted. Shpall et al. have used pharmacologic purging with escalating doses of 4-HC in a phase 1 trial.[98] Patients had metastatic breast cancer with bone or bone marrow involvement. Twenty-four patients were first treated with AFM and then marrow was harvested and the mononuclear cell fraction separated in Ficoll-Hypaque was purged. The 4-HC dose was increased in 20 mg/ml increments to a maximum of 80 mg/ml. At this dose the mean time to engraftment was 38.5 days; this was considered the maximally tolerated dose. The true effectiveness of this agent to purge breast cancer tumor cells is difficult to determine because of the lack of appropriately sensitive techniques to detect residual tumor cells.

Other techniques to render autologous bone marrow free of breast cancer cells include in vivo purging of bone marrow by chemotherapy given before stem cell harvest. Alternatively, peripheral stem cell harvest may decrease contamination with tumor cells specifically involving bone marrow. Circulating tumor cells, however, may still be harvested. Until these techniques are further developed, most investigators limit candidates for transplantation to those without evidence of overt bone marrow involvement.

Peripheral stem cell harvest

Human peripheral blood stem cells recently have been used successfully as a sole source of stem cell rescue after high-dose therapy for breast cancer. Between five and eight leukophereses are required for adequate stem cell collection. In the series investigating high-dose therapy with stem cell rescue reported from Nebraska, engraftment failed in only one patient.[60]

More recently, the combination of peripheral stem cells and bone marrow cells was used by the Milan group as part of high-dose therapy for breast cancer patients with a poor prognosis. Peripheral stem cells were harvested after high-dose single-agent cyclophosphamide therapy. This technique previously had been shown to result in transient high numbers of hematopoietic precursors in peripheral blood.[39] Patients then undergo conventional autologous bone marrow harvest and receive both products after high-dose therapy. Seven patients with inflammatory breast cancer and 26 patients with 10 or more involved lymph nodes have been treated with this regimen.[38] One patient died in the course of treatment from pulmonary edema and capillary leak syndrome felt to be related to granulocyte-macrophage colony stimulating factor (GM-CSF) infusion. All other patients tolerated the treatment well with minimal toxicity. Patients had rapid (within 12 days) complete hematopoietic re-

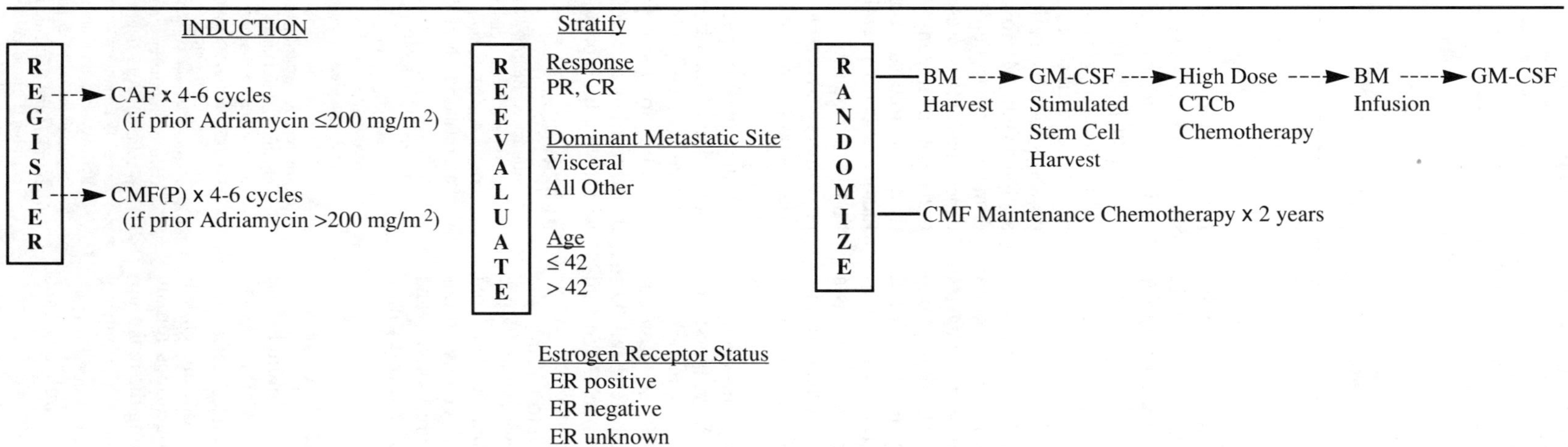

Fig. 18-2 Schema for the Philadelphia Bone Marrow Transplantation Group randomized, controlled trial for metastatic breast cancer patients.

Table 18-9 Summary of high-dose therapy in breast cancer patients

Patient status	No. pts.	Complete response (%)	Overall response (%)	Continuous complete response (%)	Death (%)
Relapsed and refractory advanced	366	16	47	0	—
Untreated advanced	53	47	75	17	9
Responding advanced	273	58	89	30	9
Responding unresectable	56	89	—	54	3
Poor prognosis resectable	89	—	—	87	4

Adapted from Antman K et al: Dose intensive therapy in breast cancer: current status. In Gale RP and Champlin RE, editors: New strategies in bone marrow transplantation, New York, Wiley Liss, 1990, pp 423-436.

covery. This intriguing observation is now under investigation at various centers. For now the role of peripheral stem cells in high-dose therapy for breast cancer remains in an area of active investigation.

Growth factors

The degree of toxicity attributed to high-dose therapy is related primarily to the duration of profound cytopenias. Recent clinical experience suggests that infections, bleeding, and even direct toxic complications of high-dose therapy may be reduced by the use of hematopoietic growth factors.[80] Granulocyte-macrophage colony stimulating factor is a major in vivo regulator of human hematopoiesis. GM-CSF has effects on early erythroid and megakaryocyte precursors as well as granulocyte and monocyte progenitors. Additionally, this agent enhances the function of mature peripheral blood leukocytes. Ongoing clinical trials are looking at GM-CSF in two areas. First, GM-CSF has been administered during peripheral blood stem cell harvest to augment progenitor cell numbers. Ten-fold increases in CFU-GM have been reported. Additionally, GM-CSF has been shown to enhance the rapidity of engraftment and decrease the incidence and severity of other toxicities when administered after bone marrow infusion. Other colony stimulating factors such as G-CSF, erythropoietin, and interleukin-3 are also under active investigation alone or in combination.

SUMMARY AND FUTURE DIRECTIONS

Antman et al.[1] have surveyed the use of high-dose therapy in breast cancer and a summary is presented in Table 18-9. Patients with advanced refractory disease are least likely to benefit from this expensive and toxic treatment. Many questions remain to be answered, however, concerning the make-up, route of administration, and dosage of the optimal high-dose regimen. Patients with advanced refractory disease should be enrolled in well designed pilot studies to answer these questions.

Patients with responding metastatic or early breast cancer with a poor prognosis now have shown high response rates and manageable toxicity with a number of high-dose therapy regimens. A number of large multicenter groups have initiated randomized trials that now will seek to compare high-dose therapy to conventional treatment approaches in these patients. A schema for the Philadelphia Bone Marrow Transplantation Group randomized, controlled trial for metastatic breast cancer patients is presented in Fig. 18-2 and illustrates one such study. These trials also will investigate the role of bone marrow purging, growth factors, and peripheral stem cell harvest. Evaluation of the quality of life and relative costs (approximately $100,000 to $200,000 for an autologous bone marrow transplant) also will be major areas of investigation.

Today, 50% of patients with breast cancer ultimately die of the disease. High-dose therapy with stem cell rescue holds great promise for increasing cure rates for these patients. Well-designed randomized trials to investigate this approach further will have a high priority for the next decade.

REFERENCES

1. Antman K, Bearman SI, Davidson N, et al: Dose intensive therapy in breast cancer: current status. In Gale RP and Champlin RE, editors: New strategies in bone marrow transplantation, New York, 1990, Wiley Liss, Inc, pp 423-436.
2. Antman K, Eder JP, Elias A, et al: High dose combination alkylating agent preparative regimen with autologous bone marrow support: The Dana-Farber Cancer Institute/Beth Israel Hospital experience, Cancer Treat Rep 71:119, 1987.
3. Antman K, Eder J, Elias A, et al: High dose cyclophosphamide, thiotepa and carboplatin intensification with autologous bone marrow support in patients with breast cancer responding to standard dose induction therapy, Proc Am Soc Clin Oncol 9:33, 1990 (abstract).
4. Antman K and Gale RP: Advanced breast cancer: high dose chemotherapy and autologous bone marrow transplantation, Ann Intern Med 108:570, 1988.
5. Ariel I: Treatment of disseminated cancer by intravenous hydroxyurea and autogenous bone marrow transplants: experiences with 35 patients, J Surg Oncol 7:331, 1975.
6. Barr RD and McBride JA: Haemopoietic engraftment with peripheral blood cells in the treatment of malignant disease, Br J Haematol 51:181, 1987.

7. Barr RD, Whang-Pong J, and Perry S: Hematopoietic stem cells in human peripheral blood, Science 190:284, 1975.
8. Bitran J, Kaminer L, and Williams S: High dose chemotherapy with autologous hematopoietic stem cell rescue in stage IV breast cancer: the Univeristy of Chicago experience. In Dicke K, Spitzer G, Jagannath S, and Evinger-Hodges M, editors: Autologous bone marrow transplantation: proceedings of the fourth international symposium, Houston, 1989, University of Texas, MD Anderson Cancer Center Press, pp. 367-371.
9. Bitran J and Williams SF: A phase II study of induction chemotherapy followed by intensification with high dose chemotherapy with autologous bone marrow rescue (ABMR) in stage IV breast cancer, Breast Cancer Res Treat 10:88, 1987 (abstract).
10. Bonodonna G: Karnofsky Memorial Lecture, J Clin Oncol 10:1386, 1989.
11. Brown R, Herzig R, Fay, J, et al: A phase I-II study of high-dose N, N1, N2 triethylenethiophosphoramide (Thio-Tepa) and autologous marrow transplantation for refractory malignancies, Proc Am Soc Clin Oncol 5:494, 1986 (abstract).
12. Cheson BD, Lacerna L, Leyland-Jones B, et al: Autologous bone marrow transplantation, Ann Intern Med 110:51, 1989.
13. Clark GM, Sledge GW, Osborne CK, and McGuire WL: Survival from first recurrence: relative importance of prognostic factors in 1,015 breast cancer patients, J Clin Oncol 5:55, 1987.
14. Clift RD, Buckner CD, Thomas CD, et al: The treatment of acute nonlymphocytic leukemia by allogeneic marrow transplantation, Bone Marrow Transplant 2:243, 1987.
15. Collins C, Mortimer J, and Livingston R: High-dose cyclophosphamide in the treatment of refractory lymphomas and solid tumor malignancies, Cancer 63:228, 1989.
16. Corringham R, Gilmore M, Prentice H, and Boesen E: High-dose melphalan with autologous bone marrow transplant: treatment of poor prognosis tumors, Cancer 52:1783, 1983.
17. Douer YD, Champlin R, Ho L, et al: High-dose combined-modality therapy and autologous bone marrow rescue for refractory solid tumors, Am J Med 71:973, 1981.
18. Dunphy FR, Spitzer G, Buzdar A, et al: High-dose therapy with ABMT in metastatic breast cancer: clinical features and prolonged progression-free survival, Proc Am Soc Clin Oncol 8:91, 1989 (abstract).
19. Dunphy FR, Spitzer G, Dicke K, et al: Tandem high-dose chemotherapy as intensification in stage IV breast cancer. In Gale RP and Champlin RE, editors: Bone marrow transplantation: current controversies, New York, 1989, Alan R. Liss, Inc., pp 245-251.
20. Eder JP, Antman K, Elias A, et al: Cyclophosphamide and thiotepa with autologous bone marrow transplantation with solid tumors, J Natl Cancer Inst 80:1221, 1988.
21. Eder JP, Antman K, Peters W, et al: High-dose combination alkylating agent chemotherapy with autologous bone marrow support for metastatic breast cancer, J Clin Oncol 4:1592, 1986.
22. Eder JP, Elias A, Shea TC, et al: A Phase I/II study of cyclophosphamide, thiotepa and carboplatin with autologous bone marrow transplantation in solid tumor patients, J Clin Oncol 8:1239, 1990.
23. Eder JP, Shea TC, Henner WD, et al: High-dose combination alkylating agent therapy with carboplatin and autologous bone marrow transplantation in solid tumors. In Bunn PA, Canetta R, Ozols RF, and Rozencweig M, editors: Carboplatin (JM-8), Philadelphia, 1990, WB Saunders Co, pp 353-360.
24. Ellis G, Ferguson M, Yamanaka E, et al: Monoclonal antibodies for detection of occult carcinoma cells in bone marrow of breast cancer patients, Cancer 63:2509, 1989.
25. Emanuel D, Cunningham I, Jules-Elysee K, et al: Cytomegalovirus pneumonia after bone marrow transplantation successfully treated with the combination of ganciclovir and high-dose intensive immunoglobulin, Ann Intern Med 109:887, 1988.
26. Fay JW, Wolff SN, Herzig RH, et al: Phase II studies of intensive thiotepa chemotherapy with autologous marrow transplantation in the treatment of neoplastic diseases, Semin Oncol 17:2, 1990.
27. Fefer A: Bone marrow transplantation for cancer. In Calabresi P, Schein PS, and Rosenberg SD, editors: Medical oncology, New York, 1985, MacMillian, pp 1371-1374.
28. Fefer A: Current status of syngeneic marrow transplantation and its relevance to autografting, Clin Hematol 15:49, 1986.
29. Fisher B, Bauer M, Wickerham DL, et al: Relationship of number of positive axillary nodes to the prognosis of patients with primary breast cancer: an NSABP update, Cancer 52:1551, 1983.
30. Fraschini G, Esparza L, Holmes F, et al: High-dose etoposide in metastatic breast cancer, Breast Cancer Res Treat 14:39, 1989 (abstract).
31. Frei E III: Curative cancer chemotherapy, Cancer Res 45:6523, 1985.
32. Frei E III, Antman K, Teicher B, et al: Bone marrow autotransplantation for solid tumors—prospects, J Clin Oncol 7:515, 1989.
33. Frei E III and Canellos GP: Dose: a critical factor in cancer chemotherapy, Am J Med 69:585, 1980.
34. Frei E III, Cucchi CA, Rosowski A, et al: Alkylating agent resistance: in vitro studies with human cell lines, Proc Natl Acad Sci USA 82:2158, 1985.
35. Frei E III, Teicher BA, Cucchi CA, et al: Resistance to alkylating agents: basic studies and therapeutic implications. In Woolley PV III and Tew KD, editors: Mechanisms of drug resistance in neoplastic cells, San Diego, 1988, Academic Press.
36. Frei E III, Teicher BA, Holden SA, et al: Effect of alkylating agent dose: preclinical studies and possible clinical correlation, Cancer Res, 1991, in press.
37. Gelman RS and Henderson IC: Analysis of dose intensity for adjuvant chemotherapy trials in stage II breast cancer, SAKK Bulletin 1:10, 1987.
38. Gianni AM and Bonadonna G: High-dose chemo-radiotherapy for sensitive tumors: is sequential better than concurrent drug delivery? Eur J Cancer Clin Oncol 25:1027, 1989.
39. Gianni AM, Siena S, Bregni M, et al: Granulocyte-macrophage colony-stimulating factor to harvest circulating hematopoietic stem cells for autotransplantation, Lancet ii:580, 1989.
40. Gisselbrecht C, Lepage E, Espie M, et al: Cyclophosphamide, total body irradiation with autologous bone marrow support for metastatic breast cancer, Proc Am Soc Clin Oncol 6:255, 1989 (abstract).
41. Gisselbrecht C, Lepage E, Extra J, et al: Inflammatory and metastatic breast cancer: cyclophosphamide and total body irradiation (TBI) with autologous bone marrow transplantation (ABMT). In Dicke K, Spitzer G, Jagannath S, and Evinger-Hodges M, editors: Autologous bone marrow transplantation: proceedings of the fourth international symposium, Houston, 1989, University of Texas, MD Anderson Cancer Center Press, pp 363-367.
42. Goldman JM, Apperby JF, Jones L, et al: Bone marrow transplantation for patients with chronic myeloid leukemia, N Engl J Med 314:202, 1986.

43. Henderson IC, Harris JR, Kinne DW, and Hellman S: Cancer of the breast. In DeVita VT, Hellman S, and Rosenberg SA, editors: Cancer principles and practice of oncology, ed 3, Philadelphia, 1989, JB Lippincott.
44. Henderson IC, Hayes DF, and Gelman R: Dose response in the treatment of breast cancer: a critical review, J Clin Oncol 6:1501, 1988.
45. Herzig R, Phillips G, Lazarus H, et al: Intensive chemotherapy and autologous bone marrow transplantation for the treatment of refractory malignancies. In Dicke K, Spitzer G, and Zander A, editors: Autologous bone marrow transplantation: proceedings of the first international symposium, Houston, 1985, University of Texas, MD Anderson Cancer Center Press, pp 197-202.
46. Hortobagyi GN: Evaluation of high-dose versus standard FAC chemotherapy for advanced breast cancer in protected environment units: a prospective randomized study, J Clin Oncol 5:354, 1987.
47. Hortobagyi GN: The role of high-dose chemotherapy with autologous bone marrow transplantation in the treatment of breast cancer, Bone Marrow Transplant 3:525, 1988.
48. Hryniuk W and Bush H: The importance of dose intensity in chemotherapy of metastatic breast cancer, J Clin Oncol 2:1281, 1984.
49. Hryniuk W and Levine MN: Analysis of dose intensity for adjuvant chemotherapy trials in stage II breast cancer, J Clin Oncol 4:1162, 1986.
50. Ingle JN, Tormey DC, and Tan KH: The bone marrow examination in breast cancer: diagnostic considerations and clinical usefulness, Cancer 41:670, 1978.
51. Jacobs S, Earle M, Shadduck R, and Stoller R: A phase I-II trial of ablative chemotherapy with cyclophosphamide, etoposide, cis-platinum and autologous bone marrow rescue in advanced solid tumors, Proc Am Soc Clin Oncol 8:53, 1989 (abstract).
52. Jones R, Shpall EJ, and Peters WP: AFM-Intensive induction chemotherapy for advanced breast cancer, Breast Cancer Res Treat 10:90, 1987 (abstract).
53. Jones R, Shpall EJ, Shogan J, et al: AFM induction chemotherapy followed by intensive consolidation with autologous bone marrow support for advanced breast cancer, Proc Am Soc Clin Oncol 7:29, 1988 (abstract).
54. Kaizer H, Ghalle R, Adler SS, et al: High dose chemotherapy and bone marrow transplantation in the treatment of metastatic breast cancer, J Cell Biochem 14A:321, 1990.
55. Kaminer L, Williams S, Beschorner J, et al: High dose chemotherapy with autologous hematopoietic stem cell support in the treatment of refractory Stage IV breast carcinoma, Breast Cancer Res Treat 12:62, 1988 (abstract).
56. Kaminer L, Williams S, Beschorner J, et al: High dose chemotherapy with autologous bone hematopoietic stem cell support in the treatment of Stage IV breast carcinoma, Proc Am Soc Clin Oncol 8:174, 1989 (abstract).
57. Kaplan HS: Evidence for a tumoricidal dose level in the radiotherapy of Hodgkin's disease, Cancer Res 26:1221, 1966.
58. Kennedy MJ, Beveridge R, Rowley S, et al: Dose-intense cytoreduction followed by high dose consolidation chemotherapy and rescue with purged autologous bone marrow for metastatic breast cancer, Breast Cancer Res Treat 14:3, 1989 (abstract).
59. Kennedy MJ, Beveridge R, Rowley S, et al: High dose consolidation chemotherapy and rescue with purged autologous bone marrow following dose-intense induction for metastatic breast cancer, Proc Am Soc Clin Oncol 8:69, 1989 (abstract).
60. Kessinger D, Armitage JO, Landmark JD, et al: Autologous peripheral hematopoietic stem cell transplantation restores hematopoietic function following marrow ablative therapy, Blood 71:723, 1988.
61. Knight WA, Page CP, Kuhn JG, et al: High dose L-pam with autologous bone marrow infusion for advanced, steroid hormone receptor negative breast cancer, Breast Cancer Res Treat 4:336, 1984 (abstract).
62. Knight WA, Page CP, Kuhn JG, et al: High dose L-pam and autologous marrow infusion for refractory solid tumors, Proc Am Soc Clin Oncol 3:150, 1984 (abstract).
63. Langieben A, Ahlgreen P, Shustik C, and Fauser A: Autologous bone marrow transplantation for metastatic breast cancer: a phase I study, Proc Am Soc Clin Oncol 7(38):149, 1988 (abstract).
64. Lazarus J, Herzig R, Graham-Pole J, et al: Intensive melphalan chemotherapy and cryopreserved autologous bone marrow transplantation for the treatment of refractory cancer, J Clin Oncol 2:359, 1983.
65. Lazarus HM, Reed MD, Spitzer TR, et al: High-dose IV thiotepa and cryopreserved autologous bone marrow transplantation for therapy of refractory cancer, Cancer Treat Rep 71:689, 1987.
66. LeMaistre CF, Herzig GP, Herzig RH, et al: High dose thiotepa and autologous bone marrow rescue for the treatment of refractory breast cancer, Breast Cancer Res Treat 10:89, 1987 (abstract).
67. Leoni M, Rosti G, Flamini E, et al: High-dose chemotherapy and ABMT in advanced breast cancer: a pilot study, Bone Marrow Transplant 3:299, 1988 (abstract).
68. Livingston R, Schulman S, Guffin B, et al: Combination chemotherapy and systemic irradiation consolidation for poor prognosis breast cancer, Cancer 9:1249, 1987.
69. Maraninchi D, Gastuat JA, Herve P, et al: High dose melphalan and autologous marrow transplantation in adult solid tumors: clinical responses and preliminary evaluation of different strategies. In McVie JG, Dalesio O, and Smith IE, editors: Autologous bone marrow transplantation and solid tumors, New York, 1984, Raven Press, pp 145-150.
70. Maraninchi D, Plana L, Blaise D, et al: Phase I and II studies of high dose alkylating agents in poor risk patients with breast cancer with autologous bone marrow transplantation. In Dicke K, Spitzer TR, and Jaggannath S, editors: Autologous bone marrow transplantation: proceedings of the third international symposium, Houston, 1987, University of Texas, MD Anderson Hospital Press, pp 475-480.
71. McCredie KB, Hersh EM, and Friereich EJ: Cells capable of colony formation in the peripheral blood of man, Science 171:293, 1971.
72. Meyers, JD, Reed EL, Shepp PA, et al: Acyclovir for prevention of cytomegalovirus infection and disease after allogeneic bone marrow transplantation, N Engl J Med 318:70, 1988.
73. Micklem HS, Anderson N, and Ross E: Limited potential of circulating haemopoietic stem cells, Nature 256:41, 1975.
74. Muggia FM and Gill I: Primary chemotherapy: concepts and trials, Principles Pract Oncol Updates 4:1, 1990.
75. Mukaiyama T, Ogawa M, Horikoshi N, et al: A study to overcome drug resistance using high-dose chemotherapy with autologous bone marrow transplantation, Jpn J Cancer Chemother 16:2013, 1989.
76. Mulder NH, Meinesz AP, Sleijfer DT, et al: High-dose etoposide with or without cyclophosphamide and autologous bone marrow transplantation in solid tumors. In McVie JG, Dalesio O, and Smith IE, editors: Autologous bone marrow transplantation and solid tumors, New York, 1984, Raven Press.
77. Mulder NH, Sleijfer DT, DeVries EG, and Willemse PH:

Intensive induction chemotherapy and intensification with autologous bone marrow reinfusion in patients with stage IIIB and IV breast cancer, Proc Am Soc Clin Oncol 7:26, 1988 (abstract).
78. Mulder POM, Sleijfer DT, Willemse PH, et al: High dose cyclophosphamide or melphalan with escalating doses of mitoxantrone and autologous bone marrow transplantation for refractory solid tumors, Cancer Res 49:4654, 1989.
79. Niederwieser D, Aulitzky W, Frommhold H, et al: Bone marrow transplantation in the treatment of haematological malignancies and solid tumors, Wien Klin Wochenschr 99:49, 1987.
80. Peters WP: The effect of recombinant human colony-stimulating factors on hematopoietic reconstitution following autologous bone marrow transplantation, Semin Hematol 26:18, 1989.
81. Peters WP, Jones R, Shpall E, and Shogan J: Dose intensification using high-dose combination alkylating agents and autologous bone marrow support for the treatment of breast cancer. In Dick K, Spitzer G, Jagannath S, and Evinger-Hodges M, editors: Autologous bone marrow transplantation: proceedings of the fourth international symposium, Houston, 1989, University of Texas, MD Anderson Cancer Center Press, pp 389-399.
82. Peters WP, Shpall EJ, Jones RB, and Ross M: High-dose combination cyclophosphamide, carboplatin and carmustine with bone marrow support as initial treatment for metastatic breast cancer with 3-6 year follow-up, Proc Am Soc Clin Oncol 9:31, 1990 (abstract).
83. Peters WP, Shpall EJ, Jones RB, et al: High-dose combination alkylating agents with autologous bone marrow support: a phase I trial, J Clin Oncol 4:646, 1986.
84. Peters WP, Shpall EJ, Jones RB, et al: High-dose combination alkylating agents with bone marrow support as initial treatment for metastatic breast cancer, J Clin Oncol 6:1368, 1988.
85. Rappeport JM, Smith BR, Parkinson R, et al: Application of bone marrow transplantation in genetic disease, Clin Haematol 12:755, 1983.
86. Redding WH, Monaghan P, Imrie SF, et al: Detection of micrometastases in patients with primary breast cancer, Lancet ii:1271, 1983.
87. Reed EC, Bowden RA, Dandliker PS, et al: Treatment of cytomegalovirus with gancyclovir and intravenous cytomegalovirus immunoglobulin in patients with bone marrow transplants, Ann Intern Med 109:783, 1988.
88. Robinson W, Hartmann D, Mangalik A, et al: Autologous nonfrozen bone marrow transplantation after intensive chemotherapy: a pilot study, Acta Haematol 66:145, 1981.
89. Rosti G, Galligioni E, Argnani M, et al: Autologous bone marrow transplantation as intensification therapy in breast cancer: an Italian cooperative experience. In Dicke K, Spitzer G, Jagannath S, and Evinger-Hodges M, editors: Proceedings of the fourth international symposium, Houston, 1989, University of Texas, MD Anderson Cancer Center Press, pp 357-363.
90. Rosti G, Tumolo S, Figoli F, et al: High dose chemotherapy and autologous bone marrow transplantation in advanced breast cancer, Breast Cancer Res Treat 10:110, 1987 (abstract).
91. Santos GW and Colvin OM: Pharmacological purging of bone marrow with reference to autografting, Clin Haematol, 15:67, 1986.
92. Saral R, Burns WH, Laskin OL, et al: Acyclovir prophylaxis of herpes-simplex virus infections, N Engl J Med 305:63, 1981.
93. Schabel FN Jr, Griswold DP Jr, and Corbett TH: Increasing therapeutic response rates to anticancer drugs by applying the basic principles of pharmacology, Pharmacol Ther 20:282, 1984.
94. Schabel FN Jr, Trader NW, Laster WRS, et al: Patterns of resistance and therapeutic synergism among alkylating agents, Antibiot Chemother 23:200, 1978.
95. Schilcher RB, Young JD, Ratanathorathorn V, and Baker LH: High dose mitomycin C and autologous bone marrow transplantation: clinical results and pharmacokinetics, Blut 45:183, 1982.
96. Schilcher RB, Young JD, Ratanathorathorn V, et al: Clinical pharmacokinetics of high dose mitomycin C, Cancer Chemother Pharmacol 13:186, 1984.
97. Shea TC, Flaherty M, Elias A, et al: A phase I clinical and pharmacological study of high-dose carboplatin and autologous bone marrow support, J Clin Oncol 7:651, 1989.
98. Shpall EJ, Best RC, and Jones W: Immunopharmacologic bone marrow purging in metastatic breast cancer (CA) patients (pts) receiving high dose chemotherapy with autologous bone marrow support, Proc Am Soc Clin Oncol 9:29, 1990 (abstract).
99. Slease RB, Benear JB, Selby GB, et al: High-dose combination alkylating agent therapy with autologous bone marrow rescue for refractory solid tumors, J Clin Oncol 6:1314, 1988.
100. Slease RB, Reitz CL, Hughes WL, et al: Autologous bone marrow transplantation for metastatic breast carcinoma: autotransplantation for breast carcinoma. In Dicke K, Spitzer G, and Jagannath S, editors: Autologous bone marrow transplantation: proceedings of the third international symposium, Houston, 1987, The University of Texas, MD Anderson Cancer Center Press.
101. Slease RB, Selby G, Saez R, et al: Autologous bone marrow transplantation for metastatic breast carcinoma in complete or partial remission, Breast Cancer Res Treat 14:58, 1989 (abstract).
102. Spitzer G, Buzdar A, Auber M, et al: High dose cyclophosphamide/VP-16/platinum intensification for metastatic breast cancer, Breast Cancer Res Treat 10:89, 1987.
103. Spitzer G, Dunphy F, Ellis J, et al: High-dose intensification for Stage IV hormonally refractory breast cancer. In Dicke K, Spitzer G, Jagannath S, and Evinger-Hodges M, editors: Autologous bone marrow transplantation: proceedings of the fourth international symposium, Houston, 1989, The University of Texas, MD Anderson Cancer Center Press, pp 399-405.
104. Stewart P: Autologous bone marrow transplantation in metastatic breast cancer, Breast Cancer Res Treat 2:85, 1982.
105. Storb R: Bone marrow transplantation. In DeVita VT, Hellman S, and Rosenberg SA, editors: Cancer principles and practice of oncology, ed 3, Philadelphia, 1989, JB Lippincott.
106. Storb R, Thomas ED, Bruckner CD, et al: Marrow transplantation for aplastic anemia, Semin Haematol 21:27, 1984.
107. Tajima T, Sonoda K, Kubnota M, et al: High-dose combination chemotherapy with autologous bone mrrow transplantation in breast carcinoma, Jpn J Cancer Chemother 10:840, 1983.
108. Tajima T, Sonoda K, Tokuda Y, et al: High-dose chemotherapy supported by autologous bone marrow transplantation in solid tumors, Tokai J Exp Clin Med 8:41, 1988.
109. Tajima T, Tokuda Y, Ohta M, et al: Role of autologous bone marrow transplantation in cancer chemotherapy, Low Temp Med 15:44, 1989.
110. Tannir N, Spitzer G, Dicke K, et al: Phase II study of high-dose amsacrine and autologous bone marrow transplantation in patients with refractory metastatic breast cancer, Cancer Treat Rep 67:599, 1983.

111. Tannir N, Spitzer G, Schell F, et al: Phase I-II study of high dose mitomycin with autologous bone marrow transplantation in refractory metastatic breast cancer, Cancer Treat Rep 68:805, 1983.
112. Tannock IF, Boyd NF, Deboer G, et al: A randomized trial of two dose levels of cyclophosphamide, methotrexate and fluorouracil chemotherapy for patients with metastatic breast cancer, J Clin Oncol 6:1377, 1988.
113. Teicher BA, Cucchi CA, Lee JB, et al: Alkylating agents: in vitro studies of cross resistance patterns in human tumor cell lines, Cancer Res 46:4379, 1986.
114. Teicher BA, Holden SA, Cucchi CA, et al: Combination thiotepa and cyclophosphamide in vivo and in vitro, Cancer Res 48:94, 1988.
115. Thomas ED, Buckner CD, Bonaji I, et al: One hundred patients with acute leukemia treated by chemotherapy, total body irradiation, and allogeneic marrow transplantation, Blood 49:511, 1977.
116. Thomas ED, Clift RD, Fefer A, et al: Marrow transplantation for the treatment of chronic myelogenous leukemia, Ann Intern Med 104:155, 1986.
117. Tobias J, Weiner F, and Griffiths C: Cryopreserved autologous marrow infusion following high-dose cancer chemotherapy, Eur J Cancer 13:269, 1977.
118. Valagussa P, Bonnadonna G, and Veronesi U: Patterns of relapse and survival following radical mastectomy: analysis of 716 consecutive patients, Cancer 40:574, 1977.
119. Vincent MD, Trevor J, Powles R, et al: Late intensification with high dose melphalan and autologous bone marrow support in breast cancer patients responding to conventional chemotherapy, Cancer Chemothr Pharmacol 21:255, 1988.
120. Wade JL, Newton B, Flournoy N, et al: Oral acyclovir for prevention of herpes simplex virus reactivation after marrow transplantation, Ann Intern Med 100:823, 1984.
121. Williams S, Mick R, Desser R, et al: High dose consolidation therapy with autologous stem cell rescue in stage IV breast cancer, J Clin Oncol 7:1824, 1989.
122. Willemse PHB, deVries EGE, Sleijfer DT, et al: Intensive induction chemotherapy and intensification with autologous bone marrow reinfusion in patients with stage IIIb and IV breast cancer, Breast Cancer Res Treat 12:163, 1988 (abstract).
123. Wolff S, Fer M, and McKay C: High-dose VP-16-213 and autologous bone marrow transplantation for refractory malignancies: a phase I study, J Clin Oncol 1:701, 1983.

19 Bilateral Breast Cancer

Lawrence J. Solin

INCIDENCE

There is a small but significant incidence of patients with bilateral carcinoma of the breast. Terms that have been used to describe the presentation of carcinoma in both breasts at the same time include "synchronous," "concurrent," or "simultaneous" breast carcinoma. Terms that have been used to describe bilateral carcinoma of the breast that presents at different times in the two breasts include "metachronous" or "sequential" breast cancer.

The crude incidence of bilateral breast cancer is shown in Table 19-1. The incidence of patients presenting with synchronous bilateral breast cancer is 1.0% overall (range: 0.1% to 8.4%), and the majority of reports give an incidence of <2.0%. The crude incidence of metachronous bilateral breast cancer is 2.7% overall (range: 1.4% to 11.8%), and most reports give an incidence of <7.0%. The total incidence of bilateral breast cancer is 3.4% overall (range: 0.4% to 9.1%).

For patients presenting with a unilateral carcinoma of the breast, the risk of developing a metachronous contralateral breast cancer is strongly related to the length of follow-up. Table 19-2 shows seven reports in which the actuarial risk of developing a metachronous contralateral breast cancer has been listed by 5-year intervals. Synchronous contralateral breast cancers have been excluded. For each of the 5-year intervals, the risk among the various series is remarkably similar. The risk appears to be relatively constant at the rate of approximately 0.75% per year of follow-up. Fisher et al.[29] and Mueller and Ames[56] also have reported a constant risk of developing a metachronous contralateral breast cancer at the rate of slightly under 1% per year of follow-up to 10 years and 15 years, respectively.

A number of larger series have evaluated the relative risk of developing a metachronous breast cancer. In patients with unilateral breast cancer, the estimated relative risk of developing a metachronous breast cancer is 1.4 to 4.5 times the risk in a normal population.[13,61,67-69,75,81]

RISK FACTORS

Many studies have attempted to evaluate the potential risk factors for the development of bilateral breast cancer. A very large number of potential risk factors have been reported (Table 19-3). There is relative agreement that young age or premenopausal status at presentation of a unilateral breast cancer is associated with a substantially increased risk for the development of a metachronous, contralateral breast cancer. Other risk factors commonly associated with bilateral breast cancer include a positive family history of breast cancer or multicentric disease in the first affected breast. A number of risk factors for the development of bilateral breast cancer may share the common mechanism of a higher probability for longer survival in the subgroup of patients with that particular risk factor. Those risk factors that may be associated with a longer period of risk for the development of a contralateral breast cancer include young age, favorable histologic subtype of carcinoma, pathologically negative axillary lymph nodes, positive estrogen receptors, and positive progesterone receptors. Other risk factors may share the common mechanism of a generalized increased diathesis for the development of breast carcinoma, and these risk factors may include a positive family history, fibrocystic disease of the breast, multicentricity, history of estrogen use, P2 or DY mammographic parenchymal pattern (according to the Wolfe criteria), and associated in situ lobular carcinoma. In this regard it is of interest that the factor of in situ lobular carcinoma associated with invasive ductal carcinoma has been found to be a significant risk factor for the development of a contralateral breast cancer.[47,76] Simultaneous bilateral carcinoma has been reported as being more common with older age at presentation.[21,76]

One area of possible concern has been the potential for the use of radiation in the management of first breast cancer to increase the risk of development of a metachronous contralateral breast cancer. A number of studies have attempted to evaluate whether or not the use of radiation increases the risk of metachronous breast cancer. These studies are summarized in Table 19-4. The studies generally can be grouped into epidemiologic studies, single-institution retrospective reviews, and prospective randomized trials. The overwhelming preponderance of evidence suggests that there is no

Table 19-1 Crude incidence of bilateral breast cancer

		Pts. with bilateral breast cancer					
		Synchronous		Metachronous		Total*	
Author	Total no. pts.	No.	%	No.	%	No.	%
Adair et al.[1]	1,458	—	—	100	6.9	—	—
Al-Jurf et al.[4]	5,608	26	0.5	78	1.4	104	1.9
Bailey et al.[7]	911	17	1.9	22	2.4	39	4.3
Basco et al.[9]	14,000	—	—	194	1.4	—	—
Bedwinek et al.[10]	235	—	—	—	—	1	0.4
Berte et al.[12]	1,036	44	4.2	17	1.6	61	5.9
Bodian and Haagensen[13]	2,551	21	0.8	163	6.4	184	7.2
Chu et al.[17]	146	—	—	—	—	8	5.5
de Ustaran and Meiss[20]	1,654	28	1.7	—	—	—	—
Devitt[21]	1,530	17	1.1	56	3.7	73	4.8
Farrow[24]	5,576	21	0.4	181	3.2	202	3.6
Fenig et al.[25]	291	—	—	6	2.1	—	—
Fisher et al.[29]	1,578	—	—	66	4.2	—	—
Fracchia et al.[30]	4,443	179	4.0	224	5.0	403	9.1
Harris and Hellman[32]	255	—	—	—	—	11	4.3
Hislop et al.[34]	9,000	100	1.1	175	1.9	275	3.1
Holmberg et al.[36]	1,423	1	0.1	66	4.6	67	4.7
Kesseler et al.[38]	967	17	1.8	18	1.9	35	3.6
Khafagy et al.[39]	4,955	—	—	82	1.7	—	—
Lawson[43]	547	11	2.0	21	3.8	32	5.9
Leis[45]	500	42	8.4	—	—	—	—
Leis et al.[46]	611	2	0.3	47	7.7	49	8.0
Lewis et al.[48]	1,865	—	—	—	—	105	5.6
Lewison and Neto[50]	490	5	1.0	31	6.3	36	7.3
Martin et al.[51]	153	—	—	6	3.9	—	—
McCredie et al.[53]	3,082	10	0.3	88	2.9	98	3.2
Michowitz et al.[54]	1,215	9	0.7	57	4.7	66	5.4
Mueller and Ames[56]	3,558	33	0.9	96	2.7	129	3.6
Parker et al.[58]	1,630	18	1.1	30	1.8	48	2.9
Pomerantz et al.[59]	187	—	—	22	11.8	—	—
Prior and Waterhouse[61]	21,967	93	0.4	306	1.4	399	1.8
Robbins and Berg[64]	1,458	4	0.3	87	6.0	91	6.2
Sarrazin et al[65]	179	—	—	11	6.1	—	—
Schell et al.[66]	2,076	39	1.9	87	4.2	126	6.1
Schenker et al.[67]	12,302	—	—	—	—	246	2.0
Schottenfeld and Berg[68]	9,792	58	0.6	248	2.5	306	3.1
Schwartz et al.[69]	17,944	—	—	624	3.5	—	—
Sears et al.[70]	268	12	4.4	7	2.6	19	7.1
Shellito and Bartlett[72]	292	3	1.0	19	6.5	22	7.5
Slack et al.[73]	2,734	—	—	52	1.9	—	—
Solin et al.[74]	1,167	11	0.9	20	1.7	31	2.7
Storm and Jensen[75]	56,237	—	—	—	—	1840	3.3
van Limbergen et al.[79]	235	—	—	—	—	3	1.3
Veronesi et al.[80]	701	—	—	34	4.9	—	—
Veronesi et al.[81]	6,986	45	0.6	189	2.7	234	3.3
Wanebo et al.[82]	500	4	0.8	33	6.6	37	7.4
Total	206,293	870	1.0†	3563	2.7‡	5380	3.4§

*Excludes series reporting only synchronous or only metachronous bilateral breast cancers.
†For evaluable series only (870/90,838 = 1.0%).
‡For evaluable series only (3563/132,864 = 2.7%).
§For evaluable series only (5380/159,959 = 3.4%).

Table 19-2 Actuarial incidence of the development of metachronous contralateral breast cancer over time[a]

Author	Total no. pts.	Contralateral breast cancer (%) 5 yr	10 yr	15 yr	20 yr	25 yr	30 yr
Adair et al.[1]	1458	3.8[b]	6.9[b]	9.8[b]	13.6[b]	16.0[b]	17.6[b]
Bodian and Haagensen[13]	1731	3	7	12	15	18	24
Chaudary et al.[16]	4656	3.4	7.2	10.1	12.2[c]	—	—
McCredie et al.[53]	1489	4.0[d]	8.7[d]	12.5[d]	21.5[d]	—	—
Robbins and Berg[64]	1458	3.3	6.4	9.0	12.6	13.7[e]	—
Sarrazin et al.[65]	179	2[f]	9	—	—	—	—
Slack et al.[73]	2734	2.2	—	—	—	—	—

[a]Synchronous contralateral breast cancers have been excluded.
[b]Reported at intervals of 0 to 4, 5 to 9, 10 to 14, 15 to 19, 20 to 24, and 25 to 29 years, respectively.
[c]Reported at 19 years.
[d]Estimated from table.
[e]Reported at 24 years.
[f]Estimated from curves.

Table 19-3 Risk factors for the development of a contralateral breast cancer

Risk factor	Positive study (reference no.)	Negative study (reference no.)
Young age	2, 6, 11, 13, 16, 26, 34, 38, 45, 61, 62, 64, 69, 73, 75, 81	21, 57
Family history of breast cancer	6, 13, 15, 20, 29, 34, 38, 45, 54, 70, 76	47
Multicentricity	29, 45, 47, 59, 76	
Histologic subtype of carcinoma		
▪ Lobular	1, 8, 22, 26, 29, 34, 40, 64, 76	20
▪ Comedo	1, 38, 45, 54, 64	
▪ Tubular	26, 29, 38, 45	
▪ Colloid	38, 45, 64	
▪ Medullary	45, 64	
▪ Papillary	45	
▪ Mucoid	54	
▪ Adenoid cystic	45	
Associated in situ lobular carcinoma	47, 76	
In situ carcinoma		20
Pathologically negative axillary lymph nodes	34, 54, 83	64, 76
Large tumor size	29, 54, 73	
Stage	38, 45	20
P2 or DY mammographic parenchymal pattern (Wolfe criteria)	45, 76	
Positive estrogen receptors	47	76
Positive progesterone receptors	37	76
Histologic grade		76
▪ High	1, 11, 64	
▪ Low	47	
Genetic predisposition	5	
Subareolar location	20	
Location by quadrant		76
Fibrocystic disease	29	
Nipple involvement	29	
Absence of sinus histiocytosis	29	
History of estrogen use	34	
Positive thermography	45	
Low parity status	54	13, 47

Table 19-4 The effect of the use of radiation in the management of the first breast cancer on the development of a metachronous contralateral breast cancer

				Contralateral breast cancer (%)		
Author	**Total no. pts.**	**Patient population**	**Type of treatments**	**Without radiation**	**With radiation**	**Statistical comparison**
Basco et al.[9]	388	Province-wide cancer registry, British Columbia, Canada	Mastectomy ± radiation	—	—	0.99 (0.76-1.30)*
Fisher et al.[28]	1665	Randomized trial, NSABP	Mastectomy ± radiation	4.2	4.6	Not stated
Hankey et al.[31]	25,724	Connecticut tumor registry	Surgery ± radiation	—	—	0.7-1.6†
Harvey and Brinton[33]	41,109	Connecticut tumor registry	Any ± radiation	—	—	1.4† (significant)
Horn and Thompson[37]	556	Connecticut tumor registry	Any ± radiation	—	—	0.9 (0.6-1.4)‡
McCredie et al.[53]	1489	London Clinic, Ontario, Canada	Mastectomy ± radiation	17§	23§	Not significant
Parker et al.[58]	1484	UCLA tumor registry	Surgery ± radiation	—	—	2.0† (not significant)
Sarrazin et al.[65]	179	Randomized trial, Institut Gustave-Roussy, France	Mastectomy vs. definitive radiation therapy	9	9	0.9†
Schell et al.[66]	2076	M.D. Anderson Hospital	Any ± radiation	7.3	3.4	Not significant
Schenker et al.[67]	12,302	Israel Cancer Registry	Any ± radiation	—	—	Not significant
Storm and Jensen[75]	56,237	Danish Cancer Registry	Any ± radiation	—	—	1.3† (significant)
Veronesi et al.[80]	701	Randomized trial, National Cancer Institute, Milan, Italy	Mastectomy vs. definitive radiation therapy	4.6	5.1	Not significant

NSABP, National Surgical Adjuvant Breast Project; UCLA, University of California at Los Angeles.
*Relative risk (95% confidence interval).
†Relative risk.
‡Adjusted odds ratio (95% confidence interval).
§Estimated from curves at 20 years.

significant increase in the incidence of contralateral breast cancers with use of radiation in the management of the first breast cancer (see Table 19-4). Only two epidemiologic studies have suggested that there is a statistically significant increased risk.[33,75] The 10-year data from two prospective, randomized trials as reported by Sarrazin et al.[65] and Fisher et al.[28] have shown no difference in the risk of developing a contralateral breast cancer when the first breast cancer was managed with vs. without radiation.

DIFFERENTIAL DIAGNOSIS

Bilateral breast cancer must be distinguished from the metastatic spread of a unilateral breast cancer across midline to the contralateral breast. Less commonly, the distinction of bilateral breast cancer from systemic metastatic disease to the contralateral breast needs to be made.

Many criteria have been used to distinguish between bilateral breast cancer and unilateral breast cancer that has metastasized to the contralateral breast. These criteria generally fall into the categories of pathologic, clinical, and mammographic characteristics. Table 19-5 details the various characteristics that have been used to distinguish bilateral breast cancer from metastatic, unilateral breast cancer. The presence of in situ carcinoma in association with invasive carcinoma strongly favors a second primary cancer, whereas the absence

Table 19-5 Characteristics useful in distinguishing a second contralateral breast cancer from a metastatic first breast cancer

Characteristic	Reference no.
Pathologic	
Histologic confirmation of cancer bilaterally	24, 29
Associated in situ carcinoma	26, 29, 45, 50, 64
Location within the breast	26, 45, 50, 64, 72
Growth pattern	26, 29, 50, 64
Different histologies	13, 26, 29, 45, 50
Grade	29, 45, 72
Axillary lymph node status	29
Clinical	
Adequate treatment of first cancer	24
Absence of relapse during interval between first and second cancers	24, 45, 50
Interval between first and second cancers	45, 49, 50
Absence of relapse during time immediately after treatment of second cancer	24, 72
Spread across midline	13, 26, 29, 33, 45, 49, 50, 64, 72
Number of lesions	26, 50, 64, 72
Tumor size	29
Mammographic	23

of an in situ component must raise the possibility of metastatic carcinoma.[26,29,45,50,64] The location of the tumor within the breast parenchyma favors a new primary carcinoma, whereas metastases to the contralateral breast may occur in fatty or subcutaneous tissues.[26,45,50,64,72] The most commonly used clinical criterion for distinguishing bilateral breast cancer from metastatic, unilateral breast cancer is the spread of the tumor across midline.[13,26,29,33,45,49,50,64,72] Medial lesions are more likely to spread across the midline, and similarly, medial lesions in the contralateral breast are more likely to be metastatic. A long disease-free interval between the first and second cancers favors bilateral breast cancer.[45,49,50] Adequate treatment of the first cancer and the absence of a relapse during the interval between the first and second cancers also favors bilateral breast cancer.[24,45,50]

Egan[23] has reported that a number of radiographic features were useful in differentiating bilateral breast carcinoma from metastatic breast carcinoma. Radiographic features favoring a primary contralateral breast carcinoma include a solitary nodule, the presence of microcalcifications, the absence of skin thickening, and the presence of skin or nipple retraction. Radiographic features favoring metastatic carcinoma in the contralateral breast include multiple nodules, the presence of diffuse skin thickening, the absence of skin or nipple retraction, and the presence of breast edema or diffuse density.

As the distinction between bilateral breast cancer and metastatic, unilateral breast cancer can be difficult, clinical, pathologic, and mammographic findings must all be considered. In uncertain cases, the prudent policy generally is to proceed as though the involvement of the contralateral breast carcinoma is a primary, not metastatic, lesion, and to treat the patient for cure.

METHOD OF DETECTION

Mammography and physical examination

Mammography has been important in the detection of early bilateral breast cancer. For patients presenting with unilateral carcinoma of the breast, bilateral mammography is a standard component of the initial evaluation in order to screen for nonpalpable, contralateral carcinoma as well as to provide a baseline for future studies.

Mammography has increased the diagnosis of synchronous bilateral carcinoma of the breast. For example, the patient who has a unilateral breast carcinoma on physical examination may be found to have a nonpalpable, contralateral lesion on mammography. Egan[23] reported an increase in the incidence of synchronous bilateral breast cancer and a reduction in the incidence of metachronous bilateral breast cancer during the first 6 years of follow-up as compared to other studies. He attributed these findings to the diagnosis of nonpalpable breast cancers that were detected mammographically. Chaudary et al.[16] found that there was a fivefold increase in the detection of synchronous bilateral breast cancer (an incidence of 2.4%) following the introduction of routine mammography. Kesseler et al.[38] also have reported that mammography has increased the detection of synchronous bilateral breast cancer.

Mammography and physical examination by the physician and by the patient are all important in the detection of a contralateral breast cancer. Egan[23] reported that the second breast cancer in patients with bilateral breast cancer was found by mammography in 46% (31/67), by patient breast self-examination in 25% (17/67), by physician examination in 13% (9/67), and by other signs and symptoms in 15% (10/67). Kesseler et al.[38] reported that the second breast cancer in patients with metachronous bilateral breast cancer was discovered by the patient in 56% (10/18), by the physician in 33% (6/18), and unknown in 11% (2/18). The mammogram was reported as being abnormal in 43% (15/35) of patients with bilateral synchronous or metachronous carcinoma of the breast. Senofsky et al.[71] found that 40% of second breast cancers were found on mammography only, and 24% were found on both mammography and physical examination. Tulusan et al.[76] reported that the detection of contralateral breast cancer was by mammography in 60% (48/80) of the patients, by clinical examination in 1% (1/80), and by both methods in 39% (31/80). Urban et al.[78] reported a positive biopsy rate of 79% (22/28) for patients with positive signs of malignancy and 12% (74/625) for patients with minimal signs of malignancy.

Blind contralateral breast biopsy

Because of the known risk of an occult synchronous contralateral breast cancer in a patient presenting with unilateral carcinoma of the breast, blind contralateral breast biopsies have been proposed as a mechanism of detecting asymptomatic, occult contralateral breast carcinomas. A number of series have evaluated the results of blind contralateral biopsies performed in asymptomatic patients presenting with unilateral carcinoma of the breast (Table 19-6). The patients studied in all of these series represent cases in which only asymptomatic patients underwent contralateral breast biopsy; cases with positive mammographic or clinical signs have been excluded. There are a number of differences among the various studies. In most series, blind contralateral breast biopsies were performed in all patients with unilateral carcinoma of the breast, whereas Donegan and Perez-Mesa[22] performed blind contralateral biopsies only in the presence of invasive lobular carcinoma or in situ lobular carcinoma. The location of most of the blind contralateral breast biopsies was either the mirror image site or the upper outer quadrant of the contralateral breast. The amount of tissue removed has ranged from very limited biopsies to removal of one quarter of the breast parenchyma. The rate of positivity for contralateral invasive carcinoma ranges from <1% to 20%, with an average of 3%. The total rate of positivity for invasive and noninvasive carcinoma is reported as 2% to 39%, with an average of 9%.

The risk of developing a metachronous contralateral breast carcinoma following a negative blind contralateral biopsy is small. Fenig et al.[25] reported that 2% (6/291) of the patients with a negative contralateral biopsy developed a metachronous contralateral carcinoma of the breast. Tulusan et al.[76] reported on the follow-up of 348 patients with a negative contralateral breast biopsy. In this group, 2.9% (10/348) of patients developed a contralateral breast cancer within 3 years of follow-up. Urban et al.[78] reported that 2.4% (20/835) of patients with a negative biopsy subsequently developed a metachronous contralateral breast cancer. Wanebo et al.[82] reported that 4.1% (2/49) of patients with a negative breast biopsy developed a metachronous contralateral breast cancer. Therefore the risk of development of a metachronous contralateral breast carcinoma after a negative blind contralateral breast biopsy is low and appears to be similar to the incidence of a metachronous, contralateral cancer developing in all patients presenting with unilateral carcinoma of the breast (see Table 19-1).

Proponents of the use of contralateral blind biopsy or contralateral mastectomy in patients with unilateral carcinoma of the breast argue that the early detection of a metachronous contralateral breast cancer remains difficult, and that many cases are diagnosed with adverse prognostic factors such as large tumor size or positive axillary lymph nodes. Further, there is a small but significant incidence of synchronous, occult contralateral breast cancer that may be detected and possibly cured with early treatment. Arguments against the routine use of contralateral biopsy or prophylactic mastectomy are as follows. First the absolute incidence of finding a contralateral carcinoma in the asymptomatic patient is low, and many of these lesions are noninvasive (see Table 19-6). Second, it is possible that the cancers that are found on blind biopsy, both invasive and noninvasive, might never develop into clinically significant disease, particularly in the face of a known contralateral invasive breast cancer. Therefore, all patients would be subjected to a contralateral biopsy or prophylactic mastectomy for the benefit of a very small number of patients. Slack et al.[73] have estimated from National Surgical Adjuvant Breast Project (NSABP) data that a prophylactic contralateral mastectomy would result in an increase of 0.8% survival at 5 years at the cost of performing unnecessary contralateral prophylactic mastectomies in 98% of the patients. Third, the majority of contralateral breast cancers subsequently detected in patients who are followed carefully with clinical examination and mammography are found to be relatively favorable lesions potentially curable with standard therapy. One final argument against prophylactic mastectomy is that the widespread use of breast-preserving surgery and definitive irradiation means that the patient with an early contralateral carcinoma

Table 19-6 Results of blind contralateral breast biopsies performed in asymptomatic patients with unilateral breast cancer

Author	Indication for biopsy	Location of biopsy	Tissue removed	Total no. pts.	Pts. with infiltrating carcinoma		Pts. with in situ carcinoma		Total positive	
					No.	%	No.	%	No.	%
Donegan and Perez-Mesa[22]	Infiltrating lobular carcinoma	Same quadrant and upper outer quadrant	Biopsy	5	1	20	0	0	1	20
	LCIS ± other histologies	Same quadrant and upper outer quadrant	Biopsy	18	3	17	4	22	7	39
Fenig et al.[25]	All patients with invasive and operable carcinoma	Mirror image	30% of the quadrant	314	13	4	10	3	23	7
Fracchia et al.[30]	150 consecutive patients	Subareolar and upper outer quadrant	Biopsy	150	—		—		19	13
King et al.[41]	All patients with potentially curative carcinoma	Mirror image and upper outer quadrant	Biopsy	109	1	1	4	4	5	5
Leis[44, 45]	NS	Mirror image and upper outer quadrant	Biopsy (4-5 cm diameter of tissue specimen)	321	10	3	14	4	24	7
Martin et al.[51]	100 consecutive patients	Mirror image	Biopsy (average 3 cm diameter of tissue specimen)	100	2	2	0	0	2	2
Pressman[60]	85 consecutive patients	Mirror image	Biopsy	85	2	2	10	12	12	14
Tulusan et al.[76]	NS	Upper outer quadrant	Biopsy (10-50 g of tissue)	234	1	<1	19	8	20	9
Urban et al.[78]	NS	Mirror image and tail of the breast	20%-25% of the breast parenchyma	301	5	2	18	6	23	8
Wanebo et al.[82]	40 consecutive patients	Mirror image and outer quadrant	20%-25% of the breast parenchyma	40	—		—		7	18
Total				1677	—	3*	—	5†	143	9

LCIS, lobular carcinoma in situ.
NS, not stated.
*For evaluable series only (38/1487 = 3%).
†For evaluable series only (79/1487 = 5%).

would be treated with a more radical surgical procedure (mastectomy) than the known ipsilateral carcinoma, which could be treated with breast preservation and definitive irradiation.

Autopsy, prophylactic mastectomy, and reduction mammoplasty

Other information relevant to the detection of contralateral carcinoma or bilateral carcinoma found in the asymptomatic patient comes from autopsies, prophylactic mastectomies, and reduction mammoplasties. Lawson[43] reported a series of 100 consecutive autopsies of women with carcinoma of the breast. Excluding eight patients who had undergone mastectomy for the carcinoma of the contralateral breast, 14% (13/92) of patients were found to have gross cancer in the contralateral breast. Nielsen et al.[57] performed autopsies on 84 consecutive women with invasive breast cancer. Excluding two patients with bilateral mastectomy for bilateral invasive breast cancer, 67% (55/82) of the patients were found to have carcinoma in the contralateral breast. Invasive carcinoma was found in 32% (26/82) of the cases, and in situ carcinoma was found in 35% (29/82) of the cases. Ringberg et al.[63] performed a prophylactic subcutaneous contralateral mastectomy for 73 patients with carcinoma of the breast, 30 with invasive carcinoma, and 43 with noninvasive carcinoma. Forty percent of the patients with invasive carcinoma were found to have contralateral carcinoma, and 44% of the patients with noninvasive carcinoma were found to have contralateral carcinoma. Overall, invasive contralateral carcinoma of the breast was found in 5% (4/73) of patients, intraductal carcinoma (with or without associated in situ lobular carcinoma) was found in 16% (12/73), and in situ lobular carcinoma was found in 21% (15/73). McCarty et al.[52] performed a prophylactic contralateral subcutaneous mastectomy in 50 patients with carcinoma of the breast. Only 6% (3/50) of the patients were found to have a contralateral unsuspected carcinoma, although the histologic subtypes were not presented. In a series of 112 prophylactic mastectomies performed in patients felt to be at increased risk for developing a contralateral breast cancer, Leis[45] found 19 (17%) unsuspected carcinomas, 12 (11%) noninvasive, and 7 (6%) invasive. In a study by de Mascarel et al.,[19] contralateral reduction mammoplasty was performed in 41 patients treated with mastectomy for carcinoma of the breast. Unsuspected carcinoma was found in 34% (14/41) overall, three (7%) invasive carcinomas, six (15%) intraductal carcinomas, and five (12%) in situ lobular carcinomas.

OUTCOME OF TREATMENT

In the majority of the reports of treatment outcomes for patients with bilateral breast cancer, the predominant local treatment has been mastectomy with or without adjuvant radiation therapy or chemotherapy. Evaluating treatment outcomes for bilateral breast cancer patients poses a number of difficulties relative to the reporting of outcome. First, patients with synchronous and nonsynchronous bilateral carcinoma of the breast should be analyzed separately. Second, for patients with metachronous bilateral carcinoma of the breast, the outcome of treatment can be reported from the time of the first breast cancer or the second breast cancer. Bodian and Haagensen[13] have recommended that the treatment outcomes for patients with nonsynchronous bilateral carcinoma of the breast be reported from the time of treatment of the second breast cancer. The reason for this recommendation is that the survival outcome from the treatment of the first breast cancer results in a bias in reporting as the patient must have lived long enough to have developed the second breast cancer. Third, few of the reports in the literature have sufficient data to separate survival by stage or by other prognostic variables. Fourth, although in many of the reports adjuvant postoperative radiotherapy is utilized, adjuvant systemic chemotherapy is rarely utilized, although it has been well established at the present time that systemic chemotherapy is beneficial in

Table 19-7 Survival rates for patients with synchronous bilateral breast cancer

Author	Total no. pts.	Actuarial survival (%) 5 yr	10 yr	15 yr	20 yr
Al-Jurf et al.[4]	26	38	20	—	—
Finney et al.[26]	15	90	20	0	0
McCredie et al.[53]	10	40	40	40	40
Veronesi et al.[81]	12	50*	8*	—	—
Wilson and Alberty[83]	39	44*	7*	3*	—

*Crude survival, not actuarial survival.

the adjuvant setting for appropriately selected women with unilateral breast cancer. Fifth, the outcome of treatment for bilateral breast cancer patients should be compared to the outcome of patients with unilateral breast cancer to establish whether or not bilateral carcinoma is an adverse prognostic factor for outcome. However, this comparison is difficult in that all of the other problems also need to be considered for such comparisons. Finally, little information is available concerning the outcome of treatment for patients with bilateral carcinoma of the breast utilizing definitive irradiation as an alternative to mastectomy for appropriately selected and staged patients.

Given all these caveats, Table 19-7 shows reported series with actuarial survival rates for patients treated with synchronous bilateral breast cancer. There is a wide variation in outcome, especially at 5 and 10 years, and these differences may be caused by differences in the patient populations. Table 19-8 shows series reporting the survival rates for patients with metachronous bilateral breast cancer. Again, there are significant differences that may relate to the patient populations within the various series. There is a tendency for those series reporting survival from the first breast cancer to have slightly more favorable results than series reporting survival from the second breast cancer, perhaps reflecting the lead time bias inherent in reporting survival from the first breast cancer.

Because of the difficulty in comparing unilateral and bilateral breast cancer based on retrospective data such as that presented in Tables 19-7 and 19-8, a number of authors have attempted to make a direct comparison of the outcome of patients with unilateral and bilateral breast cancer. These series are shown in Table 19-9. With the exception of the reports by Holmberg et al.[36] and Robbins and Berg,[64] the reports do not show a survival disadvantage for patients with bilateral carcinoma of the breast. In the report of Holmberg et al.,[36] the survival rate for patients with unilateral versus bilateral breast cancer was found to be statistically different ($p = .006$) on multivariate analysis including age, histology, and axillary lymph node status. Wanebo et al.[82] evaluated the endpoint of disease-free survival, and they reported that the prognosis was better for patients with bilateral breast cancer as compared to patients with unilateral breast cancer at 5 years (89% vs. 68%; $p = .006$) and 10 years (63% vs. 54%; $p = .09$). This apparent improvement in disease-free survival rates for patients with bilateral breast cancer is probably caused by lead time bias (see above). Schell et al.[66] reported 126 patients with synchronous or metachronous bilateral breast cancer out of a total population of 2076 stage I and stage II breast cancer patients and found no difference in the 20-year disease-free survival rates for patients with synchronous or metachronous bilateral breast cancer as compared to patients with unilateral breast cancer.

Table 19-8 Survival rates for patients with metachronous bilateral breast cancer

Author	Total no. pts.	Actuarial survival (%) 5 yr	10 yr	15 yr	20 yr	Survival calculated from 1st vs. 2nd cancer
Al-Jurf et al.[4]	78	92	74	—	—	1st
Bodian and Haagensen[13]	48[a]	88	66	51	39	2nd
Devitt[21]	56[b]	48[c]	31[c]	—	—	NS
Finney et al.[26]	50	85	50	33	20	1st
	50	50	44	8	0	2nd
Fisher et al.[29]	66	73[d]	51[d]	—	—	1st
Khafagy et al.[39]	79	70	49	—	—	NS
Leis et al.[46]	47	98	49	—	—	1st
McCredie et al.[53]	88	72[e]	62[e]	58[e]	58[e]	NS
Michowitz et al.[54]	66	—	39	—	—	2nd
Pomerantz et al.[59]	22	59	35[d]	—	—	2nd
Robbins and Berg[64]	91	54	44	30	23	2nd
Slack et al.[73]	52	71[d]	—	—	—	1st
Veronesi et al.[81]	92	79	65	—	—	1st
	92	49	33	—	—	2nd
Wilson and Alberty[83]	80	98[f]	60[f]	28[f]	—	NS

NS, not stated.
[a]Columbia classification stages A and B only.
[b]Stages I, II, and III only.
[c]Crude survival estimated from table.
[d]Estimated from curves.
[e]Estimated from table.
[f]Crude survival, not actuarial survival.

Table 19-9 Survival rates for patients with unilateral vs. bilateral breast cancer

		Actuarial survival (%)									
		Unilateral				Bilateral					
Author	Total no. pts.	5 yr	10 yr	15 yr	20 yr	5 yr	10 yr	15 yr	20 yr	Bilateral cases reported	p value
Berte et al.[12]	1036	74-86*	—	—	—	70-81*	—	—	—	M	.63-.70
Bodian and Haagensen[13]	979†	81	67	53	41	88	66	51	39	M	NS
Devitt[21]	1513	36-74	20-54	—	—	24-65	8-43	—	—	M	.1
Fisher et al.[29]	1578	70‡	50‡	—	—	73‡	51‡	—	—	M	.56
Holmberg et al.[36]	1349	67‡	—	—	—	58‡	—	—	—	M	.006§
Khafagy et al.[39]	4955	64	40	—	—	70	49	—	—	M	NS
Mueller and Ames[56]	3558	—	—	—	—	76‡	52‡	32‡	—	S, M	NS
Robbins and Berg[64]	102	77‡	69‡	64‡	53‡	51‡	45‡	40‡	31‡	S, M	Not stated
Slack et al.[73]	2734	69*	—	—	—	71‡	—	—	—	M	NS

S, synchronous; M, metachronous; NS, not significant.
*At 4 years.
†Columbia classification stages A and B only.
‡Estimated from curves.
§Multivariate analysis.

There is only limited information on patients treated bilaterally with definitive breast irradiation. Solin et al.[74] reported the outcome of 30 women treated bilaterally with definitive irradiation and breast-conserving surgery for bilateral carcinoma of the breast. The local control rate was 94% at 5 years, and the relapse-free survival and no evidence of disease (NED) survival rates were 72% and 79% at 5 years, respectively. This report showed that definitive radiation technically can be delivered with low complication rates. The rates of local control and survival were found to be similar to 1136 patients with unilateral breast cancer treated similarly. However, survival rates for the bilateral cases were reported from the time of first breast cancer. Kopelson et al.[42] reported on 34 women with bilateral breast cancer who received bilateral breast or chest wall irradiation. However, only 9 patients received bilateral definitive breast irradiation, and the remaining 25 patients were treated on one or both sides with mastectomy or for palliation. They reported three cases of subcutaneous fibrosis or necrosis in 15 patients surviving for ≥5 years after treatment.

PROGNOSTIC FACTORS

A number of studies have evaluated the relative prognostic factors for first vs. second breast cancers in patients with bilateral breast cancer. Most studies have evaluated prognostic factors in terms of tumor size, pathologic nodal status, stage, and histology. In addition to the intrinsic value of determining prognostic factors, comparison of the prognostic factors for the second breast cancer relative to the first breast cancer is useful to determine if metachronous lesions are diagnosed earlier because of careful follow-up. Generally, the prognostic factors for the second breast cancer are found to be more favorable or equivalent to the first breast cancer, but not worse. These findings generally support the theory that the second breast cancer in patients with metachronous bilateral breast cancer tends to be found slightly earlier, probably because of careful follow-up after treatment of a first breast cancer.

A number of studies have evaluated tumor size or T stage in bilateral breast cancer. Second breast cancers generally are found to be more favorable than[7,23,29,48,64,76] or similar to[3] first breast cancers. Bailey et al.[7] found that the T stage for the second primary cancer was significantly lower than the first breast cancer ($p<.01$). Lewis et al.[48] found that the mean tumor size was 2.6 cm for the first breast cancer as compared to 1.3 cm in the second breast cancer for 35 patients with metachronous bilateral carcinoma. Tulusan et al.[76] also found that the mean tumor size was smaller for second breast cancers (1.2 cm) as compared to first breast cancers (2.5 cm). Egan[23] found that there was no difference in the size of simultaneous bilateral breast cancers, but for patients with metachronous bilateral breast cancers, the second carcinoma was generally smaller than the first carcinoma, with 30% being <1 cm in size. For metachronous bilateral breast cancers, Fisher et al.[29] also found that the size of the second breast cancer was smaller than the first breast cancer (2.4 cm vs. 3.5 cm, respectively).

Pathologic axillary nodal staging is one of the strongest prognostic factors for patients with unilateral carcinoma of the breast. In series reporting pathologic nodal staging or number of positive axillary lymph nodes for patients with bilateral carcinoma of the breast, the second carcinoma is generally more favorable than[3,7,29,64,70] or similar to[4,23,38,39,48,53,83] the first breast cancer, but generally not worse. Alexander et al.[3] reported that the mean number of positive axillary lymph nodes in patients with metachronous bilateral breast cancer was 4.2 for the first breast cancer and 2.4 for the second breast cancer. Bailey et al.[7] reported that the pathologic nodal staging was statistically significantly better ($p<.01$) for second vs. first breast cancers. In a report from the NSABP, Fisher et al.[29] reported that the incidence of negative axillary lymph nodes was higher and the incidence of patients with four or more positive axillary lymph nodes was lower for the second breast cancer in patients with metachronous bilateral breast cancer as compared to the first breast cancer or as compared to patients with unilateral breast cancer. However, these differences were not statistically significant. Egan[23] found that for patients with synchronous or metachronous bilateral breast cancer, there was no difference in the presence vs. absence of axillary adenopathy or the level of axillary involvement.

The reported literature also suggests that the overall staging for second breast cancers is either slightly better than or equivalent to the overall staging for first breast cancers. Only Leis et al.[46] have reported a worse staging for second breast cancers as compared to first breast cancers for 47 patients with bilateral metachronous breast cancer (21% stages III-IV vs. 6% stage III-IV, respectively). Mueller and Ames[56] found no difference in the stage distribution for 129 patients with synchronous or metachronous bilateral breast cancer. For 38 patients with synchronous or metachronous bilateral breast cancer, Sears et al.[70] found a higher incidence of stage I presentation for the second breast cancers (47%) as compared to the first breast cancers (23%) or to all breast cancers (29%).

The histologic subtypes of carcinomas reported for first and second breast cancers tends to be similar.[4,23,29,39,46,54,64,81,83] When differences are reported, there tends to be a suggestion of more favorable histologies in the second breast cancers. Some reports have noted a possible increase in second breast cancers for the favorable histologic subtypes of noninvasive, intraductal carcinoma,[3,4] lobular carcinoma,[3,29,39,54] comedocarcinoma,[46] and intracystic carcinoma.[81]

Very little information is available relative to the status of hormone receptors in bilateral breast cancer. Holdaway et al.[35] reported the estrogen receptor (ER) status of 64 patients with synchronous and 35 patients with metachronous bilateral breast cancer. For the synchronous group, 58% had both tumors ER positive, 22% had both tumors ER negative, and 20% had one tumor ER positive and one tumor ER negative. For the metachronous group, the respective figures were 40%, 29%, and 31%. There was a significantly increased incidence of both tumors being ER positive in the synchronous group ($p<.001$), and the authors suggested that these findings were consistent with a hormonal influence on the development of bilateral breast cancer. In contrast, there was a significantly increased incidence of discordant estrogen receptors (i.e., one tumor ER positive and one tumor ER negative) for patients with metachronous carcinomas ($p<.025$), which was associated with a change in the histologic tumor type. The authors suggested that these findings inferred different mechanisms of induction for patients with synchronous vs. metachronous bilateral carcinoma. Kiang et al.[40] reported the estrogen receptor status of 11 patients with synchronous bilateral breast cancer and seven patients with metachronous bilateral breast cancer. For the synchronous group, 73% had both tumors ER positive, 18% had both tumors ER negative, and 9% had one tumor ER positive and one tumor ER negative. For the metachronous group, the respective figures were 0%, 29%, and 71%. Kiang et al.[40] suggested that these findings were consistent with a hormonal influence on the development of synchronous bilateral breast cancer, but not metachronous bilateral breast cancer. Alexander et al.[3] reported higher mean progesterone receptor levels for the second tumor as compared to the first tumor for 24 metachronous lesions (56 vs. 30, respectively) and 14 synchronous tumors (104 vs. 50, respectively). However, the estrogen receptors were similar for the metachronous lesions (48 vs. 54, respectively) and the synchronous lesions (92 vs. 95, respectively). Lesser et al.[47] reported that the estrogen receptor status for the first breast cancer was positive in 63% (64/102) of patients, borderline positive in 6% (6/102), and negative in 31% (32/102).

FOLLOW-UP FOR PATIENTS PRESENTING WITH UNILATERAL CARCINOMA OF THE BREAST

Patients presenting with unilateral carcinoma of the breast are at significant risk for the development of a metachronous contralateral breast cancer over

Table 19-10 The effect of the use of tamoxifen in the management of the first breast cancer on the development of a metachronous contralateral breast cancer

Author	Total no. pts.	Endpoint measured	Contralateral breast cancer (%) No tamoxifen	Tamoxifen	p value
Berte et al.[12]	606	Crude incidence	2.0 (4/198)	0.7 (3/408)	.32
	992	Actuarial incidence at 2 yr	0.8	0.4	.41
Breast Cancer Trials Committee[14]	1312	Crude incidence (first recurrence)	2.2 (14/651)	1.2 (8/661)	Not stated
Cuzick and Baum[18]	Not stated	Actuarial incidence at 3 yr	2.6*	0.4*	.05
Fisher et al.[27]	2644	Crude incidence	2.2 (29/1326)	1.0 (13/1318)	.0089
Horn and Thompson[37]	556	Adjusted odds ratio	—	—	0.9 (0.1-5.3)†
Nielson et al.[57]	84	Not stated	—	—	Not significant

*Estimated from curves.
†Adjusted odds ratio (95% confidence interval).

time (see Tables 19-1 and 19-2). The risk of developing a metachronous contralateral breast cancer over time is approximately 0.75% per year of follow-up (see Table 19-2). Therefore careful follow-up of patients with unilateral carcinoma of the breast is essential for the early diagnosis of a metachronous contralateral breast cancer. The components of a follow-up program for the early detection of a metachronous contralateral breast cancer include breast self-examination,[23,38,49,51,70,82] periodic examination of the patient by the physician,[49,51,54,55,64,70,71,78,82] and periodic mammography.[16,23,38,49,51,54,55,64,70-72,76-78,82]

To detect a metachronous contralateral breast cancer, current recommendations for follow-up of patients treated for unilateral carcinoma of the breast include yearly mammography. Patients are advised to perform monthly breast self-examination. Follow-up examination by the physician is performed at 3- to 4-month intervals for the first 3 years of follow-up, at 6-month intervals in years 4 and 5, and at 6- to 12-month intervals thereafter. These recommendations are for asymptomatic patients; symptomatic patients require prompt workup as indicated. The follow-up schedule in the asymptomatic patient can be modified based on clinical parameters, and patients potentially at higher risk should be followed more carefully.

PREVENTION OF METACHRONOUS CONTRALATERAL BREAST CANCER

Recent interest has focused on the possible use of tamoxifen to inhibit the development of breast cancer. Table 19-10 summarizes six studies that have evaluated the influence of tamoxifen in the treatment of a first breast cancer on the development of a metachronous contralateral breast cancer. Four of the studies reported a reduction in the incidence of contralateral breast cancers with the use of tamoxifen,[12,14,18,27] and in two of these studies, the reduction was statistically significant.[18,27] These studies suggest that the use of tamoxifen might be associated with a reduction in the risk of contralateral breast cancer. However, further studies are necessary before concluding that tamoxifen can be used routinely as a preventive agent, either for a first breast cancer or a second breast cancer. In this regard it is interesting that the report by Horn and Thompson from the Connecticut Tumor Registry also showed a reduction in the risk of contralateral breast cancer with the use of chemotherapy, particularly alkylating agents.[37]

REFERENCES

1. Adair F, Berg J, Joubert L, and Robbins GF: Long-term followup of breast cancer patients: the 30-year report, Cancer 33:1145, 1974.
2. Adami H-O, Bergstrom R, and Hansen J: Age at first primary as a determinant of the incidence of bilateral breast cancer: cumulative and relative risks in a population-based case-control study, Cancer 55:643, 1985.
3. Alexander AI, Mercer RJ, Muir IM, et al: Predicting survival in bilateral breast carcinoma, Aust NZ J Surg 59:35, 1989.
4. Al-Jurf AS, Jochimsen PR, Urdaneta LF, and Scott DH: Factors influencing survival in bilateral breast cancer, J Surg Oncol 16:343, 1981.
5. Anderson DE: Genetic study of breast cancer: identification of a high risk group, Cancer 34:1090, 1974.
6. Anderson DE and Badzioch MD: Bilaterality in familial breast cancer patients, Cancer 56:2092, 1985.
7. Bailey MJ, Royce C, Sloane JP, et al: Bilateral carcinoma of the breast, Br J Surg 67:514, 1980.

8. Baker RR and Kuhajda FP: The clinical management of a normal contralateral breast in patients with lobular breast cancer, Ann Surg 210:444, 1989.
9. Basco VE, Coldman AJ, Elwood JM, and Young MEJ: Radiation dose and second breast cancer, Br J Cancer 52:319, 1985.
10. Bedwinek JM, Perez CA, Kramer S, et al: Irradiation as the primary management of Stage I and II adenocarcinoma of the breast: analysis of the RTOG breast registry, Cancer Clin Trials 3:11, 1980.
11. Berge T and Ostberg G: Bilateral carcinoma of the female breast, Acta Chir Scand 140:27, 1974.
12. Berte E, Buzdar AU, Smith TL, and Hortobagyi GN: Bilateral primary breast cancer in patients treated with adjuvant therapy, Am J Clin Oncol 11:114, 1988.
13. Bodian C and Haagensen CD: Bilateral carcinoma of the breast. In Haagensen CD, editor: Diseases of the breast, ed 3, Philadelphia, WB Saunders Co, 1986, pp 440-461.
14. Breast Cancer Trials Committee: Adjuvant tamoxifen in the management of operable breast cancer: the Scottish trial, Lancet ii:171, 1987.
15. Chaudary MA, Millis RR, Bulbrook RD, and Hayward JL: Family history and bilateral primary breast cancer, Breast Cancer Res Treat 5:201, 1985.
16. Chaudary MA, Millis RR, Hoskins EOL, et al: Bilateral primary breast cancer: a prospective study of disease incidence, Br J Surg 71:711, 1984.
17. Chu AM, Cope O, Russo R, and Lew R: Patterns of local-regional recurrence and results in stages I and II breast cancer treated by irradiation following limited surgery: an update, Am J Clin Oncol 7:221, 1984.
18. Cuzick J and Baum M: Tamoxifen and contralateral breast cancer, Lancet ii:282, 1985 (letter).
19. de Mascarel I, Trojani M, Coindre JM, and Faucher A: The incidence of cancer in contralateral reduction mammoplasty after mastectomy and reconstruction of the removed breast, Tumori 72:183, 1986.
20. de Ustaran JK and Meiss RP: Primary synchronous bilateral breast cancer: epidemiological approach, Breast Cancer Res Treat 12:311, 1988.
21. Devitt JE: Bilateral mammary cancer, Ann Surg 174:774, 1971.
22. Donegan WL and Perez-Mesa CM: Lobular carcinoma—an indication for elective biopsy of the second breast, Ann Surg 176:178, 1972.
23. Egan RL: Bilateral breast carcinomas: role of mammography, Cancer 38:931, 1976.
24. Farrow JH: Bilateral mammary cancer, Cancer 9:1182, 1956.
25. Fenig J, Arlen M, Livingston SF, and Levowitz BS: The potential for carcinoma existing synchronously on a microscopic level within the second breast, Surg Gynecol Obstet 141:394, 1975.
26. Finney GG, Finney GG, Montague ACW, et al: Bilateral breast cancer, clinical and pathological review, Ann Surg 175:635, 1972.
27. Fisher B, Costantino J, Redmond C, et al: A randomized clinical trial evaluating tamoxifen in the treatment of patients with node-negative breast cancer who have estrogen-receptor-positive tumors, N Engl J Med 320:479, 1989.
28. Fisher B, Redmond C, Fisher ER, et al: Ten-year results of a randomized clinical trial comparing radical mastectomy and total mastectomy with or without radiation, N Engl J Med 312:674, 1985.
29. Fisher ER, Fisher B, Sass R, et al: Pathologic findings from the National Surgical Adjuvant Breast Project (Protocol No. 4). XI. Bilateral breast cancer, Cancer 54:3002, 1984.
30. Fracchia AA, Robinson D, Legaspi A, et al: Survival in bilateral breast cancer, Cancer 55:1414, 1985.
31. Hankey BF, Curtis RE, Naughton MD, et al: A retrospective cohort analysis of second breast cancer risk for primary breast cancer patients with an assessment of the effect of radiation therapy, J Natl Cancer Inst 70:797, 1983.
32. Harris JR and Hellman S: The results of primary radiation therapy for early breast cancer at the Joint Center for Radiation Therapy. In Harris JR, Hellman S, and Silen W, editors: Conservative management of breast cancer: new surgical and radiotherapeutic techniques, Philadelphia, 1983, JB Lippincott, pp 47-52.
33. Harvey EB and Brinton LA: Second cancer following cancer of the breast in Connecticut, 1935-82, Natl Cancer Inst Monogr 68:99, 1985.
34. Hislop TG, Elwood JM, Coldman AJ, et al: Second primary cancers of the breast: incidence and risk factors, Br J Cancer 49:79, 1984.
35. Holdaway IM, Mason BH, Bennett RC, et al: Estrogen receptors in bilateral breast cancer, Cancer 62:109, 1988.
36. Holmberg L, Adami HO, Ekbom A, et al: Prognosis in bilateral breast cancer. Effects of time interval between first and second primary tumours. Br J Cancer 58:191, 1988.
37. Horn PL and Thompson WD: Risk of contralateral breast cancer: associations with histologic, clinical, and therapeutic factors, Cancer 62:412, 1988.
38. Kesseler HJ, Grier WRN, Seidman I, and McIlveen SJ: Bilateral primary breast cancer, JAMA 236:278, 1976.
39. Khafagy MM, Schottenfeld D, and Robbins GF: Prognosis of the second breast cancer: the role of previous exposure to first primary, Cancer 35:596, 1975.
40. Kiang DT, Kennedy BJ, and Snover DC: Biological and histological characteristics of simultaneous bilateral breast cancer, Lancet ii:1105, 1980.
41. King RE, Terz JJ, and Lawrence W: Experience with opposite breast biopsy in patients with operable breast cancer, Cancer 37:43, 1976.
42. Kopelson G, Munzenrider JE, Doppke K, and Wang CC: Bilateral breast cancer: radiation therapy results and technical considerations, Int J Radiat Oncol Biol Phys 7:335, 1981.
43. Lawson R: Mammary cancer—the other breast, Can Med Assoc J 73:676, 1955.
44. Leis HP: Bilateral breast cancer, Surg Clin North Am 58:833, 1978.
45. Leis HP: Managing the remaining breast, Cancer 46:1026, 1980.
46. Leis HP, Mersheimer WL, Black MM, and De Chabon A: The second breast, NY State J Med 65:2460, 1965.
47. Lesser ML, Rosen PP, and Kinne DW: Multicentricity and bilaterality in invasive breast carcinoma, Surgery 91:234, 1982.
48. Lewis TR, Casey J, Buerk CA, and Cammack KV: Incidence of lobular carcinoma in bilateral breast cancer, Am J Surg 144:635, 1982.
49. Lewison EF: The follow-up examination of the contralateral breast: from the viewpoint of the surgeon, Cancer 23:809, 1969.
50. Lewison EF and Neto AS: Bilateral breast cancer at the Johns Hopkins Hospital: a discussion of the dilemma of contralateral breast cancer, Cancer 28:1297, 1971.
51. Martin JK, van Heerden JA, and Gaffey TA: Synchronous and metachronous carcinoma of the breast, Surgery 91:12, 1982.
52. McCarty KS, Kesterson GHD, Wilkinson WE, and Georgiade N: Histopathologic study of subcutaneous mastectomy specimens from patients with carcinoma of the contralateral breast, Surg Gynecol Obstet 147:682, 1978.
53. McCredie JA, Inch WR, and Alderson M: Consecutive primary carcinomas of the breast, Cancer 35:1472, 1975.

54. Michowitz M, Noy S, Lazebnik N, and Aladjem D: Bilateral breast cancer, J Surg Oncol 30:109, 1985.
55. Moffat FL, Ketcham AS, Robinson DS, et al: Breast cancer: management of the opposite breast, Oncology 2:25, 1988.
56. Mueller CB and Ames F: Bilateral carcinoma of the breast: frequency and mortality, Can J Surg 21:459, 1978.
57. Nielsen M, Christensen L, and Andersen J: Contralateral cancerous breast lesions in women with clinical invasive breast carcinoma, Cancer 57:897, 1986.
58. Parker RG, Grimm P, and Enstrom JE: Contralateral breast cancers following treatment for initial breast cancers in women, Am J Clin Oncol 12:213, 1989.
59. Pomerantz RA, Murad T, and Hines JR: Bilateral breast cancer, Am Surg 55:441, 1989.
60. Pressman PI: Bilateral breast cancer: the contralateral breast biopsy, Breast: Diseases of the Breast 5:29, 1979.
61. Prior P and Waterhouse JAH: Incidence of bilateral tumours in a population-based series of breast-cancer patients. I. Two approaches to an epidemiological analysis, Br J Cancer 37:620, 1978.
62. Prior P and Waterhouse JAH: The incidence of bilateral breast cancer. II. A proposed model for the analysis of coincidental tumours, Br J Cancer 43:615, 1981.
63. Ringberg A, Palmer B, and Linell F: The contralateral breast at reconstructive surgery after breast cancer operation—a histopathological study, Breast Cancer Res Treat 2:151, 1982.
64. Robbins GF and Berg JW: Bilateral primary breast cancers: a prospective clinicopathological study, Cancer 17:1501, 1964.
65. Sarrazin D, Le MG, Arriagada R, et al: Ten-year results of a randomized trial comparing a conservative treatment to mastectomy in early breast cancer, Radiother Oncol 14:177, 1989.
66. Schell SR, Montague ED, Spanos WJ, et al: Bilateral breast cancer in patients with initial stage I and II disease, Cancer 50:1191, 1982.
67. Schenker JG, Levinsky R, and Ohel G: Multiple primary malignant neoplasms in breast cancer patients in Israel, Cancer 54:145, 1984.
68. Schottenfeld D and Berg J: Incidence of multiple primary cancers. IV. Cancers of the female breast and genital organs, J Natl Cancer Inst 46:161, 1971.
69. Schwartz AG, Ragheb NE, Swanson GM, and Satariano WA: Racial and age differences in multiple primary cancers after breast cancer: a population-based analysis, Breast Cancer Res Treat 14:245, 1989.
70. Sears HF, Janus C, McDermott A, and Grotzinger P: Bilateral breast carcinoma: prospective evaluation of factors assisting diagnosis, J Surg Oncol 32:203, 1986.
71. Senofsky GM, Wanebo HJ, Wilhelm MC, et al: Has monitoring of the contralateral breast improved the prognosis in patients treated for primary breast cancer? Cancer 57:597, 1986.
72. Shellito JG and Bartlett WC: Bilateral carcinoma of the breast, Arch Surg 94:489, 1967.
73. Slack NH, Bross IDJ, Nemoto T, and Fisher B: Experiences with bilateral primary carcinoma of the breast, Surg Gynecol Obstet 136:433, 1973.
74. Solin LJ, Fowble BL, Schultz DJ, and Goodman RL: Bilateral breast carcinoma treated with definitive irradiation, Int J Radiat Oncol Biol Phys 17:263, 1989.
75. Storm HH and Jensen OM: Risk of contralateral breast cancer in Denmark 1943-80, Br J Cancer 54:483, 1986.
76. Tulusan AH, Ronay G, Egger H, and Willgeroth F: A contribution to the natural history of breast cancer. V. Bilateral primary breast cancer: incidence, risks and diagnosis of simultaneous primary cancer in the opposite breast, Arch Gynecol 237:85, 1985.
77. Urban JA: Bilateral breast cancer, Cancer 24:1310, 1969.
78. Urban JA, Papachristou D, and Taylor J: Bilateral breast cancer: biopsy of the opposite breast, Cancer 40:1968, 1977.
79. van Limbergen E, van den Bogaert W, van der Schueren E, and Rijnders A: Tumor excision and radiotherapy as the primary treatment of breast cancer. Analysis of patient and treatment parameters and local control, Radiother Oncol 8:1, 1987.
80. Veronesi U, Banfi A, Del Vecchio M, et al: Comparison of Halsted mastectomy with quadrantectomy, axillary dissection, and radiotherapy in early breast cancer: long-term results, Eur J Cancer Clin Oncol 22:1085, 1986.
81. Veronesi U, Rilke F, Salvadori B, et al: Bilateral cancer of the breast. In Severi L, editor: Multiple primary malignant tumours: proceedings of the Fifth Perugia Quadrenniel International Conference on Cancer, Perugia, 1973, Division of Cancer Research (Perugia University Medical School), pp 337-343.
82. Wanebo HJ, Senofsky GM, Fechner RE, et al: Bilateral breast cancer: risk reduction by contralateral biopsy, Ann Surg 201:667, 1985.
83. Wilson ND and Alberty RE: Bilateral carcinoma of the breast, Am J Surg 126:244, 1973.

20 Special Considerations

Lawrence J. Solin

PAGET'S DISEASE

The earliest clinical descriptions of Paget's disease were made in 1856 by Velpeau[36] and in 1874 by Paget.[25] Even today, the clinical descriptions of Paget's disease by Velpeau and Paget are accurate.

The incidence of Paget's disease is relatively low, comprising 0.5% to 3.2% of all female breast carcinomas.[1,2,5,8,18,19,22,27] The age at presentation generally is reported as being approximately the same as or slightly older than for other female breast carcinomas.[1,5,13,18-20,22,27,32] Of interest is that Haagensen[13] reported that the mean age at diagnosis for patients with nipple changes only (58 years) was slightly older than for patients presenting with a palpable tumor mass with or without nipple changes (51 years). This difference in the age distribution may suggest a different biology for these two clinical presentations.

The classic pathologic finding in Paget's disease is the so-called Paget cell within the nipple epidermis.[24,28] There continues to be a major controversy surrounding the origin of the Paget cell. Several hypotheses have been proposed to explain the clinical presentations and histologic features of this disease. These hypotheses generally fall into two major categories: (1) Paget's cells represent in situ or intraepidermal malignancy with possible secondary migration to the underlying breast parenchyma; or (2) Paget's cells represent an epidermotrophic migration from an underlying carcinoma to the nipple.[2,5,7,26,28] A number of investigators have used different techniques to attempt to resolve this controversy, including pathologic examination of whole breast specimens,[2,7,8,13,26,33,37] immunohistochemical studies,[2,5,23,37] and immunocytochemical detection of estrogen receptors.[35]

The difference in the two theories of the origin of Paget's disease has great practical implications. For example, if Paget's disease could arise as an intraepidermal process, then there might be selected patients for whom limited excision of the nipple and areola would be curative. Conversely, if Paget's disease could be a manifestation of underlying carcinoma within the breast parenchyma, then limited excision would be an inappropriate surgical procedure, and mastectomy or breast irradiation would be required. This controversy remains unresolved at the present time. It is possible that neither hypothesis explains all cases of Paget's disease, but that each hypothesis might be correct for a subset of patients presenting with Paget's disease. Consistent with this explanation is the observation by Haagensen[13] of a difference in age distribution for patients presenting with vs. without a palpable tumor mass (vide supra).

Mammography is indicated in the evaluation of the patient presenting with Paget's disease of the nipple. Mammography may be useful in identifying an underlying carcinoma seen as a mass or as microcalcifications.[14,15,34] Because there are relatively few cases of Paget's disease, there is relatively little information about the frequency of underlying carcinoma found on mammogram without a palpable mass. Paone and Baker[26] found that xeromammography was positive in five of six such cases. Maier et al.[18] also found that mammography was useful in patients presenting without a palpable mass. However, Edeiken[9] found that mammography was negative in all of nine cases of Paget's disease presenting without a palpable mass.

The clinical presentation for Paget's disease includes a number of symptoms related to the nipple. Such symptoms can include redness, eczemoid changes, crusting, erosion, discharge, retraction, inversion, or irritation.[1,2,18,20,22,26] Haagensen[13] has proposed the subdivision of the clinical presentations of Paget's disease into three groupings: (1) nipple involvement only; (2) nipple involvement plus a palpable tumor mass; and (3) presentation with a breast tumor but with Paget's disease seen on pathologic examination of the mastectomy specimen. Haagensen[13] reported that the incidence of these clinical presentations in 182 patients was 45.7%, 29.6%, and 24.7%, respectively. Most authors reporting large series of cases with Paget's disease generally include patients with clinical presentations of nipple involvement with or without an associated palpable mass, but not mastectomy cases with pathologic findings of Paget's disease. The incidence of patients presenting with a palpable mass generally is reported as approximately 50% to 60%, although the reported range of values is 30% to 80%.[1,2,8,13,18,20,22,27,29]

The standard treatment for patients with Paget's disease of the breast has been mastectomy. The outcome of treatment is related to a number of prognostic variables. The most significant prognostic variables in reported series of mastectomy patients are the presence vs. absence of a palpable mass, the presence vs. absence of associated invasive carcinoma, and the presence vs. absence of pathologically positive axillary lymph nodes. Table 20-1 shows the 5- and 10-year survival outcomes for patients with Paget's disease as a function of the presence vs. absence of a palpable mass and the presence vs. absence of pathologically positive axillary lymph nodes. For Table 20-1, the patients generally were treated with mastectomy, although a small number of patients were treated with other local treatment modalities.

In view of the possibility of Paget's disease presenting as noninvasive ductal carcinoma confined to the nipple, recently there has been interest in breast-conserving surgical procedures with or without definitive breast irradiation.[3,4,10,17,32] The rationale for breast-conserving surgical procedures in Paget's disease is based on observations of the limited extent of noninvasive ductal carcinoma and the low probability of axillary disease in patients without a palpable mass in the breast. There also has been recent interest in breast-conserving surgery and definitive irradiation for noninvasive, intraductal carcinoma in other areas of the breast.[11,31,38]

Fourquet et al.[10] reported a series of 20 patients with Paget's disease who presented without an associated palpable mass and who were treated with definitive irradiation. Before definitive irradiation, three patients underwent excisional biopsy, and 17 patients underwent incisional biopsy. There were three breast failures, all with only Paget's disease, and the 7-year recurrence-free survival rate was 81%. Stockdale et al.[32] reported on the outcome of 28 women treated with definitive radiation for Paget's disease. Nineteen patients had a normal mammogram and no palpable mass, and nine patients had a palpable mass, an abnormal mammography, or no mammography performed. The breast recurrence rate was 16% (3/19) for patients with a normal mammogram and no palpable tumor, but 89% (8/9) for the other patients. Bulens et al.[3] reported the results of treatment of 13 patients with Paget's disease but without an associated mass. All patients were treated with an incisional biopsy and definitive breast irradiation of 6000 to 7000 cGy. With a median follow-up of 52 months, there were no local or distant recurrences. Rissanen and Holsti[27] reported the results of eight patients treated with definitive radiation. The delivered radiation dose was only 1400 to 3100 cGy, which would be considered inadequate for breast irradiation by current standards. In five of six patients treated with excisional biopsy plus irradiation, there was no local recurrence, whereas there was local recurrence in two of two patients treated with incisional biopsy followed by definitive irradiation. Other authors also have reported on the treatment of a small number of patients with definitive irradiation.[1,5,18-20]

There have been reported very limited numbers of patients with Paget's disease treated with excision only, without definitive irradiation.[17-20,26,27] Lagios et al.[17] reported the results of five patients treated with excision only. Only one of the five patients developed a recurrence of Paget's disease at 14 months, and this patient was treated with

Table 20-1 Survival outcome for female patients with Paget's disease of the breast

	Palpable mass				Pathologically positive axillary lymph nodes			
	No		Yes		No		Yes	
Author	5 yr (%)	10 yr (%)	5 yr (%)	10 yr (%)	5 yr (%)	10 yr (%)	5 yr (%)	10 yr (%)
Ascensao et al.[1]	78	—	46	—	83	—	58	—
Ashikari et al.[2]	92	87	42	38	—	—	—	—
Haagensen[13]	—	81	—	54	—	80	—	35
Maier et al.[18]	70	—	38	—	—	—	—	—
Malak and Tapolcsanyi[19]	88	47	73	45	—	—	—	—
Nance et al.[22]	94	—	41	—	—	—	—	—
Paone and Baker[26]	100	100	46*	33	83*	44	25*	10
Rissanen and Holsti[27]	83	75	0	0	—	—	—	—
Salvadori et al.[29]	92	82	38	22	—	—	—	—

*Estimated from curves.

resection of the residual areola. Paone and Baker[26] reported the results of five cases treated with excision only, none of which have had recurrences. In a study of 32 mastectomy specimens, Chaudary et al.[5] found that there was in situ ductal carcinoma in areas other than the subareolar region in 78% (25/32) of the mastectomy specimens for patients presenting with Paget's disease. For patients with intraductal carcinoma in other areas of the breast, Lagios et al.[16] also have reported the results of treatment with excision only, and the incidence of recurrence in the breast was 10% (8/79).

At the present time, mastectomy must be considered the standard treatment for Paget's disease. Too few cases have been treated with either definitive irradiation or excisional biopsy only to justify such treatment as a standard policy. Because of the small number of cases of Paget's disease, it is unlikely that any prospective trial will be mounted to compare mastectomy with definitive irradiation. However, the results of trials of intraductal carcinoma treated with excision with or without definitive irradiation will be of interest, as these results undoubtedly will be extrapolated to the setting of Paget's disease presenting without an associated mass and without associated invasive carcinoma.

There are a number of unusual manifestations of Paget's disease. Such manifestations include Paget's disease of the male breast,[12] a presentation of Paget's disease after subcutaneous mastectomy,[30] clinical presentation with brain metastasis,[6] and a presentation of Paget's disease as the first evidence of recurrence after definitive irradiation for a primary invasive carcinoma of the breast.[21]

AXILLARY LYMPH NODE PRESENTATION

The presentation of a patient with axillary lymphadenopathy but without a detectable primary breast carcinoma is unusual. The incidence of patients with an axillary lymph node presentation is approximately 0.4% of all patients presenting with carcinoma of the breast (Table 20-2).

Clinical presentation

For the patient presenting with an axillary lymph node metastasis from a presumptive breast carcinoma, the age at presentation tends to be similar to all women with carcinoma of the breast. For series that report the age distribution of such patients, the median age at presentation is 46 to 58 years, and most series report the median age at presentation as 54 to 58 years.[40,47,49,52,54,58-60,68] The mean age at presentation is 48 to 58 years.[39,43,46,47,49,52,54,56,58,59,63,64,68,69] The youngest age at presentation in one report was 30 years,[63] and the oldest age at presentation in another report was 90 years.[54] In the report of Copeland and McBride,[44] which included both male and female patients combined, the youngest reported presentation was age 5 years.

Table 20-2 Incidence of breast cancer patients with an axillary lymph node presentation

Author	No. pts. with axillary lymph node presentation/total no. pts.
Baron et al.[40]	35/10014 [0.3]
Fitts et al.[49]	13/1300 [1.0]
Griffith et al.[52]	9/2500 [0.4]
Haagensen[54]	28/8000 [0.4]
Owen et al.[63]	27/5451 [0.5]
Total	112/27265 [0.4]

[ ], % pts.

The duration of symptoms tends to be relatively short. Most patients report symptoms for <6 to 12 months.[52,54,63,69] Haagensen[54] reported the median duration of symptoms as 2 months, and the mean duration of symptoms as 4 months. Westbrook and Gallager[69] reported the mean duration of symptoms as 9.5 weeks. However, there are a few cases reported with duration of symptoms >1 year,[54] or >2 years.[63]

Differential diagnosis

The differential diagnosis for the woman who presents with an axillary lymph node and an unknown primary site can be a challenging problem. The primary site for an adenocarcinoma in the axilla usually is presumed to be the breast, both because this is the most common site and because this is a primary site that is potentially curable. However, when the biopsy of the axillary lymph node shows adenocarcinoma or undifferentiated carcinoma, the differential diagnosis includes carcinoma of the lung, carcinoma of pancreas, carcinoma of the gastrointestinal tract, carcinoma of the thyroid, carcinoma of the ovary, melanoma, lymphoma, germ cell tumor, and renal cell carcinoma.[44,48,58,60,64,65,67] Nonmalignant etiologies for an axillary lymph node presentation also must be considered and include benign inflammatory changes, infection, and tuberculosis.[65] Careful pathologic examination is essential. The biopsy tissue should be evaluated for the presence of hormone receptors. A positive estrogen or progesterone receptor is strongly suggestive of a breast primary tumor.[67] Numerous reports have found positive hormone receptors.[40,41,53,56-58,60] However, negative hormone receptors do not preclude the diagnosis of occult carcinoma of the breast as the primary site. Bhatia et al.[41] reported that the estrogen receptor status from the axillary lymph node was strongly positive in two cases and negative in one case of three cases of occult primary breast carcinomas with positive estrogen receptors that were diagnosed with an axillary lymph node presentation. Electron microscopy and special stains are also frequently useful.[56,58,66,67]

Detection of the occult primary breast carcinoma

Mammography. For the woman who presents with an axillary lymph node but without a palpable mass in the breast, mammography is frequently useful in locating the occult breast carcinoma. The incidence of finding an occult breast lesion on mammography is 0 to 56% (Table 20-3). However, Haupt et al.[56] reported that the finding of a lesion on mammography was not always correlated with the primary carcinoma from the mastectomy specimen. Additionally, two reports noted that carcinoma was not always found within the mastectomy specimen for patients with a positive mammography.[52,64] Notwithstanding the occasional lack of correlation of a primary carcinoma with a positive mammogram, bilateral mammography should be obtained before definitive therapy. A positive mammogram can lead to the definitive diagnosis, and some of these patients might be candidates for breast-preserving treatment.

It is important to recognize that patients with an initially negative mammogram may still have a primary carcinoma of the breast. Patel et al.[64] reported that four breast carcinomas were detected in mastectomy specimens out of nine patients with negative mammograms. Westbrook and Gallager[69] reported that four of the nine patients with initially negative mammograms were found to have positive mammograms on serial examination. Griffith et al.[52] reported that two of four patients with an initially negative mammogram were found to have a breast carcinoma on clinical examination after 6 and 9 months of follow-up, respectively. Bhatia et al.[41] reported the development of a breast recurrence in two patients with initially negative mammograms at 6 and 19 months of follow-up, respectively. Detectable breast recurrences have been reported with prolonged latent periods of 48 months[61] and 64 months.[54]

Pathologic findings from mastectomy specimens. Table 20-4 shows the pathologic findings in the breast in patients who have undergone mastectomy. There are significant differences among the various studies in the use of preoperative mammography as well as in the diligence of the pathologic examination to uncover a primary breast carcinoma. Overall, the predominant finding is that of an occult invasive carcinoma. However, there are significant numbers of patients in whom an occult breast primary carcinoma is not discovered. Additionally, there is a small number of patients in whom the finding of only noninvasive carcinoma is reported. Rosen[66] also reported eight patients with the presentation of axillary lymph node metastasis with occult noninvasive carcinoma of the breast. Possible explanations for the finding of only noninvasive carcinoma include sampling error, metastasis from a contralateral breast cancer, heterotropic glandular tissue, breast tissue within the axillary fat, or the existence of benign lesions that simulate metastatic carcinoma of the breast.[66] Electron microscopy also can be useful in uncovering invasion that is not seen on routine light microscopy.[56,58,66,67]

The location of occult breast carcinomas found on mastectomy has been documented in only a small number of reports (Table 20-5). Overall, 42% of the carcinomas were in the upper outer quadrant of the breast. When cases in which the location of the occult carcinoma was unknown are excluded, 50% (35/70) of the cases were in the upper outer quadrant. There is also a significant number of lesions in the central or subareolar location.

Few series have reported the size of the occult breast carcinomas found in patients who have undergone mastectomy (Table 20-6). Although the size of the occult carcinomas generally were reported as small, 36% of the cases were noted to have tumors ≥1 cm.

The number of pathologically positive lymph

Table 20-3 Incidence of occult breast lesions found on mammography in patients with an axillary lymph node presentation

Author	No. positive/total
Ashikari et al.[39,a]	3/25 [12]
Baron et al.[40,a]	9/34 [26]
Feigenberg et al.[47]	0/7 [0]
Griffith et al.[52]	5[b]/9 [56]
Haupt et al.[56,a]	11[c]/43 [26]
Iglehart et al.[58]	0/5 [0]
Kemeny et al.[60]	1/18 [6]
Montague[62,d]	13[e]/24 [54]
Patel et al.[64]	8[f]/17 [47]
Westbrook and Gallager[69,d]	6/17 [35]

[ ], % pts.
[a]Multiple reports from a single institution.
[b]Only 3/5 positive on pathology.
[c]Not always correlated with carcinoma on pathology.
[d]Multiple reports from a single institution.
[e]Positive on first or subsequent mammograms.
[f]Only 6/8 positive on pathology.

Table 20-4 Pathologic findings in the breast on mastectomy in patients with an axillary lymph node presentation

Author	Total no. pts.	Preoperative mammography	No. positive: Invasive carcinoma	DCIS	LCIS	No. negative
Ashikari et al.[39,a]	34	Yes[b]	20	2	1	11
Baron et al.[40,a]	33[c]	Yes	18	4[d]	—	11
Bhatia et al.[41]	9	Yes	8	1	—	—
Ellerbroek et al.[46,e]	10	Yes[b]	0	0	0	10
Feigenberg et al.[47]	7	Yes	3	—	—	4
Feuerman et al.[48]	10	NS	7	—	—	3
Fitts et al.[49]	13	NS	11	—	—	2
Griffith et al.[52]	5	Yes	5	—	—	—
Haagensen[54]	15	NS	13	1	—	1
Iglehart et al.[58]	5	Yes	5	—	—	—
Kaplan and Reinstine[59]	4	NS	3	—	—	1
Kemeny et al.[60]	11	Yes	3	1	1	6
Montague[62,e]	16	Yes[b]	10	2	—	4
Owen et al.[63]	37	NS	25	—	—	12
Patel et al.[64]	29	Yes[b]	16[f]	—	—	13
Westbrook and Gallager[69,e]	8	Yes[b]	6	1	—	1

DCIS, ductal carcinoma in situ; LCIS, lobular carcinoma in situ; NS, not stated.
[a]Multiple reports from a single institution.
[b]Preoperative mammography obtained in some, but not all of the patients.
[c]Includes five patients with quadrantectomy specimens.
[d]Includes DCIS and LCIS combined.
[e]Multiple reports from a single institution.
[f]Includes all positive cases.

nodes in the axilla is shown in Table 20-7. Overall, 40% of the patients have four or more positive axillary lymph nodes; this is slightly higher than the percentage of node-positive patients with a primary breast cancer and four or more positive axillary lymph nodes found on axillary dissection for mastectomy or for breast-conserving surgery and definitive irradiation. Fitts et al.[49] reported that the distribution of the number of positive axillary lymph nodes was more favorable for patients with an occult carcinoma of the breast than for patients with a nonoccult carcinoma of the breast. Ashikari

Table 20-5 Location of occult carcinomas in the breast found on mastectomy in patients with an axillary lymph node presentation

Author	Total no. pts.	Location of occult carcinoma: UOQ	UIQ	LOQ	LIQ	Central or subareolar	Other	Unknown
Ashikari et al.[39]*	7	5	1	—	—	1	—	—
Fitts et al.[49]	11	3	—	—	2	1	2†	3
Haagensen[54]	13	4	2	1	1	3	1‡	1
Haupt et al.[56]*	17	11	1	3	—	2	—	—
Owen et al.[63]	20	6	—	—	—	9	—	5
Patel et al.[64]	16	6	1	3	—	1	—	5
Total	84	35 (42%)	5 (6%)	7 (8%)	3 (4%)	17 (20%)	3 (4%)	14 (17%)

UOQ, upper outer quadrant; UIQ, upper inner quadrant; LOQ, lower outer quadrant; LIQ, lower inner quadrant.
*Multiple reports from a single institution.
†1 in upper central and 1 in outer lateral location.
‡1 in upper central location.

Table 20-6 Size of occult carcinomas in the breast found on mastectomy in patients with an axillary lymph node presentation

Author	Total no. pts.	<1 cm	1-2 cm	>2 cm
Ashikari et al.[39]	23	*	*	*
Bhatia et al.[41]	9	4	3	2
Fitts et al.[49]	11	5	5	1
Iglehart et al.[58]	5	3	2	—
Kemeny et al.[60]	5	3	1	1
Owen et al.[63]	25	20	5	—
Total†	55	35 (64%)	16 (29%)	4 (7%)

*Approximately 1/3 for each size grouping.
†For evaluable series only.

et al.[39] reported the highest level of axillary lymph node involvement as level I in 21% (6/28), level II in 46% (13/28), and level III in 32% (9/28) of the cases.

Treatment

The outcome of treatment from multiple series is shown in Table 20-8. Because of the small number of patients in each series, various forms of treatment have been utilized, including various types of mastectomy, mastectomy plus preoperative or postoperative irradiation, definitive irradiation, and occasionally, adjuvant systemic therapy. The 5-year and 10-year actuarial survival rates are 52% to 82% and 42% to 71%, respectively. These 5- and 10-year survival rates are generally similar to the reported outcomes for pathologically node-positive primary breast cancer patients. However, some authors have suggested that the outcome of treatment for the patient with an axillary lymph node presentation possibly may be more favorable than for the patient presenting with a primary breast carcinoma and pathologically positive axillary lymph node metastases.[43,48,49,54,60,69] Although the Haagensen criteria defined the patient with a primary breast carcinoma and a lymph node >2.5 cm as inoperable, the patient presenting with an axillary lymph node without a primary breast carcinoma was defined as inoperable only if the lymph node was not movable, even if the size of the axillary lymph node was >2.5 cm.[54] Fitts et al.[49] reported that the distribution of number of positive axillary lymph nodes was more favorable for patients with an occult carcinoma than for patients with a nonoccult carcinoma, and they suggested that this more favorable distribution inferred a more favorable prognosis.

Although the predominant mode of treatment for the patient with an axillary lymph node presentation is mastectomy with or without adjuvant radio-

Table 20-7 Number of positive axillary lymph nodes in patients with an axillary lymph node presentation

		No. positive axillary lymph nodes			
Author	Total no. pts.	1	2-3	≥4	Unknown
Bhatia et al.[41]	11	—	3	7	1
Fitts et al.[49]	11	6	2	3	—
Haagensen[54]	28	4	6	11	7
High and Watne[57]	2	1	—	1	—
Iglehart et al.[58]	5	5	—	—	—
Kaplan and Reinstine[59]	4	1	1	—	2
Kemeny et al.[60]	11	2	2	7	—
Patel et al.[64]	29	11	4	11	3
Weinberger and Stetten[68]	5	3	1	1	—
Westbrook and Gallager[69]	11	3	2	6	—
Total	117	36 (31%)	21 (18%)	47 (40%)	13 (11%)

Table 20-8 Outcome of treatment for breast cancer patients with an axillary lymph node presentation

Author	Total no. pts.	5-yr survival		10-yr survival	
		Actuarial (%)	Crude (%)	Actuarial (%)	Crude (%)
Ashikari et al.[39]*	34	—	56	—	38
Baron et al.[40]*	35	75	—	55	—
Campana et al.[43]	31	76	—	71	—
Ellerbroek et al.[46]†	35	68	—	64	—
Feigenberg et al.[47]	7	69	29	—	—
Fitts et al.[49]	13	82	54	—	—
Haagensen[54]	28	52	39	42	18
Kemeny et al.[60]	18	67	22	—	—
Owen et al.[63]	18	—	50	—	50
Weinberger and Stetten[68]	5	—	40	—	—
Westbrook and Gallager[69]†	18	62	33	—	—

*Multiple reports from a single institution.
†Multiple reports from a single institution.

therapy or systemic therapy, there is a small number of cases reported of treatment with definitive irradiation and breast conservation.[40,47,54,59,62,69] Campana et al.[43] reported on 31 patients with an axillary lymph node presentation. Of the 31 patients, 30 were treated with breast radiotherapy, and one patient was treated with mastectomy. The recurrence rate in the breast was 23% (7/30), and four of the seven breast recurrences were isolated breast recurrences without nodal recurrences. Ellerbroek et al.[46] reported on 35 patients with an axillary lymph node presentation. Mastectomy was performed in 10 patients, and the breast was preserved in 25 patients. Local recurrence was 12% (2/16) with breast irradiation, but 56% (5/9) without breast irradiation.

In view of the limited number of patients reported and the variety of treatments employed, it is difficult to make firm recommendations regarding the optimal management of the patient with an axillary lymph node presentation. Most authors have recommended mastectomy as the treatment of choice.[48,49,54,56,57,59,64,68,69] Three series have reported no difference in the survival rates of patients treated with mastectomy compared to patients treated without mastectomy.[40,46,60] However, the number of patients in these reports was small. More recently, some authors have recommended breast conservation and definitive irradiation.[43,44,46,62] However, with the exception of the reports by Campana et al.[43] and Ellerbroek et al.,[46] there is minimal information about the outcome of treatment with definitive irradiation as an alternative to mastectomy. Additionally, the size of the occult carcinomas found in the breast at mastectomy reveals 36% as being ≥1 cm (Table 20-6). The dose of radiotherapy generally recommended for the definitive treatment of the whole breast in this situation is 5000 cGy,[62] and this dose is unlikely to control disease which is gross rather than microscopic.[50,51] In the report of Campana et al.,[43] the dose delivered to the midpoint of the breast was 6200 cGy (range = 5500 to 8800 cGy). The failure rate in the breast of 23% as reported by Campana et al.[43] is not inconsistent with the expected failure rate that is based on the inability to control occult, gross tumors within the breast (Table 20-6).

Our current approach to the management of the patient with an axillary lymph node presentation is to perform an axillary lymph node biopsy. Estrogen and progesterone receptor analysis is performed on the tissue. In conjunction with other specialized tests such as special stains or electron microscopy as indicated, careful pathologic examination frequently will give supporting evidence for a primary breast carcinoma and exclude other histologies and sites of primary disease. A metastatic survey is performed in the same manner as for the patient presenting with a known primary breast carcinoma. This consists of bilateral mammography, chest x-ray, bone scan, and serum liver function tests. If the lymph node histology is consistent with a primary breast carcinoma, a comprehensive radiologic search for a primary site other than the breast generally is not performed. Mastectomy and axillary lymph node dissection are performed as the initial therapeutic maneuver. Mastectomy is utilized to avoid the potential risk of breast irradiation in the setting of occult, gross disease (Table 20-6) and to attempt to identify a primary breast carcinoma pathologically (see Table 20-4). It has not been our policy to perform breast conservation and definitive irradiation in this setting. Adjuvant postoperative radiotherapy and systemic chemotherapy or hormonal therapy are added as indicated, based on the pathology findings from mastectomy. A secondary approach to the management of the axillary lymph node presentation is to perform a complete, not limited, axillary dissection plus definitive breast irradiation.

Contralateral axillary lymph node metastasis

While an axillary lymph node presentation in the de novo patient is unusual, it is important to recognize that the development of a contralateral axillary lymph node metastasis in the patient with a known primary carcinoma of the breast is not uncommon. Devitt and Michalchuk[45] reported the development of a contralateral axillary lymph node metastasis in 3.6% (52/1440) of women with carcinoma of the breast, and 1.3% (18/1440) developed a contralateral axillary lymph node metastasis as the site of first recurrence. Haagensen[55] estimated that 4% of his patients developed a contralateral axillary lymph node metastasis. Breslow[42] reported that 0.4% (6/1543) of patients who had previously been treated with mastectomy developed a contralateral axillary lymph node metastasis without evidence of other metastatic disease. On mastectomy, four of the six patients were found to have a primary breast carcinoma in the contralateral breast, and two of the mastectomy specimens showed no evidence of breast cancer. As three of the patients were alive without evidence of disease at 8 to 14 years of follow-up, Breslow[42] recommended mastectomy for the patient presenting with an isolated contralateral lymph node metastasis.

BREAST CANCER AND PREGNANCY

Breast cancer associated with pregnancy presents the clinician with difficult management problems. The optimal management of the patient with breast cancer and the optimal management of the pregnancy frequently involve opposing considerations. Therefore, the patient and her physicians often are faced with the challenging and difficult task of considering the effects of diagnostic or therapeutic interventions on these two different processes. Frequently, the breast cancer or the pregnancy must be managed in a manner that is suboptimal because of the competing demands of the other condition. Difficult choices must be made in weighing various potential diagnostic and therapeutic options when there are no perfect solutions.

The diagnosis of breast carcinoma in pregnancy represents a twofold problem for the patient. Not only is she faced with the difficulties of treatment of a breast carcinoma, but the patient also is faced with the prospect of possibly losing her pregnancy as well. The optimal choice of treatment for the breast cancer frequently raises the issue of therapeutic abortion, and such a decision only can be made by the patient in conjunction with religious and ethical considerations.

If abortion is not required, the management of the breast cancer may have to be modified to account for possible effects on the fetus. The physician faced with the treatment of breast cancer in pregnancy may be required to limit the diagnostic or therapeutic interventions in order to minimize the risk of spontaneous abortion or congenital malformations.

Hormonal and immunologic changes

There are a large number of hormonal changes that take place in the pregnant patient. Such changes include major alterations in estrogens, progesterones, corticosteroids, and prolactin.[84,86,99] Such changes may influence hormonally dependent breast cancers. Further, elevated hormone levels may give false-negative levels of measured estrogen and progesterone receptors secondary to saturation of binding sites.[95,128] Although the hormonal dependence of breast carcinomas on estrogen and progesterone is well recognized, Hobbs et al.[93] reported that 39% of all breast carcinomas also are prolactin dependent.

Pregnancy is a condition that is associated with immunosuppression.[84,85,86,99,112,128] Pregnancy also is associated with a short-term increased risk of a new breast cancer.[74,100] Janerich[100] has proposed that the immunotolerance associated with pregnancy may be the etiology for this transient increase in breast cancer risk by the tolerance of the immune system of the patient for nonpatient antigens.

Incidence

The incidence of breast cancer in pregnancy is low when considered relative to all breast carcinomas or to all pregnancies. However, the magnitude of the problem of breast cancer associated with pregnancy is increased when one considers only premenopausal or younger patients.

The overall incidence of breast carcinoma associated with pregnancy in multiple series ranges from 0.2% to 3.8%.[71,76,77,85,98,114,117,119-121,125,128,130,132] Two literature reviews found that the incidence of breast carcinoma associated with pregnancy was 2.8% and 2.9% of all breast carcinomas, respectively.[131,133] A number of studies has estimated the risk of breast carcinoma as a function of the total number of pregnancies. The risk of breast carcinoma per pregnancy has been estimated as 1 in 3300,[77] 10 to 39 in 100,000,[128] 1 in 3000,[85] 3 in 10,000,[130-132] and 2.2 in 10,000.[125]

When the incidence of breast carcinoma associated with pregnancy is considered as a function only of patients at risk (i.e., premenopausal patients or younger patients), the risk becomes much more significant. Ribeiro and Palmer[117] found that 2.8% of all breast carcinomas in women ≤45 years of age were associated with pregnancy. Nugent and O'Connell[110] found that 11% of all breast carcinomas in women <40 years of age were associated with pregnancy. Peters[114] found that 15% of all premenopausal patients with breast carcinoma were associated with pregnancy. Treves and Holleb[127] noted that 20% of all women <35 years of age with breast carcinoma had an associated pregnancy. In women ≤45 years of age, Applewhite et al.[71] found that 8% of all breast cancers were associated with pregnancy. Horsley et al.[98] found that 25% of breast carcinomas in women ≤35 years of age were associated with pregnancy. These studies suggest that the incidence of breast carcinoma associated with pregnancy in the premenopausal patient or younger patient is substantial.

Clinical presentation

Patient age at diagnosis for breast carcinoma associated with pregnancy is lower than for the overall population of patients with breast carcinoma as all pregnant patients are premenopausal by definition. The mean age at presentation in numerous series was between 29 and 38 years.[71,75,76,78,89,90,102,110,113,119-121,128] The median age at presentation was between 33 and 38 years.[96,113,126] The youngest reported patient age at diagnosis of breast cancer associated with pregnancy was 17 years.[76] The oldest reported age for a patient with breast cancer associated with pregnancy was 48 years.[75]

The diagnosis of breast cancer in pregnant patients tends to be delayed. In a number of reported series, the mean interval from symptoms to diagnosis was 1.4 to 13 months.[71,76,79,90,102,117,119,121,126] In two studies, the interval to diagnosis was reported as being longer than that for other breast cancer patients.[71,90] Only the study of Clark and Reid[80] did not find a significant delay in diagnosis of the patient with breast cancer associated with pregnancy. The relative infrequency of the diagnosis in breast carcinoma with associated pregnancy, the young age of the patients, and the difficulty of breast examination during pregnancy commonly are cited as causes of the delay in diagnosis. A number of benign breast diseases can mimmick carcinoma during pregnancy.[76,77,105,118]

The presentation of bilateral breast carcinoma associated with pregnancy is quite rare. However, bilateral breast carcinoma at presentation has been reported in multiple series.[80,119,121] A contralateral breast carcinoma also has been reported following an initial breast carcinoma associated with pregnancy.[90,96] The risk of developing a contralateral breast cancer obviously is related to the prognosis of the initial breast cancer. However, as these patients are all young, the risk period for development of a contralateral breast cancer can be quite long, particularly if the patient has a favorable prognosis for the first breast carcinoma.

Clinical and pathologic staging

Table 20-9 shows a summary of the reported series with clinical staging of patients presenting with breast cancer in pregnancy or lactation. Although there are some differences in the staging systems, these reports generally show significantly increased percentages of advanced-stage patients when compared with the distribution of all breast cancer patients. Unusual clinical presentations that have been described include inflammatory breast

Table 20-9 Clinical staging for patients presenting with breast cancer in pregnancy or lactation

Author	Staging system	Pregnancy or lactation	Total no. pts.	Clinical stage (%) I	II	III	IV
Bunker and Peters[75]	Not stated	P, L	62	26	29	35	10
Chiedozi et al.[79]	UICC 1980	P, L	36	0	17	53	30
Greene and Leis[89]	T, N, M	P, L	65	42	32	18	8
Haagensen[90]	Columbia (A, B, C, D)	P, L	59	46	20	19	15
Ribeiro and Palmer[117]	UICC 1968	P, L	88	11	56	23	10
Rissanen[119]	UICC 1960	P, L	33	15	30	40	15
Sahni et al.[121]	T, N, M	P, L	18	17	11	11	61
Tretli et al.[126]	Norwegian Cancer Registry	P, L	35	26	43	17	14

P, pregnancy; L, lactation; UICC, Union Internationale Contre le Cancer (International Union against Cancer).

Table 20-10 Pathologic axillary lymph node staging for patients presenting with breast cancer in pregnancy or lactation

Author	Pregnancy or lactation	Total no. pts.	Pathologic axillary lymph nodes			
			Negative		Positive	
			No.	%	No.	%
Applewhite et al.[71]	P, L	33	9	27	24	73
Bunker and Peters[75]	P, L	50	20	40	30	60
Byrd et al.[76]	P, L	29	11	38	18	62
Cheek[78]	P	14	3	21	11	79
Deemarsky and Neishtadt[82]	P, L	91	30	33	61	67
Greene and Leis[89]	P, L	65	27	42	38	58
Haagensen[90]	P, L	39	17	44	22	56
Holleb and Farrow[96]	P, L	117	31	26	86	74
King et al.[102]	P	63	24	38	39	62
Rissanen[119]	P, L	33	8	24	25	76
White and White[133]	P, L	37	12	32	25	68
Total		571	192	34	379	66

P, pregnancy; L, lactation.

cancer[126,131,134] and bilateral breast cancer.[80,119,121] Metastatic carcinoma of the breast to the placenta has been described.[115]

The results of pathologic axillary lymph node staging for patients presenting with breast cancer in pregnancy or lactation has been reported in a large number of series (Table 20-10). The incidence of positive axillary lymph nodes reported ranges from 56% to 79%. On average, approximately two thirds of patients present with positive axillary lymph nodes; this figure is more than double the expected incidence for all patients presenting with breast cancer.

The interval to diagnosis of carcinoma of the breast in the pregnant or lactating patient is long and has been reported as being longer than that for all patients with breast carcinoma (vide supra). The more advanced presentation as evidenced by clinical staging and pathologic nodal staging may be caused by this delay.

Only a few series have reported the findings from estrogen and progesterone receptor analysis of breast cancers associated with pregnancy or lactation (Table 20-11). Overall, only 31% of the estrogen receptors and 24% of the progesterone receptors were positive. Even though younger women are known to have a lower incidence of positive estrogen and progesterone receptors, the incidence in pregnant patients is still lower than expected. It is possible that the elevated hormonal levels associated with pregnancy may be associated with false-negative estrogen and progesterone receptors because of saturation of binding sites.[95,128] A more reliable assessment of the estrogen and progesterone receptor status in pregnant women is obtained with immunohistochemical techniques.

Table 20-11 Estrogen and progesterone receptor assays for patients presenting with breast cancer in pregnancy or lactation

Author	Pregnancy or lactation	No. pts. with positive estrogen receptors/total	No. pts. with positive progesterone receptors/total
Geggie[88]	P, L	2/11 [18]	2/11 [18]
Holdaway et al.[95]	P	0/3 [0]	0/2 [0]
	L	3/3 [100]	2/3 [67]
Nugent and O'Connell[110]	P	4/14 [29]	— —
Wallack et al.[128]	P, L	4/11 [36]	1/5 [20]
Total		13/42 [31]	5/21 [24]

P, pregnancy; L, lactation; [ ], % pts.

Risks to the fetus

Radiologic studies. The radiologic evaluation of the patient with breast cancer in pregnancy must consider the risk of radiation to the fetus. The risk to benefit ratio of diagnostic studies must be weighed carefully for the potential benefit to the patient and for the potential risk to the fetus. Judgment on the part of the physician as well as significant input by the patient are required to balance these potentially competing factors. Frequently, no course of action is ideal. Further, many of the risks to the fetus are only estimates based on limited information or theoretical concerns.

The risk to the fetus from radiation depends upon the gestational age, the total dose, and the dose rate.[72,73,91,106,108,112,124,128] During the stage of preimplantation and implantation (approximately the first 2 weeks of pregnancy) significant radiation exposure is generally lethal. The stage of organogenesis usually occurs from the third through the tenth week, and significant radiation exposure during this period generally results in malformations of major organ systems. Radiation exposure after the stage of organogenesis can result in a number of more subtle abnormalities such as growth retardation, sterility, cytogenetic abnormalities, behavioral disorders, and tumor induction. The estimated radiation dose to the fetus from commonly performed staging studies includes 1 to 8 mrad from a chest x-ray,[108,112] 99 to 180 mrad from a 15 mCi bone scan,[128,129] and 14 to 21 mrad from a liver-spleen scan.[128] Should there be any doubt as to the dose to the fetus from a diagnostic or therapeutic radiation exposure, the dose can be calculated or estimated from phantom measurements.[108,128]

Although the risk of complications from radiation rises with the dose, the indications for abortion are not well established. In the reviews by Brent,[72,73] therapeutic abortion from radiation exposure was found not to be indicated for a dose of ≤5 rad. In the review of Wallack et al.,[128] therapeutic abortion was recommended for a dose of ≥10 rad during organogenesis. A number of review articles have discussed the issue of radiation exposure in detail.[72,73,91,108,112,124,128]

Although mammography is indispensible in the nonpregnant patient, mammography in the pregnant patient poses a number of problems. The changes in the breast during pregnancy and lactation make breast imaging and interpretation difficult.[77,82,84,94] The increased tissue density can obscure malignancies. The radiation exposure to the fetus from mammography is low (<10 mrad).[108] Ultrasound may be useful in evaluating mass lesions of the breast during pregnancy.[77]

Surgery and anesthesia. Diagnostic surgical procedures of aspiration cytology or needle biopsy can be performed with local anesthetics. When a patient is to undergo general anesthesia (e.g., for mastectomy), there are a number of considerations. There are physiologic changes associated with pregnancy that affect the optimal delivery of anesthesia.[112,128] Although there are theoretical concerns about the possible teratogenic effects of anesthetic agents on the fetus, the risk is greatest during the first trimester of pregnancy, and there is probably little risk in the second and third trimesters.[85,128] General anesthesia can be delivered safely during pregnancy for mastectomy.[112,128] The risk of abortion from general anesthesia for mastectomy is approximately 1% or less.[85,128]

Chemotherapy. There are significant fetal risks associated with the use of systemic chemotherapy for the treatment of breast cancer, particularly during the first trimester of pregnancy. The risk of fetal malformations associated with systemic cytotoxic chemotherapy administered during the first trimester of pregnancy has been reported as 11.6% to 12.7% in literature reviews.[107,122,124] The risk of congenital malformations is highest for antimetabolites such as methotrexate or aminopterin.[83,107,109,116,122,124] The risk of congenital malformations associated with the use of chemotherapy during the first trimester of pregnancy has been estimated as being five times greater than normal.[122] The use of chemotherapy during the second and third trimesters of pregnancy has not been associated with an increased risk of congenital malformations, but the number of reported cases is small.[83,87,107,122,124] Delayed effects of chemotherapy exposure in utero have been described.[87,111] Spontaneous abortion also has been associated with the administration of chemotherapy during pregnancy, particularly during the first trimester.[83,101,107,123]

Recommendations for work-up and treatment

General guidelines. Recommendations for workup and treatment for the management of breast cancer presenting during pregnancy or lactation must be based on a multitude of factors, including the presentation of the breast cancer, the stage of pregnancy, and the wishes of the patient. Often, the optimal management of the breast cancer in the mother directly conflicts with the optimal management of the pregnancy. Because of the difficulty in weighing the various medical considerations, the patient must play a significant role in the management of both the breast cancer and the pregnancy.

For the management of breast cancer associated with pregnancy, only general work-up and treatment guidelines can be given (Table 20-12). However, it must be emphasized strongly that the work-up and treatment for each patient presenting with

Table 20-12 General guidelines for the work-up and treatment of breast cancer during pregnancy

	Stage of pregnancy					
	Early stage			Late stage		
Stage of breast cancer	Breast cancer work-up	Breast cancer treatment	Management of the fetus	Breast cancer work-up	Breast cancer treatment	Management of the fetus
Stage I and stage II	Bilateral vs. unilateral mammogram,† CXR,‡ bone scan, LFTs, CBC	1. Mastectomy 2. Breast-conserving surgery and definitive RT§	No abortion (abortion required only if chemotherapy or radiation therapy indicated)	Bilateral vs. unilateral mammogram,† CXR,‡ bone scan, LFTs, CBC	1. Mastectomy* 2. Breast-conserving surgery and delayed definitive RT*	No abortion
Stage III (nonmetastatic)	Bilateral vs. unilateral mammogram,† CXR,‡ bone scan, LFTs, CBC	Combined modality therapy‖ as indicated	Abortion usually required	Bilateral vs. unilateral mammogram,† CXR,‡ bone scan, LFTs, CBC	Combined modality therapy‖ as indicated	Abortion as indicated
Stage IV (metastatic)	As indicated	As indicated (usually systemic chemotherapy or hormonal therapy)	Abortion as indicated	As indicated	As indicated (usually systemic chemotherapy or hormonal therapy)	Abortion as indicated

RT, radiation therapy; CXR, chest x-ray; CBC, complete blood count; LFTs, serum liver function tests.
*Consider also giving chemotherapy if indicated.
†Consider single view mammography only. Ipsilateral mammography not required if patient to undergo mastectomy.
‡Consider single PA view only.
§Definitive RT given after abortion or delayed definitive RT given after delivery of full-term pregnancy.
‖Combined modality therapy of chemotherapy, radiation therapy, and/or surgery.

breast cancer in pregnancy be individualized as each patient will present with a unique set of considerations relative to the stage of breast cancer and to the stage of pregnancy. Therefore, the guidelines in Table 20-12 must be considered within the context of each individual patient's presentation.

Stages I and II. The workup for clinical stage I and stage II breast cancer should be reasonably complete because of the need to confirm the early stage of the disease. Obviously, a positive finding on metastatic survey or a positive finding in the contralateral breast on mammography will strongly alter the management of the patient. The estimated dose to the fetus from various radiologic studies previously has been described (see above discussion on radiologic studies). In order to minimize the radiation exposure to the fetus, consideration should be given to the use of a single posterioanterior (PA) chest x-ray, as opposed to a PA and lateral chest x-ray, as well as to single-view mammography as opposed to conventional double-view mammography. Mammography of the ipsilateral breast is not indicated if the patient is to be treated with mastectomy. A single PA chest x-ray without the lateral view may be sufficient if the PA view is normal. Although bone scan generally is required, in selective cases the bone scan may be omitted. For example, a patient with a small microinvasive carcinoma and a normal serum alkaline phosphatase level may not require a bone scan. While the radiation dose to the fetus from a bone scan is dependent on the stage of pregnancy and the dose of radioactive tracer used for the bone scan (see above discussion on radiologic studies), the risk to benefit ratio is generally in favor of obtaining a bone scan for the patient with an invasive breast carcinoma when balanced against the radiation exposure to the fetus. For the treatment of stage I or stage II invasive carcinoma of the breast, mastectomy generally has been recommended.[82,85,86,90,96,97,99,102,103,114,125,128]

Therapeutic abortion is not recommended routinely in the absence of other indications for abortion, as therapeutic abortion has not been associated with an improvement in survival (see discussion on results below).[70,75,82,85,86,96,97,99,102,110,117,119,125,130,133] Because of the survival advantage with adjuvant systemic chemotherapy in certain subsets of breast cancer patients following mastectomy, therapeutic abortion generally is indicated in patients presenting with early pregnancies who also require adjuvant systemic chemotherapy.[102,110,117,128] Alternatively, for patients who do not wish to undergo abortion, consideration could be given to delaying adjuvant systemic chemotherapy until the later stages of pregnancy, during which an increased risk of congenital malformation has not been documented. In patients requiring adjuvant systemic therapy who present in late stages of pregnancy, consideration could be given to delaying chemotherapy until after the completion of pregnancy.[102,110,117] For the patient who has undergone a mastectomy, adjuvant postoperative radiotherapy should be delivered based on the same considerations as for the nonpregnant patient. However, the adjuvant radiotherapy should be delayed until after delivery or abortion of the fetus.

In the pregnant patient who presents with an early-stage breast cancer and who is a candidate for breast-conserving surgery and definitive irradiation as an alternative to mastectomy, consideration could be given to performing the breast-conserving surgery during pregnancy and delaying the definitive irradiation until after delivery.[103,104] However, it must be remembered that a significant delay (i.e., ≥7 weeks) in starting definitive radiation treatments following breast-conserving surgery is associated with an increased rate of local failure, although not with a disadvantage in terms of survival. In particular, a suitable candidate for definitive breast irradiation who presents in the late stages of pregnancy reasonably could be treated with breast-conserving surgery during pregnancy, with a delay of the definitive breast irradiation until after term delivery; there would be a reasonable expectation of local control.

Stage III (nonmetastatic). The work-up for the patient who presents with a locally advanced, nonmetastatic stage III carcinoma of the breast generally requires a complete evaluation beause of the high risk of disseminated disease. Chest x-ray and bone scan usually are required in this setting to screen for metastatic disease. Additionally, ipsilateral mammography may be required to evaluate the extent of disease and as a baseline to measure response to further therapy. However, ipsilateral mammography is not required if the determination has been made that the patient will undergo mastectomy.

The treatment of stage III, nonmetastatic breast cancer is usually with combined modality therapy. Therapeutic abortion generally is indicated for advanced disease because of the need to deliver systemic chemotherapy and/or therapeutic radiation.[70,85,96,102,103,110,117,128] However, for selected patients presenting with stage III breast cancer during the later stages of pregnancy, therapeutic abortion could be avoided if systemic chemotherapy is delayed until the later stages of pregnancy. Therapeutic radiation should be postponed until after delivery or abortion because of the high radiation dose to the fetus.

Stage IV (metastatic). The work-up of the patient with metastatic disease during pregnancy should proceed only up to the point that there is clearly documented evidence of metastatic spread of the breast carcinoma. Therefore, selective studies for metastatic disease could be eliminated in the presence of other clearly defined evidence of metastatic disease. The required staging evaluation is dependent on whether the patient is found to have unsuspected metastatic disease or presents with symptoms suspicious for metastatic disease. Although the asymptomatic patient may be found on routine staging to have metastatic disease, the patient with symptoms can have a more limited and directed work-up based on the symptoms. For example, a patient who presents with pulmonary metastatic disease based on a positive chest x-ray obtained for pulmonary symptoms (e.g., cough or shortness of breath) might not be required to have a bone scan during pregnancy to document further evidence of metastatic disease, but can have the remaining staging studies done after abortion or delivery.

The treatment of metastatic, stage IV breast cancer is generally dependent on patient symptoms. In the asymptomatic patient who does not require immediate therapy, abortion is not required, and the patient might be allowed to continue to term delivery. However, as there are significant hormonal changes associated with pregnancy, the termination of pregnancy may have significant antitumoral effects that must be considered in view of metastatic disease. If systemic chemotherapy is indicated during the early stages of pregnancy, then therapeutic abortion is required, but abortion may not be required if systemic chemotherapy is necessary during the later stages of pregnancy. Although local-regional management of the breast and regional lymph nodes generally does not require mastectomy or radiation therapy for patients with metastatic disease, abortion is indicated when therapeutic breast irradiation is required because of the high radiation dose that will be delivered to the fetus.

Results of treatment

The outcome of treatment at 5 and 10 years by clinical stage is shown in Table 20-13. There were relatively few patients reported in each of the series, and there were significant differences between the studies with regards to staging systems used and overall treatment policies. However, the results suggest that the survival rates at 5 and 10 years are less than those for all women with breast cancer when compared on a stage by stage basis.

A number of studies have compared the results of treatment in pregnant vs. nonpregnant patients directly. Although some series have reported the survival rates as being no different between these two groups,[80,89,110] most series suggest that the probability of survival is less for the pregnant patient.[71,79,90,114,126,127,132] Haagensen[90] reported that the survival for Columbia stage A pregnant patients was 63% at 10 years, as compared to 72% at 10 years for his nonpregnant patients. The number of pregnant patients with Columbia stage B, stage C, and stage D was too small to evaluate. In a matched pair analysis, Tretli et al.[126] found that there was a significantly decreased survival rate ($p<.05$) for the pregnant patients as compared to two sets of matched controls. Although the survival rate was also lower for the patients with carcinoma presenting in lactation, the difference between the pa-

Table 20-13 Five- and 10-year survival rates for patients presenting with breast cancer in pregnancy or lactation

Author	Staging system	Pregnancy or lactation	Total no. pts.	Survival by clinical stage (%) I 5 yr	I 10 yr	II 5 yr	II 10 yr	III 5 yr	III 10 yr	IV 5 yr	IV 10 yr
Bunker and Peters[75]	Not stated	P, L	62	69	—	28	—	32	—	0	—
Greene and Leis[89]	T, N, M	P, L	65	71*	48*	71*	48*	20	0	—	—
Haagensen[90]	Columbia (A, B, C, D)	P, L	59	—	63	—	33	—	27	—	0
King et al.[102]	AJC 1978	P	63	73	—	52	—	25	—	8	—
Peters[114]	Not stated	P, L	187	60	—	39	—	18	—	0	—
Ribeiro and Palmer[117]	UICC 1968	P, L	88	90	90	37	21	15	10	0	0
Rissanen[119]	UICC 1960	P, L	33	80	80	80	78	15	22	0	0

P, pregnancy; L, lactation; AJC, American Joint Committee; UICC, Union Internationale Contre le Cancer (International Union against Cancer).
*Stages I and II combined.

tients with breast cancer presenting in lactation as compared with two groups of case controls did not achieve statistical significance. Peters[114] also showed that patients presenting with breast cancer in pregnancy had a worse survival rate compared with matched controls. Treves and Holleb[127] found that there was a difference in survival rates for pregnant patients with operable breast cancer for the node-negative group (5-year survival rates of 50% vs. 60%), but not for the node-positive group (20% vs. 21%). In summary, the bulk of the evidence suggests that the breast cancer associated with pregnancy does confer a survival disadvantage independent of other factors.

The strongest prognostic factors for outcome of treatment in breast cancers associated with pregnancy are stage (Table 20-13) and pathologic axillary lymph node status.[71,75,80-82,90,102,127] In addition to stage and axillary lymph node status, Haagensen[90] suggested that tumor grade and histology of the tumor were prognostic factors.

The use of a therapeutic abortion in most studies is not associated with an improvement in survival.[75,82,96,102,117,119,130,133] However, the number of patients reported with therapeutic or spontaneous abortions is generally quite small. In a group of 31 total patients of all stages, Rissanen[119] reported that the 5-year survival rate in patients with an abortion was 38%, compared to 43% in patients without an abortion. In a group of 24 patients, Holleb and Farrow[96] found that the 5-year survival rate was improved in patients who delivered normally as opposed to patients with an abortion (33% vs. 17%). However, Clark and Reid[80] found that patients with a therapeutic abortion did markedly worse than patients with a live birth, with 10-year survival rates of 8% vs. 23%, respectively; patients with a spontaneous abortion had a 10-year survival rate of 38%. King et al.[102] found that the 5-year survival rate of 21 patients who underwent therapeutic abortion was 43% vs. 59% for patients whose pregnancy resulted in delivery at or near term. In summary, although the numbers of reported patients is quite small, the literature suggests that there is no benefit to a therapeutic abortion. Therefore, in the absence of other diagnostic or therapeutic considerations, therapeutic abortion in the pregnant patient is not indicated for management of the breast cancer.

For patients presenting with breast cancer during pregnancy, the outcome of pregnancy rarely is reported. Table 20-14 summarizes those reports that give the outcome of pregnancies for patients presenting with breast cancer during pregnancy. A substantial number of patients had live deliveries (57% to 97%). There were significant differences in the number of patients who underwent therapeutic abortions (0 to 33%), which reflects the differences in treatment philosophies and patient wishes in the various series. Relatively few patients had a spontaneous abortion (1% to 12%) or a stillborn child or a child that died perinatally (0 to 5%).

The prognostic significance of the timing of the presentation of breast cancer as related to the stage of pregnancy remains controversial. Based on small numbers, there is some suggestion that breast cancer presenting in the first trimester or first half of pregnancy, compared to later stages of pregnancy, is associated with an improved outcome,[75,80,114,131] but this observation has not been shown in all studies.[117] Breast cancer occurring in the postpartum period may be associated with an improved rate of survival.[75,80,131]

Pregnancy after a previously treated breast cancer

In the younger patient who previously has been treated for a breast cancer, the issue frequently is raised as to when the patient may become pregnant.

Table 20-14 Outcome of pregnancies for patients presenting with breast cancer during pregnancy

		Outcome of pregnancy							
		Live delivery		Stillborn or perinatal death		Spontaneous abortion		Therapeutic abortion	
Author	Total no. of pregnancies	No.	%	No.	%	No.	%	No.	%
Bunker and Peters[75]	68	63	93	—	—	1	1	4	6
Chiedozi et al.[79]	36	35	97	—	—	1	3	—	—
Clark and Reid[80]	121	93	77	1	1	14	12	13	11
King et al.[102]	63	36	57	3	5	3	5	21	33
Ribeiro and Palmer[117]	88	73	83	2	2	1	1	12	14
Total	376	300	80	6	2	20	5	50	13

It is well established that the risk of recurrence is highest in the first few years after treatment and that the risk of recurrence decreases over time. Therefore, some authors have recommended a delay before pregnancy of some arbitrarily defined number of years corresponding to the period of highest risk. The recommended time before pregnancy has been suggested by various authors as 1 year,[114] 2 years,[102,103,110,120] or 3 to 5 years.[86,97] A number of authors have suggested that patients should be counseled differently for this delay based on the prognosis of the breast cancer, and that patients with node-positive or unfavorable breast cancers should delay pregnancy for a longer period than patients with node-negative or favorable breast cancers.[78,90]

Very little information is available about the effects of a subsequent pregnancy in a patient who has been previously treated for breast cancer. Approximately 7% of fertile women treated for breast cancer will have a subsequent pregnancy.[86] However, a subsequent pregnancy does not seem to have a deleterious effect on these women. Ribeiro and Palmer[117] compared 40 breast cancer patients with a subsequent pregnancy to 120 matched controls and found no difference in rates of survival ($p = .40$), with a follow-up of up to 14 years. Harvey et al.[92] found that the 10-year relapse-free survival rate was 80% for node-negative patients and 79% for node-positive patients. Peters[114] found that the outcomes of 96 patients with a subsequent pregnancy were better than for a group of 96 matched controls (55% vs. 27% at 10 years). In a literature review, White[131] found that the survival rate of patients with a subsequent pregnancy was no different than that of patients without a subsequent pregnancy. In a matched pair analysis, Cooper and Butterfield[81] found no statistically significant difference for patients with a subsequent pregnancy compared to patients without a subsequent pregnancy when matched for stage and pathologic nodal status. Some authors have suggested that the favorable outcome of breast cancer patients with a subsequent pregnancy is from the selection of favorable cases without recurrence.[75,84,86,96,133] There is probably no beneficial effect of therapeutic abortion in this setting.[96]

MALE BREAST CANCER

Incidence

Breast cancer is a relatively uncommon disease in men. The annual incidence is 0.7 per 100,000.[145] Male breast cancer constitutes 0.2% of all cancers in men.[202]

The annual number of newly diagnosed male breast cancer patients is slightly less than 1% of that reported for female breast cancer. The Surveillance, Epidemiology, and End Results (SEER) program[202] reported the relative male to female incidence as 0.9%. The range of values reported in various series is 0.5% to 3.2%.[137,159,166,179,186,193,197,200]

Risk factors

A large number of risk factors have been described for male breast cancer. A common pathway for many of these risk factors is consistent with a hormonal imbalance from elevated estrogens. Risk factors in this category include testicular injury, mumps orchitis, high environmental temperatures with presumed secondary testicular injury, conditions associated with elevated prolactin levels (e.g., certain drugs, brain concussions, and skull fractures), and elevated body weight with presumed secondary elevated estrogen levels.[141,176,178] Other risk factors include a prior history of irradiation,[141,142,157,171,178] family history of male or female breast cancer,[141,170,178,201] and cancer family syndrome.[157,170,201] The risk of breast cancer in males from irradiation or family history appears to be analogous to female breast cancer. Other possible risk factors that have been described include Jewish religion,[176] prior military service,[176] and prior inguinal hernia.[178]

A history of gynecomastia or swollen breast remains controversial as a risk factor for male breast cancer; both positive[172,176,178,189] and negative[141,196] studies have been reported. Gynecomastia may be difficult to determine by history. Nuttall[177] reported that palpable gynecomastia is a common finding in normal men and increases with age. Of men aged 40 to 59 years, 51% were found to have palpable gynecomastia.[177]

Klinefelter's syndrome has been associated with male breast cancer,[150,179,190,196] and patients with Klinefelter's syndrome should be screened for male breast cancer. Reports of male breast cancer have included patients with Klinefelter's syndrome. In a study by van Geel et al.,[196] the chromosomal pattern in 11 patients was evaluated, three of whom were found to have abnormalities: two with Klinefelter's syndrome (XXY) and one male hermaphrodite (XX). Scheike et al.[190] found Klinefelter's syndrome in nine out of 242 patients in a literature review. The risk of male breast cancer associated with Klinefelter's syndrome was estimated to be 20 times that in normal men and one fifth of the risk of breast cancer in females.[190]

Exogenous estrogen administration has been associated with the development of male breast cancer. Symmers[195] reported the development of male breast cancer in two 30-year-old transsexual patients, both approximately 5 years after the sex change operation. These two cases are more remarkable in view of the rarity of male breast cancer at age 30. Pritchard et al.[182] reported a case of the development of breast cancer in a 45-year-old transsexual who had received 10 years of oral estrogens. Case reports also have been documented of male breast cancer developing after the administration of estrogens for prostate cancer.[164,172,191] However, the risk of the development of male breast cancer while on estrogens for prostate cancer is thought to be small. Liechty et al.[172] reported that only one patient of 3000 patients with carcinoma of the prostate treated with estrogen therapy developed breast cancer. Holleb et al.[164] reported the results of a questionnaire in which only two cases of breast cancer were found in 17,000 cases of prostate cancer treated with estrogens.

Dao and Greiner[146] reported a study showing the importance of unopposed estrogens on the induction of breast cancer in male rats. Breast cancer developed in 16% of the rats with an ovarian graft but which had not been castrated whereas breast cancer developed in 66% of the rats with an ovarian graft but which had been castrated. These results suggested that the male breast cancer was induced by the ovarian estrogens and that the risk was increased when the estrogens were unopposed by the normal male androgen production (i.e., in the castrated rats).

Abnormal estrogen metabolism has been documented in men with breast cancer.[140,147,150] Dao et al.[147] found that urinary excretion of endogenous estrogens in seven male breast cancer patients was significantly increased as compared with controls. Calabresi et al.[140] found that the plasma estrogen levels in 17 male breast cancer patients were significantly elevated as compared to controls. However, Scheike et al.[188] found that the metabolism of estradiol-17β was not different in men with breast cancer as compared to men with other malignancies or healthy men.

El-Gazayerli and Abdel-Aziz[151] found that male breast cancer comprised 6.8% of all breast cancers in a study from Eqypt. It was postulated that the increased incidence of male breast cancer in Egypt was caused by hyperestrogenism secondary to bilharzial liver fibrosis.

Lloyd et al.[173] suggested a possible viral association for male breast cancer. In that study, 89% of male breast cancers showed murine mammary tumor virus or related antigen positivity, but there was only a 28% positivity for female breast cancers.

Clinical presentation

The predominant clinical finding in patients with male breast cancer is a lump in the breast. The clinical presentation of a lump in the breast has been reported in 71% to 100% of patients in various series.[143,159,163,166,172,183,186,197,200] Only the study by Erlichman et al.[152] reported a relatively low incidence (43%) of patients presenting with a breast mass. Other reported presentations include nipple retraction, nipple ulceration, skin ulceration, and eczema.[143,152,159,160,163,166,172,183,186,197,201] Pain is a relatively uncommon presentation, found in 2% to 16% of patients in various series.[152,160,166,172,183,186,201] Nipple discharge is also a relatively infrequent presentation.[152,159,160,163,164,166,172,186,197,200] However, the symptom of discharge, particularly bloody discharge, should make the clinician highly suspicious of an underlying carcinoma.[143,160,164] Male breast cancer is occasionally an incidental finding on routine physical examination,[166,186] and general physical examinations should include a breast examination, particularly in older males or males at high risk.

As the most common clinical presentation is a lump in the breast, the differential diagnosis for male breast cancer is most commonly gynecomastia.[143,160,164] Mammography can be useful in distinguishing gynecomastia from carcinoma.[149,168,169] Secondary signs of carcinoma, such as ulceration, pectoral muscle fixation, nipple discharge, or the presence of palpable axillary lymph nodes can help to distinguish between gynecomastia and male breast carcinoma. Although the incidence of male breast carcinoma increases with age,[145,154,166,186] the incidence of gynecomastia also increases with age.[177] Bilaterality favors gynecomastia, although rare cases of bilateral breast carcinoma have been reported.[143,164,166,179,186,194,200,201] The incidence of bilateral carcinoma of the male breast is reported as 0.6% to 3.6%.[143,164,166,179,194,200,201]

The incidence of male breast cancer increases with age. Male breast cancer rarely is reported before age 30. The Third National Cancer Survey[145] reported no cases of male breast cancer in patients <30 years of age. However, there have been a number of reported cases between ages 20 and 29 years,[143,152,159,166,179,183,185,193,196,200,201] and the youngest reported case is at age 5 years.[143]

The age at presentation for male breast cancer is slightly older than that for female breast cancer. On average, male breast cancer patients present approximately 5 to 10 years later in age than female breast cancer patients. The reported median age for presentation of male breast cancer is 59 to 66 years in multiple series.[139,152,166,179,185,193,197,201] The mean age for presentation of male breast cancer has been reported as 52 to 69 years in multiple series.[135,137,139,143,159,166,172,183,185,186,193,196,197,200]

Because of the rarity of diagnosis of male breast cancer, the duration of symptoms before diagnosis tends to be relatively long. The mean duration of symptoms is reported in a number of series as 4 to

17 months.[143,160,166,172,196,197] Symptoms were present for >1 year in 25% to 43% of patients,[166,186,196] and >2 years in 11% to 27% of patients.[166,186,197]

The work-up for male patients with breast cancer is similar to that for female patients with breast cancer. All patients should have bilateral mammography. Mammography can be useful in distinguishing gynecomastia from carcinoma.[149,168,169] The metastatic survey should include a chest x-ray, a bone scan, a complete blood count, and serum liver function tests. Other studies that may be useful include chromosome analysis for the detection of Klinefelter's syndrome[150,179,190,196] and a determination of estrogen metabolism.[140,147,150]

The pathology of breast cancer in males is similar to breast cancer in females, in that the majority of cases are invasive ductal carcinoma.[143,152,159,165,196,197] Although the number of invasive carcinomas other than ductal reported in men is small, the distribution approximates that for female breast cancer. Cases of Paget's disease of the nipple in men have been reported.[139,144,158,160,165,172,192,194,198] Although it has been stated that lobular carcinoma does not exist in men,[143,165,179,198] a small number of cases of lobular carcinoma have been reported.[156,197]

The clinical stage at presentation for male patients with breast carcinoma is shown in Table 20-15. The number of patients presenting with stage I or stage II disease ranges from 38% to 70%. These series are not directly comparable in view of the differences in staging systems used. Although approximately half of the patients present with stage I or stage II disease, there are a substantial number of patients presenting with locally advanced, nonmetastatic disease. Breast cancer might more often present in men with locally advanced disease as such breast cancers can involve chest wall or skin early in the clinical course because of the relatively small breast size.

Treatment

The management of breast cancer in men with surgery, radiotherapy, and adjuvant systemic therapy has been based mainly on extrapolation of information from female breast cancer patients. Although radical mastectomy has been abandoned as the surgical procedure of choice for breast cancer in women, radical mastectomy still is utilized widely for male breast cancer patients, based on the anatomic differences between the male and female breast as well as the historical data supporting the use of radical mastectomy for breast cancer in men.

The historical mainstay of the surgical management of male breast cancer patients has been the radical mastectomy.[160,165,183,185,196] The rationale for radical mastectomy is the small size of the male breast and the proximity of the tumor to the skin and to the underlying chest wall. In some cases, skin grafting may be required to close the surgical mastectomy defect.[143,160,165,167,194,197] Simple and modified radical mastectomies also have been utilized for management.[148,152,159,163,167,179,183,187,194,197] However, for most series in which multiple types of mastectomy were utilized, the criteria for selection of each type of mastectomy is not clear. It seems likely that only earlier lesions were treated with less than radical mastectomy. There is a trend in more recent literature to utilize less radical surgical procedures with or without postoperative radiotherapy when adequate surgical resection of the primary tumor can be accomplished.[148,183,185]

The outcome of treatment in most series is not related to the type of mastectomy performed. However, in all of these series, case selection undoubtedly influenced the type of procedure performed. Hultborn et al.[167] found that there was no difference in 10-year survival rate as a function of the type of local treatment (radical mastectomy, modified radical mastectomy, simple mastectomy, or local excision). Ribeiro[183] reported no significant differ-

Table 20-15 Clinical stage at presentation for male breast cancer patients

			Clinical stage (%)			
Author	**Total no. pts.**	**Clinical staging system**	**I**	**II**	**III**	**IV**
Haagensen[160]	62	Columbia (A, B, C, D)	55	11	5	29
Hultborn et al.[166]	122*	UICC (1978)	10	43	36	11
Ribeiro[183]	301	UICC (1968)	38	21	26	15
Scheike[187]	253	UICC (1968)	35	11	42	12
Siddiqui et al.[193]	13	UICC (1982)	23	15	0	62
Spence et al.[194]	79*	Manchester (1977)	38	32	20	10
van Geel et al.[196]	104	UICC (1982)	25	35	24	16

UICC, Union Internationale Contre le Cancer (International Union against Cancer).
*Includes only patients with known staging and excludes patients with unknown staging.

ence for local recurrence in patients treated with radical mastectomy vs. simple mastectomy and postoperative radiotherapy. Erlichman et al.[152] found that postoperative radiotherapy did not impact on survival rates at 10 years, but there was a significantly reduced local relapse rate in patients treated with postoperative radiotherapy. In a direct comparison of radical mastectomy vs. modified radical mastectomy, Ouriel et al.[179] found no difference in rates of 5-year survival for modified radical mastectomy (80% survival at 5 years) vs. radical mastectomy (75% survival at 5 years). Liechty et al.[172] found that the survival rate in node-negative patients was better with simple mastectomy, but the survival rate in node-positive patients was better with radical mastectomy. Scheike[187] reported that the 5-year survival rate was not different for simple mastectomy vs. radical mastectomy and that the rate of local-regional recurrence was not different for patients treated with mastectomy alone vs. mastectomy and postoperative radiotherapy. All of the studies cited were retrospective analyses, and surgical treatments undoubtedly were based on individual patient selection. As the number of male patients with breast cancer is small, it is unlikely that there will be any prospective, randomized trials on which to base treatment recommendations. However, the literature suggests that appropriately selected patients need not undergo radical mastectomy but could be managed with modified radical mastectomy or simple mastectomy plus postoperative radiotherapy. Robison and Montague[185] have recommended the use of adjuvant postoperative radiotherapy after mastectomy because breast cancers in male patients are predominantly central in location.

The pathologic axillary lymph node findings from mastectomy are shown in Table 20-16 for cases in which axillary staging was performed. The rate of pathologically positive axillary lymph nodes is 36% to 60%, which is substantially higher than the rate of axillary nodal positivity for female breast cancer patients. In the report of Hultborn et al.,[166] the axillary lymph nodes also were evaluated for extracapsular extension, and extracapsular extension was found in 72% of the positive axillary lymph nodes.

There are anecdotal case reports of patients treated with lumpectomy and radiotherapy as primary management.[148,167,183,193] Because of the small number of cases in each series, insufficient information is available to comment on the outcome of such treatment. Long-term control has been reported anecdotally with this method of treatment.[148]

A number of recent reports have recommended the use of adjuvant systemic therapy for selected male breast cancer patients after mastectomy.[138,139,152,183] This is based on the data from breast cancer in females showing improvement in survival with adjuvant systemic therapy for selected subsets of patients. Bagley et al.[138] reported on the results of adjuvant chemotherapy for pathologically node positive male breast cancer patients following radical or modified radical mastectomy. A regimen of cyclophosphamide, methotrexate, and 5-fluorouracil (CMF) was given for 12 cycles. Only four of 24 patients had recurrences, and the 5-year actuarial survival rate was approximately 90%. Ribeiro[183] has utilized adjuvant tamoxifen for patients with pathologically positive axillary lymph nodes or T3a lesions, and there was an improvement in survival rates with adjuvant tamoxifen as compared to historical controls.

Prognosis and survival

Long-term outcomes of treatment have been reported in a number of series. The 5-, 10- , and 15-year outcomes by stage are shown in Table 20-17. There were differences among the series for staging. Also, the patients within each study were

Table 20-16 Pathologic axillary lymph node staging in male breast cancer patients

Author	Total no. pts.	Node-negative No.	Node-negative %	Node-positive No.	Node-positive %
Erlichman et al.[152]	59	24	41	35	59
Haagensen[160]	25	16	64	9	36
Holleb et al.[165]	82	36	44	46	56
Hultborn et al.[166]	91	48	53	43	47
Liechty et al.[172]	29	14	48	15	52
Ouriel et al.[179]	38	18	47	20	53
van Geel et al.[196]	53	21	40	32	60
Vercoutere et al.[197]	43	24	56	19	44
Total	420	201	48	219	52

Table 20-17 Outcome of treatment by clinical stage for male breast cancer patient

			Survival (%)											
			Stage I			Stage II			Stage III			Stage IV		
Author	Total no. pts.	Clinical staging system	5 yr	10 yr	15 yr	5 yr	10 yr	15 yr	5 yr	10 yr	15 yr	5 yr	10 yr	15 yr
Haagensen[160]	25	Columbia (A, B, C, D)	—	55	—	—	33	—	—	0	—	—	0	—
Hultborn et al.[167]	166	UICC (1978)	89*	71*	—	75*	53*	—	42*	27*	—	0*	0*	—
Ouriel et al.[179]	50	AJC (1983)†	80	57	—	67	52	—	25	—	—	0	—	—
Ribeiro[183]	292	UICC (1968)	85*	68*	63*	58*	44*	44*	28*	5*	5*	5*	—	—
Scheike[187]	253	UICC (1968)	58	38	—	38	10	—	29	9	—	4	0	—
van Geel et al.[196]	101	UICC (1982)	67	28	—	58	33	—	63	23	—	13	—	—

UICC, Union Internationale Contre le Cancer (International Union against Cancer); AJC, American Joint Committee.
*Survival outcomes estimated from curves.
†Pathologic stage, not clinical stage.

Table 20-18 Prognostic factors correlating with outcome for male breast cancer patients

Prognostic factors	References
Pathologic axillary lymph node status	152, 159, 160, 167, 172, 196, 201
Stage	160, 167, 179, 183, 187, 196
Tumor size	152, 167, 179, 187, 201
Skin involvement	179, 196
Ulceration	201
Age	
Yes	135, 167
No	136
Nationality	135
Pathology of the primary tumor	
Yes	159, 160
No	196
Grade of the primary tumor	167, 187

treated by nonuniform methods; the type of mastectomy, use of adjuvant radiotherapy, and use of adjuvant tamoxifen all varied. However, survival is clearly stage related. Long-term survival of 10 or 15 years is very uncommon for patients with stage III and stage IV disease, although there have been case reports of >10 year survival in stage IV disease.[193,194]

One major controversy that remains unresolved is the relative survival of comparably staged male patients with breast cancer as compared to female patients with breast cancer. The data from Table 20-17 would suggest that the probability of survival for male patients with breast cancer may be slightly less than for comparably staged female patients with breast cancer. However, a number of studies have suggested that the survival rates for male vs. female breast cancer patients are not different.[136,164,196,197] In a study of four Nordic countries, Adami et al.[135] reported that the survival rate for male breast cancer patients was equal to female breast cancer patients in two of the four countries, but worse than for female breast cancer patients in the other two countries.

The prognostic factors for outcome in male breast cancer patients are listed in Table 20-18. In general, these are similar to prognostic factors described for female breast cancer patients. The strongest prognostic factors for outcome in most series are the presence vs. absence of pathologically involved axillary lymph nodes and the stage at presentation. Age was a prognostic factor for outcome in two studies,[135,167] but not a prognostic factor in a third study.[136] The pathologic subtype of carcinoma was a prognostic factor for outcome in two studies,[159,160] but not a prognostic factor in a third study.[196] Nipple involvement was not found to be a prognostic factor in the study of Yap et al.[201]

Systemic therapy for metastatic disease

Hormonal management in the form of orchiectomy has long been recognized as an effective palliative approach for metastatic breast cancer in men. A number of recent reports have shown a very high precentage of primary breast cancers in men to be hormonally sensitive as measured by estrogen and progesterone assays (Table 20-19). Further, the measured levels of estrogen and progesterone receptors are frequently very high. The hormonal maneuvers that have been reported to have response rates in metastatic male breast cancer patients include orchiectomy,[181] tamoxifen therapy,[162,174,181,184] adrenalectomy,[181] aminoglutethimide therapy,[161,174,181] estrogen therapy,[174] cyproterone acetate therapy,[174] and buserelin.[199] Serial hormonal maneuvers are frequently effective in the management of metastatic breast cancer.[174,181] Although hormonal and endocrine manipulations are the treatment of choice for male patients with metastatic breast cancer, responses to chemotherapy also have been documented.[175] The chemotherapeutic agents utilized are based on treatment regimens described for female breast cancer patients.[138,175]

BREAST CANCER ASSOCIATED WITH AUGMENTATION OR REDUCTION MAMMOPLASTY

Breast cancer associated with augmentation mammoplasty

The rate of incidental carcinoma found at the time of augmentation mammoplasty or carcinoma found in follow-up after augmentation mammoplasty is low. The low risk of breast cancer associated with augmentation mammoplasty may be related to the generally young age of such patients.[211] In a survey of 250 plastic surgeons, Snyderman and Lizardo[234]

Table 20-19 Incidence of positive hormone receptors in male breast cancer patients

Author	Pts. with positive estrogen receptors/total	Pts. with positive progesterone receptors/total
Bezwoda et al.[139]	15/23 [65]	— —
Everson et al.[153]	19/22 [86]	5/8 [63]
Friedman et al.[155]	12/12 [100]	— —
Ouriel et al.[179]	8/10 [80]	— —
Pacheco et al.[180]	7/8 [88]	6/8 [75]
Ribeiro[183]	12/16 [75]	10/16 [63]
Vercoutere and O'Connell[197]	7/7 [100]	— —
Total	80/98 [82]	21/32 [66]

[ ], % pts.

reported that only 0.3% (7/2516) of the patients were found to have carcinoma of the breast on pathologic examination of the tissue from augmentation mammoplasty. In a survey of 265 plastic surgeons, de Cholnoky[211] reported an incidence of 0.22% benign lesions and 0.007% malignant lesions in follow-up after 10,941 augmentation mammoplasties.

Imaging the breast after augmentation mammoplasty may be difficult. The breast implant can obscure significant amounts of breast parenchyma and mask an underlying carcinoma.[221,233] Routine mammographic evaluation with three views of the breast (craniocaudal, mediolateral, and axillary views) may be useful for more optimal mammographic imaging of the augmented breast.[227] Despite the problems with mammographic imaging following augmentation mammoplasty, screening mammography can be useful in detecting carcinoma.[209,227] In a series of 75 patients referred for routine screening mammography after augmentation mammoplasty, Mitnick et al.[227] found three cases with microcalcifications, two of which were intraductal carcinoma and one of which was sclerosing adenosis. Mammography can be useful in evaluating palpable masses.[221,227] Ultrasound and magnetic resonance imaging also may be useful in evaluating the breast after augmentation mammoplasty.[208,218]

It is uncertain whether or not breast cancer can be detected early in the course of follow-up of the patient with augmentation mammoplasty. Silverstein et al.[233] have suggested that the presentation of breast cancer in women after augmentation mammoplasty is more advanced than in women without augmentation mammoplasty. In that study, 20 patients with breast cancer after augmentation mammoplasty were compared to 733 patients with breast cancer without augmentation mammoplasty. All of the patients with augmentation mammoplasty presented with palpable masses, and none presented with in situ carcinoma. A comparison of patients with augmentation mammoplasty vs. those without augmentation mammoplasty showed that there was a significant difference in the incidence of in situ carcinomas (0 vs. 26%, respectively; $p<.01$), a significant difference in the incidence of occult carcinomas (0 vs. 21%, respectively; $p<.05$), and a higher percentage of cases with positive axillary lymph nodes (65% vs. 28%, respectively; $p<.001$). Conversely, Schmidt et al.[232] reported that breast cancer was detected early in patients following augmentation mammoplasty. Of 110 patients with breast implants, breast cancers were detected in follow-up in 12 patients. There were 66% with stage I disease, 17% with stage II disease, and 17% with stage IV disease. Negative axillary nodes were found in 82%.

The presence of a prosthesis for augmentation mammoplasty generally is not felt to be associated with an increased risk of carcinogenesis.[203,210,228] In an epidemiologic study of 3111 patients following augmentation mammoplasty, Deapen et al.[210] reported no increased risk of breast cancer in follow-up (9 observed cases vs. 15.7 expected cases; $p = NS$).

The management of breast cancer detected during or after augmentation mammoplasty has only been reported anecdotally.[203,207,213,217,220,225,228,230,233] The local treatment of breast cancer diagnosed during or after augmentation mammoplasty generally has been with mastectomy.[203,207,213,225,228,233] A number of recent case reports have suggested that breast-conserving surgery and irradiation can be utilized in appropriately selected patients with breast cancer diagnosed after augmentation mammoplasty.[217,220,225,230,233] Radiation therapy can be delivered following breast implantation without a significant change in the dosimetric characteristics of the radiation.[223,224,226,231] Halpern et al.[217] re-

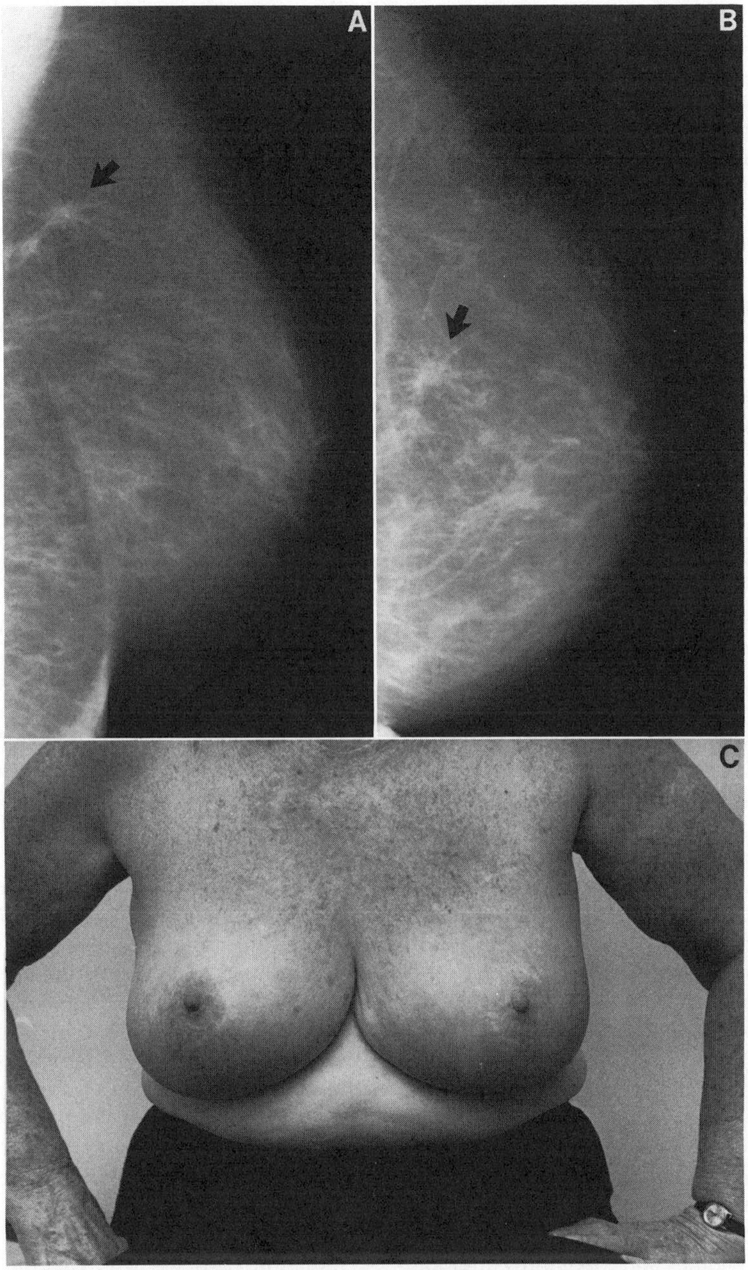

Fig. 20-1 A 72-year-old woman presented with a thickening in the upper central aspect of the left breast on physical examination 2 years after bilateral reduction mammoplasties. Angled mediolateral **(A)** and craniocaudal **(B)** film screen mammograms showed a spiculated mass *(arrow)* in the upper central aspect of the left breast. Biopsy showed infiltrating and intraductal carcinoma. Clinical and pathologic American Joint Committee (AJC) staging were both stage I. The patient was treated with breast-conserving surgery and definitive irradiation. Cosmetic outcome 30 months after definitive irradiation showed an excellent cosmetic result **(C)**.

ported the treatment of 13 patients with breast implants. The radiation doses were 4500 to 7100 cGy. Of the 12 patients with follow-up, only four had a good cosmetic outcome. Jacobson et al.[220] reported the treatment of three patients diagnosed as having carcinoma incidentally discovered at the time of augmentation mammoplasty. These three patients were treated with breast irradiation of 5000 to 6000 cGy. All three patients had no evidence of disease, and two of three had an excellent or good cosmetic outcome. In a rabbit model, Caffee et al.[206] reported that postoperative irradiation to a silastic implant did not change the development of capsular contraction at 6 months.

Bingham et al.[203] reported a case of a breast carcinoma detected after augmentation mammoplasty that was found to be attached to but not invading the prosthetic capsule. This suggested a possible barrier to spread of the carcinoma.

Two large series have evaluated the detection of local recurrence in patients treated with mastectomy and immediate breast reconstruction for malignancy.[215,222] Feller et al.[215] analyzed 100 consecutive patients treated with modified radical mastectomy and immediate reconstruction with implantation of a breast prosthesis or with a myocutaneous flap. Only five patients had a local-regional recurrence, and four of the five were clinically free of disease at the time of last follow-up. Johnson et al.[222] reported on 118 patients treated with mastectomy for breast cancer and immediate reconstruction with a silicone prosthesis. Local recurrence with or without distant disease was found in seven patients, but three of the four patients with local only recurrence subsequently died of disease.

Morgenstern et al.[228] reported that the diagnosis of malignancy on physical examination and mammography was obscured by silicone mastopathy. Pennisi[229] has reported the association of carcinoma following silicone injections and paraffin injections for augmentation. Silicone injections can be associated with mammographic microcalcifications.[221]

In a case report, Frantz and Herbst[216] reported the unusual association of carcinoma developing more than 30 years after pediatric irradiation for congenital hemangiomas and 32 months after augmentation mammoplasty for an underdeveloped breast.

Breast cancer associated with reduction mammoplasty

The incidence of carcinoma found at the time of reduction mammoplasty is low. In a survey of 250 plastic surgeons reporting 5008 reduction mammoplasties, only 19 malignancies (0.4%) were discovered, 5 (0.1%) on physical examination before operation and 14 (0.3%) on pathologic examination of the tissue specimens.[234] Bondeson et al.[204] reported the pathologic findings from 400 tissue specimens in 200 consecutive cases of bilateral reduction mammoplasties in patients without symptoms of breast carcinoma. In that study, no malignant lesion was seen in patients under age 30, and the most significant finding was in situ lobular carcinoma in 9% (6/70) of the patients aged ≥40 years.

In contrast to the findings on reduction mammoplasty for the asymptomatic patient, de Mascarel et al.[212] reported a 34% incidence (14/41) of previously unsuspected cancer in asymptomatic patients with a contralateral breast cancer undergoing reduction mammoplasty for reasons of asymmetry. Of the 14 malignancies in that study, 3 were invasive carcinoma, 6 were in situ ductal carcinoma (with or without in situ lobular carcinoma), and 5 were in situ lobular carcinoma.

The changes on mammography that are seen after reduction mammoplasty can be similar to the mammographic findings associated with carcinoma. Brown et al.[205] studied the mammographic changes over time in 42 patients following reduction mammoplasty. The mammographic changes found included periareolar changes, inferior pole alterations, asymmetrical densities, fat necrosis, and calcifications. The incidence of calcifications increased over time, whereas the incidence of soft tissue changes decreased over time. Biopsy findings from four masses were all negative for malignancy. Isaacs et al.[219] reported the biopsy findings from seven patients with masses after reduction mammoplasty. These seven cases showed fat necrosis, mammary dysplasia, hematoma, and postoperative fibrosis. In the asymptomatic patient who is to undergo reduction mammoplasty, mammographic evaluation is recommended preoperatively, postoperatively at 6 months as a baseline, and thereafter as indicated.[205,207,219]

Only a small number of cases have been reported of the management of carcinoma found incidentally at the time of reduction mammoplasty.[207,214] Although the majority of these cases have been managed with mastectomy, Cathcart and Hagerty[207] reported a case treated with wide resection and radiation. Patients who develop carcinoma of the breast subsequent to a reduction mammoplasty can be treated with breast-conserving surgery and definitive radiation (Fig. 20-1).

REFERENCES

Paget's disease

1. Ascensao AC, Marques MSJ, and Capitao-Mor M: Paget's disease of the nipple: clinical and pathological review of 109 female patients, Dermatologica 170:170, 1985.
2. Ashikari R, Park K, Huvos AG, and Urban JA: Paget's disease of the breast, Cancer 26:680, 1970.

3. Bulens P, Vanuytsel L, Rijnders A, and van der Schueren E: Breast conserving treatment of Paget's disease, Radiother Oncol 17:305, 1990.
4. Campana F, Vielh P, Fourquet A, et al: Maladie de Paget du mamelon sans tumeur mammarie associee cliniquement ou radiologiquement decelable: a propos de 51 cas traites a l'Institut Curie, J Gynecol Obstet Biol Reprod 16:1069, 1987.
5. Chaudary MA, Millis RR, Lane EB, and Miller NA: Paget's disease of the nipple: a ten year review including clinical, pathological, and immunohistochemical findings, Breast Cancer Res Treat 8:139, 1986.
6. Dawson JF, Burrows D, and Fannin T: Paget's disease of the breast presenting as a cerebellar metastasis, Clin Exp Dermatol 11:299, 1986.
7. Dockerty MB and Harrington SW: Preclinical Paget's disease of the nipple, Surg Gynecol Obstet 93:317, 1951.
8. Du Toit RS, Van Rensburg PSJ, and Goedhals L: Paget's disease of the breast, S Afr Med J 73:95, 1988.
9. Edeiken S: Mammography in the symptomatic woman, Cancer 63:1412, 1989.
10. Fourquet A, Campana F, Vielh P, et al: Paget's disease of the nipple without detectable breast tumor: conservative management with radiation therapy, Int J Radiat Oncol Biol Phys 13:1463, 1987.
11. Fowble B: Intraductal noninvasive breast cancer: a comparison of three local treatments, Oncology 3:51, 1989.
12. Gupta S, Khanna NN, Khanna S, and Gupta S: Paget's disease of the male breast: a clinicopathologic study and collective review, J Surg Oncol 22:151, 1983.
13. Haagensen CD: Paget's carcinoma of the breast. In Haagensen CD, editor: Diseases of the breast, ed 3, Philadelphia, 1986, WB Saunders Co, pp 758-781.
14. Hoeffken W and Lanyi M: Mammography, Philadelphia, 1977, WB Saunders Co, pp 178-183.
15. Kopans DB: Breast imaging, Philadelphia, 1989, JB Lippincott, pp 290-295.
16. Lagios MD, Margolin FR, Westdahl PR, and Rose MR: Mammographically detected duct carcinoma *in situ:* frequency of local recurrence following tylectomy and prognostic effect of nuclear grade on local recurrence, Cancer 63:618, 1989.
17. Lagios MD, Westdahl PR, Rose MR, and Concannon S: Paget's disease of the nipple: alternative management in cases without or with minimal extent of underlying breast cancer, Cancer 54:545, 1984.
18. Maier WP, Rosemond GP, Harasym EL, et al: Paget's disease in the female breast, Surg Gynecol Obstet 128:1253, 1969.
19. Malak G and Tapolcsanyi L: Characteristics of Paget's carcinoma of the nipple and problems of its negligency, Oncology 30:278, 1974.
20. McGregor JK and McGregor DD: Paget's disease of the breast: a twenty-year survey of cases presenting at a large general hospital, Surgery 45:562, 1959.
21. Menzies D, Barr L, and Ellis H: Paget's disease of the nipple occurring after wide local excision and radiotherapy for carcinoma of the breast, Eur J Surg Oncol 15:271, 1989.
22. Nance FC, DeLoach DH, Welsh RA, and Becker WF: Paget's disease of the breast, Ann Surg 171:864, 1970.
23. Ordonez NG, Awalt H, and Mackay B: Mammary and extramammary Paget's disease: an immunocytochemical and ultrastructural study, Cancer 59:1173, 1987.
24. Page DL and Anderson TJ: Diagnostic histopathology of the breast, New York, 1987, Churchill Livingstone, pp 184-186.
25. Paget J: On disease of the mammary areola preceding cancer of the mammary gland, St. Bartholomew's Hosp Rep 10:87, 1874.
26. Paone JF and Baker RR: Pathogenesis and treatment of Paget's disease of the breast, Cancer 48:825, 1981.
27. Rissanen PM and Holsti P: Paget's disease of the breast: the influence of the presence or absence of an underlying palpable tumor on the prognosis and on the choice of treatment, Oncology 23:209, 1969.
28. Rosai J: Ackerman's surgical pathology, ed 7, St Louis, 1989, CV Mosby Co, pp 1238-1239.
29. Salvadori B, Fariselli G, and Saccozzi R: Analysis of 100 cases of Paget's disease of the breast, Tumori 62:529, 1976.
30. Shearman CP and Watts GT: Paget's disease of the nipple after subcutaneous mastectomy for cancer with primary reconstruction, Ann R Coll Surg Engl 68:17, 1986.
31. Solin LJ, Fowble BL, Schultz DJ, et al: Definitive irradiation for intraductal carcinoma of the breast, Int J Radiat Oncol Biol Phys 19:843, 1990.
32. Stockdale AD, White WF, Brierly JD, et al: Radiotherapy for Paget's disease of the nipple: a conservative alternative, Lancet ii:664, 1989.
33. Suehiro S, Inai K, Tokuoka S, et al. Involvement of the nipple in early carcinoma of the breast, Surg Gynecol Obstet 168:244, 1989.
34. Tabar L and Dean PB: Teaching atlas of mammography, New York, 1985, Georg Thieme Verlag, p 164.
35. Tani EM and Skoog L: Immunocytochemical detection of estrogen receptors in mammary Paget cells, Acta Cytol 6:825, 1988.
36. Velpeau A: A treatise on the diseases of the breast and mammary region, London, 1856, Sydenham Society, pp 2-4.
37. Wood WS and Hegedus C: Mammary Paget's disease and intraductal carcinoma: histologic, histochemical, and immunocytochemical comparison, Am J Dermatopathol 10:183, 1988.
38. Zafrani B, Fourquet A, Vilcoq JR, et al: Conservative management of intraductal breast carcinoma with tumorectomy and radiation therapy, Cancer 57:1299, 1986.

Axillary lymph node presentation

39. Ashikari R, Rosen PP, Urban JA, and Senoo T: Breast cancer presenting as an axillary mass, Ann Surg 183:415, 1976.
40. Baron PL, Moore MP, Kinne DW, et al. Occult breast cancer presenting with axillary metastases: updated management, Arch Surg 125:210, 1990.
41. Bhatia SK, Saclarides TJ, Witt TR, et al: Hormone receptor studies in axillary metastases from occult breast cancers, Cancer 59:1170, 1987.
42. Breslow A: Occult carcinoma of the second breast following mastectomy, JAMA 226:1000, 1973.
43. Campana F, Fourquet A, Ashby MA, et al: Presentation of axillary lymphadenopathy without detectable breast primary (T_0 N_{1b} breast cancer): experience at Institut Curie, Radiother Oncol 15:321, 1989.
44. Copeland EM and McBride CM: Axillary metastases from unknown primary sites, Ann Surg 178:25, 1973.
45. Devitt JE and Michalchuk AW: Significance of contralateral axillary metastases in carcinoma of the breast, Can J Surg 12:178, 1969.
46. Ellerbroek N, Holmes F, Singletary E, et al: Treatment of isolated axillary nodal metastases in patients with an occult primary consistent with breast, Int J Radiat Oncol Biol Phys 17(suppl I):178, 1989.
47. Feigenberg Z, Zer M, and Dintsman M: Axillary metastases from an unknown primary source: a diagnostic and therapeutic approach, Isr J Med Sci 12:1153, 1976.
48. Feuerman L, Attie JN, and Rosenberg B: Carcinoma in axillary lymph nodes as an indicator of breast cancer, Surg Gynecol Obstet 114:5, 1962.

49. Fitts WT, Steiner GC, and Enterline HT: Prognosis of occult carcinoma of the breast, Am J Surg 106:460, 1963.
50. Fletcher GH: Local results of irradiation in the primary management of localized breast cancer, Cancer 29:545, 1972.
51. Fletcher GH and Shukovsky LJ: The interplay of radiocurability and tolerance in the irradiation of human cancers, J Radiol Electrol Med Nucl 56:383, 1975.
52. Griffith CDM, Christmas TJ, Elston CW, and Blamey RW: Axillary lymph node metastases from clinically occult breast carcinoma, J R Coll Surg Edinb 32:237, 1987.
53. Grundfest S, Steiger E, and Sebek B: Metastatic axillary adenopathy: use of estrogen receptor protein as an aid in diagnosis, Arch Surg 113:1108, 1978.
54. Haagensen CD: Physicians' role in the detection and diagnosis of breast disease. In Haagensen CD, editor: Diseases of the breast, ed 3, Philadelphia, 1986, WB Saunders Co, pp 516-576.
55. Haagensen CD: The natural history of breast carcinoma. In Haagensen CD, editor: Diseases of the breast, ed 3, Philadelphia, 1986, WB Saunders Co, pp 635-718.
56. Haupt HM, Rosen PP, and Kinne DW: Breast carcinoma presenting with axillary lymph node metastases: an analysis of specific histopathologic features, Am J Surg Pathol 9:165, 1985.
57. High RM and Watne AL: The axillary mass in occult breast carcinoma: case reports and overview, Am Surg 50:630, 1984.
58. Iglehart JD, Ferguson BJ, Shingleton WW, et al: An ultrastructural analysis of breast carcinoma presenting as isolated axillary adenopathy, Ann Surg 196:8, 1982.
59. Kaplan IW and Reinstine H: Occult carcinoma of the breast, Am Surg 20:575, 1954.
60. Kemeny MM, Rivera DE, Terz JJ, and Benfield JR: Occult primary adenocarcinoma with axillary metastases, Am J Surg 152:43, 1986.
61. Klopp CT: Metastatic cancer of axillary lymph node without a demonstrable primary lesion: report of a case with a 48 month latent period, Ann Surg 131:437, 1950.
62. Montague ED: Axillary metastases from unknown primary sites. In Fletcher GH, editor: Textbook of radiotherapy, ed 3, Philadelphia, 1980, Lea & Febiger, pp 582-583.
63. Owen HW, Dockerty MB, and Gray HK: Occult carcinoma of the breast, Surg Gynecol Obstet 98:302, 1954.
64. Patel J, Nemoto T, Rosner D, et al: Axillary lymph node metastasis from an occult breast cancer, Cancer 47:2923, 1981.
65. Pierce EH, Gray HK, and Dockerty MB: Surgical significance of isolated axillary adenopathy, Ann Surg 145:104, 1957.
66. Rosen PP: Axillary lymph node metastases in patients with occult noninvasive breast carcinoma, Cancer 46:1298, 1980.
67. Ultmann JE and Phillips TL: Cancer of unknown primary site. In DeVita VT, Hellman S, and Rosenberg SA, editors: Cancer: principles and practice of oncology, ed 3, Philadelphia, 1989, JB Lippincott, pp 1941-1952.
68. Weinberger HA and Stetten D: Extensive secondary axillary lymph node carcinoma without clinical evidence of primary breast lesion, Surgery 29:217, 1951.
69. Westbrook KC and Gallager HS: Breast carcinoma presenting as an axillary mass, Am J Surg 122:607, 1971.

Breast cancer and pregnancy

70. Anderson JM: Mammary cancers and pregnancy, Br Med J 1:1124, 1979.
71. Applewhite RR, Smith LR, and DiVincenti F: Carcinoma of the breast associated with pregnancy and lactation, Am Surg 39:101, 1973.
72. Brent RL: The effect of embryonic and fetal exposure to X-ray, microwaves, and ultrasound: counseling the pregnant and nonpregnant patient about these risks, Semin Oncol 16:347, 1989.
73. Brent RL: The effects of ionizing radiation, microwaves, and ultrasound on the developing embryo: clinical interpretations and applications of the data, Curr Probl Pediatr 14(9):1, 1984.
74. Bruzzi P, Negri E, La Vecchia C, et al: Short term increase in risk of breast cancer after full term pregnancy, Br Med J 297:1095, 1988.
75. Bunker ML and Peters MV: Breast cancer associated with pregnancy or lactation, Am J Obstet Gynecol 85:312, 1963.
76. Byrd BF, Bayer DS, Robertson JC, and Stephenson SE: Treatment of breast tumors associated with pregnancy and lactation, Ann Surg 155:940, 1962.
77. Canter JW, Oliver GC, and Zaloudek CJ: Surgical diseases of the breast during pregnancy, Clin Obstet Gynecol 26:853, 1983.
78. Cheek JH: Cancer of the breast in pregnancy and lactation, Am J Surg 126:729, 1973.
79. Chiedozi LC, Iweze FI, Aboh IF, and Ajabor LN: Breast cancer in pregnancy and lactation, Trop Geogr Med 40:26, 1988.
80. Clark RM and Reid J: Carcinoma of the breast in pregnancy and lactation, Int J Radiat Oncol Biol Phys 4:693, 1978.
81. Cooper DR and Butterfield J: Pregnancy subsequent to mastectomy for cancer of breast, Ann Surg 171:429, 1970.
82. Deemarsky LJ and Neishtadt EL: Breast cancer and pregnancy, Breast, Diseases of the Breast 7:17, 1981.
83. Doll DC, Ringenberg QS, and Yarbro JW: Antineoplastic agents and pregnancy, Semin Oncol 16:337, 1989.
84. Donegan WL: Mammary carcinoma and pregnancy. In Donegan WL and Spratt JS, editors: Cancer of the breast, ed 3, Philadelphia, 1988, WB Saunders Co, pp 679-688.
85. Donegan WL: Cancer and pregnancy, CA 33:194, 1983.
86. Donegan WL: Breast cancer and pregnancy, Obstet Gynecol 50:244, 1977.
87. Garber JE: Long-term follow-up of children exposed *in utero* to antineoplastic agents, Semin Oncol 16:437, 1989.
88. Geggie PHS: Breast cancer in pregnant women, Can Med Assoc J 127:358, 1982 (letter).
89. Greene FL and Leis HP: Management of breast cancer in pregnancy: a thirty-five year multi-institutional experience, Proc Am Soc Clin Oncol 8:25, 1989.
90. Haagensen CD: Diseases of the breast, ed 3, Philadelphia, 1986, WB Saunders Co, pp 924-929.
91. Hall EJ: Radiobiology for the radiologist, ed 3, Philadelphia, 1988, JB Lippincott, pp 445-465.
92. Harvey JC, Rosen PP, Ashikari R, et al: The effect of pregnancy on the prognosis of carcinoma of the breast following radical mastectomy, Surg Gynecol Obstet 153:723, 1981.
93. Hobbs JR, De Souza I, Salih H, and Raggatt P: Selection of hormone-dependent breast cancers, Br J Surg 61:785, 1974.
94. Hoeffken W and Lanyi M: Mammography, Philadelphia, 1977, WB Saunders Co, pp 72-80.
95. Holdaway IM, Mason BH, and Kay RG: Steroid hormone receptors in breast tumours presenting during pregnancy or lactation, J Surg Oncol 25:38, 1984.
96. Holleb AI and Farrow JH: The relation of carcinoma of the breast and pregnancy in 283 patients, Surg Gynecol Obstet 115:65, 1962.
97. Hornstein E, Skornick Y, and Rozin R: The management of breast carcinoma in pregnancy and lactation, J Surg Oncol 21:179, 1982.

98. Horsley JS, Alrich EM, and Wright CB: Carcinoma of the breast in women 35 years of age or younger, Ann Surg 169:839, 1969.
99. Hubay CA, Barry FM, and Marr CC: Pregnancy and breast cancer, Surg Clin North Am 58:819, 1978.
100. Janerich DT: The influence of pregnancy on breast cancer risk: is it endocrinological or immunological? Med Hypotheses 6:1149, 1980.
101. Jochimsen PR, Spaight ME, and Urdaneta LF: Pregnancy during adjuvant chemotherapy for breast cancer, JAMA 245:1660, 1981.
102. King RM, Welch JS, Martin JK, and Coulam CB: Carcinoma of the breast associated with pregnancy, Surg Gynecol Obstet 160:228, 1985.
103. Kitchen PRB and McLellan R: Breast cancer and pregnancy, Med J Aust 147:337, 1987.
104. Lichter AS and Lippman ME: Special situations in the treatment of breast cancer. In Lippman ME, Lichter AS, and Danforth DN, editors: Diagnosis and management of breast cancer, Philadelphia, 1988, WB Saunders Co, pp 407-438.
105. Majmudar B and Rosales-Quintana S: Infarction of breast fibroadenomas during pregnancy, JAMA 231:963, 1975.
106. Miller RW and Mulvihill JJ: Small head size after atomic irradiation, Teratology 14:355, 1976.
107. Murray CL, Reichert JA, Anderson J, and Twiggs LB: Multimodal cancer therapy for breast cancer in the first trimester of pregnancy: a case report, JAMA 252:2607, 1984.
108. National Council on Radiation Protection and Measurements: Medical radiation exposure of pregnant and potentially pregnant women, NCRP Report No. 54, Washington, DC, 1977.
109. Nicholson HO: Cytotoxic drugs in prenancy: review of reported cases, J Obstet Gynaecol Br Commonwealth 75:307, 1968.
110. Nugent P and O'Connell TX: Breast cancer and pregnancy, Arch Surg 120:1221, 1985.
111. Okun DB, Groncy PK, Sieger L, and Tanaka KR: Acute leukemia in pregnancy: transient neonatal myelosuppression after combination chemotherapy in the mother, Med Pediatr Oncol 7:315, 1979.
112. Orr JW and Shingleton HM: Cancer in pregnancy, Curr Probl Cancer 8(1):1, 1983.
113. Parenti JT, Amsel M, Lerner R, and Chinea F: Breast cancer associated with pregnancy, Obstet Gynecol 71:861, 1988.
114. Peters MV: The effect of pregnancy in breast cancer. In Forrest APM and Kunkler PB, editors: Prognostic factors in breast cancer, London, 1968, E & S Livingstone Ltd, pp 65-89.
115. Potter JF and Schoeneman M: Metastasis of maternal cancer to the placenta and fetus, Cancer 25:380, 1970.
116. Powell HR and Ekert H: Methotrexate-induced congenital malformations, Med J Aus 2:1076, 1971.
117. Ribeiro GG and Palmer MK: Breast carcinoma associated with pregnancy: a clinician's dilemma, Br Med J 2:1524, 1977.
118. Rickert RR and Rajan S: Localized breast infarcts associated with pregnancy, Arch Pathol 97:159, 1974.
119. Rissanen PM: Carcinoma of the breast during pregnancy and lactation, Br J Cancer 22:663, 1968.
120. Rosemond GP: Carcinoma of the breast during pregnancy, Clin Obstet Gynecol 6:994, 1963.
121. Sahni K, Sanyal B, Agrawal MS, et al: Carcinoma of breast associated with pregnancy and lactation, J Surg Oncol 16:167, 1981.
122. Schapira DV and Chudley AE: Successful pregnancy following continuous treatment with combination chemotherapy before conception and throughout pregnancy, Cancer 54:800, 1984.
123. Sutton R, Buzdar AU, and Hortobagyi GN: Pregnancy and offspring after adjuvant chemotherapy in breast cancer patients, Cancer 65:847, 1990.
124. Sweet DL and Kinzie J: Consequences of radiotherapy and antineoplastic therapy for the fetus, J Reprod Med 17:241, 1976.
125. Torres JE and Mickal A: Carcinoma of the breast in pregnancy, Clin Obstet Gynecol 18:219, 1975.
126. Tretli S, Kvalheim G, Thoresen S, and Host H: Survival of breast cancer patients diagnosed during pregnancy or lactation, Br J Cancer 58:382, 1988.
127. Treves N and Holleb AI: A report of 549 cases of breast cancer in women 35 years of age or younger, Surg Gynecol Obstet 107:271, 1958.
128. Wallack MK, Wolf JA, Bedwinek J, et al: Gestational carcinoma of the female breast, Curr Probl Cancer 7(9):1, 1983.
129. Weber DA, Makler PT, Watson EE, et al: Radiation absorbed dose from Technetium-99m-labeled bone imaging agents, J Nucl Med 30:1117, 1989.
130. White TT: Carcinoma of the breast associated with pregnancy: report of fifty-six cases followed five years or more, Northwest Med 57:477, 1958.
131. White TT: Carcinoma of the breast in the pregnant and the nursing patient: review of 1,375 cases, Am J Obstet Gynecol 69:1277, 1955.
132. White TT: Prognosis of breast cancer for pregnant and nursing women: analysis of 1,413 cases, Surg Gynecol Obstet 100:661, 1955.
133. White TT and White WC: Breast cancer and pregnancy: report of 49 cases followed 5 years, Ann Surg 144:384, 1956.
134. Zeigerman JH, Honigman FH, and Crawford RW: Inflammatory mammary cancer during pregnancy and lactation: report of a case, Obstet Gynecol 32:373, 1968.

Male breast cancer

135. Adami H-O, Hakulinen T, Ewertz M, et al: The survival pattern in male breast cancer: an analysis of 1429 patients from the Nordic countries, Cancer 64:1177, 1989.
136. Adami H-O, Holmberg L, Malker B, and Ries L: Long-term survival in 406 males with breast cancer, Br J Cancer 52:99, 1985.
137. Agbata AI and Kovi J: Carcinoma of the breast in American negro men, J Nat Med Assoc 66:404, 1974.
138. Bagley CS, Wesley MN, Young RC, and Lippman ME: Adjuvant chemotherapy in males with cancer of the breast, Am J Clin Oncol 10:55, 1987.
139. Bezwoda WR, Hesdorffer C, Dansey R, et al: Breast cancer in man: clinical features, hormone receptor status, and response to therapy, Cancer 60:1337, 1987.
140. Calabresi E, De Giuli G, Becciolini A, et al: Plasma estrogens and androgens in male breast cancer, J Steroid Biochem 7:605, 1976.
141. Casagrande JT, Hanisch R, Pike MC, et al: A case-control study of male breast cancer, Cancer Res 48:1326, 1988.
142. Cohen R and Schauer PK: Male breast cancer after repeated fluoroscopy, Am J Med 76:929, 1984.
143. Crichlow RW: Carcinoma of the male breast, Surg Gynecol Obstet 134:1011, 1972.
144. Crichlow RW and Czernobilsky B: Paget's disease of the male breast, Cancer 24:1033, 1969.
145. Cutler SJ and Young JL, editors: Third national cancer survey: incidence data, Nat Cancer Inst Monog 41, 1975.
146. Dao TL and Greiner MJ: Mammary carcinogenesis by 3-methylcholanthrene. III. Induction of mammary carcinoma and milk secretion in male rats bearing ovarian grafts, J Nat Cancer Inst 27:333, 1961.
147. Dao TL, Morreal C, and Neomoto T: Urinary estrogen excretion in men with breast cancer, N Engl J Med 289:138, 1973.

148. Davidson AT: A review of the treatment of cancer of the male breast with a case follow-up, J Natl Med Assoc 79:879, 1987.
149. Dershaw DD: Male mammography, AJR 146:127, 1986.
150. Dodge OG, Jackson AW, and Muldal S: Breast cancer and interstitial-cell tumor in a patient with Klinefelter's syndrome, Cancer 24:1027, 1969.
151. El-Gazayerli MM and Abdel-Aziz A-S: On bilharziasis and male breast cancer in Egypt: a preliminary report and review of the literature, Br J Cancer 17:566, 1963.
152. Erlichman C, Murphy KC, and Elhakim T: Male breast cancer: a 13-year review of 89 patients, J Clin Oncol 2:903, 1984.
153. Everson RB, Lippman ME, Thompson EB, et al: Clinical correlations of steriod receptors and male breast cancer, Cancer Res 40:991, 1980.
154. Ewertz M, Holmberg L, Karjalainen S, et al: Incidence of male breast cancer in Scandinavia, 1943-1982, Int J Cancer 43:27, 1989.
155. Friedman MA, Hoffman PG, Dandolos EM, et al: Estrogen receptors in male breast cancer: clinical and pathologic correlations, Cancer 47:134, 1981.
156. Giffler RF and Kay S: Small-cell carcinoma of the male mammary gland: a tumor resembling infiltrating lobular carcinoma, Am J Clin Pathol 66:715, 1976.
157. Greene MH, Goedert JJ, Bech-Hansen NT, et al: Radiogenic male breast cancer with *in vitro* sensitivity to ionizing radiation and bleomycin, Cancer Invest 1:379, 1983.
158. Gupta S, Khanna NN, Khanna S, and Gupta S: Paget's disease of the male breast: a clinicopathologic study and a collective review, J Surg Oncol 22:151, 1983.
159. Gupta S, Pant GC, and Gupta S: Male breast cancer, J Surg Oncol 16:149, 1981.
160. Haagensen CD: Carcinoma of the male breast. In Haagensen CD, editor: Diseases of the breast, ed 3, Philadelphia, 1986, WB Saunders Co, pp 976-990.
161. Harris AL, Dowsett M, Stuart-Harris R, and Smith IE: Role of aminoglutethimide in male breast cancer, Br J Cancer 54:657, 1986.
162. Hilliard DA, Wilbur DW, and Camacho ES: Tamoxifen response following no response to orchiectomy in metastatic male breast cancer: a case report, J Surg Oncol 25:42, 1984.
163. Hodson GR, Urdaneta LF, Al-Jurf AS, and Jochimsen PR: Male breast carcinoma, Am Surg 51:47, 1985.
164. Holleb AI, Freeman HP, and Farrow JH: Cancer of male breast: part I. NY State J Med 68:544, 1968.
165. Holleb AI, Freeman HP, and Farrow JH: Cancer of male breast: part II. NY State J Med 68:656, 1968.
166. Hultborn R, Friberg S, and Hultborn KA: Male breast carcinoma. I. A study of the total material reported to the Swedish Cancer Registry 1958-1967 with respect to clinical and histopathologic parameters, Acta Oncol 26:241, 1987.
167. Hultborn R, Friberg S, Hultborn KA, et al: Male breast carcinoma. II. A study of the total material reported to the Swedish Cancer Registry 1958-1967 with respect to treatment, prognostic factors and survival, Acta Oncol 26:327, 1987.
168. Kapdi CC and Parekh NJ: The male breast, Radiol Clin North Am 21:137, 1983.
169. Kopans DB: Breast imaging, Philadelphia, 1989, JB Lippincott, pp 342-350.
170. Kozak FK, Hall JG, and Baird PA: Familial breast cancer in males: a case report and review of literature, Cancer 58:2736, 1986.
171. Li FP, Corkery J, Vawter G, et al: Breast carcinoma after cancer therapy in childhood, Cancer 51:521, 1983.
172. Liechty RD, Davis J, and Gleysteen J: Cancer of the male breast: forty cases, Cancer 20:1617, 1967.
173. Lloyd RV, Rosen PP, Sarkar NH, et al: Murine mammary tumor virus related antigen in human male mammary carcinoma, Cancer 51:654, 1983.
174. Lopez M, Di Lauro L, Lazzaro B, and Papaldo P: Hormonal treatment of disseminated male breast cancer, Oncology 42:345, 1985.
175. Lopez M, Di Lauro L, Papaldo P, and Lazzaro B: Chemotherapy in metastatic male breast cancer, Oncology 42:205, 1985.
176. Mabuchi K, Bross DS, and Kessler II: Risk factors for male breast cancer, J Nat Cancer Inst 74:371, 1985.
177. Nuttall FQ: Gynecomastia as a physical finding in normal men, J Clin Endocrinol Metabol 48:338, 1979.
178. Olsson H and Ranstam J: Head trauma and exposure to prolactin-elevating drugs as risk factors for male breast cancer, J Nat Cancer Inst 80:679, 1988.
179. Ouriel K, Lotze MT, and Hinshaw JR: Prognostic factors of carcinoma of the male breast, Surg Gynecol Obstet 159:373, 1984.
180. Pacheco MM, Oshima CF, Lopes MP, et al: Steroid hormone receptors in male breast disease, Anticancer Res 6:1013, 1986.
181. Patel JK, Nemoto T, and Dao TA: Metastatic breast cancer in males: assessment of endocrine therapy, Cancer 53:1344, 1984.
182. Pritchard TJ, Pankowsky DA, Crowe JP, and Abdul-Karim FW: Breast cancer in a male-to-female transsexual: a case report, JAMA 259:2278, 1988.
183. Ribeiro G: Male breast carcinoma—a review of 301 cases from the Christie Hospital and Holt Radium Institute, Manchester, Br J Cancer 51:115, 1985.
184. Ribeiro GG: Tamoxifen in the treatment of male breast carcinoma, Clin Radiol 34:625, 1983.
185. Robison R and Montague ED: Treatment results in males with breast cancer, Cancer 49:403, 1982.
186. Scheike O: Male breast cancer. 5. Clinical manifestations in 257 cases in Denmark, Br J Cancer 28:552, 1973.
187. Scheike O: Male breast cancer. 6. Factors influencing prognosis, Br J Cancer 30:261, 1974.
188. Scheike O, Svenstrup B, and Frandsen VA: Male breast cancer. II. Metabolism of oestradiol-17β in men with breast cancer, J Steroid Biochem 4:489, 1973.
189. Scheike O and Visfeldt J: Male breast cancer. 4. Gynecomastia in patients with breast cancer, Acta Pathol Microbiol Scand [A]81:359, 1973.
190. Scheike O, Visfeldt J, and Petersen B: Male breast cancer. 3. Breast carcinoma in association with the Klinefelter Syndrome, Acta Pathol Microbiol Scand [A]81:352, 1973.
191. Schlappack OK, Braun O, and Maier U: Report of two cases of male breast cancer after prolonged estrogen treatment for prostatic carcinoma, Cancer Detect Prev 9:319, 1986.
192. Serour F, Birkenfeld S, Amsterdam E, et al: Paget's disease of the male breast, Cancer 62:601, 1988.
193. Siddiqui T, Weiner R, Moreb J, and Marsh RD: Cancer of the male breast with prolonged survival, Cancer 62:1632, 1988.
194. Spence RAJ, MacKenzie G, Anderson JR, et al: Long-term survival following cancer of the male breast in Northern Ireland: a report of 81 cases, Cancer 55:648, 1985.
195. Symmers WSC: Carcinoma of breast in trans-sexual individuals after surgical and hormonal interference with the primary and secondary sex characteristics, Br Med J 2:83, 1968.
196. van Geel AN, van Slooten EA, Mavrunac M, and Hart AAM: A retrospective study of male breast cancer in Holland, Br J Surg 72:724, 1985.
197. Vercoutere AL and O'Connell TX: Carcinoma of the male breast: an update, Arch Surg 119:1301, 1984.

198. Visfeldt J and Scheike O: Male breast cancer. I. Histologic typing and grading of 187 Danish cases, Cancer 32:985, 1973.
199. Vorobiof DA and Falkson G: Nasally administered buserelin inducing complete remission of lung metastases in male breast cancer, Cancer 59:688, 1987.
200. Williams WR, Badzioch MD, and Anderson DE: Epidemiology of male breast cancer. In Ames FC, Blumenschein GR, and Montague ED, editors: Current controversies in breast cancer, Austin, Tex, 1984, University of Texas Press, pp 589-601.
201. Yap HY, Tashima CK, Blumenschein GR, and Eckles NE: Male breast cancer: a natural history study, Cancer 44:748, 1979.
202. Young JL, Percy CL, and Asire AJ: Surveillance, epidemiology, and end results: incidence and mortality data, 1973-1977, Nat Cancer Inst Monogr 57, 1981.

Breast cancer associated with augmentation or reduction mammoplasty

203. Bingham HG, Copeland EM, Hackett R, and Caffee HH: Breast cancer in a patient with silicone breast implants after 13 years, Ann Plast Surg 20:236, 1988.
204. Bondeson L, Linell F, and Ringberg A: Breast reductions: what to do with all the tissue specimens? Histopathology 9:281, 1985.
205. Brown FE, Sargent SK, Cohen SR, and Morain WD: Mammographic changes following reduction mammaplasty, Plast Reconstr Surg 80:691, 1987.
206. Caffee HH, Mendenhall NP, Mendenhall WM, and Bova FJ: Postoperative radiation and implant capsule contraction, Ann Plast Surg 20:35, 1988.
207. Cathcart RS and Hagerty RC: Preoperative and postoperative considerations in elective breast operations, Ann Plast Surg 22:533, 1989.
208. Cole-Beuglet C, Schwartz G, Kurtz AB, et al: Ultrasound mammography for the augmented breast, Radiology 146:737, 1983.
209. Dalinka MK, Rockett JF, and Kurth RJ: Carcinoma of the breast following simple mastectomy and mammoplasty, Radiology 93:914, 1969.
210. Deapen DM, Pike MC, Casagrande JT, and Brody GS: The relationship between breast cancer and augmentation mammaplasty: an epidemiologic study, Plast Reconst Surg 77:361, 1986.
211. de Cholnoky T: Augmentation mammaplasty: survey of complications in 10,941 patients by 265 surgeons, Plast Reconstr Surg 45:573, 1970.
212. de Mascarel I, Trojani M, Coindre JM, and Faucher A: The incidence of cancer in contralateral reduction mammaplasty after mastectomy and reconstruction of the removed breast, Tumori 72:183, 1986.
213. DerHagopian RP, Zaworski RE, Sugarbaker EV, and Ketcham AS: Management of locally recurrent breast cancer adjacent to prosthetic implants, Am J Surg 141:590, 1981.
214. Dinner MI and Artz JS: Carcinoma of the breast occurring in routine reduction mammaplasty, Plast Reconst Surg 83:1042, 1989.
215. Feller WF, Holt R, Spear S, and Little JW: Modified radical mastectomy with immediate breast reconstruction, Am Surg 52:129, 1986.
216. Frantz P and Herbst CA: Augmentation mammoplasty, irradiation, and breast cancer: a case report, Cancer 36:1147, 1975.
217. Halpern J, McNeese MD, Kroll SS, and Ellerbroek N: Irradiation of prosthetically augmented breasts: a retrospective study on toxicity and cosmetic results, Int J Radiat Oncol Biol Phys 18:189, 1990.
218. Heywang SW, Eiermann W, Bassermann R, and Fenzl G: Carcinoma of the breast behind a prosthesis—comparison of ultrasound, mammography and MRI (case report), Comput Radiol 9:283, 1985.
219. Isaacs G, Rozner L, and Tudball C: Breast lumps after reduction mammaplasty, Ann Plast Surg 15:394, 1985.
220. Jacobson GM, Sause WT, Thomson JW, and Plenk HP: Breast irradiation following silicone gel implants, Int J Radiat Oncol Biol Phys 12:835, 1986.
221. Jensen SR and Mackey JK: Xeromammography after augmentation mammoplasty, AJR 144:629, 1985.
222. Johnson CH, van Heerden JA, Donohue JH, et al: Oncological aspects of immediate breast reconstruction following mastectomy for malignancy, Arch Surg 124:819, 1989.
223. Krishnan L and Krishnan EC: Electron beam irradiation after reconstruction with silicone gel implant in breast cancer, Am J Clin Oncol 9:223, 1986.
224. Krishnan L, St. George FJ, Mansfield CM, and Krishnan EC: Effect of silicone gel breast prosthesis on electron and photon dose distributions, Med Phys 10:96, 1983.
225. Lafreniere R and Ketcham AS: Breast carcinoma post-augmentation mammaplasty: therapy with limited surgery and radiation, J Surg Oncol 35:99, 1987.
226. McGinley PH, Powell WR, and Bostwick J: Dosimetry of a silicone breast prosthesis, Radiology 135:223, 1980.
227. Mitnick JS, Harris MN, and Roses DF: Mammographic detection of carcinoma of the breast in patients with augmentation prostheses, Surg Gynecol Obstet 168:30, 1989.
228. Morgenstern L, Gleischman SH, Michel SL, et al: Relation of free silicone to human breast carcinoma, Arch Surg 120:573, 1985.
229. Pennisi VR: Obscure carcinoma encountered in subcutaneous mastectomy in silicone- and paraffin-injected breasts: two patients, Plast Reconst Surg 74:535, 1984.
230. Phillips RL and Siegfried MS: Breast treatment planning using ultrasound in patient with silicone implants, Int J Radiat Oncol Biol Phys 9:1245, 1983 (letter).
231. Piontek RW and Kase KR: Radiation transmission study of silicone elastomer for mammary prosthesis, Radiology 136:505, 1980.
232. Schmidt RT, Peters GN, and Evans WP: Silicone implants and breast cancer: another perspective, Proc Am Soc Clin Oncol 7:23, 1988.
233. Silverstein MJ, Handel N, Gamagami P, et al: Breast cancer in women after augmentation mammoplasty, Arch Surg 123:681, 1988.
234. Snyderman RK and Lizardo JG: Statistical study of malignancies found before, during, or after routine breast plastic operations, Plast Reconstr Surg 25:253, 1960.

21 Psychosocial Aspects of Breast Cancer

Jeannie Pasacreta, Ruth McCorkle, and *Gerald Margolis*

"Without question, breast cancer is the most widely studied cancer with respect to its psychological impact."[85] Reasons for concern regarding psychosocial adjustment are multiple. Historically breast cancer has been the most common type of cancer in women, affecting one in every 9 (only recently has the incidence of lung cancer in women competed for first place).[3] Publicity regarding breast cancer prevalence and the lack of decline in mortality rates despite abundant investigative efforts[3] has led to fear and concern among women with and without the illness.

Growing public concern regarding the seemingly random occurrence and lack of clear-cut risk factors associated with breast cancer is evident. In addition, concern about an individual's ability to cope and possibly alter the course and progression of the illness is increasingly apparent. Frequent media events from television movies to documentaries portray the woman's struggle to adapt to uncertainty, raising important questions, ranging from which type of treatment to choose to one's ability to improve the chances for survival.

For many women, breast cancer threatens an organ that is intimately connected to self-esteem, feminine identity, and sexuality; thus its psychologic impact is of primary concern. Major changes in the understanding and treatment of breast cancer have led to a wider range of treatment options and increasing length of survival from time of diagnosis than was ever before possible. While such advances are quite positive, their impact on the emotional lives of women and families faced with complex treatment decisions and the emotional consequences of chronic illness cannot be overlooked.

In light of the fact that breast cancer poses a major public health concern in this country, health care professionals should be informed of the factors that affect psychosocial adjustment, the wide range of psychologic responses that accompany the disease during each of its phases, and the efficacy of various modes of psychosocial intervention in minimizing distress and promoting adaptation. Awareness of the psychosocial issues that accompany diagnosis and treatment for breast cancer can enhance understanding of psychosocial adjustment to other types of cancer in that the three major cancer treatment modalities (surgery, chemotherapy, and radiotherapy) often are used in conjunction to treat and control cancer of the breast.

CHANGES IN TREATMENT AND SOCIETAL ATTITUDES: ACCOMPANYING TRENDS IN PSYCHOSOCIAL ISSUES

When examining the psychosocial responses of women after the diagnosis of breast cancer, it is useful to begin with an overview of the changes that have occurred in treatment, the increased involvement of women in determining the approach to be used, and the impact that these changes have had on the emotional lives of women with breast cancer. Until the past decade, radical or modified radical mastectomy was the prescribed and standard treatment for breast cancer in the United States. An early study on the psychosocial impact of mastectomy revealed that women reacted to that surgery with symptoms associated with clinical depression, diminished self-esteem, sexual impairment, and decreased functional status.[6] The understanding of breast cancer as a systemic disease[24] has eroded the premise on which radical breast surgery had been based.[85] Randomized trials have demonstrated that breast-conserving procedures are associated with survival rates equal to those achieved through more radical approaches.[4,26,30,88] Controlled studies confirm that with small breast lesions, survival outcome for combined lumpectomy and radiation vs. radical mastectomy are equivalent.[8,25] Despite the existence of breast cancer treatment guidelines established by the National Cancer Institute, the lack of agreement among experts in the field has been publicized widely. This debate, along with the information that prognosis is uncertain regardless of treatment, has been disseminated to the public to an extent that has never before been paralleled.

Concurrent with the well-publicized advances and disagreements regarding the optimal treatment for breast cancer, dramatic changes in societal attitudes regarding the disease and encouragement for women to participate actively in decisions regarding their care have occurred. Several factors, including public disclosure by several prominent women of their personal experiences with breast cancer, and the women's movement, which advocates greater participation in making informed decisions regarding medical care in general, have produced widespread sentiment in favor of a woman's right to control what happens to her body.

The changes in treatment and society mentioned above have led to simultaneous changes in the psychosocial issues encountered by women who are faced with a diagnosis of breast cancer. As stated by Rowland and Holland[85]:

> The emotional issues are different today but equally compelling. Although fears about breast loss and threat to body image and sexual function have decreased with the introduction of breast conserving treatment techniques, fears and anxieties about having made the right treatment choice and about the likelihood of survival have increased. A change that is integral to the initial emotional burden today is the patient's increased level of participation in primary treatment decisions (p. 189).

In addition to the preceding overview of changes in treatment and in the societal attitudes toward breast cancer, the changes in professional attitudes and behaviors regarding disclosure of medical information deserve mention. The secrecy that prevailed in the 1960s and prohibited the disclosure of a cancer diagnosis by most physicians[79,81] has given way to the practice of imparting the particulars of diagnosis, treatment options, and prognosis routinely.[47,79] Despite this change, however, it has been suggested that resolution of fears and concerns among health care providers about cancer have not kept up with changes in behavioral and practice expectations. In many cases, a discrepancy between attitude and action has resulted, leading to communication of emotionally laden information in a fashion ranging from overprotective and paternalistic to blunt and matter of fact.[40]

Discrepancies between attitude and practice also have been demonstrated by nurses who have been found to avoid clear, open discussions of topics such as cancer and death, despite consistently expressed beliefs regarding the importance of openness and honesty with all mentally competent patients.[14,71] Thus, while the prevailing attitude in health care supports disclosure of medical information and the active involvement of patients in decisions that affect them, the actual behavior of health care providers is likely to reflect a more limited improvement in patient care.

In light of the discrepancies between attitude and action discussed above, clinicians should be mindful of how their personal views and concerns about cancer impact on communication with patients, which is always important, but especially so at key decision-making and transition points along the continuum of care. The initiation of and participation in staff support groups, as well as the use of peers and alternate providers to assist patients with issues and concerns that primary clinicians do not feel prepared to or comfortable dealing with, are useful strategies for insuring maximum support for patients faced with the complex decisions inherent in breast cancer treatment.

FACTORS THAT IMPACT ON PSYCHOSOCIAL ADJUSTMENT

Psychosocial responses to breast cancer vary widely. In addition to the changes in clinician's attitudes and the increased treatment choices that are available to women with breast cancer, a review of the literature regarding psychosocial adaptation points to several key factors that impact on psychosocial adjustment. These include the following:

1. Health-seeking behaviors of women
2. Previous coping strategies and emotional stability
3. The existence of social support
4. Role shifts during illness
5. Women's caregiving abilities

Health-seeking behaviors of women

Several authors have reported consistent differences in the ways that men and women use health care services. Women use physicians and hospital services more frequently than men.[73,102] These differences have been a source of considerable debate and empirical investigation over the past 10 years. Some authors maintain that women report their symptoms more often than men because they are more interested in health and are more knowledgeable about health care.[23] Gove[34] suggests that women are more willing to admit to psychosocial distress and to seek treatment for it because they place less stigma on these actions. Another explanation is greater flexibility in arranging medical appointments, although as more and more women join the work force, this is changing. Also, women suffer less cost associated with medical care in relation to time-off from work, possibly because of differences in pay structures.

Mounting evidence suggests that gender differences in health behaviors are largely a consequence of social and psychologic factors rather than biologic or genetic factors.[35,73] A consensus is emerging that sex differences in morbidity reports and the differences in the uptake of health services in Western industrial societies are a result of differences in the way symptoms are perceived, evaluated, and acted on.[40,70]

In view of their higher morbidity and utilization

rates, women should be diagnosed and treated early for diseases such as breast cancer. In fact, delay in seeking treatment for some women has been associated with such diagnoses as early stage breast cancer.[22,45] Hackett et al.[38] found that breast cancer patients overall responded rapidly in seeking health care, with nearly 75% receiving care in <1 month. Approximately 20%, however, delayed reporting symptoms for at least 1 year. Lierman[58] reported that >35% of her sample of breast cancer patients delayed seeking treatment for months and in several instances years. All of the women who delayed for over a year had a close relative with cancer. Lierman[58] defined delay as the amount of time lapse between the initial discovery of the symptom and first seeking professional assistance. Based on data from 16 women whose symptoms were discovered outside the health care system, four behavioral responses were identified:

1. Early help seeking (1 to 4 weeks)
2. Ignoring symptoms (weeks to months)
3. Wait and see (months to years)
4. Preparation for death (years)

The majority of Lierman's sample (70%) reported that their initial symptom was a breast lump, the most common presenting symptom for breast cancer.[58] However, the initial symptom in 30% of the women was an inverted nipple, nipple discharge, or a burning sensation. Bullough[12] and Gould-Martin et al.[33] reported similar findings. These findings indicate the importance of describing symptoms other than lumps when teaching breast self-examination (BSE).

Margarey et al.[60] identified five psychologic factors associated with an increased length of delay in women with breast cancer. These factors, identified as unconscious mental processes, included marked use of denial and suppression, intellectualization, isolation, anxiety, and depression. Similarly, Watson et al.[103] cited avoidance and denial as the most frequently observed coping responses in women with breast cancer. In their study, however, deniers and acceptors did not differ in the length of delay in seeking treatment.

Gould-Martin et al.[33] noted that women who found breast lumps by breast self-examination were actually more likely to delay seeking treatment than women whose lumps were discovered accidentally. Funch[27] points out conflicting evidence in the literature about the relationship of BSE and delay in seeking treatment. Her study found no significant relationship between frequency of BSE and delay in seeking treatment. Women practicing BSE were most likely to delay if they had less education, larger breasts, were older, or had a family member who had died of breast cancer.

One factor suggested for the lack of decline in death rates from breast cancer is that one third of patients diagnosed with the disease present with a tumor that is too advanced to respond to treatment.[18] Because as many as 98% of breast tumors are detected by women themselves, breast self-examination could lead to early detection of abnormalities and to a more positive prognosis.[16] It is important for health care providers to be aware of the motivating and inhibiting factors that influence a woman's decision to perform breast screenings so that these issues can be addressed through community education programs.

Previous coping strategies and emotional stability

The most important predictors of psychosocial adjustment to breast cancer are the coping strategies and emotional stability of the woman before diagnosis. Individuals with a history of poor psychosocial adjustment before developing cancer are at highest risk for emotional decompensation[95] and should be monitored closely throughout all phases of treatment. This is particularly true for women with a history of major psychiatric syndromes and/or psychiatric hospitalization.

Since an individual's coping style is determined relatively early in life and remains stable over time and across situations, it serves as a useful predictor for how an individual will adjust to breast cancer.[31] Several investigators have found specific personality characteristics, coping strategies, and/or life experiences that either enhance or inhibit positive adjustment to breast cancer. Coping strategies found to be most effective have included a "fighting spirit"[82] and having a feeling of control over events, resulting in active participation in treatment.[54] On the other hand, poor adjustment has been associated with coping strategies based on avoidance,[83] prior negative sexual experiences, body image problems, and inhibition in discussing personal and sexual problems.[91]

The existence of social support

Social support consistently has been found to influence a woman's psychosocial adjustment to breast cancer.[10,82] The ability and availability of significant others in dealing with diagnosis and treatment can affect the patient's view of herself significantly.[10]

As is the case for individuals diagnosed with all types of cancer, breast cancer patients experience a heightened need for interpersonal support. Individuals who are able to maintain close connections with family and friends during the course of illness are more likely to cope effectively with the disease than those who are not able to maintain such relationships.[50] Northouse examined fears about recurrence in breast cancer patients 1 to 4 years after mastectomy. She found less fear of recurrence among women who reported a significant social network that was responsive to discussions about their concerns, and more fear in women reporting few significant relationships.[78]

The most important sources of social support for women, in order of importance are, her spouse, her family, and her friends.[95] Particularly for single women or those with a limited social network, self-help groups such as Reach to Recovery, Can-Surmount, and others should be made known. The proliferation and usefulness of such groups are recognized widely, and referrals to such programs should be made frequently in light of the importance of social support in promoting adaptation.

Role shifts during illness

Living with cancer creates disruptions in family roles and responsibilities.[20] Adult females clearly carry a disproportionate percentage of household responsibility before illness. What is clear is that women are taking on new roles outside the home without giving up their old roles. What happens to family roles and household responsibilities during illness is less clear, and how the shifts in responsibility affect adjustment is even less well understood.

Green[37] interviewed nine families headed by nonpartnered females with breast cancer and 18 partnered families all in which the adult woman had breast cancer in order to identify the responsibilities of individual family members at the time of diagnosis and again 6 to 12 months later. Green found that women carried considerably more responsibility for household duties than did any other single family member, and often more responsibility for shopping, meal preparation, kitchen cleaning, housework, clothing upkeep, pet care, child care, coordination of children's activities, and financial management than any other family member. Partners often assisted the women with these activities, but assumed primary responsibility for outside upkeep, vehicle maintenance and repair, household repairs, and financial input. In single-parent families, the women assumed primary responsibility for these latter activities also. Women in both types of families worked outside the home.

Family responsibilities initially lessened for women after diagnosis. A portion of their workload was assumed by one or more other people. Friends and relatives, including children, became much more visible, especially in single-parent families. This redistribution of responsibility, however, was short lived. By the second interview, all families had returned to their prediagnostic patterns, and in several instances women had assumed more responsibility than they had before.

Several interesting findings emerged during the initial treatment phases. Families reported that chemotherapy and radiation therapy constituted new family activities that required additional distribution of responsibility in the weeks and months after diagnosis. Additional treatment meant that someone had to take repsonsibility for making appointments, arranging for transport, and taking the women to treatment if they needed assistance. The families stated that health care professionals assisted with these activities, but the women, their families, friends, and relatives had to assume the majority of care. For a small number of families the patient with cancer needed temporary assistance with the activities of daily living after surgery and during recovery. These new responsibilities were shared by the family group, friends, and relatives.

During the recovery period, the distribution of responsibility for some activities shifted more drastically than for others. The "high-shift" activities were defined as transfer of $\geq 15\%$ of total responsibility from one member to another. The greatest shifts for partnered families occurred in shopping, housework, coordination of children's activities, child care, and clothing upkeep. With the exception of coordination of children's activities, the same high shift in activities occurred in nonpartnered families. In addition, nonpartnered women experienced high shifts in five other activities: meal preparation, kitchen cleaning, assistance with activities of daily living, outside upkeep, and vehicle maintenance. Overall, a greater percentage of responsibility was shifted in nonpartnered families than in partnered families.

Family members and friends who took on new roles and responsibilities reported spending less time in wage-earning activities. For both types of families, the hours spent in financial input (employment responsibilities) decreased by approximately one third during the weeks after surgery. Time spent in outside upkeep decreased for both groups. In contrast, the time commitment to children and to shopping remained stable.

Although exploratory in nature, Green's study[37] provides evidence that shifts in roles and responsibilities do occur in illness. The effects of a long-term or progressive illness on the redistribution of roles and responsibilities in families have not yet been determined. Strauss[100] identified the need for health care providers to assist patients with management of treatment regimens and symptoms, and with the reduction of social isolation. These factors clearly affect a woman's ability to perform her own roles or redistribute roles to others in the family unit.

In research with lung cancer patients, individuals reported relinquishing recreational and social roles before their work roles, activities in the home, or self-care behaviors.[68] Role shifts in families seem less disruptive if the patient is a man rather than a woman. For men, being ill typically translates into staying home from work and retreating into an environment where they can be taken care of. When a woman is ill, she must confront her role as a pivotal female in the family. She cannot escape the work within the home, even if she is employed outside the home. She is expected to recuperate in the very arena in which she is seen by herself and others as a responsive and continued worker.[86] Clinicians, particularly nurses and social workers, are in a unique position to assist women by informing them of the areas where major role shifts can occur and by exploring with them ways to plan the redistribution of responsibilities.

Women's caregiving abilities

Lewis et al. state that family adaptation to breast cancer is characterized by powerlessness, ambivalence, interdependence, uncertainty, role restructuring, and resiliency.[56] In a longitudinal study of 126 families of women with breast cancer, they report that family adaptation involves not only the coordination of care for the person with cancer, but also the development of the family system. Of interest are the responses of the children to the mother's breast cancer. School-aged children (7 to 10 years of age) experienced feelings of sadness, fear, and loneliness, with worry over the integrity of the family unit highlighting the need for consistent messages to the child that the family unit will be maintained, and the child will always be cared for. Children between the ages of 10 and 13 years of age focused on the change in their lives caused by the disease, such as the family expectation of assisting more with household tasks. These children need specific information regarding the disease and its treatment Finally, adolescents between the ages of 14 and 19 years reported conflict between their desire to be "doing their own thing" and "spending time at home." The researchers emphasize that adaptation to the illness is a family phenomenon impacting on the life process of the family and, as such, the family system should be targeted for intervention.

Living with breast cancer often requires continuing care management by a team of specialists. Care usually is provided to women through follow-up visits to ambulatory or outpatient clinics and consulting rooms, rather than through hospitalization. Families are relied on to be the major provider of care outside the health care institution during treatment as well as during the advanced phases of illness. Currently, little is known about differences in caregiver abilities and responsibilities assumed by male and female family members or about differences in the ways men and women react to their caregiver roles.

Horowitz[43] studied 131 adult children identified as the primary caregiver to an older, frail parent. Sons tended to become caregivers only in the absence of an available female sibling, and they were more likely to rely on the support of their own spouses. Sons provided less overall assistance to their parents than daughters, especially with regard to "hands-on" services. Sons also reported less stressful caregiving experiences independent of their degree of involvement.

Stetz[98] documented the demands reported by 64 spouses taking care of a terminally ill spouse with cancer in the home. The majority of spouses, 12 men (32%) and 30 women (68%) reported that managing the physical care, treatment regimens, and imposed changes was the most difficult part of their spouses' illness. Other demands commonly cited were managing the household and finances, standing by, dealing with alterations in their own well-being, unmet expectations from the health care system, constant vigilance, anticipating the future, and handling alterations in their relationship with their spouses. Major differences in the caregiving demands were noted between male and female caregivers. Overall, women reported more demands on themselves than men reported. On average, each woman reported between two or three demands, whereas each man reported zero to two. Men may have reported fewer overall concerns than women because family members may be willing to offer greater assistance and support to male caregivers than to female caregivers.

Women rated "standing by" as more difficult than "managing the household and finances," while men reversed the ratings for these demands. Approximately one third of the women (n = 13) experienced alterations in their own pattern of living and health as a direct result of the caregiving experience. In addition, significantly more women whose husbands had died of cancer felt they were in poor health during the illness as compared with other widows. Thus individuals who experience alterations in their own health during the caregiving experience could be at greater risk for illness in the ensuing months. Germino[28] found that adult children were more concerned about the father's health when the mother was the patient than vice versa.

Ekberg et al.[21] in a study of 30 married couples, found that chronic illness in one partner can result in increased responsibilities for the spouse and eventually lead to spouse burnout. The authors concluded that clinicians have a responsibility to care for spouse caregivers as well as for the patient. Clinicians need to be knowledgeable about the common physical and emotional symptoms of burnout. With this knowledge clinicians are better prepared to assist the spouse in early recognition of problems and to plan interventions accordingly.

One such intervention is to arrange respite care. Respite care is designed to provide relief to family caregivers for limited time periods when long-term home health care is a noninstitutional alternative and where the nursing therapeutic regimen is brought into the patient's own home.[71] Investing in caregivers' physical, financial, and emotional well-being may be more effective than providing the care required when caregivers become "patients."[5]

CLINICAL COURSE OF CANCER

The clinical course of breast cancer, as is the case for other cancer diagnoses, follows one of several possible courses or trajectories. Fig. 21-1 outlines a scheme of clinical cancer. A number of patients respond to the curative attempt with no recurrence of disease, remain well, and are, after a period of time, considered cured (course A). Some patients have a positive response to a curative attempt but then develop recurrence or metastasis (course B). Other patients begin treatment with a hope for cure but do not respond, and progressively decline (course C). In some patients the disease is too far advanced at the time of diagnosis, and they experience a progression of their disease (course D).

The acute stress response[42] has been described as a usual response to the diagnosis of cancer occurring at each transitional point of illness (beginning treatment, recurrence, treatment failure, disease progression). The response is characterized by shock, disbelief, anxiety, depression, sleep and appetite disturbance, and difficulty performing activities of daily living. The acute stress response usually subsides within 1 to 2 weeks of onset. Emotional support, giving clear information with sensitivity to the emotional issues at hand, and enhancing a patient's control over her environment can enhance resolution and inhibit more severe and long-standing emotional sequelae.

Obviously, the stage of disease at time of diagnosis, the clinical course of illness (including medical treatments), and possible recurrence will all impact on the psychosocial profiles of women with breast cancer. To a large extent these factors will determine the emotional issues that are most pressing at any given point.

Several authors[85,90,93,101] have described the clinical course of breast cancer by stage and the common events and psychosocial issues often associated with each. Such categorizations are useful as they highlight the chronic nature of breast cancer and draw attention to key emotional vulnerabilities that may occur at particular times. The uniqueness of every woman, however, always should be kept in mind. The discrete stages highlighted in the literature should be acknowledged as useful guides and conceptual frameworks, although they are limited as a result of obvious human differences.

THE DIAGNOSIS OF CANCER

Diagnostic phase

The prediagnostic phase is the time of initial symptom discovery, usually a breast lump. This period often is characterized by fear and disbelief, and in some cases may result in denial, withdrawal, and delay in seeking treatment.[92] The health-seeking behavior of women, particularly as it relates to early or delayed reporting of symptoms already has been discussed.

The period from time of diagnosis through surgery is characterized by medical evaluation, the development of new relationships with unfamiliar medical personnel, and the need to integrate a barrage of information that is at best frightening and confusing. Within the context of this anxiety-provoking situation a decision must be made regarding treatment. As one woman aptly stated "a decision upon which my very life or death might be based." This statement illustrates the tremendous responsibility, concern, and isolation that many women experience during this period.

Meaning of cancer

Despite increased openness about cancer by health care providers and the existence of broad public education programs aimed at increasing the awareness of cancer as curable or avoidable, the reaction of the general public remains largely negative. Cancer is more dreaded than any other life-threatening disease and may be asociated with protracted pain, disability, and death.[52] Consistent with this view, individual reactions to a cancer diagnosis are characterized by shock, disbelief, depression, fear, and panic.[53,80] Initial reactions to the diagnosis have been described as similar in nature to those accompanying acute grief reactions.[41,42] A large proportion of patients retrospectively describe the diagnostic period as the most stressful of their entire cancer experience,[50] although many could not share their feelings with family, friends, or health care providers at the time.[50,62]

Few women are informed of what to expect once they are discharged from the hospital. An early study by Quint[83] found that women are poorly prepared to deal with their concerns about the future and the potential for the recurrence of disease once they are home. Current clinical practice suggests that this may still be the case. Mechanic[69] noted

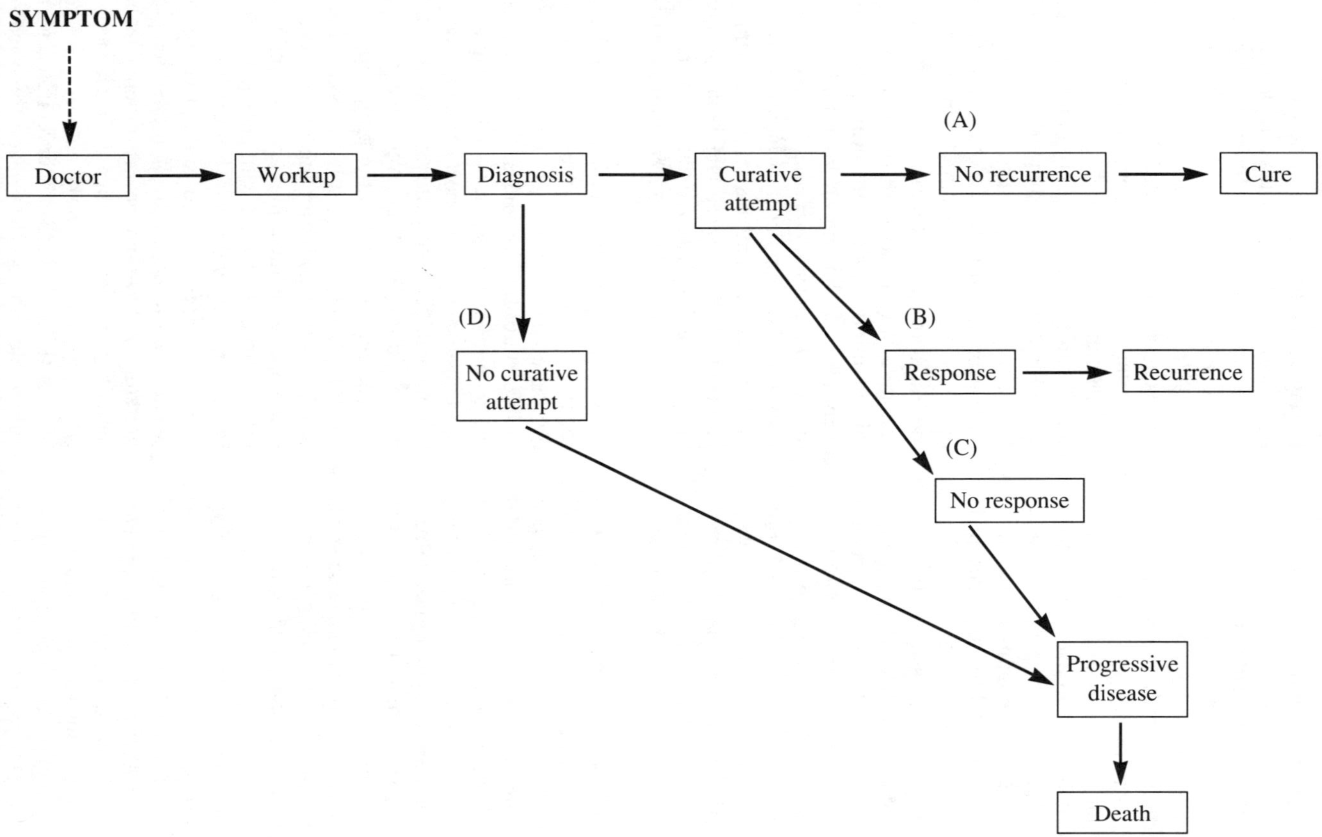

Fig. 21-1 Possible clinical courses of cancer. (From Holland J: Psychologic aspects of cancer. In Holland J and Frei E III, editors: Cancer medicine, Philadelphia, 1982, Lea & Febiger, with permission.)

that a woman's symptoms may limit her activity and interfere with her role obligations. Clinicians need to establish ongoing mechanisms to monitor patients' symptoms and assess patients' perceptions of what they think is interfering with their activities and responsibilities. The clinician is then in a position to help women to find the best solution for their situations.

Weisman and Worden describe the first 100 days following diagnosis as the period of "existential plight in cancer."[104] During this period, patient concerns focus on existential issues of life and death rather than on concerns related to health, work, finances, religion, self, or relationships with family and friends. While it is most unusual to observe extreme emotional reactions as the first response to breast cancer diagnosis, it remains important to assess the nature of the patients' reaction carefully. Initial reactions are often predictive of later adaptation.[36,76] Careful initial assessment by clinicians can help to identify individuals at risk for later adjustment problems and those in greatest need of ongoing psychosocial support.[105,108]

The initial response and adjustment to a diagnosis of breast cancer may be influenced profoundly by prior association with the disease.[85] Patients with memories of close relatives with breast cancer—particularly their mothers—may demonstrate heightened distress, especially if the relative died or had negative treatment experiences. Similarly, women with daughters may respond with excessive distress and guilt to the idea that the risk for the development of breast cancer is heightened in their offspring.[95] Women whose self-esteem depends largely on a "perfect" body can be expected to handle the prospect of breast loss poorly and may develop severe depressive symptoms irrespective of treatment.[95] These situations demonstrate the impact that life experiences and personality characteristics may have on adjustment, and stress the importance of evaluating the unique experiences and responses of women faced with a diagnosis of breast cancer.

During the diagnostic and early treatment period, patients may search for explanations or causes for their cancer and may struggle to translate clinical information into personal terms. In light of the fact that many clinicians are guarded about disclosing information until a firm diagnosis is established, patients may develop highly personal explanations that may be inaccurate and provoke intensely negative emotions. Clinicians should bear this in mind and keep patients informed throughout the diagnostic period. Ongoing involvement and information may minimize uncertainty and the development of maladaptive coping strategies based on erroneous beliefs.

While the literature clearly communicates the devastating emotional impact of a cancer diagnosis, it is also well documented that many individuals cope effectively. Positive coping strategies such as taking action and finding favorable characteristics in the situation have been reported as effective.[32] Maintaining optimism and the meaning of life[61] and having an active determination to recover[44] have been associated with positive adjustment. Contrary to the beliefs of many clinicians, denial also has been found to assist patients in coping effectively with a diagnosis of breast cancer[103] unless used to an excessive or psychotic degree. Most patients understand that the first course of treatment offers the best chance for "cure"; any sense of "fighting spirit" can be seen most prominently at this time.

With the firm establishment of the breast cancer diagnosis, planning for treatment begins. If patients have been given a clear explanation of their condition while being encouraged to maintain hope, the initial reaction of shock, fear, and desperation can give way to a sense of optimism.[41] Bearing this in mind, health care providers should view themselves as having an important role in monitoring and possibly mediating psychosocial adjustment. The most critical factors during this period are keeping patients informed, being actively involved in their care, and being aware of the unique meaning that individuals may associate with a diagnosis of breast cancer. Being alert to those women with pervasive and unyielding negative affects is always of primary importance, as they may require ongoing psychosocial intervention throughout the course of treatment and disease course.

In a study by Northouse,[77] 83% of a sample of mastectomy patients described the diagnostic phase through surgery as the most stressful time for them. "Women talked about being in an emotional upheaval during this time, yet having to make important decisions with little professional help." A study by Scott[92] revealed high levels of anxiety in women before and after breast biopsy that, when combined with incoming and unfamiliar medical information, interfered with decision-making ability in some individuals.

The need to expand supportive services for women before hospitalization is supported by the literature and would be instrumental in assisting patients and their families with decision making, stress management, early promotion of problem-solving skills, and crisis intervention at particularly vulnerable points. Expansion of such services would also acknowledge the diversity of emotional responses and the range of decision-making abilities of women diagnosed with breast cancer.

The treatment decision

Psychosocial factors cannot be ignored in considering which treatment is best for a particular patient, for even if the physician and/or the patient wish to ignore them, they will inevitably play a role in the patient's adjustment to life afterwards. Because cure rates for most cases of stage I or stage II breast cancer are the same regardless of whether the treatment is modified radical mastectomy or lumpectomy plus radiation therapy,[9,25,26] the woman should be well informed about the two treatments in order to make the best choice possible for herself. This process should include not only information about the medical and surgical aspects of the treatments, but also what is known about the psychosocial sequelae. In general, women choosing breast-conserving treatment have a greater degree of anticipatory concern regarding adverse effects on body image, disfigurement, and on their femininity than do those choosing mastectomy.[64] Women who choose breast-conserving treatment anticipate more difficulty handling the psychosocial problems that they expect mastectomy would entail. On the other hand, mastectomy patients, when making their treatment decision, tend as a group to be more afraid of death and less afraid of breast loss than those choosing lumpectomy and radiation therapy. In addition, they tend to be less likely to anticipate that mastectomy will cause problems with sexual desirability or enjoyment of sexual relations.[64]

Unfortunately, most mastectomy patients have problems in all of these areas when studied a year or more after treatment, and those receiving the breast-conserving treatment do not.[1,64,87,97] For these reasons, about half of the mastectomy patients will regret their treatment choice, whereas this is not the case for lumpectomy-radiation therapy patients. In an effort to help avoid posttreatment regrets, a thorough and unhurried discussion at the time of the cancer diagnosis regarding the likely psychosocial sequelae of mastectomy is indicated. This task is not always easy for a busy physician, but it is important enough to warrant the time required. If the diagnosing physician is unable or unwilling to do this, the patient should be referred to her primary care physician or to another member of the health care team. Generally, it is helpful for the patient to discuss treatment options with both a surgeon and a radiation oncologist to insure the communication of comprehensive information regarding treatment options.

Often, patients react to a diagnosis of breast cancer with feelings of fear and helplessness. When in such an emotional state, the patient is often looking to her primary physician for a curative treatment that will preserve her quality of life. The patient may feel threatened and think she can do nothing but rely on her doctors. Combating feelings of helplessness, to the greatest extent possible, can help to alleviate painful anxiety. This is best done by a member of the health care team who has established a treatment alliance with the patient. The health care provider should make the woman feel like a partner in everything that takes place. This is especially true regarding the decision about which treatment to choose. If a treatment alliance is forged at this point it can be used later on, during and after treatment, to help the woman adjust to the new realities of having a serious diagnosis and, in the case of mastectomy patients, a disfiguring treatment.

The postoperative period is a time when women are particularly vulnerable to a combination of anxiety and depression.[96] Concerns about whether or not the cancer was removed "completely" are prominent at this time. While attempting to deal with her own feelings, the patient also must manage and respond to the emotions and reactions of family members[30] who are often monitoring her emotional adjustment closely. Patients have reported psychosocial support from health care workers as one of the most valuable factors in their adjustment during the postoperative period.[79] Such support can be immensely influential in promoting both physiologic and psychologic adaptation.[93]

Adjuvant chemotherapy. While in the past adjuvant chemotherapy or hormonal therapy was reserved for women with stage II breast cancer (positive axillary lymph nodes), its use in treating stage I, node-negative disease is increasingly recommended, especially for women at known high risk. A recent and well-publicized randomized clinical trial was stopped abruptly because of the significant disease-free or recurrence-free survival advantage of 10% seen in node-negative women receiving adjuvant treatment over those who did not.[74] This news, although promising, presents even women with early stage disease with yet another decision to add to their already complex choice regarding surgical method. For women with more advanced illness, usually first discovered during what was hoped to be curative surgery, the news of positive lymph nodes and the need for additional treatment can be devastating.

The need for systemic treatment often elicits fears of side effects, discomfort, and deterioration. Women should be carefully educated about the specific drugs that will be used, the expected side effects, and their temporary nature. Misconceptions, often based on prior association with family and friends who received chemotherapy (and thus not specific to the disease or drugs used in the current breast cancer treatment) should be elicited and corrected before initiation of treatment.

Psychologic preparation for chemotherapy and functional support to assist in tolerating the disruption and side effects can greatly diminish adverse emotional responses.[95] Careful explanations of side effects assist women in knowing what to expect, help them to plan their lives and schedule accordingly, and add a dimension of control to the treatment experience.

Frequently experienced side effects among women receiving adjuvant treatment for breast cancer include nausea and vomiting, weight gain, alopecia, fatigue, and diminished energy. Anticipatory and posttreatment nausea and vomiting have been found to be most severe in women with high levels of anxiety.[48] Behavioral techniques such as relaxation exercises have been found to reduce the emetic effects of chemotherapy and will be discussed in greater detail later in this chapter. Antiemetic drugs such as prochlorperazine also may be effective. Weight gain of >10 lb is a frequent consequence of systemic breast cancer therapy and was demonstrated in one half of patients in a recent study.[46] Although its etiology is unclear, weight gain may be related to diminished activity during the treatment period. Efforts to minimize this effect including nutritional guidance and promotion of exercise, if tolerated, should be adopted by health care providers to reduce further risk of insult to body image and self-esteem. The expected and transient nature of alopecia should be explained to patients and efforts made to promote a positive appearance despite hair loss. The emergence of programs—such as Look Good, Feel Better, endorsed by the American Cancer Society—are increasingly available and should be made known to all women undergoing treatment. Selection and use of wigs and turbans as well as use and application of makeup to disguise skin discolorations and eyebrow loss are useful techniques to minimize the cosmetic effects of adjuvant therapies. In addition, these programs put women in touch with a support system that is eager to help, as many of the people involved have had personal experiences with breast cancer and have coped successfully with its treatment. In communities where such programs do not exist, their development should be explored and alternate providers used in the meantime.

On completion of the chemotherapy regimen, anxiety, depression, and fears of recurrence may skyrocket.[85] Anticipation of these responses and reassurance regarding the presence of frequent medical follow-up should be given. In women whose emotional distress does not subside, ongoing psychotherapeutic intervention may be indicated.

Recovery/reconstruction. Despite the availability and increased use of breast-conserving procedures, mastectomy remains a major treatment method following diagnosis for breast cancer and is associated with the occurrence of body image problems, diminished self-esteem, and adjustment difficulties.[10] Surgical breast reconstruction has been found to alleviate at least some emotional sequelae following mastectomy in certain women, particularly in diminishing fears of recurrence once the visible reminder of the mastectomy scar is removed.[95] Reconstructive surgery is becoming increasingly available through improved surgical techniques, although clinical practice suggests that women are not always informed adequately about the option.

While the need for further research to examine the psychologic benefits of breast reconstruction is clear, there is beginning evidence favoring its positive impact, especially when it is performed along with or immediately following mastectomy. One study indicated that early breast reconstruction was associated with diminished feelings of loss, disfigurement, and subsequent emotional trauma.[106] Other investigators have found early reconstruction to promote satisfaction and psychosocial adjustment in patients when compared to women who underwent mastectomy alone.[19,75,99] In contrast to the clearly positive impact of early reconstruction, Schain[89] found less than striking differences in adjustment between the immediate and delayed reconstruction groups and demonstrated that differences would likely diminish over time. Still others suggest that immediate reconstruction may inhibit the necessary grief reaction associated with breast cancer diagnosis and thus may interfere with the working through and integration of those issues.[85] Further research is obviously needed to determine the risks and benefits of early vs. delayed reconstruction and the particular subgroups of women that will best be served by each.

The need for ongoing investigation in the area of reconstructive breast surgery following mastectomy is clear. The informational needs of women, psychosocial sequelae for those who choose reconstruction as opposed to those who do not, specific subgroups who may demonstrate particular benefits from the procedure, and the risk/benefit of delayed vs. immediate reconstruction are all important areas of study.

Within the current state of knowledge, the most pressing issue is to insure that the option for breast reconstruction is communicated to all women undergoing mastectomy. One survey revealed that 43% of women learned about the availability of breast reconstruction through television and print media as opposed to their physicians.[17] The probability of securing inaccurate or incomplete information from popular media sources is high and demonstrates the need for health care providers to assume an active role in educating patients about all of their options following surgery.

Progressive/advanced disease. As mentioned earlier, the psychosocial issues faced by women with breast cancer depend in part on the clinical course of the disease process. As the disease progresses, women often report an upsetting scenario that includes frequent pain, disability, increased dependence, and diminished functional ability.[41]

The development of recurrence after a disease-free interval can be especially devastating for a woman and those close to her. The work-up for metastatic disease is often difficult and anxiety provoking,[11] and psychosocial problems experienced at the time of diagnosis frequently resurface, often with greater intensity.[41]

Investigators studying quality of life in cancer patients have demonstrated a clear relationship between an individuals' perception of quality of life and the presence of discomfort.[67] As uncomfortable symptoms increase, perceived quality of life diminishes. Thus an important goal in the psychosocial treatment of patients with advanced breast cancer centers around symptom control.

Symptoms frequently experienced include pain secondary to bone metastasis, confusion secondary to hypercalcemia in those with secondary bone disease, dyspnea secondary to lung metastasis, wound problems related to locally advanced disease, and diminished functional ability. The presence of increased physical discomfort combined with a lack of control and predictability regarding the occurrence of symptoms often enhances psychosocial distress in women with advanced disease.

Shock and depression often accompany recurrence and require the woman and her family to reevaluate the future. Chekryn studied psychosocial reactions of women and their spouses when exposed to a recurrence of gynecologic or breast cancer.[15] Eight themes emerged from interviews, including difficulties with closure, uncertainty, grief, feelings of injustice, fear and anger, existential concerns, coping, family impact, and the inability to communicate about the meaning of recurrence. Patients were shocked and surprised at the recurrence, with 50% of the patients and 30% of the spouses expecting a cure. Fears were voiced around treatment, pain, family separation, and the possibility of death.

Fear of recurrence was a predominant response of 30 women with stage I, stage II, and stage III breast cancer studied by Northouse.[78] She found that a greater fear of recurrence was associated with patients having fewer significant others (social support) ($p<.025$). Subjects identified maintaining a positive attitude and support as important coping mechanisms. However, with actual recurrence, psychosocial responses encompassed feelings of anxiety, powerlessness, and fear of death, disability, and pain.[55] The thought of undertaking additional treatment can be overwhelming. The psychosocial impact of losing one's hair is difficult with initial treatment and can be even more devastating with the commencement of additional treatment. Reliving an initial treatment experience can be a difficult experience for patients, particularly when coupled with the uncertainty of prognosis.

In spite of the overwhelming nature of the psychosocial responses, patients do indeed cope with advanced illness. Lewis et al.[57] investigated personal control in 57 late-stage cancer patients. They found that patients used several cognitive strategies to achieve feelings of control including monitoring their progress, waiting things out, refocusing by explaining and searching for meaning, and turning aspects of control over to others.

Social support appears to be a crucial aspect of coping ability. Lewis and Bloom[55] identified three sources of support: family, friends, and caregivers. Support involved sharing information, problem-solving, and assisting with communication regarding fears and concerns. Lindsey et al.,[59] in a review of social support in postmastectomy women, concluded that social support was an important factor in adjustment.

Quality of life components of those patients who present with advanced disease are similar in many respects to those who develop a recurrence; the management of symptoms is dependent on the site of metastasis, and decreased functioning leads to altered family roles. Psychosocial responses, however, are somewhat different. Weisman and Worden,[104] in their classic study of existential plight, found that patients with advanced cancer exhibited more vulnerability, were more distressed, had more mood disturbance, and were more concerned about existential, health, and work issues than those with less advanced cancer.

A final issue that repeatedly surfaces among patients, family members, and professional care providers deals with the use of aggressive treatment protocols in the presence of disseminated disease. Often patients and families ask to participate in experimental protocols even when there is little likelihood of extending survival. Controversy continues about the efficacy of such therapies and the role health professionals can play in facilitating patients' choices about participating.

The need for health care professionals to establish structured dialogues with patients, family members, and care providers regarding treatment goals and expectations is essential. The idea that certain individuals may respond to investigational treatment with increased hope, despite the existence of progressive illness, should be a consideration in treatment planning. The need to separate and clarify the values, thoughts, and emotional reactions of care providers, patients, and families about these delicate issues is important if individualized care with attention to womens' psychosocial needs is to be provided.

It is beyond the scope of this chapter to present a comprehensive overview of the psychosocial reactions of patients to the process of dying. It should be mentioned, however, that once the terminal period has begun, it is not usually the fact of dying, but the quality of dying, that seems to be the overwhelming concern.[101]

MANAGEMENT OF PSYCHOSOCIAL PROBLEMS

The increased length of survival for patients from the time of diagnosis has highlighted the need for psychotherapeutic and behavior-oriented interventions to reduce distress, promote adjustment, and improve quality of life. The pessimism of the past, often associated with the perception of cancer as a death sentence, fears of "unleashing" painful feelings, or the belief that even extreme expressions of emotional distress are "appropriate" for cancer patients, have given way to more realistic information. Such information stresses the importance and effectiveness of interventions aimed at managing and reducing the psychosocial distress associated with cancer. While the need for further research in this area is clear, numerous studies have documented the efficacy of a variety of modalities in managing psychosocial problems for the patient with breast cancer. The issues and problems that can be managed effectively include emotional distress such as anxiety and depression, problems with sexuality and body image, marital and family difficulties, compliance, pain, organic complications such as delirium and dementia induced by brain metastases and/or treatment, anticipatory and post-treatment nausea and vomiting, and anorexia and feeding problems.[41,85]

Psychotherapeutic modalities

Depending on the nature of the problem, the treatment modality may take the form of individual psychotherapy, group therapy, family therapy, marital therapy, pharmacotherapy, behavior-oriented therapies, or some combination when indicated.

Individual psychotherapy. Individual therapy has the advantage of enabling the patient to elaborate and explore her thoughts, fantasies, and distressing emotions in the confidential privacy of the psychiatric clinician's office. Patients who have adverse reactions to their diagnosis and/or treatment of sufficient severity to warrant referral often respond to a brief, focused, goal-directed form of psychotherapy. The role of the therapist will center around support and enhancement of the ability to cope with distressing feelings with a therapist who is accepting and nonjudgmental. The frequency of visits should be geared to the patient's needs, but generally once or twice a week for 10 to 20 weeks is sufficient, as the focus is on an unpleasant reality that the patient needs a more productive perspective on. Guidance, suggestions, and even advice are often useful. Very often short-term psychotherapy will be aided by combining it with pharmacotherapy and family therapy. These will be discussed briefly below, but it should be noted that in almost all situations requiring psychiatric intervention, individual psychotherapy should play an important role. Even when the focus is on group, family, or marital therapy, the patient should be given the chance to clarify feelings and enhance coping skills individually, with the help of a skilled psychotherapist.

Group therapy. Group therapy frequently is employed with breast cancer patients, particularly in a group where other patients have the same illness and are grappling with similar problems. Indeed, even for patients not requiring psychiatric referral, support groups are often a useful adjunct in promoting adjustment to breast cancer. The American Cancer Society's Reach to Recovery groups have proven useful for many patients. A recent study suggests that patients with advanced breast cancer who are in a support group live longer than those who are not.[96] Formal psychotherapy groups also offer support but usually are reserved for patients with more than usual emotional distress, and involve an attempt to offer insight as well as support.[51] These groups have the advantage of being less expensive for the patient than individual treatment and can sometimes provide rapid insights into current problems through interaction with others. Observing someone else struggle with problems that the patient herself is experiencing may be beneficial. In addition, helping others in the group to gain perspective on problems can help the patient gain a similar, personal perspective. Most of the time, patients in sufficient psychiatric distress to require referral to a psychotherapy group will also require individual psychotherapy. There is often a need to discuss matters too personal to be safely revealed in a group setting.

Marital therapy. Marital therapy can be a useful tool for many patients, most often as an adjunct to brief individual psychotherapy. Most of the time this is recommended when one or both of the following situations occur: (1) the patient is having sexual difficulties as a result of illness and/or treatment; or (2) the husband is having a great deal of difficulty coping with his wife's disease and/or treatment. In a situation where the husband is handling the matter well but the patient is upset, the psychiatric clinician may find it useful to see the husband and patient in order to enlist the husband's help in providing extra support for his spouse. For example, if a mastectomy patient is depressed over feeling disfigured and less sexually desirable, the husband may be enlisted to reassure her of his continuing love and sexual interest. Naturally this depends on the husband being a relatively stable and interested partner. In a situation where the husband is not stable or interested, utilizing him in this fashion becomes difficult. If the husband is having a great deal of difficulty coping with the illness and treatment, marital therapy also can be helpful. The focus in these situations is to enable the couple to clarify their difficulties and work together to resolve them. Individual therapy for the husband also may be necessary, particularly when the husband is having more psychologic difficulty coping than the patient is.

Pharmacotherapy. Pharmacotherapy, as an adjunct to one or more of the above psychotherapies, can be an important aid in bringing psychosocial symptoms under control. Psychopharmacologic agents for the treatment of psychiatric complications of breast cancer will be reviewed only briefly here. For a thorough review, as well as expanded treatment guidelines, the reader is referred to a comprehensive chapter by Massie and Lesko.[65]

For patients with excessive anxiety, an anxiolytic is often fast acting and effective. These drugs are best used for rapid, short-term relief in helping the patient gain temporary control over agonizing anxiety. Use of these medications also may assist the patient in making use of psychotherapy, which can provide more permanent control over symptoms. If used in this manner, problems with habituation can be avoided. Breast cancer patients often need time to adjust to the new realities brought upon them by their illness and these medications can be useful in helping them to adjust. Constant, long-term use of benzodiazepines and other chemically similar drugs can be habituating and is not recommended.

There are a number of anxiolytics available, including diazepam (Valium), chlordiazepoxide (Librium), alprazolam (Xanax), lorazepam (Ativan), clorazepate (Tranxene), and oxazepam (Serax). These drugs are all similar in their overall clinical effects. Table 21-1 compares the three anxiolytics most often recommended in clinical practice. Dosages indicated usually should be divided. Because of their shorter half-life, alprazolam and lorazepam have advantages for elderly patients because toxicity from sedating medications is more common, and withdrawal reactions may occur upon abrupt discontinuance unless the patient's dose is tapered.[51]

Buspirone is a nonbenzodiazepine that has less abuse potential than the benzodiazepines and does not cause sedation. However, as it takes 1 to 2 weeks at therapeutic doses before antianxiety effects occur, it is often not useful for the fast relief of anxiety experienced by most breast cancer patients. Benzodiazepines accomplish this better. For those patients with chronic anxiety, buspirone may be considered.

In patients who develop clinically relevant depressive syndromes a combination of psychotherapy and antidepressant medication often proves useful. The antidepressants most commonly used for cancer patients are the tricyclic antidepressants (e.g., amitriptyline, doxepin, imipramine, nortriptyline, and protriptyline). These medications are started in low doses given at bedtime (25 to 50 mg) and are increased slowly, over days to weeks, until symptoms subside. Peak dosages are usually substantially lower than those tolerated by physically healthy individuals. Antidepressant medications may take 2 to 4 weeks to produce their desired effects. Patients may need ongoing support, reassurance, and monitoring before experiencing the antidepressant effects of medication.

Table 21-1 Three anxiolytic medications commonly prescribed in the oncology setting

	Alprazolam (Xanax)	Lorazepam (Ativan)	Diazepam (Valium)
Dosage	0.25-5 mg/day	0.5-6 mg/day	2-20 mg/day
Half-life	12-15 hours	10-14 hours	20-50 hours
Oral absorption rate	Intermediate	Intermediate	Fast
Advantages	Shorter after effects	Shorter after effects	Easier to divide dosages
Disadvantages			May cause depression and/or confusion

Adapted in part from Karasu TB, editor: Treatment of psychiatric disorders, Washington, DC, 1989, American Psychiatric Association Press, p 2040.

Behavioral interventions

Behavioral interventions such as progressive muscle relaxation, guided imagery, biofeedback, and systematic desensitization add a useful dimension to the care of breast cancer patients. Self-administered behavioral techniques have been used increasingly by cancer patients, with the advantage of increasing their sense of control and participation in treatment.[66] The behavioral model emphasizes a sequential continuing process of evaluation and intervention: problem identification, formulating therapy goals, determining and implementing treatment methods, and collecting information to evaluate goal attainment.[2] The effectiveness of intervention techniques is assessed systematically after each session, and if the techniques are not helpful they are revised or discarded with input from the patient. Behavioral interventions appeal to patients because they are self-directed and enhance a sense of participation in treatment as well as feelings of self-control and mastery. The behavioral techniques mentioned above have proven to be effective in controlling many of the undesirable consequences of cancer.[84] Anxiety, pain, the fear associated with medical procedures, anticipatory and posttreatment nausea and vomiting, and feelings of helplessness often associated with depressive states in cancer patients have been reduced by the use of behavioral strategies.

During the last 10 years the development and description of behavioral techniques and their efficacy in controlling the immediate unpleasant consequences produced by cancer and its treatment have abounded in the literature. Behavior-oriented clinicians have made important gains in developing techniques aimed at managing treatment side effects and psychosomatic symptoms in cancer patients.[7,13,72,84]

The goal of behavioral therapies in cancer care is the modification of maladaptive behavior, as opposed to the uncovering of psychologic conflicts and the restructuring of defense mechanisms. Interventions are (1) focused on reduction of immediate and disturbing symptoms; (2) individualized to meet patient's preferences and individual circumstances; (3) time limited and explicitly goal directed; (4) evaluated in terms of objectively observable changes in patient's symptoms and behavior; and (5) modified or discarded based on patient response.

The use of behavioral therapies rests on the notion that illness behavior may persist long after its organic cause has disappeared.[2] Behavioral approaches have been used successfully with breast cancer patients and have demonstrated particular benefit in reducing pain, anxiety, nausea and vomiting secondary to adjuvant chemotherapy, and fear associated with medical procedures, and in enhancing personal control over emotions.[84]

Progressive muscle relaxation/guided imagery. One of the most common methods of behavior therapy is progressive muscle relaxation, originally developed as a method of treatment for insomnia, anxiety, tension, and psychosomatic disorders.[49] Passive and active methods with and without the use of guided imagery have been described. The passive method involves teaching a patient to relax all parts of the body systematically while focusing on the feelings and sensations produced by relaxation, and learning to deepen that state progressively. The active method of progressive muscle relaxation instructs the patient to tense each part of the body before relaxing it. Each procedure can be combined with the technique of guided imagery. Guided imagery involves a process whereby the clinician suggests a scene or experience that has been described as peaceful or pleasant by the patient and is used to further promote a relaxed state. All methods of progressive muscle relaxation share the goal of producing a deep state of relaxation and have been found to be equally effective.[67] The use and effectiveness of any method depends on the preferences of the patient and clinician. Taped relaxation procedures, although popular, are usually less effective than those tailored to individual patient needs, especially when the procedure is being taught for self-use.

Progressive muscle relaxation increasingly has been recognized as effective for controlling the emotional distress, pain, nausea, and vomiting associated with cancer treatment.[7,66,84,93] Successful treatment of those symptoms is based partially on the openness of the patient to the approach and a belief that it will be helpful, as well as the availability of the clinician to make frequent, unhurried visits. Several sessions are often needed to teach patients to use relaxation techniques on their own, if so desired.

Adverse reactions to relaxation techniques, although extremely rare, should be mentioned, as clinicians should be cognizant of their possible occurrence. Patients with major functional or organic psychiatric syndromes should not be managed by relaxation, which may evoke unexpected negative responses. Occasionally relaxation techniques may increase anxiety.[66] This may occur in patients with unrealistic expectations regarding the goals of the procedure, for patients with underlying personality disorders, or in patients who equate relaxation with loss of control and death. Finally, patients treated with progressive muscle relaxation for anticipatory or posttreatment nausea and vomiting may develop a conditional nausea and vomiting response to a relaxation tape or exercise.[7] The clinician may suggest that the patient do a different form of relaxation in the hospital from that used at home.

Relaxation and imagery techniques that claim to promote relaxation as well as tumor regression[94] should be avoided. At the very least, such claims are highly controversial and lack scientific merit. In addition, the development of extreme and unwarranted feelings of responsibility and control over the course of illness may result. Particularly in cases where breast cancer progresses to advanced stages, such feelings can promote guilt, despair, and diminished self-esteem and may induce a severe depressive state.

Biofeedback. Biofeedback uses specialized instrumentation to reflect changes in physiologic function to patients in such a way as to allow them to intervene and change their own internal activity. Clinical biofeedback devices are electronically sophisticated, sometimes portable instruments that present information in a variety of engaging fashions. Through skin electrodes or thermistors they monitor subtle changes in temperature, muscle activity, brain waves, sweat gland activity, blood pressure, and cardiac rate and rhythm. This information allows the patient to make internal adjustments toward a relaxed state and receive immediate rewards for having done so. The equipment externally validates the presence of internal changes, thus greatly speeding up the learning and reinforcement of those changes. Biofeedback has been used most frequently to help people learn to relax overactivity of the sympathetic nervous system. Biofeedback research and clinical application have centered on treatment of vascular and tension headaches, cardiovascular control, disorders of motor function, gastrointestinal disorders, the management of chronic pain, and the management of anxiety and treatment side effects from chemotherapy or radiation.[30] Behavioral treatment using biofeedback methods alone may be of limited value. Gains made within treatment sessions must extend and become incorporated into the patient's everyday life, so that control of physiologic responses without mechanical assistance can be attained.[109]

Biofeedback should be used as one component of a total treatment program tailored to individual symptoms and needs. Other modalities used in conjunction with biofeedback may include pharmacotherapy, progressive muscle relaxation and imagery, and promoting awareness of the antecedents to treatment side effects and/or anxiety. When used with other treatment modalities, biofeedback may contribute significantly to symptom relief by providing objective evidence of the contributory nature of emotional factors to physical distress and anxiety, thus enhancing personal control over discomfort.

Systematic desensitization. "Systematic desensitization means substituting an emotional response that is appropriate or adaptive to a given situation for one that is inappropriate or maladaptive."[2] Systematic desensitization is a form of counterconditioning and refers to any procedure that uses learning principles to train a patient to substitute one type of response for another. In desensitization, relaxation is specifically substituted for anxiety.[2]

Systematic desensitization requires using a combination of progressive muscle relaxation, autogenics, and guided imagery. The person is instructed to recall events or situations that are individually stressful, such as a chemotherapy infusion or a diagnostic test. First, the problem to be desensitized must be identified; then it is helpful to establish a sequential list of images to use in the desensitization process. The patient is instructed to move from the least to the most stressful image. Each scene in the sequence is imagined in as much vivid detail as possible. When the least stressful scene can be imagined without anxiety, the person is instructed to move on to the next scene in the sequence. If the person becomes anxious in response to an imagined scene, the clinician dismisses the scene and shifts, instead, to a relaxing scene or uses some other short relaxation technique. Once relaxation is reestablished, the scene is imagined again until it can be done without resulting in anxiety. The desensitization process is done over a series of sessions and eventually the person should be able to move from the least to most stressful image in one session. Once the person has mastered the process, she can relax when the stressful situation is encountered in real life.

PSYCHOLOGIC IMPACT OF BREAST CANCER: DIFFERENTIATING PSYCHIATRIC COMPLICATIONS FROM EXPECTED PSYCHOLOGIC RESPONSES

Most patients develop transient psychologic symptoms that are responsive to information about what to expect regarding the cancer course, its treatment, support, and reassurance. There are some who may require more aggressive psychotherapeutic intervention such as pharmacotherapy and ongoing psychotherapy. The following are some guidelines to assist the clinician in identifying patients who exhibit criteria suggesting the presence of a psychiatric syndrome.

Most patients do not react to a diagnosis and treatment for breast cancer by developing a clinically diagnosable psychiatric condition.[63] In some instances this may occur, particularly in patients who have a past history of significant psychiatric disturbance. When severe reactions do occur, prompt referral and collaboration with a psychiatric liaison service is indicated. What is much more likely is for some patients to react to diagnosis and treatment with subclinical depression,[63] which may include transient suicidal ideation and increased anxiety at the time of reexaminations. If a good treatment alliance previously has been established, it can be utilized in providing support to the patient during these difficult periods. Patients who are more upset and cannot be calmed through support and guidance by the health provider may require treatment with psychoactive medication. Benzodiazepines or tricyclics may be prescribed to alleviate excessive symptoms of anxiety and/or depression (see the previous discussion of pharmacotherapy). It remains important, however, to continue to use the therapeutic relationship to support patients during anxiety-provoking times. Using psychoactive medications alone without supportive intervention is usually counterproductive and may contribute to feelings of abandonment and helplessness, thus provoking increased anxiety.

If the patient's problems become severe—meaning that the provider feels supportive measures are insufficient and ineffective in controlling emotional distress—referral to a psychiatric clinician is indicated. Factors that may prevent adjustment to breast cancer illness and treatment include a history of significant depression, manic-depressive illness, schizophrenia, neuroses, organic mental conditions, personality disorders, lack of social support, or inadequate control of physical discomfort.

Because transient symptoms of anxiety and depression are common in women with breast cancer, the ability of health care providers to distinguish expected reactions from more severe psychiatric complications is crucial. As stated earlier, anxiety and depression are common symptoms that are particularly evident at transition points during the clinical course of cancer. Usually these symptoms subside within 2 to 4 weeks and are responsive to supportive reassurance and information regarding what to expect during the course of treatment. For a small proportion of women psychologic distress does not subside with usual interventions. Unfortunately, clinically relevant and severe psychiatric syndromes often are missed by nonpsychiatric care providers.[107] One of the reasons that it may be difficult to detect serious psychiatric reactions in patients is that several of the diagnostic criteria used to evaluate the presence of severe depression (lack of appetite, insomnia, decreased sexual interest, diminished energy) may overlap with usual disease and treatment effects. Additionally, it is not unusual for health care providers to confuse their own fears about cancer with the emotional reactions of their patients (i.e., "I too would be extremely depressed if I were in a similar situation").

The following list will provide some general guidelines to assist in recognizing patients who should be referred for evaluation by a trained psychiatric clinician.

1. Past history of psychiatric hospitalization and/or significant psychiatric/personality disorder
2. Persistent refusal, indecisiveness, or noncompliance with regard to needed treatment
3. Persistent symptoms of anxiety and depression that are unresponsive to usual support from health care providers and/or family members; the symptoms may present in the form of constant fear associated with treatment and procedures and/or excessive crying and hopelessness that worsen rather than improve over time
4. An abrupt, unexplained change in mood or behavior
5. Insomnia, anorexia, diminished energy that is out of proportion to expected treatment effects
6. Persistent suicidal ideation
7. Unusual or eccentric behavior or confusion (may be indicative of an organic mental disorder)
8. Excessive guilt and self-blame for illness

It should be stressed again that a majority of patients reveal subclinical levels of depression and do not require referral to a psychiatric clinician.

After referral to a psychiatric specialist, one or a combination of several therapeutic modalities may be employed. Breast cancer and its treatment may precipitate an exacerbation of an underlying mental illness for which the patient was already predisposed that may require extensive treatment (e.g., hospitalization for a psychosis, ongoing pharmacotherapy or psychotherapy, and the like). A discussion of these specialized forms of treatment is not warranted here, but the interested reader can consult appropriate standard texts.[51] As stated earlier, most reactions to breast cancer do not require referral to a psychiatric clinician. When they do, some form of brief psychotherapy aimed at minimizing distress and enhancing coping skills is the standard treatment of choice.

SUMMARY AND CONCLUSIONS

The psychosocial issues faced by women diagnosed and treated for breast cancer are influenced by sociocultural, medical, family, and individual factors. Rapid scientific advances as well as highly publicized, conflicting treatment philosophies among experts in the field have added a new dimension on an already emotionally charged scenario encountered by those diagnosed with breast cancer. Active participation in treatment decisions have placed new responsibilities on patients, at a time when even the most well-informed experts do not have all of the answers. Responsibility to participate in the decision-making process adds emotional "fuel" to a "fire" already laden with the fear, anxiety, and concern inherent in the diagnostic process. Although involvement in decision making is clearly a positive aspect of current breast cancer therapies, great care should be taken to insure the repeated communication of timely and relevant information that is consistent with patients' needs, tolerance, and comprehension. A multidisciplinary approach is essential to guarantee the communication of comprehensive information to all women. Women should be given the opportunity to speak with a surgeon, radiation oncologist, chemotherapist, oncology nurse, physical therapist, social worker, and other women who have experienced breast cancer treatment. Care should be taken to provide needed information from a variety of expert perspectives while respecting the unique characteristics, psychosocial profiles, needs, and desires of each individual. In treatment settings with limited resources, every effort should be made to enlist the help and support of providers and services that can assist patients with their complex treatment decisions. Referral to community resources and support services following discharge from the hospital is often helpful, even for women that cope well with initial treatment. The time immediately following surgery is often stressful, and additional support may be instrumental in promoting positive adaptation, especially for women with limited family support.

Evidence supports the fact that women adapt well to both mastectomy and lumpectomy plus radiation, but the retention of the breast appears to promote better self- and body-image and has less negative impact on sexuality. Reconstruction provides an important treatment option associated with improved social, sexual, and psychologic function. The availability of the reconstructive option should be communicated clearly to all women undergoing mastectomy. Adjuvant chemotherapy produces psychologic distress, largely because of its association with unpleasant side effects. These are temporary in nature and often are responsive to information and routine psychotherapeutic interventions. Treatment for advanced breast cancer centers on enhancing the patient's physical and emotional comfort, with the goal of maintaining symptom control and providing psychosocial support. Family members, although an important source of support for patients, are also vulnerable to the emotional effects of the cancer crisis. Every effort should be made to include them in the patient's treatment. Some women may request assistance regarding the communication of information to their children, and age-appropriate guidelines should be given. Additionally, families that have had extreme problems before cancer diagnosis may be subject to increased conflict and disorganization, particularly at transitional points along the clinical cancer course. These families should be encouraged to see a psychiatric specialist.

Most women undergoing breast cancer treatment and their families experience expected periods of emotional turmoil that occur at transitional points along the clinical course of cancer. For a small proportion of women, more severe psychiatric complications may occur, warranting referral to a psychiatric specialist. A variety of psychotherapeutic modalities are useful in helping women to work through the expected emotional responses to breast cancer, as well as more severe responses. Supportive psychotherapeutic measures should be used routinely, as they minimize distress and enhance feelings of control and mastery over self and environment. For these reasons alone their utility in the care of women with breast cancer is paramount. Again, in women who are not responsive to routine support and information, referral to a psychiatric specialist may be indicated.

Throughout the clinical course of cancer the patient's relationship with health care providers and the presence of a supportive social network are important factors in assuring successful negotiation of the many physical and psychosocial demands imposed by breast cancer diagnosis and treatment. Further investigation regarding the utility of systematically tested interventions aimed at promoting psychosocial adjustment to breast cancer are needed. Investigation aimed at enhancing understanding of the behaviors of individuals experiencing the crisis of cancer and identification of individuals in need of intensive psychosocial support also is needed. For treatments that offer equal survival benefit, inquiry regarding emotional sequelae may be useful in guiding treatment decisions. Additionally, research regarding women who delay in seeking treatment for suspected breast cancer and the association of that behavior with psychosocial variables is critical.

As scientific inquiry continues to produce vast, although sometimes conflicting information regarding etiology and treatment for breast cancer, concurrent investigations regarding the psychosocial aspects of the disease are crucial. This line of inquiry will, at the very least, assist in promoting emotional well-being in women faced with an extreme and unexpected life crisis. At best, expanding the knowledge base relative to the psychosocial aspects of breast cancer may provide some "missing links" regarding psychosocial adaptation and quality of life, as well as their impact on survival.

REFERENCES

1. Aaronson NK, Barelink H, van Dongen JA, et al: Evaluation of breast-conserving therapy: clinical, methodological, and psychosocial perspectives, Eur J Surg Oncol 14:133, 1988.
2. Abel GG, Rouleau JL, and Coyne BJ: Behavioral medicine strategies in medical patients. In Abel GG, editor: Principles of medical psychiatry, New York, 1987, Grune & Stratton, pp 329-345.
3. American Cancer Society: Cancer facts and figures—1988, New York, 1988, American Cancer Society, Inc.
4. Bader J, Lippman M, Swain S, et al: Preliminary report of the NCI early breast cancer study: a prospective randomized comparison of lumpectomy and radiation to mastectomy for Stage I and II breast cancer, Int J Radiat Oncol Biol Phys 13:160, 1987 (abstract).
5. Bader JE: Respite care: temporary relief for care-givers, Women Health 10:39, 1985.
6. Bard M and Sutherland AM: Psychosocial impact of cancer and its treatment. IV. Adaptation to radical mastectomy, Cancer, 8:652, 1955.
7. Berenson S: The cancer patient. In Zahovrek RP, editor: Relaxation and imagery: tools for therapeutic communication and intervention, Philadelphia, 1988, WB Saunders, pp 168-191.
8. Blichert-Toft M: A Danish randomized trial comparing breast preservation with mastectomy in mammary carcinoma. Proceedings of the NIH Consensus Development Conference on Early Stage Breast Cancer, Bethesda, June 1990, pp 28-31.
9. Blichert-Toft M, Brincker H, Andersen JA, et al: A Danish randomized trial comparing breast-preserving therapy with mastectomy in mammary carcinoma, Acta Oncol 27:671, 1988.
10. Bloom JR: Social support, accommodation to stress and adjustment to breast cancer, Soc Sci Med 16:1329, 1982.
11. Bope E: Follow-up of the cancer patient: surveillance for metastasis, Prim Care 14:391, 1987.
12. Bullough B: Discovery of the first signs and symptoms of breast cancer, Nurse Pract 31:31, 1980.
13. Burish TG and Lyles JN: Effectiveness of relaxation training in reducing the aversiveness of chemotherapy in the treatment of cancer, Behav Ther Exp Psychiatry 10:357, 1979.
14. Castles MR and Murray R: Dying in an institution, New York, 1979, Appleton-Century-Crofts.
15. Chekryn J: Cancer recurrence: personal meaning, communication, and marital adjustment, Cancer Nurs 7:491, 1984.
16. Clarke DE and Sandler LS: Factors involved in nurses' teaching breast self examination, Cancer Nurs 12:41, 1989.
17. Clifford E and Clifford M: Psychological perspectives of mastectomy and breast reconstruction, Res Staff Phys February, p 49, 1981.
18. Crooke CE and Jones SD: Educating women about the importance of breast screenings: the nurses' role, Cancer Nurs 12:161, 1989.
19. Dean C, Chetty U, and Forrest APM: Effects of immediate breast reconstruction on psychosocial morbidity after mastectomy, Lancet 17:459, 1985.
20. Edstrom S and Miller MW: Preparing the family to care for the cancer patient at home: a home course, Cancer Nurs 11:49, 1981.
21. Ekberg JY, Griffith N, and Foxall MJ: Spouse burnout syndrome, J Adv Nurs 11:161, 1986.
22. Elwood JM and Moorehead WP: Delay in diagnosis and long-term survival in breast cancer, Br Med J 280:1291, 1980.
23. Feldman J: The dissemination of health information, Chicago, 1966, Aldine.
24. Fisher B and Barboni P: Breast cancer. In Holland JF and Frei E, editors: Cancer medicine, ed 2, Philadelphia, 1982 Lea & Febiger, pp 2025-2056.
25. Fisher B, Bauer M, Margolese R, et al: Five-year results of a randomized clinical trial comparing total mastectomy and segmental mastectomy with or without radiation in the treatment of breast cancer, N Engl J Med 312:665, 1985.
26. Fisher B, Redmond C, Poisson R, et al: Eight year results of a randomized clinical trial comparing total mastectomy and lumpectomy with or without irradiation in the treatment of breast cancer, N Engl J Med 320:822, 1989.
27. Funch DP: The role of patient delay in the evaluation of breast self-examination, J Psychosoc Oncol 2:31, 1985.
28. Germino B: Family members' concerns after cancer diagnosis, unpublished doctoral dissertation, University of Washington, Seattle, Washington, 1984.
29. Giaquinta B: Helping families face the crisis of cancer, Am J Nurs 77(10):1585, 1977.
30. Glatsein E, Straus K, Lichter A, et al: Results of the NCI early breast cancer trial. Proceedings of the NIH Consensus Development Conference on Early Stage Breast Cancer, Bethesda, June 1990, pp 32-33.
31. Gorzynski JG, Holland JC, Katz J, et al: Stability of ego defenses and endocrine responses in women prior to breast biopsy and ten years later, Psychosom Med 42:323, 1980.
32. Gotay CC: Causal attributions and coping behaviors in early-stage cervical cancer. Presented at the Annual Meeting of the American Psychological Association, Los Angeles, 1981.
33. Gould-Martin K, Paganini-Hill A, Casagrande C, et al: Behavioural and biological determinants of the surgical stage of breast cancer, Prevent Med 11:1429, 1982.
34. Gove WP: Gender differences in mental and physical illness: the effects of fixed roles and nurturant roles, Soc Sci Med 19:77, 1984.
35. Gove WP and Hughes M: Possible causes of the apparent sex differences in physical health, Am Sociol Rev 44:59, 1979.
36. Graydon JE: Factors that predict patients' functioning following treatment for cancer, Int J Nurs Stud 25:117, 1988.
37. Green CP: Changes in responsibility in women's families after the diagnosis of cancer, Health Care Women Int 7:221, 1986.
38. Hackett TP, Cassem NH, and Raker JW: Patient delay in cancer, New Engl J Med 89:14, 1973.
39. Hibbard JH and Pope CR: Another look at sex differences in role performance, Gerontologist 25:612, 1986.
40. Holland JC: Coping with cancer: a challenge to the behavioral sciences. In Cullen JW, Fox BH, and Isom RN, editors: Cancer: the behavioral dimensions, New York, 1976, Raven Press.
41. Holland JC: Psychologic aspects of cancer. In Holland JF and Frei E III, editors: Cancer medicine, Philadelphia, 1982, Lea & Febiger pp 1175-1184.
42. Holland JC and Mastrovito R: Psychologic adaptation to breast cancer, Cancer, 46:1045, 1980.
43. Horowitz A: Sons and daughters in care-givers to older parents: differences in role performance, Gerontologist 25:612, 1985.
44. Hughes J: Emotional reactions to the diagnosis and treatment of early breast cancer, J Psychosom Res 26:277, 1982.
45. Huguley CM Jr and Brown RL: The value of breast self-examination, Cancer 47:89, 1981.
46. Huntington M: Weight gain in patients receiving adjuvant chemotherapy for carcinoma of the breast, Cancer 56:472, 1985.

47. Israel L: Conquering cancer, New York, 1978, Random House.
48. Jacobsen PB, Redd WH, and Holland JC: Parameters of chemotherapy induced anticipatory nausea in cancer patients. Presentation at the Annual Meeting of the Society of Behavioral Medicine, New Orleans, March 29, 1985.
49. Jacobson E: Progressive relaxation, Chicago, 1988, University of Chicago Press.
50. Jamison KR, Wellisch DK, and Pasnau RO: Psychosocial aspects of mastectomy. I. The woman's perspective, Am J Psychiatry 135:432, 1978.
51. Karasu TB, editor: Treatment of psychiatric disorders, Washington, DC, 1989, American Psychiatric Press.
52. Krant MJ: Problems of the physician in presenting the patient with the diagnosis. In Cullen JW, Fox BH, and Isom RN, editors: Cancer: the behavioral dimensions, New York, 1976, Raven Press, pp 269-274.
53. Krant MJ: Psychosocial impact of gynecological cancer, Cancer 48:608, 1981.
54. Levy S, Heberman R, Malvish A, et al: Prognostic risk assessment in primary breast cancer by behavioral and immunologic parameters, Health Psychol 4:99, 1985.
55. Lewis F and Bloom J: Psychosocial adjustment to breast cancer: a review of selected literature, Int J Psych Med 9:1, 1978.
56. Lewis F, Ellison E, and Woods N: The impact of breast cancer on the family, Semin Oncol Nurs 1:206, 1985.
57. Lewis F, Haberman M, and Wallhagen M: How adults with late stage cancer experience personal control, J Psych Oncol 4:27, 1986.
58. Lierman L: Discovery of breast changes: women's responses and nursing implications forthcoming, Cancer Nurs (in press).
59. Lindsey A, Norbeck J, Carrieri V, and Perry E: Social support and health outcomes in post mastectomy women: a review, Cancer Nurs 4:377, 1981.
60. Magarey CJ, Todd PB, and Blizard PF: Psychosocial factors influencing delay and breast self-examination in women with symptoms of breast cancer, Soc Sci 11:229, 1977.
61. Mages NL, Castro JR, Fobair P, et al: Patterns of psychosocial response to cancer: can effective adaptation be predicted? Int J Radiat Oncol Biol Phys 7:385, 1981.
62. Maguire PG: The psychological and social consequences of breast cancer, Nurs Mirror 140:54, 1975.
63. Margolis GJ, Goodman RL, and Rubin A: Psychological effects of breast-conserving cancer treatment and mastectomy, Psychosomatics 31:33, 1990.
64. Margolis GJ, Goodman RL, Rubin A, and Pajak T: Psychological factors in the choice of treatment for breast cancer, Psychosomatics 30:192, 1989.
65. Massie MJ and Lesko LM: Psychopharmacological management. In Holland JC and Rowland JH, editors: Handbook of psychooncology: psychological care of the patient with cancer, New York, 1989, Oxford University Press, pp 470-491.
66. Mastrovito R: Behavioral techniques: progressive relaxation and self-regulatory therapies. In Holland JC and Rowland JH, editors: Handbook of psychooncology: psychological care of the patient with cancer, New York, 1989, Oxford University Press, pp 492-501.
67. McCorkle R: A randomized clinical trial of home health nursing care for lung cancer patients, Cancer 64:199, 1989.
68. McCorkle R and Quint-Benoliel JQ: Symptom distress, current concerns and mood disturbance after diagnosis of life-threatening disease, Soc Sci Med 17(7):431, 1983.
69. Mechanic D: Sex, illness, illness behavior, and the use of health services, J Hum Stress 2:29, 1976.
70. Miller DB: Women and long term nursing care, Women Health 10:29, 1985.
71. Mood DW and Bickes JT: Strategies to enhance self care in radiation therapy, Oncol Nurs Forum, 16(suppl):143, 1987.
72. Morrow GR and Morrell BS: Behavioral treatment for the anticipatory nausea and vomiting induced by cancer chemotherapy, N Engl J Med 307:1476, 1982.
73. Nathanson CA: Illness and the feminine role: a theoretical review, Soc Sci Med 9:57, 1975.
74. National Cancer Institute: Clinical alert, May 16, 1988.
75. Noone RB, Frazier TG, Hayward CZ, et al: Patient acceptance of immediate reconstruction following mastectomy, Plast Reconstruct Surg 69:632, 1982.
76. Northouse L: The impact of cancer on the family: an overview, Int J Psychiatry Med 14:215, 1984.
77. Northouse L: A longitudinal study of the adjustment of patients and husbands to breast cancer, Oncol Nurs Forum 16:511, 1989.
78. Northouse LL: Mastectomy patients and the fear of cancer recurrence, Cancer Nurs 4(3):213, 1980.
79. Novack DH, Plumer R, Smith RL, et al: Changes in physicians' attitudes toward telling the cancer patient, JAMA 241:897, 1979.
80. Novotny E, Hyland J, Coyne L, et al: Factors affecting adjustment to cancer, Bull Menninger Clin 48:318, 1984.
81. Oken D: What to tell cancer patients: a study of medical attitudes, JAMA 175:1120, 1961.
82. Penman DT, Bloom JR, Fotopoulou S, et al: The impact of mastectomy on self concept and ego function. A combined cross sectional and longitudinal study with comparison groups, Women Health 11:3, 1986.
83. Quint JC: The impact of mastectomy, Am J Nurs 63(11):29, 1963.
84. Redd WH, Andersen GV, and Minagawa RY: Hypnotic control of anticipatory emesis in patients receiving cancer chemotherapy, J Consult Clin Psychol 50:14, 1982.
85. Rowland JH and Holland JC: Breast cancer. In Holland JC and Rowland JH, editors: Handbook of psychooncology: psychological care of the patient with cancer, New York, 1989, Oxford University Press, pp 188-207.
86. Sandelowski M: Women's health and choice, Princeton, NJ, 1981, Prentice-Hall.
87. Sanger CK and Reznikoff M: A comparison of the psychological effects of breast saving procedures with the modified radical mastectomy, Cancer 48:234, 1981.
88. Sarrazin D, Le MG, Arriagada R, et al: Ten-year results of a randomized trial comparing a conservative treatment to mastectomy in early breast cancer, Radiother Oncol 14:177, 1989.
89. Schain WS: Prophylaxis therapy and rehabilitation for the psychosocial concerns of breast cancer patients: a stage-related approach, Dis Breast 4(2):23-27, 4(3):26-31, 1978.
90. Schain WS: Sexual problems of patients with cancer. In DeVita VT, Hellman S, and Rosenberg SA, editors: Cancer: principles and practice of oncology, Philadelphia, 1982, JB Lippincott, pp 278-291.
91. Schain WS, Wellisch DK, Pasnau RD, et al: The sooner the better: a study of psychosocial factors in women undergoing immediate versus delayed breast reconstruction, Am J Psychiatry 142:40, 1985.
92. Scott DW: Anxiety, critical thinking and information processing during and after breast biopsy, Nurs Res 32:24, 1983.
93. Scott DW: Quality of life following the diagnosis of breast cancer, Topics Clin Nurs, January, p 20, 1985.
94. Simonton OC, Matthews J, Simonton S, and Creighton JL: Getting well again, New York, 1978, Bantam Books.

95. Sinsheimer L and Holland JC: Psychosocial issues in breast cancer, Semin Oncol 14(1):75, 1987.
96. Spiegel D, Bloom J, Kraemer HC, et al: Effect of psychosocial treatment on survival of patients with metastatic breast cancer, Lancet ii:888, 1989.
97. Steinbert MD, Juliano MA, and Wise L: Psychological outcome of lumpectomy versus mastectomy in the treatment of breast cancer, Am J Psychiatry 142:34, 1985.
98. Stetz K: The experience of spouse care-giving during advanced cancer. Unpublished doctoral dissertation, University of Washington, Seattle, Wash, 1986.
99. Stevens LA, McGrain MH, Druss RG, et al: The psychological impact of immediate breast reconstruction for women with early breast cancer, Plast Reconstr Surg 73:619, 1984.
100. Strauss A: Chronic illness and quality of life, St Louis, 1975, CV Mosby Co.
101. Thomas SG: Breast cancer: the psychosocial issues, Cancer Nurs 1(1):53, 1978.
102. Verbrugge LM: Female illness rates and illness behavior: testing hypothesis about sex differences in health, Women Health 4:61, 1979.
103. Watson M, Greer S, Blake S, and Sharpnell K: Reaction to a diagnosis of breast cancer: relationship between denial, delay, and rates of psychological morbidity, Cancer 53:2008, 1984.
104. Weisman A and Worden JW: The existential plight in cancer: significance of the first 100 days, Int J Psychiatry Med 7(1):1, 1976-1977.
105. Weisman AD, Worden JW, and Sobel HJ: Psychosocial screening and intervention with cancer patients: final report of the Omega Project (CA 19797), Bethesda, MD, National Cancer Institute, 1980, pp 1-203.
106. Wellisch DL, Schain WS, Noone BR, and Little JW: Psychosocial correlates of immediate versus delayed reconstruction of the breast, Plast Reconstr Surg 76:713, 1985.
107. Wells KB, Hays RD, Burnam A, et al: Detection of depressive disorder for patients receiving prepaid or fee-for-service care, JAMA 262:3298, 1989.
108. Worden JW: Psychosocial screening of cancer patients, J Psychosoc Oncol 1(4):1, 1983.
109. Young LD and Blanchard EB: Medical application of biofeedback training—a selective review. In Rachman S, editor: Contributions to medical psychology vol 2, New York, 1980, Pergamon Press, pp 215-254.

22 Rehabilitation

Mary E. Cooley and Bernadette Erikson

The diagnosis of breast cancer creates profound changes for the woman who undergoes treatment. After the diagnosis of breast cancer, life will never be the same. However, the initiation of a comprehensive approach to rehabilitation can assist the individual in successful adaptation to living with cancer. This chapter discusses the concept of rehabilitation and highlights the physical, psychologic, social, and economic issues that are critical in rehabilitation of the individual with breast cancer. In addition, community resources will be identified that are available for education and support of individuals with breast cancer.

OVERVIEW OF REHABILITATION

The first rehabilitation program that was designed specifically for individuals with cancer was at Memorial Sloan-Kettering Cancer Center in 1967.[9] Unfortunately, rehabilitation services in cancer care have been slow in gaining widespread recognition. In 1978, Lehmann et al.[27] published a landmark study which indicated that individuals with cancer have multiple rehabilitation needs which were not being addressed. Lehmann et al.[27] stated that the lack of identification of patient problems and lack of appropriate referral for patients with rehabilitation problems were the major barriers to optimal delivery of services. Recently, rehabilitation in cancer care has received increased visibility. Watson[54] predicts that the next decade will bring rehabilitation to the forefront of cancer care. The increased success of treating various cancers, coupled with increasing numbers of long-term survivors of cancer have created a dramatic need for rehabilitation services.

In order to plan for and provide rehabilitation services, a clear understanding of rehabilitation and the components of a program are necessary. Dudas and Carlson[11] define rehabilitation as a process which enables individuals to function at the maximum level of their physical, mental, emotional, and economic potential. As the above definition implies, rehabilitation services must include attention to physical limitations, as well as the resulting psychologic, social, and economic issues. There are several other factors that are essential for a rehabilitation program to be successful:

- Services should begin at diagnosis and continue throughout all phases of disease and treatment.
- The patient and family should be considered the unit of care.
- An interdisciplinary team approach is best.[4,9,41]

The process of rehabilitation should begin at diagnosis. It should be integrated into the plan of care and continue throughout all phases of disease and treatment. Dietz[9] has developed four categories for cancer rehabilitation: preventative, restorative, supportive, and palliative. As the names imply, these categories reflect the various state of the person's disease and overall goals for treatment. No matter what the goal is for rehabilitation, early implementation of a rehabilitation program helps minimize adverse consequences of decreased mobility, as well as the adverse psychosocial sequelae of disability.

The patient and family should be considered the unit of care. Patients should be actively involved with the health care team in decision-making and mutual goal-setting regarding the rehabilitation process. When developing goals for rehabilitation, it is absolutely essential to include the individual's personal goals and values and consider the impact on their life-style.[11] Goals which are established must be realistic and consistent with the individual's chance for recovery.

An interdisciplinary approach to care is strongly suggested in a comprehensive rehabilitation program. The use of this approach provides expertise from different disciplines, which helps provide optimal care. The most common members of an oncology rehabilitation team include a physician, a registered nurse, social worker, and a physical therapist. Other team members may include a psychologist, clergy, vocational counselor, occupational therapist, and a dietitian. In the case of breast cancer, a Reach to Recovery volunteer may be an additional member of the team.[19,42]

Before a rehabilitation program is begun, a thorough assessment is essential. The assessment

REHABILITATION ASSESSMENT

1. **General information**
   a. Age
   b. History of present illness
      1) Diagnosis and stage of disease
      2) Current cancer treatment
      3) X-rays and lab data
      4) Physical exam
      5) Understanding of disease
   c. Past medical history
   d. Medications
   e. Cognitive function
2. **Physical**
   a. Physical performance
   b. Mobility and endurance
   c. Ability to perform activities of daily living
3. **Psychosocial**
   a. Past psychiatric history
   b. Coping strategies
   c. Support systems
   d. Impact of cancer treatment on lifestyle
4. **Economic**
   a. Occupation
   b. Insurance coverage

should include information about physical status, as well as psychologic, social, and occupational status of the individual. Suggestions for assessment[9,41,42,54] are presented above. Upon completion of the assessment, discussion by various members of the team will identify patient problems and help develop a comprehensive plan for care.

ISSUES IN REHABILITATION

The literature concerning rehabilitation in breast cancer is scant. However, this section provides an introduction to the physical, psychosocial, and economic issues that are important in rehabilitation of breast cancer patients and provide suggestions for future research.

One of the first steps in implementing a successful rehabilitation program is the development of mutually formulated goals between the health care provider and the individual with breast cancer. Major goals when providing care to women with breast cancer are to promote optimal physical, psychosocial, and vocational function. Examples of goals and desired outcomes that may result from the rehabilitation program are provided on p. 573.[4,41,42,44]

The process of recovery from breast cancer evolves over an extended period of time. Although many milestones are achieved within the first year, particularly related to physical function, it may take several years for full recovery. Often the speed of recovery is related to an individual's age, as well as the extent of disease and surgery. Older women usually have a more difficult time with physical recovery, whereas younger women may have a more difficult time with psychologic adjustment.[53] It is important to begin interventions directed towards rehabilitation as soon as possible to promote recovery. The ideal time to begin rehabilitation interventions is before the surgery is performed. Providing information about diagnostic tests, the disease, and treatment options can be tremendously helpful for women struggling to make decisions about treatment. The time immediately after surgery is a particularly critical period for rehabilitation.[44] It is during this time that interventions must be directed toward regaining mobility and function of the affected arm, as well as integrating the change in body image.[44] Although interventions with respect to physical, psychosocial, and economic issues should be addressed simultaneously, each issue will be discussed separately here.

Physical issues

Ganz[16] conducted a study that identified the rehabilitation needs of women treated with either modified radical mastectomy or segmental mastectomy and radiation therapy the first month after primary treatment. The most frequent physical problems were limited upper extremity mobility, arm weakness, and fatigue. The limited upper extremity mobility and arm weakness often caused difficulty with household chores, physical activity, driving, and lifting. Nickkanen[32] also identified shoulder dysfunction and lymphedema as the primary physical complications following surgical treatment of breast cancer. It is interesting to note that these problems occurred with same frequency irrespective of the procedure performed.

The results of these studies demonstrate the need for an intense physical rehabilitation program. It is important to evaluate patients as early as possible, ideally before surgery, to determine their baseline functional ability and arm circumference, and to instruct them on postoperative measures to prevent shoulder limitation and the development of lymphedema. Following surgery, these patients should be further evaluated to determine their level of dysfunction, to set reasonable rehabilitation goals, to instruct and provide treatments to correct their dysfunction, and to assure follow-up intervention if necessary.

Shoulder dysfunction. There are several aspects of conventional treatment of breast cancer

GOALS FOR CARE IN BREAST CANCER

Goals	Patient outcome
Promote optimal physical function.	Participate in exercises to restore optimal physical function and mobility of affected arm and shoulder. Identify an acceptable method to restore external physical appearance. Discuss appropriate self-care management to prevent lymphedema and infection of affected arm.
Promote optimal psychosocial function.	Identify and/or utilize successful coping strategies to adapt to diagnosis of breast cancer. Develop and/or maintain satisfactory family and/or social relationships. Adjust to change in body image.
Promote optimal vocational function.	Engage in desired employment. Identify community resources that are available for women with breast cancer.

that can lead to temporary or permanent shoulder and arm dysfunction. Decreased skin mobility of the chest wall and formation of fibrous adhesions resulting from surgical dissection, radiation fibrosis and axillary scarring can cause shoulder joint dysfunction, leading to scapular substitution for proper shoulder motion, which can promote joint contracture. If allowed to progress, adhesive capsulitis or rotator cuff tendonitis can result. The shoulder joint dysfunction can cause pain, muscle spasms, immobility, and a functional loss of range of motion.

Trauma to the long thoracic nerve during axillary dissection can lead to paralysis of the serratus anterior muscle, which is a primary stabilizer of the scapula, causing functional impairment especially with reaching. If damage is due to vascular deprivation or stretching, the nerve may recover; however, paralysis will be permanent if the nerve is transected. Intermittent chest wall pain, not associated with movement or posterior upper arm pain or paresthesia can be due to cutaneous nerve regeneration or entrapment by adhesions. Prolonged spasms of the rhomboids or trapezius are most often due to overcompensation for the loss of breast weight or the high anxiety levels of the patient.[45,49] Instruction in proper posture and relaxation techniques can reduce the forward head positioning and rounded shoulders that can lead to interscapular pain, headache, and low back pain.[58]

Early physical therapy intervention is beneficial in preventing and avoiding further functional loss due to shoulder dysfunction.[59] Patients who are categorized as middle aged or older often have preexisting conditions such as osteoarthritis that can cause additional difficulties. Preoperative evaluation can often assist with setting reasonable goals for postoperative recovery. Patients often do not realize that they have a limitation in motion because they have kept their arm immobile postoperatively for fear of hurting the incision, or they simply do not move the arm through a full range of motion with their daily activities. Often the initial realization of the limited motion comes when they are unable to attain the needed positioning, e.g., for radiation therapy simulation or to close the back zipper on a dress.

An exercise program consisting of gentle stretching and active assisted motion is necessary for restoring motion. Range of motion (ROM) exercises should begin soon after surgery while the patient is still hospitalized. Initially, they should consist of active hand and elbow ROM exercises followed by hand and forearm isometrics. Active assisted ROM exercises can be started with the shoulder, avoiding incisional stretching. When the drains are removed, gentle resistance can be added. By week 3 or 4, strengthening exercises can be added for progressive resistance. Aggressive exercises with heavy weights, exercises that promote a prolonged dependent position, or substitution of other muscles or joints should be avoided. After the patients are instructed in the proper techniques of the exercises, they should be provided with a written home exercise program to be completed three times daily with 5 to 10 repetitions each. Specific exercise programs are based on individual patient deficits but most often include a combination of the following exercises: shoulder shrugs, assisted forward flexion, abduction with external rotation, internal/external rotation, internal rotation, and extension. See below for explanations.

Increased scarring and adhesions can be reduced by a combination of massage and gentle passive stretching followed by active motion exercises. Because patients may develop erythema and moist desquamation during radiation therapy, wound and skin management is important. Patients must be discouraged from using topical ointments without physician approval. If irritation develops from bra elastic, patients are encouraged to wear tube tops or cotton vests for breast support to prevent further irritation until the skin heals, approximately 2 to 3 weeks after completion of radiation therapy.

Numbness and pain associated with surgical nerve trauma or entrapment by adhesions can produce elevated anxiety levels in patients. They often perceive this sensation as edema of the axilla or chest wall when numbness is the actual problem. Various desensitization techniques can be employed to provide re-education of normal sensation as regeneration occurs. Pain can be treated with massage, stretching exercises, or with transcutaneous electrical nerve stimulation (TENS),[58] either at the site of pain or proximally along the dermatome or at the nerve root.

Decreased strength can gradually be improved by encouraging normal functional use of the arm and by active and progressive resistive exercise programs utilizing surgical tubing or Theraband, and eventually light weights, 1 to 5 lbs; however, vigorous programs with heavy weights or resistance should be avoided.

Lymphedema. Lymphedema is one of the most significant long-term complications following surgery for breast cancer. It causes physical discomfort, a decrease in the functional ability of the arm, cosmetic disfigurement, and can lead to cellulitis, lymphangitis, and lymphangiosarcoma. Reported incidence rates vary significantly from 6.7% to 62.5% following radical mastectomy[3] to 5% to 10% for modified radical mastectomy or lesser procedures.[14,45] The lymphatic system is a complex arrangement of vessels and nodes which serve to

ACTIVE ASSISTED EXERCISES

Repeat 5-10 times each, 3 times daily.

Shoulder shrug—position: sitting

Start with your arms held loosely at your sides and breathe deeply as you lift your shoulders. Breathe out as you lower your shoulders. Next, make circular motions with the tips of your shoulders, first forward, then backward.

Assisted forward flexion—position: lying on back

Begin by holding a cane with both hands on your thighs and then slowly raise the cane over your head, keeping elbows straight. The work should be done by the uninvolved arm with the involved arm remaining relaxed. Lower your arms to the original position. Relax.

Abduction with external rotation—position: lying on back

Holding the cane with both hands, raise arms overhead and then bend elbows so the cane comes to rest on the top of your head. Straighten your elbows and return arms to your side.

Internal/external rotation—position: lying on back

Place your arm out to the side with your elbow bent to 90 degrees with fingers pointing toward the ceiling. Move your hand forward to touch the mat and then backward to the mat, keeping your elbow in contact with the mat at all times.

Internal rotation—position: standing

Stand with your involved arm behind your back and your uninvolved arm over your shoulder, holding a towel between both hands. Straighten your strong elbow and raise your involved arm up your back slowly. Return to the original position.

Extension—position: standing

Grasp a cane between both hands behind your back, then raise your hands as far as possible. Slowly lower them again. Keep your elbows and back straight at all times.

return lymph and proteins from the tissue spaces to the circulatory system. Its three main functions are to return proteins from the interstitial fluid, to remove bacteria and other large particles, and to provide the pathway by which fat absorbed from the gastrointestinal tract reaches the bloodstream.[6]

The primary etiologic factors implicated in the formation of lymphedema in the breast cancer patient are the extent of surgical resection, peripheral lymphatic irradiation, and infection.[2] Postoperative lymphedema is a result of lymphatic flow insufficiency, which is usually controlled by the formation of collateral vessels and anastamoses that reroute the drainage. Following the formation of fibrosis from irradiation or scarring from infection, further blockage results in an accumulation of protein in the interstitial fluid. The decreased hydrostatic pressure results in dilatation of the lymphatic vessels, valvular incompetency, and eventual lymphostasis.[14]

Acute postoperative lymphedema occurs within the first 6 weeks following surgery. It is usually transient as lymphatic regeneration is adequate. It is pitting in nature and can generally be controlled by proper early positioning, elevation, gentle massage, and compressive bandaging.

Chronic lymphedema presents a much more severe problem as it develops weeks or even years following surgery. The risk factors associated with the development of chronic lymphedema include extensive surgical resection with ablation of the lymph nodes, axillary radiation, the development of infection or delayed wound healing, and possibly obesity and age. Chronic lymphedema is brawny and nonpitting due to increased protein content in the interstitial fluid and fibrosis of subcutaneous tissue. This can produce a sensation of heaviness due to compression which can result in decreased extremity use and an increase in venous and lymphatic obstruction.[14] Nerve entrapments can occur proximally with resultant brachial plexus neuropathy following radiation therapy or distally presenting as carpal tunnel syndrome with pain and paresthesia.[15]

In addition to the physiologic effects of lymphedema, patients must endure the weight of the affected limb which often increases postural imbalances and causes further development of musculoskeletal problems. The evident size difference of the limb hinders clothing choices and can cause the patient to feel pressured to explain her medical condition to others or anxiety that the swelling is the result of a recurrence of the cancer.[23] Early intervention for prevention and management of lymphedema is of utmost importance for the patient's physical and mental well-being.

Lymphedema management includes patient education on the prevention of lymphedema, ongoing screening for the onset of lymphedema and treatment based on the degree and duration of the swelling. The goals of treatment are to reduce tissue induration, remove excess fluid from the arm, regain the skin elasticity, reduce the risk of inflammation, increase the ROM of the extremity, increase the strength of the musculature and encourage full use of the arm.

Before patients are discharged from the hospital, they should be instructed about and provided with written information on hand and arm care to prevent the development of lymphedema. Patients should be instructed on how and why lymphedema occurs following lymph node dissection and informed that they are at risk for infection throughout their lives. Burns should be avoided by using elbow length oven mitts, wearing rubber gloves when washing dishes, keeping the extremity covered when exposed to the sun, and utilizing special care when using irons or frying pans. Patients should avoid skin punctures by refusing venipuncture in the involved arm and by using garden gloves to avoid thorns and dirt. Arm constriction from elastic clothing or tight jewelry should be avoided and blood pressure measurements should be taken on the other arm. Excessive strain to the arm should be avoided immediately after surgery by refraining from heavy lifting, pushing, or pulling. Patients must be aware of good arm hygiene and treat all cuts and scratches with a thorough washing and application of an antiseptic. Any signs of infection, redness, increased warmth, hardness, or swelling, should be reported to their physician for possible antibiotic treatment. See p. 576 for patient instructions.

The degree of lymphedema can be categorized as either mild, moderate, or severe depending on the amount of actual swelling present. There are two methods of measuring the swelling. The first is volumetric measurements using water displacement in a special cylinder. This method is technically more accurate,[24] but is less efficient for regular sequential measurements and does not permit localization of specific sites of swelling. The other is arm circumference measurements using a fiberglass tape measure, which is less likely to stretch and can be cleaned easily. Measurements should be taken by the same person if possible to reduce inaccuracy and the tape should be pulled taut without skin indentation. The arm is measured at the palmar crease; the wrist; 5, 10, and 15 cm above the wrist; at the olecranon; and 5, 10, and 15 cm above the olecranon. An increase of 1.5 to 3 cm is mild, 3 to 5 cm is moderate, and 5 cm is severe[24,31] when compared to the uninvolved extremity or prelymphedema measurements of the same extremity.

Mild lymphedema can be treated with elevation,

PATIENT INFORMATION—HAND AND ARM PRECAUTIONS

- Do not permit injections, blood samples, or vaccinations to be done on your affected arm unless specifically recommended by a physician who is aware of your surgery.
- When trimming cuticles, take extra care not to tear hangnails.
- Wear heavy gloves when gardening and digging or handling thorny plants.
- Always use a thimble when sewing to avoid pinpricks and wear rubber gloves while washing dishes.
- Protect your arm from burns especially from small appliances such as irons or frying pans and from the sun.
- Be sure your hand and arm are well protected with an elbow length mitt when reaching into a hot oven.
- Always have blood pressure measurements taken on the opposite arm.
- Avoid arm constriction from tight elastic sleeves or jewelry.
- Do not carry heavy objects—especially heavy grocery bags or luggage—or push heavy furniture.
- Apply a good lanolin cream several times daily if your skin appears dry.

Treat cuts and scratches by washing the area well and applying an antiseptic. Contact your physician if signs of infection, redness, warmth, or swelling occur.

especially at night, with the shoulder positioned at 90 degree abduction, the elbow flexed 60 to 90 degrees and the hand resting on pillows. Manual massage can be utilized distally to proximally in a centripetal fashion with the arm elevated. This is followed by the placement of elastic bandaging (Tubigrip or ace wraps) applying increased pressure distally. These should be worn during waking hours and should be monitored often for readjustments in pressure as swelling declines.

More persistent edema requires the use of pneumatic compression devices that consist of a nylon sleeve containing an air chamber that is inflated by a pneumatic pump to 40 to 70 mmHg. The pumps are available in various styles for clinic use or home rental or purchase. Uniform intermittent compression sleeves (Pression, Jobst, Flowtron) contain a single air chamber. Differential sequential compression sleeves (Wright Pump, Hemaflow, Lymphapress) range from 3 to 14 chambers. The benefits of one type over the others is widely debated.[64] Treatment times for the pumps range from 2 to 8 hours daily. Patients will also use compressive bandages to provide continued compression and to maintain decreases attained by the use of the pump and to prevent loss of skin elasticity. As significant gains are achieved using the pump, the patient is measured for a custom pressure gradient support sleeve (Jobst, Sigvaris). These sleeves are used to maintain edema reduction and should be remeasured often for elasticity and fit. Active and isometric exercises performed three to four times daily will assist with improved lymph flow.[17]

Other methods of lymphedema control include manual lymph drainage (MLD) which was first developed in the 1930s in Austria and Germany but is only recently being utilized in the United States. It is based on the theory that the area of lymphatic malfunction can be bypassed by stimulating lymphatic flow in the contralateral quadrant and then directing the excess fluid from the involved side, across the chest by lymphatic anastomoses, to the unaffected opposite quadrant.[13,23] Cold lasers are also being utilized in an experimental technique that involves applying laser teatments along the course of specific venous return, distally to proximally along the upper extremity. Both of these methods look promising in the control of this significant problem, but further research is needed to delineate their effectiveness.

Cosmetic appearance. Another aspect of care that should be addressed is the cosmetic appearance of the breast. The woman usually engages in a discussion with the physician before surgery. Options are explored and decisions made about the best approach for the individual. Treatment options usually include either a segmental mastectomy and radiation therapy or a modified radical mastectomy. Althogh segmental mastectomy and radiation often leave a better cosmetic appearance, this approach is not appropriate for all women. Therefore, a modified radical mastectomy may be performed. In the case of the modified radical mastectomy, decisions must be made about the resulting cosmetic appearance. For some women, reconstructive surgery may be an option. This type of surgery may be done immediately after the mastectomy or may be delayed until healing has occurred. This decision is usually made by the patient and physician before the surgical procedure. Since all women are not candidates for reconstruction surgery, the remaining option is the use of an external prosthesis.

Individuals who choose an external prosthesis as an option will require assistance and guidance in identifying local resources for purchasing a prosthesis and suggestions for clothing and accessories.[4,60] The American Cancer Society is especially helpful with this aspect of care. The Reach to Recovery program was developed specifically to meet the needs of women after breast surgery.[51] A volunteer who has had previous surgery, at the request of the surgeon, will visit the woman in the hospital and can provide information about local resources for a permanent prosthesis, clothing tips, and exercises to help assist in rehabilitation. A permanent prosthesis can be ordered once healing has occurred over the incision site. This is usually 6 to 12 weeks after the surgery.[60] Proper fitting is especially important. Correct fit helps prevent muscular aches and pains in the neck, shoulder, and back associated with imbalance of the breast. The women may choose from a variety of breast prostheses, including foam filled, liquid silicone filled, or custom-made sculptured.[52,60] Personal choice as well as cost may play a role in decision-making about the prosthesis. Most insurance companies will pay for the prosthesis. Another concern that may emerge is what type of clothing can be worn with the prosthesis. In general, most women can wear the same clothes after the surgery as they did before the surgery. Information about bathing suits and evening wear is available through the American Cancer Society.

Physical changes related to chemotherapy and hormonal therapy. There may be multiple physiologic changes resulting from adjuvant therapies that affect the sexuality and fertility of women treated for breast cancer. The most well known of these therapies is adjuvant chemotherapy for the premenopausal woman. Alkylating agents, especially Cytoxan, can cause ovarian dysfunction that results in decreased production of estrogen and progesterone and may cause premature menopause. The incidence of chemotherapy-induced ovarian dysfunction has been reported in as many as 75% of treated women.[5,43] Risk factors for developing menopause include patient age and dose of chemotherapy. Women over the age of 30 are at increased risk, as well as women who receive multiple courses of combination chemotherapy. Induced ovarian failure associated with chemotherapy appears to be a progressive problem rather than an abrupt change.[5] Symptoms include hot flashes, irritability, decreased libido, and decreased vaginal lubrication. It is important to inform women about these possible side effects and provide suggestions for interventions that might allay some of the discomfort. The use of water-based lubricant may be helpful to alleviate vaginal dryness. In the case of severe hot flashes, clonidine has been identified as a potential treatment.[5,26]

Women who are treated with antiestrogen therapy may experience similar problems. These women may experience severe vaginal atrophy that is associated with dyspareunia.[43] Information should be provided about the use of a water-based lubricant before intercourse.

The increased success of treating breast cancer has led to emerging issues related to fertility. Although pregnancy was generally discouraged after diagnosis and treatment of breast cancer, delayed parenthood, coupled with the success of treating breast cancer has caused a reevaluation of this stance.[20] If the patient exhibits a strong desire for parenting, it is important to discuss the risks versus benefits of pregnancy with the patient. Studies indicate that pregnancy after primary treatment for breast cancer has no adverse effect on disease recurrence.[8,10] However, the long-term risks associated with conception after chemotherapy have not been fully recognized. Although evidence shows that many women have been able to conceive and give birth to normal progeny, there is no long-term follow-up on children born to women who have received chemotherapy.[5] If the couple is committed to the idea of parenthood, it is generally suggested that parenting should be delayed for 2 years after the treatment of breast cancer. This period allows for observation of disease recurrence and evaluation of prognosis.[20] For further discussion, see Chapter 20.

Psychosocial issues

The diagnosis and treatment of breast cancer cause a myriad of psychosocial issues for women. This section discusses psychologic adaptation and issues related to body image, relationships, and social support.

Exploration of the psychologic adaptation of women to breast cancer has been one of the most extensively studied areas in the literature. It appears that the most stressful time for adaptation is immediately after discovery of the lump.[44] This high stress time seems to last for at least 2 to 3 months after primary treatment.[30]

Multiple studies have identified that mild to moderate psychologic distress persists for at least 1 to 2 years after primary treatment.[30,36,53] However, according to a recent report by Vinokur et al.,[52] patients with early stage disease who survived over 5 years attained the same levels of physical, social, and psychologic function as women who did not have breast cancer. The results of the study suggest several risk factors that adversely affected psychologic adaptation. These factors included stage of disease, physical impairment, and age. Advanced stage of disease and its consequent physical impairment posed serious risk factors for poor mental health and well-being of young women with breast cancer. Physical impairment seemed to be the most significant factor for deteriorating mental health. They suggest that greater attention should be paid to the impact of disease on younger patients' mental health and well-being. Morris et al.[29] identified other indicators of difficulty adjusting to the diagnosis of breast cancer. These factors included previous history of psychologic disturbance, evidence of depression at the time of primary diagnosis, general emotional lability, and anticipated or actual lack of social support. In general, women without prior psychiatric disturbance or suicidal ideation pose a low risk for severe anxiety disorder.[37] Careful assessment before primary therapy is essential to identify high-risk individuals and to begin appropriate interventions. Jamison et al.[22] suggest that preoperative counseling may help alleviate the emotional distress associated with surgery.

Several authors have identified areas of major concern for women undergoing primary treatment for breast cancer. These concerns include a pervasive sense of uncertainty about the situation, fear of death, worry about recurrence, sense of mutilation, and loss of feelings of femininity.[30,33,35,38,55] The two most difficult issues for women have been identified as the pervasive sense of uncertainty and fear of death and worry about recurrence. Northouse[35] identified that a sense of uncertainty was particularly stressful before surgery. Women in her study identified that having to make decisions about surgery with insufficient information during a time of emotional crisis was difficult. The author suggested that health professionals need to develop more effective links with patients during the preoperative phase to help lessen the anxiety and uncertainty surrounding these monumental decisions.

Welch-McCaffrey[55] describes fear of disease recurrence as the most powerful disrupter that patients face during cancer remission. However, according to Northouse,[34,35] social support can provide a buffer to fears of recurrence. In this study, women who reported a greater number of people with whom they could discuss mastectomy-related concerns had significantly decreased fears of recurrence. Furthermore, Northouse suggests that family members be included as an integral part of the patient's care to help facilitate communication and adaptation.

Although uncertainty about the disease and fear of death and worry about recurrence are important concerns, issues related to body image often emerge as significant issues. Recent advances in medical and surgical treatment have increased the number of options for women undergoing primary treatment for breast cancer. Segmental mastectomy and primary radiation therapy are now viable options for many women diagnosed with breast cancer. There have been several studies that have examined the effect of modified radical mastectomy versus segmental mastectomy upon body image and psychologic adjustment. It is somewhat surprising that measures of emotional distress have revealed little or no difference between women who have undergone modified mastectomy versus segmental mastectomy.[40,48,50] However, the effect of the type of procedure upon perceived body image has been somewhat more positive. Steinberg et al.[48] report that although both modified radical mastectomy and segmental mastectomy patients reported feeling less attractive and less feminine the first 6 months after surgery, the segmental mastectomy patients showed virtually no impairment of self-image at 2 years after treatment. This was in striking contrast to the persistence of negative changes in the self image of the mastectomy patients.

Patients undergoing adjuvant chemotherapy for breast cancer often experience significant alterations in body image. Side effects of chemotherapy that affect body image include: hair loss, weight gain, induced ovarian failure, and a general lack of well-being. Hair loss is often a devastating event for many women. Counseling before chemotherapy is especially important. Suggestions for minimizing hair loss should be discussed, as well as the use of wigs and turbans before actual hair loss occur.

Weight gain in women receiving adjuvant chemotherapy has been identified as a major issue. Knobf[25] identified that 70% of patients gained an average of 17 lbs. during treatment. Weight gain occurred regardless of age, menopause status, drugs, number of drug cycles, or steroids. Although the cause is unexplained, 23% of patients reported successful weight loss after a dieting program upon completion of chemotherapy. Winningham[61] and Winningham et al.[62] recently investigated the effects of aerobic exercise in patients with breast cancer who are receiving adjuvant chemotherapy. Results from the studies indicate that aerobic exercise may have a role in stabilizing body weight, as well as minimizing nausea and promoting physical well-being.

Induced ovarian failure and a general lack of well-being during chemotherapy can adversely affect body image and self-esteem.[5] As discussed in the previous section, it is especially important to provide anticipatory guidance about this problem to minimize adverse psychosocial sequelae. Suggestions to help minimize problems associated with hot flashes, irritability, decreased libido, and vaginal dryness can be helpful. Although women with breast cancer are not candidates for estrogen replacement, the use of clonidine may be useful for severe postmenopausal symptoms.[5,26,43]

Relationships are often affected by the diagnosis of breast cancer. Twenty to forty percent of marital couples express concerns about sexual adjustment after treatment for breast cancer.[29] Viewing the incision site and resumption of the sexual relationship were identified as emotionally stressful events.[35,38,57] Although most couples were able to surmount this task successfully, studies indicated a small percentage of couples who experienced difficulty. In general, the sexual adaptation was strongly predetermined by the type and quality of relationship before surgery.[57,63]

Social support has been identified as a critical element in psychosocial recovery from breast cancer. Family support has been identified as one of the most important predictors of positive adjustment after primary treatment for breast cancer.[37] Several authors have noted positive effects of social support. Woods and Earp[63] noted that social support buffered the effects of postmastectomy depression in women with few physical complications. Similarly, Northouse[33,34] identified the positive effect of social support in decreasing fears related to disease recurrence.

The concept of social support is not limited to family and friends. Other examples of social support include either one to one support through an organization or the use of support groups. The Reach to Recovery program is an excellent model of one to one support through an organization. The Reach to Recovery program[51] was developed by a former mastectomy patient. This model was adopted by the American Cancer Society and provides a woman with the opportunity to discuss issues of concern with someone who has successfully surmounted the challenge of living with cancer. Educational materials have been developed for this program to meet the specific needs of women after breast surgery.

Another type of social support is the use of support groups. It appears that support groups may be particularly useful in dealing with the stress of living with cancer.[46,47] Almost all patients benefit from contact with other patients who are exeriencing similar life experiences. Christ et al.[7] postulated three ways in which support groups are useful: (1) other patients provide insight into dealing with the cancer experience; (2) contact with other patients helps normalize the experience of cancer by decreasing the sense of isolation and loneliness; and (3) other patients help model successful recovery. A recent study by Spiegel et al.[46] provides startling evidence that social support may be an important factor in survival. Eighty-six patients with metastatic breast cancer were randomly assigned to either a treatment group or a control group. The treatment group received 1 year of intervention which consisted of weekly supportive group therapy with self hypnosis for pain. Both patient groups received routine care provided by an oncologist. Results of the study demonstrated a significant difference in survival favoring the group that received the weekly interventions.

Economic issues

The economic issues facing patients with cancer are complex. While the direct costs of cancer care can be financially devastating, the indirect costs of cancer can be equally troublesome. Two areas which can have a great impact on the successful rehabilitation of patients with cancer are problems related to employment and insurance coverage.[2,12,56] One of the greatest barriers to patients' return to employment are myths surrounding cancer. While several laws have been enacted to protect the rights of patients returning to work, more difficult issues to deal with are inaccurate perceptions and myths about the person with cancer ability to work. Mellette[28] surveyed women who were treated for breast cancer. This survey revealed that the majority of women treated for breast cancer were able to continue working. The majority of work time which was lost was related to time needed for surgery and recovery after the procedure. Results of the survey indicated that women treated with primary therapy and adjuvant chemotherapy and those with metastatic disease were able to maintain an excellent employment record. Although this group encountered relatively few problems, many felt locked into their jobs after the diagnosis of cancer.

Several authors[28,56] have noted the occurrence of other employment problems that may occur after the diagnosis of cancer. These include dismissal, demotion, or problems related to the disease state. Dismissal and demotion are severe forms of discrimination related to the cancer diagnosis. It is important to recognize that several laws may be helpful to patients who experience these difficulties. The federal Rehabilitation Act of 1973[39] protects the rights of those with a physical impairment, as well as those with a history of impairment. This law was passed to prevent discrimination against the handicapped and pertains to individuals in whom cancer is diagnosed. In addition, there may be state laws that pertain to individuals with cancer. Patients should be advised to check with either the American Cancer Society, National Coalition for

COMMUNITY RESOURCES FOR BREAST CANCER PATIENTS

Organization	Available services
American Cancer Society National Headquarters 3340 Peachtree Road, NE Atlanta, GA 30326 404-32925	Provides information Special program designed to meet needs of patients with cancer. Examples of programs which may be helpful to women with breast cancer include: ▪ Reach to Recovery program—provides information and support to women who have had breast surgery ▪ I Can Cope—8-week course that provides information about cancer, treatment, and impact on living with cancer May provide assistance such as equipment, home care, transportation, pharmacy, prosthesis
Breast Cancer Advisory Center 11426 Rockville Pike, Suite 406 Rockville, MD 20859 301-984-1020	Physician referral Information about breast cancer Library of breast cancer materials
Cancer Information Service 800-4-CANCER	Current reliable information Free publications Referrals to local sources of cancer care
Make Today Count P.O. Box 222 Osage Beach, MO 65065	Provides group and individual emotional support for cancer patients National newsletter Book entitled *Make Today Count* Community projects Workshops and seminars Social activities
National Cancer Information Clearinghouse 9000 Rockville Pike Bethesda, MD 20205 800-422-6237	Provides information Provides free searches of resources
National Coalition for Cancer Survivorship 323 8th Street, S.W. Albuquerque, NM 87102 505-764-9956	Publications Political advocacy
National Self Help Clearinghouse Graduate School and University Center City University of New York 33 W. 42nd Street New York, NY 10036	Provides information about self-help groups in specific community Provides assistance in organizing a self-help group
YWCA U.S.A. National Board* 726 Broadway New York, NY 10003 212-614-2700	Sponsers ENCORE program. ENCORE is a program that incorporates gentle land and water exercises for women after breast surgery. This program offers group support, as well as exercises.
Intimacies by Alice 3 Hudson Watch Drive Ossining, NY 10562 914-923-2010	Specialty boutiques and mail order catalog Provides sleepwear, loungewear, sportswear, and lingerie for women who have had breast surgery

*Provides information about ENCORE program available throughout the country.

COMMUNITY RESOURCES FOR BREAST CANCER PATIENTS—cont'd

Organization	Available services
Mary Catherine's 1914 Northeast 42 Avenue Portland, OR 97213 800-843-3215	Mail order catalog Intimate apparel, bras, prostheses, swimwear for women following breast surgery
Nearly Me 316 West Florence Avenue Inglewood, CA 90301 800-421-2322	Breast prostheses, mastectomy swimsuits and accessories Wide range of prices available
Y-Me Breast Cancer Support Program 18220 Harwood Homewood, IL 60430 800-221-2141	Education and support services Wig and prosthesis bank available for women with limited resources

Cancer Survivors, or an employment attorney for additional resources. Problems related to the disease state may be real problems for some individuals with cancer. Examples of these problems include decreased stamina or decrease in functional status to accomplish the job. In the case of breast cancer, precautions necessary to prevent or minimize damage to the affected arm may interfere with one's ability to perform a job. Vocational counseling and vocational rehabilitation may be helpful in these situations.

Problems related to insurance coverage pose another major rehabilitation barrier for individuals with cancer. The California Division of the American Cancer Society[18] undertook a survey on the social, economic, and psychologic needs of patients with cancer in California. Eight hundred and ten patients with cancer were surveyed, as well as 142 families of surviving cancer patients and 20 families of patients who died. Sixty percent of the sample did not have comprehensive insurance coverage. Major problems related to insurance for individuals with cancer include loss of insurance coverage, reduced health benefits, and increased health insurance premiums.[18] Unfortunately, there is no universal legal requirement that an insurance company must insure everyone.[2] As a result, many individuals with cancer are faced with a difficult situation regarding insurance coverage. An important consideration for an individual who will be out of work for a prolonged time is to consider switching from group health insurance to an individual policy. Although this will be more costly, it will help ensure continuation of health care benefits. There are time limit constraints on initiation of this process. The individual is responsible for initiation of this process so this should be done in a timely fashion.[12] Cancer survivor organizations provide an excellent source of securing up to date information about important survivor issues such as insurance coverage. Referral of individuals to these organizations may be helpful in securing resources.

COMMUNITY RESOURCES

Community resources are an important source of information and support for women with breast cancer. Information about organizations and the services that they provide is found on pp. 580-581.

SUMMARY

There are a growing number of women who have been treated successfully for breast cancer. These women face an increased number of issues related to long-term survival. To have a successful impact on the long-term quality of life of these women, a comprehensive rehabilitation program is essential. Rehabilitation programs must encompass the physical, psychologic, social, and economic issues that are important in learning to live with cancer. This chapter presented an introduction of several issues that are considered important in the rehabilitation process. However, at the present time there is a limited amount of research that has evaluated the outcomes of such a progam. The challenge to health care professionals for the next decade will be to coordinate, deliver, and measure the effectiveness of a comprehensive rehabilitation program that addresses the diverse needs of women with breast cancer.

REFERENCES

1. Aitken D and Minton J: Complications associated with mastectomy, Surg Clin North Am 63(6):1331, 1983.
2. Anderson JL: Insurability of cancer patients: a rehabilitation barrier, Oncol Nurs Forum 11:42, 1984.
3. Britton RC and Nelson PA: Causes and treatment of post-mastectomy lymphedema of the arm, JAMA 180:95, 1962.
4. Burdick D: Rehabilitation of the breast cancer patient, Cancer 36:645, 1975.
5. Chapman R: Effect of cytotoxic therapy on sexuality and gonadal function, Semin Oncol 9:94, 1982.
6. Chesney K: Function of the lymphatic system, Rehabil Oncol 7(2):20, 1989.
7. Christ G, Klein L, Loscalzo M, and Weinstein L: Community resources for cancer patients. In DeVita VT, Hellman S, Rosenberg SA, editors: Cancer: principles and practice of oncology, Philadelphia, 1989, JB Lippincott.
8. Cooper DR and Butterfield J: Pregnancy subsequent to mastectomy for cancer of the breast, Ann Surg 171:429, 1970.
9. Dietz JH: Rehabilitation of the cancer patient, Med Clin North Am 53:607, 1969.
10. Donegan WL: Breast cancer and pregnancy, Obstet Gynecol 50:244, 1977.
11. Dudas S and Carlson C: Cancer rehabilitation, Oncol Nurs Forum 15:183, 1988.
12. Fitzgerald R: Life insurance after malignant disease, Ann Intern Med 95:633, 1981.
13. Foldi E, Foldi M, and Weissleder H: Conservative treatment of lymphedema of limbs, Angiology 36:171, 1985.
14. Gahagen C: Clinical management of lymphedema, Rehabil Oncol 7(2):9, 1989.
15. Ganel A: Nerve entrapments associated with post-mastectomy lymphedema, Cancer 4:2254, 1979.
16. Ganz PA: Rehabilitation needs and breast cancer: the first month after primary therapy, Breast Cancer Res Treat 10:243, 1987.
17. Grabois M: Rehabilitation of the post-mastectomy patient with lymphedema, CA 26(2):75, 1976.
18. Greenleigh Associates: Report on the social, economic and psychologic needs of cancer patients in California. Proceedings of the Western States Conference on Cancer Rehabilitation, San Francisco, California Division of the American Cancer Society, March 1982.
19. Harvey R, Jellinek H, and Habeck R: Cancer rehabilitation: an analysis of 36 program approaches, JAMA 247:2127, 1982.
20. Hassey KM: Pregnancy and parenthood after treatment for breast cancer, Oncol Nurs Forum 15:439, 1988.
21. Holland J and Mastrovito R: Psychologic adaptation to breast cancer, Cancer 46:1045, 1980.
22. Jamison K, Wellisch D, and Pasnau R: Psychosocial aspects of mastectomy: I. The women's perspective, Am J Psychiatry 134:432, 1978.
23. Kepics J: The lymphatic system; function and dysfunction, Rehabil Oncol 7(2):6, 1989.
24. Kissen MW: Risk of lymphedema following the treatment of breast cancer, Br J Surg 73:580, 1986.
25. Knobf MT: Physical and psychologic distress associated with adjuvant chemotherapy in women with breast cancer, J Clin Oncol 4:678, 1986.
26. Laufer L, Erlik Y, Meldrum D, and Judd H: Effect of clonidine on hot flashes in post menopausal women, Obstet Gynecol 60:583, 1982.
27. Lehmann JF, Delisa J, Warren G, et al: Cancer rehabilitation: assessment of need, development, and evaluation of a model of care, Arch Phys Med Rehabil 59:410, 1978.
28. Mellette S: The cancer patient at work, CA 35:360, 1985.
29. Morris T: Silent sadness of the "cured" breast cancer patient. In Aaronson N and Beckmann J, editors: The quality of life of cancer patients, New York, 1987, Raven Press, pp 201-206.
30. Morris T, Greer H, and White P: Psychologic and social adjustment to mastectomy: a two year follow-up, Cancer 40:2381, 1977.
31. Murkowski M, Wilcox JP, and Helm PA: Lymphedema incidence after specific post-mastectomy therapy, Arch Phys Med Rehabil 62:449, 1981.
32. Nickkanen TA: Swelling of upper extremity, function and muscle strength of shoulder joint following mastectomy combined with radiotherapy, Ann Clin Res 10:273, 1978.
33. Northouse L: Mastectomy patients and the fear of cancer recurrence, Cancer Nurs 4:213, 1981.
34. Northouse L: Social support in patients' and husbands' adjustment to breast cancer, Nurs Res 37:91, 1988.
35. Northouse L: The impact of breast cancer on patients and husbands, Cancer Nurs 12:276, 1989.
36. Northouse L: A longitudinal study of the adjustment of patients and husbands to breast cancer, Oncol Nurs Forum 16:511, 1989.
37. Psychological Aspects of Breast Cancer Study Group: Psychological response to mastectomy: A prospective comparison study, Cancer 49:184, 1987.
38. Quint J: The impact of mastectomy, Am J Nurs 63:88, 1963.
39. Rehabilitation Act of 1973, 29 USC 701 et seq, Washington, DC, Government Printing Office, 1973.
40. Sanger CK and Reznikoff M: A comparison of the psychological effects of breast-saving procedures with the modified radical mastectomy, Cancer 48:2341, 1981.
41. Scanlon E and Feedman J: Rehabilitation of the breast cancer patient, Semin Surg Oncol 4:268, 1988.
42. Schmid W, Kiss M, and Hibert L: The team approach to rehabilitation after mastectomy, AORN 19:821, 1974.
43. Schouer L, Schain W, and Montague D: Sexual problems of patients with cancer. In DeVita VT, Hellman S, and Rosenberg SA, editors: Cancer: principles and practice of oncology, Philadelphia, 1989, JB Lippincott.
44. Scott D: Quality of life following the diagnosis of breast cancer, Top Clin Nurs 4(4):20, 1983.
45. Sonneland J: Post-mastectomy edema of the arm, West J Surg Obstet Gynecol 70:230, 1962.
46. Spiegel D, Bloom J, Kraemer H, and Gottheil E: effect of psychosocial treatment on survival of patients with metastatic breast cancer, Lancet ii:888, 1989.
47. Spiegel D, Bloom J, and Yalom I: Group support for patients with metastatic cancer, Arch Gen Psychiatry 38:527, 1981.
48. Steinberg M, Juliano MA, and Wise L: Psychological outcome of lumpectomy versus mastectomy in the treatment of breast cancer, Am J Psychiatry 142:34, 1985.
49. Stumm D: Rehabilitation of the breast cancer patient, Clin Management 2(1):20, 1982.
50. Taylor S, Lichtman R, Wood J, et al: Illness related and treatment related factors in psychologic adjustment to breast cancer, Cancer 55:2506, 1985.
51. Timothy F: The Reach to Recovery program in America and Europe, Cancer 46:1059, 1980.
52. Vinokur A, Threatt B, Caplan K, and Zimmerman B: Physical and psychosocial functioning and adjustment to breast cancer: long term followup of a screening population, Cancer 63:394, 1989.
53. Vinokur A, Threatt B, Caplan K, and Zimmerman B: The process of recovery from breast cancer for younger and older patients: changes during the first year, Cancer 65:1242, 1990.
54. Watson P: Cancer rehabilitation: The evolution of a concept, Cancer Nurs 13:2, 1990.
55. Welch-McCaffrey D: Cancer, anxiety and quality of life, Cancer Nurs 8:151, 1985.

56. Welch-McCaffrey D, Hoffman J, Leigh M, et al: Surviving adult cancers, part 2: psychosocial implications, Ann Intern Med 111:517, 1989.
57. Wellisch D, Jamison K, and Pasnau R: Psychosocial aspects of mastectomy: II. The man's perspective, Am J Psychiatry 135:543, 1978.
58. Willhite O: Pre and post-operative rehabilitation exercises for the mastectomy patient, Home Healthcare Nurs, Jan/Feb:34, 1984.
59. Winegate L: Rehabilitation of the mastectomy patient, Arch Phys Med Rehabil 70:21, 1989.
60. Winkler W: Choosing the prosthesis and clothing, Am J Nurs 77:1433, 1977.
61. Winningham ML: Effect of aerobic exercise on body weight and composition in patients with breast cancer on adjuvant chemotherapy, Oncol Nurs Forum 16:683, 1989.
62. Winningham ML and MacVicar MG: The effect of aerobic exercises on patient reports of nausea, Oncol Nurs Forum 15:447, 1988.
63. Woods N and Earp JA: Women with cured breast cancer: a study of mastectomy patients in North Carolina, Nurs Res 27:279, 1978.
64. Zanolla R: Evaluation of the results of three different methods of post-mastectomy lymphedema treatment, J Surg Oncol 26:210, 1984.

23 Patterns of Care of Breast Cancer

Gerald E. Hanks

The 1980s have been a decade of change in the management of breast cancer in the United States. The concept of conservative management of breast cancer that began in the 1950s[22] was supported by 30-year results from the Princess Margaret Hospital[26] and was being tested in several prospective randomized trials. The Milan trial initiated by Veronesi began in 1973, and the first results were published in 1981[37]; the World Health Organization trial accessed patients during a similar time frame with an initial publication in 1982.[33] The favorable outcome of these trials was appreciated before their results were published; this recognition supported the nonrandomized efforts of several institutions in the United States including the Joint Center in Boston, the M.D. Anderson Hospital in Houston, and the University of Pennsylvania in Philadelphia. These institutions had well-established breast conservation treatment programs in place before 1980. They played a major role in publicizing the treatment method and in defining the details of patient evaluation and surgical and radiotherapy techniques. The NSABP began a prospective trial of conservative surgery and radiation therapy, conducting the largest randomized trials in the world.[9] Through this trial many surgeons were exposed to the breast preservation approach of treating early breast cancer.

Thus we would expect the 1980s to reflect the transition from mastectomy-based care to a balanced pattern of care, including breast conservation, with an emphasis on clinical and pathologic features and with patient choice largely forming the basis for treatment decisions.

The role of chemotherapy and hormone therapy also emerged during the 1970s as a result of trials conducted in Italy by Bonadonna et al. with Cytoxan, methotrexate, and 5-fluorouracil (CMF)[2] and by Fisher et al. and the NSABP with L-PAM.[8] Bonadonna reported a survival advantage for node-positive premenopausal patients treated with CMF in 1976, and this regimen quickly was adopted at major centers in the United States, although, as we will see, it was not adopted so quickly in the medical community as a whole. The 1985 National Institutes of Health (NIH) Consensus panel concluded that adjuvant chemotherapy was appropriate for premenopausal node-positive patients. For postmenopausal node-positive patients, hormone therapy was recommended, because the panel felt that the value of chemotherapy was not yet proven in that subgroup.[5] The effect of this conference on patterns of care for chemotherapy and hormonal therapy usage clearly was seen in 1985 to 1986. In the late 1980s there were further NIH efforts to define the role of chemotherapy in node-negative patients through the Clinical Alert[23] and the 1990 Consensus Panel Conference.[28] These efforts for the most part have been directed towards increasing the number of patients who "should" receive chemotherapy.

The conclusions of the recent 1990 NIH Consensus Statement on Breast Cancer are clear and straightforward, summarizing the decade's progress in terms of local-regional treatment for early breast cancer and systemic treatment for node-negative patients.[28]

1. Breast conservation treatment is an appropriate method of primary therapy for the majority of women with stage I and stage II breast cancer, and is preferable because it provides survival rates equivalent to those of total mastectomy and axillary dissection while preserving the breast.
2. The recommended technique for breast conservation includes local excision of primary tumor with clear margins, level I to level II axillary node dissection, and breast irradiation of 4500 to 5000 cGy with or without a boost.
3. The many unanswered questions in the adjuvant systemic treatment of node-negative breast cancer make it imperative that all patients who are candidates for clinical trials be offered the opportunity to participate.
4. The majority of patients with node-negative breast cancer are cured by breast-conserving treatment or total mastectomy and axillary dissection. The rate of local and distant relapse following local therapy for node-negative breast cancer is decreased by both combination cytotoxic chemotherapy and by the use of tamoxifen. The decision to use the adjuvant treatment should follow a thorough discussion with the patient regarding the likely risk of relapse without adjuvant therapy, the expected reduction in risk with adjuvant therapy,

toxicities of therapy, and its impact on quality of life.

5. While all node-negative patients have some risk for recurrence, patients with tumors ≤1 cm have an excellent prognosis and do not require adjuvant systemic therapy outside of clinical trials.

In 1990 we can see two clear problems in the patterns of care of breast cancer in the United States: (1) many women are not being offered the option of breast preservation, which would improve their quality of life; and (2) there appears to have been no improvement in the survival statistics for breast cancer in the United States as a result of adjuvant chemotherapy/hormonal therapy, despite the demonstration in clinical trials that survival rates are improved in selected subgroups of patients.

This chapter reviews the available data concerning the overall patterns of care in breast cancer, primarily focusing on the United States. Access to care, or lack thereof, influences care and differentially affects subgroups of our population, major factors influencing access are presented. Patterns of care are then divided into (1) patterns of pretreatment evaluation with data from the Community Cancer Evaluation project (POC-CCE), the Patterns of Care Study in Radiation Oncology (PCS-RO), and the results of an ideal patient evaluation survey; (2) the pattern of local treatment (i.e., the fraction of patients receiving conservative surgery and radiation therapy) including data from the international literature, the POC-CCE project, Surveillance, Epidemiology and End Results (SEER), the American College of Surgeons, two states, and 12 individual hospitals; (3) the patterns of adjuvant chemohormonal therapy, including data from SEER, POC-CCE, PCS-RO, and others represent the changes over time in this treatment. The lack of correlation of chemotherapy administration with improved survival rates in SEER data is discussed. Last, some special problems are discussed that need solutions for us to better understand the current patterns of care.

Lay groups, physician groups, and individuals must continue to apply pressure for informed decision making regarding treatment options for women with breast cancer.

ACCESS TO CARE

In order for patients to receive state of the art care, they must have access to medical care in general and to expert cancer management once a diagnosis is established.

There is evidence since the early 1970s that the pattern of care in breast cancer in the United States is affected by access problems. The End Results Group (ERG) and the American College of Surgeons have noted important differences in access to and outcome of care for blacks as compared to whites.[14,24] Blacks present with a stage distribution weighted towards advanced disease, more commonly do not receive care for their cancers, and show a worse overall survival rate.[14,24]

Other racial or ethnic groups also have been shown by SEER data to have decreased survival rates compared to whites.[14] These include Hispanics, American Indians, Chinese, Filipinos, and native Hawaiians. The magnitude of these differences are greatest for American Indians, native Hawaiians, and blacks.

Income is associated strongly with receiving treatment across racial and ethnic borders. As family income increases, the fraction of patients not receiving care for their cancer decreases (e.g., 7% of breast cancer patients with an annual family income of ≤$15,000 did not receive treatment while only 2.4% of breast cancer patients were untreated with a family income of ≥$30,000).[14]

Population density gradients exist in each income level.[14] Inner city high-density populations less frequently receive treatment and more frequently experience an adverse survival rate compared to low-density suburban populations. The stage distribution differences at diagnosis between whites and blacks influence this outcome.

Significant delays in implementing therapy after the initial medical contact are expected to have an adverse influence, and this delay also is affected by race, stage, and age.

Health insurance influences access to care.[14] With incomes of ≥$10,000, 37% of people have no insurance, while only 4% have no insurance with annual incomes of ≥$30,000. Overall, more than 30 million persons in the United States have no health insurance, comprising 14% of all whites and 23% of all blacks.

The American College of Surgeons (ACoS) has collected data on breast cancer patients treated in the hospitals that have approved cancer programs through their accreditation program. Their more recent published data concern treatment in 1977; a second report of patients treated in the mid-1980s is scheduled for the fall of 1990.[24,35,38]

They have collected interesting data on who detected the breast cancer in 1977. Seventy-three percent of cancers were detected by the patient, 23% by their physicians, and only 4% by mammography. Older women were less likely to detect their own cancer than young women, and mammography was most effective in younger women. Black patients' cancers were detected by mammography in only 2%, significantly fewer than whites (4.6% observed in whites; p = .01).[13]

Delay in detecting and diagnosing breast cancer was greater when patients detected their own cancers. In that circumstance, 29% had a delay ≥3 months, compared to 11% with a similar delay when the cancer was diagnosed by a physician or by mammography ($p = .0001$). Larger tumors also were noted in patients with more than 3 months of delay.

The ACoS also has shown that blacks presenting with breast cancer in 1977 did so with less advanced cancer than in 1972, suggesting an improvement in access during that 5-year interval.[24]

PATTERNS OF PRETREATMENT EVALUATION

Information on patterns of pretreatment evaluation of breast cancer patients is presented from two sources, each representing a different subset of the United States population. There are no reliable data representative of the United States as a whole.

Patterns of Care—Community Cancer Evaluation (POC-CCE)[7]

The data for breast cancer were collected over 4 years, with year 1 before institution of the data accession part of the program (1982 to 1983) and the subsequent 3 years while the intervention program was active (1983 to 1984, 1984 to 1985, 1985 to 1986). The data collection interval brackets a time of important changes in adjuvant therapy and primary management, and the 1985 NIH Consensus Conference.

Sixty-two successful Community Clinical Oncology Program (CCOP) programs were divided into eight strata based on size, experience, and medical sophistication. Four were randomly selected from each stratum (32 total). Controls were selected from CCOP applicants who were approved but not funded. They were divided into four strata, and the top four institutions selected from each stratum; one stratum had only three facilities, therefore there was a total of 15 institutions.

Sampling was intended to survey a minimum of 50 breast cancers per institution per year. Other cancer sites also were studied. An advisory committee selected key items to obtain from the medical records of patients from institutions participating in this program. Table 23-1 summarizes the compliance rates for several pretreatment items.

Table 23-1 Patterns of pretreatment evaluation community cancer evaluation program—United States, 1982-1985

	Compliance (%)		
	1982-1983	1983-1984	1984-1985
Clinical stage stated			
CCOP	33	35	32
Control	23	29	24
Clinical size stated			
CCOP	78	77	76
Control	75	77	77
Liver scan/CT			
CCOP	33	33	30
Control	38	31	29
Lymph node dissection performed			
Age 0-49 yr			
CCOP	98	97	96
Control	96	98	98
≥10 nodes removed			
CCOP	85	85	84
Control	80	81	84
ER assay			
CCOP	83	85	82
Control	82	83	87
PR assay			
CCOP	70	78	78
Control	71	78	82

Little difference is observed between CCOPs and controls, with compliance generally good. The description of a clinical stage was present in only about one third of the records, the clinical size in three quarters, and the use of liver scan or computerized tomography (CT) for liver evaluation was decreasing. Progesterone receptors (PRs) were increasing in use, and good compliance is noted for obtaining the status of estrogen receptors (ERs) and progesterone receptors, performing a lymph node dissection, obtaining 10 or more nodes, and stating the clinical size in these strata of community practice.[7]

PATTERNS OF CARE STUDY IN RADIATION ONCOLOGY (PCS-RO)[34]

The patterns of care study in radiation oncology is a statistically valid sample of the entire U.S. practice of radiation oncology.[33] Data obtained are true national averages for patients treated with radiation therapy. The breast cancer survey was conducted in 1985 by on-site reviews of 191 patient records in randomly selected facilities. The patients were treated in 1983 and were selected randomly from the institution's total number of patients seen that year. The review was conducted by a radiation oncologist, a radiation physicist, and a data manager. Patients treated with conservative surgery and radiation therapy were surveyed; those with postmastectomy radiation were not studied. The pretreatment evaluation shown in Table 23-2 is relatively complete, with deficits noted in stating the clinical size of the lesion and stating the clinical stage. These same deficits were observed in the POC-CCE surveys. Mammography was obtained in only 77% of patients, a deficit with potentially serious results. Bone scans were obtained in 59% of patients, illustrating the lack of consensus concerning using that procedure as a screening test.

The patient's breast surgery for the conservative approach was appropriate in essentially all patients. Only 2% had an incisional biopsy, which has been associated with increased local recurrence rates. The axillary surgery removed six or more nodes in 84% of patients and 25% of patients had reexcision of the primary site. There was a surprisingly poor compliance rate for obtaining estrogen and progesterone receptor measurements, with only 28% and 36% compliance, respectively. This low value may be caused in part by a failure to transfer information to the radiation therapy record. The final pathologic margins were known to be negative in half the patients, positive in 9%, and unknown in 41%.

These two data sources are clearly different. The CCE data concerns all patients with breast cancer of all stages seen at institutions where 80% of patients were treated with mastectomy. The PCS-RO data only reports on patients treated with conservative surgery and radiation. In both groups the evaluation was good, although short of what we would expect in 1990. Clinical staging and stating the clinical size of the primary tumor needs the greatest improvement in the CCE institutions, while the PCS-RO data shows an inadequate use of mammography (a question not asked in the POC-CCE), and a lack of ER/PR information.

Table 23-2 Patterns of Care Study: pretreatment evaluation, conservative surgery, and radiation—United States, 1983

	Compliance (%)
History and physical	99
Menopausal status stated	91
Clinical size stated	64
Clinical stage stated	64
Clinical or pathologic stage	96
Chest x-ray	83
Chemistry panel	81
Liver scan	35
Bone scan	59
Mammography	77
Breast surgery	
Incisional	2
Excisional	71
Partial/quadrantectomy	25
Unknown	3
Pathologic size stated	83
Reexcision primary	25
Final margins	
Negative	50
Positive	9
Unknown	41
Axillary surgery	
Yes	72
≥6 nodes removed	84
≥10 nodes removed	69
Estrogen receptors	36
Progesterone receptors	28

Ideal evaluation survey

Table 23-3 lists the response of radiation oncologists at five institutions representing a spectrum of practice types and locales with respect to what tests they require in 1990 for evaluation of a 42-year-old woman with a 2-cm primary tumor, no clinically positive nodes, and a needle aspiration cytology positive for malignancy. Special tests and information contained in the pathology report are specified after excisional biopsy and limited axillary dissection.

There was remarkable agreement as to the eval-

Table 23-3 Pretreatment evaluation of breast cancer in selected facilities—1990

Pretreatment	Private hospital, West Coast	Private hospital, East Coast	Closed-panel HMO, West Coast	University hospital, West Coast	University hospital, East Coast
History and physical	Yes	Yes	Yes	Yes	Yes
Bilateral mammogram	Yes	Yes	Yes	Yes	Yes
CBS	Yes	Yes	Yes	Yes	Yes
Chemistry panel	Yes	Yes	Yes	Yes	Yes
Bone scan	No	No	No	No	Yes
CEA	No	No	No	No	No
Special studies					
ER assay	Yes	Yes	Yes	Yes	Yes
PR assay	Yes	Yes	Yes	Yes	Yes
DNA analysis	Yes	Yes	No	Yes	Yes
Cathepsin D	No	No	No	No	No
HER-2-neu	No	No	No	No	No
Epidermal growth factor	No	No	No	No	No
Pathology report					
Tumor size	Yes	Yes	Yes	Yes	Yes
Histologic subtype	Yes	Yes	Yes	Yes	Yes
Histologic and nuclear grade	Yes	Yes	Yes	Yes	Yes
Intraductal component	Yes	Yes	Yes	Yes	Yes
Lymphatic or vascular invasion	Yes	Yes	Yes	Yes	Yes
Margins	Yes	Yes	Yes	Yes	Yes
No nodes removed	Yes	Yes	Yes	Yes	Yes
No nodes positive	Yes	Yes	Yes	Yes	Yes
Level of involvement	Yes	Yes	Yes	Yes	Yes
Extranodal extension	Yes	Yes	Yes	Yes	Yes

uation requested by all locales and practice settings, as illustrated by the "yes" responses in Table 23-3. Only one institution requested a routine bone scan and one institution did not require a DNA analysis. Chest x-ray, postoperative mammograms (when microcalcifications were initially present), assessment for an extensive intraductal component, mitotic index, and pathologic knowledge of the highest node involved were all additional items requested by one or more institutions. No physician requested cathepsin, oncogene, or growth factor assays, and this finding may be related to the fact that these markers currently do not impact on the choice of local treatment.

Local treatment options

The important local treatment options for eradication of local-regional disease are mastectomy or conservative surgery and radiation therapy. This section considers the proportions of patients treated with mastectomy or conservative surgery and radiation therapy, how it varied during the 1980s, and the influences of geography, practice setting, and the like. Once again, it is important to note that there are no accurate data reflecting the patterns of practice in the United States as a whole.

Two-stage mastectomy

It is generally accepted that a two-stage mastectomy (where the mastectomy is not performed at the same time as a diagnostic biopsy) offers women an opportunity to participate in their treatment decision and to discuss options with radiation oncologists as well as their surgeons.

PATTERNS OF CARE STUDY—COMMUNITY CANCER EVALUATION PROJECT (POC-CCE)[7]

There was an increase in the use of two-stage mastectomy from 1982 to 1985. In 5400 patients the overall rates for CCOP and control institutions increased from 30% to 40%, to 40% to 50%. The use of a two-stage procedure was dependent on age, being used in about 65% of women under 44 years and in about 30% of women 75 years of age or older. From 1982 to 1985, CCOPs were more compliant than control facilities, and both types of facilities increased the fraction of two-stage mas-

SUITABILITY FOR CONSERVATIVE SURGERY AND RADIATION THERAPY

	Estimate	
Patient stage I and stage II	**Contraindications to breast conservation**	**All stages**
100 patients		100 patients
NA	Advanced disease	−20
100		80
−5	Multicentric or diffuse microcalcifications	−5
95		75
−15	Extensive intraductal component/positive margins	−15
80		60
−10	Patient preference for surgery	−10
70%		50%

tectomies over the 3-year time interval. However, these data show that more than half of women in community medical centers treated with mastectomy in the mid-1980s (1982 to 1986) had mastectomy without an interval between the diagnostic biopsy and mastectomy. It is unlikely that they were involved in a meaningful discussion of treatment options except the one used. There is no information on the use of two-stage mastectomy from SEER.

Fraction of patients expected to be treated with conservative surgery and radiation therapy

One may estimate the fraction of new breast cancer patients who could be treated with conservative surgery and radiation therapy if the option was made available to them without prejudice. This fraction can be estimated for all new patients and for restricted groups such as clinical stage I and stage II patients as shown above.

The frequencies suggested above for deletion of patients because of contraindications are high approximations based on the University of Pennsylvania experience and the literature. The percentage of patients who prefer mastectomy despite being good candidates for breast conservation is estimated to be 10%, depending, of course, on what the patient is told by her physician. For example, one author advised patients that there is a 2% local recurrence risk after modified radical mastectomy and a 15% local recurrence risk after conservative surgery and radiation therapy.[39] It is not surprising that 50% of his patients prefer mastectomy. The estimates made in Table 23-4 show that at least 50% of all patients and 70% of patients with stage I and stage II cancer should be treated with conservative surgery and radiation therapy.

INTERNATIONAL USAGE OF CONSERVATION SURGERY AND RADIATION THERAPY

No worldwide data are available for the number of patients selecting various local treatment options for their breast cancer. However, there are treatment opinion surveys from several countries including Italy, the United Kingdom, Canada, and the United States. Opinion surveys may be poor

Table 23-4 Management preference survey of British physicians for a 40-year-old patient, $T_{1\text{-}2}N_0M_0$ breast cancer[16]

Treatment	Simple mastectomy	Wide excision
Local surgery	122 (39%)	189 (61%)
Local surgery with radiation	8/122 (3%)	110/189 (58%)
Axilla		
Dissected	76/122 (62%)	84/189 (44%)
Sampled	19/122 (16%)	31/189 (16%)
None	27/122 (22%)	115/189 (61%)

approximations of reality, as these surveys commonly obtain the opinion of oncologists who do not participate in the primary management decision, and it has been shown that experts actually do not manage cancer as they say they do.[32]

Italy

In Italy, International Group for Cancer Care Evaluation[16] (GIVO) has ascertained that 39% of patients received "thorough" information on their breast cancer diagnoses, while only 11% received detailed information about the surgery. The physicians' perception of the same data was that 62% received "thorough" information. Additional survey data from the same source indicates 90% of physician respondents favored a conservative approach for a 35-year-old patient with a 2-cm primary tumor while only 66% favored the same treatment for a 2-cm lesion in a 60-year-old woman. Chemotherapy was favored by 78% of physicians for node-positive premenopausal patients.[17] Veronesi has noted that the lack of good radiotherapy centers, particularly in the south of Italy, limit the utilization of conservative surgery and radiation therapy. He has estimated that nearly one half of patients with ≤ 2 cm tumors are treated with a conservative approach, usually a quadrantectomy (alone).

United Kingdom

In a 1986 survey, Morris et al.[21] assessed the management preferences of British physicians for a 40-year-old patient with a $T_{1\text{-}2}N_0M_0$ breast cancer. The response is shown in Table 23-4 and illustrates the major differences in breast cancer management between the United States and the United Kingdom. Radical surgery was never chosen, simple mastectomy was preferred by 39%, and three quarters of those would perform an axillary dissection. Sixty-one percent of physicians preferred wide excision, 60% with axillary surgery. Seventy percent of wide excision patients would receive radiation therapy. When asked if they offered patients a choice of management, 63% did for most or all of their patients. These data show that British surgeons believe simple mastectomy is adequate for the management of local disease. There is no consistent management of the axilla, and radiation therapy is not added to local excision in 30% of patients with early disease.

Another U.K. survey in 1985 by Gazet et al.[10] concluded "no consensus among surgeons about the treatment of primary breast cancer . . . many different types of primary surgery . . . patterns of referral for postoperative radiotherapy vary widely . . . adjuvant systemic therapy given often by some surgeons and not at all by others . . . few patients are entered into controlled randomized trials."

A report of Greenberg and Stevens[13] compares hospital discharges in the United States and the United Kingdom for breast cancer surgical trends. Fig. 23-1 shows the trends by type of mastectomy in the two countries. Simple mastectomy was used in three quarters of patients in the United Kingdom vs. 25% in the United States. In the United States, modified radical mastectomy has replaced radical mastectomy and approaches 75% usage, while the radical procedures are used in <25% of patients in the United Kingdom. This report also notes an increased incidence of breast cancer surgery in the United States as compared to the United Kingdom, which was ascribed to detection of more cancers by mammographic screening.

Canada

In 1985 Deber and Thompson[6] determined that 30% of Canadian surgeons and oncologists recommended mastectomy for a hypothetical stage I patient. When comparing the two groups of surgeons (those who recommended surgery and those who recommended conservative surgery and radiation therapy) there were few differences, although those recommending mastectomy expressed more skepticism about the ability of clinical trial results to be transferred into practice, because of individual patient uniqueness.

United States

Surveillance, epidemiology, and end results.[30] Tables 23-5 to 23-7 summarize the changes in use of less radical surgery from 1983 to 1987 as tabulated by SEER. Table 23-5 shows an increase from 17% to 26% in the proportion of patients treated with less than a mastectomy for all stages of breast cancer. The increase is a result of a doubling in the number of patients treated with conservative surgery and axillary dissection. The rate of breast preservation (26%), however, is one half the ideal, and it is not known what fraction received radiation therapy.

Table 23-6 shows the change in management of stage I patients of all ages. The use of conservative surgery increased from 23% to 37% between 1983 and 1987, again because of a doubling in the number of patients treated with conservative surgery and axillary node dissection. Again, the rate of breast preservation was one half the ideal.

Table 23-7 compares the use of conservative surgery by age grouping for 1983 and 1987. There was little change in the frequency of surgery without node dissection except for patients 80 years of age and over, where it increased from 20% to 28%. All age groups showed increases in the use of con-

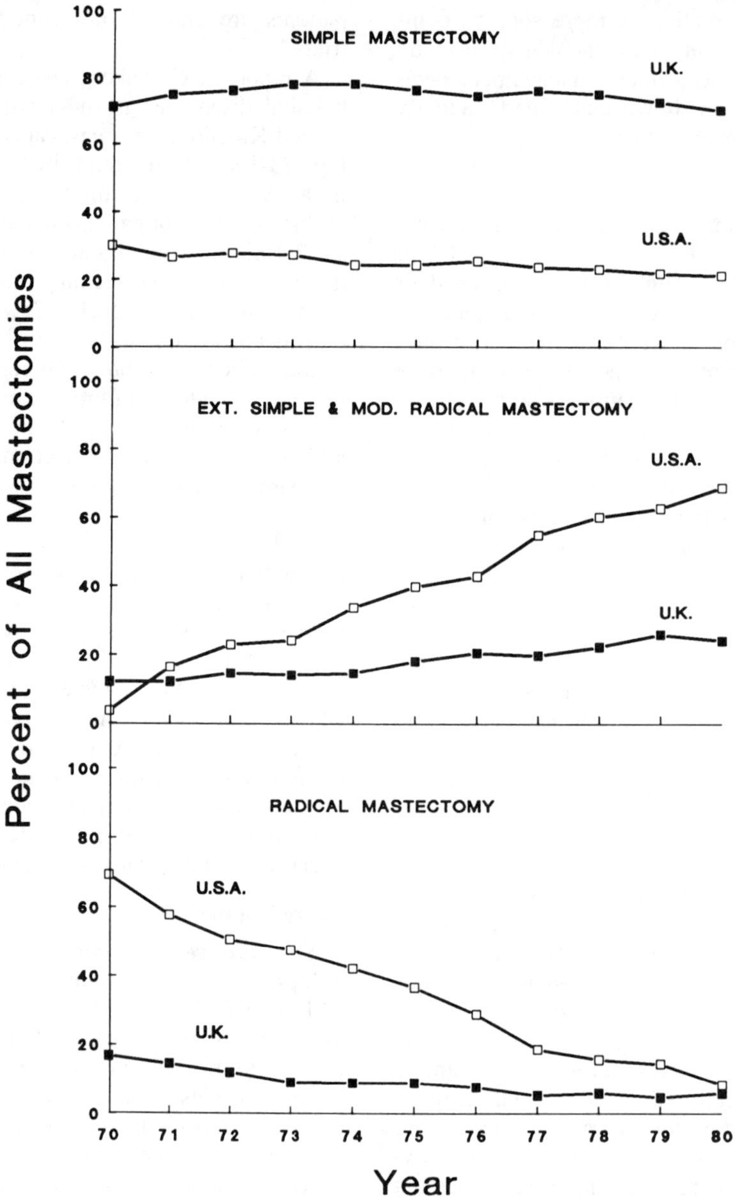

Fig. 23-1 Trends in types of mastectomy in the United States and England and Wales (U.K.). (Modified from Greenberg ER and Stevens M: Br Med J 292:1487, 1986.)

servative surgery and axillary dissection by factors of two to four, with patients 80 years of age and older showing the least increase. More than 40% of women under 60 years were treated with conservative surgery, an overall tripling of the 1983 rate, although still short of the 70% ideal.

The SEER data shows a dramatic rise in the use of conservative surgery in women of all ages during the 1983 to 1987 interval. This increase is most apparent in women under 60 years of age where the surgery is associated with axillary dissection, but it also is seen in women over 60 years of age where one half of the conservatively managed patients do not have axillary surgery.

American College of Surgeons 1985 data.[35] The American College of Surgeons published data on Patterns of Care in breast cancer from hospitals participating in their cancer accreditation programs. The most recent review was from hospitals whose patients represented 30% of all new breast

Table 23-5 Conservative surgical management of breast cancer—Surveillance Epidemiology and End Results—United States, all ages, all stages

	Pts. (%)				
Treatment	**1983**	**1984**	**1985**	**1986**	**1987**
No lymph node dissection	8.2	9.8	10.1	8.9	8.1
Lymph node dissection	8.8	10.4	16.8	17.4	18.3
Total	17.0	20.3	26.9	25.3	26.4

Table 23-6 Surgical management less than mastectomy for breast cancer—Surveillance Epidemiology and End Results—United States, all ages, stage I

	Pts. (%)				
Treatment	**1983**	**1984**	**1985**	**1986**	**1987**
No lymph node dissection	10.6	14.5	13.7	11.4	9.6
Lymph node dissection	12.7	15.3	23.7	26.9	26.9
Total	23.3	29.9	37.4	38.3	36.5

Table 23-7 Surgical management less than mastectomy for breast cancer—Surveillance Epidemiology and End Results—United States, stage I by age, 1983 vs. 1987

	Pts. (%)											
	<40 yr		**40-49 yr**		**50-59 yr**		**60-69 yr**		**70-79 yr**		**80+ yr**	
Less than mastectomy	**1983**	**1987**	**1983**	**1987**	**1983**	**1987**	**1983**	**1987**	**1983**	**1987**	**1983**	**1987**
No lymph node dissection	6.3	3.7	5.0	3.3	5.5	6.5	6.3	7.5	10.1	11.9	20.4	27.5
Lymph node dissection	16.0	38.1	12.2	38.7	9.2	35.9	8.3	26.6	5.2	18.4	5.7	11.5
Total	22.3	41.8	17.2	42.0	14.7	42.4	14.6	34.1	15.3	29.3	36.1	39.0

cancer diagnosed in the United States in 1985. Partial mastectomy was significantly more common in comprehensive cancer centers than in teaching or community hospitals. There were geographic differences; in the New England states partial mastectomy without node dissection was used more frequently compared to the rest of the country. In New England, the mid-Atlantic, Pacific coast, and Western mountain states partial mastectomy with node dissection was used more commonly than the rest of the United States. The rate of partial mastectomy usage was only 24.8% in 1985, half of the ideal, although that was an increase from 2.8% in 1976. The number of patients treated with less than mastectomy who received radiation therapy is not stated.[14] Chemotherapy and hormonal therapy was underutilized: only 43% of node-positive patients received that treatment in 1985 (Table 23-8).

Illinois. Tumor registry data from 101 hospitals are available for 5766 patients with breast cancer treated in Illinois in 1988.[15] Table 23-9 shows stage vs. treatment pattern. A lack of compliance with the modern concepts of treatment of breast cancer is evident. There is underutilization of conservative surgery, as only 26% of stage I and 14% of stage IIA patients were treated with conservative surgery. Of those treated with conservative surgery, 37% of stage I patients and 45% of stage IIA patients did not receive radiation therapy. Only 24% of patients 80 years of age or older and 54% of patients in their 70s had radiation added to their conservative surgical procedure. In this 1988 Illinois series, conservative surgery was used in 22%

Table 23-8 ACoS survey on breast cancer

Year	All stages, less than mastectomy with or without axillary dissection	Stage II chemo/hormonal therapy
1976	2.8	38%
1981	7.2	—
1982	8.5	52%
1985	24.8	43%

of early stage disease, in contrast to the 70% considered optimal.

New Mexico. Data from the New Mexico Tumor Registry for breast cancer were reviewed from 1969 to 1985,[20] demonstrating an increase in breast-conserving surgery from 6% to 25% from 1980 through 1985. However, 25% is still only one half of the optimal goal. The addition of radiation therapy to conservative surgery could not be documented in 26% of patients under 65 years of age, and 56% of patients 65 years of age or older, again identifying a significant problem in incomplete usage of both components of the conservative modality.

Major institutions. Fig. 23-2 shows the changes in use of mastectomy over the 1980s for seven major medical institutions or cancer centers. The variation is great, and ranged from the New England Medical Center,[31] where mastectomy use decreased from 79% to 38% for T_{1-3}, N_{0-1} patients over 3 years, while at Barnes Hospital in St. Louis there was a minimal (88% to 81%) reduction in the use of mastectomy for T_{1-2} N_{0-1} patients between 1981 and 1989.[19] The Jewish Hospital in St. Louis showed an initial reduction in mastectomy from 87% to 57% between 1981 and 1985, but a subsequent return to 69% mastectomy in 1989.[19] The Mayo Clinic showed a modest reduction in the use of mastectomy for all patients from 90% to 95% in the late 1970s to 80% in 1987.[27] A separate analysis of <3-cm N_{0-1} tumors treated in 1989 at the Mayo Clinic showed that 93% underwent mastectomy.[27] Memorial Hospital in New York shows a small change from 99% to 84% mastectomy,[18] while Fox Chase Cancer Center in Philadelphia had a decrease over a 7-year period from 85% mastectomy to 32% mastectomy.[25]

Community hospitals. Fig. 23-3 illustrates the variability in usage of conservative surgery and radiation therapy in community hospitals and one closed-panel HMO facility. The range is from 62% of all patients receiving conservative surgery and radiation therapy in San Pablo Hospital[4] to 25% of T_{1-2}, N_{0-1} at St. John's Hospital in St. Louis.[19] The closed panel HMO[3] quickly adopted conservative surgery and radiation therapy for about 50% of all patients in 1984.

CCE-POC.[15] Changes in segmental mastectomy with time are shown for the CCOP and control programs of the CCE-POC study in Table 23-10.

For patients with tumors ≤1 cm, 28% were treated with segmental mastectomy at the end of the 4-year observation, and of these <20% had axillary surgery performed. Similar frequencies (27%) of segmental mastectomy are associated

Table 23-9 Tumor registry data for 5766 patients from 101 hospitals—Illinois, 1988

Stage	Primary management: Total mastectomy	Partial mastectomy	Total
0	261	155 (37%)	416
I	1448	529 (26%)	1968
IIA	1687	286 (14%)	1973
	3396	961 (22%)	4357

Stage	Use of radiation therapy with partial mastectomy: Conservative surgery	Conservative surgery + radiation therapy	Total
0	111	44 (28%)	155
I	194	326 (63%)	520
IIA	128	158 (55%)	286
	433	528 (55%)	961

Modified from Imperato et al: Proc Am Soc Clin Oncol 9:102, 1990.

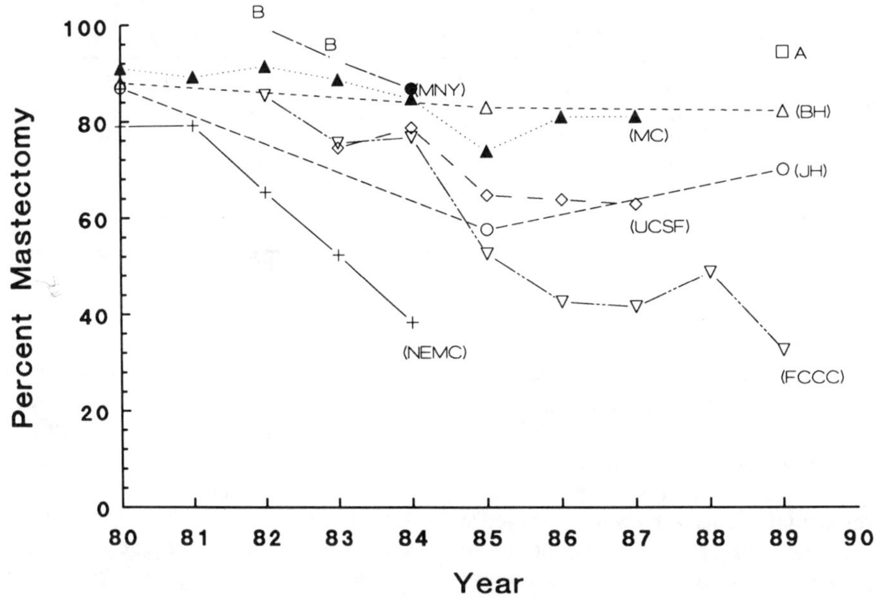

Fig. 23-2 Changing patterns of surgical management of breast cancer during 1980 to 1989 in university hospitals or cancer centers. A, Mayo Clinic, <3 cm $N_{0,1}$; BH, Barnes Hospital; FCCC, Fox Chase Cancer Center; JH, Jewish Hospital; MC, Mayo Clinic, MNY, Memorial Hospital, New York; NEMC, New England Medical Center; UCSF, University of California, San Francisco.

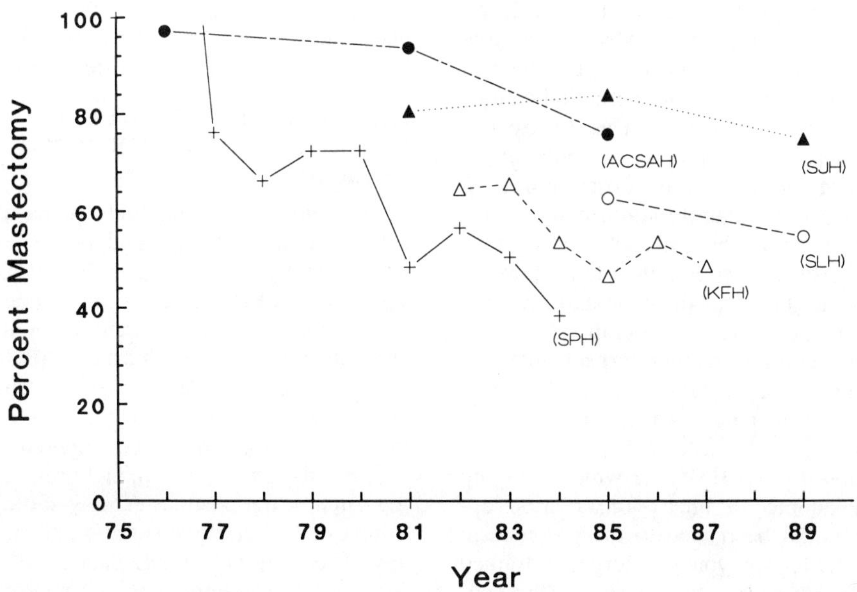

Fig. 23-3 Changing patterns of surgical management of breast cancer in community hospitals and American College of Surgeons accredited hospitals.

Table 23-10 Patterns of Care: Community Cancer Evaluation—breast and axilla surgery by primary tumor size

Primary tumor size	Facility	Segmental (%)				Axillary surgery (%)			
		1982-1983	1983-1984	1984-1985	1985-1986	1982-1983	1983-1984	1984-1985	1985-1986
≤1 cm	CCOP	19	23	32	27	18	14	29	18
	Control	12	18	42	29	0	16	41	21
>1 to ≤2 cm	CCOP	18	18	20	28	54	61	76	65
	Control	15	16	24	27	84	37	69	68
>2 to ≤5 cm	CCOP	12	13	14	17	57	55	60	65
	Control	10	13	18	22	58	56	68	65

with 1- to 2-cm tumors, but in these cases two thirds also had axillary surgery performed. About 20% of patients with 2- to 5-cm tumors had segmental mastectomy, with two thirds also having axillary surgery. These data show an increase in the use of segmental mastectomy and an increase in the use of axillary surgery, but they continue to show a major lack of use of conservative surgery and radiation therapy for patients with T_1 and T_2 cancers. The 25% rate is about a third of what is optimal for stage I and stage II.

WHY THE DIFFERENCES IN RATES OF CONSERVATIVE SURGERY AND RADIATION THERAPY

It is unlikely that the low rates of utilization of conservative surgery and radiation therapy in selected major teaching hospitals and in selected private community hospitals are caused by the referral of more patients with advanced disease, as low rates are even seen in T_1, T_2 tumors. The referral of patients to major centers with contraindications to conservation management such as diffuse microcalcifications or gross multifocal or multicentric disease could in part explain this observation, but there are no published data to confirm such a referral pattern. Some of these hospitals may be located at long distances from their referral populations, so it is not practical for patients to receive 6 weeks of outpatient radiation therapy at the surgeon's facility, and the treating surgeon may not have confidence in the radiation therapy available to the patients in their home towns and therefore may elect to perform a mastectomy.

The one closed-panel HMO for which there are data quickly adopted a breast-conservation approach. This could be related to the presence in closed-panel HMOs of younger surgeons trained in this technology and/or the absence of an economic incentive for mastectomy.

As there are no solid data, one is tempted to speculate on reasons for the low frequency of conservative surgery and radiation therapy rates for certain institutions and practice settings. Some surgeons simply have refused to participate in breast conservation management by not accurately presenting options either through lack of knowledge or disbelief in the technique. This phenomenon or bias may be more common in physicians with many years of established practice than in younger surgeons.

A multidisciplinary approach to the patient, as provided by some breast centers where the surgeon, the radiation oncologist, and the medical oncologist see the patient, may be the ideal way to present options fairly. In this setting, consistent patterns of practice can be established, and conflicts about data interpretation can be resolved between physicians without involving the patient. The patients are reassured by a unified opinion where everyone understands what the other has said, and there is less chance for incorrect perception.

PATTERNS OF ADJUVANT CHEMOTHERAPY/HORMONAL THERAPY

There is no accurate national data base that reports the use of chemotherapy and/or hormonal therapy in women with breast cancer. The use frequencies shown by SEER are felt to be inaccurate, with a larger fraction than reported receiving adjuvant chemotherapy and/or hormonal therapy.[29] The POC-CCE database is probably accurate but reflects a small sample of 47 hospitals and is limited in size and geography. There are no data indicating whether the pattern of chemohormonal therapy is the same in the postmastectomy setting compared to that of conservative surgery and radiation therapy. There are no reliable data on the sequencing patterns of radiation therapy, chemotherapy, and hormonal therapy used by physicians, or how sequencing has changed during the 1980s. The 1990

NIH Consensus Statement also showed there still is no consensus on sequencing: "No precise recommendations regarding the sequence and timing of radiation therapy and chemotherapy can be made."[28]

In a recent survey of 465 American oncologists, 80% stated they would prescribe adjuvant chemotherapy for a premenopausal woman with ER-negative, node-negative breast cancer and for a postmenopausal patient with ER-negative, node-positive disease.[1] A majority of respondents favored the choice of breast conservation or modified radical mastectomy for local treatment. The authors note that the local management decision is supported by data from clinical trials, but that chemotherapy for ER-negative, node-negative premenopausal patients is supported only by an improvement in time to recurrence and not survival, and that the treatment of postmenopausal patients with chemotherapy is not supported by randomized trials or metaanalysis. They conclude that trials have a minimal impact on practice if their results are counter to belief.

SEER chemotherapy data[11]

Fig. 23-4 shows SEER data for the use of chemotherapy in premenopausal node-positive patients since 1975. There has been an increase from 23% in 1975 to 63% in 1985. These data are felt to be inaccurate in that a larger fraction is thought actually to have received chemotherapy; efforts are underway to clarify this issue. There appears to be a 10% decrease in chemotherapy use between 1982 and 1985, although it is uncertain whether this is a real decrease or sampling error.

POC-CCE data on adjuvant chemotherapy[7]

The use of chemotherapy and tamoxifen in the POC-CCE study is shown in Table 23-11. One important difference from the SEER data is that 80% to 90% of node-positive premenopausal patients received chemotherapy over each of the 4 years of observation, a 20% higher rate than given by SEER and, perhaps, a more accurate assessment. The CCE also shows that in 1982 one half of postmenopausal patients with node-positive cancers received chemotherapy. That pattern of care dramatically decreased following the 1985 NIH Consensus Conference, at which time hormonal therapy was the recommended treatment. Also consistent with an effect of this conference was an increase in the use of tamoxifen alone from 11% to 47% for ER-positive, node-positive postmenopausal women. In contrast to Belanger's survey,[1] this study suggests an immediate responsiveness to the NIH educational effort.

The American College of Surgeons 1985 survey[35] indicated that only 43% of stage II patients

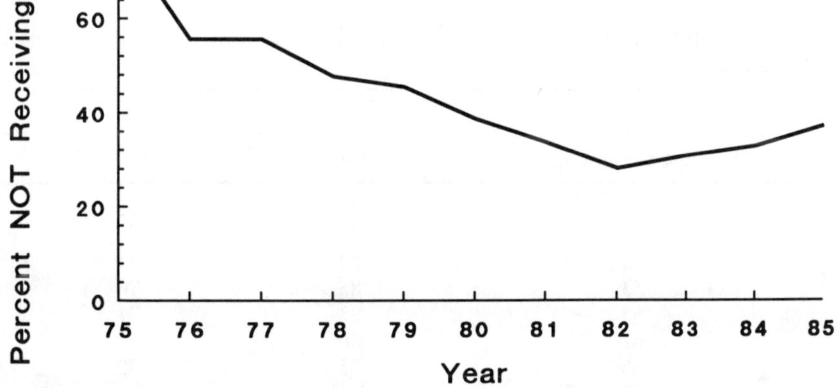

Fig. 23-4 Premenopausal node-positive stage II breast cancer patients not receiving chemotherapy. (Modified from General Accounting Office: Cancer treatment 1975-1985, January 1988.)

Table 23-11 Patterns of chemotherapy and/or tamoxifen use: Community Cancer Evaluation—breast cancer

		Node positive, ER positive or negative: chemotherapy				Node positive, ER or PR positive: tamoxifen + chemotherapy				Node positive, ER positive: tamoxifen only			
Age	Facility	1982-1983	1983-1984	1984-1985	1985-1986	1982-1983	1983-1984	1984-1985	1985-1986	1982-1983	1983-1984	1984-1985	1985-1986
0-49	CCOP	88	93	86	84	14	10	8	11				
	Control	81	87	81	84	17	5	10	6				
≥50	CCOP	55	55	49	32	36	36	44	61	11	15	22	47
	Control	60	59	46	26	38	34	39	55	11	10	23	47
≥60	CCOP	45	47	39	23	39	32	45	57				
	Control	53	43	35	17	47	38	30	67				

received chemotherapy or hormonal therapy (see Table 23-8), in contrast with the POC-CCE data, and it is unclear which is more acccurate or more representative of practice in the United States.

PCS-RO data on adjuvant chemotherapy[34]

The preceeding POC-CCE data were obtained from patients, 80% of whom were treated with modified radical mastectomy. The use of chemotherapy in patients treated with conservative surgery and radiation therapy is not clearly known, but in a group of 15 premenopausal node-positive patients from 1983 PCS-RO survey, 83% received chemotherapy, and the sequencing was equally divided before RT, during RT and after RT.

Italy

The Milan National Tumor Institute has questioned whether patients treated with chemotherapy outside of research settings have a similar beneficial effect.[36] In a group of node-positive patients not entered into protocols, 534 received adjuvant chemotherapy away from the institute, while 81 patients received their care in the Institute's medical oncology clinic. The 8-year comparison data showed a 10% difference in recurrence-free survival rates (75% versus 65%) for premenopausal patients, a 5% difference in recurrence-free survival rates for postmenopausal patients (65% vs. 60%), a 17% difference in survival rates for premenopausal patients (80% vs. 63%), and a 16% survival rate difference in postmenopausal patterns (73% vs. 57%). The better outcome always was observed in the patients treated at the Milan Tumor Institute. The authors concluded that rates of recurrence-free survival are not strikingly different, but that survival was influenced by early detection and salvage treatment in the Institute. No statistics were presented in this 81-patient vs. 534 patient comparison. It seems obvious that the recurrence-free and survival benefits of adjuvant chemotherapy were *not* observed when given outside of the research center, the same observation that perplexes us in the United States.

Table 23-12 Chemotherapy and survival of premenopausal, node-positive stage II breast cancer patients—SEER results

		Survival rate		
Year	Chemotherapy (%)	3 yr	5 yr	7 yr
1975	23	.82	.72	.64
1976	45	.85	.71	.64
1977	46	.83	.71	.64
1978	53	.83	.70	.63
1979	55	.83	.71	.65
1980	62	.86	.77	
1981	66	.83	.72	
1982	72	.84		
1983	69	.85		

Illinois chemotherapy data[15]

The 1988 Patterns of Care Study in Illinois showed a marked underutilization of conservative surgery and radiation therapy previously described, and also showed a lack of use of chemotherapy in locally advanced disease. Only half of patients with stage IIA, stage IIB, and stage IIIA breast cancers received chemotherapy. Of the patients who did receive chemotherapy, one half were <50 years of age, and one half were older. No age breakdown is available, but underutilization is apparent in premenopausal women.

SEER data on survival with chemotherapy[12]

Table 23-12 shows SEER survival data for premenopausal node-positive patients treated between 1975 and 1983. No differences in 3- to 7-year survivors are shown, despite an increase from 20% to 70% in the fraction of patients receiving adjuvant chemotherapy from 1975 to 1982 (and probably closer to 85% judging by the POC-CCE data). The General Accounting Office has concluded that this lack of improvement may result from (1) many patients not receiving chemotherapy, (2) the benefits of chemotherapy may be small and difficult to detect, and (3) it may be difficult to determine how well the treatments are implemented. The NIH is developing strategies to study this critical question further.

CONCERNS ABOUT THE PATTERNS OF CARE OF BREAST CANCER IN THE UNITED STATES

The absence of a comprehensive representative database that accurately reflects the United States as a whole, with its important geographic, ethnic, and practice subdivisions, restricts any conclusions that can be drawn regarding breast cancer treatments. National data are not available to reflect accurately pretreatment work-up, treatment details, or the use of adjuvant therapies.

There has never been a pattern of chemotherapy practice study to test the commonly held belief that dosage and schedule differences between clinical trials and community practice account for different outcomes, or that the same factors result in our failing to see a survival effect of chemotherapy usage in breast cancer in the United States.

The breast conservation approach that has been shown effective in clinical trials has not been reproduced in practice. Data from Illinois and New Mexico demonstrate that, depending on age, 25% to 50% of women do not receive radiation therapy after conservative surgery. While the NSABP trial demonstrated no adverse effect on overall survival rates with the omission of radiation, it clearly demonstrated a significantly increased risk of breast recurrence.[9]

Fewer than 5% of breast cancer patients enter clinical trials in the United States. There are important questions to answer, and we must increase patient participation in trials and the speed with which answers are found.

SUMMARY

The decade of the 1980s saw major changes in the management of breast cancer, largely in response to the results of clinical trials. Despite these advances, there is a long way to go in correctly implementing our current knowledge regarding local treatment options and the use of adjuvant chemohormonal therapy across the entire United States. All patients eligible for breast conservation management must be offered that option, all patients who may benefit from chemotherapy and/or hormonal therapy must be offered treatment, and many more patients must enter clinical trials than currently are doing so if we are to achieve timely answers to our questions. We must establish a national registry in order to measure accurately the treatment patients with breast cancer receive in the United States and to assure one level of care for all.

ACKNOWLEDGMENTS

The literature on patterns of care in breast cancer is limited, and much of the data in this chapter was either unpublished or gathered at my specific request. I am extremely grateful for permission to use both sources of data, and I offer my most sincere thanks to Leslie Ford of the National Cancer Institute, and to Polly Fiegle and Paula Diehr, both principal investigators of the Community Cancer Evaluation project. I would also like to thank Lynn Ries of the NCI (Cancer Statistics Branch) for the SEER data on patterns of surgical care of breast cancer, 1983 to 1987; Robert Kuske of Washington University for patterns of surgical care of early breast cancer treated at four institutions in St. Louis; Thomas Pizansky for patterns of surgical care at the Mayo Clinic and their management of small lesions in 1989; Francine Halberg for patterns of surgical care at UCSF; Ruth Peter for patterns of care at Fox Chase Cancer Center; Bob Kagan, Glen Tonneson, Scotte Doggett, Francine Halberg, and Larry Solin for completing a survey on patient evaluation; and David Winchester and Charles Smart for help obtaining information from the American College of Surgeons Patterns of Care Studies in Breast Cancer.

REFERENCES

1. Belanger D, Moore M, and Tannock I: How American oncologists treat breast cancer: an assessment of the influence of clinical trials, Proc Am Soc Clin Oncol 9:129, 1990.
2. Bonadonna G, Brusamelino E, Valagussa P, et al: Combination chemotherapy as an adjuvant treatment in operable breast cancer, N Engl J Med 294:405, 1976.
3. Brooks C: Personal communication, August 1990.
4. Chism SE, Brown BS, and Hoyle BA: Breast cancer treat-

ment: evolving approaches but stable results, Int J Radiat Oncol Biol Phys 12:2073, 1986.
5. Consensus Conference on Adjuvant Chemotherapy for Breast Cancer, JAMA 254:3461, 1985.
6. Deber RB and Thompson GG: Who still prefers aggressive surgery for breast cancer? Arch Intern Med 147:1543, 1987.
7. Diehr P, Chu J, Feigl P, et al: Patterns of care study, Nov 7-8, 1989, Rockville, MD.
8. Fisher B, Glass A, Redmond C, et al: L-phenylalanine mustard (L-PAM) in the management of primary breast cancer: an update of earlier findings and a comparison with those utilizing L-PAM plus 5 fluorouracil (5-FU), Cancer 39:2883, 1977.
9. Fisher B, Bauer M, Margolese P, et al: Five year results of a randomized clinical trial comparing total mastectomy and segmental mastectomy with or without radiation in the treatment of breast cancer, N Engl J Med 312:665, 1985.
10. Gazet JC, Rainsbury RM, Ford HT, et al: Survey of treatment of primary breast cancer in Great Britain, Br Med J 290:1793, 1985.
11. General Accounting Office: Cancer treatment 1975-1985. The use of breakthrough treatment for seven types of cancer, Washington, DC, 1988, U.S. General Accounting Office.
12. General Accounting Office: Breast cancer. Patient's survival. Washington, DC, 1989, U.S. General Accounting Office.
13. Greenberg ER and Stevens M: Recent trends in breast surgery in the United States and United Kingdom, Br Med J 292:1487, 1986.
14. Horm JW, Brown V, Gibbs Y, et al: Patient access to cancer care: diagnosis and treatment, Bethesda, 1990, Special Population Studies Branch, NCI.
15. Imperato JP, Sener SF, Fremgen A, et al: Breast cancer in Illinois 1988: patterns of care, Proc Am Soc Clin Oncol 9:102, 1990.
16. Interdisciplinary Group for Cancer Care Evaluation, Italy (GIVIO): What doctors tell patients with breast cancer about diagnosis and treatment: findings from a study in general hospitals, Br J Cancer 54:319, 1986.
17. Interdisciplinary Group for Cancer Care Evaluation, Italy (GIVIO): Survey of treatment of primary breast cancer in Italy, Br J Cancer 57:630, 1988.
18. Kinne DW: Primary treatment of breast cancer. In Harris JR, Hellman S, Henderson IC, and Kinne DW, editors: Breast diseases, Philadelphia, 1987, JB Lippincott, p 262.
19. Kuske R: Personal communication, July 1990.
20. Mann BA, Samet JM, Hunt WC, et al: Changing treatment of breast cancer in New Mexico from 1969 through 1985, JAMA 259:3413, 1988.
21. Morris J, Royle GT, and Taylor I: Changes in the surgical management of early breast cancer in England, J R Soc Med 82:12, 1989.
22. Mustakallio S: Conservative treatment of breast carcinoma: review of 25 years follow-up, Clin Radiol 23:110, 1972.
23. National Cancer Institute: Clinical alert, June 15, 1988.
24. Nemoto T, Vana J, Bedwani RN, et al: Management and survival of female breast cancer: results of a national survey by the American College of Surgeons, Cancer 45:2917, 1980.
25. Peter R: Personal communication, July 1990.
26. Peters MV: Wedge resection with or without radiation in early breast cancer, Int J Radiat Oncol Biol Phys 2:1151, 1977.
27. Pisanky T: Personal communication, July 1990.
28. Proceedings of the NIH Consensus Panel Conference on Early Breast Cancer, Bethesda, June 1990.
29. Ries L: Personal communication, August 1990.
30. Ries L: Personal communication, Surveillance Epidemiology End Results (SEER), August 1990.
31. Robert NJ, Cuiffo B, Marchant D, et al: "Technology transfer" in surgical treatment of primary breast cancer treatment: function of multidisciplinary assessment, Proc Am Soc Clin Oncol 7:39, 1988.
32. Sanazaro PJ: Quality assessment and quality assurance in medical care, Ann Rev Public Health 1:37, 1980.
33. Sarrazin D, Le MG, Fontaine MF, et al: Conservative treatment versus mastectomy in T-1 or small T-2 breast cancer—a randomized clinical trial. In Harris J, Hellman S, and Silen W, editors: Conservative management of breast cancer, Philadelphia, 1983, JB Lippincott.
34. Solin LJ, Fowble BL, Martz KL, et al: Results of the 1983 patterns of care process survey for definitive breast irradiation, Int J Radiat Oncol Biol Phys 20:105, 1991.
35. Sutherland CM, Winchester DM, Fink DJ, et al: Trends in diagnosis and management of breast cancer: report of the breast cancer detection awareness task force, Am Coll Surg, in press.
36. Valagussa P, Zambetti M, Moliterni A, and Bondadonna G: The impact of adjuvant chemotherapy for breast cancer when delivered outside research centers, Proc Am Soc Clin Oncol 6:232, 1987.
37. Veronesi U, Saccozzi R, Del Vecchio M, et al: Comparing radical mastectomy with quadrantectomy axillary dissection and radiotherapy in patients with small cancers of the breast, N Engl J Med 305:6, 1981.
38. Wilson RE, Donegan WL, Mettlin C, et al: The 1982 national survey of carcinoma of the breast in the United States by the American College of Surgeons, Surg Gynecol Obstet 159:309, 1984.
39. Wolberg WH, Tanner MA, Romsaas EP, et al: Factors influencing options in primary breast cancer treatment, J Clin Oncol 5(1):68, 1987.

24 Adjuvant Therapy of Breast Cancer: Current Clinical Trials and Future Directions

F. Andrew Dorr

During the last 30 years extensive clinical trial experience has evolved in the treatment of primary breast cancer (adjuvant therapy trials and trials defining the optimal local treatment) and in the treatment of locally advanced and metastatic breast cancer. This experience in breast cancer provides fertile ground for asking new questions in the clinic and for applying recent advances in molecular and cellular biology to clinical trials. Laboratory-clinical correlations will provide important leads for subsequent generations of clinical trials, both by helping to target new therapies for particular subsets of patients and by identifying prognostic groups. This chapter describes current adjuvant breast cancer trials being conducted in the National Cancer Institute–sponsored Cooperative Groups and briefly summarizes ongoing laboratory-clinical correlations.

In 1985 the National Institutes of Health (NIH) sponsored a Consensus Development Conference on Adjuvant Chemotherapy and Endocrine Therapy for Breast Cancer. The Consensus statement included recommendations for standard care for patients not entered into clinical trials (see right).[18] Recently, several large randomized adjuvant therapy trials have demonstrated superior disease-free survival for patients with node-negative breast cancer receiving systemic adjuvant therapies relative to those receiving either placebo or no adjuvant therapy. Absolute recurrence rates in these trials were reduced by 5% to 16%, with relative reductions of 25% to 50%.[7,9,19,20] This led to the conclusion at an NIH Consensus Development Conference on Early Stage Breast Cancer held in June 1990 that although "the majority of patients with node-negative breast cancer are cured by breast-conserving treatment or total mastectomy and axillary node dissection, the rate of local and distant relapse following local therapy for node-negative breast cancer is decreased by both combination cytotoxic chemotherapy and by tamoxifen."[5] No specific recommendation was made regarding standard adjuvant therapy for any subset of patients.

For patients with node-positive disease at diagnosis, the National Surgical Adjuvant Breast and Bowel Project (NSABP) has recently published results suggesting that chemotherapy (Adriamycin and cyclophosphamide) added to tamoxifen extends the survival of women over 50 compared to tamoxifen alone.[11] The Southwest Oncology Group, however, was unable to demonstrate a benefit from the addition of cyclophosphamide, methotrexate, fluorouracil, vincristine, and prednisone (CMFVP) to tamoxifen in postmenopausal women with estrogen receptor–positive tumors.[25] Thus there are a number of important questions to be resolved in the adjuvant therapy of breast cancer (see p. 602).

1985 NIH CONSENSUS DEVELOPMENT CONFERENCE—TREATMENT RECOMMENDATIONS

- For premenopausal women with positive nodes, regardless of hormone receptor status, treatment with established combination chemotherapy should become standard care.
- For premenopausal patients with negative nodes, adjuvant therapy is not generally recommended. For certain high-risk patients in this group, adjuvant chemotherapy should be considered.
- For postmenopausal women with positive nodes and positive hormone receptor levels, tamoxifen is the treatment of choice.
- For postmenopausal women with positive nodes and negative hormone receptor levels, chemotherapy may be considered but cannot be recommended as standard practice.
- For postmenopausal women with negative nodes, regardless of hormone receptor levels, there is no indication for routine adjuvant treatment. For certain high-risk patients in this group, adjuvant therapy may be considered.

UNANSWERED QUESTIONS IN THE ADJUVANT THERAPY OF BREAST CANCER

- What is the optimal timing of chemotherapy relative to the time of definitive local therapy?
- What constitutes the optimal chemotherapy regimen for each subset of patients?
- What is the role of combined chemotherapy and endocrine therapy?
- How important is dose intensity?
- What is the optimal duration of therapy?
- Can high-dose chemotherapy with autologous bone marrow rescue improve survival in poor prognosis patients?
- What prognostic factors are available to better define the need for and intensity of therapy?

CLINICAL TRIALS FOR NODE-NEGATIVE PATIENTS

The number of women with resectable breast cancer and no axillary lymph node involvement is large (about 70,000 per year) and has been increasing dramatically over the past decade. Although such patients were once believed to have a uniformly good prognosis, their biologic heterogeneity has become apparent in recent years. Groups of patients with very high risk of recurrence are beginning to be differentiated from those with very low risk. Because the majority of women with node-negative breast cancer are cured by local modalities alone, with or without adjuvant therapy, there has been increased interest and research activities on several related questions including:

1. How may patients be prognostically segregated into higher- and lower-risk groups so that therapy may be tailored appropriately?
2. How can systemic therapy be improved for the higher-risk patients?
3. How can the acute and chronic toxicities of treatment be limited for all patients, particularly those with lower risk?
4. Are there markers of treatment resistance that will suggest alternative therapy for subsets of patients?

Table 24-1 summarizes the active Cooperative Group adjuvant therapy trials for women with node-negative, invasive breast cancer. For patients with very small, invasive cancers who have not been eligible for previous cooperative group studies, the NSABP is asking whether radiation therapy is needed for local control, whether tamoxifen provides comparable local control relative to radiation therapy or whether both provide superior local control as well as long-term distant disease control. For those with larger, poorer-risk tumors, different chemotherapy and chemoendocrine regimens are being compared (Intergroup-0102 and NSABP B-19 and NSABP B-20). The objectives for each of these studies are to identify the optimal cytotoxic drug combination and/or the role of combined tamoxifen and chemotherapy. In Intergroup-0102, tamoxifen is not begun until chemotherapy is com-

Table 24-1 Breast cancer clinical trials: adjuvant studies on node-negative patients

Study	Eligibility	Design	Questions asked
Intergroup-0102	$T_{1\text{-}3a}$,N_0 ER ± Pre- or postmenopausal	CAF→ tamoxifen CAF→ placebo CMF→ tamoxifen CMF→ placebo	1. Is an Adriamycin regimen superior to a non-Adriamycin regimen? 2. Does tamoxifen add to chemotherapy, including ER −, PgR − subset?
NSABP B-18	$T_{1\text{-}3a}$,$N_{0\text{-}1}$ ER ±	AC 4→ surgery Surgery→AC 4	Is preoperative chemotherapy superior to postoperative chemotherapy?
NSABP B-19	$T_{1\text{-}3a}$,N_0 ER −	MFL CMF	Is classical CMF superior to sequential M→F plus leucovorin?
NSABP B-20	$T_{1\text{-}3a}$,N_0 ER +	Tamoxifen Tamoxifen + MFL Tamoxifen + CMF	1. Does chemotherapy add to tamoxifen in this group of patients? 2. Does classical CMF provide superior results to sequential M→F?
NSABP B-21	T_1,N_0 (occult tumors [<1 cm and too small for biochemical ER])	Tamoxifen RT + placebo RT + tamoxifen	Does tamoxifen improve disease-free and overall survival?

ER, estrogen receptor; C, cyclophosphamide; A, Adriamycin; F, fluorouracil; M, methotrexate; L, leucovorin; ER ±: estrogen receptor positive or negative.

Table 24-2 Adjuvant breast cancer trials on node-negative patients

Protocol number	Target accrual	Activation date	Accrual as of 3/31/90	Closure date at current rate of accrual
NSABP B-17	775	10/01/85	640	1990
NSABP B-18	1275	10/17/88	483	1993
NSABP B-19	1020	10/17/88	870	1990
NSABP B-20	2340	10/17/88	863	1992
Intergroup-0102	2600	07/15/89	542	1992

pleted because of the concern that tamoxifen may protect tumor cells from the cytocidal effect of chemotherapy. In addition, the role of tamoxifen in patients with estrogen receptor–negative tumors is being evaluated in this study based, in part, on the observation that tamoxifen is of benefit for this population in previous trials in the United Kingdom.[1,4]

In addition to these trials for patients with invasive cancers, the NSABP is asking whether lumpectomy alone is sufficient therapy or whether radiation therapy added to lumpectomy is more effective for patients with ductal carcinoma in situ (B-17). Clinically node-negative and node-positive patients are eligible for the NSABP B-18 trial, which is evaluating preoperative versus postoperative chemotherapy.

It should be noted that the majority of patients in these trials are offered active treatment options in addition to local therapy. The exceptions are those in NSABP B-17, who have noninvasive tumors, and one-third of those entered into NSABP B-21, who have very small tumors. Also, in Intergroup-0102, patients with tumors too small (<1 cm) for quantitative estrogen receptor measurement are registered and observed. Other patients in this study who will be followed without adjuvant therapy are those with tumors less than 2 cm in diameter that are estrogen receptor (ER)–positive and have low S-phase fractions determined by flow cytometry.

Table 24-2 summarizes the current accrual information about these studies. Several of the trials are near completion and new studies are being developed as replacements. All the studies are characterized by relatively large sample sizes which permit greater statistical precision. Accrual is efficient for most of the studies so that results will be available in an acceptable period of time.

CLINICAL TRIALS FOR NODE-POSITIVE PATIENTS

Women with tumor involving axillary lymph nodes are recognized as having a greater likelihood for distant recurrence and death from breast cancer than those without spread of tumor to the axillary nodes. Although adjuvant therapy convincingly prolongs survival for many of these patients, there is substantial room for improvement. The areas of current emphasis in the adjuvant therapy trials include studies of chemoendocrine combinations (Intergroup-0100 and Intergroup-0101) (Table 24-3), dose intensification (Cancer and Leukemia Group B [CALGB] 8541, NSABP B-22, Intergroup-0108) (Table 24-4), and the role of preoperative chemotherapy relative to postoperative chemotherapy (NSABP B-18).

The rationale for exploring dose intensity is fairly complex and includes both host and tumor considerations. Higher doses may overcome drug delivery problems related to rapid drug clearance or metabolism. In addition, higher doses may over-

Table 24-3 Adjuvant trials of chemoendocrine therapy on node-positive breast cancer patients

Study	Eligibility	Design	Planned sample size
Intergroup-0100	$T_{1\text{-}3a}$,N_1 Postmenopausal ER+ and/or PgR+	Tamoxifen CAF followed by tamoxifen CAF + concurrent tamoxifen	1410
Intergroup-0101	$T_{1\text{-}3a}$,N_1 Premenopausal ER+ and/or PgR+	CAF × 6 CAF × 6 → Zoladex × 5 yr CAF × 6 → tamoxifen + Zoladex × 5 yr	960

PgR, progesterone receptor; C, cyclophosphamide; A, Adriamycin; F, 5-fluorouracil.

come poor drug uptake across cell membranes whether through diffusion or concentration-dependent active transport systems. Once the drug has entered the cell, higher intracellular concentrations may overcome intrinsic drug resistance related to several mechanisms, including substrate affinity, drug efflux, or intracellular metabolism.[13] Retrospective reviews of the past trials support the notion that dose intensity is important.[2,14] Prospective trials, however, are necessary to confirm its value. Extending the concept of dose intensity, several recent trials have tested the feasibility of high-dose chemotherapy with autologous bone marrow rescue.[6,15,17] The merit of this approach will be tested in a randomized trial, currently being developed, for patients with high-risk disease, which likely will be defined as those with ≥10 axillary lymph nodes. Patients will be randomized to either standard adjuvant chemotherapy alone or with high-dose chemotherapy as consolidation at the completion of standard adjuvant therapy.

The trials evaluating chemoendocrine therapy will determine whether chemotherapy adds to tamoxifen for postmenopausal patients or whether endocrine therapy added to chemotherapy prolongs survival in premenopausal women. One study, Intergroup-0100, is comparing tamoxifen alone with tamoxifen combined with chemotherapy given concurrently or sequentially. This important study should definitively answer whether tamoxifen's potential inhibition of cytotoxic effect is clinically significant.

The rationale for administering chemotherapy either preoperatively or perioperatively as opposed to standard postoperative timing is based on several lines of evidence. Preoperative chemotherapy is perhaps more convenient than perioperative administration and can decrease the size of the primary tumor, possibly permitting less extensive resections. The interval from diagnosis of breast cancer to administration of postoperative adjuvant therapy is typically several weeks to several months. The tumor cell burden in undetected micrometastases continues to increase during that time. Mathematical and experimental models of tumor growth support the concept that the growth fraction is inversely correlated with tumor size.[22] The efficacy of cell cycle active chemotherapy is greatest in cells that are actively dividing. Thus the administration of chemotherapy at a time when tumor growth fraction is higher rather than lower might improve its efficacy. Although the interval from diagnosis to postoperative adjuvant therapy is short relative to the preclinical duration of tumor growth, other factors also suggest a potential benefit for early chemotherapeutic intervention. Models of tumor resistance suggest that the expansion of resistant cells is a function of the number of cells at the start of chemotherapy, the doubling time of resistant cells, and the mutation rate.[12] The parameter that can be manipulated in this model is the timing of chemotherapy initiation so that fewer resistant cells are present from the outset. A third rationale for administering preoperative chemotherapy comes from data which suggests that the growth fraction in peripheral micrometastases is increased by removal of the primary tumor. While the precise cause of this perturbation is unknown, this growth stimulation can be eliminated by perioperative or preoperative chemotherapy.[8,27]

The accrual data for studies on node-positive patients are summarized in Table 24-5. As with the studies on patients with node-negative breast cancer, there are relatively few, large studies for this

Table 24-4 Adjuvant dose intensity trials in node-positive breast cancer patients

Study	Eligibility	Design (doses mg/m²)	Relative dose intensity	Planned sample size
CALGB 8541	$T_{1\text{-}3a},N_1$	CAF (400/40/400) × 6	.54	1450
		CAF (300/30/300) × 4	.35	
		CAF (600/60/600) × 4	.81	
NSABP B-22	$T_{1\text{-}3a},N_1$	AC (60/600) × 4	.63	2100
		AC (60/1200) × 4	.51	
		AC (60 × 4/1200 × 2)	.81	
Intergroup-0108	$T_{1\text{-}3a},N_1$ ER −	CAF*	1.0	630
		CAF† + VML	1.4	

C, cyclophosphamide; A, Adriamycin; F, 5-fluorouracil; V, vincristine; M, methotrexate; L, leucovorin.
*Cyclophosphamide 100 mg/m²/day × 14 days PO q 28 days; Adriamycin 30 mg/m²/day on days 1 and 8 IV q 28 days; 5-fluorouracil 500 mg/m²/day on days 1 and 8 q 28 days.
†Cyclophosphamide 100 mg/m²/day PO on days 1-7 q 14 days; Adriamycin 40 mg/m² on day 1 q 14 days; 5-fluorouracil 600 mg/m² alternating with 300 mg/m² weekly.

Table 24-5 Node positive adjuvant breast cancer trials

Protocol	Target accrual	Activation date	Accrual as of 3/31/90	Closure date at current rate of accrual
CALGB 8541	1450	01/15/85	1327	1990
NSABP B-22	2160	06/01/89	755	1992
NSABP B-18	1275	10/17/88	483	1993
Intergroup-0100	1410	05/15/89	156	1998
Intergroup-0101	960	07/24/89	127	1997
Intergroup-0108	630	08/14/89	34	2005

higher-risk group of patients, reflecting an increasing degree of cooperation among investigators. Such collaborations are the results of National Cancer Institute and Cooperative Group initiatives to identify a prioritized, national agenda for adjuvant therapy trials.

LABORATORY-CLINICAL CORRELATIONS

The primary goal of adjuvant therapy trials is to identify improved treatment regimens relative to current standards. It is becoming increasingly possible and important to incorporate studies correlating prognostic factor evaluation with clinical outcome in adjuvant trials. Biologic characterization offers insight into tumor biology and patient prognosis, while holding promise for more targeted therapeutic interventions. This is particularly important for patients with node-negative tumors, in the majority of whom a recurrence will not occur whether adjuvant therapy is administered or not. The Cooperative Group program provides the largest resource for the conduct of such studies since patients are uniformly treated and there is reliable long-term follow-up.

Some prognostic factors are related to patient characteristics while the majority of recent work has focused on characteristics of the tumor which may uniquely define its capacity to multiply, invade, and respond to normal or abnormal growth stimuli. Several recent publications have summarized the current state of knowledge about such features as steroid hormone receptors, DNA ploidy, S-phase fraction, oncogene expression, growth factor expression, and protein expression (e.g., cathepsin D and stress response proteins).[3,10,16,23,24,26,28,29] To date, studies correlating laboratory prognostic factors have frequently been flawed by inadequate sample sizes, insufficient follow-up, or lack of concurrent examination of the multiple prognostic features. There are many potential subsets of patients that may be defined. The importance of a particular marker for a postmenopausal woman with estrogen receptor–positive, node-negative breast cancer may be distinct from its value for a premenopausal woman with node-positive disease lacking hormone receptors.

While it is possible in general to identify patients at relatively higher or lower risk of recurrence following primary therapy, there is insufficient precision to allow discrete risk group designations (Table 24-6). The expanding array of potentially important prognostic factors requires a large sample size with an extensive data base on which to be

Table 24-6 Potential prognostic factors in primary breast cancer

Factors	Lower risk	Higher risk
Axillary lymph node status	Negative	Positive
Histologic tumor type	Tubular, papillary, medullary, colloid	All others
Estrogen receptors	Positive	Negative
Primary tumor size	<2.0 cm	>2.0 cm
Nuclear grade	Good	Poor
Histologic grade	Well differentiated	Poorly differentiated
Growth fraction (S-phase, Thymidine labeling index, mitotic index)	Low	High
DNA content	Diploid	Aneuploid
Epithelial growth factor receptor	Negative	Positive
HER-2/neu oncogene amplification	Absent	Present
Cathepsin D	Low	High

Table 24-7 Laboratory-clinical correlations in adjuvant breast cancer trials

Study	Laboratory endpoint(s)	Pt. population
NSABP B-13/14	HER-2/neu, DNA histograms, histologic and nuclear grade	Node negative
EST 4189	DNA histograms, HER-2/neu, ER-ICA, PgR-ICA, haptoglobin-related protein, histologic and nuclear grade	Node-positive patients treated on past adjuvant trials
Intergroup-0011	DNA histograms, HER-2/neu	Node negative
CALGB 8861	Serum CA 15-3 antigen	Node positive
CALGB 8869	DNA histograms	Node positive
Intergroup-0104	DNA histograms	Node positive, postmenopausal, ER positive
NCCTG 86-32-52	DNA histograms	Node positive
NSABP B-18	ER-ICA, DNA histograms	Node negative and node positive

EST, Eastern Cooperative Oncology Group; NCCTG, North Central Cancer Treatment Group; ER-ICA, estrogen receptor–immunocytochemical analysis; PgR-ICA, progesterone receptor–immunocytochemical analysis.

Table 24-8 Patient accrual figures to breast cancer adjuvant therapy trials

Year	Node-negative pts.	Node-positive pts.	Total no. pts.
1985	940	1708	2648
1986	982	1730	2712
1987	906	1538	2444
1988	1679	1312	2991
1989	1685	1284	2969
1990	3103	2430	5533

tested before routine clinical decisions can incorporate them. Current and recent adjuvant therapy trials are evaluating many of these possible prognostic factors (Table 24-7). Since there will likely be new factors identified each year, the task of cataloging, comparing, and integrating will become increasingly difficult. This becomes not only a clinical trials task but also a major project in information management. Relating, weighing, and combining measurement of disparate forms and functions will require computer-assisted guidance of clinical judgment. Breast cancer may become the model for the formal integration of clinical judgment with computer-assisted risk assessment in cancer care.[21]

CONCLUSIONS

The opportunities provided by the study of breast cancer patients are enormous for both basic and clinical investigators. Since a major impediment to gaining new knowledge is the vigor of the clinical trials program, it is gratifying to note the recent trend in accrual to Cooperative Group adjuvant breast studies. As shown in Table 24-8, the number of patients projected to be accrued in 1990 is approximately 75% more than were accrued in previous years. The challenge to those who sponsor and conduct clinical trials is to continue to capitalize on these opportunities to gain insight into a common malignant disease while improving the efficiency of studies and the efficacy of treatment for these patients.

REFERENCES

1. Adjuvant tamoxifen in the management of operable breast cancer: the Scottish trial: report from the Breast Cancer Trials Committee, Scottish Cancer Trials Office (MRC), Edinburgh, Lancet ii:171, 1987.
2. Bonadonna G and Valagussa P: Dose-response effect of adjuvant chemotherapy in breast cancer, N Engl J Med 304:10, 1981.
3. Clark GM, Dressler LG, Owens MA, et al: Prediction of relapse or survival in patients with node-negative breast cancer by DNA flow cytometry, N Engl J Med 320:627, 1989.
4. Controlled trial of tamoxifen as a single adjuvant agent in the management of early breast cancer: analysis at eight years by Nolvadex Adjuvant Trial Organisation, Br J Cancer 57:608, 1988.
5. Dorr FA, ed: Proceedings of the NIH Consensus Development Conference on Early Stage Breast Cancer, NCI Monogr (in press).
6. Dunphy FR, Spitzer G, Buzdar AU, et al: Treatment of

estrogen receptor-negative or hormonally refractory breast cancer with double high-dose chemotherapy intensification and bone marrow support, J Clin Oncol 8:1207, 1990.
7. Fisher B, Costantino J, Redmond C, et al: A randomized clinical trial evaluating tamoxifen in the treatment of patients with node-negative breast cancer who have estrogen-receptor positive tumors, N Engl J Med 320:479, 1989.
8. Fisher B, Gunduz A, and Saffer EA: Influence of the interval between primary tumor removal and chemotherapy on kinetics and growth of metastases, Cancer Res 43:1488, 1982.
9. Fisher B, Redmond C, Dimitrov NV, et al: A randomized clinical trial evaluating sequential methotrexate and fluorouracil in the treatment of patients with node-negative breast cancer who have estrogen-receptor negative tumors, N Engl J Med 320:473, 1989.
10. Fisher B, Redmond C, Fisher ER, et al: Relative worth of estrogen or progesterone receptor and pathologic characteristics of differentiation as indicators of prognosis in node negative breast cancer patients: findings from National Surgical Adjuvant Breast and Bowel Project Protocol B-06, J Clin Oncol 6:1076, 1988.
11. Fisher B, Redmond C, Legault-Poisson S, et al: Postoperative chemotherapy and tamoxifen compared with tamoxifen alone in the treatment of postive-node breast cancer patients aged 50 years and older with tumors responsive to tamoxifen: results from the National Surgical Adjuvant Breast and Bowel Project B-16, J Clin Oncol 8:1005, 1990.
12. Goldie JH and Coldman AJ: A mathematical model for relating drug sensitivity of tumors to their spontaneous mutation rate, Cancer Treat Rep 63:1727, 1979.
13. Henderson IC, Hayes DF, and Gelman R: Dose-response in the treatment of breast cancer: a critical review, J Clin Oncol 6:1501, 1988.
14. Hryniuk W and Levine MN: Analysis of dose intensity for adjuvant chemotherapy trials in Stage II breast cancer, J Clin Oncol 4:1162, 1986.
15. Jones RB, Shpall EJ, Ross M, et al: AFM induction chemotherapy, followed by intensive alkylating agent consolidation with autologous bone marrow support (ABMS) for advanced breast cancer. Current results, Proc Am Soc Clin Oncol 9:9, 1990.
16. Kallioniemi OP, Blanco G, Alavaikko M, et al: Improving the prognostic value of DNA flow cytometry in breast cancer by combining DNA index and S-phase fraction, Cancer 62:2183, 1988.
17. Kennedy MJ, Beveridge R, Rowley S, et al: High dose consolidation chemotherapy and rescue with purged autologous bone marrow following dose-intense induction for metastatic breast cancer, Proc Am Soc Clin Oncol 8:19, 1989.
18. Lippman ME, ed: Proceedings of the NIH Consensus Development Conference on adjuvant chemotherapy and endocrine therapy for breast cancer, NCI Monogr 1:1, 1986.
19. Ludwig Breast Cancer Study Group: Prolonged disease-free survival after one course of perioperative adjuvant chemotherapy for node-negative breast cancer, N Engl J Med 320:491, 1989.
20. Mansour EG, Gray R, Shatila AH, et al: Efficacy of adjuvant chemotherapy in high-risk node-negative breast cancer: an intergroup study, N Engl J Med 320:485, 1989.
21. McGuire WL, Tandon AK, Allred DC, et al: How to use prognostic factors in axillary node-negative breast cancer patients, J Natl Cancer Inst 82:1006, 1990.
22. Norton L and Simon R: The Norton-Simon hypothesis revisited, Cancer Treat Rep 70:163, 1986.
23. O'Reilly SM, Camplejohn RS, Barnes DM, et al: DNA index, S-phase fraction, histological grade and prognosis in breast cancer, Br J Cancer 61:671, 1990.
24. Osborne CK: Prognostic factors in breast cancer. In DeVita VT, Hellman S, And Rosenberg SA, eds: Principles and practice of oncology, vol 4, Philadelphia, 1990, JB Lippincott, pp 1-11.
25. Rivkin S, Green S, Metch B, et al: Adjuvant combination chemotherapy (CMFVP) vs tamoxifen (tam) vs CMFVP + tam for postmenopausal women with ER+ operable breast cancer and positive axillary lymph nodes: an intergroup study, Proc Am Soc Clin Oncol 9:24, 1990.
26. Rosen PP, Groshen S, Saigo PE, et al: Pathologic prognostic factors in stage I ($T_1N_0M_0$) and stage II ($T_1N_1M_0$) breast carcinoma: a study of 644 patients with median follow-up of 18 years, J Clin Oncol 7:1239, 1989.
27. Simpson-Herren L, Sanford AH, and Holmquist JP: Effects of surgery on the cell kinetics of residual tumor, Cancer Treat Rep 60:1749, 1976.
28. Slamon DJ, Godolphin W, Jones LA, et al: Studies of the HER-2/*neu* protooncogene in human breast and ovarian cancer, Science 244:707, 1989.
29. Tandon AK, Clark GM, Chamness GC, et al: Cathepsin D and prognosis in breast cancer, N Engl J Med 322:297, 1990.

25 Medicolegal Aspects in Breast Cancer Treatment

James J. McCabe, Michele L. Hartigan, and Elise E. Singer

Nineteen state legislatures have, over the last 11 years, enacted laws that specifically address informed consent to the treatment of breast cancer. This trend reflects, in part, certain facts and figures which are beyond dispute. Breast cancer will strike one of every nine American women. The American Cancer Society's "Facts and Figures" now estimates that approximately 175,900 new breast cancer cases will be diagnosed in the United States during 1991.[1] The incidence of breast cancer has increased about 3% a year since 1980.[1] The frequency of the disease and public education programs have raised public awareness about breast cancer and heightened expectations for diagnosis, treatment, follow-up care, and cure. With the heightened awareness of breast cancer, its various methods of treatment, and its possible cure, a heightened expectation has also developed on the part of the public that a diagnosis can be equated with a cure. Unfortunately, those expectations cannot always be satisfied and those disappointed patients may express their dissatisfaction with the outcome by the initiation of legal action.

The Physicians Insurers Association of America[7] (PIAA)* recently concluded a 15-year study that investigated the circumstances surrounding the high frequency of claims for "delayed" diagnosis of breast cancer and the large financial judgments that claimants often are awarded by juries. The study, published in April 1990 showed among other things that the most expensive condition and the second most common condition resulting in claims against physicians involve malignant neoplasms of the breast.[7] In addition, the study revealed that while breast cancer has a higher incidence in older women, the delay in diagnosis of cancer in younger women results in a majority of claims having an even larger proportion of indemnity payments.[7] One would anticipate these claims having higher value given the longer life expectancy of younger women and the increased potential loss of lifetime income.

In any action for alleged medical malpractice, including those actions arising from treatment relating to breast cancer and associated issues, four basic points must be appreciated. First, the norms and standards applied to the treatment in question are the medical norms and standards. There is a common misapprehension that once named in a medical malpractice action a physician will find himself or herself in a foreign land devoid of any familiar landmarks or points of reference. In fact, the most important reference points will be the same standards and norms relied upon by the physician in the daily treatment of patients.

Second, the state of the art at issue in the legal action will be the state of the art at the time treatment is rendered, a point of particular importance in the context of breast cancer where advances are achieved and new protocols are developed annually, if not more frequently. It is important for the physician defendant to recognize that he or she will not have been required to have followed the state of the art at the time the matter is actually brought to trial, but rather, the state of the art at the time of the treatment, a date likely to be several years earlier. It is axiomatic that the best prophylaxis for avoiding a lawsuit is for the physician to remain apprised of all changes in treatment methods and to practice "state of the art medicine."

Third, it is important to recognize that a physician is not bound to follow only one school or method of treatment. This concept, commonly known as the "two schools of thought" doctrine, recognizes that on many medical issues, there is a divergence of opinion as to the appropriate treatment, therapy, or procedure and that any one of a

*The PIAA comprises 43 physician-owned professional liability companies that provide malpractice insurance to 177,000 practicing physicians. Twenty-one of the member companies agreed to participate in the study and collected and reported data on 273 closed, paid breast cancer cases. While at first glance the number of cases reported appears to be relatively small, the total paid indemnity value for these claims is $60.5 million, and in addition, member companies spent $5.3 million in allocated adjustment expenses to handle these claims. Thus, it is apparent that breast cancer claims are a significant source of loss for the medical malpractice insurer and the doctors that are insured.[7]

variety of treatments, therapies, or procedures may be pursued by the physician.[3] As long as the doctor follows a recognized school of practice which is appropriate, he will not be subject to criticism because of his failure to follow another recognized school. The appropriateness of applying this doctrine is a case by case decision of the physician's attorney depending on the facts of each case and the law of the jurisdiction.

Fourth, there must be a causal relationship between the treatment and the harm that forms the basis of the patient's complaint. Harm standing alone is not a sufficient basis for a malpractice action. In the law, an act of negligence does not create liability for damage unless it causes harm to the plaintiff. In the irreverent jargon of malpractice lawyers, the "causation defense" is sometimes referred to as the "so what" defense. For example, allegations of delay in diagnosis can often be countered by demonstrating that the alleged delay did not harm the patient since the disease metastasized before the alleged negligent act. With these four principles in mind, the malpractice action can be understood in terms that are more familiar to the defendant physician.

This chapter addresses recurrent themes in lawsuits alleging professional medical negligence in the diagnosis and treatment of breast cancer patients. A frequent allegation is that a breast mass was not promptly diagnosed as cancerous because the physician failed to palpate the mass, failed to order a mammogram, or relied on a negative mammogram despite the presence of other risk factors. The PIAA study revealed that the most common reason given for delay in diagnosis by physicians was that in 147 cases (54.7%), the physical findings at examination failed to impress the physician.[7] The PIAA study also showed that the patient most commonly found the lesion (69% of all claims).[7] The study indicated that self-discovery often may be ignored, especially in younger women where the incidence of malignancy is thought to be less than in older women.[7]

The second most common reason for delay is a negative mammogram report.[7] Somewhat surprisingly, 35% of the studied PIAA claimants had a negative mammogram report. Another 14% had equivocal mammogram results.* False-negative and equivocal results occur more frequently in women under the age of 40. These results exemplify the fact that further testing may be warranted in diagnosing breast cancer in women of all ages and that a biopsy should always follow any suspicious findings.

Another recurring theme is the allegation that the physician failed to obtain informed consent to treatment, either surgery, chemotherapy, or radiation. Late complications—such as second tumors after adjuvant radiotherapy or adjuvant chemotherapy as well as more immediate complications such as extravasation of a vesicant drug following intravenous administration—frequently form the basis of a lack of informed consent allegation. This form of action is more likely in those states which create a statutory cause of action based on lack of informed consent.

This chapter presents the legal theories of a medical malpractice claim and offers suggestions on how to anticipate and avoid problem areas. Not being physicians, the authors do not attempt to define the appropriate medical standards of care because the courts rely on medical authorities and not legal authorities for this information. In addition, the authors do not presume to offer legal advice. The complexities of each case or fact situation, as well as the applicable law of each jurisdiction, require individual guidance from the physician's attorney. However, it is the authors' hope that physicians, armed with an understanding of the law and the medical pitfalls in diagnosing and treating breast cancer, will be able to minimize their exposure to malpractice actions and necessarily conduct their practice to ensure the best possible defense. The chapter concludes with a review of the 19 state statutes regarding breast cancer treatment and informed consent and the effect these laws have on a physician's daily practice.

RECURRING LEGAL THEMES IN BREAST CANCER TREATMENT

Causation

A required element of any medical malpractice action is for the plaintiff to establish "causation," that is, that the defendant physician's actions or failure to act resulted in some harm to the patient. One method of refuting the allegation of medical malpractice is to focus on the causation element of the plaintiff's case and contend that the action or failure to act on the part of the physician did not cause the harm that is the basis of the patient's complaint. Three possible approaches are the "doubling time" defense, the "so what" defense, and a defense that focuses on the patient's own contribution to the unfavorable outcome. It must be remembered that application of any of these theories depends on the facts of each case and the law of each jurisdiction.

"Doubling time" defense. In a case that focuses on a failure to diagnose, the plaintiff must show that the delay proximately caused a shortening in

*It should be remembered that the PIAA data were collected over the last 15 years. The imaging technology in 1975 was not as sophisticated as it is today. The technical performance of mammograms has improved dramatically in recent years. In fact, one of PIAA's member companies reports that they have not had a single claim for delayed breast cancer diagnosis in the last two years.[7]

her life expectancy. The doubling-time defense can be employed to suggest that the disease had metastasized before the alleged negligent act and, as a result, no damages resulted from a failure to diagnose a cancerous breast mass promptly. In essence, this defense seeks to establish that there is no diminished life expectancy.

The theory of the doubling time defense. In establishing the doubling time defense, the jury must be presented an easily understood explanation of how tumors grow and the relationship of growth to tumor size. Terms and concepts that are familiar to the physician will be foreign to the jury to whom the concept of binary division of cancer cells must be explained. The jury must be taught that the time it takes for one cell to become two or two to become four is known as the doubling time of a cancer and in theory is considered constant. The jury must be told that an average breast cancer cell measures 1000th of a cubic micron or 1/1000th of a millimeter. The jury will have to understand that a tumor in its thirtieth doubling has approximately 2^{30} cells and, if considered spherical, will have a diameter of 1 cm. Once this groundwork is laid, the jury can be expected to appreciate that a 1-cm breast cancer tumor is generally the minimum clinical size that can be detected by palpation or physical examination and to understand as well that a tumor that is 1 cm in diameter, which is in its thirtieth doubling and contains approximately one billion cells, has been growing in the patient's breast for nearly 8 years (100 days $\times$ 30 doublings $=$ 3000 days).[4]

Based on these scientific facts, the argument can be advanced that the tumor is more likely to have metastasized before the alleged negligent act than during the alleged delay between the defendant's first opportunity to diagnose and the time that the tumor was finally diagnosed. If the jury is convinced that this breast cancer has been present much longer than any delay in diagnosis and has metastasized before the first opportunity to detect, they may well also accept the conclusion that no diminution in life expectancy can be based on the alleged delay in diagnosis.*

*It is well established that any breast cancer that reaches its fortieth doubling is nearly always fatal. Therefore, the amount of time between the first possible clinical detection of the tumor and the most likely date of death for the patient is approximately only 3 years (10 doublings at 100 days), compared with a preclinical history of 8 years. This medical fact may be used to explain the patient's frequent contention that from the time she first felt a mass in her breast until the time that it was removed, it seemed to grow very rapidly. The explanation of this phenomenon by means of the doubling time theory is that tumor growth is exponential. The seemingly rapid burgeoning of the tumor in its clinical phase is no more than the normal constant doubling time being applied to the tumor when it has finally reached a fairly large and palpable proportion.

Application of the doubling time defense. The following is an application of the doubling time defense in a typical missed diagnosis of breast cancer case.[4] A 43-year-old woman visits her gynecologist complaining of what she describes as a "lump" in her right breast. The physician performs an examination but cannot palpate a distinct "lump." There are no skin changes, no palpable axillary nodes, and no evidence of distant metastasis. There is no prior nor familial history of any cancer. The physician records these results as a "fullness in the upper outer quadrant." The physician's clinical impression is fibrocystic breast disease. Nonetheless, he recommends a bilateral mammogram. The radiologist reports: "No calcifications seen in either breast. Both breasts are rather dense suggesting fibrocystic disease. There is no definite evidence of malignancy." The gynecologist relates these findings to the patient and instructs her that she merely has fibrocystic breast disease, she should not worry, but she should return if the size or characteristics of the lump change in any way.

The patient returns 15 months later stating that the lump feels larger. Upon examination, the physician notes a well-circumscribed mass measuring approximately 3.5 cm in diameter. There are still no palpable lymph nodes and no signs of distant metastasis. A repeat mammogram shows an area of increased density in the upper outer quadrant suspicious for carcinoma. A breast biopsy is performed and the pathology report reveals poorly differentiated infiltrating ductal carcinoma.

A modified radical mastectomy is performed. The axillary lymph node dissection reveals four of nine axillary nodes are positive. The largest cancerous axillary lymph node is 1.2 cm in diameter. Within 9 months, bone metastasis is found. Within 2 years, the patient has diffuse metastatic disease with a life expectancy of less than 1 year.

The legal issue for the defense is, did the 15 month delay cause a decrease in the patient's life expectancy? The defense expert's testimony should demonstrate in clear, simple terms, that according to the doubling time defense, the answer is no. The defense expert can testify that according to established medical literature, the primary breast tumor has an average doubling time of approximately 100 days. In this example, the primary tumor was approximately 3 cm in diameter; it can be demonstrated to be in approximately its thirty-fourth doubling and be present for approximately 9 years. The expert can also demonstrate that approximately five doubling times elapsed in the 15 months prior to surgery. At the time of the initial examination, the primary tumor of the breast would have been in approximately its twenty-ninth doubling and would have been less than 1 cm in size. It is generally accepted in the medical literature that a lesion is not clinically palpable until the tumor is at least 1 cm in diameter. If this argument is successful, the jury will be convinced that this breast cancer had been present and metastasized before the initial examination, requiring the conclusion that no diminution of life expectancy can be based on the alleged delay in diagnosis.

Furthermore, the defense expert can testify that the bony metastasis 9 months after surgery is significant. If it is assumed that the metastatic lesion is approximately 1 cm in diameter, its size corresponds to the thirtieth doubling. Since according to the medical literature, a metastasis does not start from one cell but rather from a bolus of cells ranging from 10,000 to 60,000 cells, the metastasis did not start until the sixteenth to eighteenth doubling. The expert could conclude that it took between 12 and 14 doublings for the bony metastasis to reach its size when found 1 year after the surgery. At a 100-day doubling time 12 to 14 doublings correspond to approximately 4 years. The bony metastasis found 9 months after the surgery or 24 months after the alleged negligent act can by this basis be established to have started growing at least 2 years before the initial examination.

It is by this process of education that a jury can be led to conclude that the failure to diagnose the cancer at the time of the initial examination played no role in the ultimate unforunate outcome of the patient's treatment. It must be stressed, however, that each element of this defense requires a careful and clear presentation of concepts and principles that are not familiar to a lay jury. If great care is not taken in the presentation of these concepts to the jury, they cannot be expected to accept the proposition that the failure to diagnose the cancer at the initial examination did not result in a decrease in the patient's life expectancy.

"So what" defense. When the plaintiff's action is predicated upon the failure of the physician to palpate a lump or perform a breast examination, the defendant physician faces significant exposure. As discussed above, the defendant physician is required to conform his treatment to the norms and standards of his specialty, one of which has long been that the physician should perform a breast examination on the occasion of the patient's annual check-up. As also mentioned above, however, there must also be causation between the treatment and the harm. If a physician fails to perform an examination, that failure takes on significance only if it can be established that there was, in fact, a lump present that could have been palpated had the examination been performed. Unfortunately, from the patient's perspective, if the lump is palpable, there is also a significant possibility that the cancer has already metastasized at the time of the examination, reducing the patient's chances of survival considerably. The fact that the patient was unlikely to survive even had the lump been palpated at the time of the exam can then be employed as a possible defense to that action.

The patient's own role in the treatment. Another defense that is available argues that the patient is in fact responsible for the unfortunate result and focuses on the patient's role in her treatment. A failure to keep appointments, for example, can take on particular significance in the context of a patient who now suggests that her physician failed to provide adequate medical care. A patient's refusal to follow the suggested therapy, be it surgery, chemotherapy, or radiation, can be of great importance when her chosen mode of treatment fails. A patient who fails to perform monthly self-examinations or who does not follow the physician's recommendation for an annual mammogram after age 50 can be argued to have played a primary role in an unfavorable outcome. While some care must be taken in the presentation of this defense as the jury may be sympathetic to a patient who may have terminal cancer, the jury can be expected to appreciate that a patient can play a significant role in her own treatment.

Norms and standards

General obligations. The norms and standards for the diagnosis and treatment of breast cancer are constantly changing. For example, over the last 10 years, the surgical approach to breast cancer treatment has evolved from radical mastectomy to modified mastectomy to lumpectomy plus radiation therapy. Similar changes have occurred over the last 5 years concerning the use of adjuvant chemotherapy in node-positive patients and, as recently as June 1990, in node-negative patients. Physicians who fail to remain informed of new developments could find themselves exposed to a medical malpractice action if the treatment they recommend is outdated or if the treatment is so different from the majority that it is not acceptable.

The practicing physician is frequently faced with clinical updates regarding breast cancer treatment that often leave practitioners wondering what if any legal effect these updates have on their daily practice. For example, in 1985, the National Cancer Institute (NCI) held a consensus conference to review the use of chemotherapy and endocrine therapy as an adjuvant to surgery and radiotherapy in the treatment of early-stage breast cancer. The consensus panel agreed that while there was sufficient evidence in 1985 to recommend chemotherapy for all node-positive premenopausal women, the evidence was insufficient to recommend the routine use of adjuvant chemotherapy for most node-negative patients. This opinion generated concern in the physicians who were already administering adjuvant therapies to select node-negative patients.

In May 1988, the NCI distributed a "Clinical Alert" to cancer specialists throughout the United States notifying physicians of the benefit of adjuvant therapy for node-negative breast cancer patients. The distribution of the "Alert" was unprecedented; this was the first attempt to distribute information on clinical studies before journal publication. A follow-up assessment of the effectiveness of the "Alert" was conducted by the NCI. Although the survey revealed a generally positive response to the "Alert," with a majority of the responding physicians changing their treatment of node-negative patients, many responding physicians expressed concern that the "Alert" set a dangerous precedent as it was equivalent to mandating a standard of care, not yet supported by published studies, that could only be violated at the peril of a malpractice action.

Most recently, in June 1990, the NCI again convened a consensus development conference on the treatment of early-stage breast cancer to evaluate the developing results of breast conservation, adjuvant therapy of node-negative breast cancer, and clinical prognostic factors. Once again, practicing physicians must apprise themselves of the panel's findings and decide whether to incorporate the panel's recommendations into daily practice.

The panel concluded, among other things, that breast conservation treatment is an appropriate method of primary therapy for the majority of women with stage I and II breast cancer and is preferable because it provides a survival equivalent to total mastectomy while also preserving the breast. Physicians performing radical mastectomy without explaining the option of a lumpectomy followed by radiation therapy may find themselves in a lawsuit claiming unnecessary surgery and lack of informed consent.

The consensus panel also addressed the role of adjuvant therapy for patients with node-negative breast cancer. The panel stated that there is clear evidence that the rate of local and distant recurrence is decreased by both adjuvant cytotoxic chemotherapy and by tamoxifen.[6] Consequently, the panel found it imperative that all patients who are candidates for clinical trials of adjuvant therapy be offered the opportunity to participate.[6] The panel also recommended that while all node-negative patients have some risk for recurrence, patients with tumors ≤ 1 cm have an excellent prognosis and do not require adjuvant systemic therapy outside of clinical trials.[6]

In assimilating the constantly changing treatment picture into daily practice, the physician must understand that no single statement, including the NCI Clinical Alert and the NCI Consensus Conference recommendations, is, in itself, legally binding. The "two schools of thought" doctrine provides that it is improper for a jury to be assigned to decide which of "two schools of thought" as to proper surgical or medical procedure should have been followed in any particular case, when both schools have respected advocates and followers in the medical profession.[3] Under this doctrine, a physician will not be held liable for exercising judgment in following a course of treatment supported by a reputable and respected body of medical experts, even if another body of expert medical opinion would favor the use of a different procedure. However, the physician must be well apprised of the current acceptable methods of treatment to avoid becoming a "majority of one."*

Maintenance of records. An obstetrician-gynecologist is often the primary physician for women, and consequently, is frequently at risk for this type of litigation.† As the standards of the profession have established, the primary physician must listen to the patient's chief complaint, perform a careful examination, make a judgment regarding the findings, and order appropriate clinical studies. The physician's best legal defense to any allegation of malpractice is thorough documentation of each visit, including the patient's complaint in her own words, physical findings, and, if a mass is found, the use of a diagram to describe its location. Similarly, any referral of the patient should be carefully documented. The referred physician's name and the purpose of the referral (i.e., second opinion or biopsy) should be noted. Any results of diagnostic studies, performed by the primary or referred physician, should be included in the patient's record along with notes indicating that the patient has been informed of the results. If a patient declines an annual mammography, the physician should carefully document that the patient was informed and understood the American Cancer Society's recommendations and that the patient has chosen not to follow the recommendations.

A surgeon usually becomes involved in a breast cancer patient's care through a consultation for biopsy or for a second opinion. If a surgeon recommends a biopsy and the patient requests time to

*The "two schools of thought" doctrine is not applicable in all jurisdictions. The physician's attorney must make an independent decision regarding its application after reviewing the facts of each case and the law of the jurisdiction.

†In fact, obstetrician-gynecologists were the specialists most frequently claimed against and had the highest average indemnity payment in the PIAA study.[7] Family–general practice physicians had the second highest incidence followed by the surgical specialties and internal medicine.[7]

think about the recommendation, it is prudent to follow-up with a reminder letter to the patient which states the date of the initial visit, the name of the referring physician, the clinical impression and recommendations of the surgeon, and stresses that any significant delay in decision-making may adversely affect the ultimate prognosis. Some leading breast surgeons send the follow-up letter by registered mail with a return receipt requested. This practice provides the best evidence that the physician fulfilled his or her responsibility to the patient and took every precaution to ensure that the patient was not "lost to treatment."

A consistent routine of documentation and clinical practice can avoid a potential malpractice action. Not to be overlooked in this process is the quality of the physician-patient relationship. A patient who perceives her physician as knowledgeable and caring will be more likely to understand that an undesirable outcome is not the product of malpractice.

Mammography. A potential point of controversy for physicians is the decision to order a mammography. It is now well known by the general public that a baseline mammography should be obtained between the age of 35 and 40, and that studies should be repeated biannually until age 50 and annually thereafter. A failure to follow that standard may subject the physician to criticism. It is obvious, however, that gray areas do exist. One such area may be the initial decision to order the mammography. While it has been argued in the past that mammography itself exposes the patient to radiation and its attendant risks, that perspective, like many other shifting standards in this area, carries less weight with the development of new films that permit clearer images at significantly reduced rates of exposure. As a result, studies which formerly called into question the efficacy of mammographies are now subject to criticism and may no longer be available as a defense to a failure to order the study. The study once obtained, however, may raise as many questions as it resolves.

For example, a physician orders a mammogram either on a routine basis or to confirm the conclusion that no lump is present and then receives a report from the radiologist recommending biopsy; the physician's clinical judgment is thus at odds with the radiologist whose report may appear more accurate to a jury than a physician's manual examination. If the physician concludes that monitoring is warranted without a biopsy, careful documentation of the reason for this choice and an explanation for that conclusion to the patient should be documented in the records with routine follow-up.

A physician also encounters the decision of recommending biopsy of a suspicious mass even though the mammogram is negative. The physician is then placed between the desire not to alarm the patient and subject her to unnecessary surgery and wanting to promptly diagnose any suspected cancerous lesion. The presence of a palpable mass warrants a biopsy. If a distinct mass is palpable and the mammogram is negative, the physician must explain to the woman that false-negative rates for mammography have varied from 5% to 30%, with the false-negative rate probably averaging about 15% for all patients shown to have cancer. The physician must stress to the patient that it is to her benefit to have the mass biopsied, even if the radiologist suggests a repeat mammogram at a later date. If the physician is unsure of the findings on manual examination, such as a "fullness" versus a distinct lump, and there are no other risk factors present, such as family history, the physician may have the patient return on a routine basis, perhaps even monthly, until the physician is assured that no tumor is present and a repeat mammogram, 3 to 6 months later, remains negative. Again, however, the process by which the decision is reached should be fully explained to the patient and recorded contemporaneously in the records.

Most importantly, any physician who performs a breast examination and suspects cancer should never minimize the possibility of cancer. Many patients will have the natural tendency to deny this possibility; any indication from the physician that there is no need to pursue a definitive diagnosis diligently may result in an allegation from the patient that her physician's lack of urgency caused her to believe that she could delay following his recommendations.

Informed consent

What is informed consent? Early common law recognized the intentional touching or striking of another without consent, called a "battery," as unlawful. The concept of informed consent in medical law evolved from this basis. In order for certain treatment to be consensual, a physician has the duty to disclose to a patient all relevant information concerning a proposed course of treatment, including the material risks involved with that treatment, the hazards of foregoing it, and available alternative treatments. The purpose of the disclosure is to inform a patient completely so that the "consent" to the elected treatment will be informed and the result of an intelligent choice. Physicians defending malpractice actions often find themselves responding to allegations that although patients have signed a consent form, they did not receive sufficient information from their physicians and had adequate disclosure of the risks been made by the physicians, the patients would not have consented to the treatment which resulted in harm.

Since 1980, 19 states have enacted some form of breast cancer informed consent legislation. The trend towards a statute governing informed consent reflects in a part a recognition of the physical and psychologic ramifications of the procedure. The laws vary widely; some require the physician to provide specific printed information while other statutes require specific procedures to obtain patient's consent to surgery.*

The early momentum to pass additional informed consent laws has slowed in the past few years.† The National Alliance of Breast Cancer Organizations[5] and the American Medical Society, Department of State Legislation,[2] suggest that reduced lobbying for laws on informed consent specific to breast cancer treatment results from passage of general medical informed consent laws that also cover treatment for breast cancer. These general laws require, for example, that a physician provide "reasonable disclosure" of relevant facts when discussing courses of medical treatment with a patient. In practice, however, this "reasonable disclosure" concept leaves many physicians confused as to their obligations to patients.

The requirements of disclosure. Physicians are frequently surprised to find that adequate disclosure is not measured by a medical standard permitting the physician to decide what the patient needed to know in order to be adequately informed. Rather, the law generally requires that the disclosure be that which a "reasonable patient" would require. As might be expected, the reasonable patient's requirements of disclosure may not be what a reasonable physician would disclose.‡ A simpler way of stating this is that the "reasonable patient" test requires the doctor to provide all information which could be significant for the reasonable patient to make a decision.

Causation in informed consent cases. One issue in informed consent cases is whether the failure to disclose adequate information caused injury to the patient. The law requires a patient to demonstrate that had adequate disclosure been made the patient would have declined treatment. The adequacy of the disclosure is determined by looking to what a reasonable physician knew or should have known about the risks involved with the contemplated procedures.*

The fundamentals of informed consent. In most cases, a physician or a member of the treating team should completely inform the patient. The pretreatment discussion should address relevant facts about the patient's condition and treatment options, including associated risks of any procedure, hazards if the condition is left untreated, and treatment alternatives available. It is crucial that the discussion and the patient's choice be carefully documented by the person who provided the information.

Most institutions have their own rules regarding the timing of consent. In some instances, state law specifies when consent should be obtained. As a general rule, consent should be obtained within a reasonable time before the treatment is performed or whenever the course of treatment will be substantially altered. In all cases, as a minimum, the hospital procedure manual should be consulted.

Once a patient has chosen a specific method of treatment, documenting the choice and the informed consent discussion is essential. Documentation of the surgical, radiological, or chemotherapeutic choice can have many forms. The most basic form is to note briefly in the medical records, "procedure discussed, patient consented." A more sound procedure is to write an extensive note describing the discussion and election process in detail and listing the risks, benefits, and alternatives.

A consent form provides a third option and is required if surgery or radiation is the chosen form of treatment. These forms may prove inadequate if a physician relies on a preprinted form as a substitute for the physician-patient discussion, and allows the preprinted signed form to speak as proof of the quality of the informed consent discussion. The most prudent practice is to include an executed consent form and a detailed note regarding the discussion in the patient's records. Contemporaneous documentation of the physician-patient conference is crucial to defend an informed consent claim as those documents, created before the dispute arose, are viewed by juries as more truthful than subsequent testimony on that same point.

Physicians must provide their breast cancer patients with complete information in order to ensure

---

*A detailed listing of the requirements of the laws of those states who have adopted legislation governing informed consent issues in the area of treatment of breast cancer may be found at the end of this chapter. It is strongly urged that the physician who practices in this area become familiar with the requirements of the states in which he practices.

†The most recent legislative effort is a currently pending federal bill, HR200, which would require each state to enact laws requiring physicians to inform their breast cancer patients of alternative methods of treatment in order to qualify for certain federal funding.

‡For a discussion of the standards and policy behind the "reasonable patient" standards, see *Cooper v. Roberts,* 220 Pa. Super. 260, 265, 286 A.2d 647, 650 (1971).

*See *Canterbury v. Spence,* 464 F.2d 772 (D.C. Cir.), *cert. denied,* 409 U.S. 1064 (1972) (holding physicians liable for nondisclosure only if the physician knew or should have known to disclose risks).

that each patient's decision is an "informed choice." Meticulous documentation of the discussion between the patient and the physician—specifically noting the information provided, alternatives discussed, any diagrams used, the patient's emotional state, and the ultimate choice of the patient—is essential. Consent by better informed but no less fearful and dependent patients will ultimately serve the best interests of both the patient and the physician.

Specific state laws. Some state laws require that the patient receive specific information before a choice is presented, while others require the patient to sign a prescribed form for a written consent before treatment. A few states require that the patient acknowledge, in writing, their receipt of this information and the physician must include this acknowledgment in the patient's medical record. Certain state statutes provide for no penalty if violated, while other states consider a violation to be a misdemeanor. A brief discussion of each state's law follows.

California. Enacted in 1980, the California statute[8] became the first law requiring disclosure of specific information to breast cancer patients. The law provides that a physician's or surgeon's failure to inform a breast cancer patient constitutes unprofessional conduct. The physician must use a standardized summary written in layperson's language that describes alternative methods of treatment, including surgical, radiological, or chemotherapeutic treatments. Physicians comply with the statute when they give the written summary to the patient. The standardized summary is available to physicians through the California Board of Medical Quality Assurance.

A 1988 amendment to the law requires a physician, before a biopsy, to note on the patient's chart that the patient has received the written summary.

Florida. The Florida statute[9] became effective in January 1985. This statute contains a unique provision requiring that both actual and high-risk breast cancer patients be informed of the treatment alternatives and associated risks. A physician can comply with the law by providing the information orally or by giving the patient a copy of a written summary prepared by the Florida Cancer Control and Research Advisory Board.

The law allows a physician to exercise discretion when providing the information by considering the emotional and physical state of the patient and the patient's ability to understand the information.

The physician is required to write a note on the patient's medical record indicating that the patient received the necessary information. Violation of the Florida statute is a misdemeanor.

Georgia. Georgia's statute,[10] enacted in 1984, requires the State Board of Medical Examiners to distribute to all physicians an informational booklet on breast cancer and its treatment. The booklet summarizes the most recent information and discusses the generally accepted and widely prevailing methods of treatment, as well as the associated risks.

A 1986 amendment provides for distribution of the booklet to also include those patients with "suspected" breast disease.

Hawaii. A Hawaii resolution[11] provided for the preparation of a Breast Cancer Treatment Alternatives Information Sheet. The Information Sheet describes the risks and procedures in treating breast cancer and is written in easily understandable language. In addition, the Hawaii Medical Association developed a model consent form which physicians can use to verify that their patients have received, read, and understood the Information Sheet.

Hawaii's general informed consent statute also has a subsection specifically addressing breast cancer. Effective January 1, 1984, the law requires the Board of Medical Examiners to establish standards for physicians to follow when giving information to a patient in order to ensure that the patient's consent to a mastectomy is an informed one.*

Illinois. The Illinois law,[12] effective July 1, 1989, requires the Department of Public Health to publish a booklet written in layperson's language, outlining the methods for early detection and diagnosis of breast cancer. The summary also includes information about the alternative methods of treatment and the advantages and risks of the various treatments. The statute states that the brochure is not meant to serve as a substitute for the sound professional advice of the physician. The booklet is not intended to alter, in any way, the existing physician-patient relationship or the existing professional obligations of the physician in caring for the patient.

Kansas. The Kansas legislature requires the State Board of Medical Examiners to distribute a standardized summary of the alternative methods of treatment of breast "disease" and the risks associated with each method.[13] The statute applies to any patient suffering from any abnormality of the breast tissue for which surgery is a recommended form of treatment.

The Kansas law specifically provides that the statute is not to be construed to authorize the board to restrict the physician's right to recommend a method of treatment or a patient's right to select a

---

**See also* H. Res. 321 (1983).

treatment method. Noncompliance with the statute is grounds for revocation, suspension, or limitation of a physician's medical license.

Kentucky. Kentucky's law,[14] enacted in 1984, also requires a booklet to be distributed to physicians that must be provided to breast cancer patients and that describes, in layperson's terms, the advantages, risks, and nature of procedures for all alternatives of breast cancer treatment.

Louisiana. Louisiana has merely adopted a Resolution[15] "urging and requesting" all physicians to advise their patients, orally and in writing, of the alternatives to a radical mastectomy before performing surgery. The Resolution also "urges and requests" the physician to include a form in the patient's record signed by the patient which acknowledges receipt of the written advisement. The Resolution is not legally binding on physicians. The Resolution's "urging and requesting" is equivalent to a suggestion. However, Louisiana does have a general informed consent statute which is applicable to breast cancer treatment.[16]

Maine. Effective in June 1989, the Maine statute[17] requires a physician to inform a patient, orally and in writing, about alternative methods of treatment, including surgical, radiologic, or chemotherapeutic, as well as the advantages and the most usual and frequent risks of each. The physician must also have the patient sign a form indicating receipt of the oral information and a copy of the written summary. This form is to be included in the patient's medical record.

The signed consent form offers the physician a degree of protection against litigation. The statute provides that a patient who has signed the form is barred from bringing a civil action based on failure to obtain informed consent, but only in regard to information pertaining to alternative forms of treatment of breast cancer and the advantages and risks of each method.

Maryland. The Maryland law,[18] effective July 1, 1987, requires physicians, before beginning treatment, to educate the patient about alternative methods of treatment that may be medically practicable. The State Department of Health and Mental Hygiene provides a standardized summary, written in layperson's language, that lists all effective methods of treatment. A physician complies with the law by providing a patient with the summary and having the patient sign a form statement acknowledging receipt of the summary.

Massachusetts. The Massachusetts Patient Bill of Rights was amended in 1985 to state that any patient suffering from any form of breast cancer is entitled to complete information on all alternative treatments that are medically viable.[19] The law does not authorize the development of any standardized information booklet nor does the statute impose a penalty for noncompliance.

Michigan. The Michigan law,[20] effective in November 1986, requires that the primary physician inform the patient orally and in writing about alternative methods of treatment for breast cancer. A standardized written brochure available through the Michigan Board of Medicine can be used by a physician to comply with the law. A statement signed by the patient, indicating that the patient has received a copy of the brochure or the physician's own written summary, must be included in the patient's medical record.

A patient who signs a form is barred from bringing a civil action against the physician, but only in reference to information pertaining to alternative forms of treatment of breast cancer and the advantages and risks of each method.

Violation of the Michigan law is grounds for an investigation of the licensee to determine whether discipline is appropriate. The law also had a sunset provision so that it was repealed July 1, 1989. However, investigation of several leading Michigan medical centers revealed that the form is still in use despite the repeal.

Minnesota. The Minnesota legislature, in 1984, amended the Minnesota Patient Bill of Rights to include a paragraph in the "Information about Treatment" section which specifically addresses breast cancer patients and informed consent.[21] The physician must fully inform a patient of all alternative methods of treatment and associated risks of which the treating physician is knowledgeable. The statute does not require a specific group to distribute an information booklet nor does it require the use of a specific consent form.

New Jersey. In New Jersey, a physician must obtain written consent on a prescribed form which allows the patient to (a) give consent only for a biopsy; (b) give consent to the performance of any necessary operation or procedure, including breast removal, where the patient has a malignant tumor; or (c) give consent for both a biopsy and the additional operation or procedure, if necessary.[22] A physician is subject to disciplinary action if he or she fails to comply.

New York. The New York statute,[23] effective January 1986, requires a standardized written summary in plain nontechnical language be provided by a physician at the time of diagnosis to each person under his or her care for the treatment of breast cancer. The summary should explain the alternative methods of treating breast cancer and the associated risks. The New York statute also specifically states that nothing in the statute should be construed to create a cause of action for lack of informed consent.

Pennsylvania. The Pennsylvania law,[24] effective February 1985, states that before a physician operates on a patient for a breast tumor the patient must sign a consent form which contains two options. The first option permits biopsy only. The second option permits biopsy and any other operation or procedure, including breast removal that are deemed necessary. Failure to comply, in addition to civil proceedings, subjects the physician to disciplinary action.

Texas. The Texas statute,[25] effective September 1990, requires the Texas Department of Health to develop a standardized summary, written in layperson's language, outlining the advantages and risks of all alternatives for the treatment of breast cancer. Any physician who treats a patient for any form of breast cancer should provide the patient with a copy of the standardized written summary.

Virginia. The 1985 Virginia law[26] requires the informed consent form to contain paragraphs that allow a patient to sign for a biopsy only or, if it is determined that the tumor in the breast is malignant, then to authorize the surgeon to perform such operation or procedures, including breast removal, that are deemed necessary. Similar to New Jersey and Pennsylvania, the Virginia statute merely requires a specific wording of the consent form and does not address the content of the informed consent discussion.

Wisconsin. The Wisconsin law,[27] effective May 7, 1982, applies to all informed consent situations including breast cancer patients. The statute requires any physician who treats a patient to inform the patient about the availability of all alternate modes of treatment and all associated benefits and risks.

The statute does not require disclosure of (1) information beyond what a reasonably well-qualified physician in a similar medical classification would know; (2) detailed technical information that in all probability a patient would not understand; (3) risks apparent or known to the patient; (4) extremely remote possibilities that might falsely or detrimentally alarm the patient; (5) information in emergencies where failure to provide treatment would be more harmful to the patient than treatment; and (6) information in cases where the patient is incapable of consenting. Violation of the Wisconsin law constitutes unprofessional conduct punishable by a reprimand, suspension, or revocation of any professional license.

REFERENCES

1. American Cancer Society: Cancer facts and figures, Atlanta, 1990, ACS.
2. American Medical Association, Department of State Legislation: Breast Cancer Informed Consent Statutes, May 1985.
3. Cherry G: The "two schools of thought" Doctrine, Penna. Bar Institute, 1990, Advanced Issues in Medical Malpractice.
4. Michels P et al: Attacking the doubling time defense in breast cancer cases, Medical Trial Tech Q, 28:301, 1981 (Winter).
5. National Alliance of Breast Cancer Organizations News: Vol. III, No. 3, July 1989.
6. National Institute of Health, Consensus Development Conference Statement, June 18-21, 1990.
7. Physician Insurers Association of America, Breast Cancer Study, March 1990.
8. California Health and Safety Code, Section 1704.5 (1980).
9. Florida Statutes Annotated, Vol. 14A, Section 381. 3812(m) (1985).
10. Georgia Code, Section 43-34-21(g) (1984).
11. Hawaii Revised Statutes, Section 671-3(c) (1983).
12. Illinois Statutes Annotated, chapter 127, Section 55.49 (1989).
13. Kansas Statutes Annotated, Section 65.2836(o) (1984).
14. Kentucky Revised Statutes, Vol. 1, Section 311.935 (1984).
15. H. Con. Res. 125 (1983).
16. Louisiana Revised Statutes, Sections 40:1299.40, 40: 1299.50
17. Maine Revised Statutes Annotated, Title 24, Section 2905-A (1985).
18. Annotated Code of Maryland, Health-General, Section 20-113 (1987).
19. Annotated Laws of Massachusetts, Chapter III, Section 70E (h) (1985).
20. Michigan Compiled Laws Annotated, Sections 333.16221, 333.17013, 333.17513 (1986).
21. Minnesota Statutes Annotated, Section 144.651 (1984).
22. New Jersey Statutes Annotated, Title 45:9-22.2 and 45: 9-22.3.
23. New York Consolidated Laws Service, Public Health, Article 24, Section 2404 (1986).
24. Purdon's Pa. Consolidated Statutes, Title 35, Sections 5641 and 5642 (1985).
25. Texas Senate Bill 1345, March 10 (1989).
26. Virginia Code Annotated, Section 54.1-2971 (1985).
27. Wisconsin Statutes Annotated, Sections 448.02(3), 448.30 (1982).

BIBLIOGRAPHY

American Medical Association, Department of State Legislation: Breast cancer informed consent statutes, May 1985.

Frable WJ: Medical and legal aspects of breast cancer, Defense Research Institute, Medical Malpractice Seminar January 21-22, 1988.

Harness JK et al: Breast cancer—collaborative management, 1988, Lewis Publishers, Inc.

Henderson IC and Danner D: Legal pitfalls in the diagnosis and management of breast cancer, Hematol/Oncol Clin North Am, vol 3, no 4, December 1989.

Marchant DJ: Breast disease, New York, 1986, Churchill Livingstone.

Seidelson DE: Lack of informed consent in medical malpractice and product liability cases: the burden of presenting evidence, Specialty Law Digest, Health Care, no 122. April 1989.

Index

C

E

J

K

L

O

S

U

V

W

X

Y

Z